Thieme

Vitreoretinal Disease

Diagnosis, Management, and Clinical Pearls

Ingrid U. Scott, MD, MPH
Jack and Nancy Turner Professor of Ophthalmology
Professor of Public Health Sciences
Penn State Eye Center
Penn State College of Medicine
Hershey, Pennsylvania

Carl D. Regillo, MD, FACS
Director, Retina Service
Wills Eye Hospital
Professor of Ophthalmology
Thomas Jefferson University
Philadelphia, Pennsylvania

Harry W. Flynn, Jr., MD
The J. Donald M. Gass Distinguished Chair in Ophthalmology
Professor of Ophthalmology
University of Miami Health System
Bascom Palmer Eye Institute
Miami, Florida

Gary C. Brown, MD, MBA
Retina Service
Wills Eye Hospital
Professor of Ophthalmology
Thomas Jefferson University
Philadelphia, Pennsylvania

609 illustrations

Thieme
New York • Stuttgart • Delhi • Rio de Janeiro

Executive Editor: William Lamsback
Managing Editor: Elizabeth Palumbo
Editorial Assistant: Haley Paskalides
Director, Editorial Services: Mary Jo Casey
Production Editor: Sean Woznicki
International Production Director: Andreas Schabert
Editorial Director: Sue Hodgson
International Marketing Director: Fiona Henderson
International Sales Director: Louisa Turrell
Director of Institutional Sales: Adam Bernacki
Senior Vice President and Chief Operating Officer: Sarah Vanderbilt
President: Brian D. Scanlan
Printer: King Printing

Library of Congress Cataloging-in-Publication Data

Names: Scott, Ingrid U., editor. | Regillo, Carl D., editor. | Flynn, Harry W., editor. | Brown, Gary C., 1949- editor.
Title: Vitreoretinal disease / [edited by] Ingrid U. Scott, MD, MPH, Professor of Ophthalmology and Public Health Sciences, Penn State Hershey Eye Center, Penn State College of Medicine, Hershey, PA, Carl D. Regillo, MD, Director, Retina Service, Wills Eye Hospital, Philadelphia, PA, Harry W. Flynn, Jr., MD, J. Donald M. Gass Chair of Ophthalmology, Professor of Ophthalmology, University of Miami Health System, Bascom Palmer Eye Institute at Miami, Miami, FL, Gary C. Brown, MD, MBA, Chief and Director, Wills Eye Institute Retina Service, Professor of Ophthalmology Jefferson Medical College Mid Atlantic Retina Plymouth Meeting, PA.
Description: Second edition. | New York : Thieme, [2018] | Includes bibliographical references and index.
Identifiers: LCCN 2016015842 (print) | LCCN 2016023064 (ebook) | ISBN 9781626231337 | ISBN 9781626231320
Subjects: LCSH: Retina–Diseases. | Vitreous body–Diseases. | Choroid–Diseases.
Classification: LCC RE551 .V57 2016 (print) | LCC RE551 (ebook) | DDC 617.7/35–dc23
LC record available at https://lccn.loc.gov/2016015842

Thieme Publishers New York
333 Seventh Avenue, New York, NY 10001 USA
+1 800 782 3488, customerservice@thieme.com

Thieme Publishers Stuttgart
Rüdigerstrasse 14, 70469 Stuttgart, Germany
+49 [0]711 8931 421, customerservice@thieme.de

Thieme Publishers Delhi
A-12, Second Floor, Sector-2, Noida-201301
Uttar Pradesh, India
+91 120 45 566 00, customerservice@thieme.in

Thieme Publishers Rio de Janeiro,
Thieme Publicações Ltda.
Edifício Rodolpho de Paoli, 25º andar
Av. Nilo Peçanha, 50 – Sala 2508
Rio de Janeiro 20020-906 Brasil
+55 21 3172-2297 / +55 21 3172-1896

Cover design: Thieme Publishing Group
Typesetting by DiTech Process Solutions

Printed in the United States of America by King Printing 5 4 3 2 1

ISBN 978-1-62623-133-7

Also available as an e-book:
eISBN 978-1-62623-132-0

Important note: Medicine is an ever-changing science undergoing continual development. Research and clinical experience are continually expanding our knowledge, in particular our knowledge of proper treatment and drug therapy. Insofar as this book mentions any dosage or application, readers may rest assured that the authors, editors, and publishers have made every effort to ensure that such references are in accordance with **the state of knowledge at the time of production of the book.**

Nevertheless, this does not involve, imply, or express any guarantee or responsibility on the part of the publishers in respect to any dosage instructions and forms of applications stated in the book. **Every user is requested to examine carefully** the manufacturers' leaflets accompanying each drug and to check, if necessary in consultation with a physician or specialist, whether the dosage schedules mentioned therein or the contraindications stated by the manufacturers differ from the statements made in the present book. Such examination is particularly important with drugs that are either rarely used or have been newly released on the market. Every dosage schedule or every form of application used is entirely at the user's own risk and responsibility. The authors and publishers request every user to report to the publishers any discrepancies or inaccuracies noticed. If errors in this work are found after publication, errata will be posted at www.thieme.com on the product description page.

Some of the product names, patents, and registered designs referred to in this book are in fact registered trademarks or proprietary names even though specific reference to this fact is not always made in the text. Therefore, the appearance of a name without designation as proprietary is not to be construed as a representation by the publisher that it is in the public domain.

FSC
www.fsc.org
100%
Paper from well-managed forests
FSC® C103101

To our families for their never-ending support and encouragement.

Contents

Foreword ... x

Preface ... xi

Contributors ... xii

I Anatomy and Physiology

1 Anatomy of the Vitreous, Retina, and Choroid ... 2
Hermann D. Schubert and Marilyn C. Kincaid

2 Retinal and Retinal Pigment Epithelial Physiology ... 14
Michael F. Marmor and Loh-Shan B. Leung

II Diagnostic Techniques

3 Examination of the Fundus ... 30
Allen Chiang and William E. Benson

4 Fundus Angiography ... 40
Suqin Yu and Lawrence A. Yannuzzi

5 Optical Coherence Tomography ... 52
Jay S. Duker and Gregory D. Lee

6 Ultrasonography ... 66
Cathy DiBernardo

7 Electrophysiology and Miscellaneous Noninvasive Tests ... 83
Lauren S. Taney and Elias Reichel

III Diseases of the Vitreous, Retina, and Choroid

8 Arterial Occlusive Disease ... 99
Gary C. Brown

9 Retinal Venous Occlusive Disease ... 121
Amol D. Kulkarni, Michael S. Ip, and Ingrid U. Scott

10 Diabetic Retinopathy ... 136
Jennifer K. Sun and Lloyd Paul Aiello

11 Cystoid Macular Edema ... 160
Stephen J. Kim and Ingrid U. Scott

12 Retinopathy of Prematurity ... 171
Yoshihiro Yonekawa and R. V. Paul Chan

13 Miscellaneous Retinal Vascular Conditions ... 184
Frank S. Siringo, Ingrid U. Scott, Naresh Mandava, and Lawrence A. Yannuzzi

14 **Age-Related Macular Degeneration** 206
Ashleigh L. Levison, Paula E. Pecen, and Peter K. Kaiser

15 **Miscellaneous Macular Degenerations** 227
Samuel K. Steven Houston III and Allen C. Ho

16 **Central Serous Chorioretinopathy** 241
M. Ali Khan and Jason Hsu

17 **Macular Holes** 250
John T. Thompson

18 **Epiretinal Membrane and Vitreomacular Traction** 267
Kevin R. Tozer and Mark W. Johnson

19 **Macular Dystrophies** 276
Anita Agarwal

20 **Hereditary Retinal Degenerations** 296
Angela M. Herro and Byron L. Lam

21 **Sickle Retinopathy** 313
Royce W. S. Chen, Harry W. Flynn Jr., Sharon Fekrat, and Morton F. Goldberg

22 **Retinal Manifestations of Metabolic Disease** 324
Katherine E. Talcott, James D. Palmer, and Shizuo Mukai

23 **Hyaloideoretinopathies** 342
William Tasman

24 **Infectious Chorioretinal Inflammatory Conditions** 352
Janet L. Davis

25 **Noninfectious Chorioretinal Inflammatory Conditions** 369
Mariana Cabrera, Nidhi Relhan, and Thomas A. Albini

26 **Choroidal Nevus and Melanoma** 392
Carol L. Shields and Jerry A. Shields

27 **Retinoblastoma** 404
Carol L. Shields and Jerry A. Shields

28 **Other Retinal, Retinal Pigment Epithelial, and Choroidal Tumors** 421
Carol L. Shields and Jerry A. Shields

29 **Retinal Tears and Rhegmatogenous Retinal Detachments** 443
Stephen G. Schwartz, Harry W. Flynn Jr., William F. Mieler, and James S. Tiedeman

30 **Exudative and Tractional Retinal Detachments** 457
Matthew D. Cooke, Robert A. Mittra, and Dennis P. Han

31 **Degenerative Retinoschisis** 469
David C. Reed and Sunir J. Garg

32 **Blunt and Penetrating Ocular Injuries** 475
Liliya Shevchenko, Thomas M. Aaberg, Jr., and Paul Sternberg, Jr.

33 **Posterior Segment Manifestations of Systemic Trauma** 499
Jason Hsu and Carl D. Regillo

34 **Drug and Light Ocular Toxicity** 505
Michael T. Andreoli, Robert A. Mittra, and William F. Mieler

35 **Posterior Segment Complications of Anterior Segment Surgery** 522
Thalmon R. Campagnoli, William E. Smiddy, and Harry W. Flynn Jr.

36 **Congenital Fundus Abnormalities** 543
Gary C. Brown

IV **Vitreoretinal Procedures**

37 **Intravitreal Injections** 562
Ingrid U. Scott and Harry W. Flynn Jr.

38 **Posterior Segment Drug Delivery** 568
Sumit Sharma and Glenn J. Jaffe

39 **Laser for Vitreoretinal Diseases** 576
Yannis M. Paulus and Mark S. Blumenkranz

40 **Vitreous Surgery** 597
Thanos D. Papakostas, Dean Eliott, and Ingrid U. Scott

Index 612

Foreword

Tell me and I forget. Teach me and I remember. Involve me and I learn.

- *Benjamin Franklin*

Life all around is a kind of sporting event and the best any of us can do is to try continually to improve our game.

- *Harvey Cushing to his son Bill*

This authoritative new edition of *Vitreoretinal Disease*, comprehensively updated from the classic of 1999 with the addition of the latest in cutting edge diagnostic and therapeutic technology, manages to both admirably fulfill Franklin's criteria for learning, and knock Cushing's sports metaphor out of the park. Well-written, clearly organized and engaging, it teaches and involves, capturing the reader in a voyage of exploration into all things vitreoretinal. And it helps all of us improve our game!

Carefully curated, this volume equips the practicing comprehensive ophthalmologist, resident, and fellow with a very accessible and practical clinical overview of the latest in vitreoretinal knowledge, while also satisfying the subspecialist's need for a focused and selected review and reference volume.

Vitreoretinal Disease has a game-winning guarantee in large part due to its winning hand of four editorial aces, Scott, Regillo, Brown and Flynn, whose extraordinary professional depth and the eminence of the colleagues they have martialled to selectively but comprehensively summarize the state of the art in our field represent a ne plus ultra of retina knowledge and experience.

Both teaching and engaging, this latest edition of a landmark text from the ophthalmic archives should inspire a new generation of eye physicians and surgeons, to the benefit of our profession, and our patients. In the final analysis, this book is for them.

Julia A. Haller, MD
William Tasman, MD endowed chair and
Ophthalmologist-in-Chief
Wills Eye Hospital
Professor and Chair
Department of Ophthalmology
Jefferson Medical College
Philadelphia, Pennsylvania

Preface

The field of vitreoretinal disease continues to evolve rapidly, and has expanded into a complex practice of medicine and surgery that utilizes a wide range of diagnostic and therapeutic modalities. From case reports to phase 3 multicenter clinical trials, published data accumulate in exponential fashion. As a result, it is increasingly difficult for the clinician dealing with vitreoretinal disease, both generalist and specialist alike, to synthesize and apply the amassed information to patient care.

This textbook is primarily intended to provide the practicing comprehensive ophthalmologist and ophthalmology resident with an up-to-date, clinically oriented source that covers the full spectrum of medical and surgical vitreoretinal diseases. Subspecialists in the field should also find it useful as a review and selected reference.

Although this text is meant to be comprehensive, we have tried to highlight the essential, clinically important aspects of vitreoretinal medical and surgical practice. Chapters dealing with disease states emphasize clinical features, diagnosis, and management. Entire chapters are devoted to the most commonly encountered problems. Clinical "pearls," special considerations, and controversial points are made to stand out in colored boxes.

The text is divided into four general parts. The first part provides a basic overview of posterior segment anatomy and physiology. The second part reviews the spectrum of diagnostic tools used in the field, from the relatively low-technology indirect ophthalmoscope to the latest, high-technology optical coherence tomography test. The third and largest part deals exclusively with the disease states and is subdivided by disease category. The fourth part covers specific vitreoretinal procedures. Since the last edition, each chapter has been revised and updated by experts in the field. Given the widespread integration of optical coherence tomography into vitreoretinal clinical practice since the first edition of this textbook was published in 1999, this new edition of the textbook devotes an entire chapter to optical coherence tomography and its applications in the management of vitreoretinal diseases. Due to advances in diagnostic techniques, the new edition also includes sections on multifocal electroretinography, scanning laser ophthalmoscopy, fundus autofluorescence, and adaptive optics. Since the first edition of the textbook was published, the intravitreal injection procedure has become the most commonly performed procedure by vitreoretinal specialists; accordingly, this new edition of the textbook devotes an entire chapter to the intravitreal injection procedure. Finally, many figures included in the revised edition have been updated to color.

Assembling a multiauthor textbook that attempts to have the chapters be both current and detailed in content along with being uniform in layout requires a special effort from all the contributors to adhere to strict guidelines; we are grateful to all those invited to participate in the writing of this textbook for these efforts. We wish to acknowledge the support of the staff and our colleagues at Penn State Eye Center, Wills Eye Hospital, and Bascom Palmer Eye Institute. The faculty, residents, fellows, and patients at our institutions always deserve credit as they are continued sources of inspiration for academic endeavors. We also wish to thank the editorial team at Thieme Publishers for their dedicated guidance and expertise. Finally, we thank our families for their unwavering and enthusiastic support and encouragement.

Ingrid U. Scott, MD, MPH
Carl D. Regillo, MD
Gary C. Brown, MD
Harry W. Flynn Jr, MD

Contributors

Thomas M. Aaberg Jr., MD
Retina Specialist
Retina Specialists of Michigan
Grand Rapids, Michigan

Anita Agarwal, MD
Professor of Ophthalmology
Retina, Vitreous and Uveitis
Vanderbilt Eye Institute
Vanderbilt University School of Medicine
Nashville, Tennessee

Lloyd Paul Aiello, MD, PhD
Director, Beetham Eye Institute
Boston, Massachusetts
Vice President of Ophthalmology
Joslin Diabetes Center
Boston, Massachusetts

Thomas A. Albini, MD
Associate Professor of Clinical Ophthalmology
University of Miami Health System
Bascom Palmer Eye Institute
Miami, Florida

Michael T. Andreoli, MD
Fellow in Vitreoretinal Surgery
Department of Ophthalmology
University of Illinois College of Medicine
Chicago, Illinois

William E. Benson, MD
Wills Eye Hospital Retina Service
Professor of Ophthalmology, Thomas Jefferson University
Mid Atlantic Retina
Philadelphia, Pennsylvania

Mark S. Blumenkranz, MD
HJ Smead Professor and Chairman
Department of Ophthalmology
Director, Byers Eye Institute at Stanford
Palo Alto, California

Gary C. Brown, MD, MBA
Retina Service
Wills Eye Hospital
Professor of Ophthalmology
Thomas Jefferson University
Philadelphia, Pennsylvania

Mariana Cabrera, MD
Ophthalmologist
Fundación Oftalmológica Nacional
Bogotá, Colombia

Thalmon R. Campagnoli, MD
Research Fellow
Bascom Palmer Eye Institute
Miami, Florida

R. V. Paul Chan, MD, FACS
Professor of Ophthalmology and Visual Sciences
Vice Chair, Global Ophthalmology
Director, Pediatric Retina and ROP Service
Illinois Eye and Ear Infirmary
UIC Department of Ophthalmology and Visual Sciences
Chicago, Illinois

Royce W. S. Chen, MD
Helen and Martin Kimmel Assistant Professor of Ophthalmology
Edward S. Harkness Eye Institute
Columbia University Medical Center
New York, New York

Allen Chiang, MD
Wills Eye Hospital Retina Service
Assistant Professor of Ophthalmology, Thomas Jefferson University
Mid Atlantic Retina
Philadelphia, Pennsylvania

Matthew D. Cooke, MD
Fellow
Dean McGee Eye Institute
The University of Oklahoma College of Medicine
Oklahoma City, Oklahoma

Janet L. Davis, MD
Professor of Ophthalmology
Bascom Palmer Eye Institute
University of Miami Miller School of Medicine
Miami, Florida

Cathy DiBernardo, CDOS, ROUB
Owner
Ophthalmic Ultrasound Services of the Carolinas
Charlotte, North Carolina
Consultant and Clinical Associate Professor
Department of Ophthalmology
UNC School of Medicine
Cornelius, North Carolina

Jay S. Duker, MD
Director, New England Eye Center
Boston, Massachusetts
Professor and Chair of Ophthalmology
Tufts University School of Medicine
Boston, Massachusetts

Dean Eliott, MD
Stelios Evangelos Gragoudas Associate Professor of Ophthalmology
Associate Director of the Retina Service
Massachusetts Eye and Ear
Harvard Medical School
Boston, Massachusetts

Sharon Fekrat, MD FACS
Vitreoretinal Surgeon
Associate Professor of Ophthalmology and Surgery
Duke University School of Medicine
Associate Chief of Staff for Surgery, Durham VA Medical Center
Durham, North Carolina

Harry W. Flynn, Jr., MD
The J. Donald M. Gass Distinguished Chair in Ophthalmology
Professor of Ophthalmology
University of Miami Health System
Bascom Palmer Eye Institute
Miami, Florida

Sunir J. Garg, MD, FACS
Professor of Ophthalmology
Thomas Jefferson University
Philadelphia, Pennsylvania
The Retina Service
Wills Eye Hospital
Philadelphia, Pennsylvania

Morton F. Goldberg, MD
Director Emeritus, Wilmer Eye Institute
Johns Hopkins University School of Medicine
Johns Hopkins Hospital
Baltimore, Maryland

Dennis P. Han, MD
Professor of Ophthalmology
Chief, Retina Service
The Eye Institute
Medical College of Wisconsin
The Eye Institute
Milwaukee, Wisconsin

Angela M. Herro, MD
Neuro-Ophthalmologist
Horizon Eye Specialists & Lasik Center
Phoenix, Arizona

Allen C. Ho, MD, FASC
Director, Clinical Retina Research Unit
Wills Eye Hospital
Philadelphia, Pennsylvania

Samuel K. Steven Houston III, MD
Florida Retina Institute
Orlando, Florida

Jason Hsu, MD
Co-Director of Retina Research
Wills Eye Hospital
Associate Professor of Ophthalmology
Thomas Jefferson University
Philadelphia, Pennsylvania

Michael S. Ip, MD
Professor of Ophthalmology
David Geffen School of Medicine
University of California - Los Angeles
Doheny Eye Institute
Medical Director
Doheny Image Reading Center
Pasadena, California

Glenn J. Jaffe, MD
Robert Machemer Professor of Ophthalmology
Chief
Vitreoretinal Division
Director
Duke Reading Center
Duke University Eye Center
Durham, North Carolina

Mark W. Johnson, MD
Professor of Ophthalmology and Visual Sciences
University of Michigan Medical School
Ann Arbor, Michigan
Chief of Vitreoretinal Service
W. K. Kellogg Eye Center
Ann Arbor, Michigan

Peter K. Kaiser, MD
Chaney Family Endowed Chair in Ophthalmology Research
Cleveland Clinic Cole Eye Institute
Cleveland, Ohio

M. Ali Khan, MD
Assistant Professor of Ophthalmology
Doheny and Stein Eye Institutes
David Geffen School of Medicine at UCLA
Los Angeles, California

Stephen J. Kim, MD
Department of Ophthalmology and Visual Sciences
Vanderbilt University School of Medicine
Nashville, Tennessee

Marilyn C. Kincaid, MD
Retired
Part Time Clinical Professor
Department of Opthalmology and Pathology
St. Louis University
St. Louis, Missouri

Amol D. Kulkarni, MD
Retina Specialist, Dean Clinic/ SSM Health, Madison, WI
Clinical Adjunct Assistant Professor
Department of Ophthalmology and Visual Sciences,
University of Wisconsin, Madison
Madison, Wisconsin

Byron L. Lam, MD
Professor
Robert Z. and Nancy J. Greene Chair
Bascom Palmer Eye Institute
University of Miami School of Medicine
Miami, Florida

Gregory D. Lee, MD
Retina Fellow
University of Kentucky/Retina Associates of Kentucky
Lexington, Kentucky

Loh-Shan B. Leung, MD
Clinical Assistant Professor
Stanford University School of Medicine
Byers Eye Institute
Palo Alto, California

Ashleigh L. Levison, MD
Retinal Specialist
Retinal Consultants of Arizona
Phoenix, Arizona
Adjunct Clinical Assistant Professor of Ophthalmology
University of Southern California
USC Eye Institute
Los Angeles, California

Naresh Mandava, MD
Sue Anschutz-Rodgers Chair in Retinal Diseases
Professor and Chair, Department of Ophthalmology
Vitreoretinal Diseases and Surgery
University of Colorado School of Medicine
Aurora, Colorado

Michael F. Marmor, MD
Professor of Ophthalmology
Stanford University School of Medicine
Byers Eye Institute
Palo Alto, California

William F. Mieler, MD
Cless Family Professor and Vice-Chairman
Director Residency and Vitreoretinal Fellowship Training
Department of Ophthalmology & Visual Sciences
University of Illinois at Chicago
Chicago, Illinois

Robert A. Mittra, MD
Retinal Surgeon
Vitreoretinal Surgery, PA
Minneapolis, Minnesota

Shizuo Mukai, MD
Associate Professor
Department of Ophthalmology
Massachusetts Eye and Ear Infirmary and Harvard Medical School
Boston, Massachusetts

James D. Palmer, MD
Retinal Specialist
Northern California Retina Vitreous Associates, Inc.
Mountain View, California

Thanos D. Papakostas, MD
Vitreoretinal Fellow
Massachusetts Eye and Ear
Harvard Medical School
Boston, Massachusetts

Yannis M. Paulus, MD
Assistant Professor
Retina and Uveitis
Department of Ophthalmology and Visual Sciences
Department of Biomedical Engineering
Kellogg Eye Center
University of Michigan
Ann Arbor, Michigan

Paula E. Pecen, MD
Assistant Professor of Ophthalmology, Vitreoretinal Surgery
University of Colorado School of Medicine
Rocky Mountain Lions Eye Institute
Aurora, Colorado

David C. Reed, MD
Attending Physician
Ophthalmic Consultants of Boston
Boston, Massachusetts

Elias Reichel, MD
Director
Vitreoretinal Diseases and Surgery Service
Professor of Ophthalmology
New England Eye Center
Tufts Medical Center
Boston, Massachusetts

Carl D. Regillo, MD, FACS
Director, Retina Service
Wills Eye Hospital
Professor of Ophthalmology
Thomas Jefferson University
Philadelphia, Pennsylvania

Nidhi Relhan, MD
Research Fellow—Retina and Uveitis
Department of Ophthalmology
Bascom Palmer Eye Institute
University of Miami Miller School of Medicine
Miami, Florida

Hermann D. Schubert, MD
Professor of Clinical Ophthalmology and Pathology
Columbia University
New York, New York

Stephen G. Schwartz, MD, MBA
Associate Professor of Ophthalmology
Bascom Palmer Eye Institute
University of Miami Miller School of Medicine
Medical Director, Bascom Palmer Eye Institute at Naples
Naples, Florida

Ingrid U. Scott, MD, MPH
Jack and Nancy Turner Professor of Ophthalmology
Professor of Public Health Sciences
Penn State Eye Center
Penn State College of Medicine
Hershey, Pennsylvania

Sumit Sharma, MD
Trainee
Vitreoretinal Fellowship Program
Duke Ophthalmology
Duke University School of Medicine
Durham, North Carolina

Liliya Shevchenko, DO
Ophthalmologist
Retina Specialists of Michigan
Grand Rapids, Michigan

Carol L. Shields, MD
Co-Director
Ocular Oncology Service
Wills Eye Hospital
Philadelphia, Pennsylvania
Attending Surgeon
Wills Eye Hospital
Philadelphia, Pennsylvania
Professor of Ophthalmology
Thomas Jefferson University
Philadelphia, Pennsylvania

Jerry A. Shields, MD
Co-Director
Ocular Oncology Service
Wills Eye Hospital
Philadelphia, Pennsylvania
Attending Surgeon
Wills Eye Hospital
Philadelphia, Pennsylvania
Professor of Ophthalmology
Thomas Jefferson University
Philadelphia, Pennsylvania

Frank S. Siringo MD, OD
Assistant Professor, Vitreoretinal Diseases and Surgery
Department of Ophthalmology
University of Colorado School of Medicine
Aurora, Colorado

William E. Smiddy, MD
Professor
Bascom Palmer Eye Institute
University of Miami, Miller School of Institute
Miami, Florida

Paul Sternberg Jr., MD
Professor and Chairman
Vanderbilt Eye Institute
Nashville, Tennessee

Jennifer K. Sun, MD
Assistant Professor
Harvard Medical School
Boston, Massachusetts
Ophthalmologist
Beetham Eye Institute
Joslin Diabetes Center
Boston, Massachusetts

Katherine E. Talcott, MD
Director, Ocular Trauma Service
Massachusetts Eye and Ear
Boston, Massachusetts

Lauren S. Taney, MD
Retina Specialist
Washington Eye Physicians and Surgeons
Chevy Chase, Maryland

William Tasman, MD
Director of Retina Research
Wills Eye Hospital
Professor of Opthalmology
Thomas Jefferson University
Philadelphia, Pennsylvania

John T. Thompson, MD
Partner
Retina Specialists
Assistant Professor
The Wilmer Institute of The Johns Hopkins University
Associate Clinical Professor
University of Maryland Department of Ophthalmology
Baltimore, Maryland

James S. Tiedeman, MD
Ophthalmologist
RetinaCare of Virginia
Fishersville, Virginia

Kevin R. Tozer, MD
Ophthalmologist
Minnesota Eye Consultants
Minneapolis, Minnesota

Lawrence A. Yannuzzi, MD
Vitreous Retina Macula Consultants of New York
New York, New York

Yoshihiro Yonekawa, MD
Retina Service, Department of Ophthalmology
Massachusetts Eye and Ear Infirmary
Boston, Massachusetts
Harvard Medical School
Boston, Massachusetts

Suqin Yu, MD
Ophthalmologist
Department of Ophthalmology
Shanghai Jiao Tong University Affiliated First People's Hospital
Shanghai, China

Part I

Anatomy and Physiology

1 Anatomy of the Vitreous, Retina, and Choroid *2*

2 Retinal and Retinal Pigment Epithelial Physiology *14*

I

1 Anatomy of the Vitreous, Retina, and Choroid

Hermann D. Schubert and Marilyn C. Kincaid

1.1 Introduction

It is a truism that the anatomy of an organ, structure, or system provides the substrate for the types of pathologic processes that can affect it. This is particularly true for the retina and its associated structures, the vitreous and choroid. Understanding their structures allows the clinician to better understand diseases that can affect them and to appreciate the studies used to elucidate those diseased conditions.

1.2 Vitreous

The vitreous is a clear gel occupying the bulk of the eye, extending posteriorly from behind the lens and adhering to the internal limiting membrane of the retina (▶ Fig. 1.1). This connective tissue comprises 80% of the total volume of the globe, about 4 mL. Normal vitreous allows visible light to pass to the retina without alteration or scatter. It also acts as a stabilizer, pressure regulator, shock absorber, and metabolic sink supporting the retina.

On clinical examination, the collagenous vitreous is not homogeneous. Centrally, Cloquet's canal, a space about 1 to 2 mm in diameter, extends from just behind the lens posteriorly to the optic nerve head. It is a remnant of the embryonic hyaloid vascular system. This canal has an S-shaped course from anterior to posterior, making a dip inferiorly before rising back to the nerve head. Anteriorly, it widens as Berger's space to form the back surface of the patellar fossa.

The anterior cortical gel of the vitreous is the vitreous surface adjacent to the lens zonules and the posterior lens capsule. Biomicroscopically, the borders and structures of the gel may resemble a membrane, but ultrastructurally it consists of denser aggregations of collagen fibers.[1] The hyaloideocapsular ligament of Wieger is a circular attachment between the orbiculoposterior zonular fibers and the posterior surface of the lens capsule. It is not a true ligament,[1] and the attachments become weaker with age. The potential space formed between the lens and the patellar fossa bounded by Wieger's ligament is called *Berger's space*. A separation of Wieger's ligament from the lens represents an anterior vitreous detachment.

Posteriorly, the canal widens to cover the *area of Martegiani*, which corresponds to the surface of the optic nerve head. The vitreous is firmly attached to the margin of the area, although with age the firmness of this attachment becomes attenuated. If the vitreous detaches completely, the glial peripapillary attachment is sometimes visible as a partial or complete ring suspended in the midportion of the eye, sometimes referred to as a *Weiss ring*.

The vitreous consists of about 99% water; the remaining compounds include hyaluronic acid and collagen, as well as inorganic salts and ascorbic acid.

Most of the vitreous collagen is concentrated peripherally in the vitreous body, adjacent to lens, retina, and optic nerve head. This denser portion of the vitreous is called the *vitreous cortex*. The remainder of the nuclear vitreous, located more centrally, has less collagen. The vitreous collagens are similar, although not chemically identical, to collagens elsewhere in the body.[2]

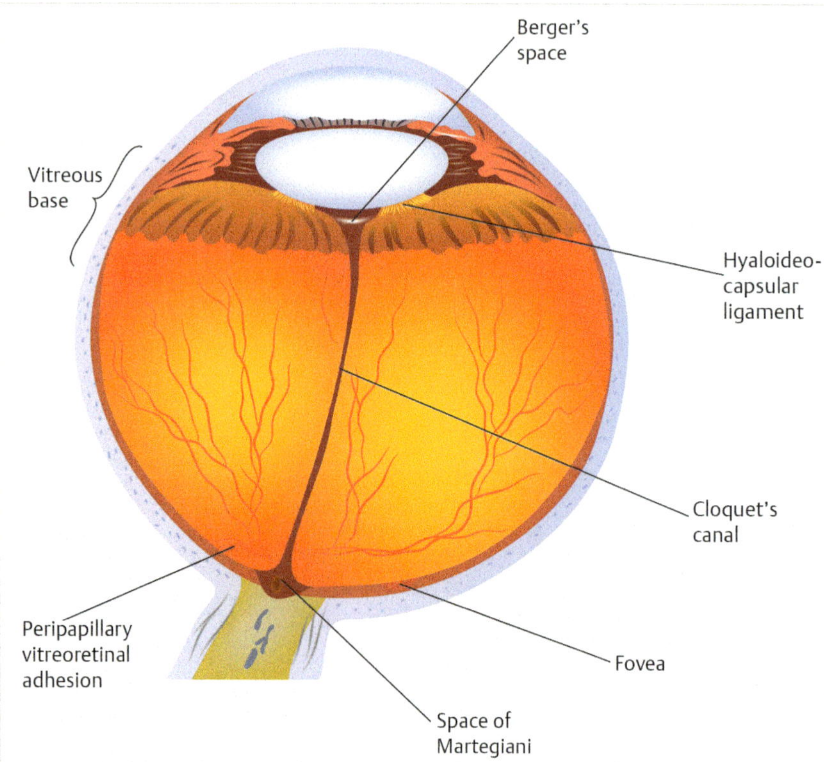

Fig. 1.1 Normal, youthful vitreous gel and associated landmarks.

The principal collagen component is type II; this is similar to the type II collagen of cartilage and suggests a support function. Type IX collagen is a minor component, also similar to the type IX collagen of cartilage.

Unlike collagen, the concentration of hyaluronic acid and other compounds is constant throughout the vitreous. The hyaluronic acid acts as a cross-link interposed between parallel fibrils of collagen forming a gel. Within the vitreous, especially in the cortex, are oval-to-spindle-shaped cells called *hyalocytes*. These cells contain organelles of synthesis and transport; in particular, they have abundant Golgi apparatus. The hyaluronic acid is believed to be synthesized in hyalocyte granules and secreted by these cells.[1]

The vitreous base overlies the posterior aspect of the pars plana and adjacent anterior aspect of the ora serrata of the retina, and is thus a ring 4 to 6 mm in width. The vitreous collagen and its attachments are most dense at the vitreous base. Traction in this area may tear the peripheral retina and adjacent pars plana epithelium.[3] The ophthalmoscopically visible phenomena of white-without-pressure and white-with-pressure appear, in some cases, to be caused by the alignment of the collagen fibrils and their insertions. Adhesions between vitreous and retina have also been observed posterior to the base, particularly in older eyes.[3] Ultrastructurally, collagen fibers insert into the basal lamina of nonpigmented ciliary epithelium and into focal breaks in the retinal internal limiting membrane.[4]

Controversial Points

- The ophthalmoscopically visible phenomena of white-without-pressure and white-with-pressure in the retinal periphery may be caused by the alignment of the cortical vitreous collagen fibrils and their insertions onto the retina in the region of the vitreous base.

The vitreous is also attached to the internal limiting membrane of the retina around the center of the foveola and alongside the larger retinal vessels; however, these attachments are not visible clinically under normal conditions. Vitreous fissures are found in front of retinal vessels and a vitreous pocket is found in front of the papilla, connecting with the premacular bursa.[5] With age, as the formed vitreous detaches and collapses anteriorly, the resultant traction on the posterior vitreous base may cause tears in the retina, sometimes accompanied by a vitreous hemorrhage if a vessel is torn.

Recently, this classic concept of posterior attachment sites has been reexamined using in vivo swept-source optical coherence tomography, corroborating and extending findings based on postmortem injections.[6] Experimental studies suggest that the vitreous is more diffusely attached in the posterior pole, at least in younger people.[7] In a study of postmortem human eyes, the vitreous was mechanically lifted away from the retina. In older eyes, the vitreous detached smoothly from the retina, leaving the internal limiting membrane intact. Ultrastructurally, the vitreal side of the membrane remained smooth. In eyes younger than 20 years, the internal limiting membrane in the posterior pole region tended to detach along with the vitreous away from the underlying retinal layers, showing the vitreous–internal limiting membrane attachment to be stronger than intraretinal attachments.

1.3 Retina

The retina is the neuroepithelium of the eye responsible for receiving light and converting it into neural impulses, which are interpreted by the cerebral cortex. It is derived from the embryonic forebrain, and is part of the central nervous system.[8] The retina is a layered and highly ordered structure. The sensory retina is transparent, except for blood vessels, so the apparent color of the fundus is derived from the retinal pigment epithelial melanin, the melanin of the choroidal melanocytes, and the choroidal vessels.

Often, the terms *retina* and *sensory retina* are used interchangeably. The term *retina* properly includes the retinal pigment epithelium as well. Both the sensory retina and retinal pigment epithelium are derived from the bilayer of the optic cup.[9] Reflecting the embryonal invagination of the optic vesicle, the cells of Müllerian glia and retinal pigment epithelium are arranged apex to apex, with the respective basement membranes (inner limiting membrane and inner aspect of Bruch's membrane) at opposite bases.

The outer neuroectodermal layer, the retinal pigment epithelium, remains a monolayer. It is discontinuous at the optic nerve head and continuous anteriorly with the pigment epithelium of the ciliary body.

The inner neuroectodermal layer proliferates, thickens, and differentiates to become the sensory retina. Except for the nerve fiber layer, the axons of which comprise the optic nerve, all layers of the sensory retina are discontinuous at the optic nerve head.

The sensory retina extends from the optic disc anteriorly to the ora serrata, where it is continuous with the nonpigmented ciliary epithelium. The ora serrata is located 6 mm behind the limbus, approximately at the insertion points of the rectus muscles, following the imaginary spiral of Tillaux.[10] The configuration of the ora serrata is discussed in more detail later.

1.3.1 Retinal Pigment Epithelium

The retinal pigment epithelium is one of the most biologically active tissues of the body. It is deeply pigmented, having become completely melanized by the sixth gestational week. Moreover, the degree of pigmentation is independent of race, unlike the pigmentation of the uveal tract, skin, and hair.[11] Biomicroscopically, this tissue is responsible for much of the color of the fundus. The macula appears darker, in part because the cells of this region are taller and narrower.

As seen in a flat preparation, the retinal pigment epithelium is a monolayer consisting of hexagonal cells with central round nuclei. Occasional cells have two nuclei, and such cells increase in number with age. Also, with age, the uniformity seen in young eyes gives way to cells more variable in size and shape.[12]

Retinal pigment epithelial cells are polar—that is, each cell has a discernible base and apex (▶ Fig. 1.2). Microvillous processes emerge from the apex of the retinal pigment epithelial cells to surround the photoreceptor outer segments. Some are fingerlike and slender, whereas others are broader and surround the outer segment like a bowl.[1] The cell nuclei are approximately spherical and lie just above the base of the cell. The unit membrane of the base is highly convoluted.

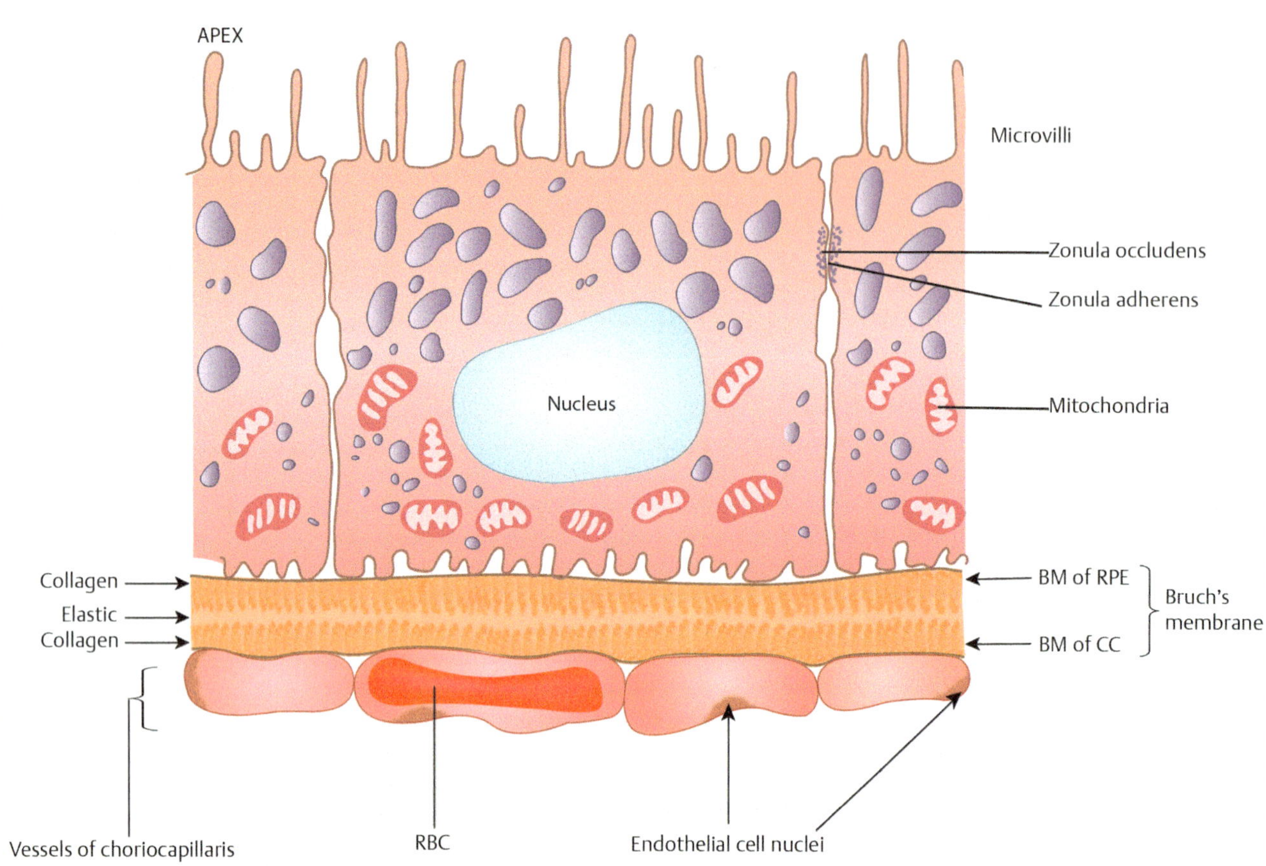

Fig. 1.2 Retinal pigment epithelial cells and the underlying Bruch's membrane. BM, basement membrane; RBC, red blood cell; RPE, retinal pigment epithelium.

A variety of conditions, such as uveitis, trauma, and retinal detachment, can stimulate the retinal pigment epithelium to proliferate. The hyperplastic retinal pigment epithelium nonetheless retains its cytologic polarity, creating tubules, acini, and rows of cells, with accompanying basement membrane formation.[13] Peripherally, the retinal pigment epithelium may proliferate in various patterns in the aging eye.[14]

Special Considerations

- A variety of pathologic conditions, such as uveitis, trauma, and retinal detachment, can stimulate the retinal pigment epithelium to proliferate. Some degree of retinal pigment epithelial proliferation is also evident in the peripheral fundus of the otherwise normal aging eye, perhaps reflecting chronic tractional forces at the vitreous base.

Each retinal pigment epithelial cell is attached to adjacent cells by tight junctions. Ultrastructurally, these junctions include a zonula adherens and an adjacent zonula occludens, both situated near the apex of the cell and encircling it.[12] The zonula adherens is a gap junction. The unit membranes of two adjacent cells are close together, but each can be separately identified. The zonula occludens, as the name implies, has no intercellular space. The peripheral margins of the unit membrane appear fused. The result is that small molecules, such as fluorescein, travel inward from the choroidal circulation only as far as the apices of the pigment epithelial cells. This barrier is referred to as the *outer blood–retinal barrier*.[15] When the junctions are lost, leakage of fluid from the choroid may be clinically evident as an exudative retinal detachment.[16]

In contrast to the convoluted unit membrane configuration at the base of the retinal pigment epithelial cell, the basement membrane is flat. It is the innermost component of Bruch's membrane, a complex consisting of five layers discerned at the ultrastructural level (▶ Fig. 1.2).[17] Extending outward from the retinal pigment epithelial side, these layers include the basement membrane of the retinal pigment epithelium, followed by a thick inner collagenous layer, an elastic layer, a thin outer collagenous layer, and the basement membrane of the choriocapillaris. Bruch's membrane thickens with age[18] and also becomes somewhat more disrupted, so that individual layers become more difficult to discern.

Special Considerations

- Ultrastructurally, Bruch's membrane has five distinct layers. However, with age, a variable degree of membrane thickening and lipid deposition make these layers less distinct.

The retinal pigment epithelium is one of the most metabolically active tissues of the body. Reflecting this, numerous organelles of synthesis and transport are seen ultrastructurally in the pigment epithelium. Mitochondria are abundant, especially in the basal half of the cell, underneath its nucleus. Smooth and rough endoplasmic reticulum, free ribosomes, and Golgi apparatus are also evident.[1]

A striking aspect of the pigment epithelium is its melanin pigment, mostly located in the apical cytoplasm of the cells. Two types of pigment granules are present in the retinal pigment epithelium- melanin and lipofuscin. Melanin is a dark brown to black pigment that is chemically poorly understood. The precursor is tyrosine, which is oxidized and polymerized through a series of enzymatic and nonenzymatic steps. Melanosomes, the site of melanogenesis, are round-to-oval membrane-bound granules morphologically similar to those of the uveal tract. In addition, there are elongated, lancet-shaped melanosomes. These granules are present in some of the apical microvilli; thus, they are in close proximity to the outer segments of the photoreceptors.[19] Recent evidence indicates that the epithelial cells do not produce additional pigment after birth, at least not through the tyrosinase enzymatic pathway. However, they do avidly take up free pigment in tissue culture.[20]

Retinal pigment epithelial hypertrophy is usually congenital. The pattern can be either solitary or grouped; the latter is sometimes called "bear tracks." The additional pigment is in the form of large, round melanosomes.[21,22]

The concentration of melanin varies regionally and also with age. The amount of melanin is actually greater at the equator than at the macula, where it is stacked up in taller and thinner cells, increasing optical density. With age, the melanin in peripheral pigment epithelium decreases, whereas that in the posterior pole remains constant for different age groups, resulting in overall greater optical density centrally.[23]

Photoreceptor outer segments are shed daily and regenerated constantly throughout life, at a rate dependent on incident light.[24,25] The shed material is engulfed and digested by the retinal pigment epithelium. However, this material is not completely digestible.[25] Lipofuscin- a complex of indigestible end products- is a golden yellow material distributed widely in the body. It is composed chiefly of vitamin A aldehyde adducts, although the composition varies even within the same tissue. With increased age, lipofuscin accumulates in the retinal pigment epithelium within secondary lysosomes due to ongoing phagocytosis. The melanosomes are displaced apically as the lipofuscin granules accumulate at the base. Complex granules containing both melanin and lipofuscin are called *melanolipofuscin granules*; in advanced age, these can be more numerous than the melanosomes. In the retinal periphery, this accumulation of lipofuscin and loss of melanin appears to be responsible for certain age-associated pigmentary patterns. Retinal pigment epithelial lipofuscin is also increased in recessive Stargardt's disease and in age-related maculopathies.[24,26]

Pearls

- Accumulation of lipofuscin- with loss of melanin- in pigment epithelial cells of the retinal periphery appears to be responsible for certain age-associated pigmentary patterns.

There are no structural junctions between the retinal pigment epithelial cells and the photoreceptors. This is in contrast to the numerous tight junctions present between the corresponding two neuroepithelial layers of the ciliary body and the iris.[1] Instead, the epithelioretinal interspace contains a glycosaminoglycan matrix. Further, the retinal pigment epithelium constantly pumps fluid out of this space, creating a net negative pressure, to maintain photoreceptor apposition. This active transport accounts for about 70% of the total forces responsible for retinal apposition.[13,24]

In addition, interphotoreceptor matrix proteins act as a glue to keep the cells apposed. These protein adhesions are surprisingly strong in the freshly enucleated, and presumably in the living, eye. In experimental studies, the sensory retina was peeled from underlying pigment epithelium in freshly enucleated human and monkey eyes. If done within 1 minute of enucleation, the cone photoreceptor sheaths- components of the interphotoreceptor matrix- stretched to twice their normal size before their attachment to the pigment epithelium broke.[27]

1.3.2 Sensory Retina

The sensory retina is distinctive for its highly ordered architecture, seen by light microscopy and optical coherence tomography (▶ Fig. 1.3). Even at low microscopy power, three distinct bands of nuclei are readily evident, separated by tissue containing few or no cell nuclei.

Photoreceptor cells, both rods and cones, are unique, elongated cells; their nuclei comprise the outer nuclear layer of the retina. There are approximately 120 million rods and 6 million cones in the human retina.[28] Both rods and cones have specialized light-gathering ends- the outer segments- which represent specialized sensory cilia.

The rods are so named because the outer segment is cylindrical in shape. The stacked discs of the rods contain rhodopsin, the visual pigment for scotopic vision. The discs are separated

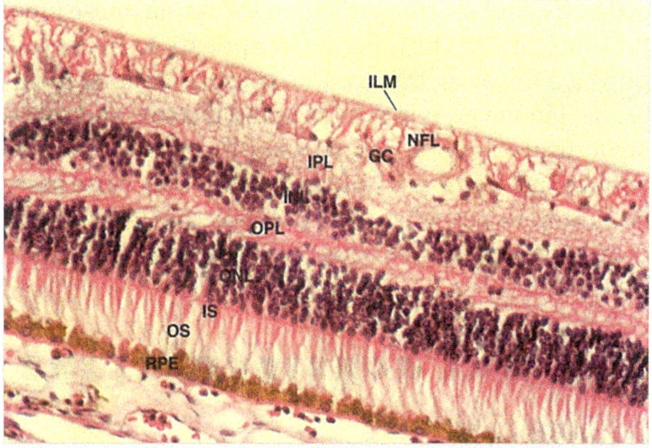

Fig. 1.3 The sensory retina and retinal pigment epithelium (RPE). The photoreceptor outer segments (OS) and inner segments (IS) have their cell nuclei within the outer nuclear layer (ONL). They synapse with the neurons of the inner nuclear layer (INL) in the outer plexiform layer (OPL). These neurons, in turn, synapse with the ganglion cells (GC) in the inner plexiform layer (IPL). Axons from the ganglion cells form the nerve fiber layer (NFL). The internal limiting membrane (ILM) is the inner margin of the sensory retina. Hematoxylin and eosin, × 156.

from the surrounding unit membrane of the cell. The outer ends of the outer segments are constantly shed, taken up by the retinal pigment epithelium, and regenerated at the proximal end.[29]

The cone outer segments are shorter than those of the rods, and thus they do not extend as closely to the pigment epithelial layer. The outer segment is tapered, giving the cone its name. However, in the fovea, the cones are not tapered, but instead are long, slender, and cylindrical in shape, allowing for tight packing. The stacked discs in cone photoreceptors generally remain continuous with the cell membrane. Cone discs are also shed and regenerated.

There are three types of cones, each type with its own spectral sensitivity; the light-sensitive proteins for these likewise reside in the stacked membranes of the outer segments. The proteins are chemically similar to opsin, the rod visual protein.

Connecting each outer segment to the inner segments is a nonmotile cilium. The inner segments, which connect the outer segments with their discs to the cell bodies, are filled with numerous mitochondria and other organelles of synthesis and transport.[29] The outer portion of the inner segment, containing the mitochondria, is called the *ellipsoid*. The inner portion of the inner segment is called the *myoid*. It contains smooth and rough endoplasmic reticulum and many microtubules. The inner segments of the cones are similar to those of the rods, but the ellipsoids are much larger and the mitochondria are several times more numerous. The presence of these organelles demonstrates the high metabolic activity and oxygen requirements of these cells.[1]

The photoreceptor cells and adjacent Müller's cells form tight junctions with each other. Because of the ordered cellular arrangement of the retina, these junctions are in line, forming what appears to be- at low power or on optical coherence tomography- a linear membrane, the external limiting membrane. However, it is not a true membrane, and ultrastructural examination reveals it to be a series of zonulae adherentes in a linear array. This close association between photoreceptors and Müller's cells may be important for inner-segment metabolism.[1]

Special Considerations

- The external limiting membrane of the retina is not a true membrane. It represents a linear array of tight junctions (zonulae adherentes) located between the photoreceptor cells and adjacent Müller's cells.

Synapses between photoreceptors and the cells of the inner nuclear layer occur in the outer plexiform layer. The synapsing end of the rod is called the *spherule*, and the much larger, broader end of the cone is called the *pedicle*. In addition, both cones and rods have lateral extensions near their synapsing ends; these extensions connect with adjacent rods and cones, but apparently without synaptic vesicles.[1]

The inner nuclear layer is populated by the cell bodies of horizontal, bipolar, interplexiform, and amacrine cells. Horizontal cells tend to be located at the outer margin of the inner nuclear layer. Bipolar cells stretch along the thickness of the inner nuclear layer, forming synapses with both the photoreceptors and the ganglion cells. Amacrine and interplexiform cells align along the inner margin of the inner nuclear layer. Interplexiform cells also have processes within both plexiform layers.[8]

Synapses with the next order of neurons, the ganglion cells, occur in the inner plexiform layer. However, in addition to centripetal synapses- from photoreceptors to occipital cortex- it is also evident that synapses occur between different cells within the inner nuclear layer.[8]

The ganglion cell layer is the innermost layer of cell nuclei. These cells are generally relatively large, with abundant cytoplasm. In the peripheral retina, this layer consists of only a single layer of cells. The anatomic macula is defined as the circular area where the ganglion cell layer consists of two or more layers of cells; more centrally at the foveal margin, it thickens to comprise up to seven or eight layers of cells. Ganglion cells have from one to several dendrites and have been classified into several different functional types.[1]

Pearls

- In conditions that result in swelling and opacification of the ganglion cell layer, such as storage disorders and central retinal artery occlusions, retinal opacification is most prominent in the macular region because the ganglion cell layer is thickest in the macula but not in the foveola where the ganglion cell layer is discontinuous—hence the "cherry red spot" appearance in the central macula in such conditions.

The ganglion cells each send a single axon through the nerve fiber layer to the optic nerve. Thus, this is the only retinal layer that is not discontinuous across the optic nerve head. As one would expect, the nerve fiber layer is thickest adjacent to the disc and thinnest at the ora serrata. As measured in quadrants adjacent to the nerve, the nerve fiber layer is thickest superiorly and thinnest in the papillomacular bundle, temporal to the disc.[30]

The axons synapse at the lateral geniculate body. Those originating in the temporal half of the retina remain ipsilateral, while those from the nasal half cross at the optic chiasm. However, there appears to be some intermingling along this vertical dividing line, so that some temporal fibers cross and some nasal fibers do not; this may explain evidence of macular sparing in unilateral occipital cortical disease.[31]

Controversial Points

- "Macular sparing" in unilateral occipital cortical infarct may be, at least in part, explained by the finding that not all ganglion cell axons from the temporal retina remain uncrossed at the optic chiasm and not all axons from the nasal retina cross at the chiasm.

Müller's cells extend virtually the entire thickness of the retina. The outermost apical portion of the cells is bound by zonulae adherentes to the photoreceptors, and the cells have delicate processes- fiber baskets- that extend even further outward, reaching the interphotoreceptor matrix. Müller's cells extend inward to the inner limiting membrane. They have lateral processes that surround adjacent cells in the nuclear and plexiform layers, acting as a support. Their nuclei reside in the inner nuclear layer and processes surround the retinal capillary plexus in a so-called bipolar arrangement, nourishing neurons. Müller's cells spread out laterally and help to form the internal limiting membrane, which is a true basement membrane. The internal limiting membrane is attenuated in areas where large blood vessels in the nerve fiber layer displace these cells.[1] Other types of glial cells, including microglia and astrocytes, are also present in the retina.[8]

1.3.3 Retinal Circulation

The retina receives a dual circulation of blood. The inner half of the sensory retina, extending outward to include approximately the inner third of the inner nuclear layer, is supplied by the retinal vasculature. The outer half receives its nourishment by diffusion from the choroidal circulation.

The retinal vessels, like those of the brain, are end vessels and do not anastomose except under pathologic circumstances. Also, like those of the brain, and unlike those elsewhere in the body, the retinal capillaries are impermeable to relatively small molecules, such as fluorescein.

Pearls

- The retinal vessels, like those of the central nervous system, are end vessels and do not normally anastomose. Similar to those of the brain, the retinal capillary endothelial cells have tight junctions, which make the vessels impermeable to relatively small molecules, such as fluorescein.

Vascularization of the retina begins during the 16th week of gestation at the optic nerve head,[32] and normally reaches the ora serrata nasally at the time of birth. It is not quite complete temporally at term because the distance from the optic nerve head to the ora is greater.

The vessels of the retinal circulation emerge at the optic disc and almost immediately divide to form four branches. The two temporal vessels run superiorly and inferiorly to the macula in an arcuate configuration, whereas the superonasal and inferonasal vessels run more directly peripherally. As the vessels proceed peripherally, they further branch and taper in size. The specific pattern of the retinal vessels is unique to each individual.

The large arterioles and venules travel in the nerve fiber layer and ganglion cell layer. (Despite the fact that the central retinal vessels remain histologically arteries and veins for only a short distance from the optic disc, peripherally becoming arterioles and venules, respectively, the terms *artery* and *vein* are used clinically and histologically to designate the respective vessels and their diseases.) The veins accompany the arteries, and the vessels may cross each other multiple times as they proceed peripherally. Where they cross, they share a common adventitial sheath. With increasing age and the development of arteriosclerosis, the crossings can become accentuated, with compression of the less resilient vein. Branch retinal vein occlusions typically occur at crossings where the artery crosses over the vein.[33]

Pearls

- Retinal arteries and veins share a common adventitial sheath where they cross. Increasing atherosclerosis can cause the artery to impinge on the underlying, less resilient vein, and this appears to explain why branch retinal vein occlusions tend to occur where the artery crosses over the vein.

The smaller vessels, including the capillaries, extend outward at the level of the nerve fiber layer and the inner nuclear layer. Close to the foveal avascular zone, the capillaries form a single layer, but elsewhere the capillaries are present in two or more distinct layers.[34] The most peripheral millimeter or so of the sensory retina is avascular.

Frequently, the retina receives some blood supply from an artery originating in the choroid that travels around the margin of Bruch's membrane at the margin of the optic nerve head (▶ Fig. 1.4). In one clinical study, about half of all the patients studied had at least one cilioretinal artery in one eye, and about a third had such vessels bilaterally.[35] Most were seen at the temporal margin of the disc, and many such vessels supplied at least a portion of the macular circulation. Such vessels are supplied by the short posterior ciliary arteries, like the choroidal vessels. Thus, they fill before the central retinal artery and can be recognized on fluorescein angiography.[35]

As noted earlier, the retinal capillaries, including those of any cilioretinal vessels, are impermeable to relatively small molecules. This so-called inner blood–retinal barrier is the vascular endothelium. The site of the barrier is the specialized tight junctions (zonulae occludentes) between individual endothelial cells. Also, in contrast to that of the choriocapillaris, the capillary endothelium of the retina does not have pores.[15]

The sympathetic nervous system is responsible in most parts of the body for regulation of vascular tone. However, the retinal vessels are an exception; regulation is mediated by a number of vasoactive substances secreted by the vascular endothelium.[36]

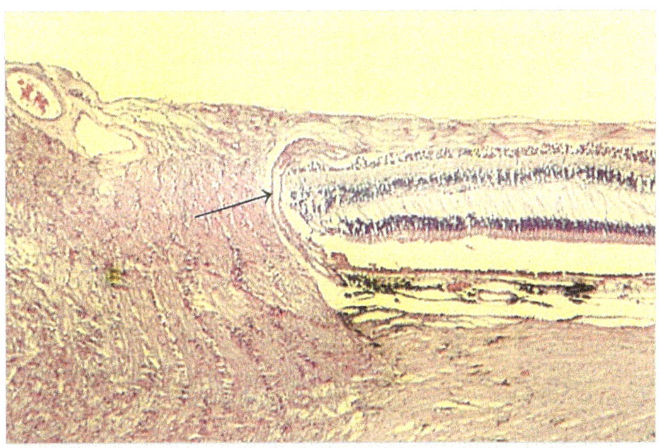

Fig. 1.4 A cilioretinal artery (arrow) originates from the choroid and proceeds inward around Bruch's membrane, retinal pigment epithelium, and outer retina to enter the nerve fiber layer. Hematoxylin and eosin, × 62.

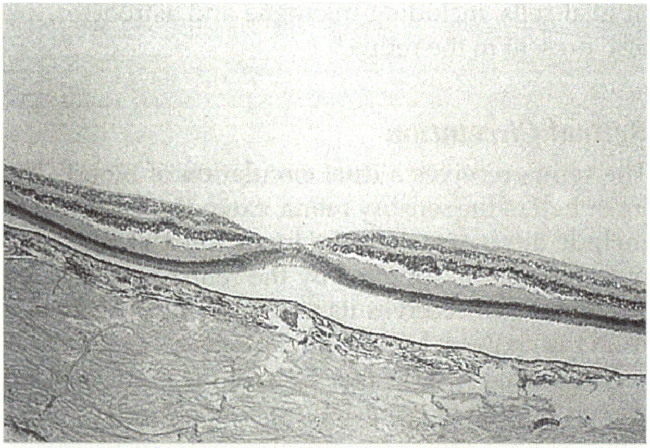

Fig. 1.5 Low-power view of the macula. Even at this magnification, the thickness of the ganglion cell layer is clearly visible. The sensory retinal detachment is an artifact. Hematoxylin and eosin, × 16.

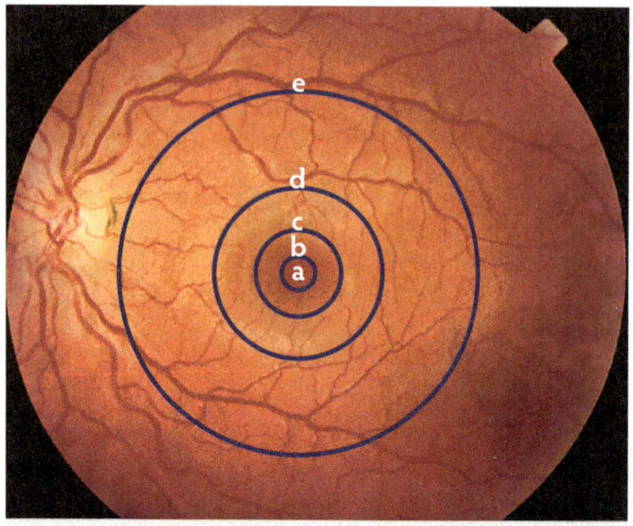

Fig. 1.6 Terms for central area of the posterior pole with approximate sizes. (**a**) Foveola: 0.35 mm diameter; (**b**) fovea: 1.5 mm diameter; (**c**) parafovea: 0.5 mm ring; (**d**) perifovea; 1.5 mm ring. The area centralis thus has a diameter of 5.5 mm: 1.5 + 2 × 0.5 + 2 × 1.5 = 5.5 mm.

1.3.4 Macula

The macula, or area centralis, is a specialized region of the retina.[37] The terms *macula* and *fovea* are used in different ways by the anatomist and the clinician because clinical landmarks have no precise anatomic counterpart, and vice versa. Anatomically, the macula includes the entire area of the retina where the ganglion cell layer is more than a single cell layer in thickness (▶ Fig. 1.5). It corresponds to the clinician's posterior pole and is about 5.5 mm in diameter, approximately bounded by the superior and inferior temporal vascular arcades (▶ Fig. 1.6). Superficial capillaries supplying the nerve fiber layer are oriented radially and are called the radial peripapillary capillary net.[38] They do not extend beyond the near periphery or fovea and cause cotton wool spots when occluded. These radial capillaries are angiographically distinct from the deeper two plexuses, the superficial one on the inner aspect of the inner nuclear layer and the deep capillary plexus on the outside. Radicular vessels-some right angled- dip deep down into the retina to supply these plexus.[39] Focal intraretinal periarteriolar transudates or paracentral acute middle maculopathies may result from deeper intraretinal (pre)capillary leakage or occlusion.[40,41]

What is clinically referred to as the fovea[42] is a central depression about 1.5 mm in diameter, approximately the size of the optic disc. In younger people, the boundary of this central depression- the margo foveae- often produces a horizontally oriented, slightly oval light reflex. With age, this reflection dims. More centrally from this boundary is the limit of the capillary network, or the foveal avascular zone, about 500 to 600 µm (0.5–0.6 mm) in diameter. The foveola measures about 350 µm (0.35 mm) in diameter and is the floor of the anatomic fovea. Particularly in younger people, a tiny bright dot of light overlying the center of this pit can sometimes be seen. This is a virtual image formed by the configuration of the retina in this region. The foveola and the foveal clivus act as a minute parabolic mirror, reflecting the incident light.

The *foveola* is populated with specialized cones, and rods are entirely absent.[1] Morphologically, the cones are long, slender, and rodlike, allowing tighter packing, particularly in the central 200-µm area, the umbo. The floor of the foveola consists only of the cones and Müllerian glial cell processes, the remaining layers of the sensory retina having been displaced peripherally (▶ Fig. 1.7). To synapse with the next order of neurons, the inner fibers of the cones in the foveola must be oriented obliquely, forming *Henle's fiber layer*. Fluids collect more easily in the outer plexiform layer around the foveola because of the oblique orientation of the photoreceptor fibers here compared to their more vertical orientation peripherally.

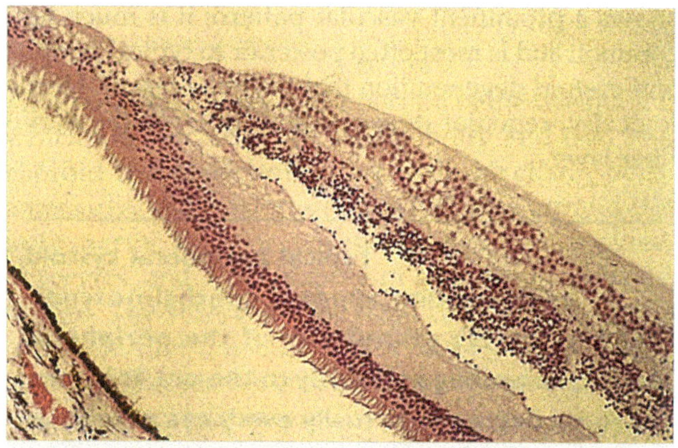

Fig. 1.7 Medium power view of the macula shows the foveola at the upper right, populated only by cone photoreceptors. Immediately adjacent, all nuclear layers are about equally thick. The split between the outer plexiform layer and the inner nuclear layer is an artifact. Hematoxylin and eosin, × 62.

A yellow coloration gives the *macula lutea* its name. This pigment is not well seen with white light, but with red-free light or with blue light photography, it is more obvious. It is present in all the retinal layers inward to the outer nuclear layer, especially in both plexiform layers.[43] Its highest concentration is in the foveola, where it is theorized to function as an optical filter. The pigment is dissolved out with routine histologic fixation, but its location has been analyzed in fresh-frozen sections and with specialized fixatives. Chemically, it is a carotenoid called *lutein*.[44]

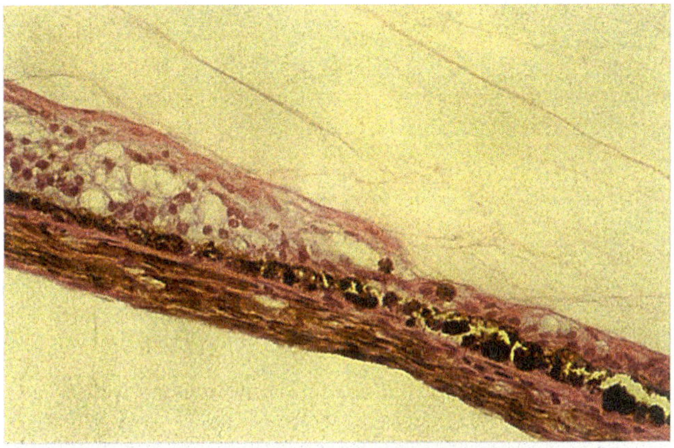

Fig. 1.8 The ora serrata region shows relatively disorganized layers in the sensory retina, to the left. There is an abrupt transition to nonpigmented ciliary epithelium, to the right. There are strands of vitreous visible overlying this region, the vitreous base. Hematoxylin and eosin, × 156.

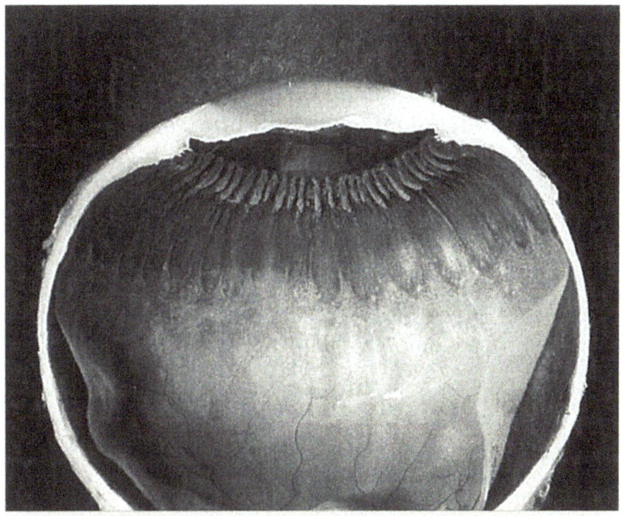

Fig. 1.9 The teeth and bays of the ora serrata are readily seen in the nasal portion of the eye.

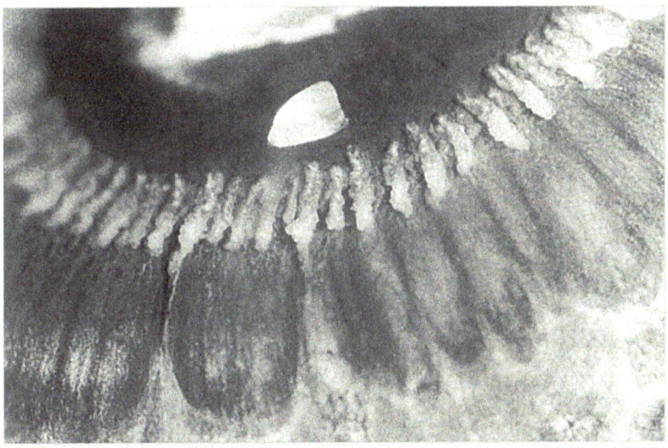

Fig. 1.10 Two meridional complexes.

Pearls

- Fluids collect more easily in the outer plexiform layer around the foveola because of the oblique orientation of the photoreceptor fibers here compared to their more vertical orientation peripherally.

1.3.5 Retinal Periphery

Anatomically, the retinal periphery includes all portions of the retina that are not part of the anatomic macula, or, otherwise stated, that part of the retina where the ganglion cell layer is a single cell layer thick. The ora serrata is the junction between the sensory retina and the nonpigmented ciliary epithelium (▶ Fig. 1.8). The ora serrata is, as the name implies, serrated in configuration. This serration is most obvious, with deep bays and more pronounced teeth, in the superonasal region (▶ Fig. 1.9).[45] Elsewhere, the teeth and bays are less distinct.

The preequatorial retina has particular anatomic structures and variations. *Meridional folds* are linear elevations in the peripheral retina that appear as tented-up ridges, with the folds arranged meridionally. They can occur anywhere from the ora-within a tooth or bay- to a region about 6 mm posterior to the ora. About four-fifths arise in a tooth. If folds arise in a dentate process that is aligned so that it meets with a ciliary process anteriorly, the structure is called a *meridional complex* (▶ Fig. 1.10). In a large autopsy study, meridional folds and complexes occurred with equal frequency in all decades of life; thus, they are congenital, not degenerative, lesions. Racial prevalence was equal, but they were more frequent in men.[45]

Ora serrata pearls are small, spherical, glistening bodies seen within retinal teeth, or just posterior to them, in aging eyes. They may appear opalescent, giving them their name. Sometimes they are brown to black. They may be multiple, extending in a line along the tooth. They are formed beneath the retinal pigment epithelium and may thus be a type of druse. Subsequently, they work their way to the retinal surface and may even end up within overlying vitreous.[46]

An oral bay may extend posteriorly to be unusually deep. Typically, such a bay is bounded by two unusually large teeth, called *giant teeth*. If the bay is closed by the fusion of two adjacent teeth, it is called an *enclosed oral bay* (▶ Fig. 1.11). The enclosed area appears clinically and histologically as an "island" of pars plana with retinal tissue both anterior and posterior to the island. These findings occur independently of age and appear to be congenital variations.[45]

With increasing age, *cystoid degeneration* occurs at the ora serrata, particularly in the temporal region. Typical peripheral cystoid degeneration involves the outer plexiform layer, resulting in spaces that contain an acid mucopolysaccharide. Clinically, it appears as a coarsely granular change in the peripheral retina, extending anteriorly to the ora serrata. Posteriorly, there is an abrupt boundary with normal-appearing peripheral retina. Typical peripheral cystoid degeneration is seen to some degree in virtually every eye of individuals older than 20 years. Reticular degeneration, in contrast, appears more finely

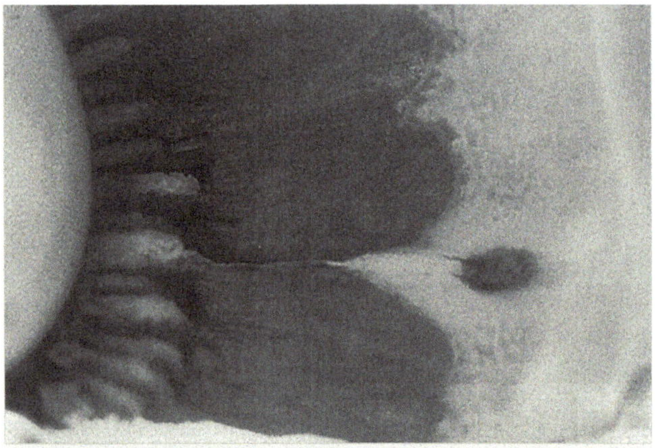

Fig. 1.11 Enclosed oral bay. Two retinal teeth enclose an island of ciliary body epithelium.

granular and shows a prominent vascular pattern; it is much less common and is most often posterior to typical peripheral cystoid degeneration that may be present. Histologically, reticular degeneration involves the nerve fiber layer.

> **Pearls**
>
> - Typical peripheral cystoid degeneration appears ophthalmoscopically as coarse granularity of the peripheral retina, extending anteriorly to the ora. It is seen to some degree in virtually every eye of individuals older than 20 years.

Both types of peripheral cystoid degeneration may progress to degenerative schisis, arbitrarily defined as spaces that extend radially for 1.5 mm or more. Typical degenerative retinoschisis tends to remain flat and be nonprogressive, whereas reticular degenerative retinoschisis shows a bullous elevation of the inner aspect of the split and has a tendency to extend posteriorly.[47]

Several types of focal elevations of retinal tissue, called *retinal tufts*, have been identified. Noncystic retinal tufts occur at the vitreous base and- by virtue of their location- do not lead to retinal detachment. Cystic retinal tufts are more posterior, and appear as 0.1- to 1.0-mm whitish elevations. They are present in all age groups and in all quadrants of the retina. There can be associated pigment changes at the base of the tuft, as well as small holes or tractional tears. Histologically, there is microcystic change within and around the tuft, and frequently vitreous condensations are present on the surface.[48]

Zonular traction tufts can also lead to retinal detachment. These are congenital lesions that extend over the pars plana from the peripheral retina and become continuous with a zonular fiber. The retina at the base of the tuft is tented up and tends to show cystoid degeneration. The tuft is composed of a thin glial strand, and rarely embryonal epithelium. For unexplained reasons, about 80% are nasal, and three-quarters occur in male subjects.[49]

Because the nonpigmented ciliary epithelium is attached to the pigmented ciliary epithelium by tight junctions between

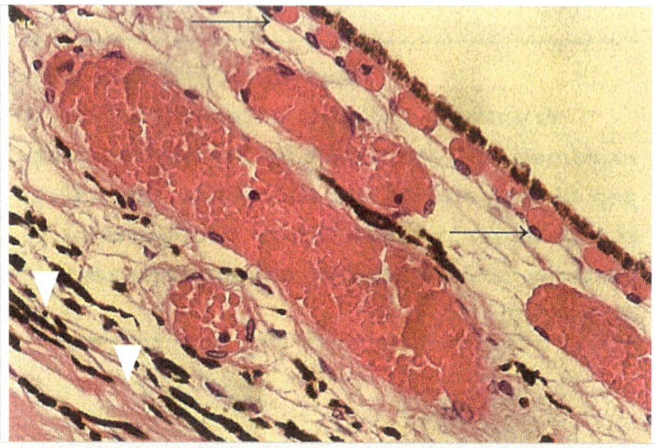

Fig. 1.12 The choroidal vasculature. Beneath the retinal pigment epithelium and Bruch's membrane (inconspicuous in this infant eye) is the choriocapillaris (arrows). There is increased pigmentation in the region of the lamina fusca (arrowheads) where choroid joins sclera. Hematoxylin and eosin, × 125.

cells, sensory retinal detachment does not usually progress anteriorly to the ora. However, tears may occur at the anterior vitreous base, perhaps triggered by iatrogenic pars plana penetration.

> **Pearls**
>
> - Sensory retinal detachments do not usually progress anteriorly to the ora because in the pars plana the nonpigmented ciliary epithelium is attached to the pigmented ciliary epithelium by tight junctions.

1.4 Choroid

The choroid is the posterior portion of the uveal tract, which also includes the ciliary body and iris. Anteriorly, the choroid is continuous with the ciliary body, and posteriorly it terminates at the glial border tissue of Jacoby around the optic nerve. It is composed of uveal melanocytes, fibrocytes, and a rich supply of anastomosing blood vessels. The vessels are the most conspicuous aspect of the choroid (▸ Fig. 1.12). When congested, they substantially thicken the choroidal parenchyma and give it a spongy consistency.

The blood supply of the uveal tract comes from several sources, although all are ultimately derived from the ophthalmic artery. Some 15 to 20 short posterior ciliary arteries enter perpendicularly through the peripapillary sclera and supply prelaminar the optic nerve and the choroid. Vessels traverse the suprachoroidal space, then branch in the choroid and extend anteriorly beyond the equator.

The two long posterior ciliary arteries enter the sclera obliquely at the foveal horizontal meridian posteriorly, proceeding anteriorly in the suprachoroidal space to the supraciliary space (▸ Fig. 1.13). They branch at about the level of the ora serrata to join the major iridal circle and supply much of the

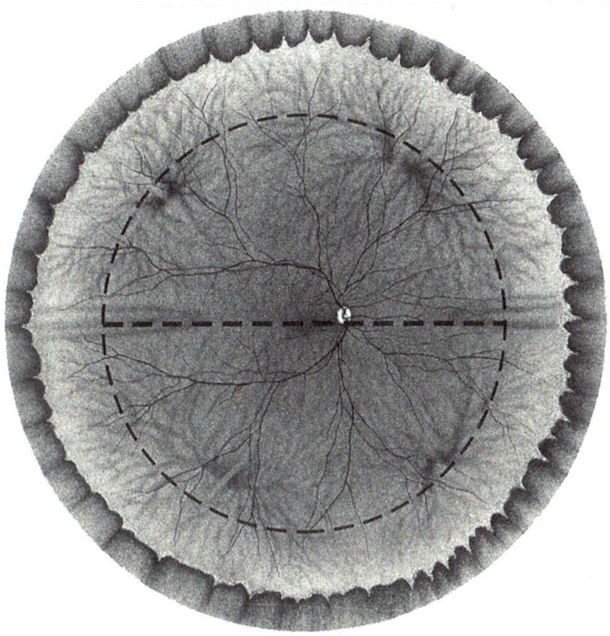

Fig. 1.13 Landmarks of the peripheral retina. The vortex vein ampullae lie just posterior to the equator (dotted circle), and the long posterior ciliary arteries and nerves mark the location of the foveal horizontal meridians (dashed line).

anterior uveal circulation, but some branches also loop back into the anterior choroid. In addition, a total of seven anterior ciliary arteries travel within the four rectus muscles, entering the sclera as major perforating branches at the rectus muscle attachments anterior to the equator. Each rectus muscle has two anterior ciliary arteries- except for the lateral rectus, which has one- derived from the lacrimal artery. In addition to supplying the iris and ciliary body via anastomoses with the major iridal circle, these vessels make contributions to the limbus and palisades of Vogt. Episcleral branches form the superficial marginal plexus and the peripheral corneal arcades. Both are prominent and hyperemic in iritis.

The choroid is drained by vortex veins. These vessels are clinically visible, particularly in blond fundi, as irregular, star-shaped, sometimes protruding structures (▶ Fig. 1.13). Venules come together and drain into a dilated structure- the vortex ampulla- from which the vortex vein pierces the sclera and exits the eye. Although schematic drawings like ▶ Fig. 1.13 show four of these vortex vein ampullae, just posterior to the equator superonasally, superotemporally, inferotemporally, and inferonasally, the number actually varies in different eyes, averaging about seven per eye; they are more numerous nasally.[1]

Pearls

- The vortex vein ampullae and the long posterior ciliary artery–nerve complexes are good clinical fundus landmarks. There are one or more vortex vein ampullae in each quadrant, all in a location just posterior to the equator. There are two long posterior ciliary artery–nerve complexes, and they are consistently located in the foveal horizontal meridians.

Within the choroid itself, the largest vessels are closest to the sclera, and the choriocapillaris is the innermost layer. The outermost layer is called *Haller's layer*, and the middle layer, consisting of medium-sized pre- and postcapillary vessels, is *Sattler's layer*. The choriocapillaris is a monolayer of interlacing capillaries and is distinctive for consisting of the largest capillaries in the body, measuring up to 20 µm in diameter in the macula and up to 50 µm peripherally.[1] The density of the choriocapillaris decreases with age.[18]

Although it appears anatomically that the capillaries of the choriocapillaris form a diffuse network throughout the choroid, evidence from postmortem studies and fluorescein angiography indicates that in the posterior pole the capillaries are arranged in a lobular pattern, with a feeding precapillary arteriole in the center of each lobule and several postcapillary venules draining the lobule peripherally.[50] The arterioles taper rapidly to form multiple capillaries, and this accounts for the high rate of blood flow through the capillary bed. This high flow rate appears to function at least in part as a heat-dissipating mechanism.[51] There are also numerous arteriole–arteriole anastomoses, particularly in the posterior pole.[52]

In the far periphery, the choroidal vessels are arranged more meridionally, so that the arteries and veins are more parallel, connected by capillaries in a manner suggesting a ladder. At the equator, the configuration is a transition between these two arrangements, a spindle configuration.[53] In this region, the venules tend to be more central and the arterioles more peripheral.[54]

The capillaries have fenestrations, or pores, which are most numerous on their inner aspect, toward the pigment epithelium. This allows diffusion of metabolites to and from the pigment epithelium and outer aspect of sensory retina. Ultrastructurally, these fenestrations consist of small, circular areas 60 nm in diameter in the unit membrane of the capillary endothelium. Like capillaries elsewhere, individual endothelial cells are joined together by zonulae occludentes.[55]

The retinal pigment epithelium and the outer half of sensory retina are nourished through diffusion from the choroidal circulation. Occlusion of the choroidal circulation occurs commonly in the far periphery, resulting in focal loss of pigment epithelium and outer retinal layers. Clinically, this is termed *cobblestone degeneration*.

The choroid is innervated by the short posterior ciliary nerves. These enter and travel with the short posterior ciliary arteries. They remain myelinated for a short distance within the eye, and then become unmyelinated. They appear to supply sympathetic innervation to the blood vessels.[1]

The long posterior ciliary nerves enter the peripapillary sclera obliquely at the foveal horizontal meridians, along with the long posterior ciliary arteries. The nerves travel in the suprachoroidal space, between choroid and sclera, and remain myelinated until arriving in the ciliary body.[1]

The choroidal melanocytes, like those of the rest of the uveal tract, skin, and hair, are derived from neural crest. They are star-shaped and have many long, delicate processes. They contain numerous small, round-to-oval melanosomes[1] and retain the ability to synthesize melanin throughout life. It is hypothesized that the melanin of both the choroid and pigment epithelium serve to absorb excessive light.[20] Other cells present in the choroid include scattered fibrocytes.

The choroid is attached to the sclera by means of long, interconnecting collagen fibers called lamina fusca. Within this suprachoroidea are melanocytes and nerve plexuses.[1] The attachments between choroid and sclera are essentially perpendicular posteriorly, keeping the choroid relatively tightly bound, but they become more obliquely oriented anteriorly. Thus, suprachoroidal fluid preferentially collects anteriorly.

Pearls

- Suprachoroidal fluid preferentially collects anteriorly. This is explained, at least in part, by the way the collagen fibers connect the choroid to the sclera; the stronger, perpendicular configuration is posterior and the weaker, oblique arrangement is anterior.

1.5 Acknowledgment

Janet Sparrow, PhD, provided materials and suggestions for section "Retinal Pigment Epithelium."

References

[1] Hogan MJ, Alvarado JA, Weddell JE. Histology of the Human Eye. Philadelphia, PA: WB Saunders; 1971

[2] Fine BS, Tousimis AJ. The structure of the vitreous body and the suspensory ligaments of the lens. Arch Ophthalmol. 1961; 65:95–110

[3] Hogan MJ. The vitreous, its structure, and relation to the ciliary body and retina. Proctor award lecture. Invest Ophthalmol. 1963; 2:418–445

[4] Foos RY. Anatomic and pathologic aspects of the vitreous body. Trans Am Acad Ophthalmol Otolaryngol. 1973; 77(2):OP171–OP183

[5] Worst JGF, Los LI. Cisternal Anatomy of the Vitreous. Amsterdam: Kugler; 1995

[6] Schaal KB, Pang CE, Pozzoni MC, Engelbert M. The premacular bursa's shape revealed in vivo by swept-source optical coherence tomography. Ophthalmology. 2014; 121(5):1020–1028

[7] Sebag J. Age-related differences in the human vitreoretinal interface. Arch Ophthalmol. 1991; 109(7):966–971

[8] Dowling JE. The Retina: An Approachable Part of the Brain. Cambridge, MA: Belknap Press of Harvard University Press; 1987

[9] Sadler TW. Langman's Medical Embryology. 12th ed. Philadelphia, PA: Lippincott Williams & Wilkins; 2012

[10] White MH, Lambert HM, Kincaid MC, Dieckert JP, Lowd DK. The ora serrata and the spiral of Tillaux. Anatomic relationship and clinical correlation. Ophthalmology. 1989; 96(4):508–511

[11] Weiter JJ, Delori FC, Wing GL, Fitch KA. Retinal pigment epithelial lipofuscin and melanin and choroidal melanin in human eyes. Invest Ophthalmol Vis Sci. 1986; 27(2):145–152

[12] Friedman E, Ts'o MOM. The retinal pigment epithelium. II. Histologic changes associated with age. Arch Ophthalmol. 1968; 79(3):315–320

[13] Duvall J. Structure, function, and pathologic responses of pigment epithelium: a review. Semin Ophthalmol. 1987; 2:130–140

[14] Bastek JV, Siegel EB, Straatsma BR, Foos RY. Chorioretinal juncture. Pigmentary patterns of the peripheral fundus. Ophthalmology. 1982; 89(12):1455–1463

[15] Cunha-Vaz J. The blood-ocular barriers. Surv Ophthalmol. 1979; 23(5):279–296

[16] Eagle RC, Jr. Mechanisms of maculopathy. Ophthalmology. 1984; 91(6):613–625

[17] Nakaizumi Y. The ultrastructure of Bruch's membrane. I. Human, monkey, rabbit, guinea pig, and rat eyes. Arch Ophthalmol. 1964; 72:380–387

[18] Ramrattan RS, van der Schaft TL, Mooy CM, de Bruijn WC, Mulder PG, de Jong PT. Morphometric analysis of Bruch's membrane, the choriocapillaris, and the choroid in aging. Invest Ophthalmol Vis Sci. 1994; 35(6):2857–2864

[19] Feeney-Burns L. The pigments of the retinal pigment epithelium. Curr Top Eye Res. 1980; 2:119–178

[20] Smith-Thomas L, Richardson P, Thody AJ, et al. Human ocular melanocytes and retinal pigment epithelial cells differ in their melanogenic properties in vivo and in vitro. Curr Eye Res. 1996; 15(11):1079–1091

[21] Champion R, Daicker BC. Congenital hypertrophy of the pigment epithelium: light microscopic and ultrastructural findings in young children. Retina. 1989; 9(1):44–48

[22] Regillo CD, Eagle RC, Jr, Shields JA, Shields CL, Arbizo VV. Histopathologic findings in congenital grouped pigmentation of the retina. Ophthalmology. 1993; 100(3):400–405

[23] Schmidt SY, Peisch RD. Melanin concentration in normal human retinal pigment epithelium. Regional variation and age-related reduction. Invest Ophthalmol Vis Sci. 1986; 27(7):1063–1067

[24] Sparrow JR, Hicks D, Hamel CP. The retinal pigment epithelium in health and disease. Curr Mol Med. 2010; 10(9):802–823

[25] Sparrow JR, Gregory-Roberts E, Yamamoto K, et al. The bisretinoids of retinal pigment epithelium. Prog Retin Eye Res. 2012; 31(2):121–135

[26] Young RW. Pathophysiology of age-related macular degeneration. Surv Ophthalmol. 1987; 31(5):291–306

[27] Hageman GS, Marmor MF, Yao XY, Johnson LV. The interphotoreceptor matrix mediates primate retinal adhesion. Arch Ophthalmol. 1995; 113(5):655–660

[28] Pycock CJ. Retinal neurotransmission. Surv Ophthalmol. 1985; 29(5):355–365

[29] Bok D. Retinal photoreceptor-pigment epithelium interactions. Friedenwald lecture. Invest Ophthalmol Vis Sci. 1985; 26(12):1659–1694

[30] Varma R, Skaf M, Barron E. Retinal nerve fiber layer thickness in normal human eyes. Ophthalmology. 1996; 103(12):2114–2119

[31] Bunt AH, Minckler DS. Foveal sparing. New anatomical evidence for bilateral representation of the central retina. Arch Ophthalmol. 1977; 95(8):1445–1447

[32] Garner A. Retinal angiogenesis: mechanism in health and disease. Semin Ophthalmol. 1987; 2:71–80

[33] Weinberg D, Dodwell DG, Fern SA. Anatomy of arteriovenous crossings in branch retinal vein occlusion. Am J Ophthalmol. 1990; 109(3):298–302

[34] Iwasaki M, Inomata H. Relation between superficial capillaries and foveal structures in the human retina. Invest Ophthalmol Vis Sci. 1986; 27 (12):1698–1705

[35] Justice J, Jr, Lehmann RP. Cilioretinal arteries. A study based on review of stereo fundus photographs and fluorescein angiographic findings. Arch Ophthalmol. 1976; 94(8):1355–1358

[36] Brown SM, Jampol LM. New concepts of regulation of retinal vessel tone. Arch Ophthalmol. 1996; 114(2):199–204

[37] Polyak SL. The Retina. Chicago, IL: University of Chicago Press; 1941

[38] Michaelson IC. Retinal Circulation in Man and Animals. Springfield, IL: Charles C Thomas; 1954

[39] His W. Abbildungen über das Gefäßsystem der menschlichen Netzhaut und derjenigen des Kaninchens. Arch f Anat u Entwicklungsg. 1880:224

[40] Hayreh SS, Servais GE, Virdi PS. Fundus lesions in malignant hypertension. IV. Focal intraretinal periarteriolar transudates. Ophthalmology. 1986; 93(1):60–73

[41] Rahimy E, Sarraf D, Dollin ML, Pitcher JD, Ho AC. Paracentral acute middle maculopathy in nonischemic central retinal vein occlusion. Am J Ophthalmol. 2014; 158(2):372–380.e1

[42] Orth DH, Fine BS, Fagman W, Quirk TC. Clarification of foveomacular nomenclature and grid for quantitation of macular disorders. Trans Sect Ophthalmol Am Acad Ophthalmol Otolaryngol. 1977; 83(3, Pt 1):OP506–OP514

[43] Nussbaum JJ, Pruett RC, Delori FC. Historic perspectives. Macular yellow pigment. The first 200 years. Retina. 1981; 1(4):296–310

[44] Snodderly DM, Brown PK, Delori FC, Auran JD. The macular pigment. I. Absorbance spectra, localization, and discrimination from other yellow pigments in primate retinas. Invest Ophthalmol Vis Sci. 1984; 25(6):660–673

[45] Spencer LM, Foos RY, Straatsma BR. Meridional folds and meridional complexes of the peripheral retina. Trans Am Acad Ophthalmol Otolaryngol. 1969; 73(2):204–221

[46] Lonn LI, Smith TR. Ora serrata pearls. Clinical and histological correlation. Arch Ophthalmol. 1967; 77(6):809–813

[47] Foos RY. Senile retinoschisis. Relationship to cystoid degeneration. Trans Am Acad Ophthalmol Otolaryngol. 1970; 74(1):33–51

[48] Byer NE. Cystic retinal tufts and their relationship to retinal detachment. Arch Ophthalmol. 1981; 99(10):1788–1790

[49] Foos R. Zonular traction tufts o the peripheral retina in cadaver eyes. Arch Ophthalmol. 1969; 82(5):620–632

[50] Ernest JT. Choroidal circulation. In: Ryan SJ, ed. Retina. 2nd ed. St Louis, MO: CV Mosby; 1994:76–80
[51] Parver LM, Auker C, Carpenter DO. Choroidal blood flow as a heat dissipating mechanism in the macula. Am J Ophthalmol. 1980; 89(5):641–646
[52] Woodlief NF, Eifrig DE. Initial observations on the ocular microcirculation in man: the choriocapillaris. Ann Ophthalmol. 1982; 14(2):176–180
[53] Yoneya S, Tso MOM. Angioarchitecture of the human choroid. Arch Ophthalmol. 1987; 105(5):681–687
[54] McLeod DS, Lutty GA. High-resolution histologic analysis of the human choroidal vasculature. Invest Ophthalmol Vis Sci. 1994; 35(11):3799–3811
[55] Spitznas M, Reale E. Fracture faces of fenestrations and junctions of endothelial cells in human choroidal vessels. Invest Ophthalmol. 1975; 14(2):98–107

2 Retinal and Retinal Pigment Epithelial Physiology

Michael F. Marmor and Loh-Shan B. Leung

2.1 Introduction

Many retinal disorders have a selective effect on particular cells or metabolic systems within the retina and retinal pigment epithelium (RPE). Effective management of these disorders, which include conditions as diverse as retinitis pigmentosa (RP), central serous chorioretinopathy (CSC), and congenital color blindness, requires an understanding of retinal physiology and of the interaction between the retina and RPE. The physiology of the retina cannot be separated from that of the RPE, especially in a clinical context, because the RPE actively supports and facilitates retinal function and is also a frequent site of damage in disorders of the ocular fundus.[1]

2.2 Retinal Pigment Epithelium

Although the RPE is derived embryologically from the same neural tube tissue as the neurosensory retina, the RPE cells differentiate into a monolayer epithelium that behaves functionally more like the lining of the gallbladder than like central nervous system tissue. The cells are linked by tight junctions and show anatomic and physiologic membrane specializations on the apical and basal surfaces (▶ Fig. 2.1). These enable the RPE to control water and nutrient access to the subretinal space, which is critical to the viability of the photoreceptors. Major functions of the RPE are outlined in the following text box.

Selected Functions of the Retinal Pigment Epithelium

- Pigment functions
  - Light adaptation and screening
  - Detoxification and binding
  - Lipofuscin accumulation
  - Antigenic properties
- Environment and metabolic control
  - Blood–retinal barrier
  - Transport of nutrients and ions
  - Dehydration of subretinal space
  - Synthesis of enzymes, growth factors, and pigments
  - Interaction with endocrine, vascular, and proliferative factors
- Visual pigment cycle
  - Capture and storage of vitamin A
  - Isomerization of all-*trans* to 11-*cis* vitamin A
- Retinal adhesion and interphotoreceptor matrix (IPM)
  - Matrix domains surrounding rods and cones
  - Metabolic control of adhesiveness
- Photoreceptor phagocytosis and aging
  - Phagocytosis of outer segment tips
  - Digestion and recycling of membrane material
  - Aging effects: lipofuscin, drusen
  - Deposits and alterations in Bruch's membrane
- Electrical activity
  - Response to light-induced ionic changes: c-wave, fast oscillation
  - Response to light-induced chemical signals: electro-oculogram (EOG)
  - Nonphotic responses to chemical agents
- Repair and reactivity
  - Repair and regeneration
  - Immunologic interactions
  - Scarring and pigment migration
  - Role in modulating fibrovascular proliferation

2.2.1 Pigments and Optical Functions of the Retinal Pigment Epithelium

The RPE is so named because of its content of *melanin*, a large polymeric molecule synthesized in cytoplasmic granules called *melanosomes*. The RPE is the first tissue in the body to become pigmented, and some degree of melanogenesis continues throughout life. However, in older eyes, many melanin granules fuse with lysosomes and break down, and the elderly fundus typically appears rather depigmented. It has long been assumed that a major function of melanin was the absorption of stray light, to minimize scatter within the eye. This is understandably true in animals such as the frog, in which long pigment-containing processes extend up between the photoreceptors. However, the RPE processes around rods are rather short in humans, and in general the RPE is less pigmented than the choroid (most racial differences in fundus appearance reflect pigmentation of the choroid rather than of the RPE). There is no difference in visual acuity between blond and heavily pigmented fundi. The loss of acuity in albinism is a result of poor foveal cone organization rather than of light scatter.

Melanin may also serve a protective function in the eye, as a free radical scavenger and as an agent that can bind toxins. This latter role is controversial, however, because it is not clear whether the binding of certain retinotoxic drugs, such as chloroquine and thioridazine, protects the retina by removing the toxic agents from the cytoplasm or enhances their toxicity by concentrating the agents near the retina.

As the eye ages, there is accumulation of another RPE pigment, *lipofuscin*. This is an aging pigment, present throughout the nervous system, but it may have special significance within the eye. Lipofuscin in the RPE is thought to be derived from lipids of the photoreceptor outer segments and metabolic by-products of the visual pigment regeneration cycle that have been ingested and digested by the RPE through the process of outer segment renewal (see later), including membrane fragments that may have been damaged by light absorption or oxidation. A major component is *N*-retinylidene-*N*-retinyl-ethanolamine, or A2E, a toxic by-product of all-*trans*-retinal binding that is controlled in part by the *ABCA4* (Stargardt's disease) gene.[2,3] Lipofuscin can be identified even in the RPE of children, but it does not become prominent until adulthood. With aging,

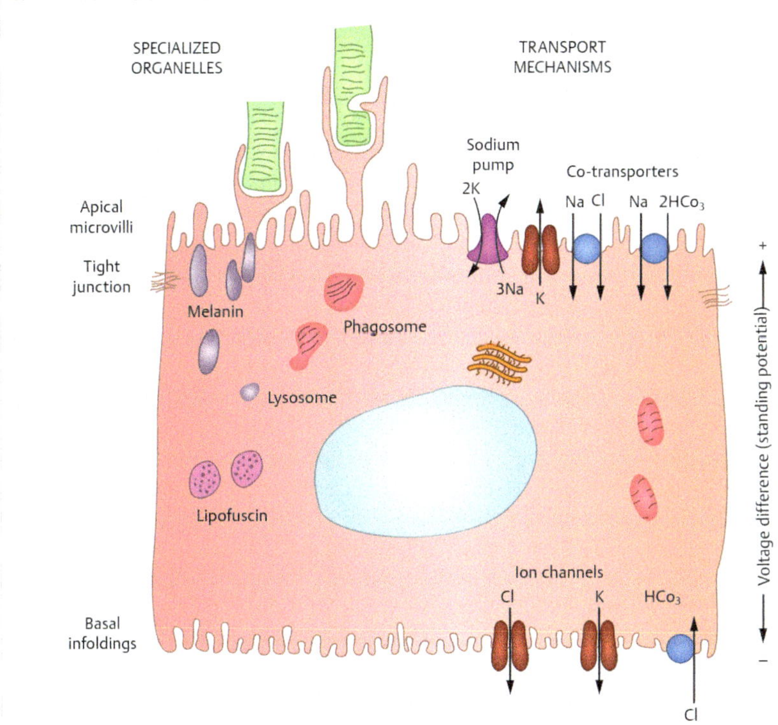

Fig. 2.1 RPE cell showing the major anatomic specializations and some of the membrane transport mechanisms. The apical region (with long microvilli ensheathing the photoreceptors) is separated by tight junctions from the basal region (with small but numerous infoldings). Lysosomes can merge with other granules to form phagolysosomes or melanolysosomes. Different ion channels and cotransporter systems are found in the apical and basal membranes, and the electrogenic sodium pump is on the apical membrane. These transport systems generate a voltage (standing potential) across the cell.

the RPE cells are often clogged massively with the golden autofluorescent pigment.

Controversial Points

- Melanin in the RPE may have a protective function in scavenging free radicals and binding toxins. However, this latter role is controversial, as it is not clear whether binding of certain drugs, such as chloroquine and thioridazine, protects the retina or enhances toxicity by concentrating the agents near the retina.

A2E is a component of the lipofuscin-like material that accumulates in the RPE of eyes with Stargardt's disease, fundus flavimaculatus, and Best's disease (vitelliform dystrophy).[4] The autofluorescent pigment in these disorders clogs cells throughout the retina, even at younger ages, and not just in the macular region, where fundus pathology of these disorders is most prominent clinically. However, we still have much to learn about these disorders. For example, although a Stargardt's disease phenotype can by caused by *ABCA4* mutations, defects in the same gene can also cause cone dystrophy or even retinitis pigmentosa. Furthermore, there can be phenotypic variations within a family, and the relationship to A2E is not always clear.

2.2.2 Control of the Subretinal Space

The neurosensory retina is embryologic brain tissue, and as such it requires the same environmental protection as tissue in the brain. A blood–brain or *blood–retinal barrier* is provided in part by the intrinsic retinal blood vessels, which have tight junctions like cerebral vessels (*inner* blood–retinal barrier). However, the choroidal vessels, which provide nutrition to the outer retina, are leaky, and the other part of the blood–retinal barrier is provided by the tight junctions of the RPE (*outer* blood–retinal barrier). Secreted factors, such as vascular endothelial growth factor (VEGF), play an important role in fluid homeostasis in the subretinal space and maintenance of this outer blood–retinal barrier (see later). The apical and basal RPE membranes contain a variety of selective ion channels and a variety of active and facilitative transport systems that control the movement of ions and water and the transport of metabolites, such as glucose and amino acids.[5] The amino acid taurine, for example, is essential for photoreceptor function and is concentrated by the RPE; D-glucose but not L-glucose is transported into the subretinal space. There are different channels and transporters on the apical and basal surfaces, such as an electrogenic sodium–potassium pump on the apical membrane and a chloride–bicarbonate exchange transporter on the basal membrane. The asymmetry between the apical and basal membranes accounts for the development of a voltage (called the *standing potential*) across the RPE, and it also results in a net movement of ions away from the subretinal space that drives the transport of water.

Special Considerations

- The blood–retinal barrier is provided by the tight junctions of the retinal blood vessels (inner barrier) and the tight junctions of the RPE (outer barrier). For proper protection and function of the neurosensory retina, the barrier needs to be intact at both levels.

The RPE active transport mechanisms for water are very powerful. If a large retinal detachment is buckled without drainage, fluid can clear within 24 hours. The RPE can remove water from the subretinal space against a substantial gradient of hydrostatic or osmotic pressure, even when the subretinal fluid contains protein.[6] It is important to recognize that it is the presence of tight junctions between the RPE cells that necessitates this active transport. Passive transport mechanisms, such as intraocular pressure against the retina and osmotic pressure from the choroid, also tend to drive fluid *out* of the subretinal space—but water movement is normally restricted by the RPE barrier. When the RPE barrier is damaged, fluid actually leaves the subretinal space *faster* than under normal conditions. In other words, a normal eye will not accumulate fluid in the subretinal space just because the RPE barrier is disrupted.

These observations have relevance for clinical disorders such as serous detachments. They show that the presence of a defect in the RPE is not by itself sufficient to cause serous detachment, even though it may be necessary.[7] There must be a pressure head within the choroid, such as a neovascular membrane or an area of ischemic or inflammatory injury, to drive fluid in the retinal direction. This explains the fluid that accumulates over areas of inflammation and RPE damage in Harada's disease or over regions of choroidal ischemia in accelerated hypertension or preeclampsia, or the local fluid that accumulates over choroidal neovascularization in age-related macular degeneration. However, this does not explain why fluid spreads far beyond a small focal leak in disorders such as idiopathic CSC (▶ Fig. 2.2), as one would expect the RPE to remove such fluid rapidly. These conditions probably involve a diffuse impairment of fluid transport across larger regions of RPE, which prevents rapid absorption. This could result from RPE disease, but may more often be a result of choroidal disease. For example, indocyanine green angiography of eyes with CSC typically shows broad areas of choroidal hyperperfusion and hyperpermeability, and high-resolution optical coherence tomography shows choroidal thickening in the central macula. The leak itself may be something of an epiphenomenon—but when a leak develops in a susceptible eye, fluid can accumulate and the disease becomes symptomatic (see Chapter 16).

2.2.3 Visual Pigment Regeneration

Another critical metabolic interaction between the retina and RPE is the visual pigment cycle. The RPE serves to capture vitamin A from the bloodstream, and it stores esterified vitamin A within its cytoplasm. Specific binding proteins (e.g., *interphotoreceptor retinoid-binding protein, IRBP*) serve to transport vitamin A across the subretinal space to be incorporated into rhodopsin in the photoreceptors. After rhodopsin is activated by light, the desensitized (*all-trans*) vitamin A is transported back to the RPE to be stored and isomerized to the 11-*cis* conformation (▶ Fig. 2.3). Many of the enzymes involved in this process have been found to cause human disease when missing or abnormal.[8]

This cycle of rhodopsin regeneration can take upward of a half-hour in a normal eye and is a basis of the clinical test of dark adaptometry. After an extensive exposure to bright light, the cones recover to maximum sensitivity in 6 to 8 minutes in the dark, whereas the rods require close to 30 minutes. The significance of this regenerative process is apparent to all of us as the time it takes to adjust to the darkness inside a movie theater or on a moonlight walk.

The *RDH5* gene in RPE causes a disorder called *fundus albipunctatus*,[9,10] which shows white dots throughout the posterior fundus associated with a curious form of night blindness. Affected individuals cannot find their seats going into a movie theater but may see well by the end of a double feature. The problem is not a *lack* of rod function but a striking *delay* in dark adaptation. After 4 hours in the dark, patients with fundus albipunctatus can have normal sensitivity and a normal rod

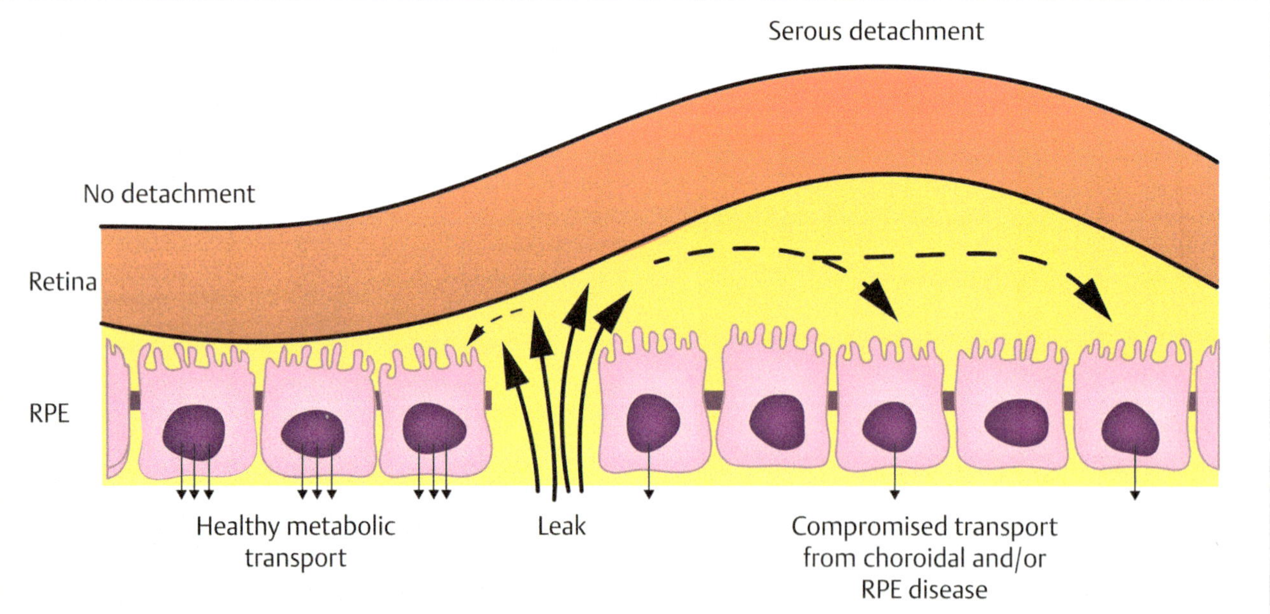

Fig. 2.2 A small site of RPE leakage. To the left, where the choroid and RPE are healthy and water transport is normal, there is no detachment. To the right, where vascular and/or RPE dysfunction compromises transport (and retinal adhesiveness as well), a serous detachment has developed beyond the site of leakage. (Modified from Marmor.[13])

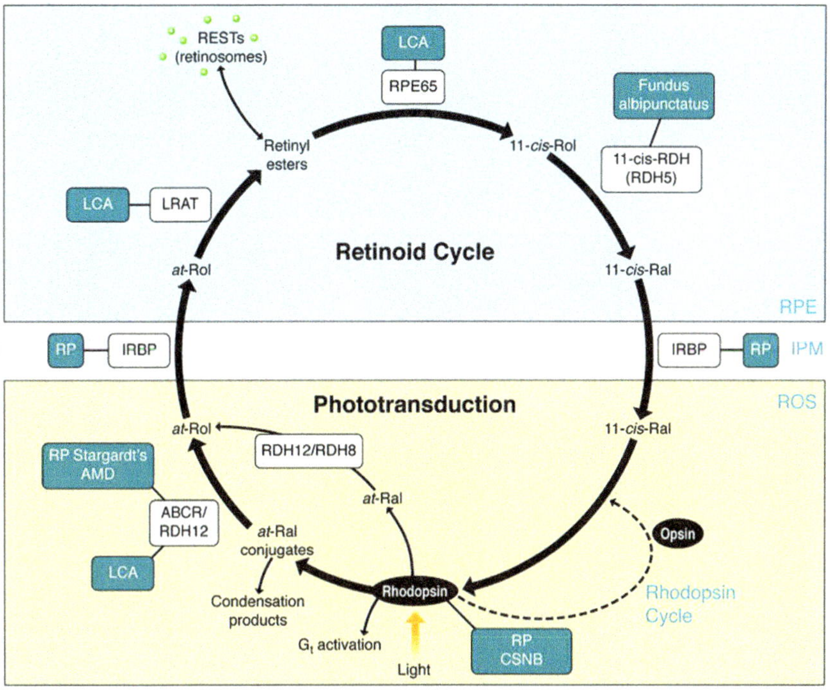

Fig. 2.3 Visual pigment regeneration cycle. The absorption of a photon by rhodopsin changes the coupled 11-*cis*-retinal to all-*trans*-retinal. This chromophore releases from the opsin and must be bound for transport to the RPE where it is esterified, stored, and then reisomerized to 11-*cis* before transported back to the outer segment where it couples again with opsin to make rhodopsin. The diagram shows some of the critical enzymes that control different phases of this cycle and that are known to cause human disease. (Reprinted with permission by Elsevier from von Lintig J et al.[8])

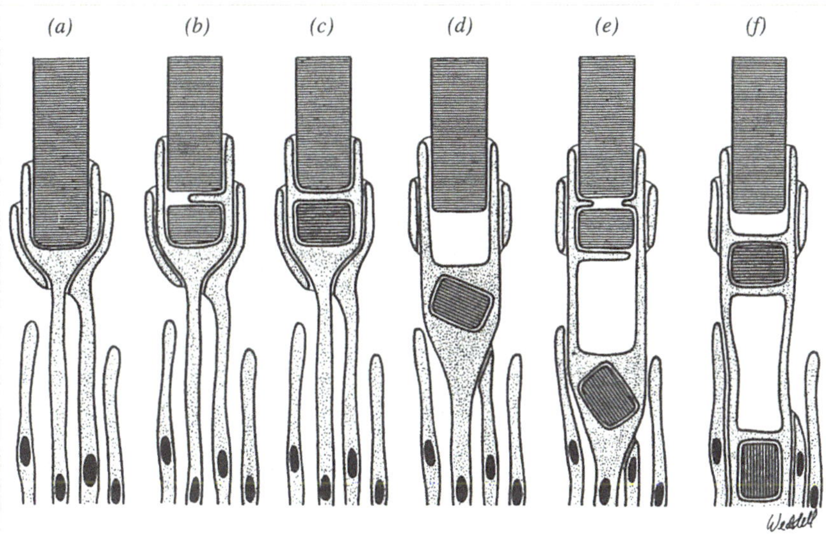

Fig. 2.4 Phagocytosis of outer segment tips by the microvilli of the RPE. (Reprinted with permission from Steinberg RH, Wood I, Hogan MJ. Pigment epithelial ensheathment and phagocytosis of extrafoveal cones in human retina. Philos Trans R Soc Lond B Biol Sci. 1977; 277(958): 459–474)

electroretinography (ERG). Loss of the RPE genes *LRAT* or *RPE65* will disrupt rod function severely and cause a form of Leber's amaurosis (essentially an early-onset severe RP).

2.2.4 Photoreceptor Regeneration and Phagocytosis of Outer Segments

The photoreceptor outer segments are exposed to radiant energy on a regular basis, and they exist in a high-oxygen environment by proximity to the choriocapillaris. Both light absorption and oxygen facilitate the production of free radicals, which damage lipid membranes. Cells in the skin would not last a lifetime without renewal, and the same is true for the photoreceptor outer segments. Thus, every day more than 100 discs at the distal end of each photoreceptor outer segment are phagocytosed by the RPE (▶ Fig. 2.4), and new discs are synthesized continually to replace them.[11] The cones tend to shed more vigorously at the onset of darkness and the rods at the onset of morning light, but some phagocytosis takes place continually. The phagocytosed disc material becomes encapsulated in bodies called *phagosomes*, which merge with lysosomes to facilitate digestion. Residual material is eventually egested across the basal RPE membrane. Some necessary fatty acids are retained and recycled back into the synthetic process. The metabolic demands of this process are impressive; each RPE cell ingests and digests upward of 4,000 discs daily. The *ABCA4* protein is believed to be a transporter within the photoreceptor disc membrane involved in the recycling process of all-*trans*-retinal. Defects lead to accumulation of A2E (discussed earlier) within the discs and subsequently within the RPE cells that phagocytose them.

A form of RP has been identified which depends on this process. Defects in the *MERTK* gene leads to a failure of RPE phagocytosis, followed by degeneration of the overlying rods and cones.[12] Pathology of the phagocytic process could, in theory, be relevant to excessive lipofuscin formation or to other aspects of aging and age-related macular degeneration.

2.2.5 Retinal Adhesion and the Interphotoreceptor Matrix

The RPE contributes to the formation of the IPM and to its effectiveness as a bond between the retina and RPE. It is important to recognize that the IPM is not just a viscous "goo" but has an elaborate structure based on segregated chemical domains that contain different glycosaminoglycans and related molecules. By binding fluorescent lectins to these molecules, one can identify discrete matrix sheaths that surround the cones and rods independently and bond to both RPE and outer segment membranes.

Adhesion of the retina to the RPE is a complex physiologic function; it appears to involve several complementary systems that keep the retina firmly in place unless a positive force (such as vitreous traction) pulls it off.[13] Retinal apposition is facilitated by intraocular pressure on the retina, by the draw of choroidal osmotic pressure, and by the presence of a formed vitreous gel. The RPE microvilli also wrap tightly around the tips of the outer segments for the purpose of phagocytosis, but there are no anatomic connections between the RPE microvilli and the outer segments. The IPM forms a viscous bond between the two layers, but this fluid connection is probably of lesser importance than the structural and chemical bond that is formed by the IPM by means of specific receptors where the matrix is in contact with the outer segment and RPE membranes. For example, these matrix domains can be seen to stretch dramatically when the retina is peeled away from the RPE (▶ Fig. 2.5), which demonstrates the firm attachment of the IPM to both the retinal and RPE surfaces.[14]

The structural and bonding characteristics of the IPM are affected by its degree of hydration and its ionic content, both of which are controlled by the transport characteristics of the RPE. Thus, the strength of retinal adhesion is highly dependent on metabolic activity, which governs RPE ion and water transport.[13] For example, retinal adhesive strength drops within minutes after death or after occlusion of the ocular circulation. This metabolic dependence of retinal adhesion may explain, in part, the greater susceptibility to detachment in older eyes (or perhaps highly myopic eyes), in which the vascular supply may be less functional as a result of age (or ocular expansion).

Retinal adhesive strength can be modulated osmotically and metabolically in experimental models. Systemic osmotic agents dehydrate the subretinal space and IPM and increase retinal adhesion to a modest degree, and a similar increase in adhesive strength can be produced by acetazolamide and other carbonic anhydrase inhibitors because they increase the rate at which fluid is transported out of the subretinal space. These agents could, in theory, prove helpful in the management of detachment disorders, but to date no such applications have been demonstrated.

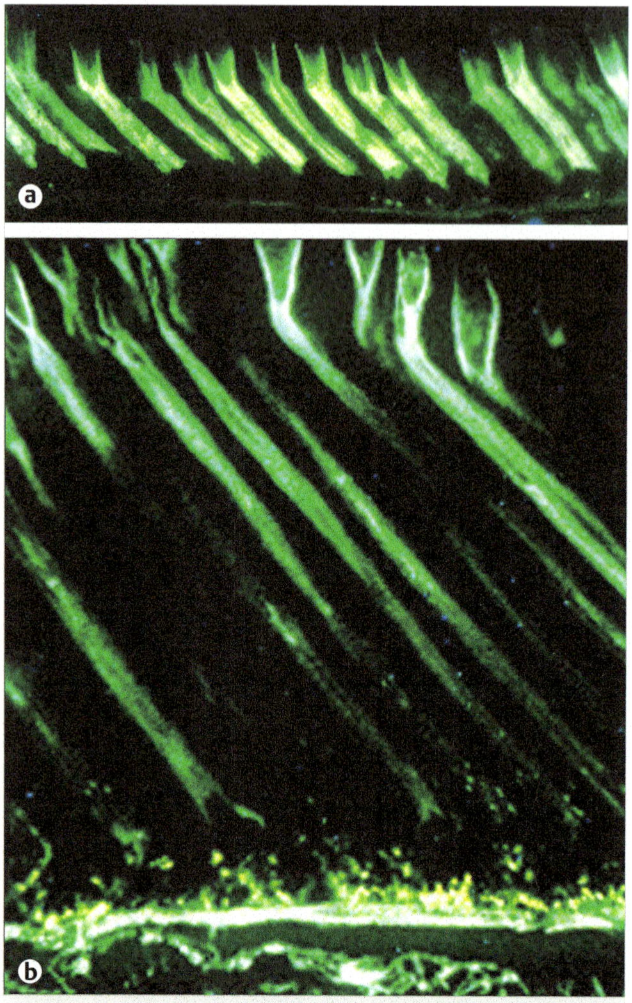

Fig. 2.5 Cone matrix sheaths of the interphotoreceptor matrix in rabbit (labeled with fluorescent peanut agglutinin). The retina is above and the RPE below. (**a**) Normal tissue with compact sheaths. (**b**) Tissue in which the retina is partially pulled away from the RPE. The cone matrix sheaths are stretched enormously, indicating strong attachment to both sides of the subretinal space. (Reprinted with permission from Hageman GS, Marmor MF, Yao X-Y, Johnson LV. The interphotoreceptor matrix mediates primate retinal adhesion. Arch Ophthalmol. 1995; 113 (5):655–660)

Pearls

- The IPM plays a significant role in the normal adhesion of the neurosensory retina to the RPE. The structural and bonding characteristics of the IPM are affected by its degree of hydration and its ionic content, both of which are controlled by the RPE. Therefore, conditions that affect the metabolic activity of the RPE can, in turn, affect the strength of retinal adhesion.

Carbonic anhydrase inhibitors might also seem relevant to the absorption of fluid in serous detachments, although anecdotally they seem to have little effect. The reason may lie with the fact that carbonic anhydrase inhibitors must act on RPE transport systems to be effective, and if the RPE is damaged by detachment, ischemia, inflammation, or disease such as CSC, there may not be a substrate on which the drug can work. Carbonic anhydrase inhibitors have been shown to reduce cystoid macular edema in some patients with conditions such as aphakia/pseudophakia and RP.[15] Significant benefits have not been found in diabetic retinopathy or other types of retinal edema.

2.2.6 Electrical Activity of the Retinal Pigment Epithelium

The RPE interacts electrically with the retina. The RPE is not a photoreceptive tissue and generates no direct response to light, but RPE cells respond electrically to ionic changes in the subretinal space or to chemical substances released as a result of photoreception. There are three basic light-induced responses of the RPE membranes.[16] As a result of photoreception, there is, for a few seconds, a drop in the potassium concentration of the subretinal space; an effect that is recordable as the *c-wave* of the ERG. This potassium change is then transmitted slowly through the RPE cell, and roughly 1 minute later the basal membrane of the RPE hyperpolarizes and produces a small negative dip in the standing potential that is called the *fast oscillation*. This response involves basal chloride channels and can be abnormal in some patients with cystic fibrosis. Light activation of the photoreceptors also causes the release of a messenger substance (as yet unknown, but possibly dopaminergic) to produce a slow basal depolarization of the RPE that does not reach its peak until 5 to 10 minutes after the onset of light. This voltage, called the *light response of the standing potential*, is the physiologic basis of the clinical EOG.

The bestrophin-1 protein, encoded by the *BEST1 (VMD2)* gene responsible for Best's vitelliform macular dystrophy, regulates a basal calcium and chloride channel in the RPE that seems responsible for the light response.[17,18] However, the visual role of these bestrophin channels is unclear, and Best's disease patients have a normal ERG. Thus, the clinical EOG is derived from the RPE, but is not necessarily a broad measure of RPE function.

Interestingly, basal RPE membrane polarization can also be induced pharmacologically by the intravenous injection of hyperosmolar agents, acetazolamide, or sodium bicarbonate. These "nonphotic" responses are specific for the RPE because they can be induced exclusive of retinal function, but their clinical significance remains to be determined.

2.2.7 Secretion

PEDF and VEGF

The RPE secretes a number of growth factors in both physiologic and pathologic states. Among the most important are pigment epithelium-derived factor (PEDF) and vascular endothelial growth factor (VEGF). Despite its name, PEDF is found in many different types of tissues and is widely conserved across species.[19] It acts as a cell cycle regulator, has antiapoptotic effects, and is likely a protective factor against agents of cellular and oxidative stress such as peroxide and glutamate. Additionally, PEDF serves as a potent inhibitor of angiogenesis, and is secreted preferentially at the RPE cell apical surface into the IPM.[20]

In contrast, the role of VEGF as an angiogenic agent is well known; initially described in the context of tumor growth, VEGF is upregulated in a variety of disease states. VEGF acts in opposition to PEDF, and the VEGF/PEDF ratio in a tissue determines whether angiogenesis takes place.[21] Its primary actions are to stimulate vascular endothelium to form new capillaries, and to increase vascular permeability. While these functions are particularly relevant to diseases such as diabetic retinopathy, macular edema, and age-related macular degeneration, VEGF also has an important physiologic role. Secreted constitutively by the RPE at the basolateral surface, VEGF maintains the fenestrations in the choriocapillaris and helps the RPE to regulate fluid resorption and serve as an outer blood–retinal barrier. VEGF activity rises when PEDF activity is depressed, which may occur with oxidative stress and complement activation and be relevant for age-related macular degeneration.[22]

2.3 Retina

Some aspects of retinal physiology are outlined in the following text box.

Selected Functions of the Retina

- Transduction
  - Rhodopsin activation
  - G-protein amplification cascade
  - Cyclic guanosine monophosphate (cGMP) control of sodium channels
  - Receptor potential generation
  - Recovery mechanisms
- Retinal integration
  - Horizontal and bipolar cell interactions
  - Center-surround receptive fields
  - Sensitivity to contrast more than brightness
  - On- and off-pathways
  - Parallel neural pathways for resolution, color and, motion/spatial orientation
- Adaptation
  - Chemical—pigment regeneration cycle
  - Neural—photoreceptors and neural adjustments
  - Increment threshold sensitivity
- Color vision
  - Trichromacy—cone photoreceptor pigments
  - Color opponency—center-surround organization (red vs. green, blue vs. yellow)
  - Special characteristics of blue-sensitive cones
- Electrical responses
  - Early receptor potential
  - Receptor potential—ERG a-wave
  - Bipolar and Müller cells responses—ERG b-wave
  - Integrative neurons—ERG oscillatory potentials
  - Ganglion cells—pattern ERG wave
  - Macular cones—multifocal ERG

2.3.1 Photoreception and Transduction

Vision takes place because of the existence of photopigments and photoreceptive cells that can transform (transduce) radiant energy (light) into a neural response. The earliest animal photoreception occurs in one-celled organisms such as *Euglena*, which have photopigments at the base of the flagellum; the absorption of light modifies swimming behavior and the organisms can move toward or away from light. With evolution, entire cells became specialized as photoreceptors and gradually evolved into a photosensitive tissue (retina) within an optical framework (eye).

The human photoreceptor is a specialized cilium in which the inner segment of the cell contains metabolic machinery to synthesize protein and maintain ionic homeostasis; the outer segment is a massive collection of cell membrane that is studded with visual pigment. Both cone and rod visual pigments consist of 11-*cis* vitamin A aldehyde (*retinal*) bound to a large protein that determines the spectral sensitivity of the pigment. Rhodopsin is most sensitive to (i.e., most likely to capture a photon from) light at 500 nm (blue-green), whereas the three cone pigments peak, respectively, at about 426, 520, and 560 nm. Note that this spectral sensitivity of a photoreceptor does not mean that it can distinguish between different colors of light, but simply that it will statistically capture more photons at the wavelength of its peak sensitivity than at a different wavelength. Once captured, the effect of a photon is identical regardless of its wavelength. In other words, rods are much more sensitive to blue light than to red, but once captured, a red photon is just as effective a stimulus as a blue one.

The fundamental process of *transduction* is similar in rods and cones, although the cone pigments are able to regenerate chemically much faster than rhodopsin (discussed earlier). The electrical responses generated by cones are also faster than those in rods, and there are major differences in saturation and adaptation that will be considered later. Some of these differences may relate to the structural qualities of rods and cones. As new rod membranes are synthesized, the "discs" become internalized within the outer cell membrane. By contrast, many of the cone discs remain in continuity with the outer cell membrane.

An ideal photoreceptor should respond to a minimum amount of light with an electrical response large enough to trigger synaptic transmission. This is achieved through a chemical amplification cascade, similar to the enzymatic cascade that governs certain hormonal responses. When a photon strikes a rhodopsin molecule, the 11-*cis*-retinal is transformed to *all-trans*-retinal, which alters the stability of the rhodopsin molecule and leads to a sequence of conformational changes. Within about 1 millisecond after absorbing a photon, the rhodopsin has changed to metarhodopsin II, and the transduction cascade is activated. Further chemical changes in the rhodopsin molecule lead to the visual pigment regeneration cycle, with eventual splitting off of the vitamin A moiety and its transport to the RPE for storage and reisomerization (▶ Fig. 2.3). However, all these later chemical changes are irrelevant to the perception of that photon and may take place during many minutes after the visual event has passed.

Activated rhodopsin initiates the transduction cascade (▶ Fig. 2.6) by activating an outer segment protein called *transducin*, a type of G-protein.[23] One rhodopsin molecule activates about 500 transducin molecules, each of which in turn activates *phosphodiesterase*, which catalyzes the breakdown of thousands of molecules of cGMP within the outer segment cytoplasm. cGMP acts on the outer segment to hold open the sodium channels in the cell membrane and keep the photoreceptor

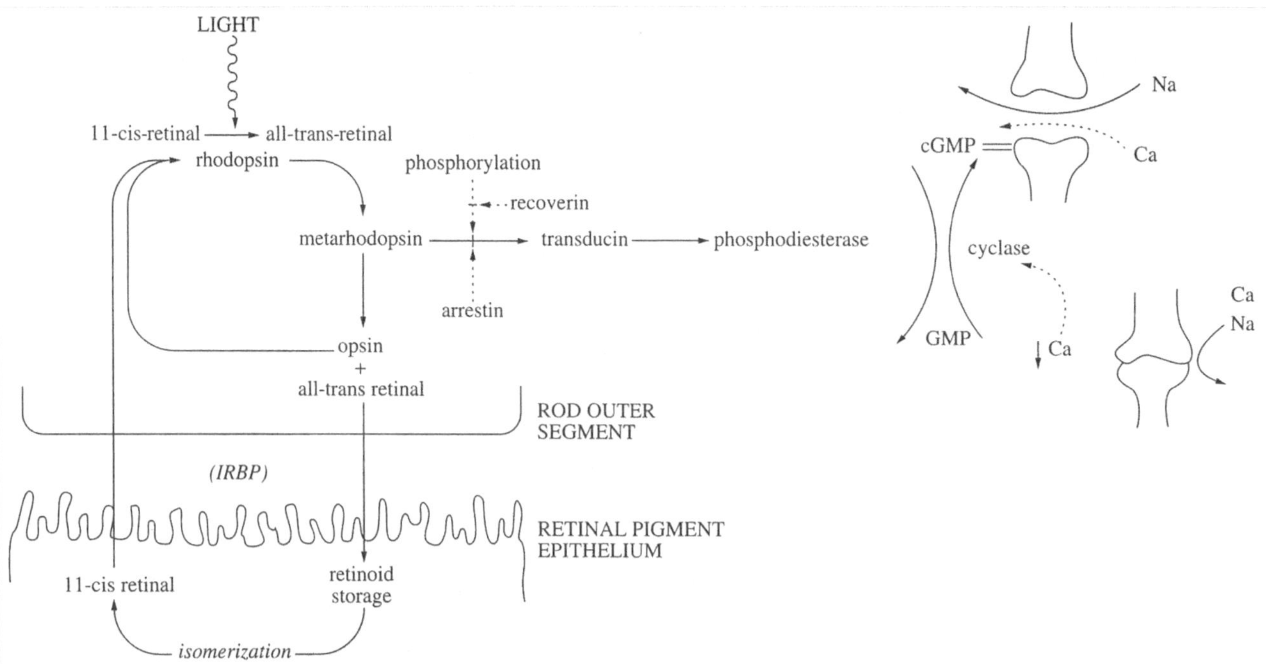

Fig. 2.6 Transduction cascade and visual pigment regeneration cycle. When light changes 11-*cis*-retinal to all-*trans*-retinal, it activates two cycles of chemical activity. The early conformational change to metarhodopsin initiates a G-protein cascade that breaks down cyclic guanosine monophosphate, closes sodium channels, and generates the receptor potential. Quite independently, the metarhodopsin continues to change chemically, eventually breaking down into retinal and opsin that recycle slowly (in part through the retinal pigment epithelium) to restore rhodopsin to the outer segments. IRBP, interphotoreceptor retinoid-binding protein.

depolarized. As light reduces the concentration of cGMP, the sodium channels close and the photoreceptor hyperpolarizes (a response called the *receptor potential*). A single photon can block the entry of more than a million sodium ions, and the resulting voltage change modulates the release of neurotransmitters at the synaptic endings of the photoreceptor to begin the neural process of vision. The receptor potential then turns off because activated rhodopsin is phosphorylated and an outer segment protein called *arrestin* binds the phosphorylated rhodopsin and prevents activation of transducin and phosphodiesterase.[24] Also, transduction causes a fall in the cytoplasmic calcium concentration that in turn activates a GMP cyclase that generates new cGMP to reopen the sodium channels.

This electrical system may seem puzzling, insofar as most nerve cells respond to stimulation by an opening of sodium channels and depolarization. The difficulty is not with the photoreceptor, however, but with our anthropomorphic notion that light must be the stimulus. If you think of a photoreceptor as a cell at rest in the light, then stimulation with a shot of darkness produces a typical depolarizing sensory response. The propensity of photoreceptors to be "stimulated" in the dark is, in fact, very important to understand their metabolism. Because the photoreceptors spend extended periods of time with open sodium channels in a state of depolarization, the cells would swell and die unless there were a means to remove the sodium as fast as it comes in. This is accomplished by an electrogenic sodium–potassium pump in the membrane of the inner segment. The energy demands of this pump give the photoreceptor one of the highest metabolic rates in the body. The choriocapillaris has one of the highest flow rates per unit area of any vascular tissue to supply a surplus of oxygen for this metabolic activity.

A number of human disorders have been recognized that involve components of the photoreceptive cascade (▶ Fig. 2.3 and ▶ Fig. 2.6).[25] A small percentage of families with RP have been found to have abnormalities in the transduction protein, *phosphodiesterase*. This leads to excess GMP within the cell and eventual photoreceptor degeneration. The most common genetic abnormality that has been identified in dominant RP is a structural change in the *rhodopsin* molecule. Well over 50 different single amino acid defects in rhodopsin have been described to date among dominant RP families, some causing very severe RP and some rather mild disease. The mechanism by which these defects lead to gradual photoreceptor decompensation remains to be shown. RP families have also been identified with defects in peripherin, an outer segment protein of uncertain role in the visual process. Abnormalities in *arrestin* have been shown to be responsible for Oguchi's disease,[26] a rare form of congenital night blindness having the curious property that patients require many hours to adapt to the dark but can lose their dark sensitivity with only a very brief exposure to light (that is insufficient to bleach most of the visual pigment). The explanation of this curious symptomatology is that without normal arrestin, the transduction process cannot be turned off quickly, and rods that are activated remain hyperpolarized with a loss of sensitivity. Another rod protein, called (somewhat inappropriately) *recoverin*, blocks rhodopsin phosphorylation in the presence of high calcium concentrations. Thus, it prevents shutoff of the cascade and may help to regulate internal calcium. Antibodies to recoverin are found in some cases of cancer-associated retinopathy.[27] The ATP-binding cassette protein, produced by the *ABCA4* gene, although not classically part of the phototransduction cascade, also plays an important role in the removal of toxic metabolites and the regeneration of retinal in the visual cycle. Its role in the context of Stargardt's macular dystrophy has been described earlier.

Pearls

Several retinal disorders are known to involve specific components of the photoreceptive cascade and visual pigment regeneration cycle. These conditions and their corresponding defective component(s) include the following:

- RP: rhodopsin, phosphodiesterase, peripherin
- Oguchi's disease: arrestin
- Cancer-associated retinopathy: recoverin
- Stargardt's disease: *ABCA4*
- Leber's amaurosis: *RPE* genes *LRAT* and *RPE65*
- Fundus albipunctatus: RDH5

2.3.2 Adaptation

Because the recovery process begins shortly after the onset of transduction, the receptor potential falls back rapidly from its peak within a period of milliseconds. In other words, the response of a photoreceptor to the onset of light is much larger than to a light that is maintained over time. This is one type of adaptation. There are other types of adaptation that occur at the photoreceptor level. At very dim light levels (scotopic illumination), only rods are functional, but as the background light gets brighter and brighter the rod response gets progressively saturated until rods can no longer respond at all. This occurs at moderate levels of light, at which we begin to see colors (mesopic illumination). Only cones are functional at higher levels of light (photopic illumination), but cones can adjust (adapt) over a large range of brightness without saturating, which is fortunate and allows us to function outside on a sunny day.

This *neural adaptation* of cones is critical to vision in the real world. The process of *chemical adaptation*, which was described earlier, is necessary to gain maximum sensitivity in a dark environment, but it would be dysfunctional in the real world if we had to wait 20 or 30 minutes every time we entered a dimly lit room. In contrast, cones can adapt to changes in ambient brightness within seconds, although we only have a limited range of black-to-white discrimination at any point in time. As the cone sensitivity shifts, what appeared white indoors will seem black in the sunlight. Thus, a tunnel seems black as we approach it on a sunny day, but when we enter, the eye resets its gray scale very quickly so that we can see the road. This adaptation to different environments also allows us to enjoy photographs and art, which cannot duplicate (on the wall of a gallery) the true brightness of either a dark room or a sunny outdoor scene. We recognize the scene because the *range* of brightness in the picture mirrors what our eyes would see in that environment

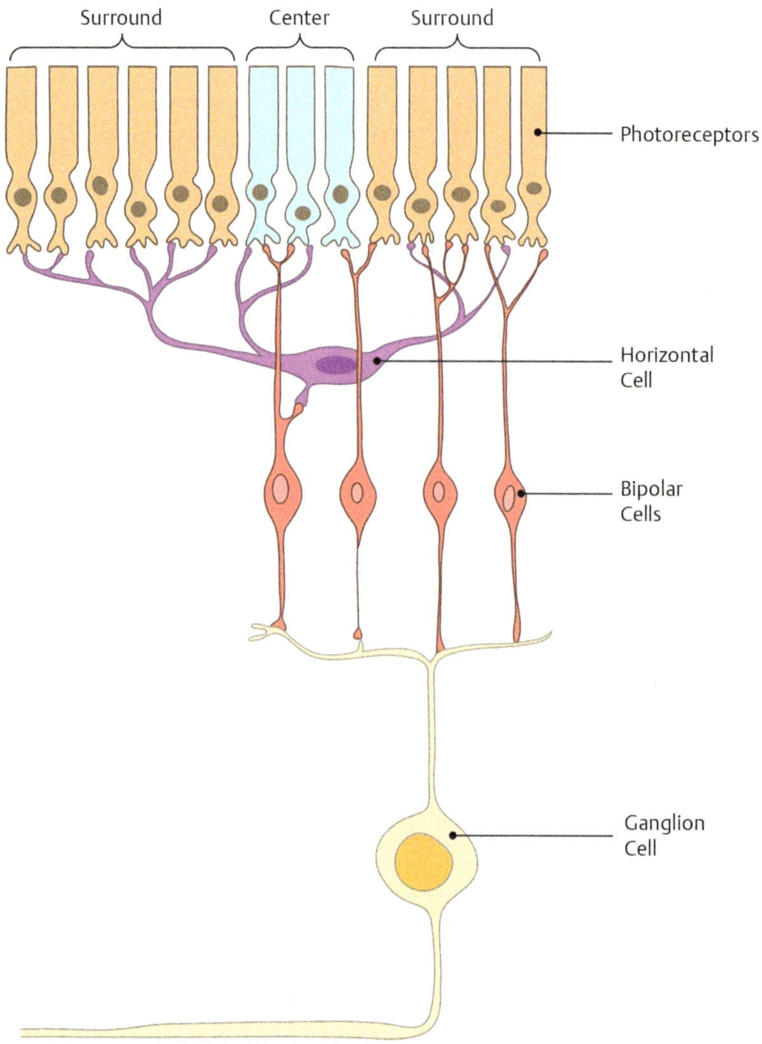

Fig. 2.7 Simplified diagram of retinal circuitry showing how center-surround (excitatory-inhibitory) receptive fields are generated in bipolar cells. The excitatory center represents direct input from overlying photoreceptors, and the surround represents inhibitory input from horizontal cells that have synaptic connections with more distant photoreceptors. (Modified from Marmor.[33])

2.3.3 Retinal Integration and the Recognition of Contrast

There are roughly 120 million rods and 6 million cones in the retina, but only 1 million optic nerve fibers. This means that it is impossible for the eye to transmit to the brain a 1:1 map of the photoreceptor image. The retina must simplify and code visual information so that all necessary spatial and color information can be transmitted through nerve fibers that are numerically less than 1% of the photoreceptive elements. The basic mechanism by which the retina accomplishes this is a neural organization that is wired to recognize contrasts and edges rather than absolutes of brightness or color.

Embryologically, retina is brain, and contains three strata of neurons that begin to process visual signals (▶ Fig. 2.7). This circuitry is very complex, as there are many different specialized types of bipolar, horizontal, amacrine, and ganglion cells (large, small, fast, slow, "on" responsive, "off" responsive, etc.) to serve different components of vision such as color, movement, depth, resolution, and so forth. This brief chapter does not allow a full description of such complexity, and what follows is merely an example of how a neural cascade can begin to code photoreceptor input into recognition of edges and contrast. It is highly simplified, and should not be construed as describing "retinal organization."

The *receptive field* of a retinal neuron is the portion of the visible world in which light can stimulate that particular cell. For each photoreceptor, this area is quite small, but the receptive fields of bipolar cells or ganglion cells can be much larger, to the extent that there is convergence of multiple photoreceptors on each bipolar cell and possibly further convergence of bipolar cells on ganglion cells. Convergence is at a minimum for the cone cells within the fovea, and close to 1:1 transmission is necessary to achieve the high resolution that we need for sharp visual acuity. However, there is considerable convergence among cones in the periphery and even more convergence within the rod system, which is designed to capture light and perceive motion rather than to resolve small objects.

The recognition of contrast begins at the bipolar cell level. The receptive fields of bipolar cells are doughnut-shaped, with an excitatory response to light in the center and an inhibitory response to light in the surround (*on-center cells*), or vice versa (*off-center cells*). This organization results from the confluence of bipolar cell and horizontal cell synaptic processes at the base of the photoreceptor (▶ Fig. 2.7). The central portion of the receptive field is determined by the photoreceptors that feed directly onto the bipolar cell. Sensitivity to the surround is determined by horizontal cells; these cells ramify over a much larger area (corresponding to the surround), and make *inhibitory* contact with the photoreceptor–bipolar synapses in the center. Thus, light falling on the center of the receptive field of an on-center bipolar cell has a direct (e.g., excitatory) effect, whereas light falling on the surround comes through horizontal cells and has an inhibitory effect on the bipolar cell. In "off-center" bipolar cells, the effects are reversed.

How does this receptive field organization generate *contrast sensitivity*? Illumination that evenly covers both the center and surround regions of the bipolar cell receptive field is relatively ineffective as a stimulus, because the center and surround regions offset each other (▶ Fig. 2.8). An edge crossing the receptive field, however, will stimulate only part of the surround and thus create an imbalance that is a powerful stimulus to the cell. Because of adaptation, it is also necessary that these edges sweep continually across the retina to maintain activation of the neurons. Vision would fade within seconds if the eyes were held absolutely still, and thus our eyes are always jiggling very slightly with microsaccades. This center-surround, contrast-sensitive organization of the bipolar cells is passed on to the ganglion cells, and eventually to cortical neurons (which develop more sophisticated receptive fields). This organization of the retina means that our eyes are exquisitely sensitive to edges and differences in brightness but are relatively disinterested in steady illumination. We see objects by their borders, and the brain fills in the centers if there is no new pattern to create a stimulus. This is why we do not perceive our own blind spot.

The powerful sensitivity of the retina to contrast accounts for many common illusions of brightness. A gray circle on a white background appears dark, whereas the same gray on a black background will appear quite light. A related phenomenon was described by the physicist/psychologist Ernst Mach.[28] At a junction between two levels of gray, we tend to perceive an extra band of lightness on the lighter side, and a band of darkness on the darker side, of the edge. These *Mach bands* are quite

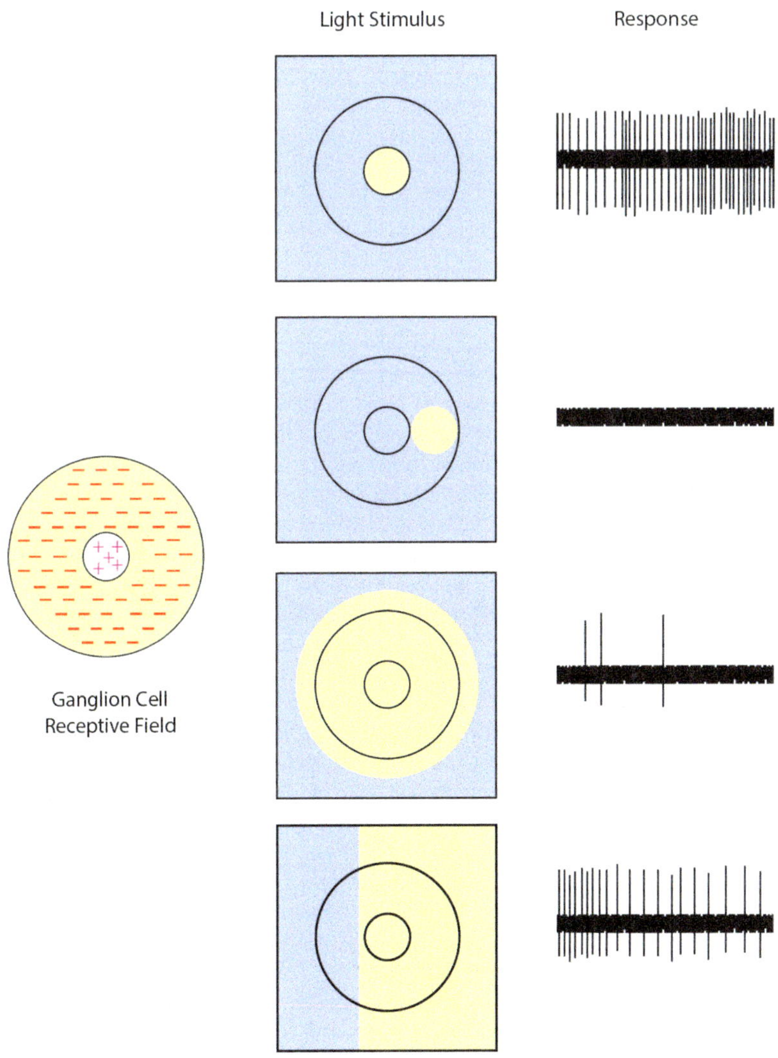

Fig. 2.8 Ganglion cell receptive fields showing why edges and contrast are critical to vision. The cell is activated by stimulation of the center area and inhibited by stimulation of the surround area, but it responds only minimally to diffuse light because the center and surround offset each other. An edge is an effective stimulus because when it covers the center, it covers only a part of the surround, and the balance of effects is excitatory. (Modified from Marmor.[33])

Fig. 2.9 Illusion of darkness and lightness produced by the presence of Mach bands. The line beneath the shaded figure shows the relative brightness at each point. Each of the three regions is equally bright, except at the junctions. The central area appears lighter because of a light-to-dark junction on either side of it. Holding a pencil over the junctions will show that all three regions are the same.

involuntary perceptions because they are hard-wired in the neural organization of our retina. Conversely, if one creates a light–dark junction within an evenly gray surface, our eyes and brain can be fooled into dividing the whole surface into perceived regions of light and dark (▶ Fig. 2.9). These illusions are powerful evidence that the human eye is an instrument for contrast detection rather than an instrument for the recognition of absolute levels of illumination.

It was noted earlier that bipolar cells may be on-center or off-center. Rods feed only into on-center cells, the so-called depolarizing bipolar cell pathway. Cones, however, feed into both depolarizing and hyperpolarizing bipolar cells. Because the hyperpolarizing cells depolarize to the *offset* of light, these pathways are sometimes called *on-* and *off-pathways*. The functional significance of the on- and off-pathways for visual perception is complex, but some human diseases have already been identified that involve these pathways selectively.[29] In the most common form of congenital stationary night blindness (CSNB), affected individuals are born without the ability to see in the dark and without any rod b-wave on ERG. The rod a-wave is present, however, and the disease was thought for a long time to represent a synaptic blockage between rods and bipolar cells. However, CSNB is actually a congenital lack of the on-pathway (of both rods and cones) rather than a specific rod disease. Retention of the cone off-pathway seems sufficient to allow relatively normal visual acuity and color perception in most of these patients.

The conscious perception of our world is far more complex than just the recognition of light and dark, or edge and center, as we also distinguish qualities such as motion, texture, color, shape, and depth. To some degree, these various perceptions begin with systems of distinct bipolar and ganglion cells that work parallel to one another within the visual system and feed into brain areas that perceive these qualities.[30] In general, the larger ganglion cells are concerned with light detection, motion, depth, and spatial orientation. These cells respond to brightness rather than color, but are sensitive to subtle contrasts and can respond rapidly even in dim light. The smaller ganglion cells form two additional parallel systems within the retina and central nervous system. One contains our color-sensitive neurons, which have moderate spatial resolution. The second contains neurons that are specialized for high spatial resolution and fine acuity. These small cell systems require good lighting and high degrees of contrast. Although these *parallel pathways* remain relatively independent up to the visual association areas of the cerebral cortex, interaction and crosstalk between these systems helps to produce an integrated perception of the world.

2.3.4 Color Vision

Mammals are almost universally red-green color-blind, with the exception of higher apes and humans. For example, cats and dogs have only short-wavelength-sensitive cones (S cones) and long-wavelength-sensitive cones (L cones). This permits them to distinguish between the blue and yellow ends of the spectrum. However, they cannot make the full range of color distinctions that are visible to most humans. The development of human trichromatic vision is a relatively recent phylogenetic event, when the long-wavelength pigment in some Old World apes mutated into a red-sensitive (L) and green-sensitive (M = middle) cone pigment. Whereas our S cone pigment shows only 43% homology in amino acid sequences with the long-wavelength pigments, there is 95% homology between the M and L pigments. The S cone pigment is coded on a somatic chromosome, but the M and L pigment genes are on the X chromosome.[31]

Although three cone pigments are necessary to perceive a full spectrum of colors, the bipolar and ganglion cells do not transmit spectral information directly (▶ Fig. 2.10). Rather, these cells are organized into center-surround receptive fields based on contrast between red and green, or blue and yellow. Some ganglion cells have a red excitatory center and green inhibitory surround, or vice versa, so that they recognize the relative levels of stimulation of the M and L cones. Blue- and yellow-sensitive ganglion cells recognize contrast between the S cones and the combined long-wavelength (M and L) system, which would be a phylogenetically older set of contrasts. Because of this cellular organization in the retina, we ultimately recognize colors by their relationships to each other as much or more than by the absolute wavelengths. One implication of this is that we can maintain a sense of color constancy under a variety of lighting conditions. We tend to see most colored objects as the same, for example, in bluish daylight or yellow incandescent light. However, the fact that form and depth are perceptions that depend on brightness means that we will have trouble distinguishing objects that differ in color but not in brightness. Color is essentially superimposed upon our brightness-based recognition of shapes, movement, and depth.

There are physiologic differences between the short-wavelength and long-wavelength cones. For example, the S cones are quite rodlike in some of their electrical and temporal characteristics. There are a much smaller number of S cones than M and L cones within the retina, and there are no S cones at all in the absolute center of the fovea. If a blue dot is tiny enough, and in

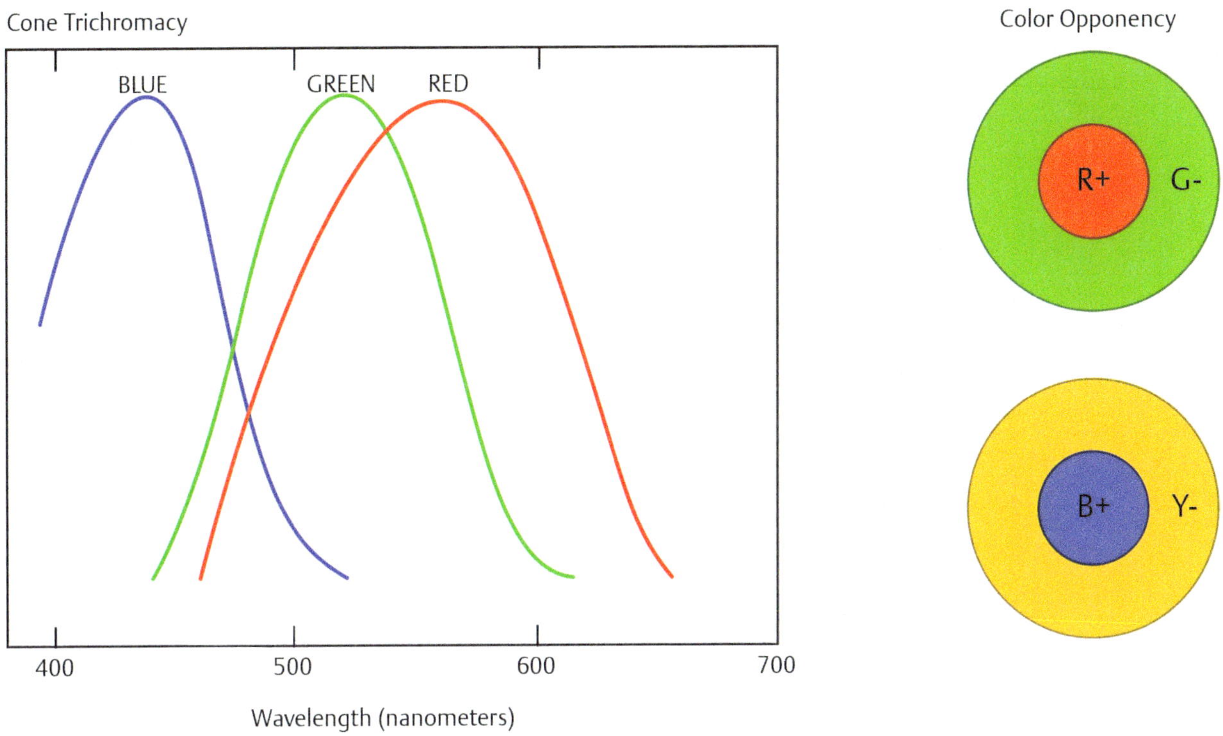

Fig. 2.10 Trichromacy and color opponency in the retina. Three cone types, with blue-, green-, and red-sensitive pigments, have the spectral sensitivities shown on the graph. However, horizontal and bipolar cell interactions lead to center-surround receptive fields at the ganglion cell level (and higher in the central nervous system) that contrast either green and red, or blue and yellow. Color perception is ultimately a matter of contrast recognition more than of absolute wavelength.

the exact center of gaze, we cannot recognize it as blue—but in reality we see blue colors just off center and our brain assumes that the color remains constant across the center of the visual field. Possibly because of their smaller numbers or because of metabolic differences, the S cones may be more susceptible to retinal disease and they can be selectively damaged in retinal degenerations and dystrophies, glaucoma, and diabetic retinopathy. Patients with all these disorders tend to have subtle deficiencies in blue-yellow discrimination.

Pearls

- The S cone system is more susceptible to retinal disease than the M or L cone system. It can be selectively damaged in retinal degenerations and dystrophies, glaucoma, and diabetic retinopathy. Therefore, patients with these disorders tend to have subtle deficiencies in blue-yellow discrimination.

2.3.5 Electrical Responses of the Retina

Clinical electrophysiologic tests are discussed in Chapter 7, but it is important to understand the cellular origin of retinal electrical signals (▶ Fig. 2.11). When a bright light is turned upon a dark-adapted eye, the eye produces a sequence of retinal and RPE voltage changes that may oscillate for hours. Within the first few milliseconds, there is a small negative wave called the early receptor potential, which is generated by conformational changes in the visual pigment molecules during transduction. A very bright flash is required to elicit this response, which seems to be dominated by cones rather than rods; although it has been recorded in humans, it is not of general use clinically. The *receptor potential*- the primary hyperpolarization of the photoreceptors in response to light- occurs within 5 to 10 milliseconds. It generates the initial negative deflection of the ERG a-wave, and the downward slope of the *a-wave* is a good measure of photoreceptor integrity. A-wave amplitude is not as precise because it also depends on the speed and magnitude with which the positive-going *b-wave* develops and cuts off the a-wave. In normal eyes, the b-wave is the largest ERG response; it peaks at 30 to 50 milliseconds and appears to be generated electrically by both Müller cells (responding passively to ionic changes in their environment) and bipolar cells. Physiologically, the b-wave represents neural activity in the inner retina. The *oscillatory potentials* on the rising phase of the b-wave are also generated in the inner retina, possibly by feedback circuits involving amacrine cells and other integrative neurons.

If electrical recording is continued after the b-wave diminishes, one observes a few *seconds* later another positive wave, called the *c-wave*. This represents a passive response by the apical membranes of the RPE and Müller cells to the fall in potassium concentration of the subretinal space that follows transduction. This ocular voltage then dips during the next *minute* to generate the *fast oscillation*, and then rises during 5 to 10 *minutes* as the *light response* of the standing potential.

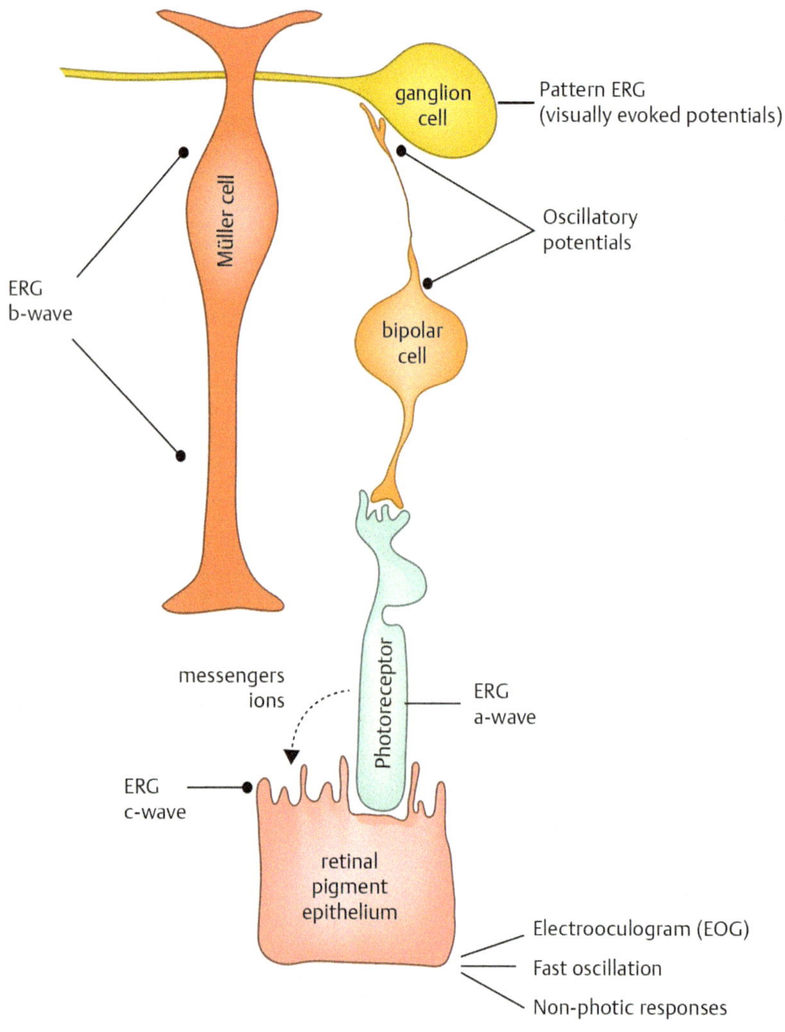

Fig. 2.11 Clinical electrical responses from the retina and retinal pigment epithelium (RPE). The RPE responses require stimulation of the photoreceptors or administration of pharmacologic agents because the RPE is not itself photosensitive. The retinal responses localize to different cellular layers as shown. ERG, electroretinogram.

These are RPE-generated responses, and their mechanism has been discussed earlier. The ocular voltage may continue to oscillate slowly during 1 to 2 hours, but these late fluctuations have not been used clinically.

All the responses noted so far come from cellular elements that are, to a large degree, oriented radially within the eye (e.g., photoreceptors, bipolar cells, RPE cells) and can summate in parallel to generate a large extraocular signal. The ganglion cells are oriented circumferentially, however, and thus produce a much smaller signal with external (corneal) recordings. Nevertheless, a small negative response arises from ganglion cells that can be elicited with strong red or yellow flashes on a blue rod-suppressing background (photopic negative response) or an alternating checkboard stimulus that minimizes luminance signals (pattern electroretinogram). These responses are reduced in glaucoma, for example, but have not yet been refined to the point that they are used much for individual patients.

The full-field ERG is dominated by the retinal periphery, even for cones (cones are most densely packed in the fovea, but 90% of cones are outside the macula). To record a macular ERG is tricky, since light scatter within the eye from a focal stimulus can overwhelm the response. A technique called multifocal ERG (mfERG) overcomes this problem by presenting a computerized stimulus of small hexagons that are scaled in size to match cone density, and that flicker on and off in a seemingly random fashion. The computer calculates how much signal correlates with each stimulus hexagon, and prints an array of small cone ERG responses from different regions of the macula. The mfERG is now widely used to assess macular pathology.

2.4 Conclusion

The primary photoreceptive tissue in the eye is the retina, which not only captures radiant energy but also codes visual input into contrast-sensitive receptive fields to maximize the visual information that can be transmitted through a limited number of optic nerve fibers. The photoreceptors are responsible for transduction, many aspects of adaptation, and the initial ability to perceive a full spectrum of colors. However, the integrative circuits of the retina, which produce contrast sensitivity, are the foundation for how objects are ultimately recognized and perceived. The retina cannot function without close apposition to the RPE and without the various support functions carried out by the RPE, which include visual pigment regeneration, phagocytosis of outer segment material, control of the subretinal space, and the maintenance of retinal adhesion. Loss of these functions through aging may contribute to a variety of diseases. A number of ocular disorders have been discovered with genetic defects in specific aspects of the transduction or integrative pathways of the retina. Physiologic tests, such as dark adaptation, the ERG, and the EOG, reflect retinal physiology and can provide the clinician with information about the status of individual cell types within the retina or about the depth and regional distribution of retinal disease.

References

[1] Marmor MF, Wolfensberger TJ, eds. The Retinal Pigment Epithelium: Function and Disease. New York, NY: Oxford University Press; 1998

[2] Allikmets R, Singh N, Sun H, et al. A photoreceptor cell-specific ATP-binding transporter gene (ABCR) is mutated in recessive Stargardt macular dystrophy. Nat Genet. 1997; 15(3):236–246

[3] Liu J, Itagaki Y, Ben-Shabat S, Nakanishi K, Sparrow JR. The biosynthesis of A2E, a fluorophore of aging retina, involves the formation of the precursor, A2-PE, in the photoreceptor outer segment membrane. J Biol Chem. 2000; 275(38):29354–29360

[4] Bakall B, Radu RA, Stanton JB, et al. Enhanced accumulation of A2E in individuals homozygous or heterozygous for mutations in BEST1 (VMD2). Exp Eye Res. 2007; 85(1):34–43

[5] Hughes BA, Gallemore RP, Miller SS. Transport mechanisms in the retinal pigment epithelium. In: Marmor MF, Wolfensberger TJ, eds. The Retinal Pigment Epithelium: Function and Disease. New York, NY: Oxford University Press; 1998:103–134

[6] Marmor MF. Control of subretinal fluid and mechanisms of serous detachment. In: Marmor MF, Wolfensberger TJ, eds. The Retinal Pigment Epithelium: Function and Disease. New York, NY: Oxford University Press; 1998:420–438

[7] Marmor M. On the cause of serous detachments and acute central serous chorioretinopathy. Br J Ophthalmol. 1997; 81(10):812–813

[8] von Lintig J, Kiser PD, Golczak M, Palczewski K. The biochemical and structural basis for trans-to-cis isomerization of retinoids in the chemistry of vision. Trends Biochem Sci. 2010; 35(7):400–410

[9] Marmor MF. Long-term follow-up of the physiologic abnormalities and fundus changes in fundus albipunctatus. Ophthalmology. 1990; 97(3):380–384

[10] Iannaccone A, Tedesco SA, Gallaher KT, Yamamoto H, Charles S, Dryja TP. Fundus albipunctatus in a 6-year old girl due to compound heterozygous mutations in the RDH5 gene. Doc Ophthalmol. 2007; 115(2):111–116

[11] Young RW. Visual cells and the concept of renewal. Invest Ophthalmol Vis Sci. 1976; 15(9):700–725

[12] Gal A, Li Y, Thompson DA, et al. Mutations in MERTK, the human orthologue of the RCS rat retinal dystrophy gene, cause retinitis pigmentosa. Nat Genet. 2000; 26(3):270–271

[13] Marmor MF. Mechanisms of normal retinal adhesion. In: Ryan SJ, ed. Retina. 2nd ed. St. Louis, MO: Mosby; 1994:1931–1953

[14] Hageman GS, Marmor MF, Yao X-Y, Johnson LV. The interphotoreceptor matrix mediates primate retinal adhesion. Arch Ophthalmol. 1995; 113 (5):655–660

[15] Cox SN, Hay E, Bird AC. Treatment of chronic macular edema with acetazolamide. Arch Ophthalmol. 1988; 106(9):1190–1195

[16] Gallemore RP, Maruiwa F, Marmor MF. Clinical electrophysiology of the retinal pigment epithelium. In: Marmor MF, Wolfensberger TJ, eds. The Retinal Pigment Epithelium: Function and Disease. New York, NY: Oxford University Press; 1998:199–223

[17] Marmorstein AD, Marmorstein LY, Rayborn M, Wang X, Hollyfield JG, Petrukhin K. Bestrophin, the product of the Best vitelliform macular dystrophy gene (VMD2), localizes to the basolateral plasma membrane of the retinal pigment epithelium. Proc Natl Acad Sci U S A. 2000; 97(23):12758–12763

[18] Strauß O, Müller C, Reichhart N, Tamm ER, Gomez NM. The role of bestrophin-1 in intracellular Ca(2+) signaling. Adv Exp Med Biol. 2014; 801:113–119

[19] Dawson DW, Volpert OV, Gillis P, et al. Pigment epithelium-derived factor: a potent inhibitor of angiogenesis. Science. 1999; 285(5425):245–248

[20] Becerra SP, Fariss RN, Wu YQ, Montuenga LM, Wong P, Pfeffer BA. Pigment epithelium-derived factor in the monkey retinal pigment epithelium and interphotoreceptor matrix: apical secretion and distribution. Exp Eye Res. 2004; 78(2):223–234

[21] Bouck N. PEDF: anti-angiogenic guardian of ocular function. Trends Mol Med. 2002; 8(7):330–334

[22] Bandyopadhyay M, Rohrer B. Matrix metalloproteinase activity creates proangiogenic environment in primary human retinal pigment epithelial cells exposed to complement. Invest Ophthalmol Vis Sci. 2012; 53(4):1953–1961

[23] Stryer L. Biochemistry. 4th ed. New York, NY: WH Freeman; 1995:332–339

[24] Baylor D. How photons start vision. Proc Natl Acad Sci U S A. 1996; 93 (2):560–565

[25] Dryja TP, Li T. Molecular genetics of retinitis pigmentosa. Hum Mol Genet. 1995; 4(Spec No):1739–1743

[26] Fuchs S, Nakazawa M, Maw M, Tamai M, Oguchi Y, Gal A. A homozygous 1-base pair deletion in the arrestin gene is a frequent cause of Oguchi disease in Japanese. Nat Genet. 1995; 10(3):360–362

[27] Adamus G, Guy J, Schmied JL, Arendt A, Hargrave PA. Role of anti-recoverin autoantibodies in cancer-associated retinopathy. Invest Ophthalmol Vis Sci. 1993; 34(9):2626–2633

[28] Marmor MF. The bands of Ernst Mach: edge effects in art. In: Marmor MF, Ravin JG, eds. The Eye of the Artist. St. Louis, MO: Mosby-Year Book; 1997:60–69

[29] Sieving PA. Photopic ON- and OFF-pathway abnormalities in retinal dystrophies. Trans Am Ophthalmol Soc. 1993; 91:701–773

[30] Livingstone M, Hubel D. Segregation of form, color, movement, and depth: anatomy, physiology, and perception. Science. 1988; 240(4853):740–749

[31] Nathans J, Thomas D, Hogness DS. Molecular genetics of human color vision: the genes encoding blue, green, and red pigments. Science. 1986; 232 (4747):193–202

[32] Steinberg RH, Wood I, Hogan MJ. Pigment epithelial ensheathment and phagocytosis of extrafoveal cones in human retina. Philos Trans R Soc Lond B Biol Sci. 1977; 277(958):459–474

[33] Marmor MF. The eye and art. In: Marmor MF, Ravin JG, eds. The Eye of the Artist. St. Louis, MO: Mosby-Year Book; 1997:2–25

Part II

Diagnostic Techniques

3 Examination of the Fundus 30

4 Fundus Angiography 40

5 Optical Coherence Tomography 52

6 Ultrasonography 66

7 Electrophysiology and Miscellaneous Noninvasive Tests 83

II

3 Examination of the Fundus

Allen Chiang and William E. Benson

3.1 Peripheral Retinal Examination

3.1.1 Indirect Ophthalmoscopy

Principles and Advantages

The standard technique for examining the retina is binocular indirect ophthalmoscopy. With this method, reflected light from the patient's fundus is focused by a lens into an intermediate image, which is then viewed by the observer (▶ Fig. 3.1). The image that is created is upside down and inverted (▶ Fig. 3.2). The headpiece of the binocular indirect ophthalmoscope is constructed so that the light from either a high-intensity incandescent or light-emitting diode bulb is focused onto a mirror that reflects the light into the patient's eye and onto the retina (▶ Fig. 3.3). Because the mirror is mounted above the view box, the beam of light entering the patient's eye (illumination beam) is separated from the light rays that are viewed by the examiner (observation beams). This arrangement prevents the corneal light reflex of the illumination beam from interfering with viewing. The view box contains prisms that provide stereoscopic vision. These prisms optically "narrow" the examiner's pupillary distance; otherwise, the light rays exiting from the patient's pupil could not reach both of the examiner's pupils (▶ Fig. 3.4).

The indirect ophthalmoscope offers several advantages over other techniques for examining the fundus and is indispensable in the evaluation of retinal detachment and other peripheral vitreoretinal pathology.[1,2,3,4,5,6] The strong illumination provided by the head lamp plus the light-gathering capability of the handheld lens enables the examiner to see through hazy media. When combined with scleral depression, indirect ophthalmoscopy provides the best view of the peripheral retina. It is a dynamic technique that allows for a broad area of the retina to be visualized at one time, thereby helping to ensure that no abnormalities will be missed.

Technique

Several aspheric condensing lenses are available for use with indirect ophthalmoscopy. The 14-diopter lens has the highest magnification of the commonly used lenses (3.6x), but it is difficult to use because of its long focal length (7 cm). The 30-diopter lens (f = 3.3 cm) is often preferred by beginners because it is easy to use, especially in patients with small pupils, but it does not provide adequate magnification (1.5x) for finding small breaks or other subtle retinal lesions. Most clinicians prefer the 20-diopter lens (f = 5 cm), which is relatively easy to use and provides a reasonable magnification of 2.3x. Any lens should be held with the more convex surface toward the examiner (▶ Fig. 3.1). It is slightly tilted to move the two light reflexes (one from each surface of the lens) away from the examiner's viewing axis. To minimize the corneal light reflex, the mirror should be adjusted so that the illumination beam is in the top of the field of view of the eyepieces. For small pupils, the light must be directed still higher (▶ Fig. 3.5).

The patient should be reclining comfortably and have a widely dilated pupil. Initially, the transformer rheostat should be set at a low voltage. Higher light intensities can be tried later if the patient becomes less light-sensitive. Bilateral cycloplegia combined with topical anesthesia reduces photophobia and enhances cooperation. The superior periphery should be examined first because photophobia is minimized in upgaze and because the periphery is less sensitive to light than the posterior pole. Some patients are intolerant of bright light and attempt to close their eyes, inducing Bell's phenomenon and making examination of the inferior retina difficult, if not impossible. To counteract this tendency, the ophthalmologist must constantly encourage the patient to keep both eyes open. Sometimes, a fixation target such as the patient's thumb or a mark on the ceiling is helpful.

Pearls

- In examination of the retina with indirect ophthalmoscopy, the superior periphery should be examined first because photophobia is minimized in upgaze and because the periphery is less sensitive to light than the posterior pole.

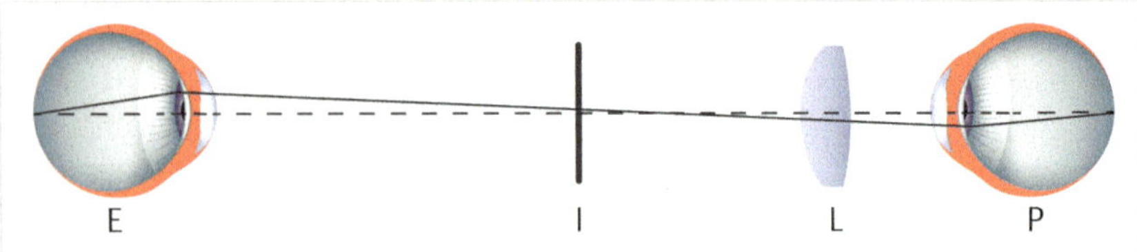

Fig. 3.1 Indirect ophthalmoscopy: Rays from a point in the patient's fundus (P) are focused by a lens (L) into an intermediate image (I), which is viewed by the examiner (E).

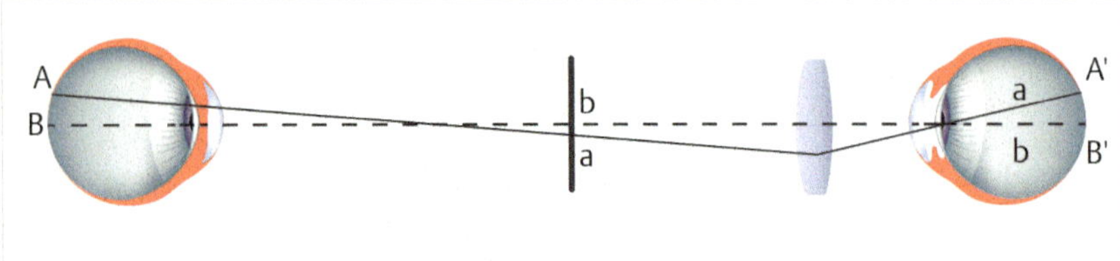

Fig. 3.2 The relative positions of rays of light a and b from points A' and B' in the patient's fundus are reversed at the intermediate image (I), so that a strikes the examiner's superior retina at A. Because the examiner's inferior visual field is "seen" by his superior retina, A appears to be inferior to B.

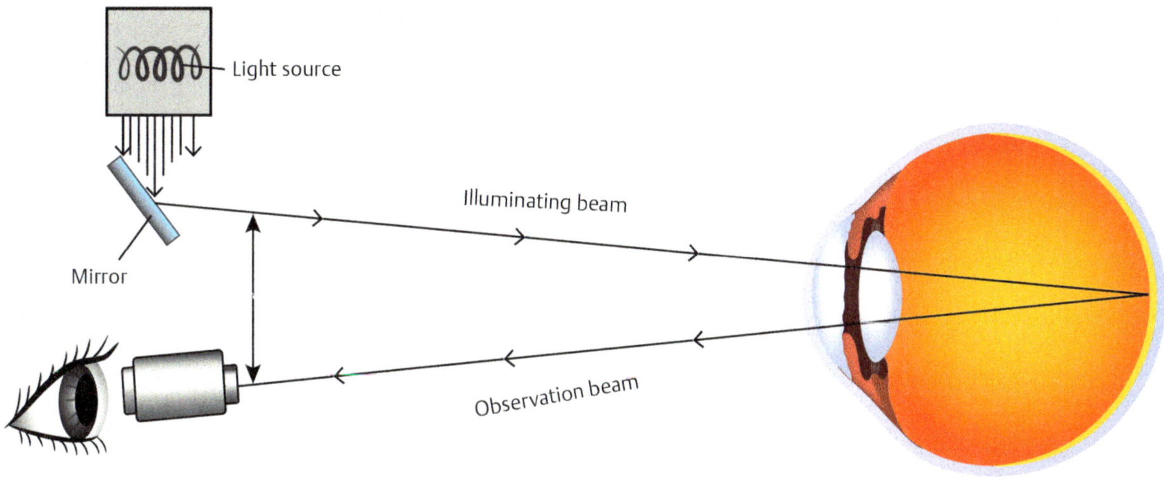

Fig. 3.3 The path of rays of light entering the eye (illumination beam) is separated from those leaving it (observation beam), minimizing corneal light reflexes.

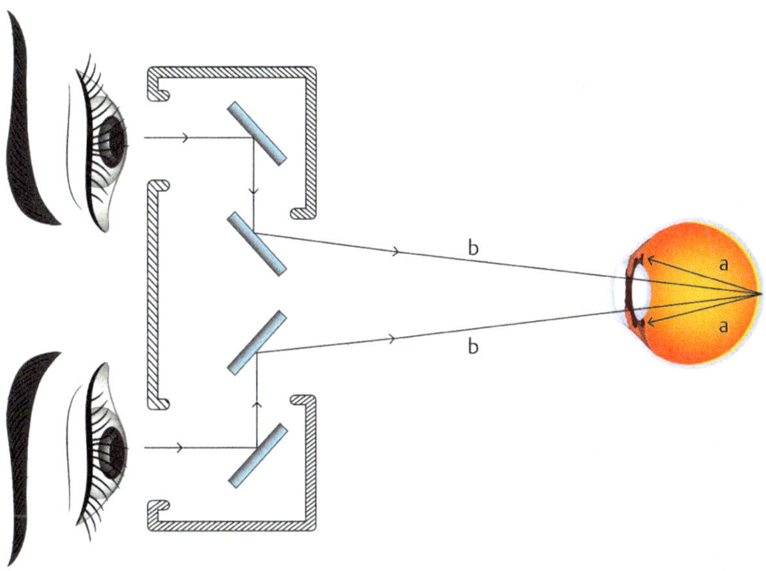

Fig. 3.4 Prisms in the view box of the binocular indirect ophthalmoscope "narrow" the examiner's pupillary distance. Therefore, from points in the patient's fundus, an observation beam (b) can reach each of the examiner's eyes. Without the view box, binocular vision would be impossible because light rays (a), aimed at each of the examiner's eyes, could not exit through the pupil.

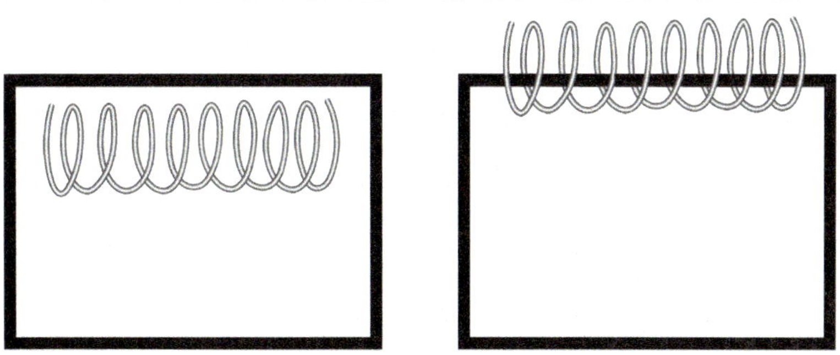

Fig. 3.5 For viewing through adequately dilated pupils (left), the reflected light (*filament*) should be at the top of the examiner's field of vision (*enclosed area*). For viewing through small pupils (right), the mirror is positioned so that only a small strip of light is seen at the top of the field of vision.

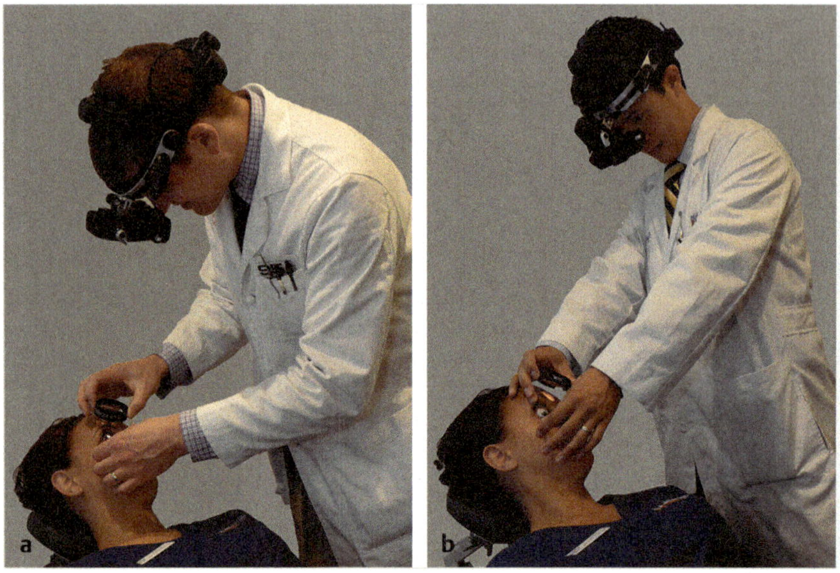

Fig. 3.6 (a) Inexperienced examiner standing too close to a patient with a small pupil. (b) Correct extension of the arm to allow examination through the small pupil. (Photo by Wm. Romano.)

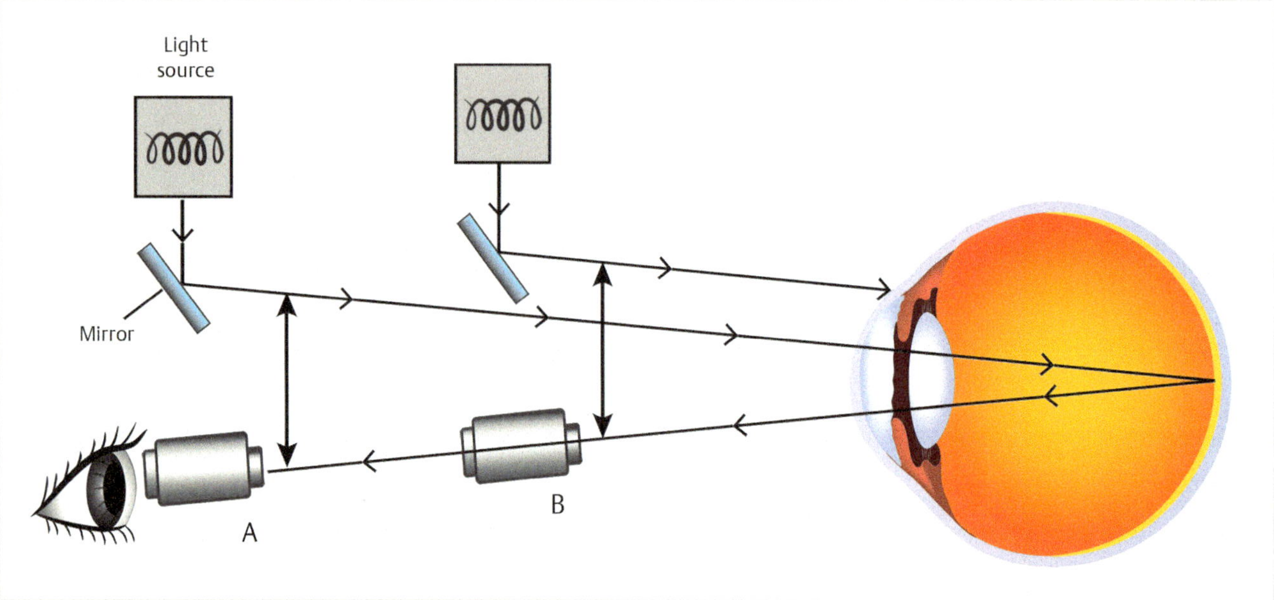

Fig. 3.7 The distance between the illumination beam and the observation beam(s) is fixed (*double-headed arrows*). When the examiner stands at position A, the illumination beam can enter the patient's pupil and the observation beam(s) can exit. At position B, the illumination beam (*open arrow*) cannot enter the eye. If the examiner lowered his head, the eye would be illuminated, but the observation beam(s) could not exit.

If the pupil is large, the examiner can increase magnification by moving closer to the eye. However, if the pupil is small, it is much easier to obtain a clear fundus image if the examiner's arm is extended. Beginners frequently make the error of standing too close to the patient (▶ Fig. 3.6 and ▶ Fig. 3.7).

The examiner's head should be held to look directly into the quadrant being examined. For example, during examination of the nasal periphery, the examiner should stand on the same side as the eye being examined (▶ Fig. 3.8 and ▶ Fig. 3.9), and for the temporal periphery, on the opposite side (▶ Fig. 3.6 and ▶ Fig. 3.10). The hand lens is shifted from the right to left hand as necessary to avoid clumsy maneuvering, especially during scleral depression. The nose becomes less of an obstacle to viewing the temporal periphery when the patient's head is rolled toward the examiner while the patient looks temporally.

The pupillary aperture appears elliptical when the examiner looks at the peripheral retina. This makes stereoscopic viewing more difficult and decreases the amount of light that can enter the eye. The voltage of the light source must be increased and the examiner's head must be tilted slightly so that part of the illumination beam can enter the eye and one of the observation beams can exit (▶ Fig. 3.11). This achieves only a monocular view, a necessary compromise to achieve an adequate image.

When a patient has a small pupil, it is easier to focus on the retina if the examiner first looks at the pupil through the lens while holding the lens away from the eye at a distance greater than its focal length. The examiner then slowly moves the lens toward the pupil. Newer ophthalmoscopes come with smaller illumination beams and adjustable prisms to enhance viewing through small pupils. Furthermore, higher-diopter condensing

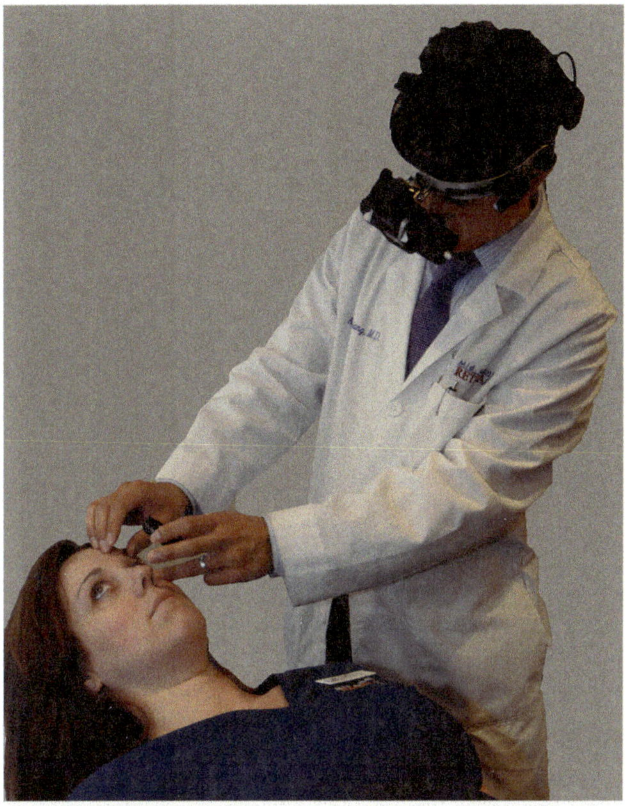

Fig. 3.8 Examination of the superonasal periphery, left eye: The patient keeps both eyes open and looks up and to the right. The examiner's arm is extended. The examiner stands on the patient's left and holds the lens in his left hand, steadying it by resting his finger on the patient's face. (Photo by Wm. Romano.)

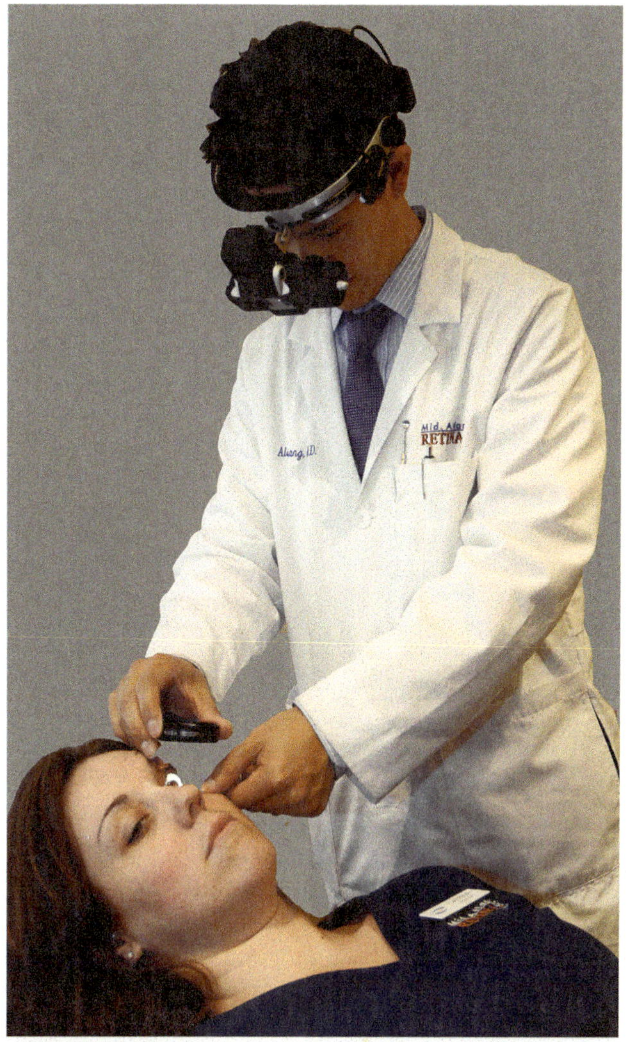

Fig. 3.9 Examination of inferonasal periphery, left eye: Patient looks down and right. The examiner remains on the patient's left but holds the lens in his right hand. (Photo by Wm. Romano.)

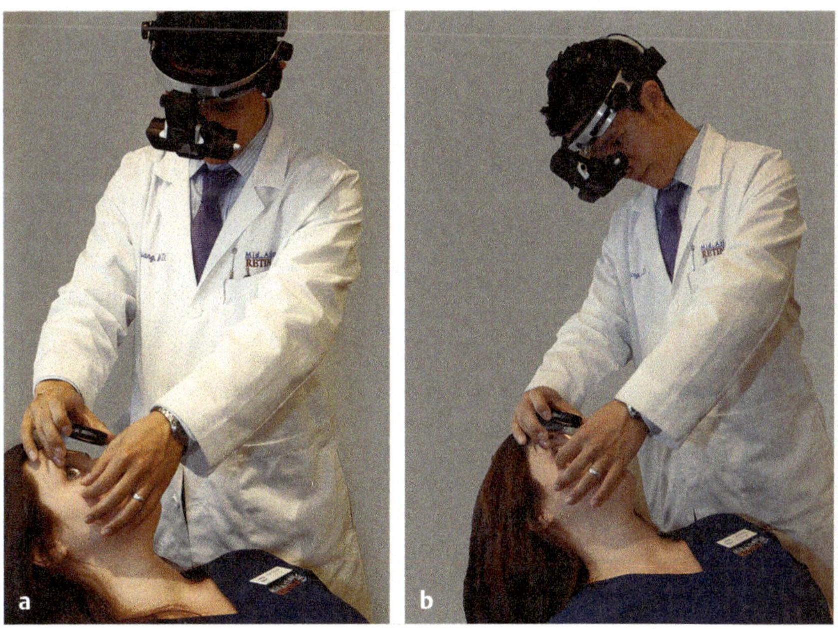

Fig. 3.10 **(a)** Examiner's head is positioned incorrectly for examination of the temporal periphery in a patient with a small pupil. **(b)** Examiner's head is properly tilted so that the eye is well illuminated and a monocular image can be seen. (Photo by Wm. Romano.)

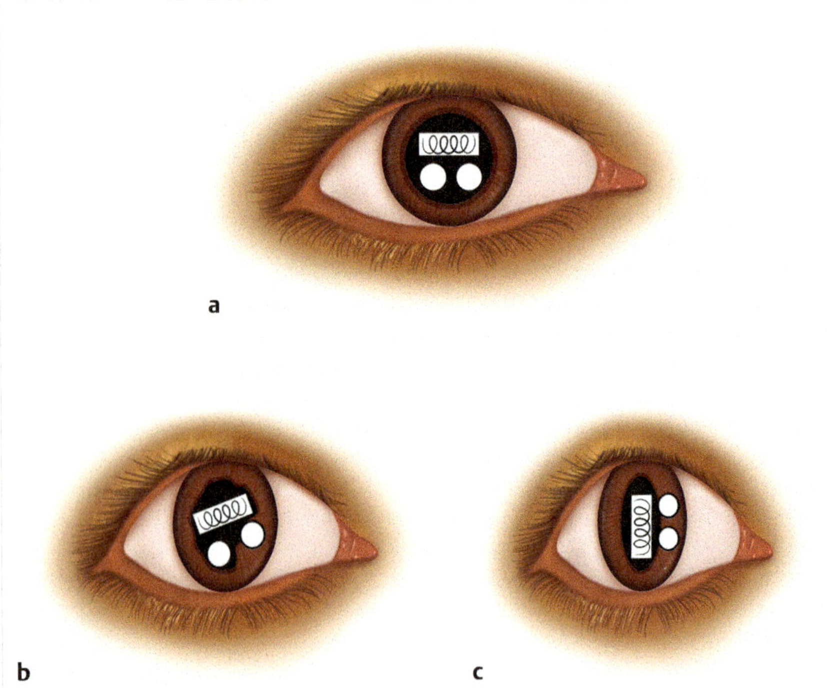

Fig. 3.11 **(a)** Viewing the posterior pole through a large pupil: The illumination beam *(filament)* enters through the top, leaving ample room for the observation beams (*white circles*) below. Binocular vision is provided. **(b)** The pupillary aperture becomes elliptical when the examiner tries to see the far periphery. If the examiner does not tilt his head, the illumination beam can enter the eye, but the observation beams cannot emerge. **(c)** The examiner must tilt his head so that part of the illumination beam can enter the eye. Often, only a monocular view of the fundus is possible, as only one of the observation beams can emerge from the eye.

lenses (e.g., 25, 28, or 30 diopters) also facilitate obtaining a good view in this setting.

Pearls

Techniques to facilitate viewing the fundus through a small pupil include the following:

- Holding the condensing lens slightly farther away from the eye
- Extending one's arm during the examination (increase the working distance)
- Using one of the higher-diopter condensing lenses (e.g., 28 or 30 diopters)
- Using an ophthalmoscope with a small illumination beam and adjustable prisms (i.e., small pupil feature found on some ophthalmoscopes)

Fundus Drawing

There are two ways to correct for the inverted and reversed image of the indirect ophthalmoscope. The first is to observe the retina, then mentally rotate the image, drawing the findings as they are, not as they are seen. The second is to invert the drawing pad and then draw the findings as they are seen. When the drawing is finished, the findings will be positioned correctly.

To examine the fundus completely, the examiner may start at the optic nerve and follow each of the retinal vessels to the periphery or systematically and circumferentially scan the periphery, followed by the posterior pole. Keeping his/her eyes and the condensing lens aligned, the examiner swings his/her gaze along the periphery (▸ Fig. 3.12). This serves two purposes. First, the entire retina is examined. Second, in cases of retinal detachment, holes can be recognized when a sudden change in the brightness of the subretinal layers is noted. A hole is perceived as a discontinuity in the nearly uniform translucency of the detached retina; when the observer's gaze is moving, the discontinuity becomes easier to see because of the contrast between the detached retina and the now-visible layers underneath. Slightly wiggling the lens from side to side produces a prism effect, which also helps to reveal discontinuities in the retina.

No matter what the patient's complaint, it is essential that the fellow eye be carefully examined. For example, in patients with retinal detachment, the examiner must look for retinal breaks or other abnormalities that might require prophylactic treatment.[7] Examining both eyes also helps to detect subtle unilateral abnormalities, such as diffuse choroidal hemangiomas.

Scleral Depression

In patients with retinal detachment or posterior vitreous detachment- after the retina has been thoroughly scanned- the peripheral retina should be examined with scleral depression to detect small holes, especially those near the ora serrata. In some patients, this region cannot be seen at all without indentation. Beginners should not attempt scleral depression until they are adept at viewing the retina anterior to the equator without it. Otherwise, the scleral depression will afford little or no information and the patient will have suffered needlessly.

Although a variety of metal scleral depressors are available, a simple cotton-tipped applicator or even a large paper clip can also be used.

Scleral depression helps in four ways to detect small breaks. First, it increases the contrast between the intact retina and the break. The indented choroid/retinal pigment epithelium (RPE) is darker than the unindented choroid/RPE and darker still than the intact retina, enabling the examiner to locate the break, which appears as a dark spot. Second, the decreased retinal translucency that results from scleral depression may increase

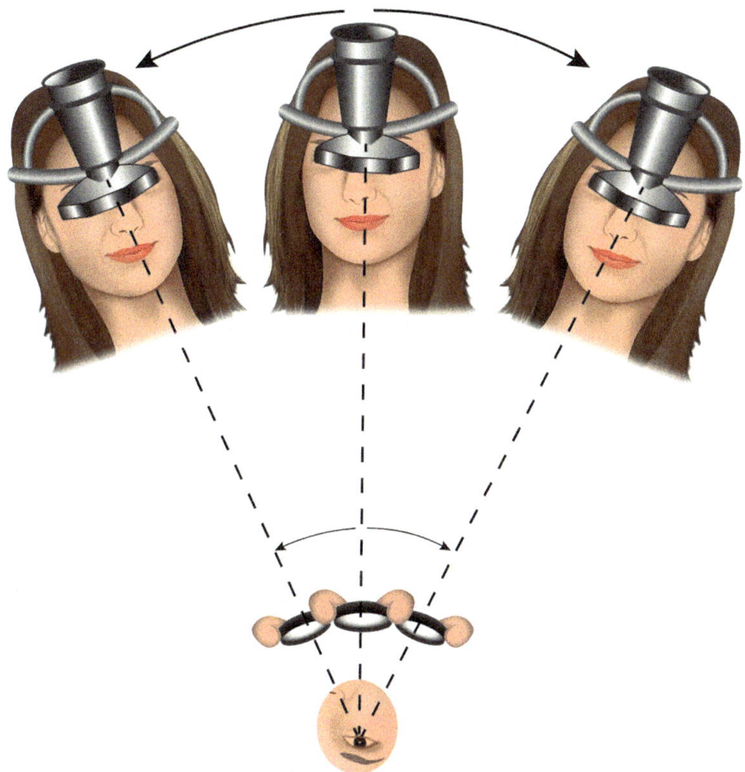

Fig. 3.12 Scanning technique for examining the retina: The examiner keeps her eyes and lens aligned while viewing the retina.

the contrast between the hole and the retina, allowing the hole to be seen. The retina appears less translucent because it is seen at a more acute angle. Moreover, the increased angle may aid the examiner to see the posterior edge of a break. Third, the flaps of tiny breaks at the posterior vitreous base can sometimes be seen as the sclera is indented. In all cases, dynamic movement of the scleral depressor maximizes the chances of finding a small break. Fourth, and finally, in patients with small pupils, depression can bring the peripheral retina into view.

There are very few contraindications to scleral depression. It should be avoided only in patients who have undergone recent intraocular surgery or who have had trauma with hyphema. Scleral depression may cause pain. It raises the intraocular pressure and is therefore especially painful in eyes with a high initial pressure. Glaucoma patients must be examined very carefully and gently, particularly if they have had glaucoma filtration surgery. Also, the examination stretches and compresses the eyelids and may thereby cause discomfort, depending on the eyelid anatomy and tissue laxity. To minimize this, scleral depression should be started superiorly because the upper lid is looser and more flexible than the lower.

Special Considerations

- Scleral depression should be avoided with eyes that have undergone recent intraocular surgery or eyes with a traumatic hyphema.

The patient looks down and the examiner places the depressor near the lid margin, following the eyelid up as the patient looks up. Beginners should hold the depressor vertically so that the indentation can be found easily with the indirect ophthalmoscope. The examiner merely follows the shaft of the depressor down into the eye. If the indentation is not seen, one should scan the fundus, moving one's head from side to side. Holding the depressor vertically also simplifies the problem of orienting one's movements in the inverted, upside-down field of the indirect ophthalmoscope (▶ Fig. 3.13). Anterior-posterior movements are easily made. If one wants to examine further posteriorly, one simply moves the depressor toward the optic nerve. However, in doing so it is important to realize that there will be less discomfort if the eye is not in an extreme position of gaze. Circumferential movements are more difficult, but they become automatic with practice. The beginner simply has to remember that the depressor should be moved opposite to the direction suggested by the view of the retina. It is essential to maintain alignment of one's head, depressor, handheld lens, and the patient's eye, with the eye acting as the fulcrum.

If the superior ora serrata is to be viewed, the patient should look as far superiorly as possible (▶ Fig. 3.14). Beginners will see the ora serrata most easily in highly myopic eyes. If areas of the superior retina posterior to the equator are to be examined, the patient must look slightly inferiorly (▶ Fig. 3.15).

Scleral depression is most difficult at the 9 o'clock and 3 o'clock positions because the eyelid is shorter here and because the canthal ligaments resist the posterior movement of the

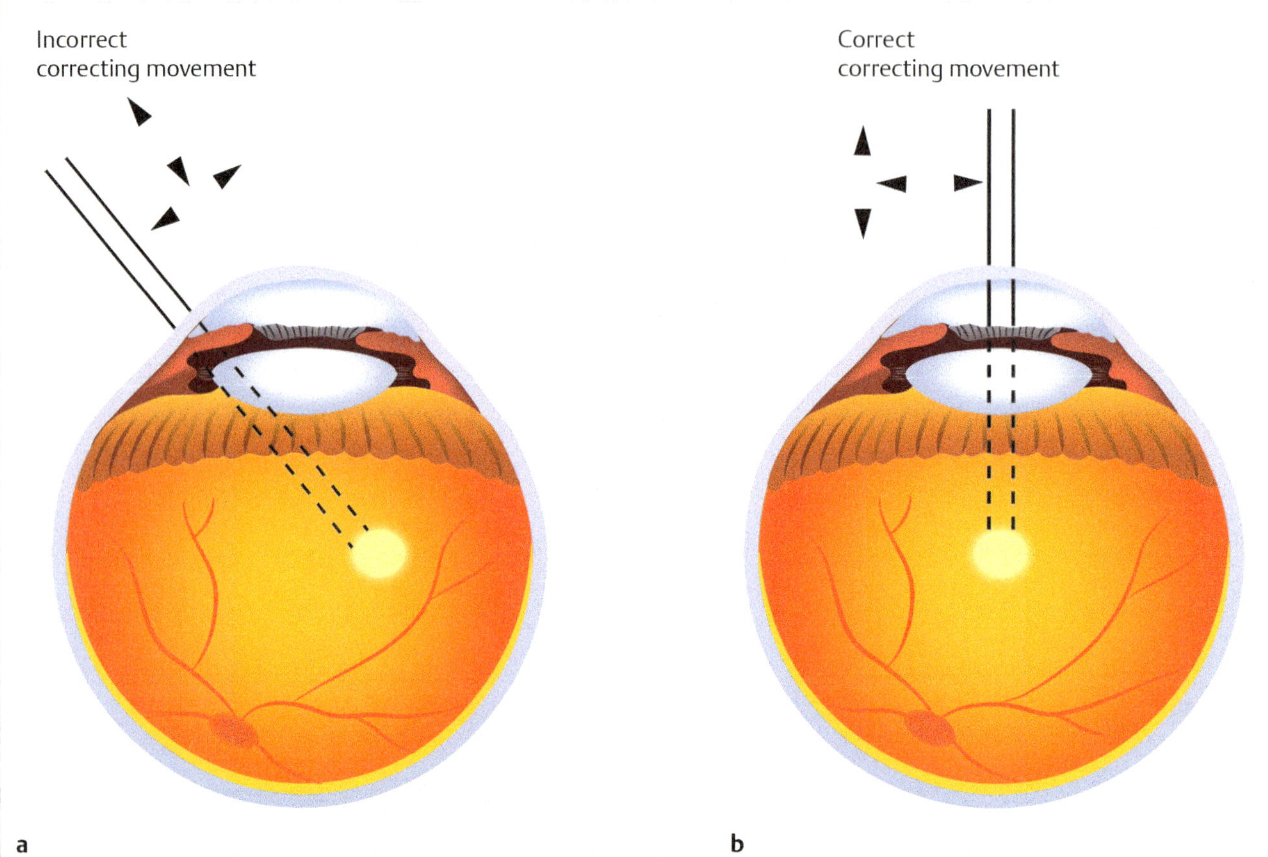

Fig. 3.13 **(a)** Incorrect technique for scleral depression: It is difficult to make diagonal correcting movements because of the upside down and backward image of the indirect ophthalmoscope. **(b)** Correct technique for scleral depression. The depressor is held vertically so that horizontal and vertical correcting movements can be made easily.

depressor. Direct scleral depression at the canthus is painful. Moreover, the depressor may slip off the eyelid and strike the patient's eye. The following techniques help to avoid these problems. First, the depressor is placed on the superior eyelid, above the horizontal axis. It is then rotated downward toward the canthus, carrying the eyelid down with it. The lid becomes more slack when the patient- head rolled away from the examiner- is not looking into an extreme position of gaze.[8] Second, a cotton-tipped applicator- being blunter and softer than a metal depressor- may be better tolerated. Finally, if the above techniques have been unsuccessful, the examiner can easily depress directly on the conjunctiva after topical anesthesia has been administered.

Pearls

- Scleral depression over the canthal areas can be both difficult to perform and painful for the patient. It is often easier to perform depression in the horizontal meridians by directly depressing the globe after placing a drop of topical anesthesia.

3.1.2 Goldmann's Three-Mirror Lens

The Goldmann's three-mirror lens may be used to view the peripheral retina when high magnification is required. The main uses are in patients with retinal detachment in whom it is difficult to find breaks with indirect ophthalmoscopy and in patients in whom it is difficult to determine whether a retinal break is of full or partial thickness. Although nearly all breaks can be found with indirect ophthalmoscopy and scleral depression, in some cases, tiny breaks may be found with the Goldmann's three-mirror lens. The lens can also be used to apply peripheral laser photocoagulation spots, such as to treat a retinal tear. However, it has not been used as often for this purpose since the advent of the laser indirect ophthalmoscope system.

3.1.3 Wide-Field Contact Lenses

The main use of wide-field contact lenses is for performing panretinal photocoagulation and other midperipheral laser treatments. However, they can also be very useful diagnostically, as in eyes with retinal detachment that have undergone cataract extraction with implantation of a posterior chamber

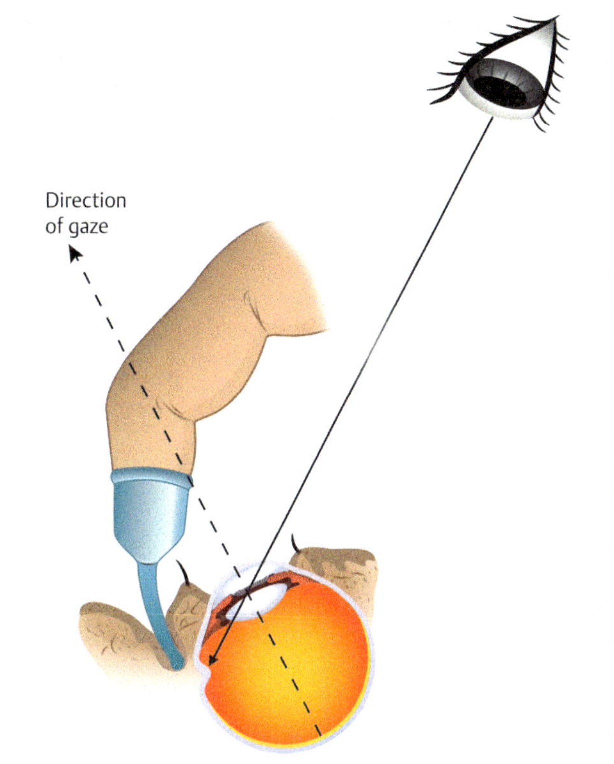

Fig. 3.14 The ora serrata can be seen best when the patient looks as far superiorly as possible.

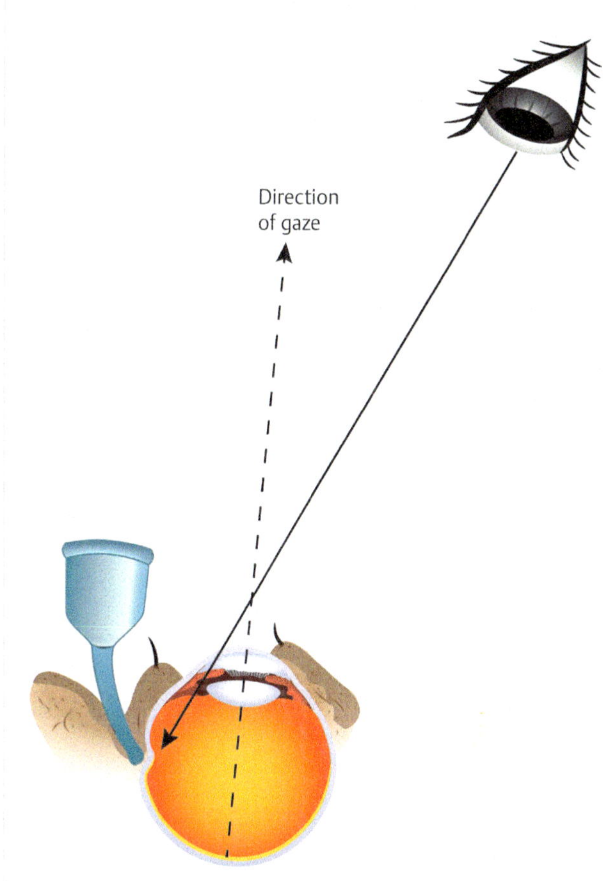

Fig. 3.15 To view the midperiphery, the examiner should have the patient look slightly inferiorly.

lens. In these eyes, opacification of the posterior capsule or shrinkage of the remaining anterior capsule may make visualization of the peripheral retina very difficult with indirect ophthalmoscopy. If yttrium-argon-garnet laser capsulotomy fails to help with visualization, the various wide-field contact lenses may be tried next. To see the retina anterior to the equator well with these lenses, there usually needs to be some combination of ocular rotation, lens tilting, and scleral depression.[9,10]

3.2 Macular Examination

The wide field of view of the indirect ophthalmoscope frequently also allows one to make the diagnosis of various macular conditions. After the peripheral retina has been examined, the patient then looks towards the light source for the examiner to view the posterior pole. With a normal macula, one should see the foveal depression and the central light reflex (▶ Fig. 3.16). Often, there is a diffuse superficial sheen as well. Sometimes, one can see large choroidal vessels. When the normal macular appearance is not present, the examiner should suspect macular pathology and examine the area with a macular lens of some type (see later). Some conditions, such as arterial occlusion, commotio retinae, and venous occlusion, are more easily diagnosed with indirect ophthalmoscopy than with macular lenses, as the wide field of view may allow one to appreciate more easily the "forest" instead of just the trees. Other conditions often can be easily diagnosed as well. For example, a focal serous elevation of the retina, as in central serous chorioretinopathy, can be diagnosed by observing the color contrast between the area of serous elevation and the normal retina (▶ Fig. 3.17). Diabetic macular edema can be suspected when the macula has a pale appearance and the foveal depression and light reflex are absent (▶ Fig. 3.18).

In most cases, however, higher magnification is needed to study the details of macular and optic nerve abnormalities. Therefore, various "macular" lenses are used in conjunction with slit-lamp biomicroscopy to permit accurate diagnosis and management of problems such as clinically significant diabetic macular edema and choroidal neovascularization. They are also essential for macular laser photocoagulation treatment. There are advantages and disadvantages to all of the various macular lenses. Just as a condensing lens is necessary for indirect ophthalmoscopy, lenses are needed to view the macula with the slit lamp.[11,12]

3.2.1 Hruby Lens

The Hruby lens is a 55-diopter plano concave noncontact lens mounted on the slit-lamp biomicroscope. Although it provides an upright image and contact with the cornea is not required, a disadvantage is that it requires a widely dilated pupil and has a very narrow field of view. Its use has been supplanted by handheld aspheric lenses.

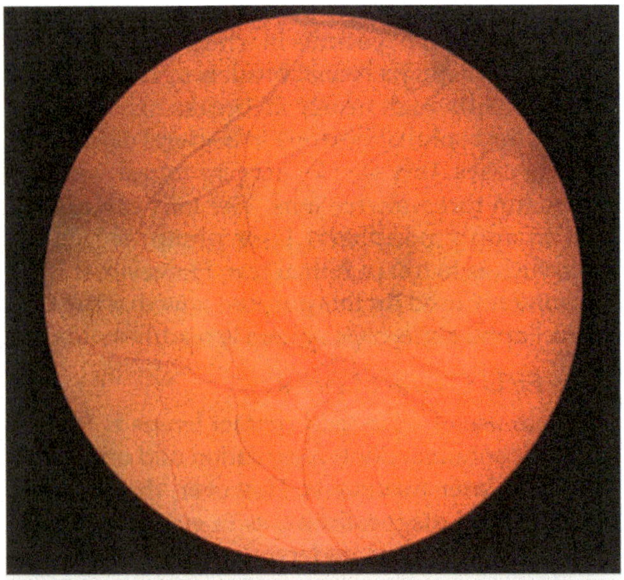

Fig. 3.16 Normal macula: There is a diffuse sheen to the area between the arcades. The foveal depression is easily seen. There is a foveal light reflex.

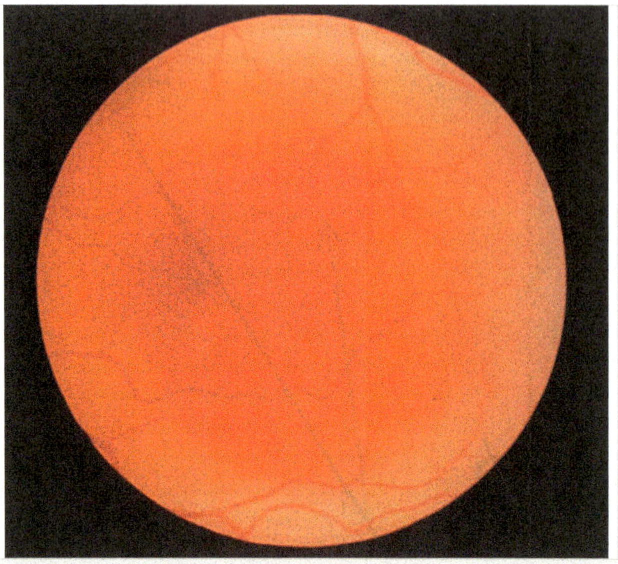

Fig. 3.17 Idiopathic central serous chorioretinopathy: Even without stereopsis, the diagnosis can be made because the area of subretinal fluid can be identified by the color change in the fundus, and the foveal depression and light reflex are lost.

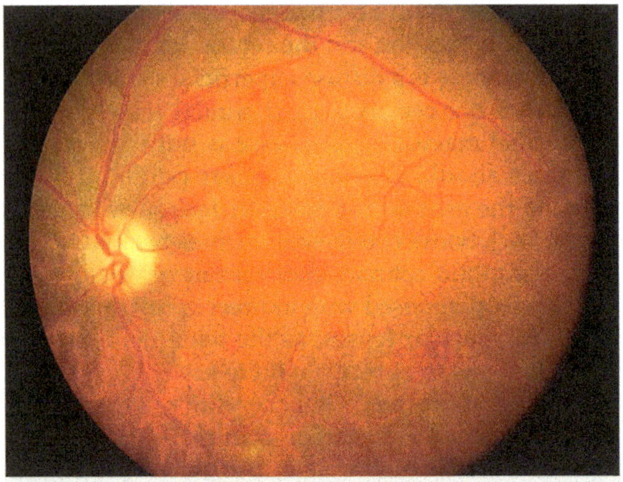

Fig. 3.18 Background diabetic retinopathy with macular edema: Macular edema can be suspected because of loss of the normal choroidal background pattern and absence of the foveal depression and light reflex.

3.2.2 Goldmann's Fundus Contact Lens

The Goldmann's fundus contact lens is a 64-diopter plano concave lens that provides a virtual, upright image. Although one is nearly always able to detect diabetic macular edema or subretinal fluid from various causes with a hand-held lens, the Goldmann's posterior pole contact lens provides the best view of the macula. For this reason it was often utilized in the past, when laser photocoagulation was the mainstay of treatment for choroidal neovascular membranes. Not to be confused, the Goldmann's three-mirror contact lens is a different lens that has a clear central portion for viewing the posterior pole, but additionally incorporates three internal mirrors to permit viewing of the patient's midperipheral retina, peripheral retina, and iridocorneal angle as well.

3.2.3 Mainster Posterior Pole Lens

The Mainster posterior pole lens (standard) is a contact lens based on principles similar to those of indirect ophthalmoscopy. It yields a high-resolution view of the macula similar to that provided by hand-held aspheric lenses, but has the disadvantage of requiring contact with the cornea. It is still commonly used for focal and grid macular laser photocoagulation.

3.2.4 Hand-Held Lens

Hand-held aspheric lenses are high-powered, biconvex condensing lenses used with slit-lamp biomicroscopy. They project a real, inverted image of the posterior pole with unparalleled convenience and ease of use. The 90-diopter aspheric lens is ideal for examining eyes with small pupils and for screening the macula in conditions such as exudative macular detachment, idiopathic central serous chorioretinopathy, age-related macular degeneration, and diabetic macular edema. In patients with retinal detachment, it is especially helpful when looking for posterior breaks. When more magnification is required, a 60-diopter lens is available. Intermediate between the two in terms of magnification and field of view is the 78-diopter lens.

References

[1] Havener WH, Gloeckner S. Atlas of Diagnostic Techniques and Treatment of Retinal Detachment. St. Louis, MO: CV Mosby; 1961:2–53

[2] Hovland KR, Elzeneiny IH, Schepens CL. Clinical evaluation of the small-pupil binocular indirect ophthalmoscope. Arch Ophthalmol. 1969; 82(4):466–474

[3] Rosenthal ML, Fradin S. The technique of binocular indirect ophthalmoscopy. Highl Ophthalmol. 1967; 9:179–257

[4] Rubin ML. The optics of indirect ophthalmoscopy. Surv Ophthalmol. 1964; 9:449–464

[5] Schepens CL. A new ophthalmoscope demonstration. Trans Am Acad Ophthalmol Otolaryngol. 1947; 51:298–301

[6] Schepens CL. Progress in detachment surgery. Trans Am Acad Ophthalmol Otolaryngol. 1951; 55:607–615

[7] Kramer SG, Benson WE. Prophylactic therapy of retinal breaks. Surv Ophthalmol. 1977; 22(1):41–47

[8] Curtin VT. Management of retinal detachment. In: Duane TD, ed. Clinical Ophthalmology. Hagerstown, MD: Harper & Row; 1978:2

[9] Lincoff H, Kreissig I. Finding the retinal hole in the pseudophakic eye with detachment. Am J Ophthalmol. 1994; 117(4):442–446

[10] Lincoff H, Gieser R. Finding the retinal hole. Arch Ophthalmol. 1971; 85 (5):565–569

[11] Tate GW, Safir A. The slit lamp: history, principles, and practice. In: Tasman W, Jaeger EA, eds. Duane's Clinical Ophthalmology. Vol. 1. Philadelphia, PA: JB Lippincott; 1996:1–44

[12] Colenbrander A. Principles of ophthalmoscopy. In: Tasman W, Jaeger EA, eds. Duane's Clinical Ophthalmoscopy. Vol. 1. JB Philadelphia, PA: JB Lippincott; 1996:1–21

4 Fundus Angiography

Suqin Yu and Lawrence A. Yannuzzi

The unique optical properties of the eye permit a more detailed noninvasive examination of human vasculature than in any other tissue. As the ocular fundus represents the most easily visualized capillary bed in the human body, examination of its angiographic pattern can yield information not only useful for ophthalmic practice but also of interest in the study of associated systemic pathology. There are two intravenous angiographic dyes- sodium fluorescein and indocyanine green (ICG)- used in fundus angiography. Although these two dyes produce significantly distinct angiographic patterns as a result of their different physical and chemical properties, angiography is performed in a similar fashion and interpretation of the image follows similar schema. They are discussed in a comparative way.

4.1 Brief History

4.1.1 Fluorescein Angiography

Von Baeyer[1] first synthesized sodium fluorescein in 1871 and its use in the diagnosis of corneal conditions followed shortly thereafter. In 1882, Ehrlich[2] demonstrated the intraocular presence of fluorescein dye in a rabbit eye following parenteral administration. In 1960, MacLean and Maumenee[3] reported on the intravenous use of fluorescein in humans. They performed angioscopy at the slit lamp with a cobalt blue filter but did not photograph the results. While useful for diagnosis, this technique did not result in permanent images that could be used for comparison, discussion, or documentation. Simultaneous advances in fundus photography, especially the advent of the electronic flash, permitted Novotny and Alvis[4] to perform the first successful human fluorescein angiogram. In the ensuing 35 years of clinical use, fluorescein angiography has become an essential tool in the diagnosis and management of many retinal disorders.

4.1.2 Indocyanine Green Angiography

Indocyanine Green (ICG) was used for fundus angiography much later than sodium fluorescein. It was originally used in cardiac and liver function tests. It has been used for over 30 years, but its early use in fundus imaging was limited by the low sensitivity of the film-based systems utilized at the time. With the refinement of camera, filters, and techniques, by 1972, Flower and Hochheimer had performed ICG angiograms in humans.[5,6] In 1986, Hayashi et al[7] reported improved image acquisition using infrared digital fundus videoangiography. In the early 1990s, Guyer et al[8] and Yannuzzi et al[9] demonstrated higher quality images using newer high-resolution (1,024 lines) digital systems. At the same time, scanning laser ophthalmoscope (SLO)-based systems also emerged and have since been shown to produce comparable quality ICG angiogram images.[10]

4.2 Properties of the Dye

Differences between the two dyes are shown in ▶ Table 4.1. Sodium fluorescein is a highly water-soluble yellow-red dye with peak absorption in the blue spectrum (490 nm) and emission in the yellow-green spectrum (525 nm) (▶ Fig. 4.1). This difference in excitation and emission spectra permits coupled photographic filters to separate incoming and exiting light. Once injected, the dye is 60 to 80% bound to plasma proteins. Sodium fluorescein does not cross intact retinal endothelial tight junctions (inner blood–retinal barrier) or intact zonula occludens of the retinal pigment epithelium (RPE) (outer blood–retinal barrier). However, the fenestrations of the choroidal capillaries permit free leakage of the dye into the choroidal extracellular space.

ICG is a water-soluble dark-green dye with peak absorption between 790 and 805 nm and emission at 835 nm (see ▶ Fig. 4.1).[11] Its large molecule size, high affinity for serum proteins, and fluorescence in the near-infrared spectrum make it a useful adjunct to sodium fluorescein. Chemically, the ICG molecule has both lipophilic and hydrophilic characteristics. It is approximately 98% protein-bound in the circulation—80% to globulins and 20% to alpha1-lipoprotein and albumin.[12] Therefore, less dye penetrates the fenestrations of the choriocapillaris, allowing enhanced imaging of choroidal vessels. Its near-infrared spectral properties allow greater penetration through retinal pigment epithelial pigmentation, macular xanthophyll, and blood. The combination of less leakage and greater penetration of fluorescence through overlying pigments makes ICG ideal for angiographic examination of the choroid and choroidal-based abnormalities.

Table 4.1 Properties of sodium fluorescein and indocyanine green dyes

	Sodium fluorescein	Indocyanine green
Chemical structure	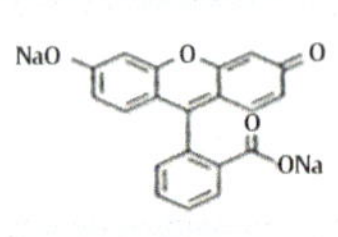	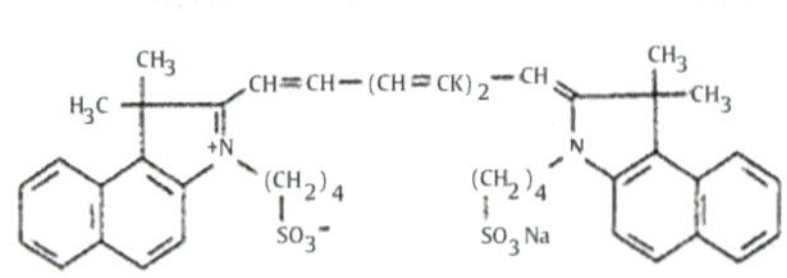
Molecular formula	$C_{20}H_{10}O_5Na_2$	$C_{43}H_{47}N_2O_6S_2Na$
Molecular weight	377 Da	775 Da
Peak absorption	465 nm	790 nm
Peak emission	525 nm	805 nm
Serum protein binding	60–80%	98%

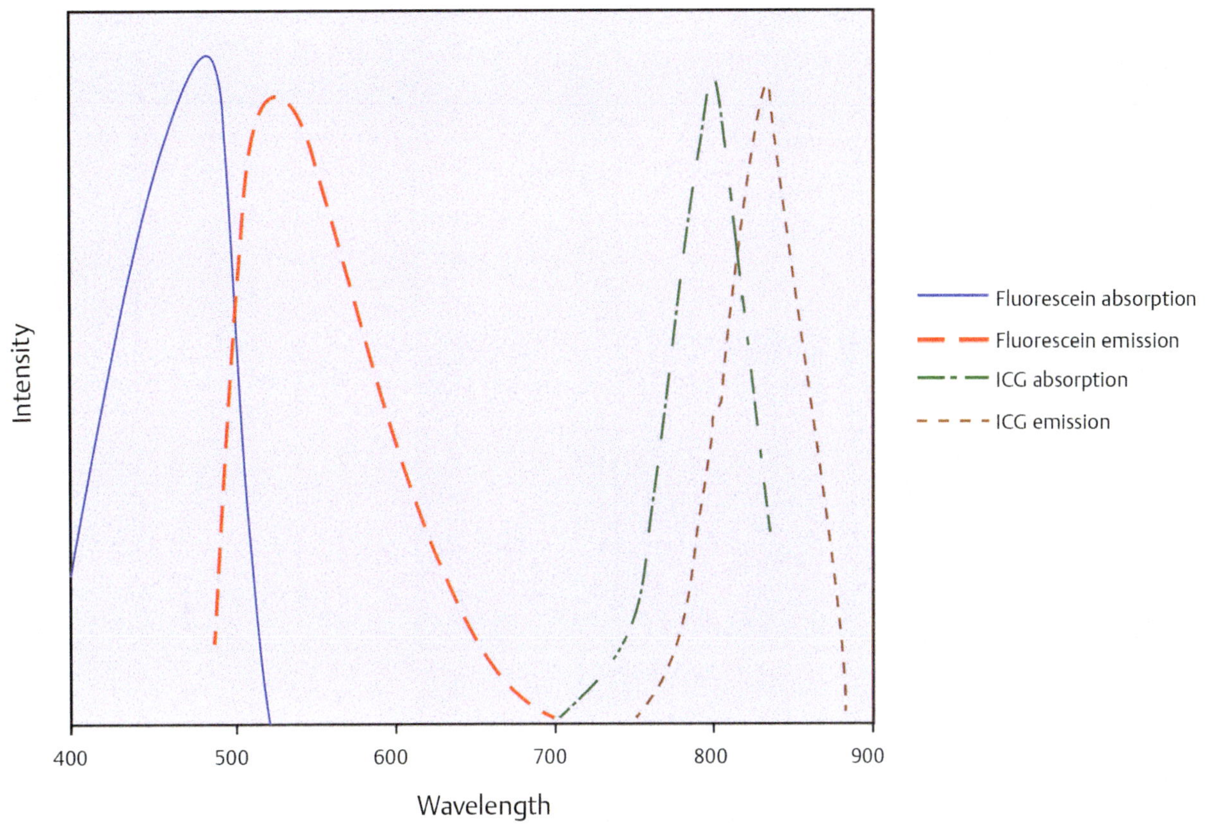

Fig. 4.1 The absorption and emission spectra of fluorescein and indocyanine green (ICG).

4.3 Technique of Angiography

Although different exciter and barrier filter settings are needed for the imaging system due to different peak absorption and emission wavelength between the two dyes, fluorescein angiography and ICG angiography are performed in a similar way.

After informed consent is obtained, color and red-free fundus photographs are usually taken. Since the first few seconds of the angiogram are often clinically useful, the dye is usually injected through a butterfly-type needle with the patient still seated at the fundus camera. After the needle is inserted, blood should be refluxed into the tubing to ensure intravascular injection since extravasation is painful and can lead to tissue necrosis. The antecubital vein is the preferred injection location. Once the dye is injected, the timer is started. Video or photographs are taken rapidly for the first several seconds and then at approximately 1-minute intervals for several more minutes to cover the complete filling of both the choroidal and retinal vascular systems. The entire photographic process- extending from 5 to 10 minutes- is usually enough for fluorescein angiography. However, ICG angiography usually needs up to 30 minutes. Middle phase photographs are taken between 8 and 12 minutes after injection and then the final photographs are taken approximately 20 to 30 minutes from the time of injection. Some examiners inject a small amount of dye during the late phases to better visualize the retinal and choroidal vessels.[13]

During fluorescein angiography, administration of sodium fluorescein is performed in a bolus fashion using either 2 to 3 mL of 25% solution or 5 mL of 10% solution. The dye is circulated and eliminated rapidly, primarily by the kidneys. Patients should be warned of transient changes in skin and urine color. During the period of skin discoloration, patients may have increased photosensitivity; thus, lightly pigmented patients should be urged to avoid excessive sun exposure for 24 to 36 hours. During ICG angiography, a 25-mg bolus of the ICG dye is injected. Since the dye is excreted by the liver,[14] there will be no urine color change afterwards.

Special Considerations

- The transient skin discoloration that occurs after intravenous injection of sodium fluorescein dye may make some patients more photosensitive. Lightly pigmented patients should be advised to avoid excessive sun exposure for 24 to 36 hours after fluorescein angiography.

4.4 Adverse Reactions to the Dyes

The incidences of adverse reaction to the two dyes are shown in ▸ Table 4.2. Although generally safe overall, angiography has a small but significant rate of adverse reactions. These reactions can be mild, medium, or severe, and can even cause death.[15] Mild reactions, such as pruritus, nausea, and vomiting, are described as transient reactions and not requiring treatment. Manifestations of more serious reactions are urticaria, syncope, pyrexia, and local tissue necrosis. Often, oral or intramuscular diphenhydramine is useful in relieving these symptoms. Severe

Table 4.2 The incidences of adverse reaction to the dye

Adverse reactions	Sodium fluorescein	Indocyanine green
Mild	1–10%	0.15%
Moderate	1.6%	0.2%
Severe	0.05%	0.05%
Death	1:222,000	1:333,333

Table 4.3 Main differences between the two normal angiograms

	Fluorescein angiogram	Indocyanine green angiogram
Optic disc	Bright	Dark
Macula	Dark	Isofluorescence
Retinal small vessels	Clear delineation	Unapparent
Choroid vessels	Unapparent	Clear delineation

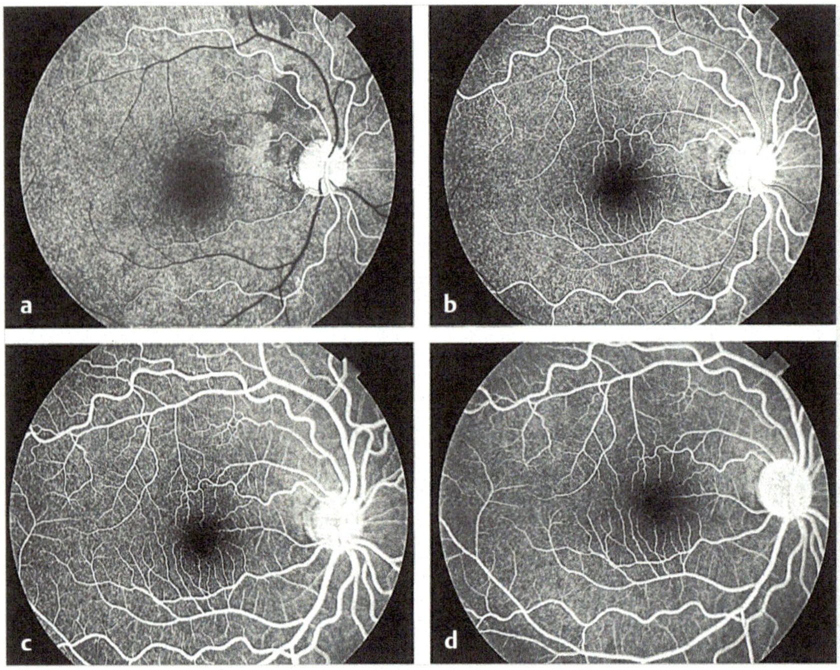

Fig. 4.2 Standard fluorescein angiogram phases: (**a**) arterial phase, (**b**) laminar venous filling phase, (**c**) full venous phase, and (**d**) recirculation phase.

reactions may involve cardiac, pulmonary, or nervous system. These reactions, such as anaphylaxis, seizures, shock, and myocardial infarction, require intensive medical intervention. For this reason, emergency resuscitative equipment should be available. Extravasation of dye can cause local tissue irritation and tenderness, but no significant permanent tissue damage is likely. The results of laboratory tests performed after fluorescein angiography may be erroneous because of interference by intravenous fluorescein.[16] The adverse reaction rate (including the death rate) to ICG is lower than that to sodium fluorescein. In general, ICG is better tolerated than sodium fluorescein. Since the preparation contains sodium iodide, the use of ICG is contraindicated in patients with iodine or shellfish sensitivities. It is also contraindicated in patients with significant liver or renal disease, as the adverse reactions have been observed to be more common and severe in these individuals. Although no reports of adverse effects during pregnancy have been reported,[17,18] until further safety studies are undertaken, use in pregnant women should be avoided unless absolutely critical for diagnosis or management.

4.5 Interpretation of Fundus Angiography

The interpretation of the two types of angiograms follows a similar schema. The schema follows a logical progression beginning with the initial determination of abnormal *hypo*fluorescence or *hyper*fluorescence on the angiogram. Using a similar medical algorithm, utilizing successive single decisions may lead to the solution of the problem and correct diagnosis. Since the ICG molecule has a higher protein-bound rate, and penetrates the fenestrations of choriocapillaris less than fluorescein, the ICG angiogram enhances the image of choroidal vessels and the optic nerve is always dark during the ICG angiogram due to lack of choroidal vessels. On the other hand, the dark area of the macula seen in fluorescein angiograms cannot be seen in ICG angiograms because the near-infrared spectral properties of the latter allow greater penetration through RPE pigmentation and macular xanthophyll. The main differences between the two normal angiograms are summarized in ▶ Table 4.3.

4.5.1 Normal Fundus Angiogram

Fluorescein Angiogram

Fluorescein angiograms are typically divided into prefilling, transit, recirculation, and late phases. The transit phase is subdivided into arterial, laminar venous, and full venous filling phases (▶ Fig. 4.2). As discussed previously, prior to injection, several color and red-free photographs are taken. These are useful for identifying landmarks and correlating areas of clinically evident pathology with their angiographic features.

Table 4.4 Fluorescein angiogram transit times (seconds)

	Normal range	Abnormal
Arm to choroid	10 to 15	> 30
Complete choroidal filling[a]	3 to 5	> 5
Arteriovenous transit[b]	8 to 12	> 15

[a]Initial appearance of dye in the choroid to uniform choroidal fluorescence.

[b]Initial appearance of dye in the retinal arteries to complete venous filling.

After the excitation and emission filters are inserted, photographs are taken to help identify areas of pseudofluorescence and autofluorescence. *Pseudofluorescence* results from mismatching of these photographic filters and is rarely encountered nowadays with improvements in angiography equipment. *Autofluorescence* results from tissues that behave similarly to fluorescein in that they emit light in the yellow-green spectrum when illuminated by blue light even in the absence of the dye.[19] These include optic nerve head drusen, flecks associated with fundus flavimaculatus, astrocytic hamartomas, deposits of lipofuscin, and Best's vitelliform lesions.[20] Autofluorescence of the lens has been related to metabolic control in diabetics.[21]

Pearls

- Abnormal fundus findings which may show hyper-autofluoresce include optic nerve head drusen, flecks associated with fundus flavimaculatus, astrocytic hamartomas, deposits of lipofuscin, and Best's vitelliform lesions.

After the fluorescein dye is injected into the antecubital vein, it is first visualized in the choroid and optic nerve head within 10 to 15 seconds (▶ Table 4.4). The time interval between injection and the choroidal flush depends on the speed of injection, the patient's age, and the patient's systemic circulatory status and is, therefore, highly variable. Delayed filling can be an indicator of circulatory or carotid disease. The choroid fluoresces in a patchy and mottled fashion due to sequential filling of choroidal lobules and variable blockage by the RPE, respectively (▶ Fig. 4.2a). This fluorescence is first noted in the posterior pole and spreads quickly anteriorly to the ora serrata. A uniform choroidal "flush" is normally seen within 3 to 5 seconds of the first appearance of dye in the choroid. The cilioretinal artery, present in approximately 32% of individuals, fills at the same time as the choroid.[22]

Special Considerations

- The time interval between injection and the choroidal flush depends on the speed of injection, the patient's age, and the patient's cardiovascular circulatory status, and can be highly variable.

Within 1 to 3 seconds after the onset of choroidal filling, the central retinal artery fills and the dye spreads to the precapillary arterioles, the capillaries, and the postcapillary venules in the early arteriovenous phase. The retinal veins then begin to fill and, at first, demonstrate laminar filling as the dye is concentrated toward the vessel walls by the faster flow of blood and concentration of erythrocytes in the central lumen (▶ Fig. 4.2b). The normal arteriovenous transit time, defined as the period from the first appearance of dye in the retinal arteries to complete filling of the retinal veins, is 8 to 12 seconds (▶ Table 4.4). The juxtafoveal capillaries fluoresce maximally during the arteriovenous transit phase. They stand out strongly against the relatively dark background of the heavily pigmented macula (▶ Fig. 4.2c).

The recirculation phase begins at about 30 seconds after the dye is injected and lasts about 2.5 minutes (▶ Fig. 4.2d). Leakage and staining of various retinal and choroidal abnormalities are usually first observed during the recirculation phase. The kidneys remove the majority of fluorescein during the first pass, so the fluorescence of the recirculation phase is considerably less intense than the transit phases. As the study continues, the concentration of extracellular fluorescein in the choroid exceeds the concentration in the choroidal vessels. Combined with staining of the outer choroidal layers and inner sclera, this produces a relatively bright background against which the choroidal vessels devoid of dye are silhouetted. This silhouetting is especially apparent in lightly pigmented fundi or in disease states that result in loss of the RPE, such as retinitis pigmentosa (▶ Fig. 4.3). By 30 minutes, essentially all fluorescein has been eliminated from the ocular circulation.

Indocyanine Green Angiogram

As with fluorescein angiography, the ICG angiogram is divided into three phases (▶ Fig. 4.4). The first or "early" phase demonstrates maximal fluorescence of both the retinal and choroidal vasculature and, unlike fluorescein angiography, there is clear delineation of medium and large choroidal vessels. However, the small retinal vessels are not demonstrated clearly. As the study progresses into the "middle" phase after about 6 minutes, the choroidal fluorescence begins to fade and any abnormalities that retain the dye and show up as relative hyperfluorescence can usually first be observed at this stage. Approximately 20 minutes into the study, during the "late" phase, the choriocapillaris is uniformly (but very mildly) fluorescent, the choroidal vessels are hypofluorescent, the retinal vessels are unapparent, and the optic nerve head is dark. During this phase, abnormal hyperfluorescent areas are visualized most easily because they stand out in contrast to the very minimal background fluorescence that remains. The ICG dye does not remain solely within the choroidal intravascular space but extravasates into the choroidal stroma and accumulates within the RPE. During the very late phase, more than 30 minutes after the dye is injected, the RPE–Bruch's membrane complex is uniformly brightly fluorescent, and abnormal hypofluorescent lesions are visualized most easily at this time.[23]

4.5.2 Abnormal Fundus Angiograms

The analysis of fundus angiograms is facilitated greatly by determining whether given abnormalities demonstrate relative hypofluorescence or hyperfluorescence.[24,25,26] By definition, hypofluorescent areas are those that display less than

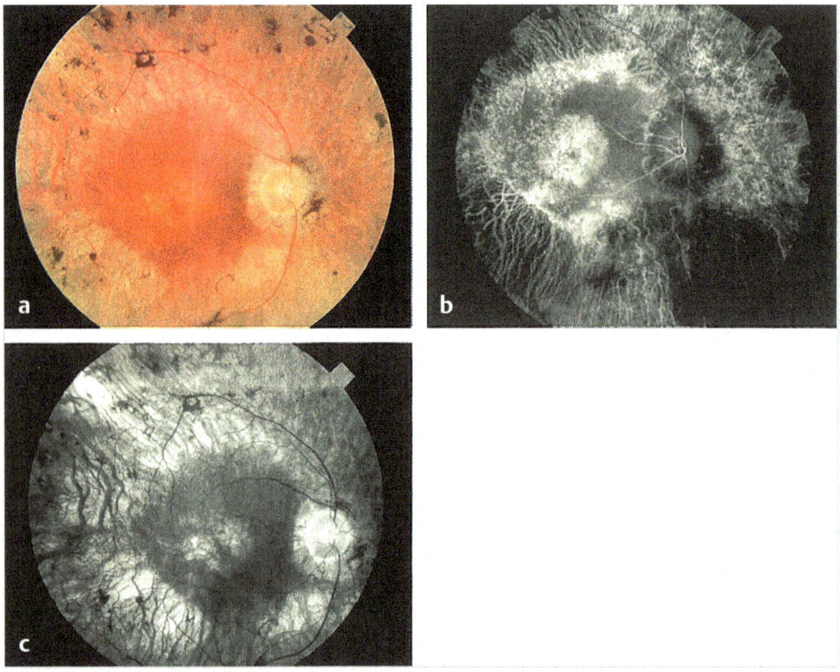

Fig. 4.3 (**a**) An eye with retinitis pigmentosa and characteristic peripheral retinal pigment epithelial loss along with some pigmentary disruption in the central macular area. (**b**) Relatively early in the fluorescein angiogram, the larger choroidal vessels in the periphery are easily seen. (**c**) In the late stages of the angiogram, the choroidal vessels appear as hypofluorescent channels against the background hyperfluorescence, which is the result of residual dye in the extravascular choroid and some scleral staining.

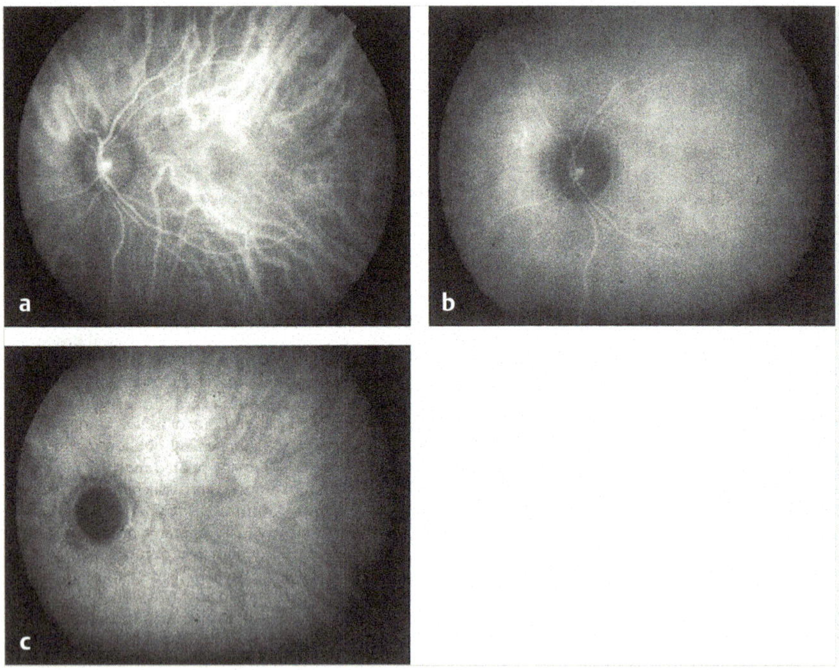

Fig. 4.4 (**a**) Early, (**b**) mid, and (**c**) late phases of indocyanine green (ICG) angiogram (*normal eye*). Note the good choroidal vascular detail in the early phase.

anticipated normal fluorescence, while hyperfluorescent areas are those that have increased fluorescence or fluorescence where it is normally absent. It is worth noting that the same lesion may demonstrate disparity between fundus camera and SLO angiography.[27] For example, serous pigment epithelial detachment appears bright throughout the fundus camera but dark throughout the SLO angiography due to SLO's suppressing scattered light.

Hypofluorescence

The causes of hypofluorescence can be divided into blockage and vascular filling defects. Blockage occurs when an overlying relatively opaque substance masks underlying fluorescence (▶ Fig. 4.5). Blood, inflammatory cells, melanin, lipofuscin, fibrin, and media opacities are frequent causes of hypofluorescence. The blockage effect in an ICG angiogram is not as obvious as in a fluorescein angiogram since ICG dye has greater penetration through these opaque substances. However, hypofluorescence due to blockage can become apparent in late-phase ICG images, in which the RPE–Bruch's membrane complex is uniformly brightly fluorescent. In addition to identifying the blocking substance, determining its anatomic location is crucial to proper fluorescein angiogram interpretation. The location of the large retinal vessels and precapillary arterioles in the nerve fiber layer and the capillaries and postcapillary venules in the

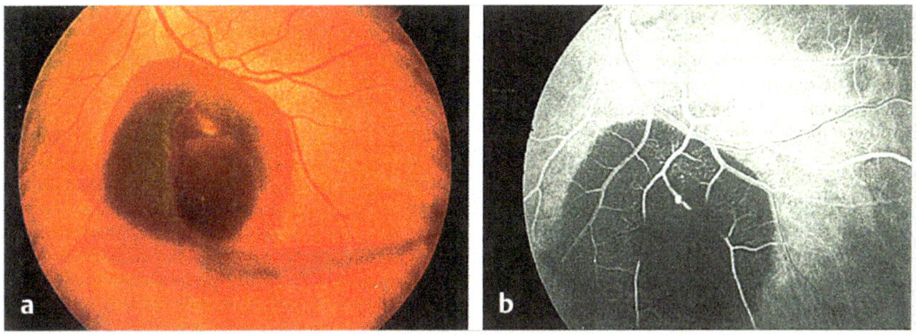

Fig. 4.5 (a) Fundus and (b) corresponding arteriovenous phase fluorescein angiogram photographs of a retinal arterial macroaneurysm with preretinal, intraretinal, and subretinal hemorrhage.

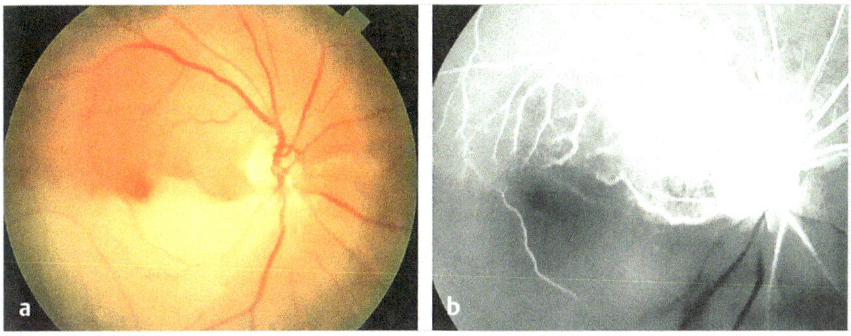

Fig. 4.6 (**a**) Acute hemiretinal branch artery obstruction with characteristic retinal whitening in the inferior retina and (**b**) hypofluorescence on the fluorescein angiogram of both the retina and retinal vessels of the affected area.

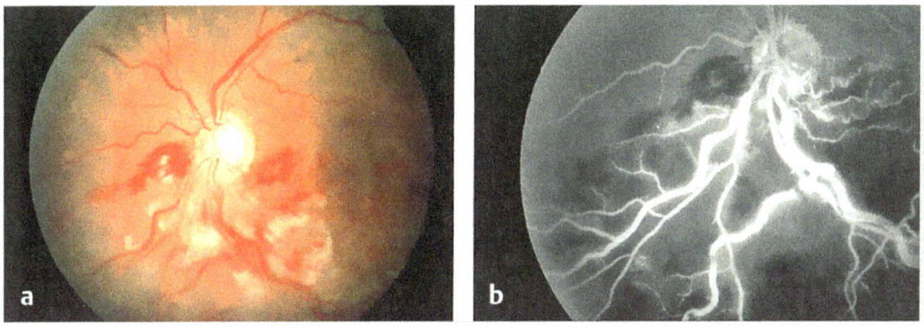

Fig. 4.7 (**a**) Inferior, ischemic branch retinal vein obstruction with intraretinal hemorrhages and cotton-wool spots in the affected area. (**b**) The corresponding fluorescein angiogram shows both blocked fluorescence (*absolute hypofluorescence*) from the patches of hemorrhage and confluent capillary nonperfusion (*relative hypofluorescence*) elsewhere inferiorly.

inner nuclear layer can help determine the depth of a lesion. For example, a flame-shaped hemorrhage, which is located in the nerve fiber layer, will block all retinal vasculature, while a deeper dot or blot hemorrhage will block capillary fluorescence but not the fluorescence of the larger retinal vessels.

Blockage of deeper choroidal fluorescence can occur not only with any of the above retinal lesions but also by subretinal substances. Common examples of this include subretinal blood, lipofuscin deposits of fundus flavimaculatus and Best's disease, hyperpigmentation associated with chorioretinal scars, and congenital hypertrophy of the RPE.

Vascular filling defects can occur at any level of the retinal or choroidal circulation. Retinal vascular occlusion will produce hypofluorescence of the retinal vessels and retina distal to the occlusion (▶ Fig. 4.6). Capillary nonperfusion such as that caused by diabetic or radiation retinopathy and retinal vein occlusions will result in relative hypofluorescence of the affected area compared with the adjacent normal capillary fluorescence and, when severe, frank "pruning" of the small vessels can be seen (▶ Fig. 4.7). However, in ICG angiography, because the ICG molecule is much bigger than sodium fluorescein and cannot reach the very small vessels, retinal capillaries are unapparent. In fluorescein angiograms, choroidal vascular filling defects are more subtle because of blockage caused by the variably pigmented RPE. Occlusion of the larger choroidal vessels can cause wedge-shaped defects in choroidal fluorescence. More commonly, choroidal hypoperfusion resulting from causes such as toxemia of pregnancy, lupus choroidopathy, and malignant hypertension will produce more diffuse zones of hypofluorescence.

Hyperfluorescence

It is useful to classify hyperfluorescence into two categories: areas with increased intensity of normally present fluorescence and areas that normally do not fluoresce. The absence of the usual blocking pigment from the RPE is the most common cause of increased intensity of normal fluorescence and is referred to as a "window defect" (▶ Fig. 4.8). This increase in transmitted fluorescence is seen in conditions such as geographic atrophy of macular degeneration, drusen, chorioretinal scars, and full-thickness macular holes.

Just as perfusion defects can cause hypofluorescent areas, excessive perfusion will manifest as abnormal hyperfluorescence. Because there is some degree of leakage occurring, the hyperfluorescence intensifies or expands into the late phases of the fluorescein angiographic study. Leakage can come from new vessels (i.e., not normally present) such as retinal neovascularization of diabetic retinopathy or from preexisting normal vessels that become incompetent such as seen in cystoid

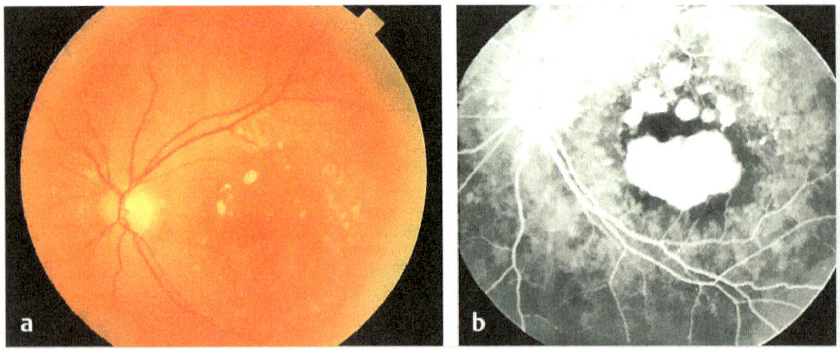

Fig. 4.8 (**a**) Fundus and (**b**) fluorescein angiogram photographs of an eye with dry age-related macular degeneration and multiple soft drusen along with a relatively large patch of geographic atrophy. Note the "window defect" hyperfluorescence with sharp borders corresponding to the areas of atrophy.

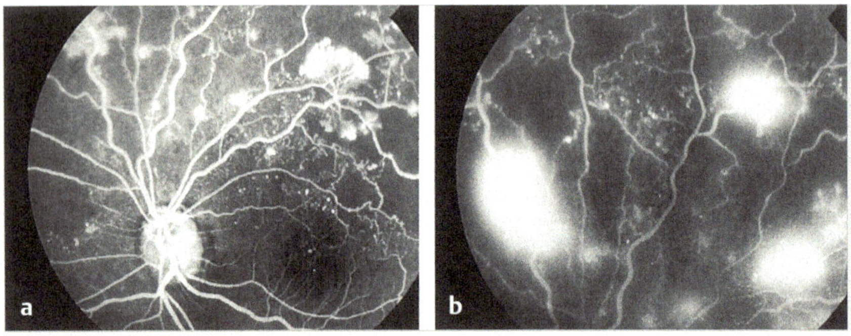

Fig. 4.9 (**a**) Early and (**b**) late-phase fluorescein angiogram photographs of an eye with advanced proliferative diabetic retinopathy. There is extensive peripheral capillary nonperfusion and multiple fronds of retinal neovascularization that show as bright, leaking hyperfluorescent foci.

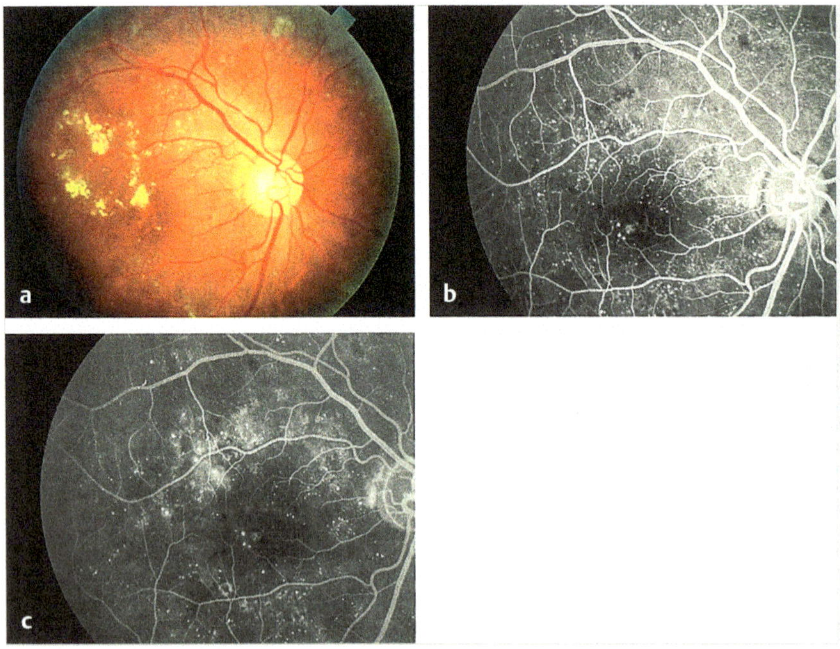

Fig. 4.10 Background diabetic retinopathy with macular edema. (**a**) The fundus photograph shows lipid exudate in the macula along with scattered dot and blot hemorrhages. The corresponding (**b**) early and (**c**) late-phase fluorescein shows multiple leaking microaneurysms, most of which are clustered in the region of lipid exudate.

macular edema. Retinal neovascularization can be identified angiographically by intense late leakage of dye emanating from the surface of the retina (▶ Fig. 4.9). Choroidal neovascularization (CNV), seen in conditions such as ocular histoplasmosis or age-related macular degeneration, will show varying degrees of hyperfluorescence and leakage from under the retina. Unlike fluorescein angiography, since less ICG dye can penetrate abnormal vessels, hyperfluorescence due to leakage is usually not so obvious in ICG angiography.

Leakage of dye from vessels that are normally present can be seen in background diabetic retinopathy or in disease states associated with ocular inflammation or vasculitis. Diabetic macular edema presents angiographically as intraretinal hyperfluorescence from leaking microaneurysms (▶ Fig. 4.10). Postoperative or uveitis-induced cystoid macular edema demonstrates leakage of dye from incompetent perifoveal capillaries; cystoid spaces of the outer plexiform layer form and result in the classic "petaloid" pattern of hyperfluorescence

(▶ Fig. 4.11). Leakage into the subretinal space takes on various patterns depending on the source of fluid. Both neurosensory and pigment epithelial detachments will result in extravasated dye pooling subretinally. The character and speed of such pooling can offer clues as to the exact anatomic location and etiology. For example, central serous chorioretinopathy, which represents mainly a neurosensory detachment, will result in slow accumulation of dye as it passes through small defects in the RPE (▶ Fig. 4.12). The pigment epithelial detachments of macular degeneration, on the other hand, display much more rapid pooling, as there is no effective barrier to the highly permeable choriocapillaris (▶ Fig. 4.13).

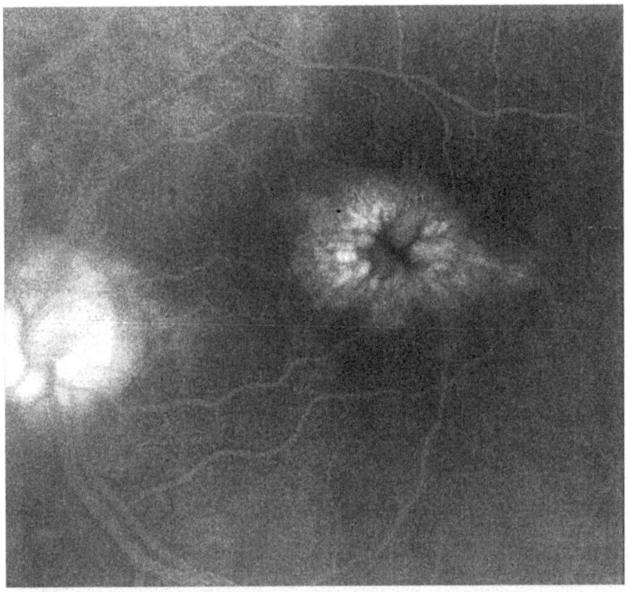

Fig. 4.11 Late-phase fluorescein angiogram photograph of postoperative cystoid macular edema with the classic petaloid pattern of dye leakage from the perifoveal capillaries.

Fluorescein dye can also stain both healthy and abnormal ocular tissues and result in hyperfluorescent areas. Disciform scars, regressed neovascular complexes, and damaged Bruch's membrane may display late staining. The normal staining of the sclera can also present as hyperfluorescence if the overlying RPE is attenuated such as in highly myopic eyes, lightly pigmented fundi, or eyes affected by diseases such as serpiginous chorioretinopathy or gyrate atrophy.

As discussed earlier, the physical-chemical properties of ICG make it an ideal substance for studying choroidal pathology, especially vascular-based abnormalities. Several investigators have demonstrated the superiority of ICG in the diagnosis and management of CNV in age-related macular degeneration. Studies by Yannuzzi et al[9] and Regillo et al[28] found that ICG angiography was able to show more clearly CNV in many cases where fluorescein angiography showed "occult" or ill-defined CNV. Up to 87% of cases of exudative macular degeneration do not have well-defined CNV on fluorescein angiography. However, on ICG angiography, the abnormal vessels of CNV can be identified clearly (▶ Fig. 4.14). Some particular structures including polypoidal choroidal vasculopathy (PCV) and retinal angiomatous proliferation can be recognized as well (▶ Fig. 4.15 and ▶ Fig. 4.16).[29,30]

ICG angiography has been shown to be useful in the diagnosis and management of other choroidal-based diseases. Shields and colleagues[31] have presented an extensive description of ICG angiography patterns of ocular tumors and demonstrated a relatively unique pattern of fluorescence with circumscribed choroidal hemangiomas (▶ Fig. 4.17). Several investigators have

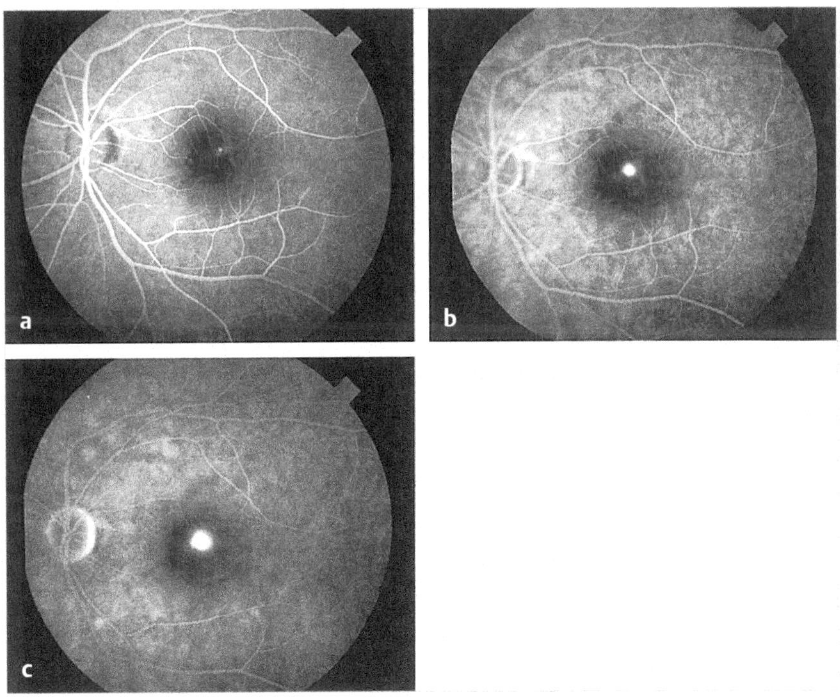

Fig. 4.12 (**a**) Early, (**b**) mid, and (**c**) late fluorescein angiogram phases of an eye with central serous chorioretinopathy and a neurosensory retinal detachment in the macula. The area of detached retina is not evident angiographically. All that is seen is a pinpoint leaking focus of dye emanating from the level of the retinal pigment epithelium.

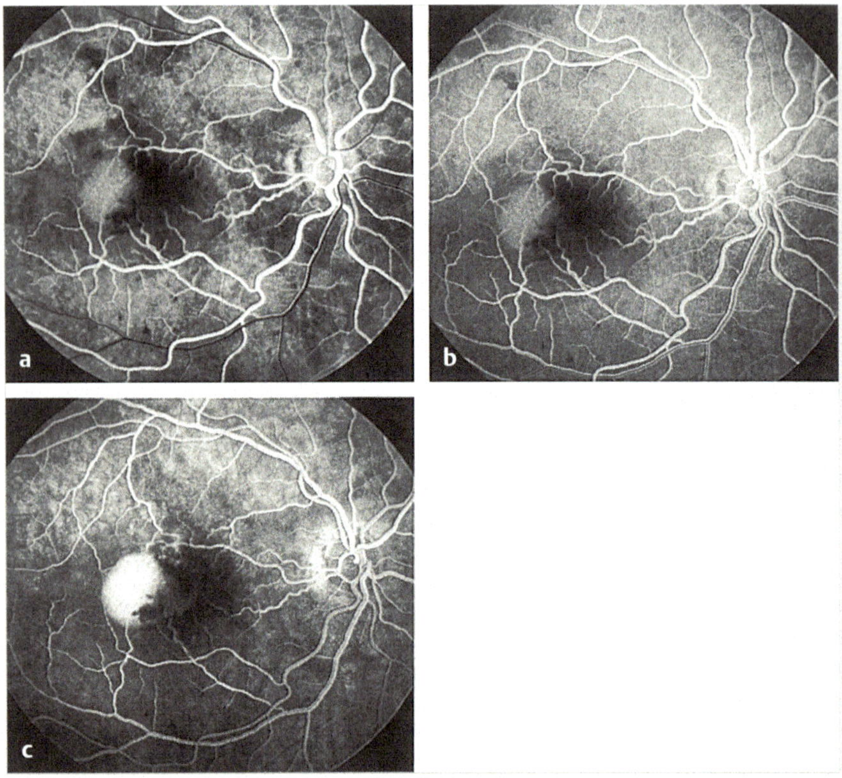

Fig. 4.13 (a) Early, (b) mid, and (c) late fluorescein angiogram phases of an eye with age-related macular degeneration and a serous pigment epithelial detachment (PED). Note the relatively rapid-appearing uniform hyperfluorescence of the entire PED.

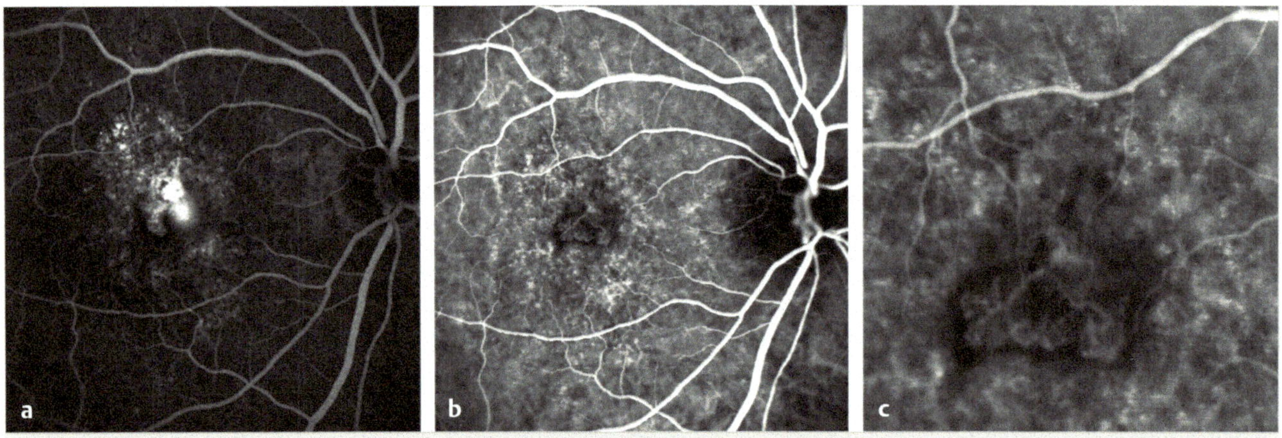

Fig. 4.14 An eye with exudative, age-related macular degeneration. (a) Fluorescein angiogram shows obvious leakage in the macula. (b) The corresponding ICG angiogram shows better delineation of the choroidal neovascularization (CNV). (c) Magnified image reveals more details of CNV.

reported on the ICG angiogram findings of central serous chorioretinopathy[7,32] as well as acute posterior multifocal placoid pigment epitheliopathy,[33] multiple evanescent white dot syndrome,[34] and idiopathic PCV.[35,36] Data from these reports have helped not only to aid in the diagnosis and management of diseases, but also to better understand the pathophysiology of diseases. Details are discussed in the chapters that cover the individual conditions.

4.6 Future of Fundus Angiography

In recent years, more and more noninvasive functional imaging tools have been developed. Laser Doppler flowmetry, scanning laser Doppler flowmetry, and Doppler optical coherence tomography (OCT) have been used to measure large (arteries and veins) retinal vascular blood flow.[37,38,39] OCT angiography with split-spectrum amplitude-decorrelation angiography has also been developed to measure local microcirculation (arterioles, venules, and capillaries).[40] More recently, adaptive optics scanning laser ophthalmoscopy and adaptive optics OCT have been used to image retinal microcirculation as well.[41,42] These new techniques may be useful for the study of ocular physiology and pathophysiology in the future.

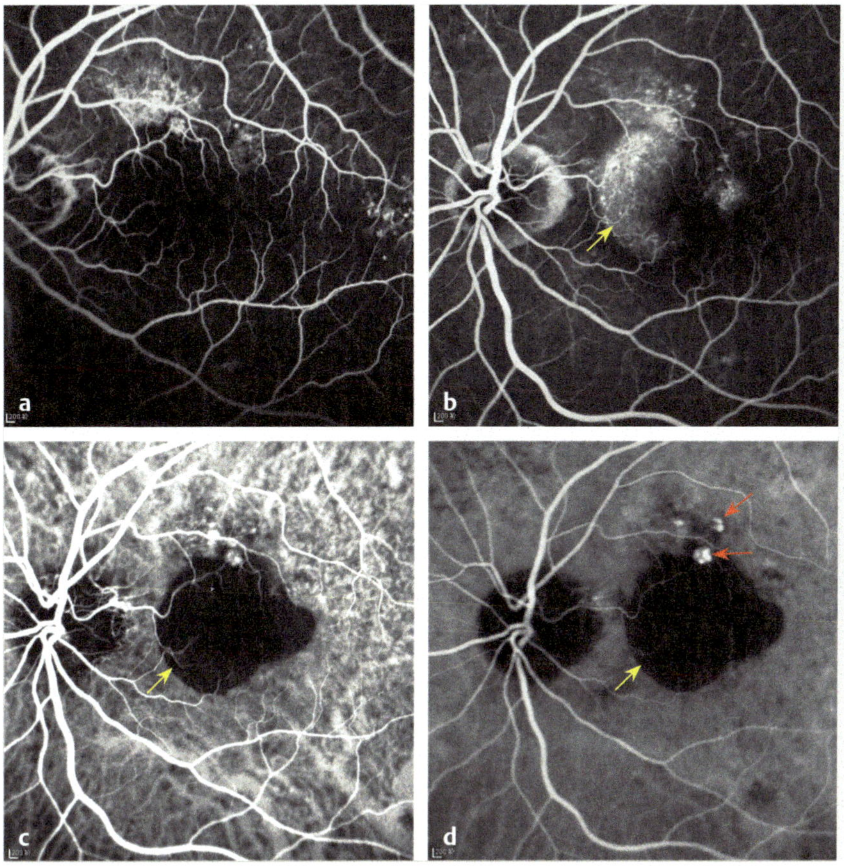

Fig. 4.15 An eye with polypoidal choroidal vasculopathy. (**a**) Early and (**b**) late fluorescein angiogram phases show poorly delineated leakage and late pooling (yellow arrow) in the macula (*occult choroidal neovascularization*). The corresponding (**c**) mid and (**d**) late ICG angiogram phases reveal polys (red arrows) at the edge of hypofluorescent area due to PED (yellow arrow).

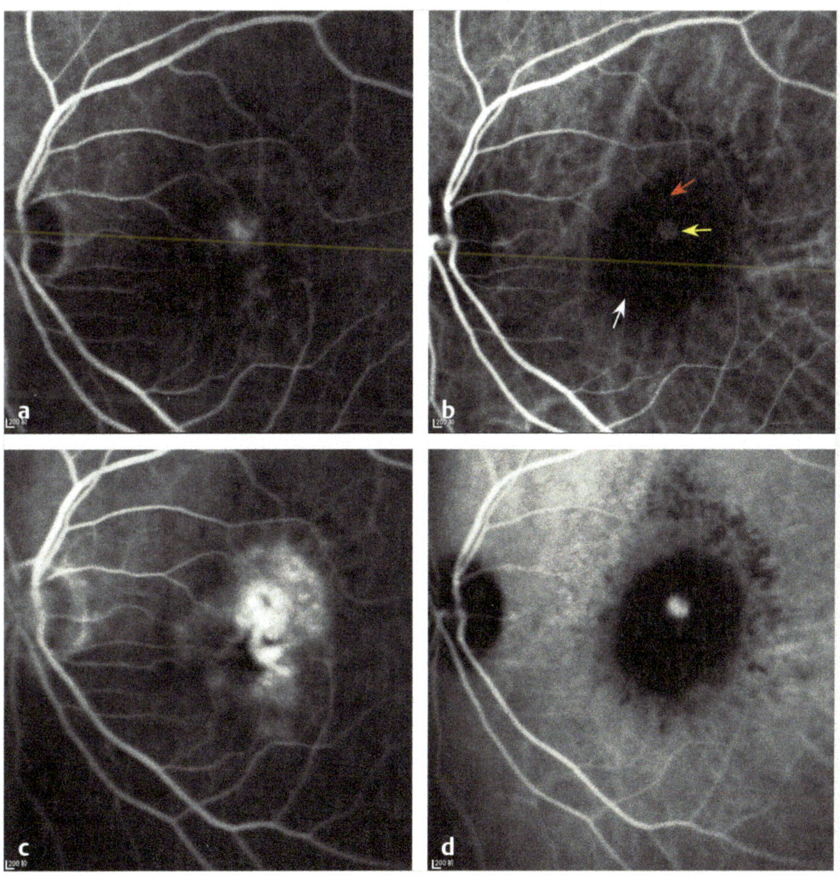

Fig. 4.16 Simultaneous fluorescein and ICG angiography of an eye with retinal angiomatous proliferation. (**a**) Early and (**c**) late fluorescein angiogram phases show poorly delineated leakage in the macula. The simultaneous (**b, d**) ICG angiograms show not only a hot spot (yellow arrow) but also an anastomosing retinal vessel to this lesion (red arrow). The well-demarcated abnormal hypofluorescence beneath the hot spot is PED (white arrow).

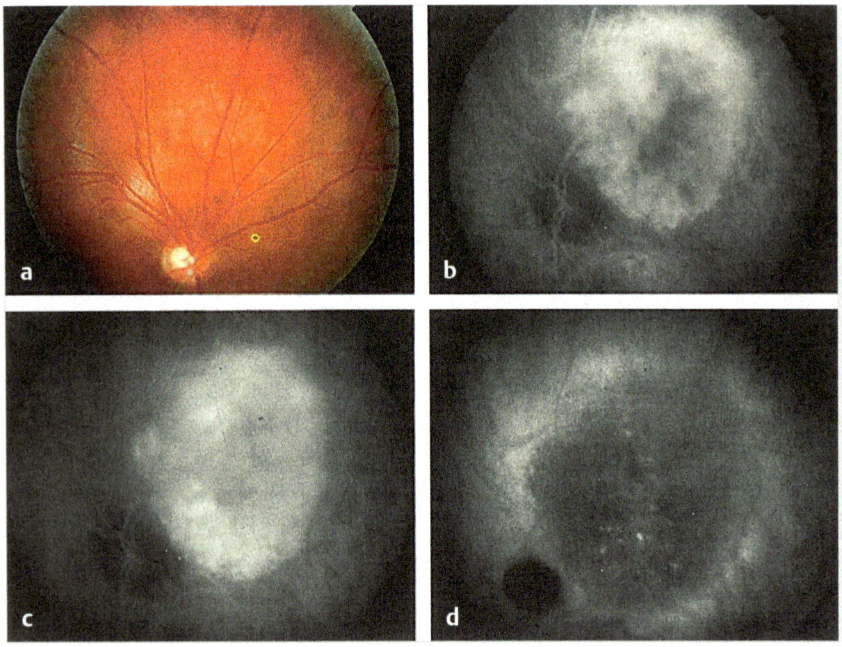

Fig. 4.17 Circumscribed choroidal hemangioma. (**a**) Fundus photograph and corresponding (**b**) early, (**c**) mid, and (**d**) late ICG angiogram phases show rapid, intense hyperfluorescence followed by late clearing of the dye from the lesion with resultant hypofluorescence. (Image courtesy of Jerry Shields, MD.)

References

[1] Von Baeyer A. Uber ein neue Klasse von farbstoffen. Der Deutschen Chem Ges. 1871; 4:555–558

[2] Ehrlich P. Über provicirte fluorescenzerscheinungen am Auge. Dtsch Med Wochenschr. 1882; 8:21–22

[3] MacLean AL, Maumenee AE. Hemangioma of the choroid. Am J Ophthalmol. 1960; 50:3–11

[4] Novotny HR, Alvis DL. A method of photographing fluorescence in circulating blood in the human retina. Circulation. 1961; 24:82–86

[5] Flower RW, Hochheimer BF. Clinical infrared absorption angiography of the choroid. Am J Ophthalmol. 1972; 73(3):458–459

[6] Flower RW, Hochheimer BF. A clinical technique and apparatus for simultaneous angiography of the separate retinal and choroidal circulations. Invest Ophthalmol. 1973; 12(4):248–261

[7] Hayashi K, Hasegawa Y, Tokoro T. Indocyanine green angiography of central serous chorioretinopathy. Int Ophthalmol. 1986; 9(1):37–41

[8] Guyer DR, Puliafito CA, Monés JM, Friedman E, Chang W, Verdooner SR. Digital indocyanine-green angiography in chorioretinal disorders. Ophthalmology. 1992; 99(2):287–291

[9] Yannuzzi LA, Slakter JS, Sorenson JA, Guyer DR, Orlock DA. Digital indocyanine green videoangiography and choroidal neovascularization. Retina. 1992; 12(3):191–223

[10] Wolf S, Wald KJ, Elsner AE, Staurenghi G. Indocyanine green choroidal videoangiography: a comparison of imaging analysis with the scanning laser ophthalmoscope and the fundus camera. Retina. 1993; 13(3):266:269

[11] Fox IJ, Wood EH. Indocyanine green: physical and physiologic properties. Proc Staff Meet Mayo Clin. 1960; 35:732–744

[12] Wipper SH. Validation of Fluorescence Angiography for Intraoperative Assessment and Quantification of Myocardial Perfusion [dissertation]. LMU München: Faculty of Medicine; 2006:18–23

[13] Brucker AJ, Brant A, Nyberg W. "Landmark injection" for localization of choroidal lesions using indocyanine green angiography. Retina. 1993; 13 (2):169–171

[14] Caesar J, Shaldon S, Chiandussi L, Guevara L, Sherlock S. The use of indocyanine green in the measurement of hepatic blood flow and as a test of hepatic function. Clin Sci. 1961; 21:43–57

[15] Yannuzzi LA, Rohrer KT, Tindel LJ, et al. Fluorescein angiography complication survey. Ophthalmology. 1986; 93(5):611–617

[16] Bloom JN, Herman DC, Elin RJ, et al. Intravenous fluorescein interference with clinical laboratory tests. Am J Ophthalmol. 1989; 108(4):375–379

[17] Halperin LS, Olk RJ, Soubrane G, Coscas G. Safety of fluorescein angiography during pregnancy. Am J Ophthalmol. 1990; 109(5):563–566

[18] Greenberg F, Lewis RA. Safety of fluorescein angiography during pregnancy. Am J Ophthalmol. 1990; 110(3):323–325

[19] Schatz H, Burton TC, Yannuzzi LA, Rabb MF. Interpretation of Fundus Fluorescein Angiography. St. Louis, MO: Mosby; 1978:8

[20] Miller SA. Fluorescence in Best's vitelliform dystrophy, lipofuscin, and fundus flavimaculatus. Br J Ophthalmol. 1978; 62(4):256–260

[21] Larsen M, Kjer B, Bendtson I, Dalgaard P, Lund-Andersen H. Lens fluorescence in relation to metabolic control of insulin-dependent diabetes mellitus. Arch Ophthalmol. 1989; 107(1):59–62

[22] Justice J, Jr, Lehmann RP. Cilioretinal arteries. A study based on review of stereo fundus photographs and fluorescein angiographic findings. Arch Ophthalmol. 1976; 94(8):1355–1358

[23] Chang AA, Morse LS, Handa JT, et al. Histologic localization of indocyanine green dye in aging primate and human ocular tissues with clinical angiographic correlation. Ophthalmology. 1998; 105(6):1060–1068

[24] Rabb MF, Burton TC, Schatz H, Yannuzzi LA. Fluorescein angiography of the fundus: a schematic approach to interpretation. Surv Ophthalmol. 1978; 22 (6):387–403

[25] Schatz H. Letter: flow sheet for the interpretation of the fluorescein angiograms. Arch Ophthalmol. 1976; 94(4):687

[26] Schatz H, Burton TC, Yannuzzi LA, Rabb MF. Interpretation of Fundus Fluorescein Angiography. St. Louis, MO: Mosby; 1978

[27] Flower RW, Csaky KG, Murphy RP. Disparity between fundus camera and scanning laser ophthalmoscope indocyanine green imaging of retinal pigment epithelium detachments. Retina. 1998; 18(3):260–268

[28] Regillo CD, Benson WE, Maguire JI, Annesley WH, Jr. Indocyanine green angiography and occult choroidal neovascularization. Ophthalmology. 1994; 101(2):280–288

[29] Spaide RF, Yannuzzi LA, Slakter JS, Sorenson J, Orlach DA. Indocyanine green videoangiography of idiopathic polypoidal choroidal vasculopathy. Retina. 1995; 15(2):100–110

[30] Yannuzzi LA, Negrão S, Iida T, et al. Retinal angiomatous proliferation in age-related macular degeneration. Retina. 2001; 21(5):416–434

[31] Shields CL, Shields JA, De Potter P. Patterns of indocyanine green videoangiography of choroidal tumours. Br J Ophthalmol. 1995; 79(3):237–245

[32] Scheider A, Nasemann JE, Lund OE. Fluorescein and indocyanine green angiographies of central serous choroidopathy by scanning laser ophthalmoscopy. Am J Ophthalmol. 1993; 115(1):50–56

[33] Dhaliwal RS, Maguire AM, Flower RW, Arribas NP. Acute posterior multifocal placoid pigment epitheliopathy. An indocyanine green angiographic study. Retina. 1993; 13(4):317–325

[34] Ie D, Glaser BM, Murphy RP, Gordon LW, Sjaarda RN, Thompson JT. Indocyanine green angiography in multiple evanescent white-dot syndrome. Am J Ophthalmol. 1994; 117(1):7–12

[35] Spaide RF, Yannuzzi LA, Slakter JS, Sorenson J, Orlach DA. Indocyanine green videoangiography of idiopathic polypoidal choroidal vasculopathy. Retina. 1995; 15(2):100–110

[36] Phillips WB, II, Regillo CD, Maguire JI. Indocyanine green angiography of idiopathic polypoidal choroidal vasculopathy. Ophthalmic Surg Lasers. 1996; 27 (6):467–470

[37] Wang Y, Fawzi AA, Tan O, Zhang X, Huang D. Flicker-induced changes in retinal blood flow assessed by Doppler optical coherence tomography. Biomed Opt Express. 2011; 2(7):1852–1860

[38] Riva CE, Falsini B, Logean E. Flicker-evoked responses of human optic nerve head blood flow: luminance versus chromatic modulation. Invest Ophthalmol Vis Sci. 2001; 42(3):756–762

[39] Falsini B, Riva CE, Logean E. Flicker-evoked changes in human optic nerve blood flow: relationship with retinal neural activity. Invest Ophthalmol Vis Sci. 2002; 43(7):2309–2316

[40] Jia Y, Tan O, Tokayer J, et al. Split-spectrum amplitude-decorrelation angiography with optical coherence tomography. Opt Express. 2012; 20(4):4710–4725

[41] Pinhas A, Dubow M, Shah N, et al. In vivo imaging of human retinal microvasculature using adaptive optics scanning light ophthalmoscope fluorescein angiography. Biomed Opt Express. 2013; 4(8):1305–1317

[42] Zawadzki RJ, Jones SM, Pilli S, et al. Integrated adaptive optics optical coherence tomography and adaptive optics scanning laser ophthalmoscope system for simultaneous cellular resolution in vivo retinal imaging. Biomed Opt Express. 2011; 2(6):1674–1686

5 Optical Coherence Tomography

Jay S. Duker and Gregory D. Lee

5.1 Introduction

Optical coherence tomography (OCT) is a noninvasive diagnostic imaging technology that renders in vivo cross-sectional images of light-scattering media with micron resolution. OCT is based on the principles of optical interferometry, which is a technique of extracting information about waves based on constructive or destructive inference patterns when two waves are superimposed.

5.2 Brief History

OCT was first reported in 1991 through a collaboration between clinicians, engineers, researchers, and students.[1] After further development of the software and hardware, in vivo retinal imaging was reported in 1993 at Tufts Medical Center, New England Eye Center, Boston, MA.[2,3,4] Carl Zeiss Meditec introduced the first commercial OCT device in 1996 and a second-generation device in 2000, with successive advances in both hardware and software capabilities. It was in 2002 with the release of the Stratus OCT (Carl Zeiss Meditec) that the technology became widely accepted in the ophthalmologic community. In 2006, the first spectral-domain OCT (SD-OCT) device was released by Optovue, Inc., allowing for higher resolution scans and faster scanning speed compared to the Stratus OCT. Over the next few years, several other manufacturers released various SD-OCT devices with differing scanning parameters, speeds, and software capabilities.

Over time, OCT has become integral in elucidating in vivo microscopic changes in ocular structures, particularly with retinal pathology. The influence of the technology is demonstrated by the number of reports and publications on OCT, with approximately 3,500 publications in 2013 alone and more than 17,000 publications from 2000 until the present time.

5.3 Principles

The initial OCT prototype was based on the Michelson interferometer in which a source emits low-coherence light into a beam splitter, with one arm directed to a reference mirror and the other arm to the sample of interest, or tissue. The resulting backscattered lights from the tissue and reference mirror are combined and analyzed for interference patterns of intensity, providing measurements of the depth and reflectivity of tissue structures at a given point (A-scan). Low-coherence light is utilized to decrease the distance over which interferometric signals are able to be detected, from meters to micrometers. However, the use of low-coherence light also requires the backscattered lights from the reference mirror and sample to be of comparable length, within one wavelength, in order to detect interferometric signals. Multiple A-scans are combined along a linear path to create a cross-sectional slice of the tissue (B-scan, or "line scan"), and likewise multiple B-scans can be combined to provide three-dimensional images (C-scan).

Three methods for the detection of interferometric signal have been developed into commercial systems.

5.3.1 Time-Domain OCT

Time-domain (TD) systems acquire interferometric signals by mechanically moving the reference mirror to correspond to the length of backscattered light in the tissue sample for each individual A-scan. TD-OCT systems were able to achieve rates of 400 A-scans per second with axial resolutions of 8 to 10 µm.[5]

5.3.2 Spectral-Domain OCT

SD technology, a type of Fourier-domain OCT, utilizes a fixed reference arm and a broadband light source to produce a spectrum of wavelengths of backscattered light, which is measured by a high-speed spectrometer in the detection arm of the interferometer.[6] This information is converted by inverse Fourier transformation to provide multiple A-scans with a single exposure. The collection of data simultaneously from each location improved sensitivity and sampling speed, generating 18,000 to 70,000 A-scans per second with axial resolution of 5 to 7 µm, several orders of magnitude faster and more sensitive than TD-OCT.[7,8]

5.3.3 Swept-Source OCT

Also referred to as time-encoded frequency-domain OCT, this technology utilizes a tunable frequency swept laser light source instead of a reference mirror to sweep through a broad range of frequencies. The interferometric signals are detected on a single or small number of receivers as a function of time and undergo inverse Fourier transformation to generate A-scan information. Speeds of up to 400,000 A-scans per second have been achieved with swept-source OCT (SS-OCT).

5.3.4 Comparison of OCT types

TD-OCT

The Stratus OCT (Carl Zeiss Meditec) is the primary commercially available scanner, which was released in 2002. It is the device with the longest history of use and has been utilized in the largest number of published studies of all OCTs available. However, being a TD-OCT system, it scans at a slower rate, resulting in more motion artifacts and covering a smaller portion of the retina. Additionally, the lower resolution of TD-OCT compared to SD-OCT and SS-OCT does not permit visualization of finer retinal structures or pathology, particularly the outer photoreceptor layers, retinal pigment epithelium (RPE), or choroid. It also suffers from lower interscan repeatability compared to SD-OCT.[9]

The main retinal scan output for this device consists of six radial line scans, centered on the fovea, separated 30 degrees apart. Owing to the amount of spacing between each line scan, retinal pathology falling in between line scans can easily be missed. The system outputs retinal thickness measurements, which have been reported in numerous studies. However, thickness measurements on the Stratus cannot be directly compared to SD-OCT scanners since the segmentation of the outer retina is different between the two types of scanners.[9]

SD-OCT

There are many commercially available SD-OCT scanners, with various scanning patterns, scanning speed, resolution, and additional modes (e.g., anterior segment OCT). The higher speed of SD-OCT scans decreases motion and blink artifacts seen with TD-OCT. Additionally, the higher scan speeds allow for denser sampling of the retinal area, decreasing the chance of missing retinal pathology. The improved resolution allows for better visualization of retinal structures such as the outer photoreceptor bands from the RPE as well as subtle retinal pathology.

Hand-held, portable SD-OCT devices have been developed, which are useful for intraoperative scanning or for patients who have positioning difficulties.[10,11] An intraoperative OCT device that attaches to the operating microscope has been developed.[12]

SS-OCT

SS-OCT provides higher scanning speeds (typically between 100,000 and 250,000 A-scans per second) than SD-OCT and has less loss of sensitivity with depth changes, allowing for improved visualization of both deep structures (i.e., choroid) and the vitreoretinal interface.[13,14] Additionally, the faster scan speeds and increased depth range allow for a larger peripheral range than SD-OCT and TD-OCT.

5.4 Types of Scans

Multiple analyses and outputs are available across the various systems and software packages, with several general scan patterns available across all commercially available devices. Variables such as B-scan density, speed, length of scan, and pixel density are programmable depending on the machine used. In current practice, there are two main types of scans, macular scans (cube, raster, star patterns) and line scans, as well as other additional scans (detailed later), for analyzing various layers of the retina in specific diseases.

5.4.1 Cube Scan

Macular cube scans are compilations of a series of B-scans to create a volumetric cube of data, similar to computed tomography scans. The scans generally cover a 6 × 6 mm area centered on the fovea and are of lower resolution than line scans in order to decrease the total scan time required. The center of the scan can be manually moved to a different area of the retina by the operator and can be output as a topographic map with a color-coded Early Treatment Diabetic Retinopathy Study (ETDRS) grid (▶ Fig. 5.1). Various scanners use different protocols, with some offering lower density B- and C-scans as "fast" options. A more significant difference that plays a role in analysis is the type of grid scan used.

5.4.2 Raster Scan

Raster scans involve a rectangular grid consisting of closely spaced parallel B-scans of the area of interest. This type of scan acquires a uniform amount of information of the area scanned, with an equal density of B-scans in the fovea and the outer macula.

5.4.3 Grid Scan

The MM5 protocol of the RTVue device is a mix of vertical and horizontal B-scans to create a grid, rather than a series of parallel B-scans. Specifically, the scan is composed of a less dense 11 × 11 B-scan grid over a 5 × 5 mm area, with each line composed of 668 A-scans, and a denser inner grid of 6 × 6 B-scans covering a 3 × 3 mm area, with each line composed of 400 A-scans. This pattern requires the least amount of interpolation between individual line scans, thereby minimizing the chances of missing pathology.

5.4.4 Radial Scan

Radial scans consist of either 6 or 12 radial high-resolution 6-mm line scans, all of which pass through the fovea. This was the primary scanning pattern of the Stratus TD-OCT and is offered on the RTVue, Topcon 3D, and Heidelberg Spectralis devices. The advantage compared to raster scanning is that with a given number of B-scans, the individual line scans are more closely spaced in the foveal area where visually significant pathology is likely located. This is similar to grid scanning, but has a speed advantage since additional scans do not need to be taken to increase the density of line scans in the foveal area. However, the disadvantage is that the software interpolates between each radial scan and may miss pathology located in the outer macular area where the radial line scans are farther apart.

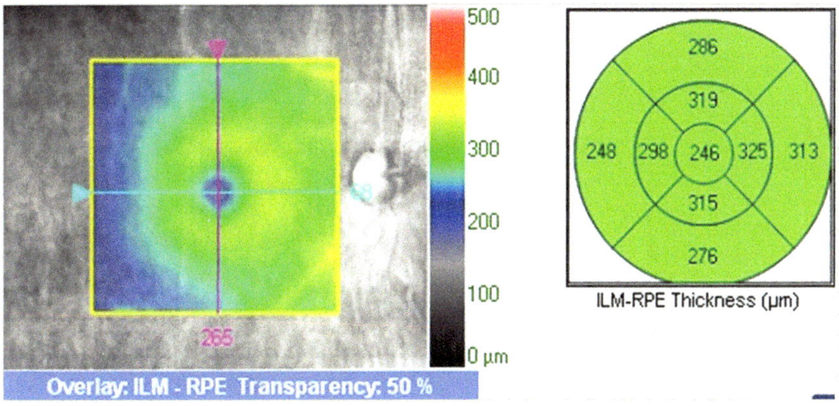

Fig. 5.1 Macular cube scan with topographic map (left) and ETDRS grid showing retinal thickness (right).

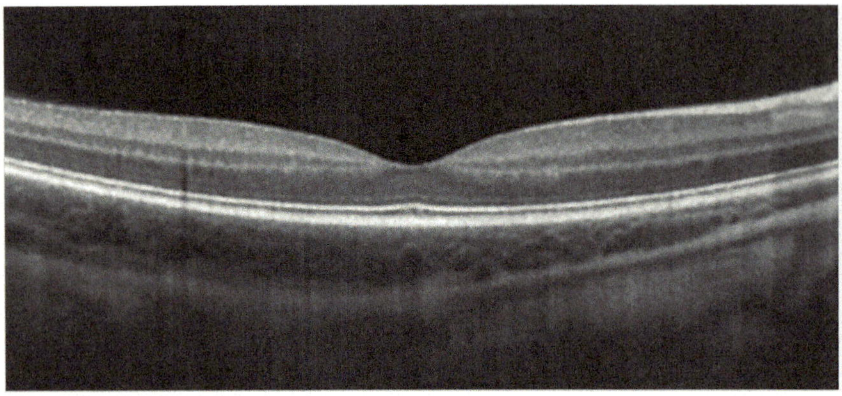

Fig. 5.2 SD-OCT line scan of a normal eye.

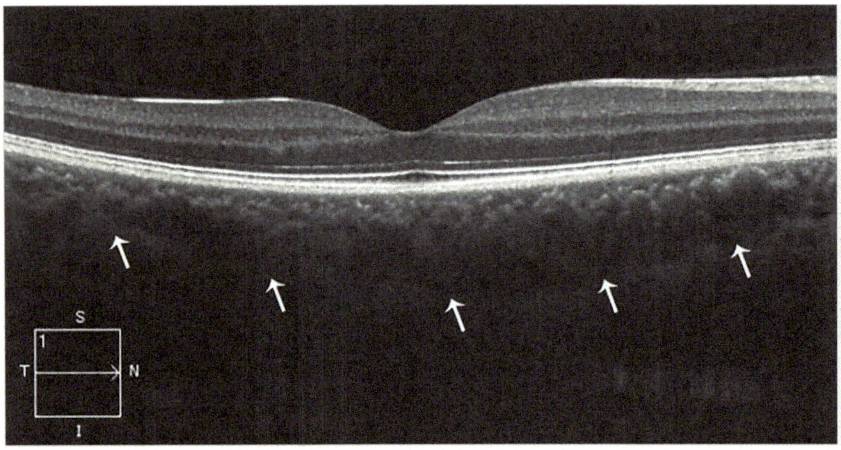

Fig. 5.3 SD-OCT using EDI to better visualize the scleral–choroidal border *(arrows)*.

5.4.5 Line, High-Definition Line, and Cross-Line Scans

Line scans (▶ Fig. 5.2) are individual B-scans composed of a higher density of A-scans compared to cube scans, resulting in higher resolution. This is particularly useful for delineating specific retinal layers and identifying subtle pathology in a known area of interest. The Zeiss Cirrus features a 6-mm five-line raster, with each line sampled four times and averaged. Additionally, the five lines can be collapsed into one line with an average of 20 samples to create a "high-definition" OCT line scan by image averaging. Image averaging averages multiple B-scans of the same retinal location to increase the signal-to-noise ratio. The RTVue system additionally features a cross-line scan, consisting of horizontal and vertical line scans, like a higher definition mesh scan. The Heidelberg Spectralis features a seven-line raster scan.

5.4.6 Enhanced Depth Imaging

Enhanced depth imaging (EDI) was first reported by Spaide et al in 2008 and is now available in all commercial OCT devices.[15] EDI better visualizes the scleral–choroidal border (▶ Fig. 5.3, arrows), allowing for measurements of choroidal thickness and analysis of lesions affecting the choroid, which would not be visible on standard line scans due to the attenuating effects of the RPE. EDI is a method of scanning in which the objective of the lens of the OCT is placed closer to the eye of the patient, resulting in an inverted image and centering the zero-delay line closer to the choroid rather than the retina.

5.4.7 Layer Specific

Various devices feature the ability to analyze specific layers of the retina using algorithms to determine the inner and outer borders of those layers. For accurate identification of the borders of the retinal layer of interest, a high-quality scan with high signal strength is required. Two analyses in particular have been reported and are used to follow specific diseases: retinal nerve fiber layer (RNFL) analysis and ganglion cell layer (GCL) analysis.

Retinal Nerve Fiber Layer

The retinal nerve fiber layer (RNFL) analysis measures the RNFL circumferentially at a radius of 1.7 mm centered on the optic nerve. It is used primarily to follow glaucoma progression, but is also used in diseases of the optic nerve such as optic neuritis, optic atrophy, nonarteritic optic neuropathy, and papilledema.[16,17,18,19,20] The output is displayed as segmented measurements of nerve fiber layer thickness as well as a color-coded graph with a comparison to age-matched controls (▶ Fig. 5.4).

Ganglion Cell Layer

The GCL analysis is an algorithm-based measurement of the GCL and inner plexiform layer extrapolated from a macular

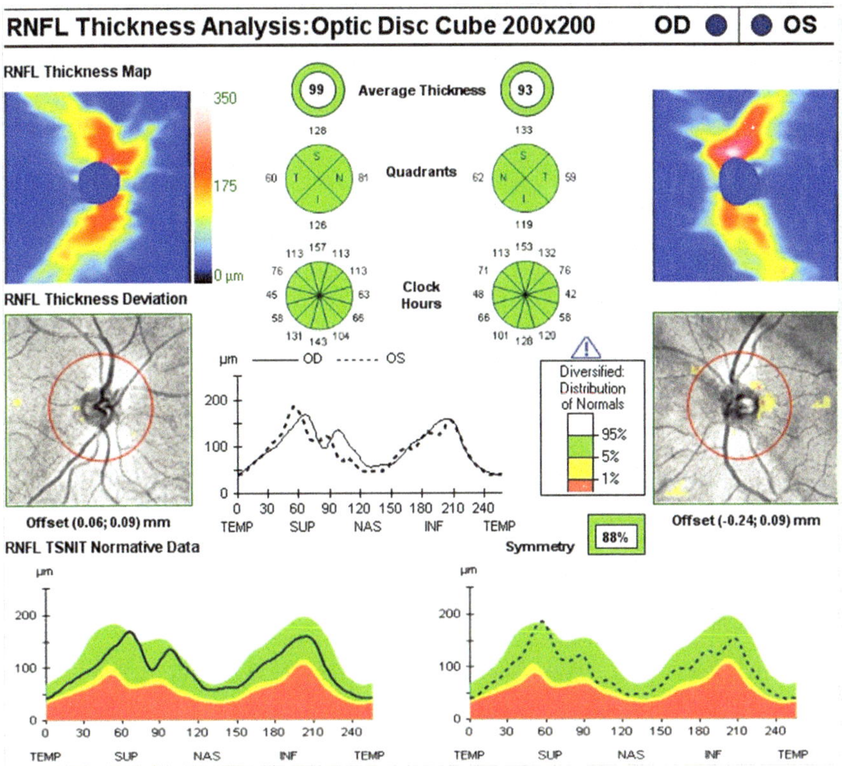

Fig. 5.4 SD-OCT retinal nerve fiber layer analysis with numerical values above and color-coded chart of nerve fiber layer thickness compared to a regular population database.

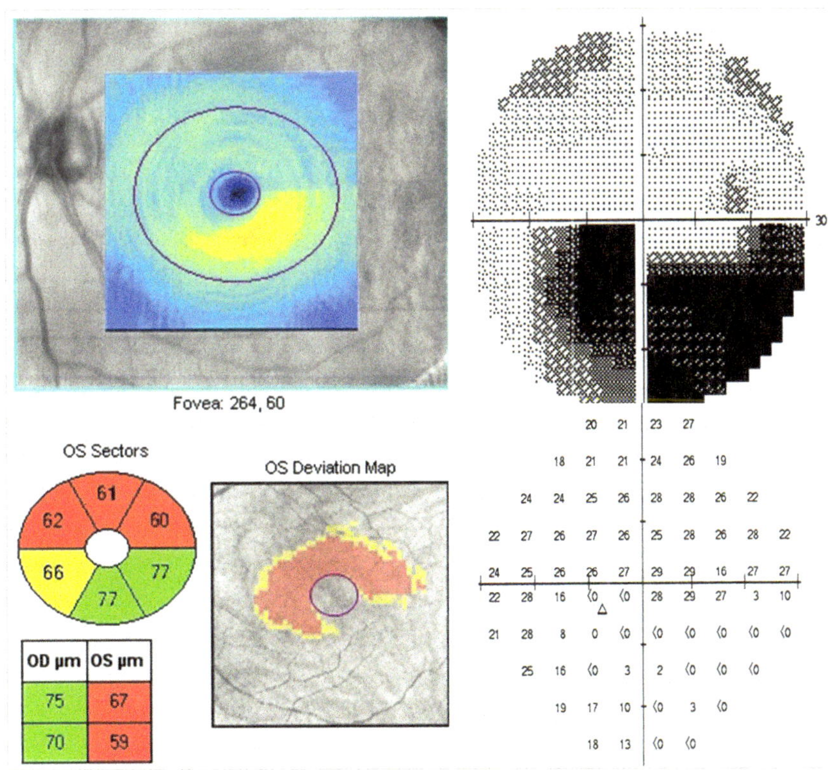

Fig. 5.5 Ganglion cell layer analysis in patient with nonarteritic anterior ischemic optic neuropathy with corresponding visual field.

cube scan. It has been used in nonarteritic optic neuropathy, intracranial compressive lesions, optic neuritis, and other diseases of the optic nerve. The output in this analysis is displayed as a color-coded map and has been shown to have a high correlation with areas of visual field loss[21,22] (▶ Fig. 5.5).

5.4.8 En Face

This output is available on all SD-OCT devices except the Heidelberg and is a summation of all B-scans to create a C-scan, which looks like a red-free image of the retina. It is also known as an OCT fundus image. Advancements in software and data

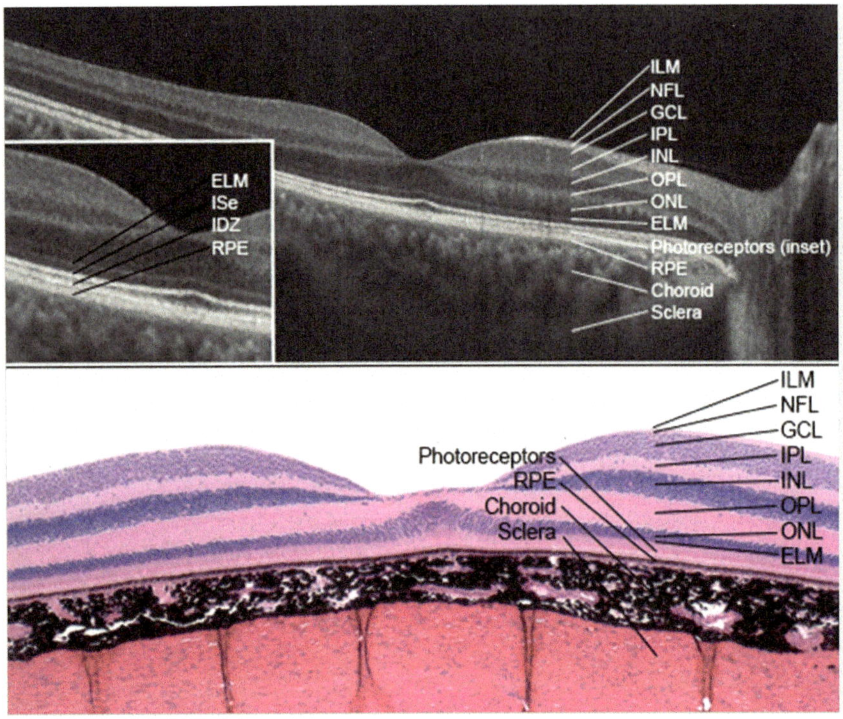

Fig. 5.6 SD-OCT line scan with labelled layers with histologic slide of the macula from another patient.

processing have allowed for the en face view of retinal or choroidal structures at varying depths set by the operator.

Currently, SS-OCT devices are being investigated to analyze en face imaging of the choroid and choriocapillaris, which may be useful in diseases such as age-related macular degeneration or diabetic retinopathy.[23,24] The enhanced visualization of the vitreoretinal interface on swept-source imaging, along with the faster scanning speed, may allow for development of en face vitreoretinal adhesion maps to elucidate pathophysiologic changes involved in macular holes, epiretinal membranes, vitreomacular traction/adhesion, and rhegmatogenous retinal detachment.

5.5 Normal Retinal OCT Scans

OCT line scans have been referred to as an "in vivo optical biopsy" because of its high correlation with the histologic appearance of the macula. Increased resolution with SD-OCT has allowed for accurate imaging of pathologic and histologic structures in the retina.[25] When light travels through the retinal tissue, it can be reflected, scattered, or absorbed, and this creates the multilayered pattern of the retina. The angle of incidence of the light, motion artifacts, speckled noise, and image contrast can affect the axial resolution of the retinal imaging. Therefore, one-to-one correspondence of histology with OCT images cannot be expected.

5.5.1 Layers on OCT

The histologic layers have corresponding layers on OCT, with a normal SD-OCT macular line scan through the fovea as shown in ▶ Fig. 5.6 with labelled layers.

Varying reflectivity properties of layers give rise to hyperreflective or hyporeflective structures on line scans. Highly reflective structures typically have more pigment or are oriented horizontally to the direction of incoming light (e.g., nerve fiber layer, GCL, plexiform layers, and RPE) (see Table 5.1 for reflectivity of normal and pathologic structures). Three bands of significance are the outermost bands, just inside the highly reflective RPE. From inner to outer, they correspond to the external limiting membrane, photoreceptor ellipsoid zone, and the photoreceptor interdigitation zone. Anatomically, these correspond to the footplates of the Müller cells, the ellipsoid portion of the inner segments of the photoreceptor cells, and the interdigitations of photoreceptor outer segments with villi from the RPE, respectively.[26] The ellipsoid and interdigitation zone bands have also historically been referred to as the inner segment/outer segment (IS/OS) layer.

5.6 Interpretation

Both qualitative and quantitative analyses are required for accurate interpretation of OCT scans.

5.6.1 Qualitative Analysis

Qualitative analysis involves interpretation of individual line scans of the areas of interest, with attention focused on pathologic findings and changes over time. A thorough knowledge of normal retinal anatomy and OCT appearance is vital in accurate identification of subtle pathology.

Devices can output the line scans in a grayscale image or color-coded image, with different colors representing the reflectivity of structures in the retina. However, the color-coded image may make it difficult to discern finer retinal details or subtle pathology (▶ Fig. 5.7). For practical purposes, grayscale imaging is recommended in analyzing line scans (compare to ▶ Fig. 5.2).

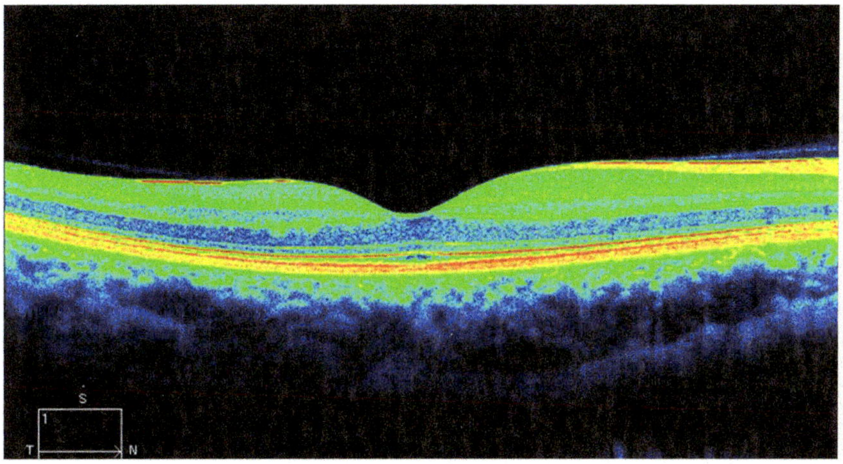

Fig. 5.7 SD-OCT color-coded line scan.

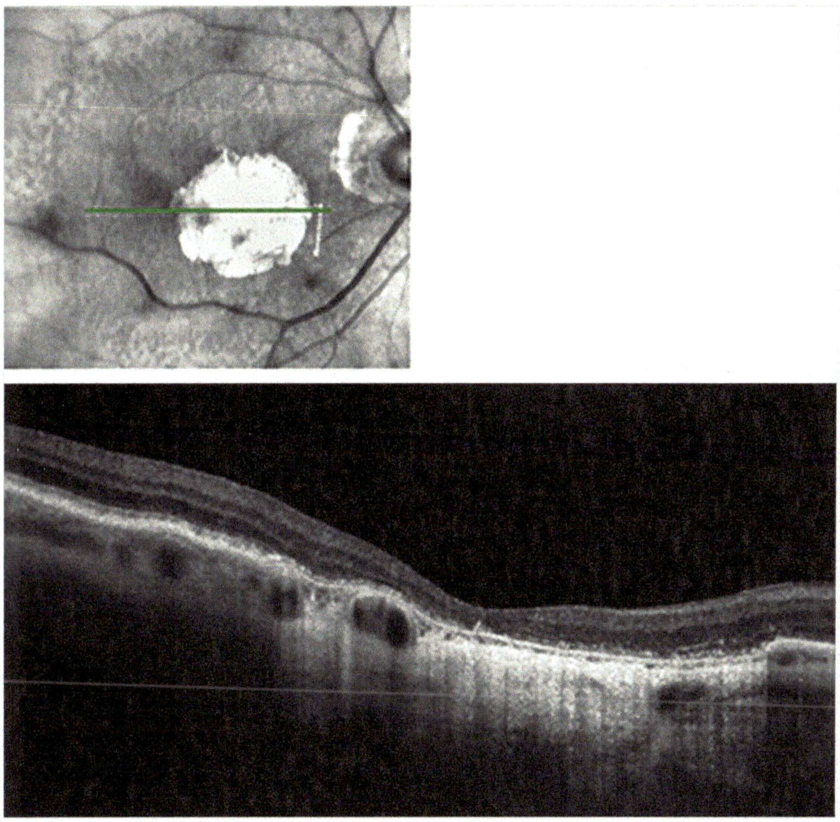

Fig. 5.8 Geographic atrophy with windowing in a patient with dry age-related macular degeneration. Note the thin choroid. Green line on (a) the accompanying infrared image corresponds to (b) the cross-sectional line scan shown

Qualitatively, pathologic lesions in an OCT scan can be described as hyperreflective or hyporeflective as described in the following section (Table 5.1). On the grayscale imaging, hyperreflective lesions appear whiter, while hyporeflective lesions appear blacker. *Shadowing* occurs when hyperreflective material or tissue blocks the transmission and reflection of light to more posterior structures. This results in decreased visualization of deep structures and may be mistaken for pathologic changes in the posterior structures. Alternatively, *windowing*, or *reverse shadowing*, occurs when there is loss of pigmented or hyperreflective structures (e.g., geographic atrophy) and increased transmission light to deeper structures, with concurrent increased reflected signal. This results in enhanced reflectivity and visualization of those deeper structures (see ▶ Fig. 5.8).

In certain diseases, it is important not only to identify pathology but also to observe changes over time. All SD-OCT devices allow for *registration*, in which retinal structures such as blood vessels are used by the device to align the scanner so that the same area of interest can be scanned accurately over subsequent visits. This allows the clinician to observe response to treatment for conditions such as diabetic macular edema or wet age-related macular degeneration.

5.6.2 Quantitative Analysis

Quantitative analysis allows for objective numerically based analysis of retinal pathology. This type of analysis depends on the software and algorithms of the OCT device to identify and calculate retinal thickness measurements. The process of

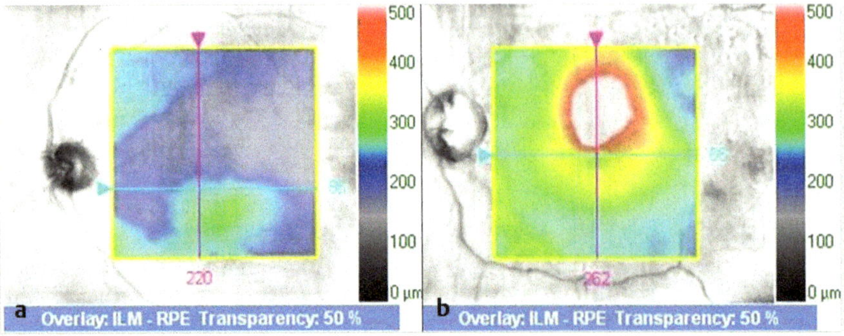

Fig. 5.9 Macular cube topographic map showing (**a**) decreased thickness from retinal atrophy in a patient with dry age-related macular degeneration and (**b**) increased thickness from macular edema in a patient with diabetic macular edema.

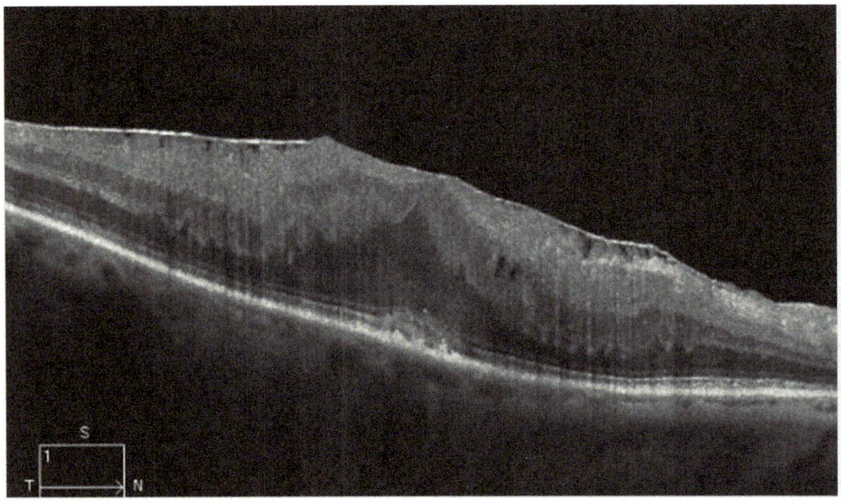

Fig. 5.10 Epiretinal membrane causing thickening and distortion of the retinal surface.

identifying and measuring sublayers (NFL, GCL) is known as *segmentation* and is dependent on a scan of adequate signal strength to identify individual layers accurately.

Macular cube, or map, analysis displays retinal thickness (RPE to vitreoretinal interface) measurements as a topographical map accompanied by numerical averages in the different segments of the Early Treatment of Diabetic Retinopathy Study grid (▶ Fig. 5.1). Both TD-OCT and SD-OCT produce this analysis, but the numerical values cannot be compared across the two types of scanning modalities since the TD-OCT typically has difficulty distinguishing the RPE from the IS/OS junction accurately, resulting in decreased thickness measurements compared to SD-OCT.

The topographic map displays retinal thickness by color scale. It is useful in visualizing decreased thickness in conditions causing retinal atrophy (▶ Fig. 5.9a) and increased thickness in conditions causing edema or elevation (▶ Fig. 5.9b).

5.7 OCT Pathology

Similar to normal retinal structures having higher or lower reflectivity profiles, pathologic changes in the retina can exhibit hyperreflectivity or hyporeflectivity. Generally, substances or materials with higher densities or pigmentation are hyperreflective. Common appearances of pathologic findings on OCT are demonstrated in ▶ Fig. 5.8 and ▶ Fig. 5.10–▶ Fig. 5.18. Examples of terminology used to interpret these scans are included in the captions.

Reflectivity profiles of normal retinal layers and pathologic findings

- High
  - Pigment (retinal pigment epithelium, choroidal nevus)
  - Scar
  - Hard exudate
  - Drusen
  - Hemorrhage
  - Neovascular membrane
  - Epiretinal membrane
  - Nerve fiber layer
  - External limiting membrane
  - Photoreceptor ellipsoid layer (IS/OS junction)
  - Photoreceptor/retinal pigment epithelium interdigitation
  - Choroid
- Medium
  - Retinal edema (commotio retinae, cotton-wool spots)
  - Fibrin
  - Inner and outer plexiform layers
  - Posterior vitreous
- Low
  - Fluid (subretinal, intraretinal, cysts, pigment epithelial detachment)
  - Ganglion cell layer
  - Vitreous

Abbreviation: IS/OS, inner segment/outer segment.

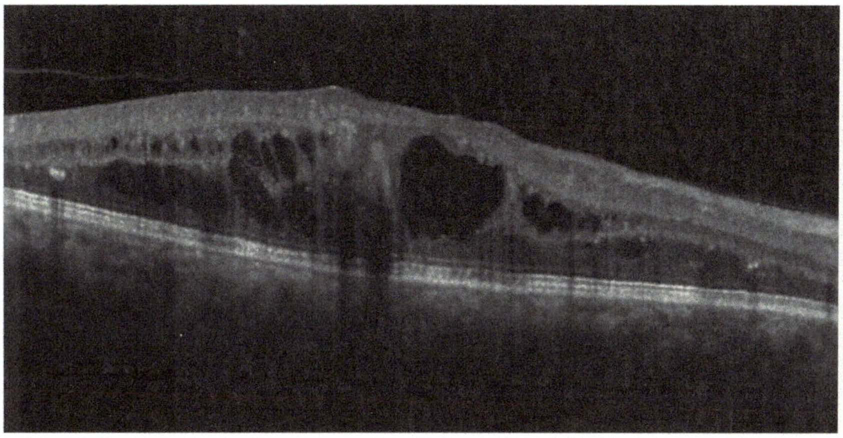

Fig. 5.11 Macular edema and intraretinal cysts. Increased retinal thickness, intraretinal cysts, and exudates in a patient with diabetic macular edema.

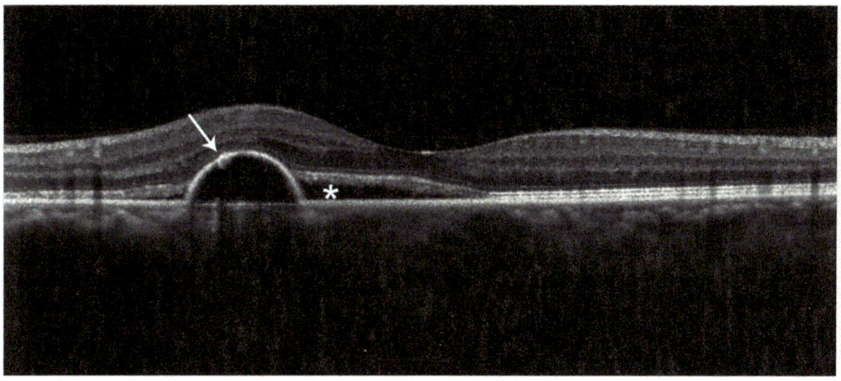

Fig. 5.12 Pigment epithelial detachment and subretinal fluid. Pigment epithelial detachment (arrow) with adjacent subfoveal subretinal fluid (*) in a patient with central serous chorioretinopathy.

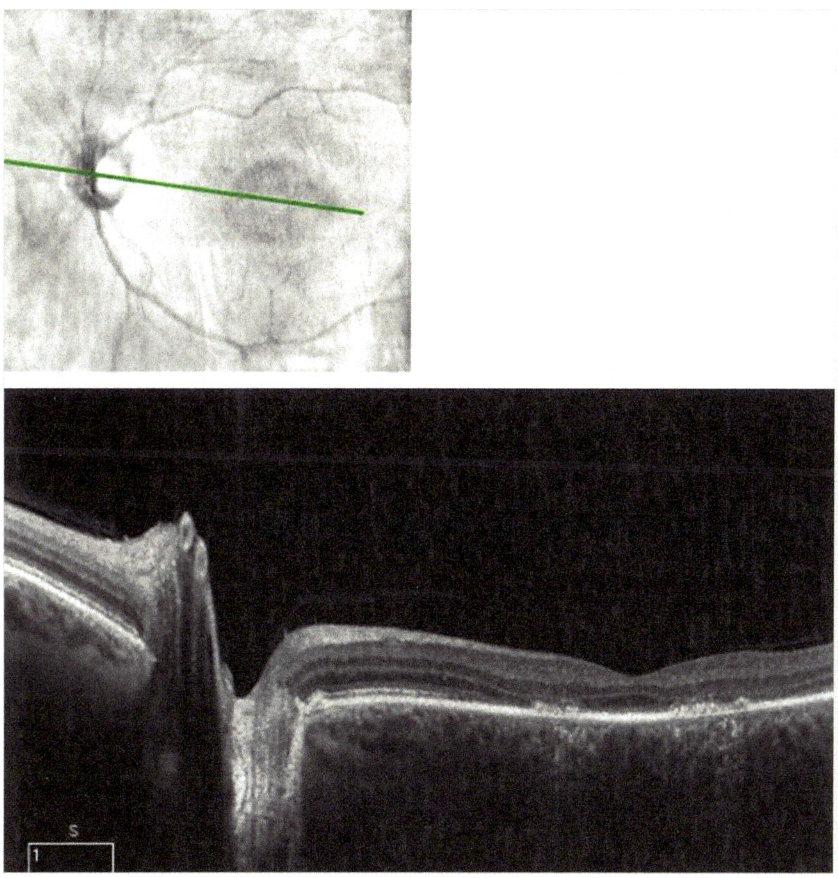

Fig. 5.13 Outer photoreceptor loss. Parafoveal outer photoreceptor loss in a patient with hydroxychloroquine toxicity. Corresponding en face C-scan demonstrates bull's eye maculopathy. Green line on (a) the accompanying infrared image corresponds to (b) the cross-sectional line scan shown

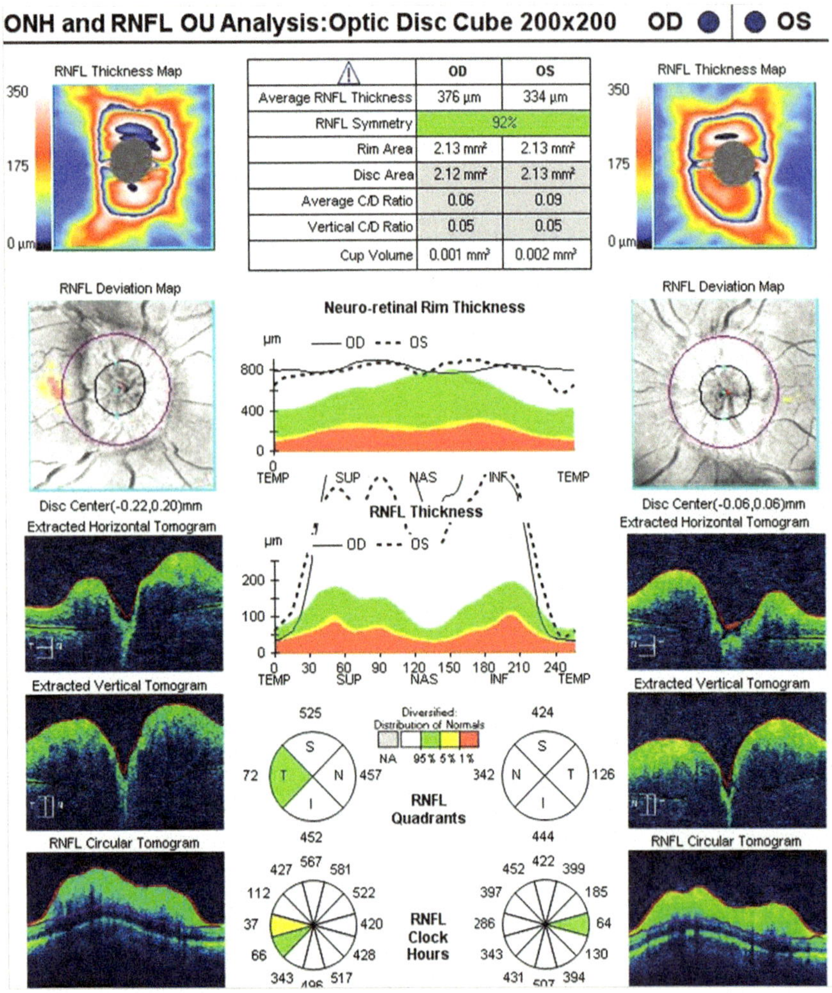

Fig. 5.14 Optic nerve swelling. RNFL scan showing increased RNFL of both eyes in a patient with papilledema from pseudotumor cerebri.

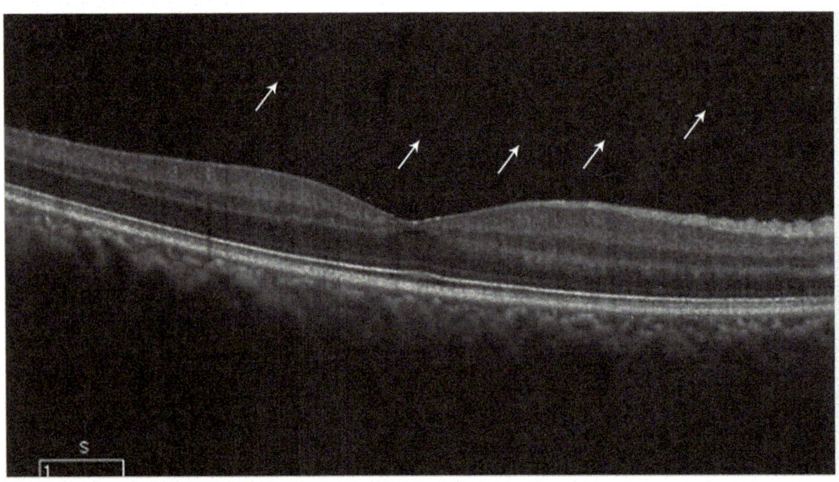

Fig. 5.15 Line scan showing normal retinal architecture with vitreous cells in a patient with intermediate uveitis (arrows).

Special Considerations

- Shadowing of Vessels
  - In an extramacular line scan, blood vessels may be scanned in cross-section, and although fluid-filled, the pigmented blood inside the vessels causes them to appear hyperreflective with shadowing underneath.

Pearls

- Windowing may occur in areas where normally hyperreflective structures have been pathologically altered, causing the underlying structures to have a higher reflectivity profile.

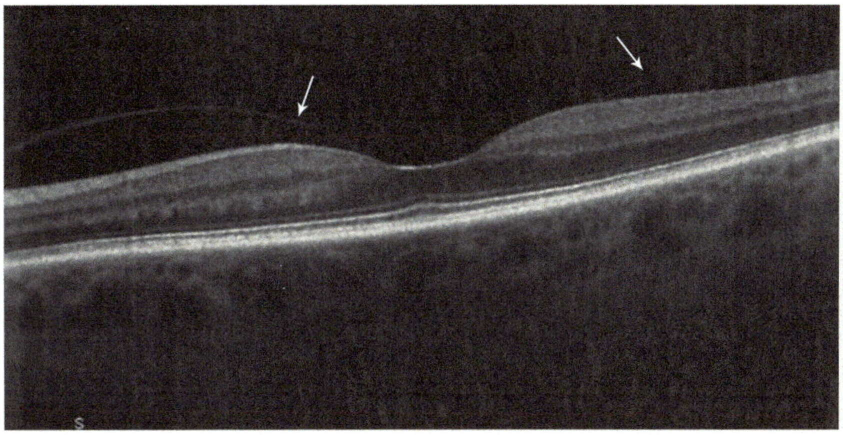

Fig. 5.16 Vitreomacular adhesion with arrows showing the posterior vitreous.

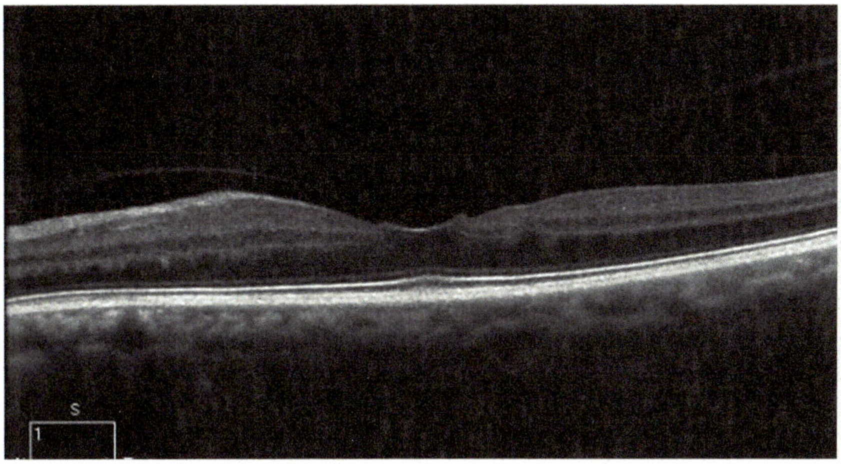

Fig. 5.17 Vitreomacular traction with broad attachment and mild perifoveal retinal distortion.

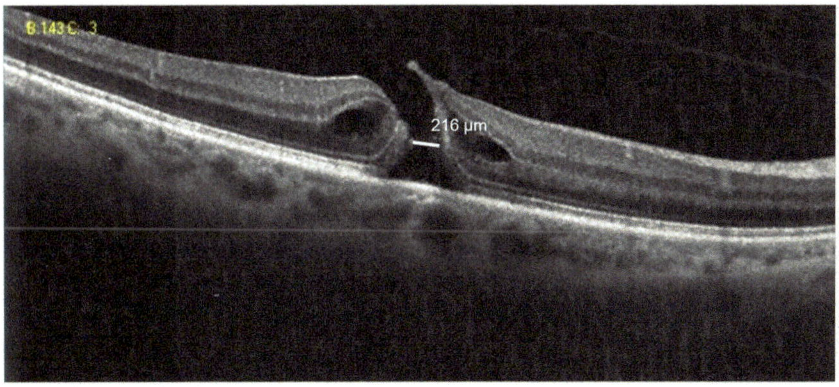

Fig. 5.18 Full-thickness macular hole with associated focal vitreomacular traction. Aperture size measured with calipers on OCT device shown in white.

5.7.1 Vitreoretinal Interface

In 2013, a panel called the International Vitreomacular Traction Study Group defined a classification system for describing the vitreoretinal interface in conditions of vitreomacular adhesion, vitreomacular traction, and macular hole using OCT-based criteria.[27] Further discussion regarding the pathology and treatment of these three conditions can be found in Chapters 17 and 18.

Vitreomacular adhesion is a perifoveal vitreous detachment without retinal abnormalities (▸ Fig. 5.16). This attachment can be broad (> 1,500 µm) or focal (< 1,500 µm), which can be measured using the caliper tool built into OCT software systems.

Vitreomacular traction is a perifoveal vitreous detachment with associated retinal distortion or abnormalities. Similar to vitreomacular adhesion, vitreomacular traction can be further delineated as broad or focal by the same parameters (▸ Fig. 5.17).

Full-thickness macular hole is an anatomic defect in the fovea extending from the nerve fiber layer to the RPE. Macular holes are further delineated by size of hole aperture, which is measured with the OCT device caliper (small, < 250 µm; medium, 200–400 µm; and large, > 400 µm). Additionally, there may be associated broad or focal vitreomacular traction (▸ Fig. 5.18).

5.8 Errors and Artifacts

OCT scans can be complicated by various errors in the scanning process, which may lead to erroneous interpretation of pathologic findings.

Special Considerations

- A high signal strength is difficult to achieve through an undilated pupil, but experienced scanning personnel can scan reliably through undilated pupils with moderately cooperative patients, particularly for RNFL OCTs.

5.8.1 Scan Quality

The first measure to note in interpreting the quality of the scan is the signal strength. Signal strength reflects the amount of light transmitted from the OCT device to the tissue of interest with the subsequent reflection back, which is measured on interferometry. Higher signal strength reflects a higher quality scan with a higher likelihood of imaging fine pathologic details. Signal strength is influenced by optical clarity of the structures between the scanner and the tissue of interest. Typical causes of decreased signal strength are corneal opacities, cataracts, vitreous cells/hemorrhage, and poor dilation.

Pearls

- Particularly with macular scans and scans requiring algorithm identification of individual retinal layers (i.e., RNFL or GCL), the algorithm can misinterpret the boundaries of the specific layer of interest if the signal strength is too low.

5.8.2 Software Error

In certain conditions, the software can misinterpret the inner or outer boundaries of retinal layers, leading to incorrect measurements of overall or layer-specific thickness. ▶ Fig. 5.19 shows a GCL analysis of the same eye with failure of the algorithm to correctly identify the individual layers due to scan quality (▶ Fig. 5.19a) and a higher quality scan with correct identification (▶ Fig. 5.19b).

5.8.3 Misalignment

Software associated with OCT devices will attempt to locate the fovea automatically based on thickness measurements to center the scan. However, in eyes with pathology resulting in thickness variance, the automatic centration may misalign the foveal center, resulting in an erroneous retinal thickness map, as seen in ▶ Fig. 5.20 with the OCT-assigned map (▶ Fig. 5.20a) and a corrected manually adjusted map (▶ Fig. 5.20b). Note the correct foveal architecture seen in the corresponding line scan in ▶ Fig. 5.20b.

5.8.4 Patient Related Errors

There are several patient-related errors that may occur, leading to abnormal-appearing scans. ▶ Fig. 5.21 to ▶ Fig. 5.24 show scans of the same eye with simulated artifacts.

Blink Artifact

Blink artifact (▶ Fig. 5.21) occurs when the patient blinks at any point during the acquisition of a scan. This type of artifact may be subtle but can be identified as a linear disruption in the scan (▶ Fig. 5.21a). The en face composite photo often shows this type of artifact as a horizontal linear abnormality with misalignment of structures immediately above and immediately below the line, as seen in the RNFL en face scan (arrows, ▶ Fig. 5.21b).

Mirror Artifact

Mirror artifact occurs when imaging is attempted on structures located too close to the zero-delay line of the OCT device,

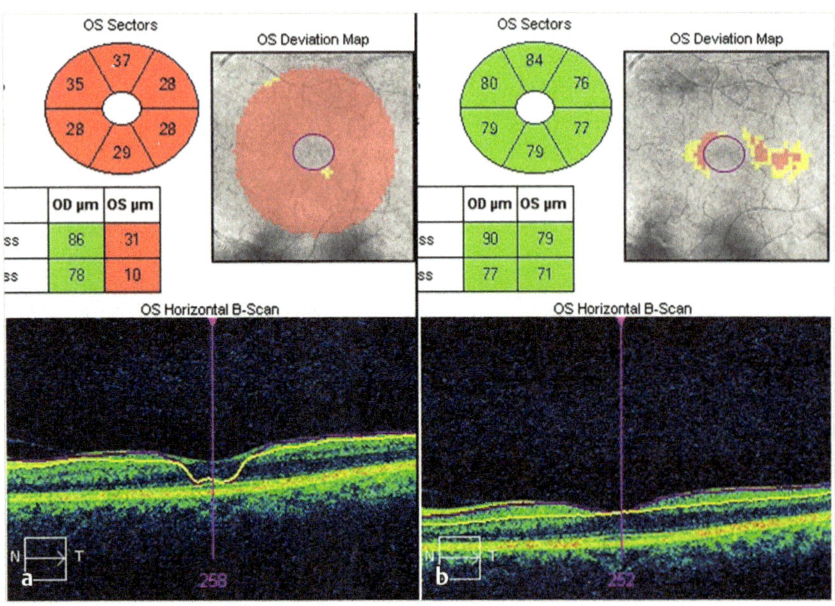

Fig. 5.19 A ganglion cell layer analysis of the same eye with (**a**) failure of the algorithm to correctly identify the individual layers due to scan quality and (**b**) higher quality scan with correct identification.

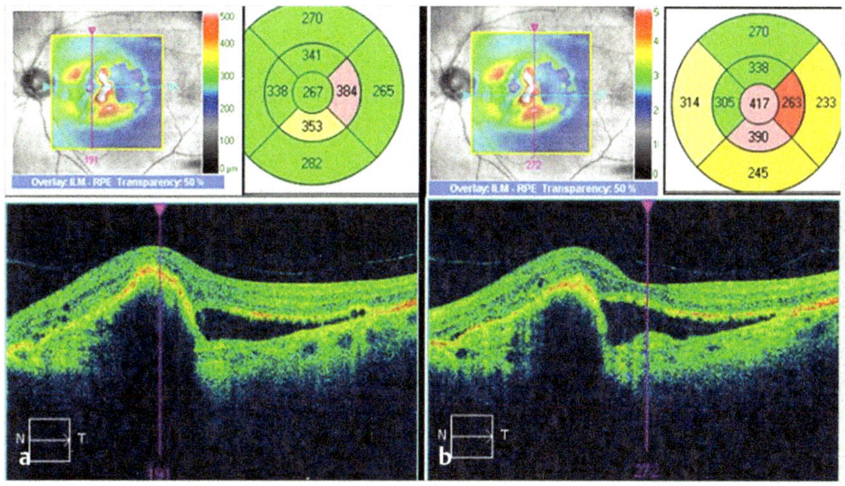

Fig. 5.20 Decentration. The macular cube scan of the same eye with severe macular edema and pigment epithelial detachment has an algorithm failure in identifying the foveal center, resulting in an erroneous retinal thickness map, as seen in the comparison with the (**a**) OCT-assigned map and (**b**) a corrected manually adjusted map. Note the correct foveal architecture seen in the corresponding line scan in b.

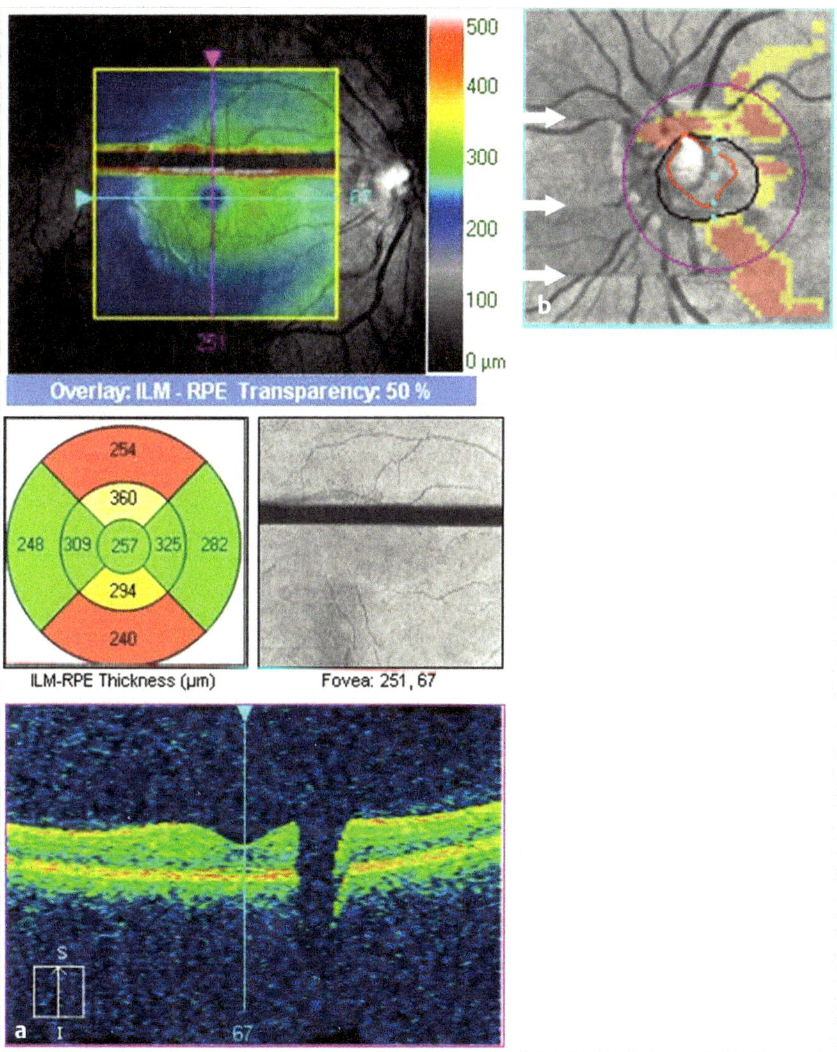

Fig. 5.21 Blink artifact. (**a**) Macular cube scan with a linear absence of signal from when the patient blinked. (**b**) En face composite photo of an RNFL scan with horizontal linear abnormality and misalignment of structures immediately above and immediately below the line (arrows).

resulting in an inversion of the structures in the scan that are outside the depth range of the OCT scan. This may occur in cases where the pathology spans a large depth range, such as retinal detachment, large choroidal tumors, retinoschisis (▶ Fig. 5.22), or peripheral lesions.

Motion Artifact

Patients may move their eye or change fixation during the scan, resulting in either loss of areas in the scan or duplication of already scanned areas (▶ Fig. 5.23).

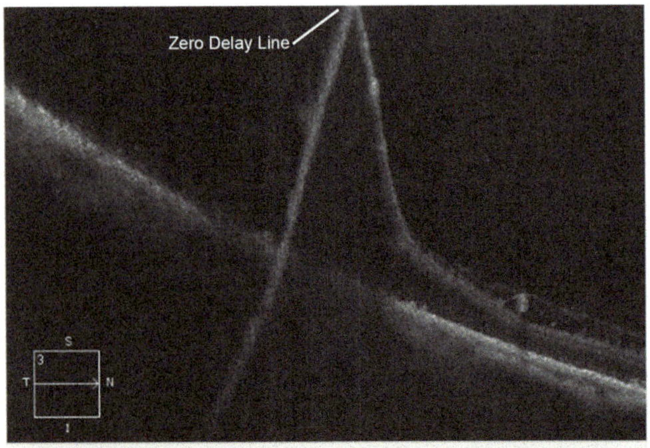

Fig. 5.22 Line scan with mirror artifact in a patient with peripheral retinoschisis.

Vignetting Artifact

This artifact results from blockage of the OCT scanning beam, most commonly by the iris in a patient with poorly dilated pupils or surgically altered pupils that do not allow for normal dilation. As a result, the scan strength of blocked areas is very low, while it is high in areas of unblocked transmittance (▶ Fig. 5.24).

5.9 Conclusion

OCT as an imaging modality has greatly enhanced the ability to visualize anatomy and pathology in the retina. The technology has given insight into pathologic processes such as vitreoretinal interface abnormalities, macular holes, serous retinal detachments, choroidal thickness in various conditions, and choroidal neovascularization, among numerous others. OCT imaging is

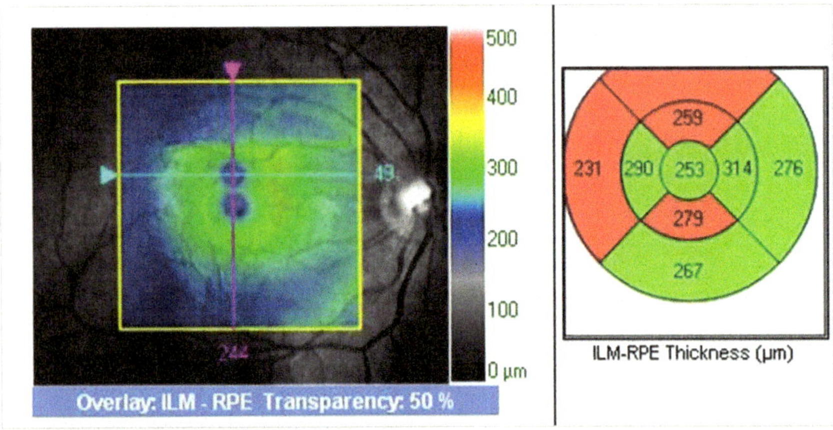

Fig. 5.23 Macular cube scan demonstrating motion artifact with recreation of the fovea in a patient with a normal macula.

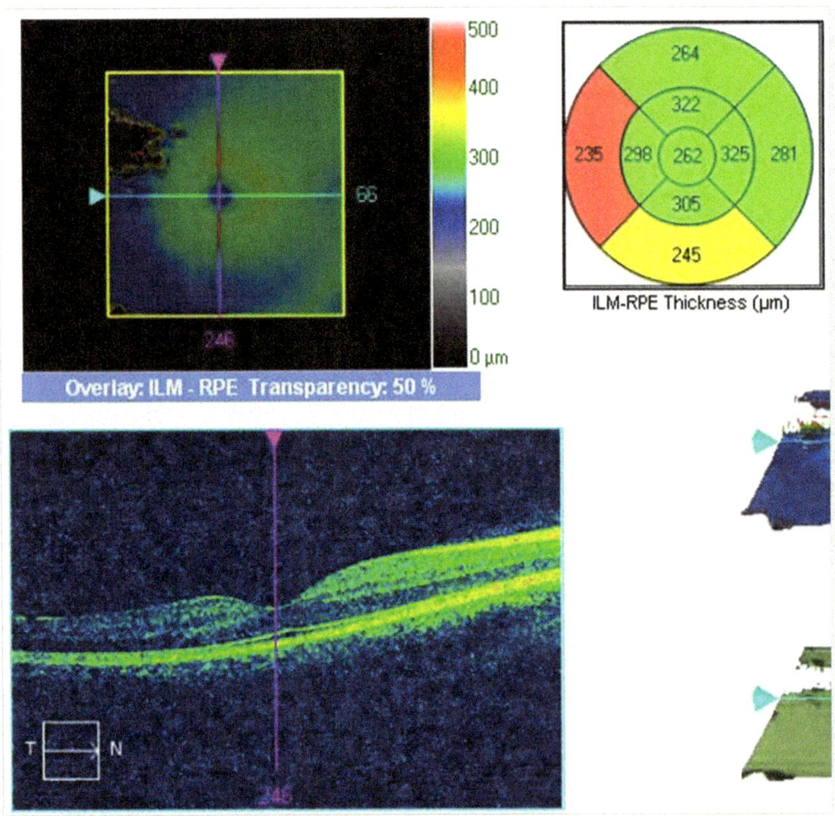

Fig. 5.24 Macular cube scan with vignetting seen as poor signal strength and algorithm failure temporally due to a poorly dilated pupil.

now an integral part of diagnosis and management of certain conditions, including diabetic macular edema, wet age-related macular degeneration, and macular holes. Both quantitative and qualitative analyses are important for accurate interpretation of OCT scans to aid in clinical decision making. Development of newer devices and investigation of the capabilities of SS-OCT may provide further insights into the pathophysiology of diseases and enhance the clinical decision making of ophthalmologists.

References

[1] Huang D, Swanson EA, Lin CP, et al. Optical coherence tomography. Science. 1991; 254(5035):1178–1181

[2] Swanson E, Huang D. Ophthalmic optical coherence tomography market: past, present, and future. Optical Coherence Tomography News. March 2009. Available online at: www.octnews.org

[3] Fercher AF, Hitzenberger CK, Drexler W, Kamp G, Sattmann H. In vivo optical coherence tomography. Am J Ophthalmol. 1993; 116(1):113–114

[4] Hee MR, Izatt JA, Swanson EA, et al. Optical coherence tomography of the human retina. Arch Ophthalmol. 1995; 113(3):325–332

[5] Sull AC, Vuong LN, Price LL, et al. Comparison of spectral/Fourier domain optical coherence tomography instruments for assessment of normal macular thickness. Retina. 2010; 30(2):235–245

[6] Wojtkowski M. Phase sensitive interferometry in optical coherence tomography. Proc. SPIE 4515, Light and Optics in Biomedicine; 2001:250

[7] de Boer JF, Cense B, Park BH, Pierce MC, Tearney GJ, Bouma BE. Improved signal-to-noise ratio in spectral-domain compared with time-domain optical coherence tomography. Opt Lett. 2003; 28(21):2067–2069

[8] Leitgeb R, Hitzenberger C, Fercher A. Performance of Fourier domain vs. time domain optical coherence tomography. Opt Express. 2003; 11(8):889–894

[9] Leung CK, Cheung CY, Weinreb RN, et al. Comparison of macular thickness measurements between time domain and spectral domain optical coherence tomography. Invest Ophthalmol Vis Sci. 2008; 49(11):4893–4897

[10] Ehlers JP, Kernstine K, Farsiu S, Sarin N, Maldonado R, Toth CA. Analysis of pars plana vitrectomy for optic pit-related maculopathy with intraoperative optical coherence tomography: a possible connection with the vitreous cavity. Arch Ophthalmol. 2011; 129(11):1483–1486

[11] Tao YK, Ehlers JP, Toth CA, Izatt JA. Intraoperative spectral domain optical coherence tomography for vitreoretinal surgery. Opt Lett. 2010; 35 (20):3315–3317

[12] Ray R, Barañano DE, Fortun JA, et al. Intraoperative microscope-mounted spectral domain optical coherence tomography for evaluation of retinal anatomy during macular surgery. Ophthalmology. 2011; 118(11):2212–2217

[13] Liu JJ, Witkin AJ, Adhi M, et al. Enhanced vitreous imaging in healthy eyes using swept source optical coherence tomography. PLoS ONE. 2014; 9(7): e102950

[14] Ruiz-Medrano J, Flores-Moreno I, Peña-García P, Montero JA, Duker JS, Ruiz-Moreno JM. Macular choroidal thickness profile in a healthy population measured by swept-source optical coherence tomography. Invest Ophthalmol Vis Sci. 2014; 55(6):3532–3542

[15] Spaide RF, Koizumi H, Pozzoni MC. Enhanced depth imaging spectral-domain optical coherence tomography. Am J Ophthalmol. 2008; 146(4):496–500

[16] Schuman JS, Hee MR, Puliafito CA, et al. Quantification of nerve fiber layer thickness in normal and glaucomatous eyes using optical coherence tomography. Arch Ophthalmol. 1995; 113(5):586–596

[17] Fisher JB, Jacobs DA, Markowitz CE, et al. Relation of visual function to retinal nerve fiber layer thickness in multiple sclerosis. Ophthalmology. 2006; 113 (2):324–332

[18] Barboni P, Savini G, Parisi V, et al. Retinal nerve fiber layer thickness in dominant optic atrophy measurements by optical coherence tomography and correlation with age. Ophthalmology. 2011; 118(10):2076–2080

[19] Deleón-Ortega J, Carroll KE, Arthur SN, Girkin CA. Correlations between retinal nerve fiber layer and visual field in eyes with nonarteritic anterior ischemic optic neuropathy. Am J Ophthalmol. 2007; 143(2):288–294

[20] Scott CJ, Kardon RH, Lee AG, Frisén L, Wall M. Diagnosis and grading of papilledema in patients with raised intracranial pressure using optical coherence tomography vs clinical expert assessment using a clinical staging scale. Arch Ophthalmol. 2010; 128(6):705–711

[21] Aggarwal D, Tan O, Huang D, Sadun AA. Patterns of ganglion cell complex and nerve fiber layer loss in nonarteritic ischemic optic neuropathy by Fourier-domain optical coherence tomography. Invest Ophthalmol Vis Sci. 2012; 53(8):4539–4545

[22] Shon K, Sung KR. Assessment of macular ganglion cell loss patterns in neurologic lesions that mimic glaucoma. Korean J Ophthalmol. 2014; 28(4):314–322

[23] Srinivasan VJ, Adler DC, Chen Y, et al. Ultrahigh-speed optical coherence tomography for three-dimensional and en face imaging of the retina and optic nerve head. Invest Ophthalmol Vis Sci. 2008; 49(11):5103–5110

[24] Ferrara D, Mohler KJ, Waheed N, et al. En face enhanced-depth swept-source optical coherence tomography features of chronic central serous chorioretinopathy. Ophthalmology. 2014; 121(3):719–726

[25] Drexler W, Sattmann H, Hermann B, et al. Enhanced visualization of macular pathology with the use of ultrahigh-resolution optical coherence tomography. Arch Ophthalmol. 2003; 121(5):695–706

[26] Spaide RF, Curcio CA. Anatomical correlates to the bands seen in the outer retina by optical coherence tomography: literature review and model. Retina. 2011; 31(8):1609–1619

[27] Duker JS, Kaiser PK, Binder S, et al. The International Vitreomacular Traction Study Group classification of vitreomacular adhesion, traction, and macular hole. Ophthalmology. 2013; 120(12):2611–2619

6 Ultrasonography

Cathy DiBernardo

6.1 Introduction

During the past couple of decades, ophthalmic ultrasound has become an important and often necessary tool to aid in the diagnosis and management of intraocular pathology. Whenever ophthalmoscopic evaluation is limited or obscured, ophthalmic ultrasound should be utilized to evaluate the posterior segment.

Common indications for diagnostic ultrasound include opacification of the cornea, cataract, vitreous hemorrhage secondary to systemic disease or trauma, and evaluation and differentiation of noted pathology, such as mass lesions.[1,2] This chapter describes the echographic evaluation and findings in vitreoretinal disease using the techniques of standardized echography.[3,4]

Standardized echography was first introduced in ophthalmology in the early 1970s by Dr. Karl Ossoinig. It is considered to be the combination of a contact B-scan and standardized A-scan in which a set of prescribed examination techniques is used.[4] Ophthalmic ultrasound (both B- and A-scan) utilizes a relatively high frequency (8–10 MHz), which produces improved resolution in superficial structures.[1] As the sound travels through the eye, it is reflected by the intraocular structures, and signals or echoes are returned to the screen. B-scan or brightness modulation provides two-dimensional images of a series of dots and lines (▶ Fig. 6.1a). A-scan or amplitude modulation provides a one-dimensional image of vertical deflections from a baseline (▶ Fig. 6.1b). The brightness or height of the signals returned depends on the density of the structure producing the signal, the angle of incidence of the sound beam, the acoustic impedance of the tissues through which it is passing, and the gain (decibel) level used on the machine.[1,2,3,4]

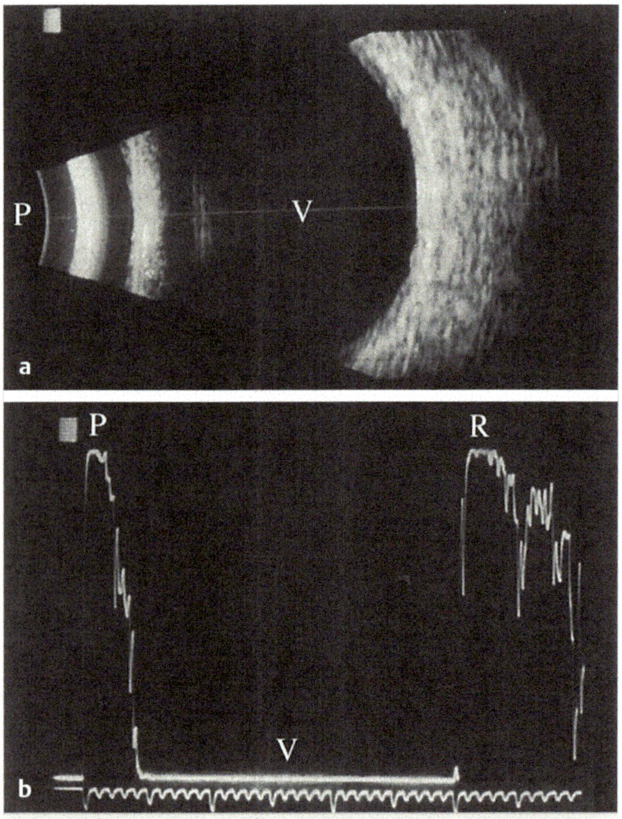

Fig. 6.1 Normal echograms. **(a)** Transverse B-scan. P, probe on the eye; V, vitreous cavity. **(b)** Standardized A-scan. P, probe on the eye; V, vitreous; R, retina and other fundus and orbit signals.

Special Considerations

The brightness or height of the signals returned depends on the following:

- Density of the structure producing the signal
- Angle of incidence of the sound beam
- Acoustic impedance of the tissues through which it is passing
- Gain (decibel) level used on the machine

B-scan provides the topographic information about intraocular structures. This includes shape, location, extension, and mobility and frequently a gross estimation of height or thickness of tissue can be obtained. The standardized A-scan has a specially designed S-shaped amplifier that allows for differentiation of tissue.[5,6] The standardized A-scan provides information necessary to secure a diagnosis, including structure (size and distribution of cells), reflectivity (height of spikes), sound attenuation (absorption), mobility, and vascularity.

6.2 Basic Screening Techniques

It is best to begin with a maximum gain setting on the B-scan for evaluating the vitreous. Evaluation at a decreased decibel level may lead to misdiagnosis because scattering of the reflected sound occurs secondary to the small size of opacities that may be present relative to the diameter of the sound beam.

Pearls

- It is best to begin with a maximum gain setting on the B-scan for evaluating the vitreous.

As mentioned previously, using a consistent screening sequence aids the echographer in obtaining a reliable, thorough examination. It also helps the screener feel confident in understanding what probe position correlates with the area of the eye being examined.

The best resolution is obtained when the probe is placed directly on the globe, as opposed to an examination through the lids. Every interface that the sound travels through decreases the amount of energy that enters the globe. Performing the examination on the globe also enables the echographer to control the patient's gaze.

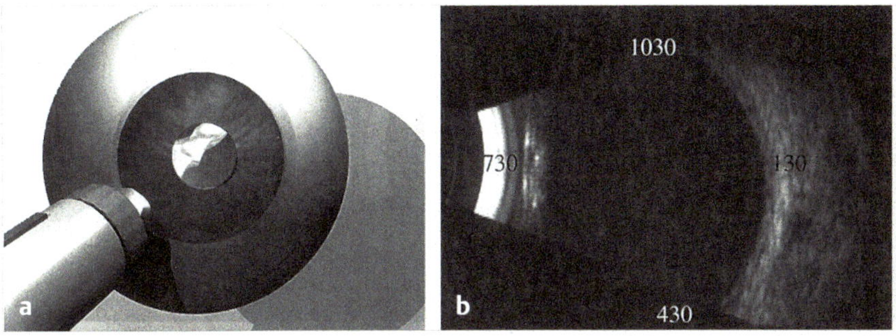

Fig. 6.2 (**a**) Schematic computer image showing the correct placement of the probe and marker when an oblique transverse scan is performed. (**b**) Oblique transverse B-scan. The probe is placed inferotemporally (7:30) with the sound beam directed superonasally (1:30). The marker is directed at 10:30 (top of screen) and opposite is 4:30 (bottom of screen).

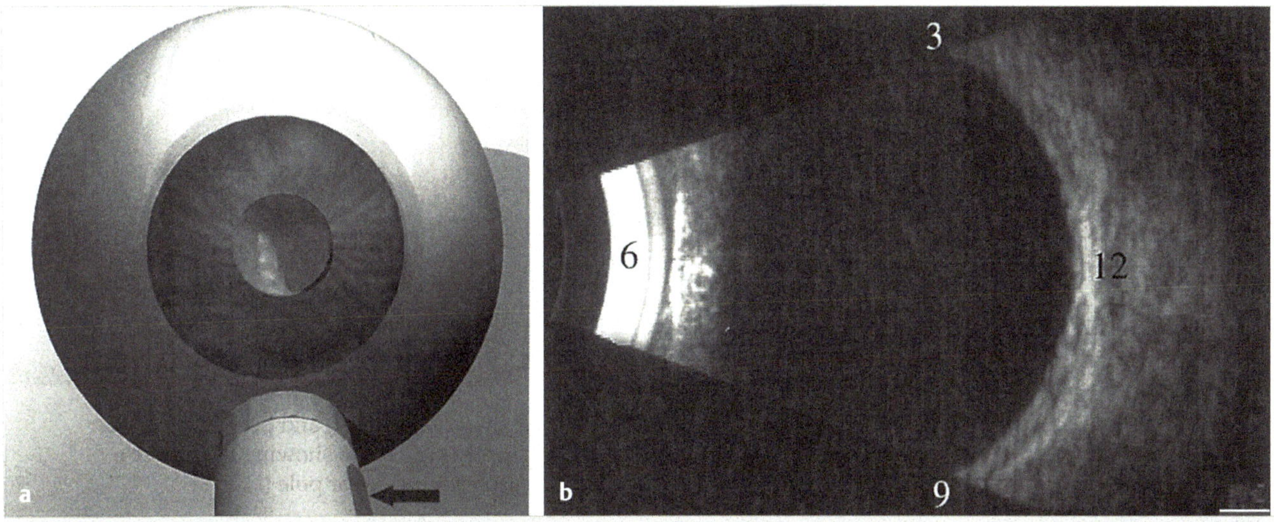

Fig. 6.3 (**a**) Schematic computer image showing placement of the probe to perform a horizontal transverse scan to evaluate the superior fundus of the right eye. The marker is directed nasally (*arrow*). (**b**) B-scan of the superior fundus. Identification of the echogram should be the meridian and the location along the meridian. The probe is placed interiorly (6), the sound is directed superiorly (12), and the marker is directed nasally and represents the upper portion of the echogram (3) and opposite is temporal (9). The sound is sweeping across the superior fundus from 9:00 to 3:00.

The probe is placed on the globe opposite the area to be examined, and the initial line on the B-scan corresponds to the probe on the eye. The marker on the probe acts as the orientation point and corresponds to the upper portion of the echogram. To evaluate the superior and inferior fundus, the marker should be directed toward the nose (horizontal transverse). To evaluate the nasal and temporal fundus, the marker should be directed up toward 12 o'clock position (vertical transverse). The best detail of pathology is obtained in the central portion of the echogram. If the pathology is not located at one of the major meridians (12, 3, 6, or 9 o'clock position), an oblique transverse scan can be used to center the pathology in the echogram. With these cuts, the marker should be directed up at an angle (▸ Fig. 6.2). With transverse scans, the sound beam is aligned perpendicularly to the fundus. This type of scan allows for the evaluation of a thin cross-section of tissue of six clock hours (▸ Fig. 6.3).

Pearls

- The best detail of pathology is obtained in the central portion of the echogram. If the pathology is not located at one of the major meridians, an oblique transverse scan can be used to center the pathology.

To be sure that all regions of the globe are evaluated adequately, the screening of each quadrant should begin with the probe face directed at the limbus for evaluation of the posterior pole. As the echographer slowly shifts the probe into the fornix, the entire fundus to the periphery is visualized. Once cross-sectional evaluation of the eye has been obtained, it is useful to evaluate any areas of interest using a longitudinal (radial) approach; in this type of scan, the sound beam is aligned parallel to the fundus. Longitudinal scans allow for evaluation of a single meridian from its most posterior aspect to the far periphery (▸ Fig. 6.4). This is accomplished by directing the marker at the corneal limbus opposite the area to be examined. Axial scans provide a pleasing, generally understandable picture; however, the information obtained from these scans can be limited, and because they require placing the probe directly on the cornea, the risk for abrasion increases with their use (▸ Fig. 6.5).

Once the eye has been screened with the B-scan, it may be necessary to incorporate the standardized A-scan, particularly if pathology is present that cannot be differentiated with the B-scan alone. To evaluate normal and abnormal tissue accurately with the standardized A-scan, the gain should be set at a decibel level known as *tissue sensitivity*.[5,6,7] Each probe and machine combination has a separate, standard tissue setting that makes the equipment sensitive to variations in tissue and

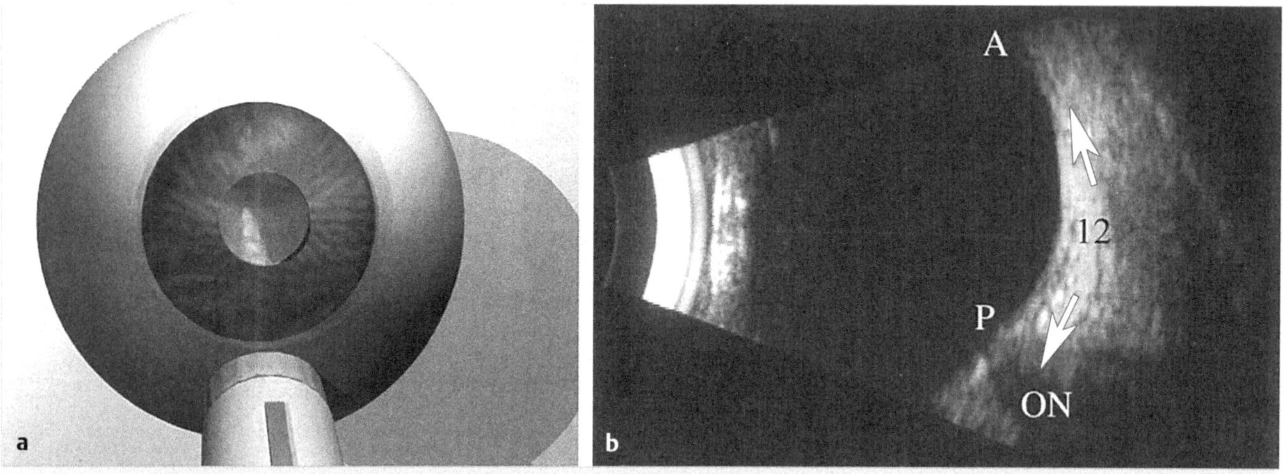

Fig. 6.4 (a) Schematic computer image showing the correct placement of the probe and the marker to evaluate the superior fundus in longitudinal view. (b) Longitudinal B-scan of the 12 o'clock meridian (12, *arrows*) from the optic nerve (ON) to the periphery (A).

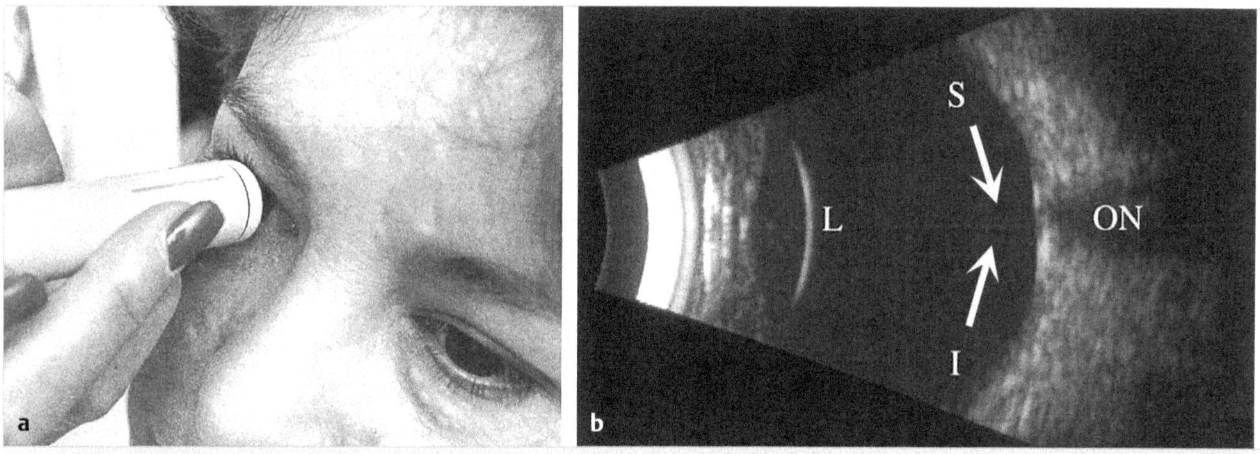

Fig. 6.5 (a) Photograph showing the correct gaze (primary) and probe and marker placement to perform a vertical axial scan. (b) Vertical axial B-scan showing the lens (L), optic nerve (ON), superior posterior pole (S), and inferior posterior pole (I).

allows for differentiation from one tissue type to another. Tissue sensitivity is determined either by the echographer using a tissue model that mimics live tissue or by the manufacturer of the equipment.

As with the B-scan, the A-scan probe is placed on the eye opposite the area to be examined. There is no marker on the A-scan because the sound beam is a parallel beam (as opposed to the B-scan, which has a focused beam). However, it should still be shifted from the limbus to the fornix for adequate evaluation of the fundus. As stated previously, the A-scan produces a single-dimension image that consists of a series of deflections (spikes) from a baseline. The height of the spikes produced as the sound encounters an interface is directly related to the density of the interface. Consequently, a maximally high spike indicates a dense interface. The space between the spikes indicates the time it takes for the sound to encounter an interface and return the signal back to the probe. This time value is then converted into distance, and measurements in millimeters can be obtained.

When mass-like lesions are evaluated, the surface of a tumor will display a maximally high signal. If signals or spikes are obtained from within the lesion, the structure and reflectivity are evaluated. The *structure* of a lesion can be categorized as either regular or irregular and is determined by aiming the sound through the lesion in different directions. If the height and distribution of the internal spikes remain consistent, the lesion is regularly structured (e.g., melanoma). If the height of the spikes varies when the sound beam is aimed through different areas, the lesion is irregularly structured (e.g., metastatic tumor).

The internal *reflectivity* of a mass lesion can be classified in various ways (low, medium-low, medium, medium-high, high, and irregular) and is determined by the density, size, and shape of interfaces within the lesion. Melanomas are comprised of small, densely compact cells of uniform proportion and distribution.[8] As sound passes through these small cells, little reflection of the sound occurs, so that reflectivity is low. Conversely, choroidal hemangiomas have large cells (blood-filled cavities) and the walls of these cavities are more reflective, producing high reflectivity.[8] Metastatic carcinomas have erratically dispersed large and small cells and interfaces, thus causing irregular reflectivity.[8]

A quick comment about B-scans with a "vector" A-scan image superimposed over the B-scan image. While almost all equipment currently on the market has this "vector" capability, those performing ultrasound examinations should be aware that this technique holds no diagnostic value and, therefore, should not be utilized to evaluate the reflectivity of structures. The vector A-scan is simply a one-dimensional duplication of the B-scan image. If the gain is turned up, the spikes will be high, and conversely if the gain is decreased, the spikes will be low.

Pearls

- The internal reflectivity of a mass-like structure is determined by the density, size, and shape of interfaces within the lesion.

The kinetic properties of pathologic structures are features that are evaluated during the dynamic portion of the examination using both the B- and A-scans. Mobility (aftermovement) is most obvious and appreciated during the B-scan screening when patients move their eyes in the same direction that the sound beam is moving (up and down for vertical transverse and left or right for horizontal transverse). If the patient has trouble with eye movement or the pathology does not readily move, the patient's head position can be shifted. Vascularity may be noted on the B-scan when large vessels are present. Detection of fast, flickering motion in the valleys of spikes on A-scan may be the best way to determine the presence of blood flow.

6.3 Evaluation of the Vitreous

A maximally high gain (decibel level) should be used to evaluate the vitreous cavity. It is important to note that dispersed opacities and dispersed hemorrhage appear identical acoustically. Having accurate clinical information can help in the distinction of one from the other. For instance, if a patient presents with an anterior chamber hyphema and opacities are noted within the vitreous cavity on ultrasound examination, the probability that opacities are red blood cells is increased and the echographer can feel comfortable reporting the echographic findings as vitreous hemorrhage. If, on the other hand, a patient presents with a dense cataract and the clinical history is limited but opacities are noted within the vitreous echographically, the echography report should describe the findings as simply "vitreous opacities."

Special Considerations

- Dispersed opacities and hemorrhage in the vitreous cavity appear identical acoustically.

6.3.1 Normal Vitreous

In a normal globe, especially that of a child or young adult, the vitreous cavity is devoid of any acoustic signals and appears black or echolucent on the B-scan. On standardized A-scan, the baseline remains flat throughout the scan (▶ Fig. 6.1).[6] During the normal aging process, the vitreous gel begins to solidify and opacities in varying amounts may form (▶ Fig. 6.6). There may be significant contracture of the vitreous gel and the posterior hyaloid surface may separate from the retina.

6.3.2 Asteroid Hyalosis

Asteroid hyalosis is a unilateral condition characterized by the formation of calcium soaps within the vitreous gel. These soaps appear as bright, round signals on B-scan. On standardized A-scan, each opacity produces its own echo spike (▶ Fig. 6.7). Generally these opacities exhibit distinct singular movement on both A- and B-scans.[9]

6.3.3 Endophthalmitis

This infection in the eye can be fungal or bacterial in nature and is most often seen following surgery or penetrating injury.[10] Patients may present with pain and decreased vision, and clinically a hypopyon is noted in the anterior chamber. Echographically, the findings vary depending on the severity of the infection. Generally, opacities are noted and membrane formation is present. In the most severe cases, retinal detachment and/or choroidal detachments may be present (▶ Fig. 6.8).[11] Serial ultrasounds may be useful in cases of endophthalmitis to evaluate and confirm the progression of the infection or in cases in which differentiation of pathology is difficult and confirmation of the findings is necessary.

6.3.4 Vitreous Hemorrhage

Patients with vitreous hemorrhage secondary to trauma or systemic disease probably account for the majority referred for ultrasound examination. Hemorrhage in the vitreous appears as small, white echoes on B-scan, and generally, the more echoes seen, the greater the density. It is possible to differentiate fresh hemorrhage (▶ Fig. 6.9) from clotted hemorrhage (▶ Fig. 6.10).[11,12] When a posterior vitreous detachment is present, it appears as an extensive, smooth membrane on B-scan. Although the posterior hyaloid face can produce a significant spike on standardized A-scan, it is generally less than 100% tall. It is important for the echographer to note any areas of the fundus where the posterior hyaloid remains adherent to the

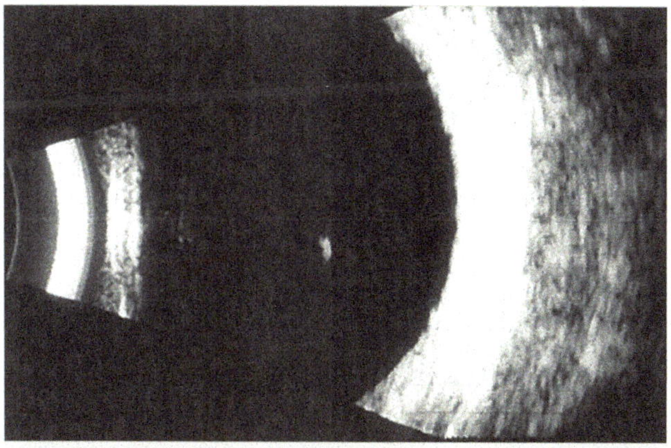

Fig. 6.6 B-scan showing a relatively clear vitreous body with a single opacity.

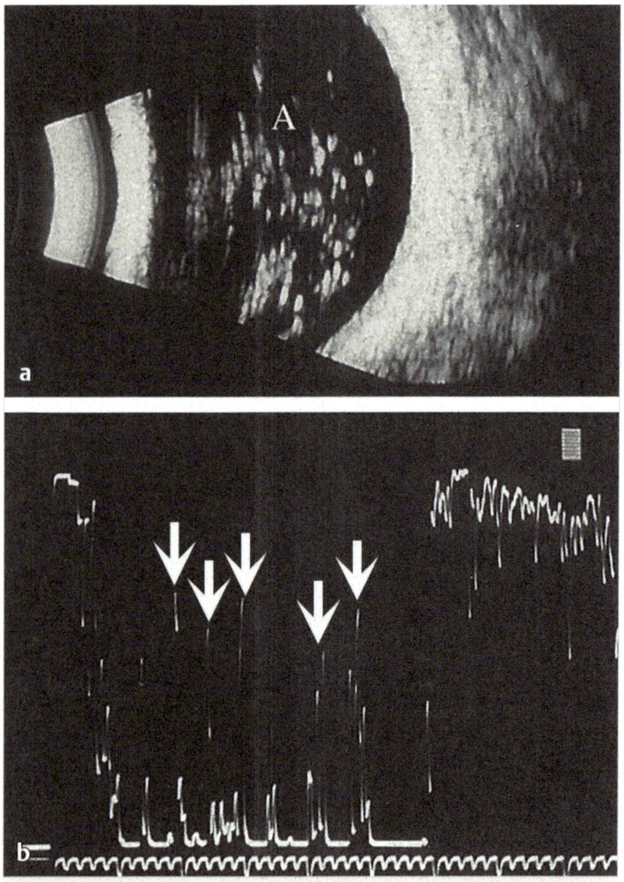

Fig. 6.7 Asteroid hyalosis. (**a**) Transverse B-scan section showing mild, dispersed asteroid hyalosis bodies (A) within the vitreous gel. (**b**) Standardized A-scan showing multiple, moderately reflective spikes produced by the dispersed asteroid bodies (*arrows*).

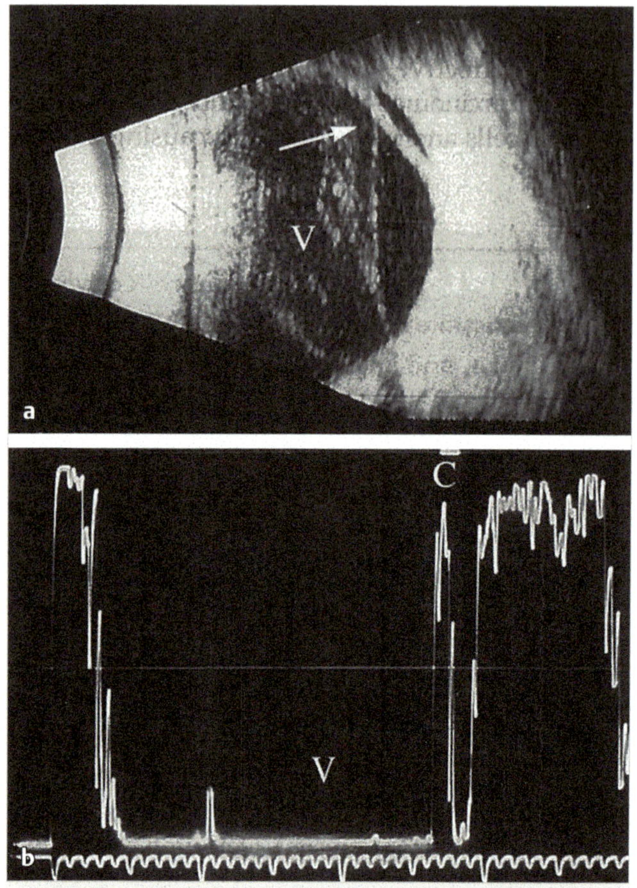

Fig. 6.8 Endophthalmitis. (**a**) Longitudinal B-scan section showing dispersed opacities and membranes within the vitreous cavity (V). Arrow shows shallow, localized choroidal detachment. (**b**) Standardized A-scan shows very low reflective spikes from the vitreous opacities (V) and a double-peaked, highly reflective spike from the shallow choroidal detachment (C).

retina. Frequently, blood may collect beneath the posterior hyaloid (▶ Fig. 6.11). This subhyaloid blood can be dispersed or clotted, and having patients move their eyes or turn their head will move the blood away from the pooled area so retinal detachment can be ruled out.[9,11]

Pearls

- Although the posterior hyaloid face can produce a significant spike on standardized A-scan, it will generally be *less than* 100% tall. This is in contrast to the spike of a detached retina, which is almost *always* 100% tall.

6.4 Evaluation of the Retina

The retina is a somewhat dense membrane, and when the direction of the sound beam is perpendicular to it, it produces a steeply rising, high (100% tall compared with the initial spike) spike.[9,11,13] On B-scan, the typical echographic features of an extensive or total retinal detachment include the following: a dense, thick, often folded membrane that inserts into the optic disc (when totally detached).[9,11,13] Generally, the retina will exhibit some mobility, depending on the length of time it has been detached. The longer the detachment has been present, the less mobile and more folded it becomes. Dense vitreous membranes and retinal detachment can look very similar echographically, so it is very important for the echographer to recognize the findings that can help to distinguish one from the other (▶ Fig. 6.12).[14]

6.4.1 Retinal Tears

When a patient presents with sudden onset of decreased vision secondary to vitreous hemorrhage, ultrasound can be useful in detecting small retinal tears.[9,15] Small tears are most frequently located in the superior quadrant, but they can be noted anywhere in the peripheral fundus.[9,15] On B-scan, small tears appear as highly reflective tufts of elevated tissue. In almost all cases, a thin vitreous membrane adherent to the flap can be detected.[15] On standardized A-scan, the flap tear will produce a maximally high spike separate from the other fundus spikes (▶ Fig. 6.13). It is important to note if the adjacent retina is detached (▶ Fig. 6.14). Observation while the blood clears is generally the treatment of choice, followed by cryotherapy or laser treatment once the view improves. Ultrasound-guided cryotherapy may be a viable early treatment option in some patients.[15,16]

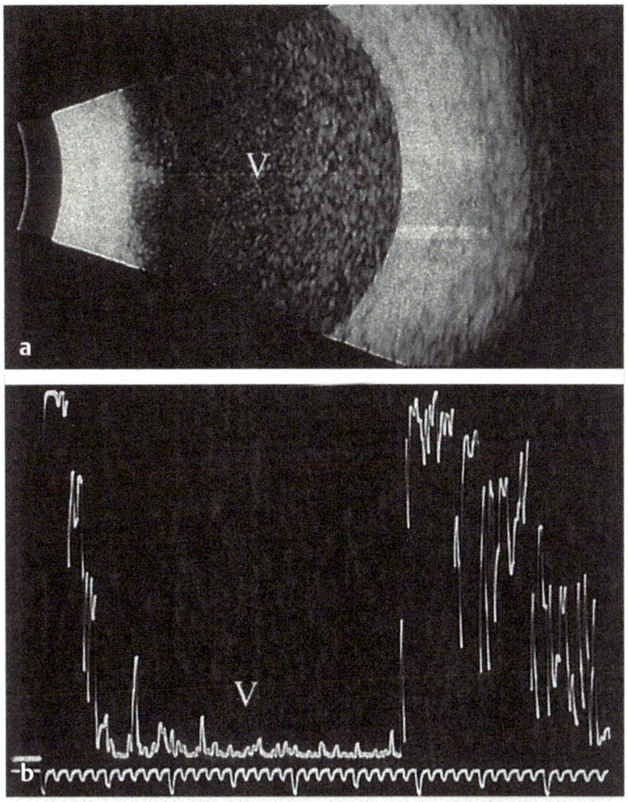

Fig. 6.9 Vitreous hemorrhage. (**a**) Transverse B-scan showing dense, dispersed hemorrhage filling the vitreous cavity (V) of an eye after vitrectomy. (**b**) Standardized A-scan showing a low chain of spikes along the vitreous baseline produced by the dispersed red blood cells (V).

Pearls

- When a patient presents with sudden onset of decreased vision secondary to vitreous hemorrhage, ultrasound can be useful in detecting relatively small retinal tears.

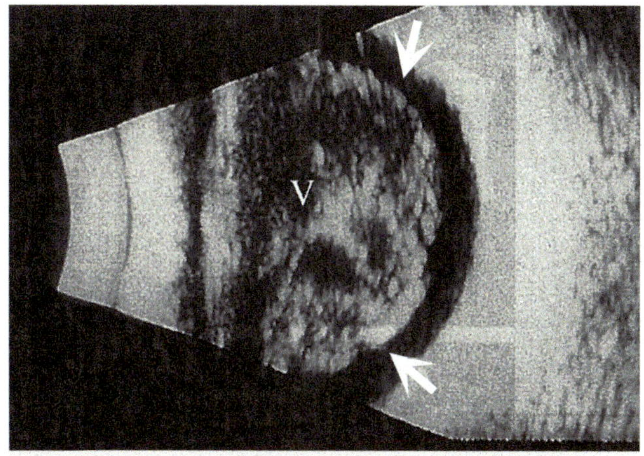

Fig. 6.10 Vitreous hemorrhage. Transverse (cross-section) B-scan showing very dense, clotted hemorrhage (V) confined within a posterior vitreous detachment (*arrows*).

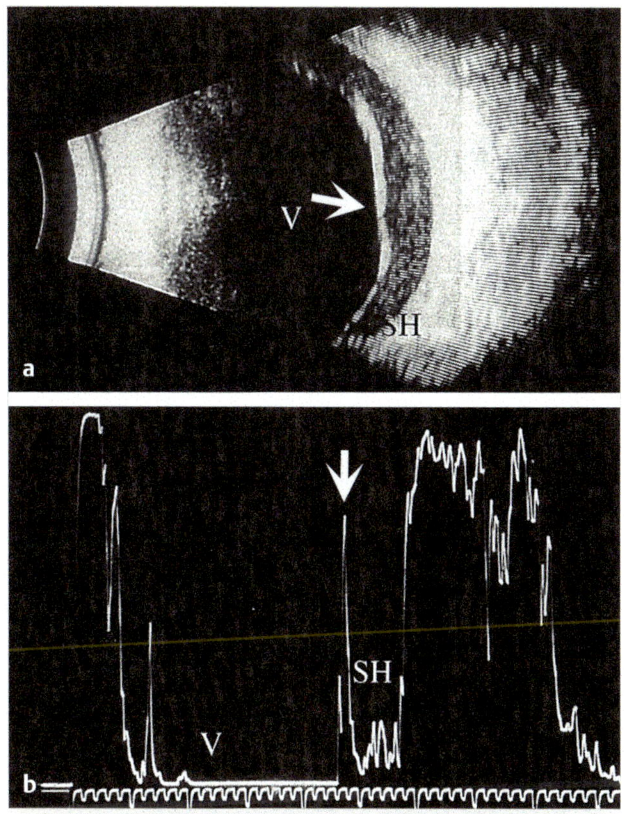

Fig. 6.11 Subhyaloid hemorrhage. (**a**) Transverse B-scan shows a relatively clear vitreous body (V) and dense posterior vitreous detachment (*arrow*) with dispersed subhyaloid hemorrhage (SH). (**b**) Standardized A-scan; the vitreous baseline is flat (V), a moderately high signal is produced from the posterior vitreous detachment (*arrow*), and a low chain of spikes is produced from the subhyaloid hemorrhage (SH).

6.4.2 Traction Retinal Detachment

Traction retinal detachment is a common finding in patients with diabetic disease or trauma, but it can also be seen in other disease processes. It is caused by the strong adherence and exertion of vitreous membranes, bands, or the posterior hyaloid face to areas of the retina. As the posterior vitreous moves away from the retina, elevation occurs. The adhesions can be focal, causing a "tentlike" traction (▶ Fig. 6.15), or broad, causing "tabletop" traction (▶ Fig. 6.16).[9,11] These types of detachments are most readily seen with the B-scan, although in some instances, when the elevation of the retina is minimal, the standardized A-scan can be useful in confirming detachment.

6.4.3 Localized Retinal Detachment

The retina can be detached in localized areas. Differentiation between retinal detachment and vitreous membrane formation becomes vital in these cases. The B-scan can be most helpful in mapping the extent of detachment when both transverse and longitudinal scans are used. The standardized A-scan should be used for confirmation of retinal detachment based on the height of the spike produced when the sound beam is aimed

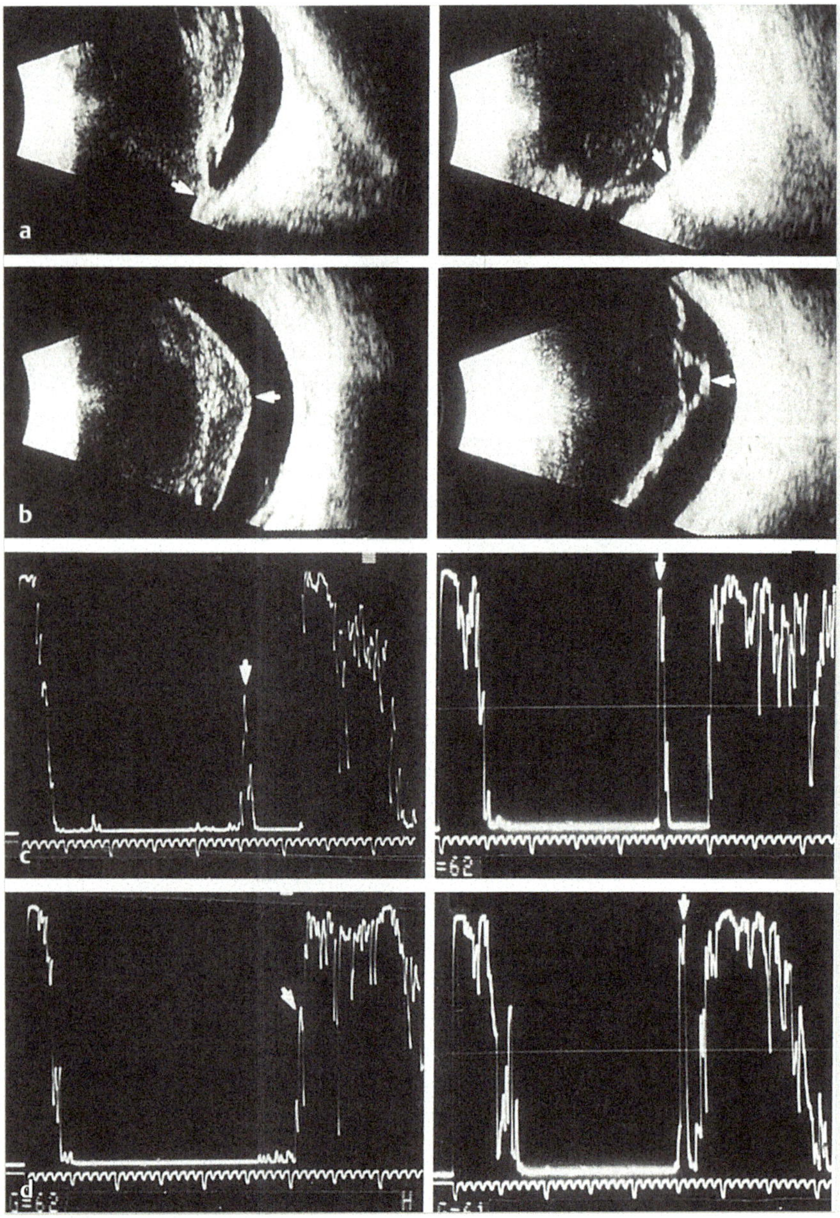

Fig. 6.12 The echographic findings in eyes with dense vitreous membrane formation can often be confusing, even to the most experienced echographer. Certain features of retinal detachment and dense vitreous membranes can assist the echographer in distinguishing between the two. (a) It is not uncommon for vitreous membranes to insert into or close to the optic disc (*left, arrow*). Retina almost always inserts into the disc (*right, arrow*). (b) B-scans: The posterior vitreous generally has a smooth consistency (*left, arrow*), whereas the retina is more folded (*right, arrow*). (c) A-scans: Although the vitreous membrane appears to be dense on B-scan, it does not produce a high-amplitude signal on A-scan (*left, arrow*). The retina almost always produces a maximally high signal (*right, arrow*). (d) The vitreous has a very weak insertion into the fundus in the region of the ora (*left, arrow*), whereas the retina maintains a maximally high signal at the ora (*right, arrow*).

perpendicularly to the retina. There can be focal detachment of the retina involving the macula or extensive detachment of the peripheral retina sparing the posterior pole.

6.4.4 Total Retinal Detachment

When there is a limited view of the posterior segment, ultrasonography can help determine the extent and duration of retinal detachment. Based on certain echographic features, a long-standing detachment can be differentiated from one that has occurred recently. In fresh detachments, the retina may be quite mobile and only slightly folded (▶ Fig. 6.17). As time passes, the vitreous space becomes limited and membranes may form and adhere to the retina from all sides, causing proliferative vitreoretinopathy (▶ Fig. 6.18).[13,17] B-scan is an excellent way to view the topography of total retinal detachments. When the retina is completely detached, it almost always remains adherent to the optic disc. It will also remain attached to the peripheral fundus near the ora. The A-scan can be useful in some cases in which multiple membranes are noted, but the diagnosis can generally be made with the B-scan. Other features, such as cysts (▶ Fig. 6.19), and subretinal opacities, such as blood (▶ Fig. 6.20), can also be documented with ultrasound.[9,11]

Pearls

- When the retina is completely detached, it almost always remains adherent to the optic disc.

6.4.5 Retinopathy of Prematurity

Retinopathy of prematurity is most commonly a bilateral condition characterized by vitreous membranes and peripheral traction retinal detachments. The amount of detachment varies

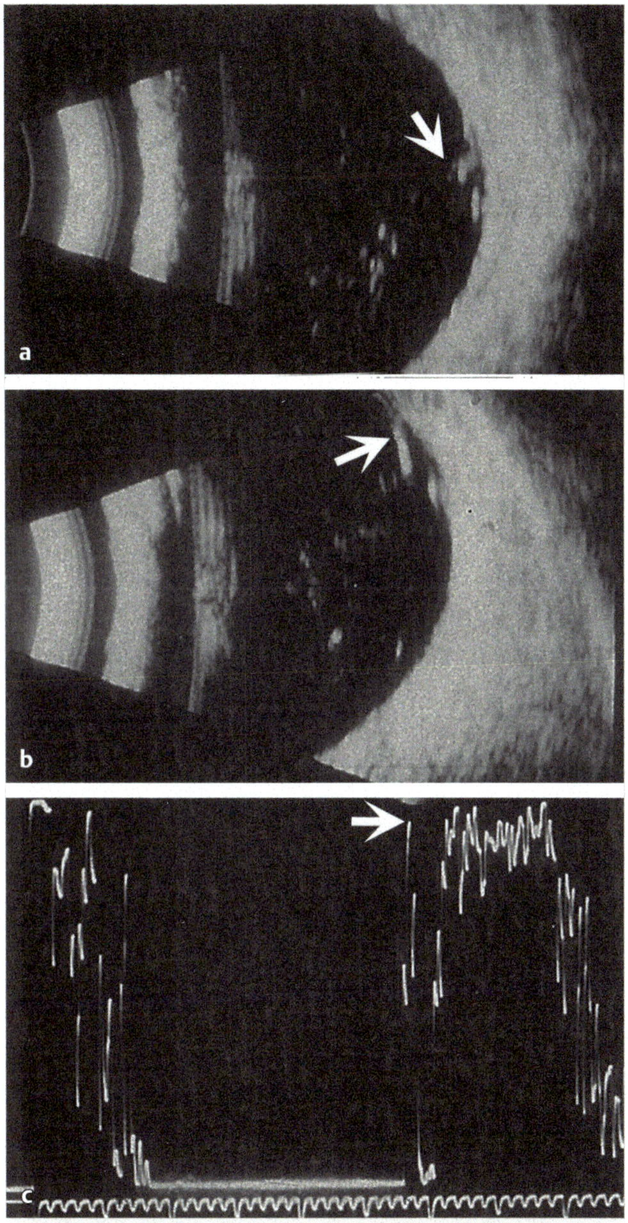

Fig. 6.13 Retinal tears. (**a**) Transverse B-scan shows mild vitreous hemorrhage (*V*) with a focal vitreoretinal adhesion and highly reflective tuft of elevated tissue (*arrow*). (**b**) Longitudinal B-scan shows the peripheral location of the flap tear (*arrow*). (**c**) Standardized A-scan. When a tear is large enough or the flap is elevated, a highly reflective spike can be obtained from the area of the tear (*arrowhead*).

with classification of the disease. In the most severe stage (stage V), total detachment in a narrow, funnel-shaped configuration is usually detected. Peripheral troughs may be formed by traction from a dense retrolental membrane. Other findings include subretinal hemorrhage and decreased axial length (▸ Fig. 6.21).[18]

6.4.6 Persistent Fetal Vasculature

Persistence of the hyaloid artery and related structures, also known as *persistent hyperplastic primary vitreous*, is most often a unilateral condition. Echographically, the globe may be small, and a vitreous band that extends from the posterior lens surface to the posterior pole is noted. This band can be very thin and difficult to image, or markedly thickened.[9,19] Peripapillary traction retinal detachment is a finding in the most severe cases (▸ Fig. 6.22).[9,19]

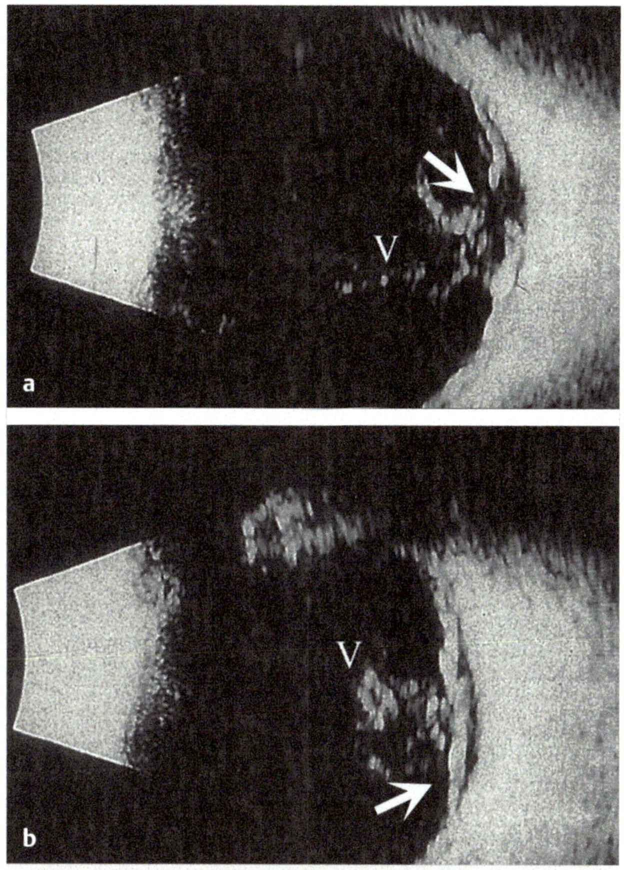

Fig. 6.14 Retinal tears and detachment. (**a**) Transverse scan showing vitreous hemorrhage (V) overlying a significant retinal tear (*arrow*). (**b**) Longitudinal scan shows vitreous hemorrhage (V) and the extent of localized shallow retinal detachment (*arrow*).

6.5 Evaluation of the Traumatized Eye

Echography can be a great help to the ophthalmologist in the evaluation of the traumatized eye. Following ocular trauma, indirect ophthalmoscopy is frequently not possible because of opacified media, as in hyphema, cataract, or vitreous hemorrhage, or because of edematous eyelids and decreased patient cooperation. Echography can supplement the clinical examination by permitting evaluation of the intraocular structures to facilitate treatment.

An attempt at a complete ophthalmoscopic evaluation is necessary before echographic evaluation to determine whether the globe has been ruptured. Surgical repair of the rupture site is generally performed before ultrasonography is attempted. However, in some instances, when a foreign body is suspected and the exact location cannot be confirmed with either plain

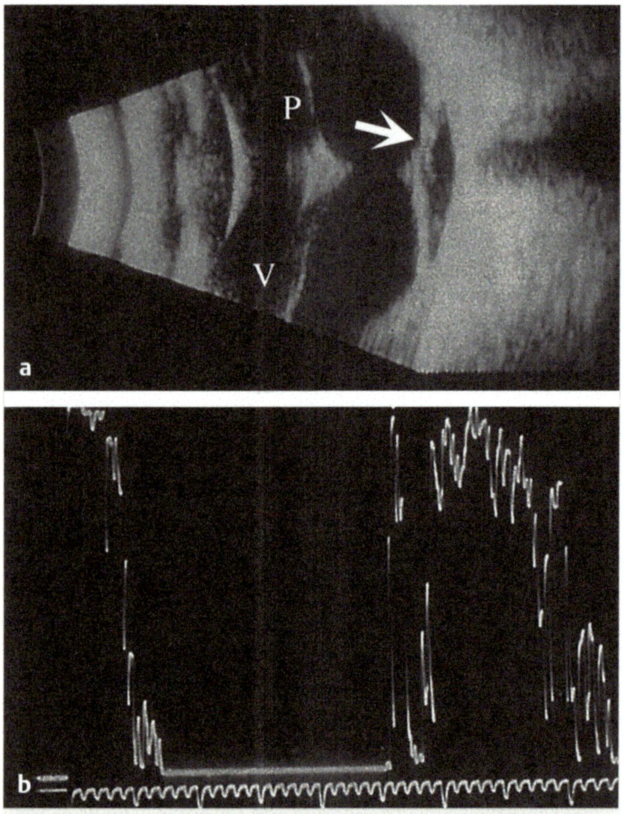

Fig. 6.15 Traction retinal detachment. (**a**) Axial B-scan showing vitreous hemorrhage (V). The posterior hyaloid is detached anteriorly (P) but is still adherent to the posterior retina, causing a tentlike traction retinal detachment (*arrow*). (**b**) A-scan demonstrates a dense, maximally high signal produced by the retinal detachment (*arrow*).

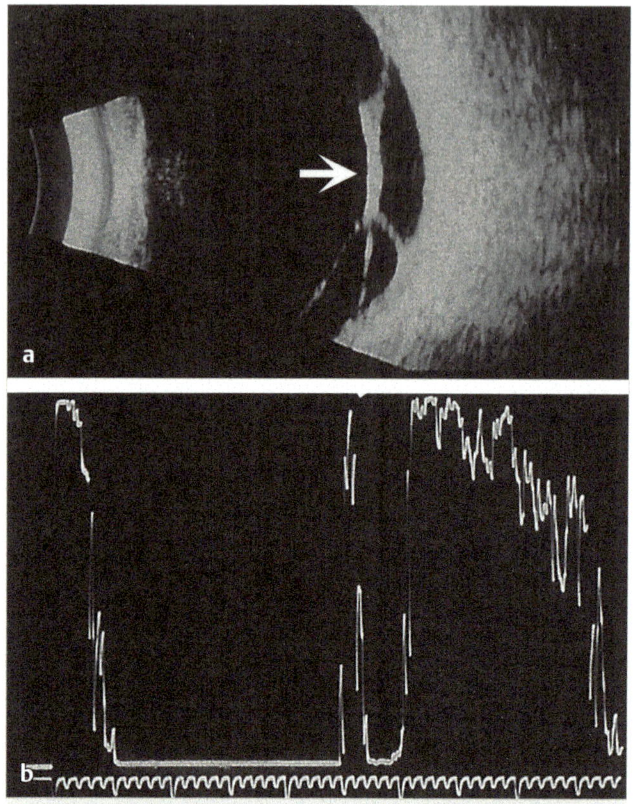

Fig. 6.16 Traction retinal detachment. (**a**) Cross-section B-scan of a very broad area where the vitreous remains adherent to the retina, causing a localized "tabletop" traction retinal detachment (*arrow*). (**b**) A-scan showing the typical, maximally high spike from the surface of the traction retinal detachment (*arrow*).

films or computed tomography, very gentle ultrasound examination through the lids, in the hands of an experienced echographer, may yield the necessary information to assist in the removal of the foreign body. This can be done in the operating room using sterile techniques.

When ultrasound examination is performed through the lids, a generous amount of methylcellulose is needed as a coupling agent to allow the echographer to apply minimal pressure on the globe and simultaneously obtain informative echograms. Increasing the system sensitivity or gain counterbalances some of the sound attenuation that occurs from the eyelids. Serial echographic studies as swelling and hemorrhage resorb may be necessary to confirm the initial echographic findings in selected cases.

Controversial Points

- Surgical repair of a ruptured globe is generally performed *before* ultrasonography is attempted. Occasionally, when an intraocular foreign body (IOFB) is present, ultrasound may be employed preoperatively (with caution) if other tests, such as computed tomography, do not provide all the information needed to plan the surgical approach.

6.5.1 Dislocated Lens

Following severe blunt or penetrating trauma, the lens can be displaced posteriorly or detached from the zonules and be seen floating in the vitreous or lying against the retina. Stands of vitreous may be attached to the dislocated lens (▶ Fig. 6.23).

6.5.2 Penetrating and Perforating Injury

When any sharp foreign object (e.g., pencil, knife, or needle) penetrates the vitreous gel, hemorrhage will line up along the tract left by the foreign body. Hemorrhagic tracts may end in the vitreous or strike the retina but not exit through the other side of the globe (▶ Fig. 6.24).[9,11] However, in some instances, when a foreign body enters the globe anteriorly and exits posteriorly, a tract usually will lead to the posterior exit site (▶ Fig. 6.25). Vitreous may become incarcerated into the wound both anteriorly and posteriorly.[9,11]

6.5.3 Intraocular Foreign Body

In most cases, IOFBs are easily detected by ultrasound. Even if radiologic studies are performed initially for localization of a foreign body, ultrasound can be a useful adjunct to determine the precise location as well as the extent of damage done to the structures within the eye.

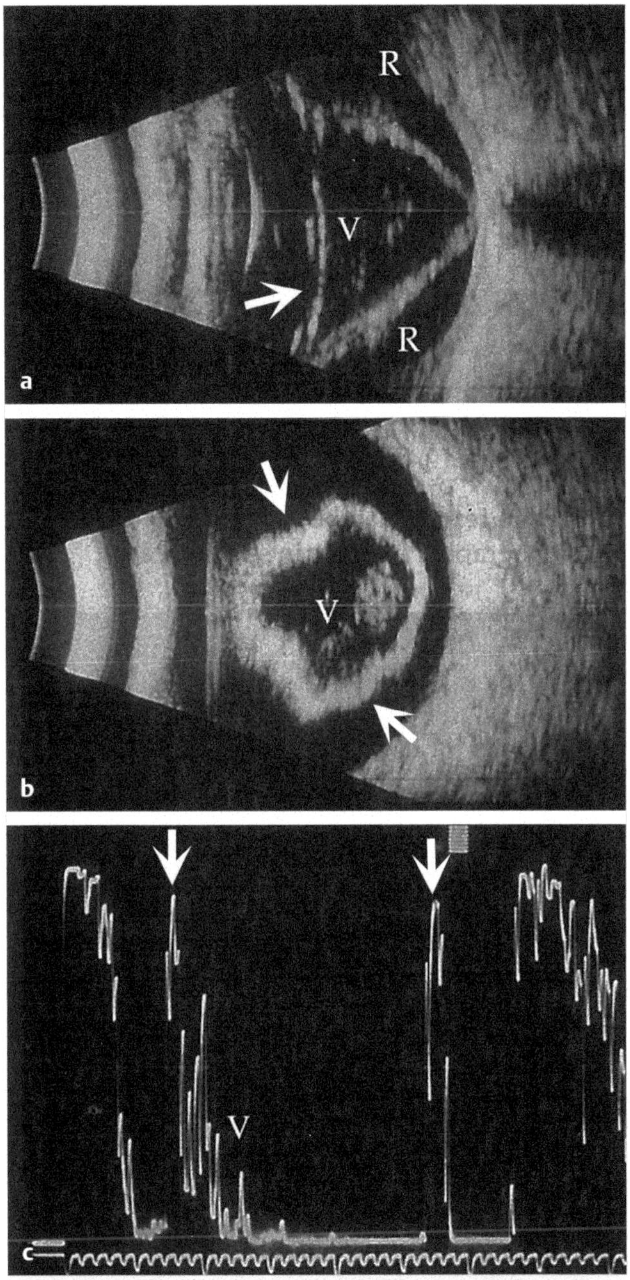

Fig. 6.17 Open funnel, total retinal detachment. (**a**) Axial B-scan showing a bridging anterior membrane (*arrow*), mild vitreous hemorrhage (V), and a wide-open funnel-shaped retinal detachment (R). (**b**) Transverse B-scan of funnel-shaped retinal detachment (*arrows*). The opacities inside the funnel represent the vitreous hemorrhage (V). (**c**) A-scan showing two maximally high spikes from the leaves of the retinal detachment (*arrows*). The chain of spikes adjacent to the first spike is produced by the hemorrhage confined within the funnel (V).

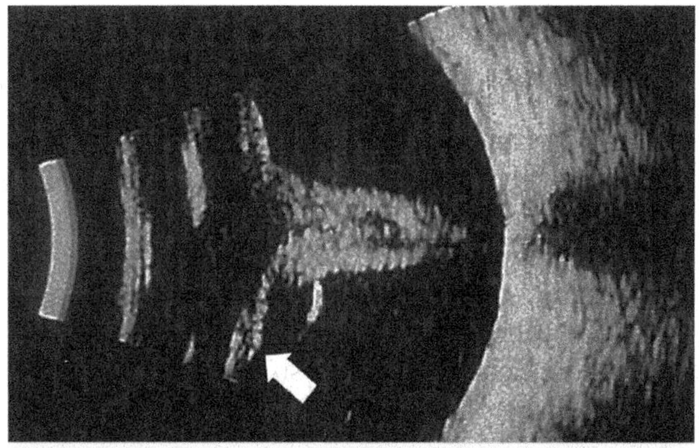

Fig. 6.19 Retinal macrocyst. Vertical axial B-scan shows a closed funnel-shaped retinal detachment and a retinal cyst interiorly (*arrow*).

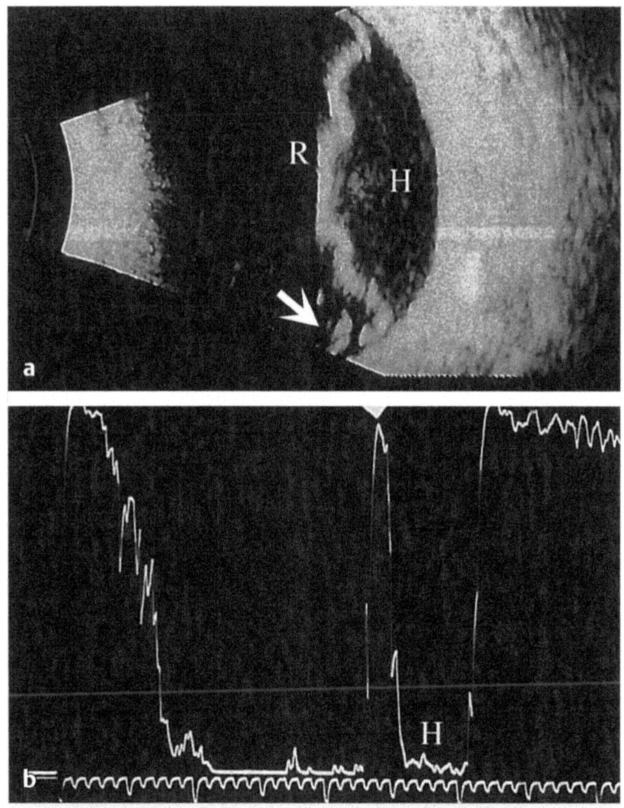

Fig. 6.20 Subretinal hemorrhage. (**a**) Transverse B-scan shows a localized, bullous retinal detachment (R) with dispersed subretinal hemorrhage (H) and a small retinal tear at the superotemporal edge (*arrow*). (**b**) A-scan shows a high spike from the retinal detachment (*arrow*) and a low chain of spikes produced by the subretinal hemorrhage (H).

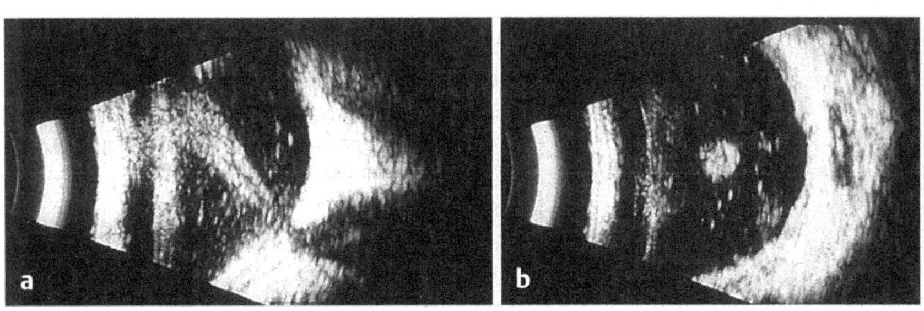

Fig. 6.18 Closed funnel, total retinal detachment. (**a**) Longitudinal B-scan showing closed funnel-shaped membrane inserting onto the optic disc. Opacities are noted beneath the funnel. (**b**) The round structure in the center of the vitreous cavity is a cross section of the closed funnel retinal detachment.

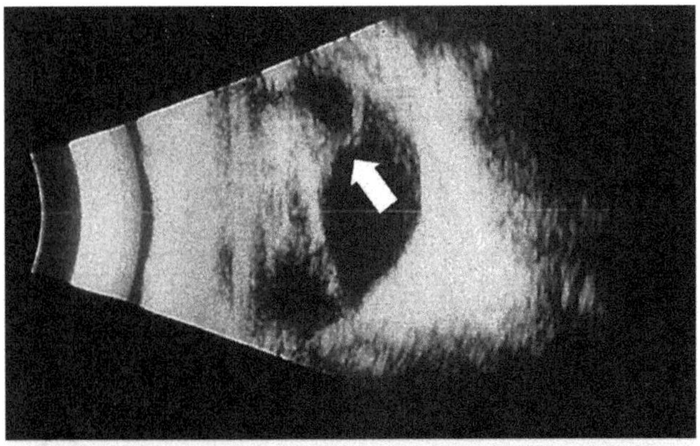

Fig. 6.21 Stage V retinopathy of prematurity. Longitudinal B-scan of an eye from an infant with stage V retinopathy of prematurity. The echographic characteristics commonly detected show dense anterior membrane formation and a narrow, closed funnel-shaped retinal detachment. Often, large peripheral troughs can be seen (*arrow*).

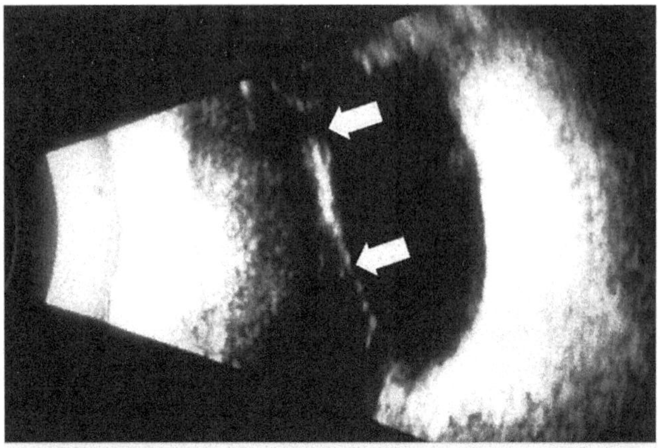

Fig. 6.22 Persistent hyperplastic primary vitreous (persistent fetal vasculature). Longitudinal B-scan showing a dense band (*arrow*) extending from the posterior lens surface to the optic disc.

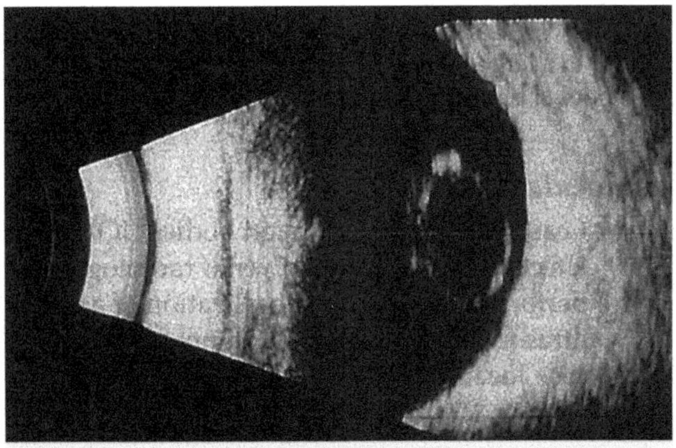

Fig. 6.23 Dislocated lens. Transverse B-scan shows the round echolucent lens in the vitreous cavity.

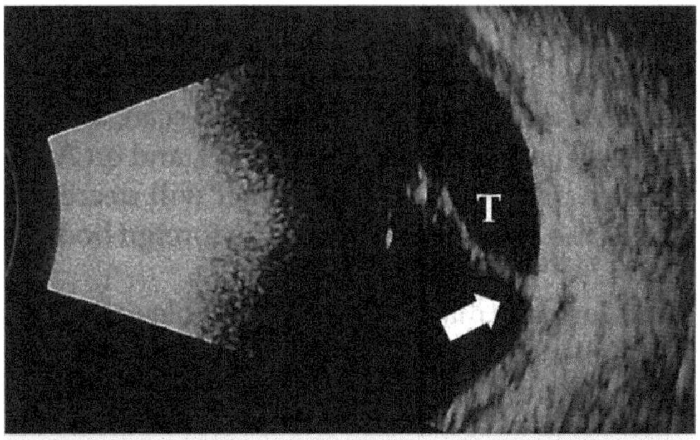

Fig. 6.24 Traumatic vitreous tract. A small metal wire entered the eye, went through the vitreous cavity, and struck the posterior globe wall before the patient pulled it out. The longitudinal scan shows the hemorrhagic tract produced by the wire (T). There is a focal area of fundus thickening at the posterior impact site (*arrow*).

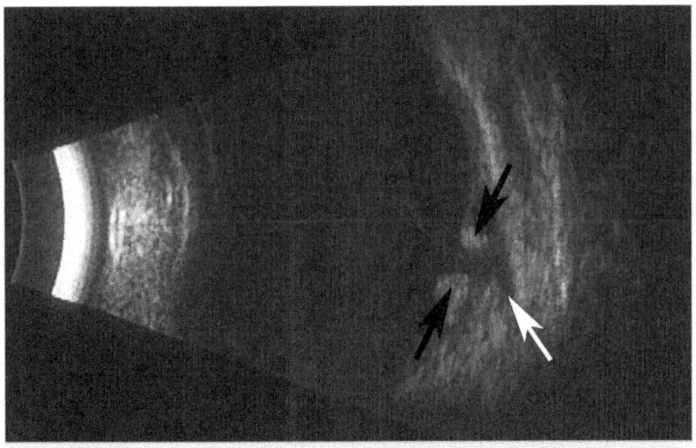

Fig. 6.25 Posterior scleral rupture. B-scan taken through the lids of a small child who sustained a penetrating eye injury after falling on a steak knife. A primary repair was performed. Ultrasound was ordered postoperatively to rule out posterior segment pathology. Ultrasound revealed a dense hemorrhagic track (*white arrow*) leading to a large posterior rupture (*black arrows*) and a large pool of blood in the orbit.

Metallic foreign bodies produce very bright signals on B-scan and very tall spikes on standardized A-scan. The composition of metallic foreign bodies may vary. However, when the sound beam is aimed at the foreign body, much of the sound is absorbed by the foreign body, thus causing a shadowing artifact in the orbit adjacent to its location (▸ Fig. 6.26).[9,11,20] Round foreign bodies produce a reverberation artifact on both B-scan and standardized A-scan. On B-scan, a chain of multiple signals will be noted (▸ Fig. 6.27), and on A-scan, the spikes produced by the artifact will decrease in height as the sound travels past the foreign body into the orbit.[9,11,20]

Glass, organic material, and air bubbles are slightly more challenging for the echographer, but they can be detected and differentiated. Follow-up ultrasound examination should be suggested whenever differentiation is difficult.

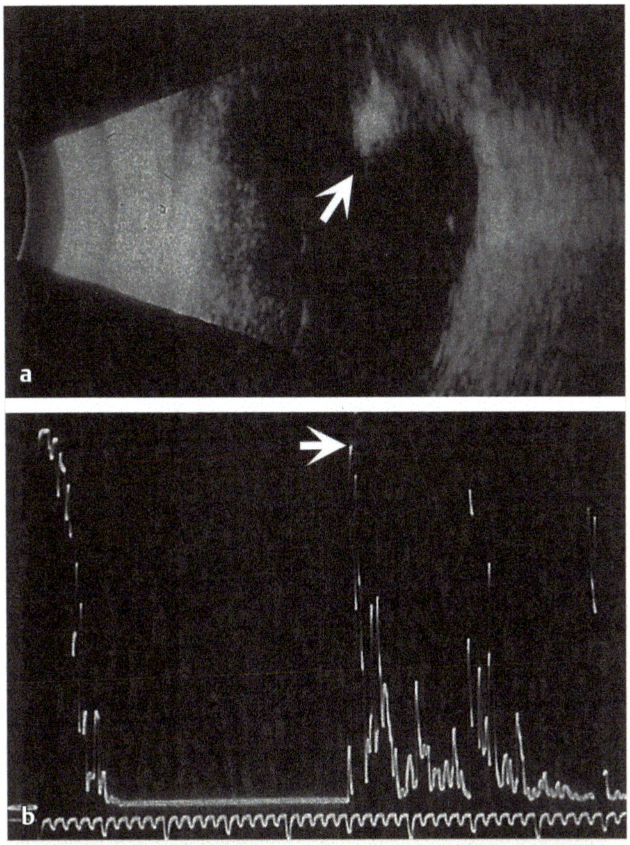

Fig. 6.26 Metallic intraocular foreign body. (**a**) Longitudinal B-scan showing a large intraocular foreign body (IOFB) (*arrow*). (**b**) A-scan taken from the region of the IOFB. The first spike (*arrow*) represents the metal fragment. Most of the sound is being absorbed by the foreign matter, causing shadowing of the orbital signals.

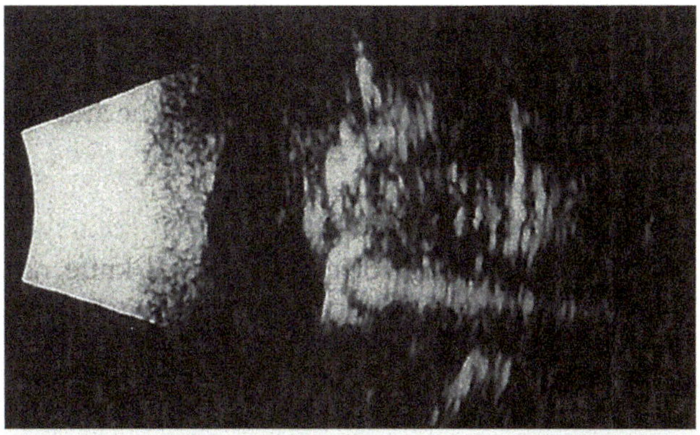

Fig. 6.27 Spherical intraocular foreign body. The "comet tail" artifact commonly seen with spherical foreign bodies.

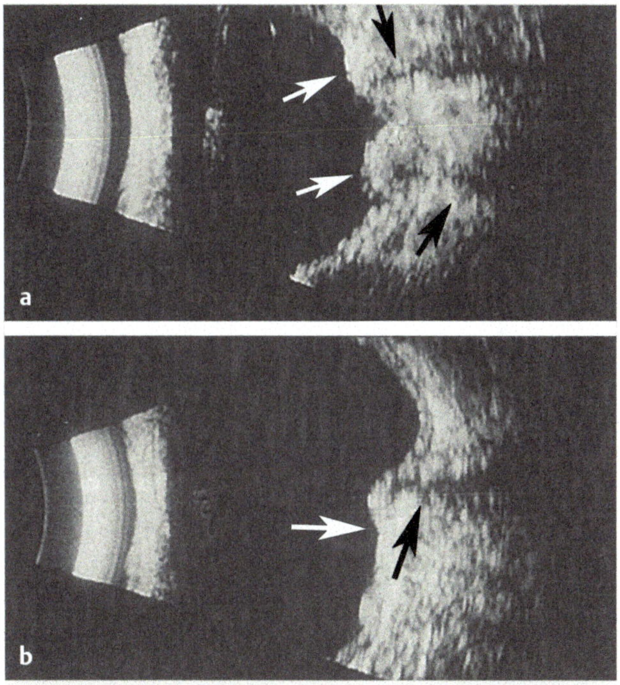

Fig. 6.28 Scleral fold. (**a**) Transverse B-scan showing multiple scleral folds (*arrows*). (**b**) Orbital shadowing is produced from the highly reflective sclera (*black arrows*).

6.5.4 Scleral Folds

Penetrating or perforating trauma can be so severe that the intraocular contents extrude from the wound and the globe wall partially or totally collapses, causing scleral infolding. Echographically, scleral folds can be mistaken for IOFBs because orbital shadowing may occur adjacent to the fold (▶ Fig. 6.28). If a scleral fold is suspected, follow-up ultrasound is useful because the fold will disappear once the eye becomes reformed.

Pearls

- Scleral folds on ultrasonography can be mistaken for IOFBs because orbital shadowing may occur adjacent to the fold.

6.6 Evaluation of the Choroid

6.6.1 Choroidal Thickening

Thickening of the choroid can be localized or diffuse and has been associated with a number of conditions, ranging from edema, in which the thickening is highly reflective (e.g., uveal effusion syndrome; ▶ Fig. 6.29), to infiltration secondary to inflammatory processes such as lymphoid hyperplasia, sympathetic ophthalmia, and Harada disease (▶ Fig. 6.30). The choroidal thickening in these latter instances is most commonly of low to medium reflectivity.[9,21] Bacterial infection from Lyme disease causes similar echographic characteristics. Diffuse choroidal thickening in the presence of mass lesions such as metastatic carcinoma, diffuse melanoma, or even lymphoma may prove difficult to differentiate echographically.[11] Follow-up examination may be useful in these cases to secure a diagnosis.

6.6.2 Choroidal Detachment

Choroidal detachments occur most commonly following an injury or during or after surgical trauma. Rarely, the choroid can detach spontaneously; therefore, access to clinical information is necessary before echographic evaluation. The echographic characteristics of choroidal detachment are usually

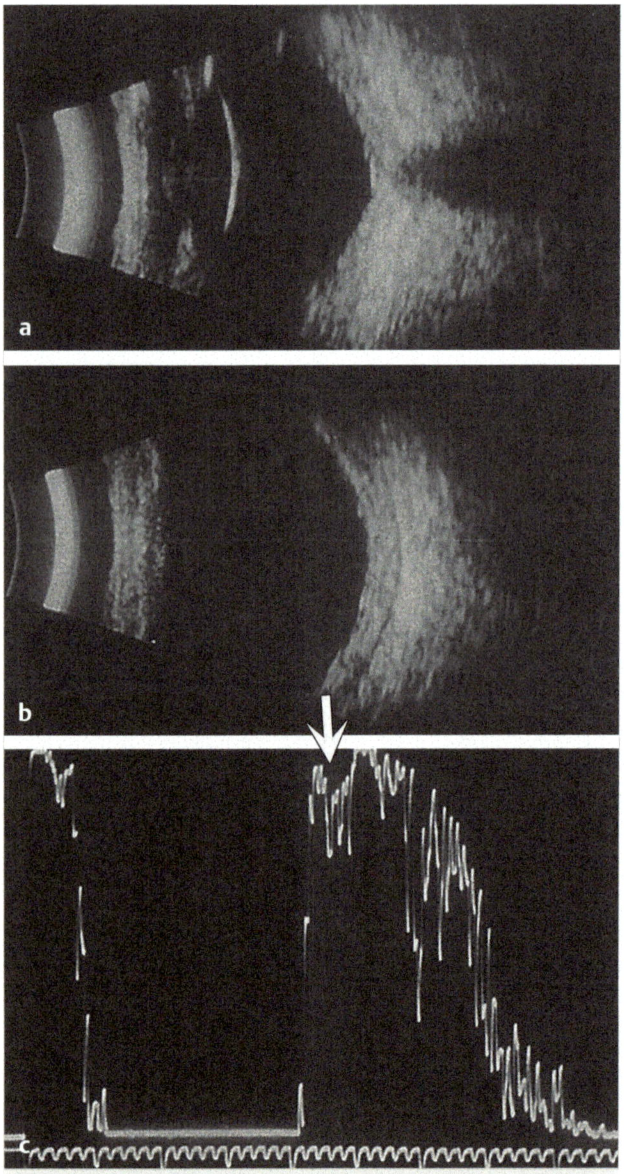

Fig. 6.29 Uveal effusion syndrome. (a) Axial-B scan shows the relatively small globe. (b) Center: Transverse B-scan shows thickening of the choroid. (c) A-scan shows the high reflectivity from the choroid (*arrowhead*).

straightforward, making the diagnosis of this pathology relatively simple.

On B-scan, a choroidal detachment presents as a smooth, dome-shaped, thick membrane that does not insert into the optic disc. The detachment may be localized or involve the entire fundus, in which case a classic scalloped appearance is seen (▶ Fig. 6.31).[9,11] During the B-scan evaluation, it is important to note the appearance of the suprachoroidal space to determine if the nature of the detachment is serous or hemorrhagic. Serous detachment will show an echolucent area beneath the surface of the detached choroid (▶ Fig. 6.31). If hemorrhage is present, the suprachoroidal space will be echodense. It is also helpful to determine if the suprachoroidal hemorrhage is more fluid in consistency or if clots have formed. Fluid hemorrhage has a similar appearance to dispersed hemorrhage in the vitreous. Clotted hemorrhage appears as extremely dense, white opacities on B-scan (▶ Fig. 6.32).[21] Often, when bullous detachment of the choroid occurs, band formation can be noted in the suprachoroidal space. This band formation is thought to be a stretched vortex vein.[9,11] The maximal elevation is another important feature to evaluate when choroidal detachments are present. If there is extensive detachment, noting the amount of vitreous space remaining between the surfaces of the choroid is important. The presence of "kissing" choroidal detachments lowers the visual prognosis, especially if they are persistent.

Pearls

- A choroidal detachment on B-scan ultrasonography appears as a smooth, dome-shaped, thick membrane that does not insert into the optic disc.

On standardized A-scan, the choroid (when detached) produces a maximally high (100% tall), thick, double-peaked (retina and choroid together) spike.[9,11] This spike exhibits little or no aftermovement. If the choroidal detachment is serous, a flat baseline will be present between the choroidal spike and the sclera (▶ Fig. 6.31). Fluid hemorrhage beneath the choroid produces a low reflective chain of spikes, and clotted blood produces a high reflective chain of spikes (▶ Fig. 6.32). The extent and location of any retinal detachment overlying the choroidal detachment should also be reported.

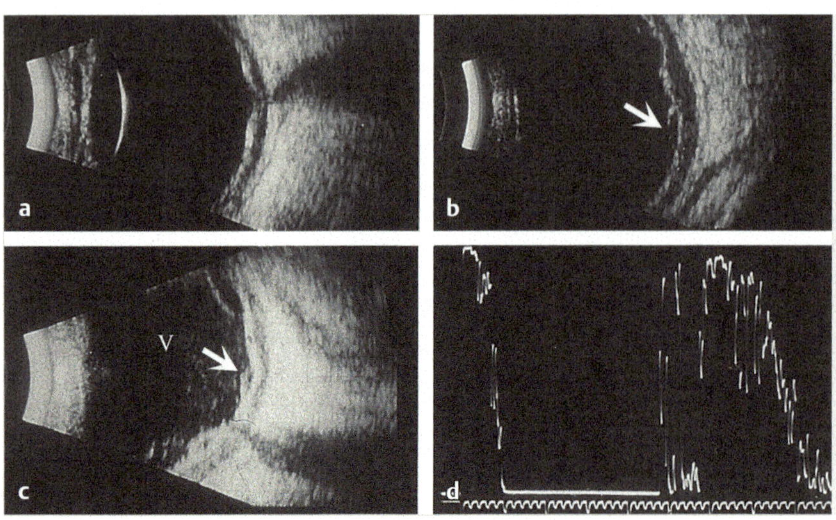

Fig. 6.30 Choroidal thickening from Harada disease. **(a)** Horizontal axial B-scan shows low reflective infiltration of the choroid in the right eye of this patient. **(b)** Transverse scan shows the choroidal infiltration in the left eye and a focal elevation of the retina overlying it (*arrow*). **(c)** Longitudinal B-scan showing dispersed vitreous opacities (V), focal macular detachment (*arrow*), and low reflective choroidal thickening. **(d)** A-scan corresponding to the top right echogram showing the spikes produced by the focal retinal detachment and choroidal thickening.

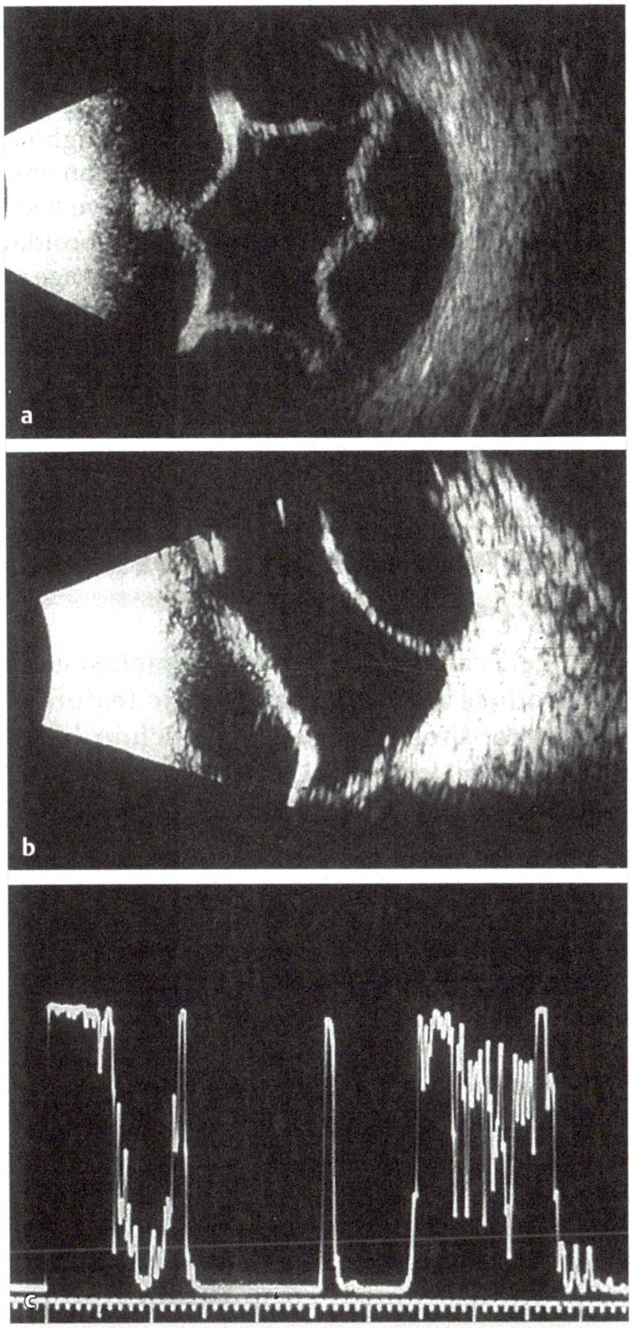

Fig. 6.31 Choroidal detachments. (a) Cross-section B-scan shows the typical scalloped appearance of 360-degree serous choroidal detachments. (b) Radial-section B-scan shows the dome shape of the choroidal detachments. Choroidal detachments may extend posteriorly but do not insert into the optic disc. (c) A-scan showing the 100% tall spikes produced by the surface of the choroid.

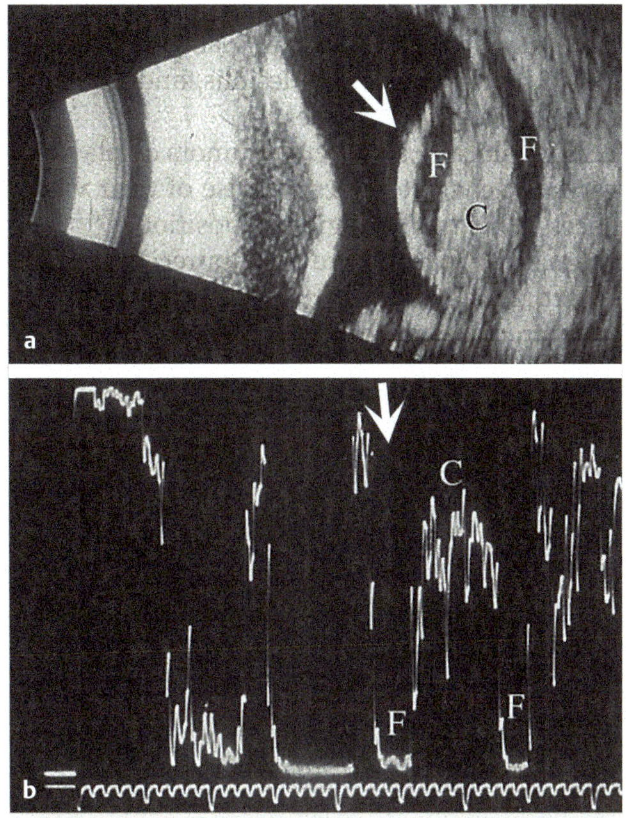

Fig. 6.32 Hemorrhagic choroidal detachments. (a) Transverse B-scan showing bullous choroidal detachments (*arrow*) and subchoroidal hemorrhage, partially fluid (F), partially clotted (C). (b) Corresponding A-scan showing the high choroidal spike (*arrow*) and irregular reflectivity with areas of both high (C) and low (F) internal spikes produced by the clotted and fluid hemorrhage, respectively.

6.7 Evaluation of Intraocular Tumors

Many intraocular tumors are easily distinguishable from one another ophthalmoscopically when the media are clear. Some mimic each other and are more difficult to differentiate, and if the media are not clear, ophthalmoscopic differentiation may be impossible. Standardized echography plays a large role in confirming the diagnosis, obtaining accurate measurements of newly discovered lesions, and monitoring changes in lesions over time.

Echographically, intraocular tumors display different acoustic characteristics because of their vast differences in histopathologic composition.[1,5,6,22] These distinguishing features are best appreciated with the standardized A-scan at "tissue sensitivity" and include structure, reflectivity, vascularity, and height.[1] The B-scan provides the topographic features—the shape, location, and extension. In many instances, ultrasound is the only imaging study performed when an intraocular mass is suspected, so careful evaluation of the orbital area adjacent to the lesion is important to rule out the possibility of extrascleral extension.

Pearls

- In many instances, ultrasound is the only imaging study performed when an intraocular mass is suspected, so careful evaluation of the orbital area adjacent to the lesion is important to rule out the possibility of extrascleral extension.

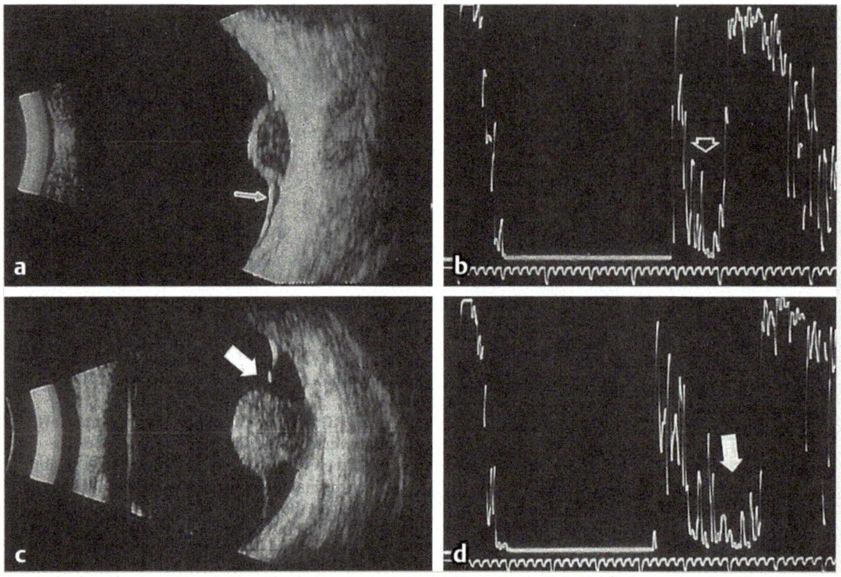

Fig. 6.33 Choroidal melanoma. (**a**) Transverse B-scan of a dome-shaped choroidal tumor with shallow retinal detachment at the inferior edge of the lesion (*arrow*). (**b**) A-scan shows the high spike from the surface of the lesion (*arrow*) and the low internal reflectivity (*arrow*). (**c**) Transverse B-scan showing the retinal detachment (*arrow*) adjacent to the collar button-shaped lesion. (**d**) Tissue sensitivity A-scan showing low internal reflectivity (*arrow*).

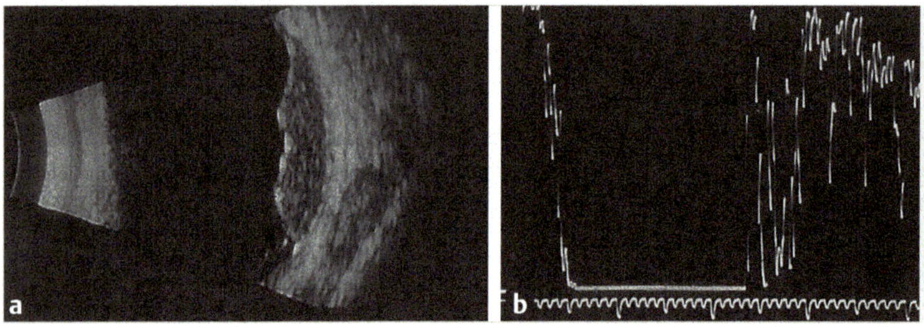

Fig. 6.34 Choroidal metastasis. (**a**) Transverse B-scan showing the lobulated shape of the metastatic lesion as well as the lateral dimensions. (**b**) A-scan at tissue sensitivity showing the irregular internal reflectivity.

6.7.1 Melanoma

Malignant melanomas are usually primary tumors of the choroid. Typically, they are comprised of small, densely compact cells of uniform distribution. Echographically, they present as solid, regularly structured, vascular lesions of low to medium reflectivity. The most common shapes are a dome or collar button (▸ Fig. 6.33); however, they can be diffused.[22,23,24] It is not uncommon for large melanomas to have a slightly irregular structure. This may be caused by necrotic tissue within the tumor. Melanomas that involve the ciliary body may also exhibit an irregular structure.[1,9,22,25]

Pearls

- Echographically, choroidal melanomas are solid, regularly structured, vascular lesions of low to medium reflectivity. In contrast, metastatic lesions are solid, irregularly structured masses with little or no detectable vascularity.

6.7.2 Metastatic Carcinoma

Echographically, choroidal metastases are solid, irregularly structured lesions. Little or no vascularity is detected (▸ Fig. 6.34).[6] Histopathologically, they generally are shown to have both large and small cells and interfaces that are erratically dispersed throughout the lesion. The shape is usually a dome with an area of central excavation. Metastatic lesions have been associated with retinal detachment and choroidal detachment,[26] but rarely with vitreous hemorrhage or subretinal hemorrhage. Small-cell carcinoma may produce atypical echographic features similar to those found with melanoma, making it difficult to differentiate one from the other.[9,27] A complete history and echographic follow-up may be useful to increase the likelihood of a correct diagnosis.

Controversial Points

- Small-cell carcinoma choroidal metastasis may produce atypical echographic features similar to those found with choroidal melanoma, making it difficult to differentiate one from the other echographically.

6.7.3 Choroidal Hemangioma

The diagnosis of choroidal hemangioma can almost always be made clinically because of the orange-colored appearance of the lesion.[28] Echographic confirmation and measurements are suggested. Common echographic characteristics include a dome shape, regular structure, and high internal reflectivity (▸ Fig. 6.35). These lesions are not ultrasonographically vascular. Retinal detachment and/or calcification at the surface of these lesions have been reported.[9]

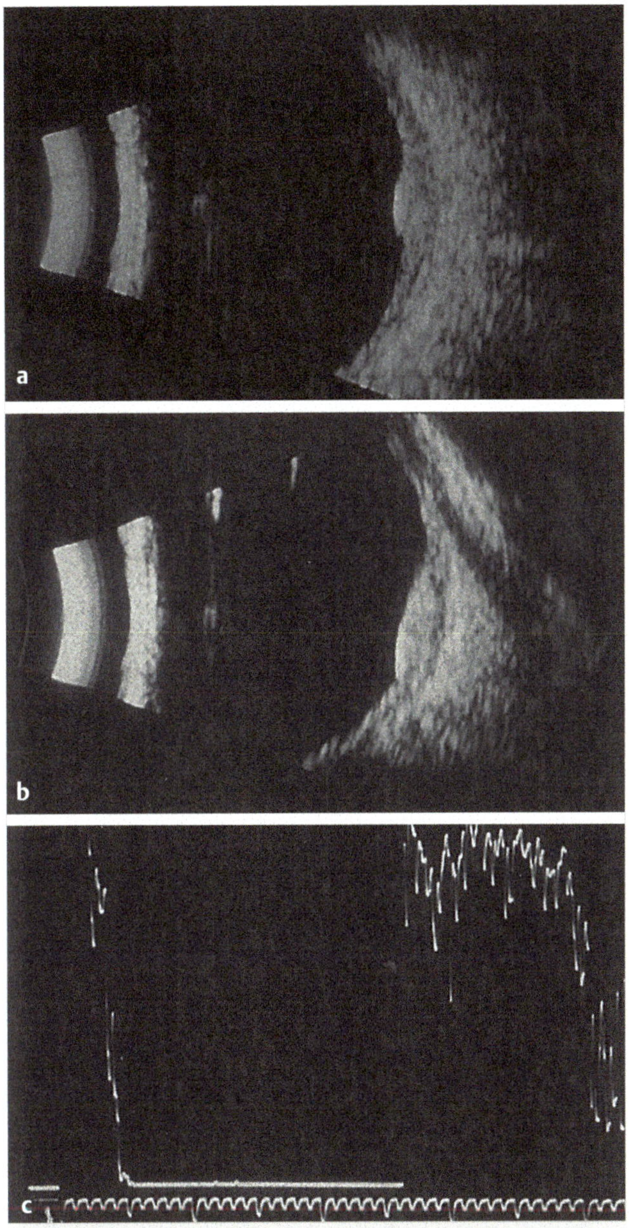

Fig. 6.35 Choroidal hemangioma. (**a**) Transverse B-scan showing the slightly dome-shaped elevation of the posterior fundus. (**b**) Longitudinal B-scan used to determine the radial dimension. (**c**) Standardized A-scan at tissue sensitivity showing the highly reflective internal structure.

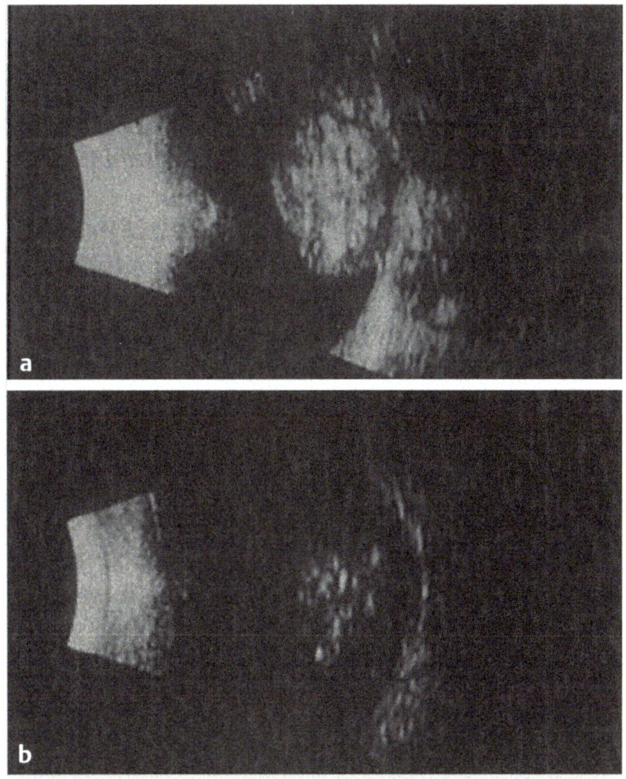

Fig. 6.37 Retinoblastoma. (**a**) B-scan at a high gain shows what appears to be areas of calcification within this large tumor. (**b**) B-scan at a decreased gain confirms the punctate areas of calcification.

6.7.4 Choroidal Osteoma

Choroidal osteomas are most commonly unilateral and appear plaque-like and minimally elevated on B-scan.[6,9,28] On standardized A-scan, they are extremely highly reflective.[6] Marked shadowing can be noted on both B- and A-scans (▸ Fig. 6.36).

6.7.5 Retinoblastoma

These childhood tumors can be unilateral or bilateral and vary in size and shape. The echographic findings most frequently associated with these tumors include an irregular shape, extremely high reflectivity when calcification is present (▸ Fig. 6.37), and low to medium reflectivity if no calcium is noted; vascularity may or may not be detected.[9,29]

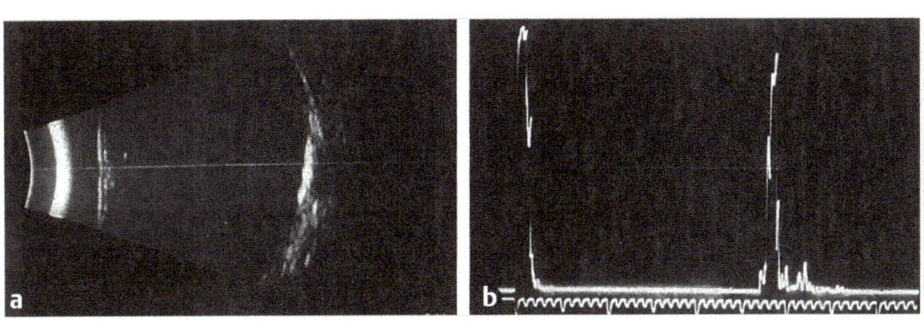

Fig. 6.36 Choroidal osteoma. (**a**) Transverse B-scan at a decreased gain setting showing the lateral extent of a plaque-like, calcified lesion with orbital shadowing. (**b**) A-scan at a reduced gain. All the sound is being absorbed by the calcified mass, producing a maximally high spike with no signal behind it.

References

[1] Ossoinig KC. Standardized echography: basic principles, clinical applications, and results. Int Ophthalmol Clin. 1979; 19(4):127–210

[2] Byrne SF. Standardized echography of the eye and orbit. In: Naidich TB, Quencer R, eds. Clinical Neurosonography: Ultrasound of the Central Nervous System. Berlin, Springer-Verlag; 1987:252–272

[3] Ossoinig KC. Basics of clinical echo-ophthalmography. IV: clinical standardization of equipment and techniques. In Bock J, Ossoinig KC, eds. Ultrasonographia Medica. Vienna, Wiener Med Akademie; 1971:83–118

[4] Ossoinig KC. The first standardized system for echo-ophthalmolography. In Massin M, Poujol J, eds. Diagnostica Ultrasonica in Ophthalmologia. Paris, Centre National d'Ophthalmologie des Quinze-Vingts; 1973:131

[5] Ossoinig KC, Patel JH. A-scan instrumentation for acoustic tissue differentiation. II: Clinical significance of various technical parameters of the 7200 MA unit of kretztechnik. In: White D, Brown RE, eds. Ultrasound in Medicine. Vol. 3B. New York, Plenum Press; 1977:1949–1953

[6] Patel JH, Ossoinig KC. A-scan instrumentation for acoustic tissue differentiation. I: signal processing in the 7200 MA unit of kretztechnik. In White D, Brown RE, eds. Ultrasound in Medicine. Vol. 3B. New York, Plenum Press; 1977:1939–1947

[7] Till P, Ossoinig KC. First experience with a new solid tissue model for the standardization of A- and B-scan instruments used in tissue diagnosis. In White D, Brown RE, eds. Ultrasound in Medicine. Vol. 3B. New York: Plenum Press; 1977:2167–2178

[8] Freyler H, Egerer I. Echography and histological studies in various eye conditions. Arch Ophthalmol. 1977; 95(8):1387–1394

[9] Byrne SF, Green RL. Ultrasound of the Eye and Orbit. St. Louis, MO: CV Mosby; 1992

[10] Dacey MP, Valencia M, Lee MB, et al. Echographic findings in infectious endophthalmitis. Arch Ophthalmol. 1994; 112(10):1325–1333

[11] Green RL, Byrne SF. Diagnostic ophthalmic ultrasound. In: Ryan SJ, ed. Retina. Vol. 1. St. Louis, MO: CV Mosby; 1989

[12] Coleman DJ, Franzen LA. Vitreous surgery; Preoperative evaluation and prognostic value of ultrasonic display of vitreous hemorrhage. Arch Ophthalmol. 1974; 92(5):375–381

[13] Blumenkranz MS, Byrne SF. Standardized echography (ultrasonography) for the detection and characterization of retinal detachment. Ophthalmology. 1982; 89(7):821–831

[14] Ossoinig KC, Islas G, Tamayo GE, et al. Detached retina versus dense fibrovascular membrane: standardized A-scan and B-scan criteria. In: Ossoinig. KC, ed. Ophthalmic Echography. Dordrecht: Dr W Junk; 1987:275–284

[15] DiBernardo C, Blodi BA, Byrne SF. Echographic evaluation of retinal tears in patients with spontaneous vitreous hemorrhage. Invest Ophthalmol Vis Sci. 1991; 32:878–879

[16] Kelley LM, Walker JP, Wing GL, Raskauskas PA, Schepens CL. Ultrasound-guided cryotherapy for retinal tears in patients with vitreous hemorrhage. Ophthalmic Surg Lasers. 1997; 28(7):565–569

[17] McLeod D, Restori M. Ultrasonic examination in severe diabetic eye disease. Br J Ophthalmol. 1979; 63(8):533–538

[18] Pulido JS, Byrne SF, Clarkson JG, Di Bernardo CL, Howe CA. Evaluation of eyes with advanced stages of retinopathy of prematurity using standardized echography. Ophthalmology. 1991; 98(7):1099–1104

[19] Goldberg MF. Persistent fetal vasculature (PFV): an integrated interpretation of signs and symptoms associated with persistent hyperplastic primary vitreous (PHPV). LIV Edward Jackson Memorial Lecture. Am J Ophthalmol. 1997; 124(5):587–626

[20] Sawada A, Fraser SL, Ossoinig KC. The role of ultrasound in the management of ocular foreign bodies. In: White D, Brown RE, eds. Ultrasound in Medicine. Vol. 3A. New York: Plenum Press; 1977:1003

[21] Forster DJ, Cano MR, Green RL, Rao NA. Echographic features of the Vogt-Koyanagi-Harada syndrome. Arch Ophthalmol. 1990; 108(10):1421–1426

[22] Ossoinig KC, Bigar F, Kaefring SL. Malignant melanoma of the choroid and ciliary body. A differential diagnosis in clinical echography. Bibl Ophthalmol. 1975; 83(83):141–154

[23] Goldberg MF, Hodes BL. Ultrasonographic diagnosis of choroidal malignant melanoma. Surv Ophthalmol. 1977; 22(1):29–40

[24] Shields JA. Diagnosis and Management of Intraocular Tumors. St. Louis, MO: CV Mosby; 1983

[25] Coleman DJ, Lizzi FL, Jack RL, et al. Ultrasonography of the Eye and Orbit. Philadelphia, PA: Lea & Febiger; 1977

[26] Sneed SR, Byrne SF, Mieler WF, Nicholson DH, Olsen K, Hughes JR. Choroidal detachment associated with malignant choroidal tumors. Ophthalmology. 1991; 98(6):963–970

[27] Verbeek AM. A choroidal oat-cell carcinoma metastasis mimicking a choroidal melanoma. In: Thijssen JM, Verbeek AM, eds. Ultrasonography in Ophthalmology. Dordrecht: Dr W Junk; 1981:131–133

[28] Gass JDM. Stereoscopic Atlas of Macular Disease: Diagnosis and Treatment. 3rd ed. Vol. 1. St. Louis, MO: CV Mosby; 1987

[29] Ossoinig KC, Cennomo G, Green RL, et al. Echographic results in the diagnosis of retinoblastoma. In: Thijssen JM, Verbeek AM, eds. Ultrasonography in Ophthalmology. Dordrecht: Dr W Junk; 1981:103–107

7 Electrophysiology and Miscellaneous Noninvasive Tests

Lauren S. Taney and Elias Reichel

7.1 Introduction

Noninvasive testing of the retina is essential for the diagnosis of retinal disorders. Such noninvasive tests may include electrophysiologic testing, psychophysical testing, and other imaging techniques.

Electroretinography (ERG) and electrooculography (EOG) have classically constituted electrophysiologic testing. Dark adaptometry and color vision testing are forms of psychophysical testing. Both electrophysiologic and psychophysical testings are used to evaluate the functional integrity of the retina, and they are discussed in the following paragraphs. Visually evoked cortical potential (VECP) recording is a technique used to measure a gross electrical signal generated at the visual cortex in response to visual stimulation and, therefore, records activity of the entire sensory visual pathway from the retina to the occipital cortex. Because it is administered infrequently by ophthalmologists, VECP will not be discussed here. Imaging modalities such as scanning laser ophthalmoscopy (SLO), fundus autofluorescence (FAF), and adaptive optics (AO) are newer techniques that are useful for the diagnosis and monitoring of a variety of retinal conditions, and they will be discussed in this chapter.

7.2 Electroretinography

ERG measures the electrical response generated by the retina following stimulation with light. The two most commonly used types of ERG are full-field ERG and multifocal ERG (mfERG). Full-field ERG employs diffuse illumination to elicit a response from the entire retina. Ganzfeld dome stimulation illumination remains the standard technique for eliciting a full-field ERG response. mfERG utilizes a flickering array of hexagonal elements to generate multiple (typically 61 or 103) local ERG responses within the cone-dominant retina; a topographic map which reflects local ERG responses is then created. Other specialized forms of ERG which are beyond the scope of this discussion include macular or focal ERG, pattern ERG, early receptor potential, scotopic threshold response, direct-current ERG, long-duration light-adapted ERG, double-flash ERG, chromatic stimulus ERG, dark-adapted and light-adapted luminance-response analyses, and saturated a-wave slope analysis.

7.2.1 Full-Field Electroretinography

Introduction

Full-field ERG measures the summative electrical response generated by the whole retina following exposure to a light stimulus. Full-field ERG responses are described according to two principal parameters: (1) state of light adaptation and (2) strength of flash stimuli.[1] The International Society for Clinical Electrophysiology of Vision (ISCEV) has standardized full-field ERG to include a total of five responses[2]:

1. Dark-adapted 0.01 ERG (rod response)
2. Dark-adapted 3.0 ERG (combined rod–cone response; maximal response)
3. Dark-adapted 3.0 oscillatory potentials
4. Light-adapted 3.0 ERG (cone response)
5. Light-adapted 3.0 flicker (30-Hz flicker)

Practical Considerations

Pupillary dilation should be performed prior to ERG testing, and maximal pupil size should be noted before testing begins. Dark adaptation for a period of at least 20 minutes should be achieved by darkening the room and placing multiple adhesive patches over both eyes to achieve total occlusion of light. Ideally, it is best to avoid ERG testing following fluorescein angiography and fundus photography, but if this is not possible, dark adaptation for at least 60 minutes should be performed following photography.

After a topical anesthetic is placed on the eyes, "active" electrodes that contact the cornea or limbal bulbar conjunctiva should then be placed underneath the eyelids; this can be performed under dim red illumination. Some consider contact lens electrodes such as the Burian-Allen or ERG-jet electrodes to provide the most stable recordings, but these also require use of nonviscous ionic conductive solution (no more than 0.5% methyl cellulose). Alternative electrode materials include conductive fibers and foils, conjunctival loop electrodes, and corneal wicks. A single ground electrode is placed with electrode paste either on the patient's forehead or ear. A reference or "inactive" electrode may be contained within each contact lens–speculum unit or may be placed temporally to the lateral orbital rims. The "active," ground, and reference electrodes all connect to a junctional box. The difference in voltage between the "active" corneal electrode and the reference electrode is then recorded by a differential amplifier.

The Grass xenon arc photostimulator with flash duration of 10 µs has been commonly used to obtain ERGs over a range of stimulus intensities. A Ganzfeld dome is necessary to standardize the white flash stimulus for full-field ERG.[3] The strength of flash stimuli, as measured at the surface of the Ganzfeld dome, is measured in units of candela-seconds per meter squared ([cd·s]/m^2). Although chromatic stimuli may be used in certain cases, white flashes should be used for standard ERG. Protocol dictates whether a stimulus may be repeated and, if so, at what interval between stimuli.

Under scotopic conditions, a series of ERG recordings is obtained using different light intensities, denoted by the number ([cd·s]/m^2) in the ERG description: 0.01 ERG, 3.0 ERG, and 3.0 oscillatory potentials. The patient is then light-adapted, which is defined as exposure to white background luminance of

30 candela per meter squared (cd/m^2) for at least 10 minutes, and this standardized luminance is delivered using the Ganzfeld dome. Under photopic conditions, the 3.0 ERG and 3.0 flicker are then completed.

The full-field ERG can be affected by a variety of conditions unrelated to the function of the retina. It is important to be aware of these confounding variables when establishing the normalcy or abnormalcy of an ERG test result. The type and position of the corneal electrode being used can affect the quality of the ERG. Media opacities, including cataract, vitreous hemorrhage, and vitreous debris, can cause both a reduction in ERG amplitude and a prolonged implicit time. Age and myopia can decrease the ERG amplitude but will not typically affect implicit time. Pupil size can also affect the amplitude of the ERG and may account for the decline in ERG amplitude associated with age. Patient compliance and the presence or absence of sedation or anesthesia may also impact test results and should, therefore, be documented.

Purpose

Full-field ERG testing is particularly useful in determining the abnormalcy of what appears to be a "normal" retina on examination. ERG testing may elucidate whether visual dysfunction can be attributed to rods, cones, or both, and it can readily document the extent of visual dysfunction while tracking changes over time. In this fashion, ERG testing can distinguish between stationary forms of night blindness and progressive degenerations such as retinitis pigmentosa. ERG may prove essential in establishing the etiology of retinal degeneration due to hereditary, toxic-metabolic, retinal vascular, or inflammatory etiologies. ERG testing may also be particularly instrumental in investigating specific patient complaints such as difficulty with peripheral vision, unexplained loss of central vision, and night blindness. Additionally, full-field ERG testing may help establish underlying retinal function in pediatric or nonverbal patients as well as in eyes in which the media is obscured.

Beyond its use in establishing pathologic conditions, ERG also reassures both the patient and physician when normalcy of retinal function is demonstrated. In such cases, alternative explanations for visual loss such as the optic nerve, central nervous system, and nonorganic visual loss should be entertained.

While instrumental in defining loss of function, a proper diagnosis can only be made when ERG testing is performed in conjunction with a complete ophthalmic examination and thorough medical evaluation. Genetic testing may be a useful adjunct in further classifying certain degenerative conditions.

Special Considerations

- Only in conjunction with a careful history and ocular examination does full-field electroretinographic testing provide for a complete evaluation and accurate diagnosis.

Interpretation

A normal ERG consists of three major components: a-wave, b-wave, and c-wave. The photoreceptors generate the initial, cornea-negative component or a-wave of the ERG, and the Müller's cells and bipolar cells are responsible for the later, cornea-positive b-wave of the ERG. The c-wave appears to be generated from the retinal pigment epithelium (RPE), although it also depends on rod photoreceptor activity. Measurement of the c-wave is difficult and highly variable; thus, it has very limited clinical application.

The character of the waveform should be examined closely and compared with an example of normal ERG, ideally one generated by the same ERG system. An identifiable a-wave and b-wave may not always be distinctly present, but when possible, the amplitude and implicit time of the a-wave and b-wave should be measured. The a-wave amplitude is measured from baseline to a-wave trough. The b-wave amplitude is measured from a-wave trough to b-wave peak. Implicit time for a-wave and b-wave is measured, respectively, from the time of the flash to the trough of the a-wave and to the peak of the b-wave. Physiological significance should be taken into account in all cases, also bearing in mind the possibility of erroneous measurements due to poor electrode contact with the cornea or improper calibration.

Normal values for ERG results depend on stimulus conditions and patient variables, as discussed earlier. These considerations need to be factored into proper interpretation of an ERG. As an approximation, a bright white flash intensity should result in a dark-adapted b-wave amplitude of at least 350 µV in patients younger than 50 years and with normal axial lengths. The normal amplitude of the 30-Hz flicker stimulus is at least 50 µV. For patients with dramatic visual dysfunction, computer-averaging techniques and narrow bandpass filtering allow for the detection of ERG responses below 1 µV.

When evaluating patients with retinal degeneration, it is important to quantify the function of both the rod and cone systems. The full-field ERG is used to establish generalized loss of rod or cone function, or both. In general, diseases associated with predominantly abnormal rod responses include congenital stationary night blindness, early retinitis pigmentosa, rod dystrophies, and rod–cone dystrophies. Diseases associated with predominantly abnormal cone responses include achromatopsia (both rod monochromatism and blue cone monochromatism), cone dystrophies, and cone–rod dystrophies. Conditions such as advanced retinitis pigmentosa, Leber's congenital amaurosis, gyrate atrophy, choroideremia, total retinal detachment, and retinal aplasia cause dramatic abnormalities in both cone and rod function.

The rod-isolated response is achieved by dark-adapting the patient, and a dim white (or blue, although this is not a part of the standardized recommendations) flash below cone threshold is used to stimulate the retina, resulting in a waveform that has almost no detectable a-wave but a large b-wave (▶ Fig. 7.1a). Using a bright white flash in the dark-adapted state causes maximal stimulation of both rods and cones and results in large a- and b-waves with oscillatory potentials in the ascending b-wave (▶ Fig. 7.1b). Although this combined rod–cone response is both rod and cone mediated, 80% of this response is attributable to rods, and the remaining 20% results from cones. Thus, if cone dysfunction is mild, the combined scotopic rod–cone response waveform, amplitude, and implicit time may all appear normal. Oscillatory potential (▶ Fig. 7.1c) is also assessed in a state of dark adaptation, but oscillatory potentials are less critical in assessing rod function. Rather, oscillatory potentials are believed to be the result of inhibitory influences effected by amacrine cell input on the b-wave and are characteristically diminished when retinal ischemia is present. Reduced oscillatory potentials may also be associated with some forms of congenital stationary night blindness.

Cone responses are obtained in a light-adapted state, as light adaptation suppresses rod responses such that they do not contribute to the waveforms generated by the 3.0 ERG and 3.0 flicker (30-Hz flicker) (▶ Fig. 7.1d, e). Both the 3.0 ERG and 3.0 flicker use a white flash at a strength of 3.0 ([cd·s]/m^2). A red flash may also be used to isolate a cone response, but this is not a part of standardized recommendations. Mild reductions in cone amplitudes may be observed when macular scarring covers an area of at least four disc diameters, although the scotopic 0.01 ERG, 3.0 ERG, and 3.0 oscillatory potentials will be affected minimally in such cases of macular disease because of the disproportionate number of rods as compared to cones in the human retina.

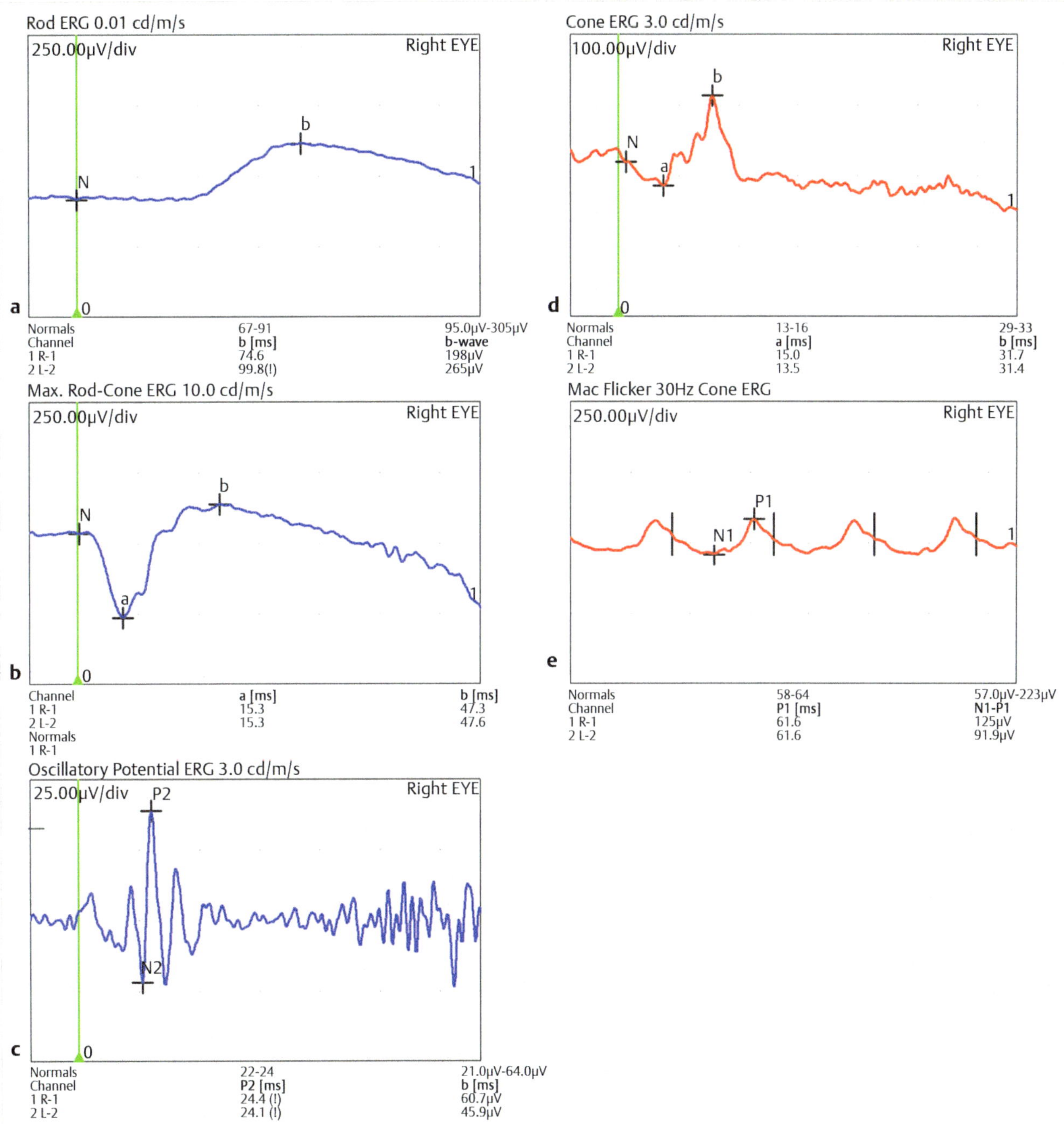

Fig. 7.1 (a) Normal full-field, dark-adapted 0.01 electroretinography (ERG) (rod response) with an undetectable a-wave but a large b-wave. (b) Normal full-field, dark-adapted 10.0 ERG (combined rod–cone response). The descending a-wave is followed by the ascending b-wave. Oscillatory potentials can be seen on the ascending b-wave. (Vertical and horizontal scales represent 250 μV per unit and 20 ms per unit, respectively.) (c) Normal full-field, dark-adapted 3.0 oscillatory potential. (d) Normal full-field, light-adapted 3.0 ERG (cone response). (e) Normal full-field, light-adapted 3.0 flicker (30-Hz flicker).

Pearls

- To observe a reduction in a-wave or b-wave amplitude, a large area of retinal tissue must be affected. Isolated macular disorders do not alter the full-field electroretinogram. Optic nerve disorders and cortical conditions likewise do not affect the full-field ERG.

Many conditions display loss of retinal function. Therefore, a careful history and ophthalmoscopic examination are necessary for establishing a diagnosis in conjunction with ERG testing. Testing retinal function is critical when considering the diagnosis of the following conditions (see the following list): hereditary retinal degenerations (such as retinitis pigmentosa, cone–rod dystrophies, stationary forms of night blindness), metabolic disorders, acquired retinal ischemia (due to retinal artery occlusion, retinal vein occlusion, or diabetic retinopathy), toxic retinopathy (such as siderosis or medication-related toxicity: chloroquine, hydroxychloroquine, chlorpromazine, thioridazine, quinine), autoimmune/paraneoplastic retinopathy (including cancer-associated retinopathy and melanoma-associated retinopathy), vitamin A deficiency, retinal detachment, media opacities, and unexplained vision loss.

Disorders Affecting Full-Field Electroretinography

- Photoreceptor degenerations
- Stationary night blindness
- Hereditary vitreoretinopathies
- Retinal artery and vein obstructions
- Diabetic retinopathy
- Toxic retinopathies
- Cancer-associated retinopathy
- Vitamin A deficiency
- Retinal detachment
- Media opacities, including cataract and vitreous hemorrhage

Laboratory testing is often needed to confirm the presence of an inherited or acquired metabolic condition (e.g., hypovitaminosis A) or to rule out the possibility of cancer-associated retinopathy. Genetic testing may be useful to confirm the presence of an inherited retinal degeneration.

A comprehensive discussion of characteristic ERG abnormalities is beyond the scope of this chapter, but a few representative points are discussed here. In early retinitis pigmentosa, individuals may display delayed cone b-wave implicit times suggestive of more diffuse retinal dysfunction; b-wave amplitudes are variably affected in early stages of retinitis pigmentosa.[4] Cases of advanced retinitis pigmentosa are usually accompanied by markedly reduced rod and cone responses to a bright flash (▶ Fig. 7.2a) and markedly reduced cone responses to a 30-Hz flicker as well as a light-adapted 3.0 ERG (▶ Fig. 7.2b). The ERG of patients with advanced choroideremia may similarly show striking reduction in rod and cone responses to a bright flash (▶ Fig. 7.2c).

Pearls

- Delayed cone implicit times are suggestive of widespread retinal disease even when cone amplitudes are normal.

The term "negative ERG" specifically refers to an abnormal waveform variant of the combined rod–cone response in which the amplitude of the b-wave is smaller than that of the a-wave (▶ Fig. 7.2d). A negative ERG can be recorded in the setting of acquired severe retinal circulatory disturbance (such as central retinal artery occlusion, ischemic central retinal vein occlusion, or proliferative diabetic retinopathy), acquired retinal diseases (such as melanoma-associated retinopathy, birdshot choroidopathy, ocular siderosis, quinine retinopathy, or methanol toxicity), or inherited retinal diseases (such as complete- and incomplete-type congenital stationary night blindness, X-linked juvenile retinoschisis, juvenile-onset neuronal ceroid lipofuscinosis, Goldmann–Favre's syndrome, and infantile Refsum's disease).[5] An extinct combined rod–cone response can be seen in advanced stages of retinitis pigmentosa, gyrate atrophy, choroideremia, and cancer-associated retinopathy.

ERG testing can play a role in the evaluation of retinal ischemia resulting from central retinal vein obstruction and diabetic retinopathy; it may be useful in deciding which patients with these conditions are the best candidates for panretinal laser photocoagulation in attempting to prevent iris or retinal neovascularization. ERG can also be helpful in differentiating an old central retinal artery obstruction from an old optic neuropathy. The ERG will show a reduced b-wave on the affected side with the former condition but be totally normal with the latter condition.

7.2.2 Multifocal Electroretinography

Introduction

Sutter and Tran developed the multifocal ERG (mfERG) in 1992, and this enabled the measurement of multiple isolated focal ERG responses.[6] In contrast to full-field ERG, mfERG measures retinal responses generated by the 40 to 50 degrees surrounding central fixation. This translates into a focus on cone-predominant retina within the macula. Depending on the clinical indication, mfERG may represent a useful primary or adjunctive test for measuring macular function. When conditions such as hydroxychloroquine toxicity, Stargardt's disease, acute zonal occult outer retinopathy, and occult macular dystrophy are suspected, mfERG is helpful for diagnosis.

Practical Considerations

mfERG is performed on light-adapted patients after pupillary dilation. Refractive error should be taken into account prior to beginning testing, and, if need be, appropriate correction should be provided. It is best not to perform mfERG following ophthalmoscopy or fundus photography, but a recovery period of 15 minutes after either may be used if necessary. mfERG is performed on one eye at a time, and the eye not being tested should be patched to minimize blinking.

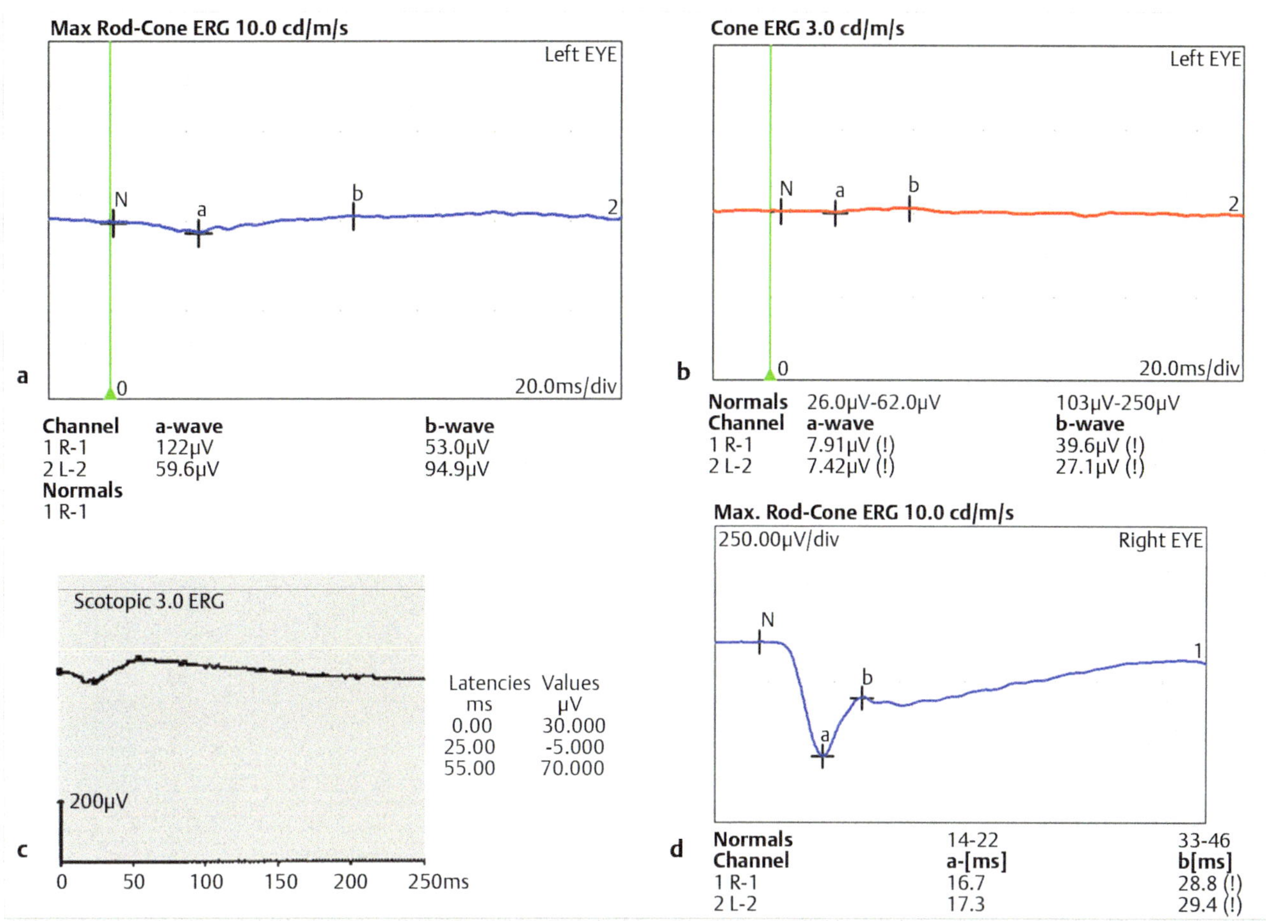

Fig. 7.2 (**a**) Abnormal full-field, dark-adapted 10.0 electroretinography (ERG) in a patient with advanced retinitis pigmentosa. The a-wave and b-wave amplitudes are dramatically reduced. (**b**) In the same patient with advanced retinitis pigmentosa, there is an abnormal full-field, light-adapted 3.0 ERG with grossly abnormal waveform. (**c**) Abnormal full-field ERG, dark-adapted 3.0 ERG in a patient with choroideremia. (**d**) Negative ERG in a patient with melanoma-associated retinopathy. In this dark-adapted 10.0 ERG, the b-wave amplitude is smaller than the a-wave amplitude.

After topical anesthetic is instilled, active, reference, and ground electrodes are placed in the fashion described for full-field ERG. As is the case for full-field ERG, the active electrode must contact the cornea or adjacent bulbar conjunctiva, and contact lens, foil, or fiber electrodes may be employed.

Either a cathode ray tube or a liquid crystal display may be used to generate the mfERG stimuli. The stimuli consist of alternating light (white) and dark (black) hexagonal elements that are smallest centrally (surrounding fixation) and larger peripherally within the overall arrangement. The luminance of the light elements should be at least 100 cd/m^2, with the dark elements dim enough to provide at least 90% contrast.[7] At any point in time, approximately 50% of the hexagonal elements are illuminated. Traditionally, either 61 or 103 element arrays are used, with testing of one eye taking at least 4 minutes to complete when 61 elements are being used and at least 8 minutes to complete when 103 element arrays are being used. Testing with 103 element arrays provides better spatial resolution than testing with 61 elements, but it takes longer to perform and results in a decreased signal-to-noise ratio.

Interpretation

The flickering hexagonal elements generate a continuous ERG signal, from which individual focal ERG signals are mathematically derived by way of correlation with the sequence of stimuli. The waveform of the mfERG response is referred to as the first-order response or first-order kernel, and it consists of a biphasic waveform with an initial negative deflection (N1) followed by a positive excursion (P1) and again a negative deflection (N2). Photoreceptors are responsible for the N1 signal, while Müller's cells and bipolar cells contribute to the N2 response.

Although the colorful topographic three-dimensional (3D) response density plot immediately draws attention, the array of mfERG traces (▶ Fig. 7.3a) should first be examined for evidence of appropriate fixation as well as the shape, amplitude, and timing of waveforms. Quantitative measurements vary from one machine to another; therefore, the amplitude of waveforms should be compared with age-adjusted normal examples from the same machine. The 3D response density plot (▶ Fig. 7.3b) represents the signal strength per unit area of retina and is particularly useful for determining the location and size of the

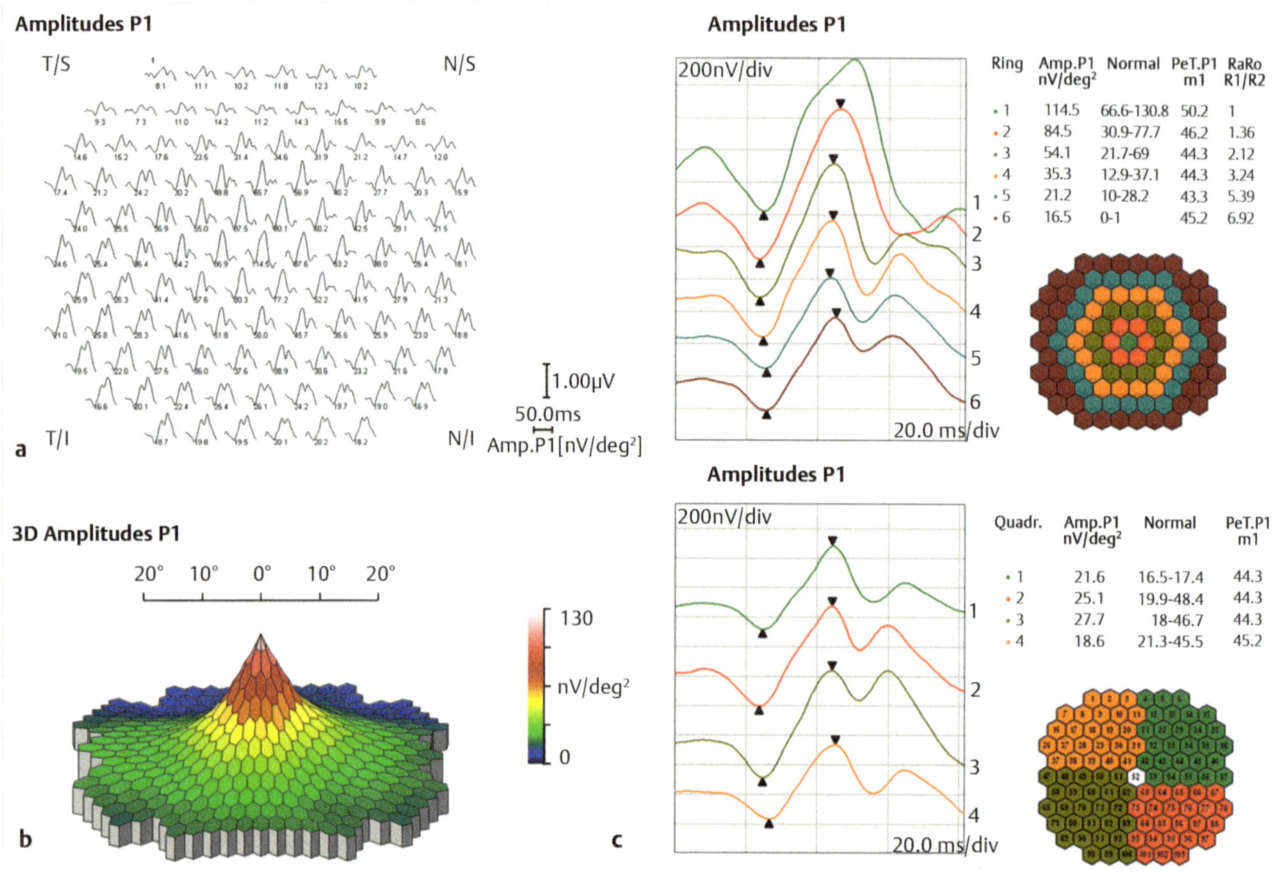

Fig. 7.3 (a) Normal multifocal electroretinography (mfERG): trace array. (Vertical and horizontal scales represent 1 µV and 50 ms, respectively.) (b) Normal mfERG: topographic (3D) response density plot. (c) Normal mfERG: ring response plots.

physiologic blind spot; it should never be used exclusively to interpret an mfERG because it can be misleading. Ring response plots (▶ Fig. 7.3c) may help draw attention to regional abnormalities, as ring response plots represent averaged trace arrays.

The fundamental use of mfERG is identification of the precise location of retinal functional abnormalities. It is of diagnostic utility to know whether discrete retinal abnormalities are located in the macula, paramacula, or more peripheral retina. For example, a bull's eye maculopathy such as that associated with hydroxychloroquine toxicity causes retinal dysfunction that is most pronounced in the parafoveal rings (▶ Fig. 7.4a). In retinitis pigmentosa, the central foveal waveform is often preserved until very advanced stages of the disease, while paramacular and more peripheral waveforms are attenuated (▶ Fig. 7.4b). In Stargardt's disease, macular and paramacular retina are most affected with more normal peripheral waveforms.

Pearls

- The fundamental use of mfERG is identification of the precise location of retinal functional abnormalities.

7.3 Electrooculography

Electrooculography (EOG) measures the standing potential generated by the RPE. In 1865, Holmgren identified a constant standing, or resting, potential between the cornea and the back of the eye. This resting potential could be altered by changes in retinal illumination. In 1951, Marg coined the term electro-oculogram for the measurement of this potential.[8]

The eye can be compared to a battery. There is a measurable voltage between the cornea, acting as the positive electrode, and the back of the eye, which serves as the negative electrode. The corneal-fundal potential is the source of voltage. The tight junctions between the RPE cells provide resistance, and a standing potential develops on either side of the RPE. All ERG components are superimposed on the standing potential of the eye. When the eye is exposed to light, the contribution of the electrical potential from the RPE increases, and EOG detects this light rise.

EOG indirectly measures the amplitude of this standing potential in the dark as well as in the light.[9] The light-to-dark ratio, or Arden ratio, is calculated by taking the peak EOG amplitude in the light and dividing it by the trough EOG amplitude during dark adaptation.[10] Normal individuals have an EOG that is at least 1.7 times greater in amplitude in the light than in the dark.

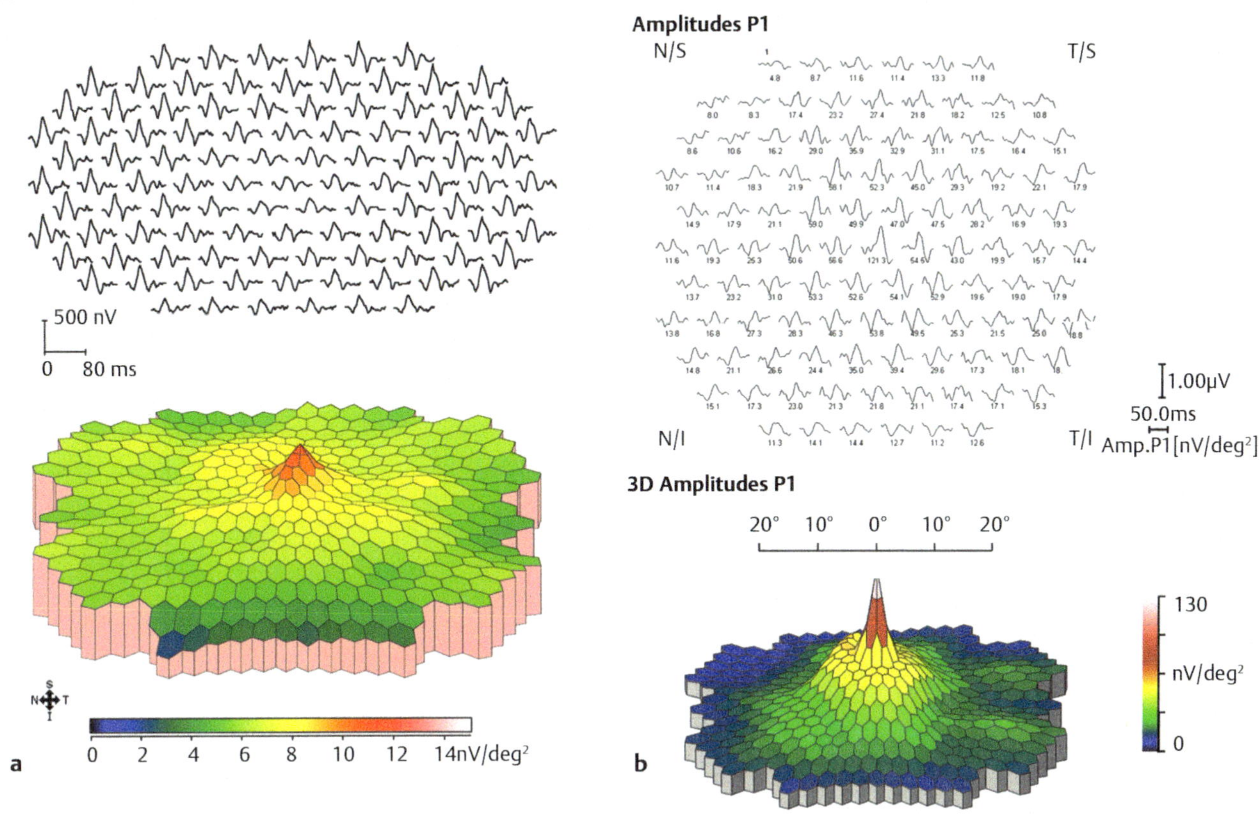

Fig. 7.4 (**a**) Subnormal multifocal electroretinography (mfERG) in a patient with hydroxychloroquine toxicity. There is pronounced reduction in the amplitude of foveal and parafoveal signals. (**b**) Subnormal mfERG in a patient with retinitis pigmentosa. The waveforms of the peripheral rings are most affected, which is most apparent in the trace array.

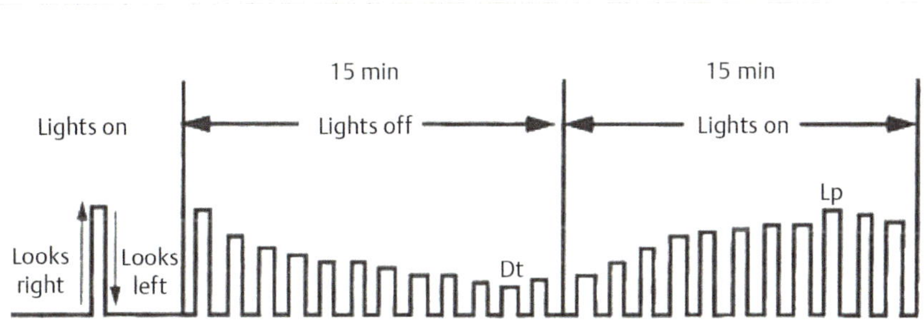

Fig. 7.5 Schematic electro-oculogram from a normal subject.

EOG recording depends on eye movement. Electrodes placed at the side of the nose and near the outer canthi measure changes in the corneal-fundal potential as the eyes move horizontally. When the positive cornea moves closer to one of the electrodes, that electrode becomes more positive than the other electrode. From a practical standpoint, the EOG is recorded at 2-minute intervals during 15 minutes of dark adaptation followed by 15 minutes of light adaptation (▶ Fig. 7.5).

The EOG is a difficult test to administer and requires patient cooperation. Young children may have difficulty with the test. In addition, reduced visual acuity can result in spurious results, so the test is generally not performed if the visual acuity is worse than 20/100.

The EOG is most useful for diagnosing Best's disease. If the EOG light-to-dark ratio is less than 1.5, the ERG result is normal, and the characteristic fundus findings are observed, then one can be fairly confident that Best's disease is present. There have been some reports of subnormal light-to-dark ratios in individuals with pattern dystrophies and adult-onset foveomacular dystrophy or pseudovitelliform macular dystrophy, again in conjunction with normal ERG results. It is possible that overlap exists between Best's disease and these other conditions on the basis of genetic heterogeneity. The EOG is less sensitive for the various forms of photoreceptor degenerations (e.g., retinitis pigmentosa) and stationary night blindness; in general, ERG is the evaluation technique of choice for these other conditions, and EOG testing is not needed.

Pearls

- Best's disease characteristically demonstrates a subnormal electro-oculogram (light-to-dark ratio of less than 1.5) in the setting of a normal electroretinogram. If this is found in any individual, then the diagnosis of Best's disease must be considered, and other family members should be evaluated.

7.4 Dark Adaptometry

Dark adaptometry is the measurement of both the rod and the cone mechanisms to recover sensitivity following exposure to light. Although cones recover more quickly than rods, rod photoreceptors have a greater sensitivity than cones.

Dark adaptation can be evaluated by plotting threshold sensitivities over time. The patient is exposed to an intense preadapting light for approximately 5 minutes, and the light is then turned off so that subsequent stimulus measurements take place in the dark. A stimulus 1 or 2 degrees in diameter is placed 15 degrees temporal to the fovea. At 1-minute intervals, the intensity of the light stimulus that produces a response from the patient is recorded.

The Goldmann–Weekers' dark adaptometer can be used to measure thresholds at various locations on the retina and can ascertain focal abnormalities in retinal function. Cone and rod thresholds to luminance are generally plotted over a 40-minute time period. Alternatively, final rod thresholds can be measured at the conclusion of dark adaptation. Typically, when threshold luminance is plotted over time, there is a decrease in threshold luminance (or a rise in sensitivity) that plateaus in approximately 5 minutes. This represents the cone sensitivity. A second rapid decline in threshold luminance plateaus in 40 minutes. This recovery plateau is attributed to the rods. The break of the second decline is called the *rod–cone break*.

Certain rare retinal conditions have characteristic findings with respect to dark adaptation profiles (see the following list). Cone degenerations show elevations of the cone threshold with normal final rod thresholds. Congenital stationary night blindness shows no evidence of a rod–cone break, with the final threshold representing cone function alone. Oguchi's disease is an unusual form of stationary night blindness. In Oguchi's disease, dark adaptation profiles reveal normal cone adaptation; rod adaptation is markedly delayed but reaches normalcy over a prolonged period of time (up to 24 hours). Fundus albipunctatus typically shows a delayed dark adaptation profile for both the rod and the cone segments.

7.4.1 Conditions Associated with Characteristic Abnormalities of Dark Adaptation

- Congenital stationary night blindness
- Cone degenerations
- Oguchi's disease
- Rod monochromatism
- Cone monochromatism
- Fundus albipunctatus

7.5 Color Vision Testing

Tests used for the evaluation of color vision in the clinical setting include screening tests, tests of color discrimination, and tests of color matching. The most common color vision abnormalities observed in the practice of ophthalmology include congenital abnormalities of color vision that affect approximately 8% of men and 1% of women. Acquired abnormalities of color vision are more difficult to characterize and are not typically evaluated on a regular basis.

Ishihara or pseudoisochromatic plate tests are the most common screening tests. Pseudoisochromatic plates have a figure of colored dots hidden among a background of differently colored dots. Pseudoisochromatic plate tests enable the clinician to identify approximately 95% of patients with congenital color defects. If a screening test identifies a defect that is not clearly classifiable, the Farnsworth–Munsell's 100-hue test or the Farnsworth panel D-15 can be used to characterize the defect further.

Pearls

- Acquired color vision defects are difficult to classify using color vision testing and are typically associated with loss of visual acuity.

Discrimination ability is tested using arrangement tests such as the Farnsworth–Munsell 100-hue test or the Farnsworth panel D-15. Although the former test can evaluate fine chromatic discrimination, the latter can be used for screening of discrimination.[11] Although these tests are easy to administer, they require manual dexterity as well as the ability to perform ordering tasks. Persons with congenital color vision defects make characteristic errors on arrangement tests such that a particular axis is weakened or lost. This is caused by the loss of chromatic discrimination resulting from their hereditary abnormality. Discrimination tests can be used to distinguish between protan (red) and deutan (green) abnormalities of color vision.[12]

Color matching is done using an anomaloscope, which allows the test subject to adjust primary colors to match a control color. In testing red–green abnormalities, red and green are mixed to match yellow. Anomaloscopes are difficult to use. Typically, they are used in research centers and not in the clinical practice setting.

7.6 Scanning Laser Ophthalmoscopy

The scanning laser ophthalmoscope was first described by Webb and Hughes in 1981.[13] A flying-spot scanning laser source, typically light in the infrared spectrum, is used to scan the fundus in a raster pattern. Light returning from the retina is then processed, and a monochromatic, en face image is generated.[14] Use of a pinhole which is confocal, or conjugate to the laser focus, is referred to as a confocal scanning laser ophthalmoscope (cSLO). cSLO provides higher contrast images than conventional fundus cameras because it reduces the amount of scattered light returning to the photodiode detector.[15,16] By optimizing contrast, cSLO may generate images that conventional fundus cameras cannot ordinarily resolve because of poor contrast.[17]

SLO uses a minimal amount of light to scan a given section of the retina and is well tolerated by patients, although a SLO image does take longer to generate than a conventional single-flash fundus photograph. Another benefit of the SLO is that it can be performed through an undilated or minimally dilated pupil, particularly in a 40-degree field of view. SLO can provide real-time, in vivo video images of the retina and, as such, is well suited to performing fluorescein and indocyanine green angiography. SLO can also operate in autofluorescence and infrared modes, and AO technology may be integrated with SLO to enhance image resolution. It also offers quantitative 3D analysis capabilities, unlike standard fundus photography.

Given these functions, many studies have undertaken to examine the role of SLO in imaging retinal pathology: macular cysts, neovascularization in age-related macular degeneration, drusen, pigment epithelial detachments, macular holes, and discontinuities in the vitreous (▶ Fig. 7.6a–c).[18,19,20,21,22,23] They have all demonstrated a role for SLO in imaging the posterior segment in such cases. As a versatile, in vivo retinal imaging technique, SLO may be used in conjunction with more traditional fundus photography.

7.7 Fundus Autofluorescence

Delori and colleagues first used a fundus spectrophotometer to measure retinal autofluorescence, and they postulated that lipofuscin in the RPE was the fluorophore with a characteristic excitation and emission at 510 and 630 nm, respectively.[24] von Rückmann and colleagues subsequently described use of a prototype cSLO to image autofluorescence in both normal eyes and eyes with retinal disease. In normal eyes, they noted hypoautofluorescence of the optic nerve and retinal vessels. They also found that absent autofluorescence corresponded with areas of retinal atrophy in diseased eyes, while hyperautofluorescence characterized the images of patients with diseases attributed to excess RPE lipofuscin, such as Best's disease and pattern dystrophy.[25] Limited access to, and the high cost of, cSLO led to the subsequent development of fundus camera–based systems for imaging autofluorescence, which involves using filters on existing fundus cameras to minimize competing autofluorescence from the crystalline lens.[26]

At this point, both cSLO and fundus camera–based FAF are commercially available and widely used. Heidelberg retina angiograph/Heidelberg Spectralis and OPTOS are the most widely used cSLO FAF imaging systems. In FAF using cSLO, fluorophores are excited using continuous, low-intensity blue light (488 nm) in a raster pattern, and image processing with pixel averaging then takes place. Because multiple scans are acquired and a mean image is then calculated, cSLO FAF takes longer to perform (about 2.5 seconds) which may limit its use in patients with difficulty fixating or remaining still. In FAF using a fundus camera, a single non-confocal flash of high-intensity light in the green spectrum is used to excite fluorophores, and bandwidth filters are employed to capture excitation within the yellow-orange emission spectrum. Image acquisition using fundus camera–based FAF is faster (1/60 s) than cSLO, but a main challenge with fundus camera–based FAF remains light scattering, particularly from the anterior segment.[27] Contrast needs to be adjusted manually, so image quality is more operator dependent in fundus camera–based FAF. A recent study comparing images from SLO and fundus camera–based FAF revealed an overall qualitative autofluorescence agreement rate of 86%.[28]

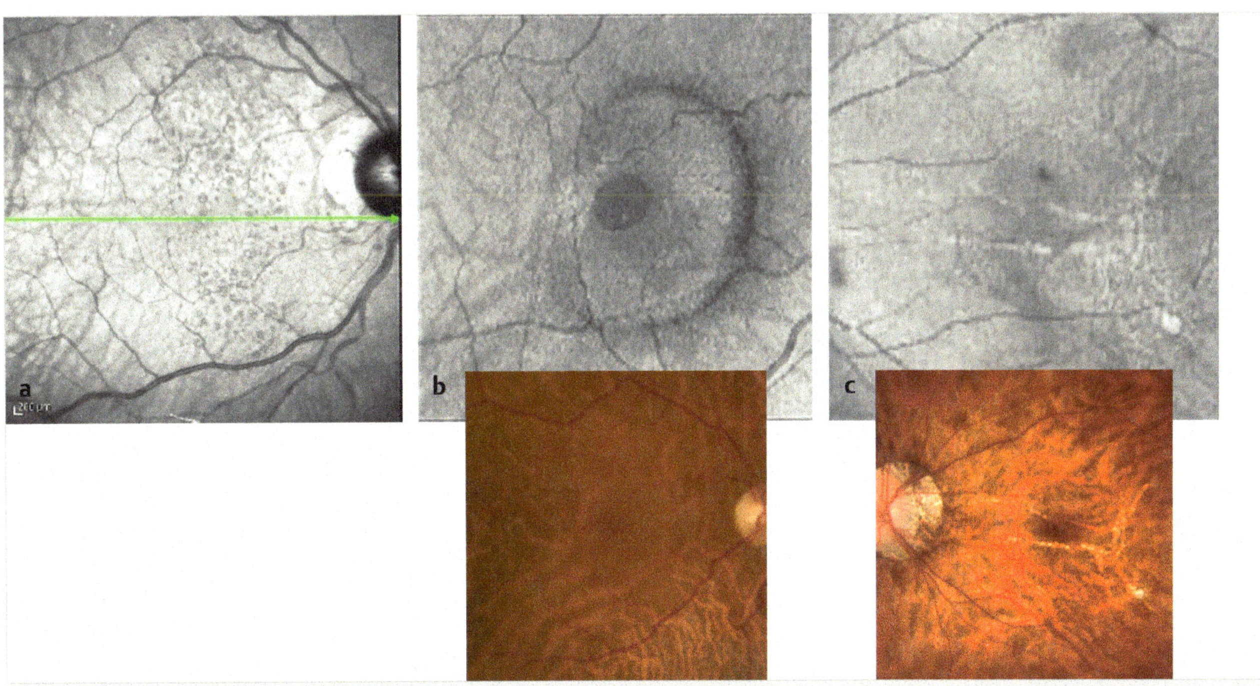

Fig. 7.6 (a) Scanning laser ophthalmoscopy (SLO) (Spectralis; Heidelberg Engineering) image of reticular pseudodrusen. (b) SLO (Cirrus; Carl Zeiss Meditech) and color image of pigment epithelial detachment and full thickness macular hole in a patient with idiopathic juxtafoveal telangiectasis type II. (c) SLO (Cirrus; Carl Zeiss Meditech) and color images of lacquer cracks in a patient with myopic degeneration.

Lipofuscin is a heterogeneous collection of molecules, many of which are by-products of the visual cycle such as shed photoreceptor outer segment disks. In normal eyes, there is a diffuse FAF signal over the posterior pole with a characteristic minimum in the fovea (which is thought to be the result of lutein and zeaxanthin absorption of short wavelength light).[29] An accumulation of lipofuscin in RPE lysosomes, as is the case in diseases such as Best's disease or pattern dystrophy, often signifies dysfunction of the underlying RPE. Because autofluorescence is an inherent property of lipofuscin, areas of lipofuscin accumulation and associated RPE dysfunction appear hyperautofluorescent on FAF. On the other hand, complete absence of autofluorescence/hypoautofluorescence is pathologic as well and may reflect RPE atrophy or death, which is usually accompanied by loss of overlying photoreceptors and concomitant visual dysfunction. The utility of FAF hinges on its ability to map the degree and distribution of RPE dysfunction qualitatively—based on the presence of hypoautofluorescent, isoautofluorescent, and hyperautofluorescent signals. Quantification of autofluorescence intensity remains a challenge and should not be used for intra- or interpatient comparison.

From a diagnostic standpoint, FAF can be essential, and its use in diagnosis of several clinical entities is discussed briefly later. Basal laminar drusen may be difficult to appreciate on ophthalmoscopic examination and using conventional fundus photography; however, FAF readily enables visualization of basal laminar drusen and is less invasive than fluorescein angiography.[30] In such cases, it may also help distinguish an associated pseudovitelliform detachment from choroidal neovascularization, as the former may exhibit hyperautofluorescent material layered inferiorly within the subretinal space (▶ Fig. 7.7a). Depending on their position within the optic nerve, optic nerve head drusen may also be visualized well using FAF, as they will exhibit characteristic hyperautofluorescence.[31] Pattern dystrophy and Best's disease, in various stages of evolution, may also be diagnosed using FAF (▶ Fig. 7.7b, c). FAF can also play a critical role in the identification of angioid streaks arising from pseudoxanthoma elasticum or other causes.[32] Additionally, early RPE damage in the setting of hydroxychloroquine or chloroquine use may be detected by using FAF, so baseline and annual FAF may be appropriate in certain patients (▶ Fig. 7.7d).[33]

In addition to its role in diagnosis, FAF may also be used to visualize qualitative changes over time in certain patients. This role is particularly evident in diseases which involve RPE dropout either primarily or secondarily—such as in retinitis pigmentosa, Stargardt's disease (▶ Fig. 7.7e), central areolar choroidal dystrophy (▶ Fig. 7.7f), choroideremia, or geographic atrophy in the setting of dry age-related macular degeneration (▶ Fig. 7.7g). In many cases, the borders of choroidal nevi or choroidal melanomas may be better appreciated using FAF as compared with standard fundus photography, although absolute margins must be interpreted with caution. By allowing visualization of the pattern and extent of RPE changes, the boundaries of either previous or existing subretinal fluid may be appreciated using FAF as is the case for choroidal nevi, choroidal melanomas (▶ Fig. 7.7h), or central serous chorioretinopathy. In chronic central serous chorioretinopathy, descending tracts of variable hyper- and hypo-autofluorescence may be present.[34]

7.8 Adaptive Optics

In the past 25 years, advancements in adaptive optics (AO) have translated into new techniques for imaging the human retina. Prior to the use of AO, aberrations in the optics of the human visual system limited transverse resolution of the retina, such that individual photoreceptors could not be visualized adequately using more conventional retinal imaging devices. AO imaging systems now enable acquisition of high-quality images of individual photoreceptor cells (▶ Fig. 7.8a).

The basis of an AO platform is the presence of a sensor that detects optical aberrations and a device that corrects for such optical aberrations.[35] In most cases, a Hartmann–Shack wavefront sensor detects optical aberrations, and either a deformable mirror or liquid crystal array adjusts for such detected aberrations.[36] These two elements comprise a system which compensates for a given patient's unique optical aberrations and, therefore, is considered *adaptive*. AO technology can be layered on a number of existing retinal imaging systems, including conventional flood-illuminated fundus photography, SLO, and optical coherence tomography (OCT).[37,38,39] AO used with SLO or OCT is, respectively, denoted as AO-SLO or AO-OCT. At this time, commercially available AO retinal imaging systems have been developed by four companies: Imagine Eyes; Boston Micromachines Corporation; Canon, Inc.; and Physical Sciences, Inc.[40]

Real-time, in vivo imaging of the human retina has enhanced understanding of its structure and function in both normal and pathologic states. AO systems image cones more easily than rods, though both have been imaged successfully using AO. Recently, developments in AO have also enabled imaging of the retinal nerve fiber layer as well as the RPE. In a normal eye, foveal and parafoveal cones are packed hexagonally, and cone photoreceptor packing is densest within a radius of 0.5 mm from the foveal center (where cone diameter is also smallest). Measured cone packing density may vary slightly depending on the software used to quantify the cone mosaics, but the average cone density at 0.5 mm from the fovea ranges from 30,000 to 37,000 cones/mm^2.[41,42,43] Cone density decreases with increasing distance from the foveal center, although it appears that cone density decreases at a higher rate along the vertical, as compared with the horizontal, meridian. This results in an elliptical isodensity contour, also referred to as a horizontal cone streak. AO has identified rods within 190 µm temporal to the foveal center, in accordance with what is known to be the case histologically.[44]

AO studies have yielded conflicting results on the question of whether cone photoreceptor density decreases with age. If an age-related decrease in cone density does exist, it may be most prominent within 0.5 mm of the foveal center.[45] The impact of axial myopia on cone photoreceptor density, however, has been well established by AO. Cone photoreceptor packing density has been shown to be lower in myopic eyes than in emmetropic eyes.[46] The same study revealed that cone packing density is lowest in the inferior meridian in both myopic and emmetropic eyes.

A number of studies have used AO platforms to examine the photoreceptors in eyes with a spectrum of pathology, including diabetes (▶ Fig. 7.8b), branch retinal vein occlusion, fundus albipunctatus, chloroquine maculopathy, retinitis pigmentosa, age-

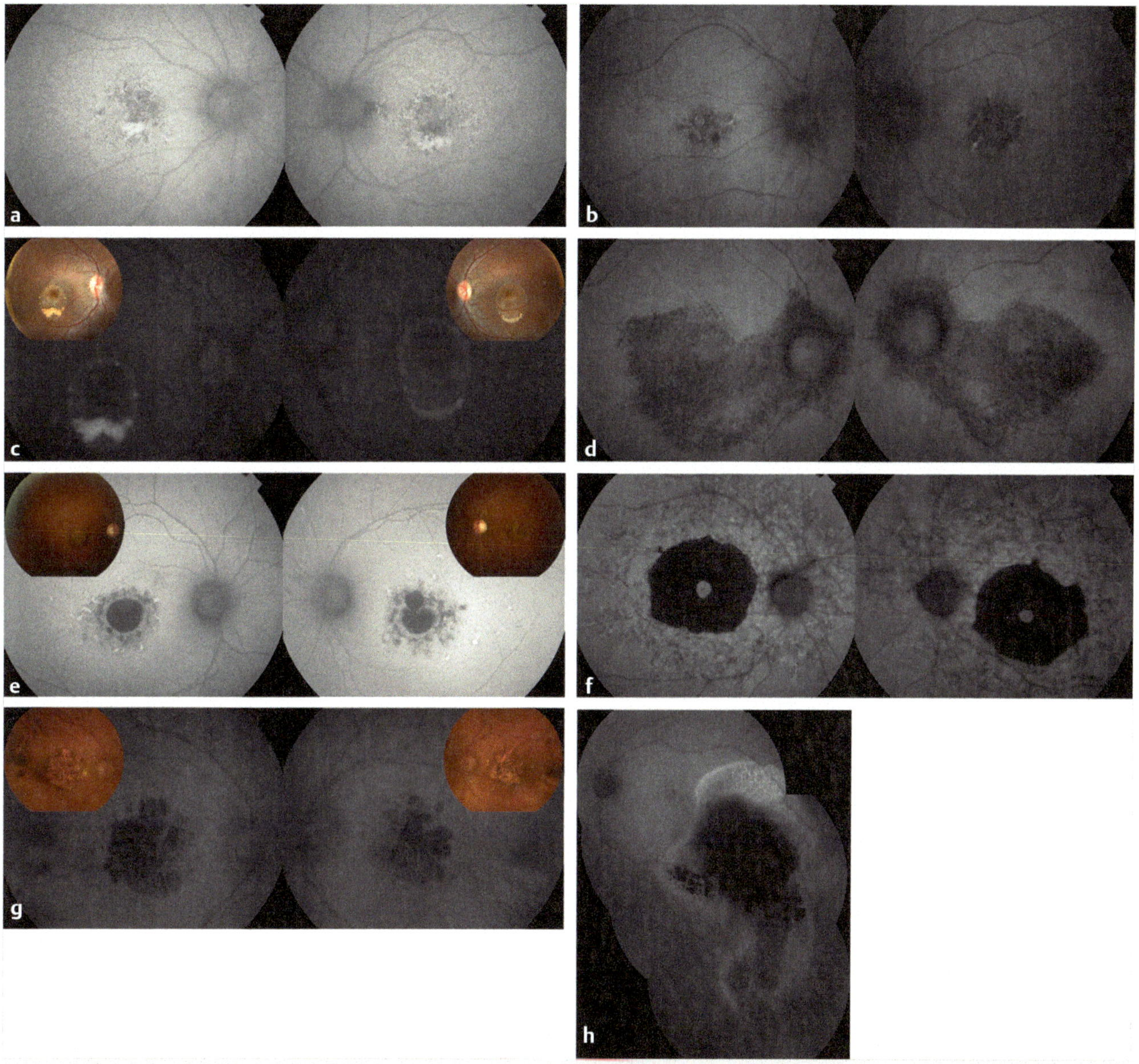

Fig. 7.7 (**a**) Fundus autofluorescence (FAF) (TRC-50DX, Topcon Medical Systems) of basal laminar drusen. The basal laminar drusen appear as a central circular area of hypoautofluorescence with a surrounding ring of hyperautofluorescence; they are present within and beyond the macula and impart a sense of graininess to the photographs. Notice the hyperautofluorescent material in both maculas, suggesting the presence of lipofuscin. (**b**) FAF (TRC-50DX) of pattern dystrophy. There are hyperautofluorescent reticular changes in both maculas. (**c**) FAF and color fundus photographs (TRC-50DX) of Best's disease/vitelliform macular dystrophy type 2. The yellowish subretinal material has primarily layered inferiorly and is intensely hyperautofluorescent. (**d**) FAF (TRC-50DX) of hydroxychloroquine toxicity. Hypoautofluorescence in the macula and peripapillary area corresponds to areas of RPE and overlying retinal atrophy. There is relative sparing of the fovea in both eyes. (**e**) FAF and color fundus photographs (TRC-50DX) of Stargardt disease. The central area of hypoautofluorescence demonstrates the distribution of RPE and overlying retinal atrophy. Pisciform flecks in both maculas are hyperautofluorescent, suggestive of underlying RPE dysfunction. (**f**) FAF (TRC-50DX) of central areolar choroidal dystrophy. Note the dramatic, confluent area of hypoautofluorescence in both maculas, with sparing of a small foveal island. There are also extensive adjacent RPE changes which extend beyond the arcades and nasal to the optic nerve in both eyes. (**g**) FAF and color images (TRC-50DX) of geographic atrophy in a patient with dry age-related macular degeneration. Well-delineated areas of hypoautofluorescence in the macula correspond to areas of RPE loss. Choroidal vessels can be visualized in the zones of RPE dropout. (**h**) FAF mosaic (Spectralis; Heidelberg Engineering) of a choroidal melanoma. The central area of confluent hypoautofluorescence corresponds with RPE loss overlying the choroidal melanoma. Adjacent zones of variable hyperautofluorescence and hypoautofluorescence suggest associated RPE changes, most likely due to chronic subretinal fluid. Guttering of subretinal fluid is suggested by the changes inferior to the choroidal melanoma.

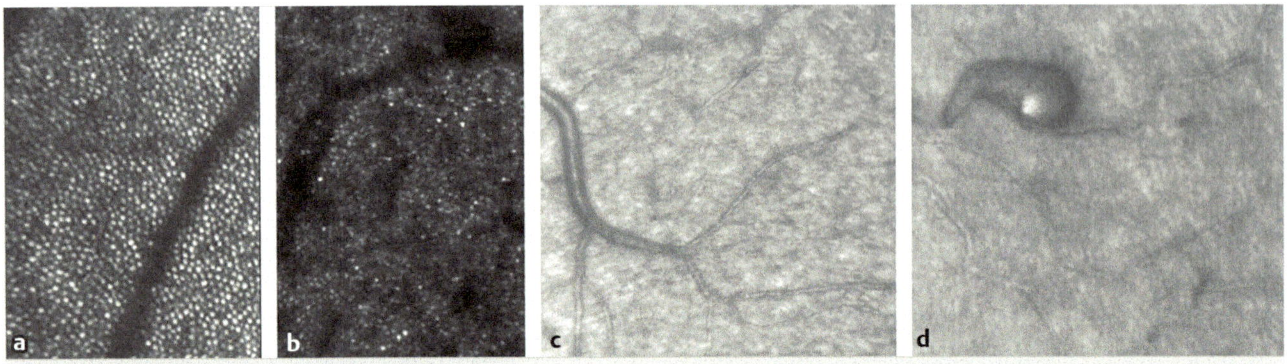

Fig. 7.8 (**a**) Adaptive optics-scanning laser ophthalmoscopy (AO-SLO) image (Apaeros Retinal Imaging System; Boston Micromachines Corporation) of a normal cone mosaic. White circles are individual cone photoreceptors. (**b**) AO-SLO image which shows loss of the normal cone mosaic in a patient with diabetic retinopathy. Black patches correspond to disturbances of the cone mosaic within 4 degrees of the fovea; this may be due to either cone dropout or a shadowing effect from microaneurysms or hemorrhages in more superficial retinal layers. (**c**) AO-SLO imaging of normal retinal vasculature. (**d**) AO-SLO image of a microaneurysm in a patient with diabetic retinopathy. (C 2014 Beetham Eye Institue, Joslin Diabetes Center. All Rights Reserved. Courtesy of J.K. Sun, MD, MPH)

related macular degeneration, geographic atrophy, reticular pseudodrusen, idiopathic macular telangiectasis type I and II, central serous chorioretinopathy, acute posterior multifocal placoid pigment epitheliopathy, and macular holes. Specific findings are beyond the scope of this discussion, but visualization of individual photoreceptor elements promises to further understanding of the mechanisms of disease.

While the focus of AO technology seems to be on visualization of individual photoreceptor elements, AO may also be useful for optimizing visualization of microvasculature (▶ Fig. 7.8c) and for providing quantitative measurements of small vessel blood flow based on erythrocyte or leukocyte movement.[47] In patients with nonproliferative diabetic retinopathy due to type I diabetes, for example, a flood-illuminated AO retinal camera revealed a significantly narrower retinal capillary lumen caliber in diabetic patients as compared with nondiabetic controls.[48] Use of AO-SLO has also shed light on microscopic features of retinal microaneurysms in the setting of diabetes (▶ Fig. 7.8d), hypertension, and retinal vascular occlusions, leading to the proposal of a new morphologic classification scheme.[49] Computer algorithms can be used with AO-SLO to determine the optical density of retinal vascular segments, which may then be used to calculate oxygen saturation.[50]

In addition to its emerging role in imaging retinal microvasculature, AO affords a sophisticated approach to understanding the interaction between the photoreceptor matrix and visual function and complements existing retinal imaging techniques.

References

[1] Marmor MF, Arden GB, Nilsson SE, Zrenner E, International Standardization Committee. Standard for clinical electroretinography. Arch Ophthalmol. 1989; 107(6):816–819

[2] Marmor MF, Fulton AB, Holder GE, Miyake Y, Brigell M, Bach M, International Society for Clinical Electrophysiology of Vision. ISCEV standard for full-field clinical electroretinography (2008 update). Doc Ophthalmol. 2009; 118 (1):69–77

[3] Cleary TS, Reichel E. Electrophysiology. In: Yanoff M, Duker JS, eds. Ophthalmology. 3rd ed. Philadelphia, PA: Mosby/Elsevier; 2009:54554–54559

[4] Hood DC, Holopigian K, Greenstein V, et al. Assessment of local retinal function in patients with retinitis pigmentosa using the multi-focal ERG technique. Vision Res. 1998; 38(1):163–179

[5] Miyake Y, Shinoda K. Clinical Electrophysiology. In: Ryan SJ, Sadda SR, Hinton DR, eds. Retina. 5th ed. Philadelphia, PA: Elsevier/Saunders; 2013:202–226

[6] Sutter EE, Tran D. The field topography of ERG components in man—I. The photopic luminance response. Vision Res. 1992; 32(3):433–446

[7] Hood DC, Bach M, Brigell M, et al. International Society For Clinical Electrophysiology of Vision. ISCEV standard for clinical multifocal electroretinography (mfERG) (2011 edition). Doc Ophthalmol. 2012; 124(1):1–13

[8] Marg E. Development of electro-oculography; standing potential of the eye in registration of eye movement. AMA Arch Opthalmol. 1951; 45(2):169–185

[9] Arden GB, Kelsey JH. Changes produced by light in the standing potential of the human eye. J Physiol. 1962; 161:189–204

[10] Marmor MF, Brigell MG, McCulloch DL, Westall CA, Bach M, International Society for Clinical Electrophysiology of Vision. ISCEV standard for clinical electro-oculography (2010 update). Doc Ophthalmol. 2011; 122(1):1–7

[11] Smith VC, Pokorny J, Pass AS. Color-axis determination on the Farnsworth-Munsell 100-hue test. Am J Ophthalmol. 1985; 100(1):176–182

[12] Pokorny J, Smith VC, Verriest G, Pinckers AILG, eds. Congenital and Acquired Color Vision Defects. New York, NY: Grune & Stratton; 1979

[13] Webb RH, Hughes GW. Scanning laser ophthalmoscope. IEEE Trans Biomed Eng. 1981; 28(7):488–492

[14] Yannuzzi LA, Ober MD, Slakter JS, et al. Ophthalmic fundus imaging: today and beyond. Am J Ophthalmol. 2004; 137(3):511–524

[15] Webb RH, Hughes GW, Delori FC. Confocal scanning laser ophthalmoscope. Appl Opt. 1987; 26(8):1492–1499

[16] Hammer DX, Ferguson RD, Mujat M, et al. Multimodal adaptive optics retinal imager: design and performance. J Opt Soc Am A Opt Image Sci Vis. 2012; 29 (12):2598–2607

[17] Woon WH, Fitzke FW, Bird AC, Marshall J. Confocal imaging of the fundus using a scanning laser ophthalmoscope. Br J Ophthalmol. 1992; 76(8):470–474

[18] Beausencourt E, Remky A, Elsner AE, Hartnett ME, Trempe CL. Infrared scanning laser tomography of macular cysts. Ophthalmology. 2000; 107(2):375–385

[19] Elsner A, Miura M, Burns S, et al. Multiply scattered light tomography and confocal imaging: detecting neovascularization in age-related macular degeneration. Opt Express. 2000; 7(2):95–106

[20] Diniz B, Ribeiro RM, Rodger DC, Maia M, Sadda S. Drusen detection by confocal aperture-modulated infrared scanning laser ophthalmoscopy. Br J Ophthalmol. 2013; 97(3):285–290

[21] Kunze C, Elsner AE, Beausencourt E, Moraes L, Hartnett ME, Trempe CL. Spatial extent of pigment epithelial detachments in age-related macular degeneration. Ophthalmology. 1999; 106(9):1830–1840

[22] Beausencourt E, Elsner AE, Hartnett ME, Trempe CL. Quantitative analysis of macular holes with scanning laser tomography. Ophthalmology. 1997; 104 (12):2018–2029

[23] Elsner AE, Burns SA, Weiter JJ, Delori FC. Infrared imaging of sub-retinal structures in the human ocular fundus. Vision Res. 1996; 36(1):191–205

[24] Delori FC, Dorey CK, Staurenghi G, Arend O, Goger DG, Weiter JJ. In vivo fluorescence of the ocular fundus exhibits retinal pigment epithelium lipofuscin characteristics. Invest Ophthalmol Vis Sci. 1995; 36(3):718–729

[25] von Rückmann A, Fitzke FW, Bird AC. Distribution of fundus autofluorescence with a scanning laser ophthalmoscope. Br J Ophthalmol. 1995; 79(5):407–412

[26] Spaide RF. Fundus autofluorescence and age-related macular degeneration. Ophthalmology. 2003; 110(2):392–399

[27] Fleckenstein M, Schmitz-Valkenberg S, Holz F. Autofluorescence Imaging. In: Ryan SJ, Sadda SR, Hinton DR, eds. Retina. 5th ed. Philadelphia, PA: Elsevier/Saunders; 2013:111–132

[28] Park SP, Siringo FS, Pensec N, et al. Comparison of fundus autofluorescence between fundus camera and confocal scanning laser ophthalmoscope-based systems. Ophthalmic Surg Lasers Imaging Retina. 2013; 44(6):536–543

[29] Schmitz-Valckenberg S, Fleckenstein M, Scholl HP, Holz FG. Fundus autofluorescence and progression of age-related macular degeneration. Surv Ophthalmol. 2009; 54(1):96–117

[30] Meyerle CB, Smith RT, Barbazetto IA, Yannuzzi LA. Autofluorescence of basal laminar drusen. Retina. 2007; 27(8):1101–1106

[31] Sato T, Mrejen S, Spaide RF. Multimodal imaging of optic disc drusen. Am J Ophthalmol. 2013; 156(2):275–282.e1

[32] Sawa M, Ober MD, Freund KB, Spaide RF. Fundus autofluorescence in patients with pseudoxanthoma elasticum. Ophthalmology. 2006; 113(5):814–20.e2

[33] Marmor MF, Kellner U, Lai TY, Lyons JS, Mieler WF, American Academy of Ophthalmology. Revised recommendations on screening for chloroquine and hydroxychloroquine retinopathy. Ophthalmology. 2011; 118(2):415–422

[34] Spaide RF, Klancnik JM, Jr. Fundus autofluorescence and central serous chorioretinopathy. Ophthalmology. 2005; 112(5):825–833

[35] Liang J, Williams DR, Miller DT. Supernormal vision and high-resolution retinal imaging through adaptive optics. J Opt Soc Am A Opt Image Sci Vis. 1997; 14(11):2884–2892

[36] Williams DR. Imaging single cells in the living retina. Vision Res. 2011; 51 (13):1379–1396

[37] Miller DT, Williams DR, Morris GM, Liang J. Images of cone photoreceptors in the living human eye. Vision Res. 1996; 36(8):1067–1079

[38] Roorda A, Romero-Borja F, Donnelly Iii W, Queener H, Hebert T, Campbell M. Adaptive optics scanning laser ophthalmoscopy. Opt Express. 2002; 10 (9):405–412

[39] Kitaguchi Y, Fujikado T, Bessho K, et al. Adaptive optics fundus camera to examine localized changes in the photoreceptor layer of the fovea. Ophthalmology. 2008; 115(10):1771–1777

[40] Lombardo M, Serrao S, Devaney N, Parravano M, Lombardo G. Adaptive optics technology for high-resolution retinal imaging. Sensors (Basel). 2013; 13 (1):334–366

[41] Chui TY, Song H, Burns SA. Adaptive-optics imaging of human cone photoreceptor distribution. J Opt Soc Am A Opt Image Sci Vis. 2008; 25(12):3021–3029

[42] Ooto S, Hangai M, Sakamoto A, et al. High-resolution imaging of resolved central serous chorioretinopathy using adaptive optics scanning laser ophthalmoscopy. Ophthalmology. 2010; 117(9):1800–1809, 1809.e1–1809.e2

[43] Song H, Chui TY, Zhong Z, Elsner AE, Burns SA. Variation of cone photoreceptor packing density with retinal eccentricity and age. Invest Ophthalmol Vis Sci. 2011; 52(10):7376–7384

[44] Dubra A, Sulai Y, Norris JL, et al. Noninvasive imaging of the human rod photoreceptor mosaic using a confocal adaptive optics scanning ophthalmoscope. Biomed Opt Express. 2011; 2(7):1864–1876

[45] Park SP, Chung JK, Greenstein V, Tsang SH, Chang S. A study of factors affecting the human cone photoreceptor density measured by adaptive optics scanning laser ophthalmoscope. Exp Eye Res. 2013; 108:1–9

[46] Chui TY, Song H, Burns SA. Individual variations in human cone photoreceptor packing density: variations with refractive error. Invest Ophthalmol Vis Sci. 2008; 49(10):4679–4687

[47] Chui TY, Gast TJ, Burns SA. Imaging of vascular wall fine structure in the human retina using adaptive optics scanning laser ophthalmoscopy. Invest Ophthalmol Vis Sci. 2013; 54(10):7115–7124

[48] Lombardo M, Parravano M, Serrao S, Ducoli P, Stirpe M, Lombardo G. Analysis of retinal capillaries in patients with type 1 diabetes and nonproliferative diabetic retinopathy using adaptive optics imaging. Retina. 2013; 33(8):1630–1639

[49] Dubow M, Pinhas A, Shah N, et al. Classification of human retinal microaneurysms using adaptive optics scanning light ophthalmoscope fluorescein angiography. Invest Ophthalmol Vis Sci. 2014; 55(3):1299–1309

[50] Li H, Lu J, Shi G, Zhang Y. Measurement of oxygen saturation in small retinal vessels with adaptive optics confocal scanning laser ophthalmoscope. J Biomed Opt. 2011; 16(11):110504

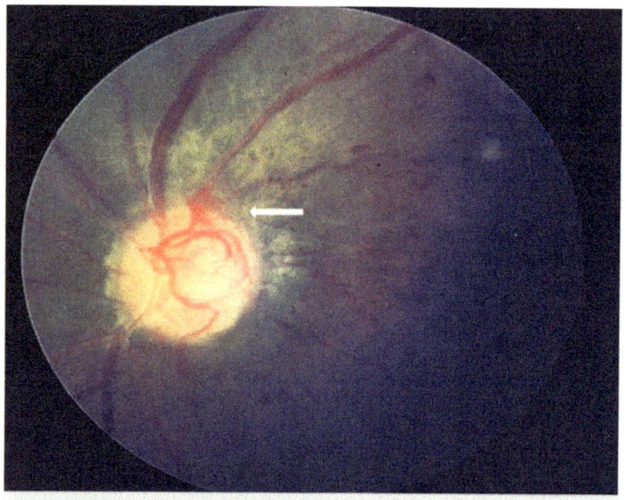

Fig. 8.6 Neovascularization of the optic disc (arrow) in the right eye of an 80-year-old, nondiabetic man with right ocular ischemic syndrome and bilateral 95% internal carotid artery stenosis.

(▶ Fig. 8.7b). As is the case with retinal capillary nonperfusion associated with other entities, it is not reversible.

Microaneurysms are often present, most commonly in the retinal periphery. In the posterior pole, they can leak and contribute to macular edema.[7] The macular edema is often more pronounced with fluorescein angiography (▶ Fig. 8.8) than clinically, and marked cystic changes are usually absent. Despite the fact that eyes with OIS and macular edema routinely demonstrate hyperfluorescence of the optic disc with fluorescein angiography, the disc generally appears normal ophthalmoscopically. Telangiectatic vascular changes may be present.

Cotton-wool spots are found in approximately 4% of affected eyes, as are spontaneous retinal arterial pulsations.[3] The arterial pulsations are most pronounced over the optic disc and extend to one to two disc diameters from the edge of the disc. Although spontaneous retinal arterial pulsations are also seen with cardiac valvular disease and increased intraocular pressure, their presence in a person older than 50 years should strongly arouse suspicion of OIS. Ischemic optic neuropathy, characterized by acute visual loss and optic disc swelling, has been observed in 1 to 2% of cases.[8]

If spontaneous retinal arterial pulsations are not present, light digital pressure on the lid will often induce them, which is not usually the case with CRVO. This can be a helpful method to differentiate between the two diseases.

A list of the key clinical features seen with OIS is shown in ▶ Table 8.1

Pearl

- 90% of eyes with the OIS have dilated, but not tortuous, retinal veins, while 80% have peripheral, midperipheral, or posterior pole dot and blot retinal hemorrhages.

8.2.7 Ancillary Tests

Fluorescein angiography reveals delayed filling of the choroid in approximately 60% of OIS eyes (▶ Fig. 8.9).[3] Normally, the choroid is completely filled within 5 seconds after the first appearance of dye within it. A marked delay in choroidal filling is perhaps the most specific fluorescein angiographic sign of the OIS. Delayed retinal arteriovenous transit time (time from the first appearance of dye within the temporal retinal arteries until the corresponding retinal veins are completely filled; normally less than 11 seconds) is found in 95% of affected eyes, but this is not as specific for OIS as is delayed choroidal filling. It can also be seen with central retinal artery occlusion (CRAO), diabetic retinopathy, and central retinal vein occlusion. Staining of the retinal vessels (▶ Fig. 8.10), often more so the arteries than the veins, is seen in about 85% of OIS eyes, probably as a consequence of endothelial cell ischemia.

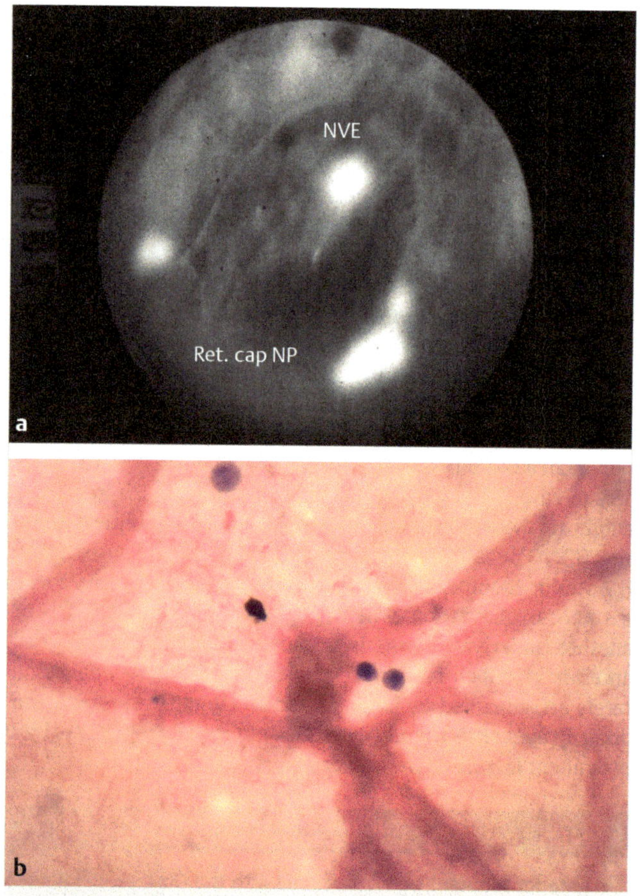

Fig. 8.7 (**a**) Fluorescein angiogram of an eye with ocular ischemic syndrome at approximately 1 minute after fluorescein injection discloses inferior retinal capillary nonperfusion associated with three hyperfluorescent areas of neovascularization of the retina. (**b**) Trypsin digest microphotograph of the retinal blood vessels in an area of retinal capillary nonperfusion. The vessels are acellular tubules without endothelial cells or pericytes. Such areas of retinal capillary nonperfusion do not typically reperfuse. Hematoxylin and eosin, × 100. (Images courtesy of W. Richard Green, MD.)

Pearls

- The fluorescein angiographic signs associated with the OIS include (1) delayed choroidal filling, (2) increased arteriovenous transit time, and (3) late staining of the retinal arteries and arterioles.

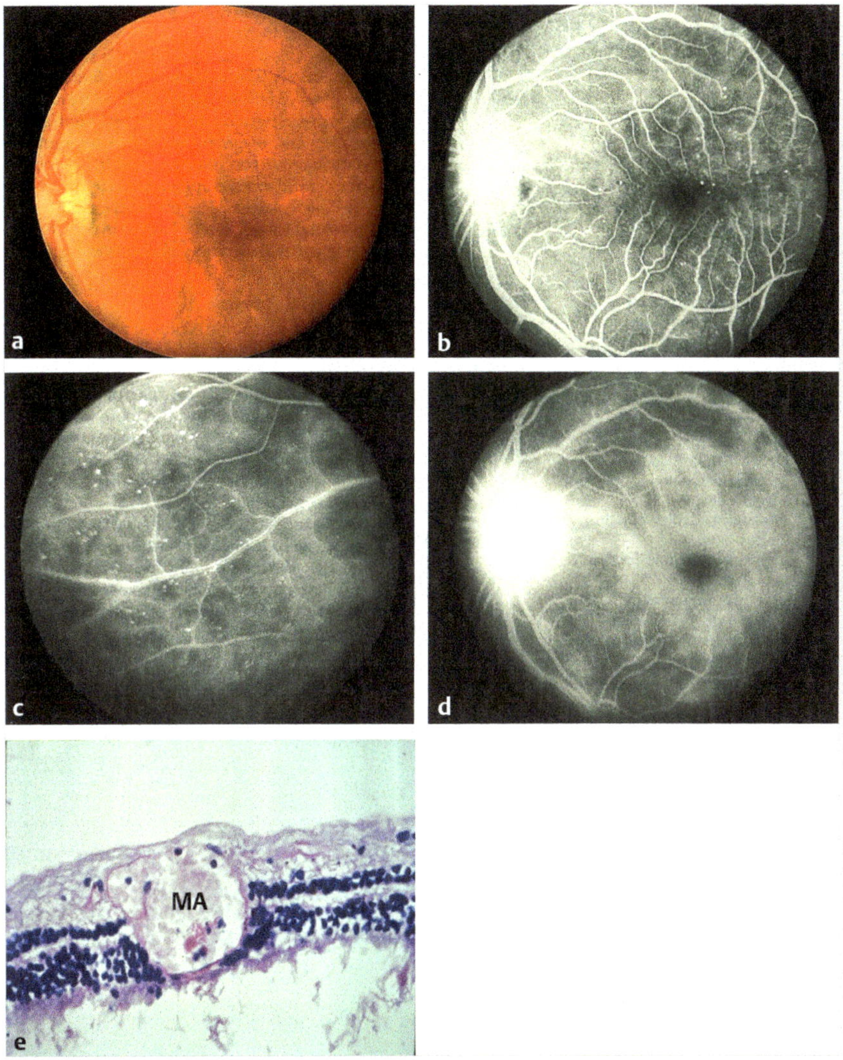

Fig. 8.8 (a) Macular cyst in an ocular ischemic syndrome eye of a patient with an ipsilateral 100% internal carotid artery occlusion. The visual acuity was 20/40. (b) Fluorescein angiogram of the eye shown in (a) at 70 seconds after injection reveals numerous hyperfluorescent foci corresponding to retinal microaneurysms in the macular region. (c) At 270 seconds after injection, numerous retinal microaneurysms can be seen in the midperiphery. (d) At 446 seconds after injection, there is marked intraretinal leakage of dye, as well as hyperfluorescence of the optic disc. (e) Light histopathologic photograph of a microaneurysm (MA) from an eye with the ocular ischemic syndrome. Note that the vascular abnormality occupies the full thickness of the retina. Rupture of such microaneurysms likely leads to the retinal hemorrhages encountered with the ocular ischemic syndrome. Periodic acid–Schiff, × 63. (Images courtesy of W. Richard Green, MD.)

Electroretinography often reveals diminution of the amplitudes of the a- and b-waves (▸ Fig. 8.11), corresponding to outer and inner retinal ischemia, respectively.[3] Histopathology reveals damage to both the inner and outer retinal layers (▸ Fig. 8.12). While retinal pigment epithelial (RPE) disturbance is often a long-term feature of the acute choroidal ischemia encountered with acute ophthalmic artery occlusion, it is not typically a manifestation of the OIS.

Carotid noninvasive testing, particularly duplex scanning (real-time B-mode arterial imaging with a pulsed Doppler to record blood flow velocity, or color duplex ultrasound), has been shown in a meta-analysis to have a 98% sensitivity and 88% specificity in detecting angiographic carotid stenoses of =50% and a 90% sensitivity and 94% specificity for identifying stenosis =70%.[10] Computed tomography (CT) angiography and magnetic resonance angiography (MRA) can be employed as confirmatory tests. In instances in which the carotid arteries appear normal with noninvasive testing, color Doppler ultrasonography of the eye and orbital vessels, in addition to CT angiography and MRA, can be helpful in identifying an underlying ophthalmic artery occlusion.

8.2.8 Differential Diagnosis

The OIS is most commonly confused with mild CRVO and diabetic retinopathy.[2] Differentiating features are shown in ▸ Table 8.2.

Diabetic retinopathy, in particular, can be confused with the OIS. This occurs because more than 50% of patients with the OIS also have diabetes mellitus, a known risk factor for increased atherosclerosis. In some instances, both diabetic retinopathy and the OIS are present concomitantly.

Features more suggestive of diabetic retinopathy than the OIS include bilaterality, the presence of hard exudate, thick macular edema, and numerous microaneurysms in the posterior pole. While it may occur without diabetes, We are unaware of a clinical case of the OIS in which hard exudate is present in the fundus unless the patient also has diabetes mellitus and a component of diabetic retinopathy. In cases of severely asymmetric diabetic retinopathy (nonproliferative disease in one eye and high-risk proliferative disease in the other eye), carotid artery occlusion has not been demonstrated convincingly to have a protective or exacerbating effect on the diabetic retinopathy.[11] Notwithstanding, there are anecdotal cases in which

Table 8.1 Clinical features of the ocular ischemic syndrome[3,9]

	Frequency
Symptoms	
• Decreased vision	90%
• Abrupt	12%
• Pain ("ocular angina")	40%
• Amaurosis fugax	10%
• Prolonged recovery to light exposure	Uncertain
Signs	
Anterior segment	
• Iris neovascularization	67%
• Anterior chamber flare	>67%
• Anterior chamber cells	20%
• Increased cataract	Uncommon
Posterior segment	
• Narrowed retinal arteries	>90%
• Dilated retinal veins	>90%
• Microaneurysms	Common
• Tortuous retinal veins	Rare
• Retinal hemorrhages	80%
• Neovascularization of optic disc	35%
• Macular edema	15%
• Neovascularization of retina	8%
• Cotton-wool spots	4%
• Spontaneous retinal arterial pulsations	4%
Fluorescein angiography	
• Delayed choroidal filling	60%
• Increased retinal arteriovenous transit time	95%
• Late arterial staining	85%
Electroretinography	
• Decreased a- and b-waves	Most
Carotid artery occlusion	
• Ipsilateral = 85–90%[a]	100%
• 100% ipsilateral	50%
• 100% bilateral	10%
Five-year mortality[9]	40%

[a]Chronic ophthalmic artery occlusion can also cause the ocular ischemic syndrome.

severe unilateral carotid artery occlusion has markedly worsened ipsilateral proliferative diabetic retinopathy.

Eyes with mild CRVO usually demonstrate venous tortuosity and prominent retinal edema, both features rarely seen with OIS. Additionally, ophthalmoscopic optic disc swelling is rarely seen with the OIS, but is common with CRVO.

While spontaneous retinal arterial pulsations are seen in only 4% of OIS eyes, light digital pressure on the upper lid of these eyes usually produces arterial pulsations. Because OIS is unilateral in 80% of cases,[3] the amount of pressure needed to cause pulsations in the affected eye can be compared with that in the contralateral eye. Ophthalmodynamometry better helps to quantitate the differences. The pulsations are best seen on the optic disc, but can extend outward for several disc diameters from the disc. With CRVO and diabetic retinopathy, substantial digital pressure must be exerted to cause retinal arterial pulsations.

8.2.9 Associated Systemic Diseases

Since marked atherosclerosis is generally not an isolated phenomenon, there is a high prevalence of diseases associated with systemic atherosclerosis in patients with OIS.[12] More than one-half of patients with OIS have diabetes mellitus and nearly one-half have ischemic cardiac disease. Approximately one-fourth of patients have had a previous cerebrovascular accident, and almost one-fifth have required peripheral bypass surgery before the discovery of OIS.

The 5-year mortality rate in patients with OIS is 40%.[12] Despite a stroke rate of 0.4% per year in patients with OIS (more than four times that of an age-matched population), the leading cause of death is cardiac disease. Thus, cardiac evaluation should be considered, depending on the clinical circumstances.

8.2.10 Management and Course

Local therapy for OIS is usually temporizing.[13] Eyes with iris neovascularization and an open anterior chamber angle can be considered for panretinal laser photocoagulation, which is successful in eradicating the new vessels in about 35% of cases.[13] The use of intraocular vascular endothelial growth factor (VEGF) inhibitors in OIS eyes with iris neovascularization should be undertaken with caution. In one series, the authors noted that two of four eyes (50%) receiving intravitreal bevacizumab developed CRAO.[9]

Although no clinical trials have evaluated surgical therapy for vision in OIS, carotid endarterectomy appears to be beneficial for maintaining or improving vision in select cases.[13] Unfortunately, once iris neovascularization is present, more than 90% of eyes are legally blind at the end of 1 year, with or without surgery.[13]

Overall, carotid endarterectomy has been proved to be of benefit in preventing disabling stroke in symptomatic patients (those with amaurosis fugax, hemispheric transient ischemic attack, or nondisabling stroke) with 70 to 99% carotid artery stenosis. The North American Carotid Endarterectomy Trial Collaborators[14] found the stroke rate in endarterectomy patients by 2 years was 0.9% at institutions that frequently performed the surgery. This compares with 26% in a control group using aspirin. Surgical benefit appears to be best in men aged 75 years or older and those who undergo surgery within 2 weeks of an

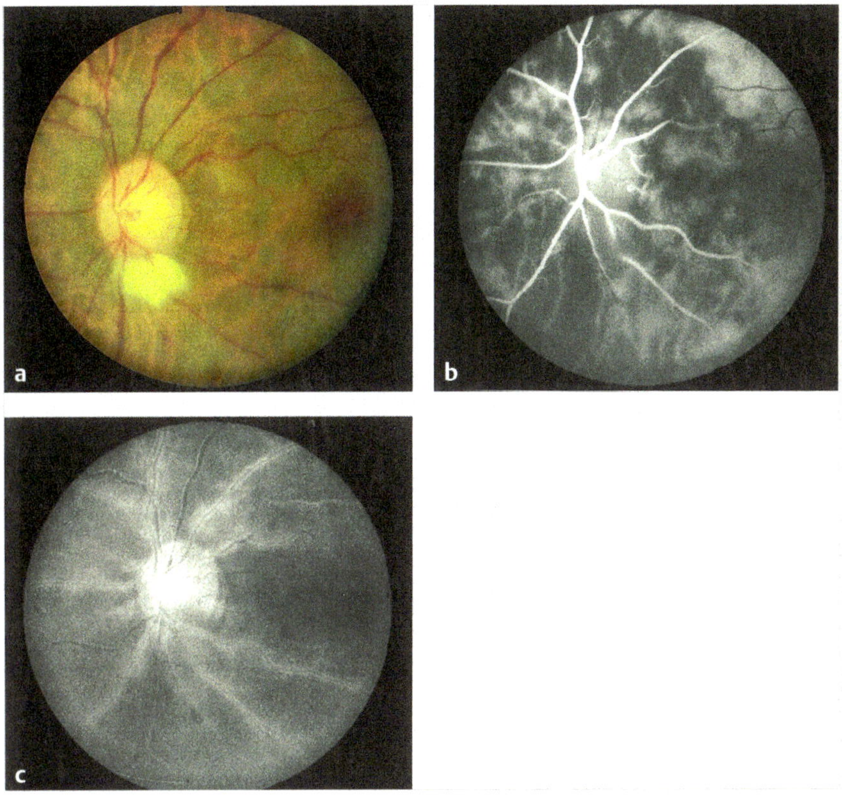

Fig. 8.9 (a) Eye with the ocular ischemic syndrome demonstrates narrowed retinal arteries and dilated retinal veins. The myelinated nerve fibers at the inferior aspect of the optic disc are unrelated to the ischemic process. (**b**) Fluorescein angiogram corresponding to (**a**) at approximately 1 minute after injection reveals a marked delay in filling of the choroid and retinal arteries. (**c**) At more than 7 minutes after injection, there is marked staining of the large retinal vessels, particularly the arteries. (Images provided courtesy of Larry E. Magargal, MD.)

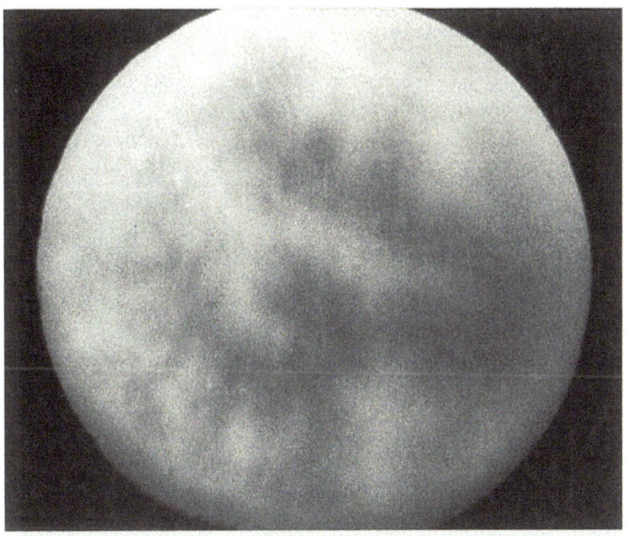

Fig. 8.10 Late fluorescein angiogram of an eye with the ocular ischemic syndrome (OIS) reveals staining of the midperipheral retinal vessels.

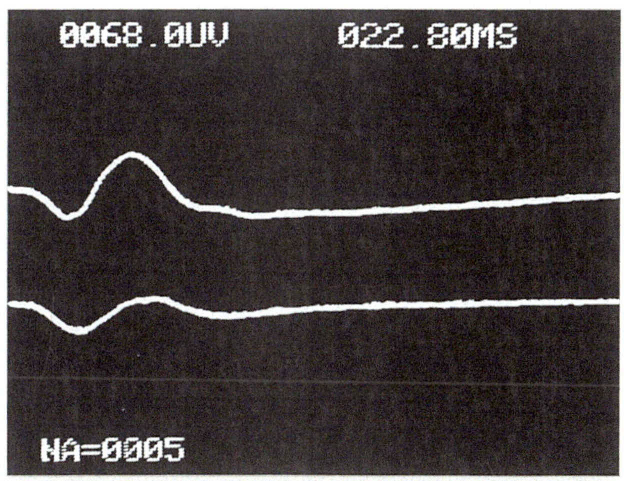

Fig. 8.11 Electroretinogram of an ocular ischemic syndrome eye discloses, in the lower tracing, diminution of the amplitudes of both the a-wave and the b-wave, indicating outer and inner layer retinal ischemic, respectively. The normal upper tracing was taken in the unaffected contralateral eye.

ischemic event.[15] A Cochrane review[15] of carotid endarterectomy for symptomatic patients found that those with an associated 0 to 29% stenosis had an increased 5-year risk of ischemic stroke with endarterectomy (absolute risk reduction [ARR] = –2.2%, $p = 0.05$), those with a 30 to 49% stenosis had no significant effect (ARR = 3.2%, $p = 0.60$), those with a 50 to 69% stenosis had marginal benefit (ARR = 4.6%, $p = 0.04$), and those with a 70 to 99% stenosis had a considerable benefit (ARR = 16.0%, $p < 0.001$).[15] Thus, many patients with symptoms from ulcerated carotid plaques fare just as well with aspirin therapy as with endarterectomy.

In asymptomatic patients with a carotid artery stenosis randomized to endarterectomy versus medical management, the 5-year stroke rate is 6.4 versus 11.8% (ARR = 5.4%, $p < 0.0001$).[16] The benefit was more pronounced in those with greater stenosis (70–90%) on ultrasonography.

In a large analysis from the Society for Vascular Surgery, the 30-day incidence of death, stroke, and/or myocardial infarction

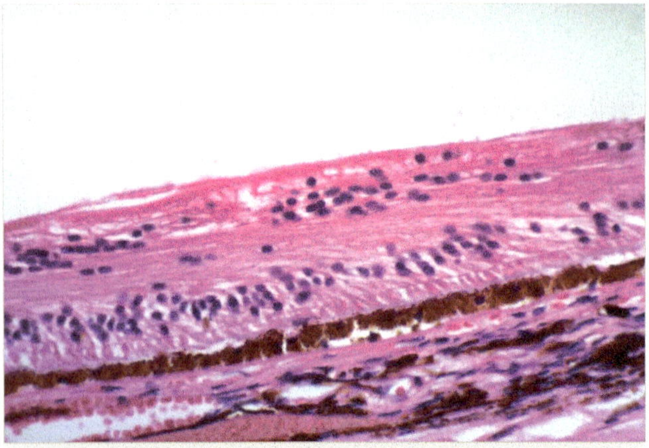

Fig. 8.12 Light microscopic section of the retina from an ocular ischemic syndrome eye reveals loss of cellularity of the ganglion cell layer (inner retinal layer ischemia), as well as photoreceptor loss (outer retinal layer ischemia). The retinal pigment epithelium is intact. Hematoxylin and eosin, × 40. (Image courtesy of W. Richard Green, MD.)

was 7.1% in symptomatic stented patients and 3.8% in endarterectomy patients. For asymptomatic patients, the comparative rates were 4.6 and 2.0%, respectively.[17] Additional follow-up data were similar.[18] Thus, stenting had a higher postoperative complication rate in patients aged 65 years or older. Refinement of comparative data outcomes will surely follow.

Treatment of symptomatic carotid stenosis is less clear. A consortium of professional medical societies[19,20] suggests carotid endarterectomy is reasonable "in asymptomatic patients who have more than 70% stenosis of the internal carotid artery if the risk of perioperative stroke, MI (myocardial infarction), and death is low." Nonetheless, it has been shown that high-dose statins decrease stroke among patients with high-risk cardiovascular disease by one-third.[21] A meta-analysis of 30 studies showed the stroke rate in patients with symptomatic internal carotid disease before the year 2000 was 2.83%, versus 1.13% after the year 2000.[22] Since this has likely occurred, in large part, due to statin therapy, the aggressive use of the most effective statins, rosuvastatin and atorvastatin, can be considered. These drugs have been shown to decrease atherosclerosis that has already formed.[23]

When a 100% carotid artery stenosis is present, a thrombus usually propagates distally, typically precluding successful endarterectomy. In such instances, extracranial to intracranial (e.g., superficial temporal artery to middle cerebral artery) bypass has been attempted. Although it may help vision transiently, at 1 year there appears to be no long-term visual advantage over observation for OIS patients.[13] Additionally, this procedure has been shown in a clinical trial not to be more beneficial than aspirin in preventing stroke[24,25] or improving cognition.[26]

Pearls

- Signs arousing suspicion of the OIS include (1) iris or posterior segment neovascularization with no obvious cause, (2) spontaneous retinal arterial pulsations, and (3) delayed choroidal filling and/or later retinal arterial (arteriolar) staining on fluorescein angiography.

Table 8.2 Differentiating features of the ocular ischemic syndrome

	OIS	Diabetic retinopathy	CRVO
Venous tortuosity	–	–	+
Retinal edema clinically	–	±	+
Retinal edema on fluorescein angiography	±	+	+
Hard exudate	–	+	–
Retinal arterial pulsations	±	–	–
Optic disc edema	–	–	+
Arterial pulsations with light pressure	+	–	–
Delayed choroidal filling	+	–	–
Bilaterality	20%	+	–

Abbreviations: CRVO, central retinal venous occlusion; OIS, ocular ischemic syndrome.

8.3 Acute Ophthalmic Artery Occlusion

Approximately 5 to 10% of cases of acute CRAO are probably acute ophthalmic artery occlusion.[27]

Acute ophthalmic artery occlusion is characterized by sudden, severe visual loss. The vision is no light perception (NLP) in 90% of cases, and there is marked opacification of the retina in the macular region and sometimes more peripherally (▸ Fig. 8.13).[27] The NLP vision is an important feature for differentiating acute ophthalmic artery occlusion from acute CRAO; the latter is typically associated with counting fingers to hand-motion vision in the far temporal field.[28]

The ischemic retinal opacification seen with acute ophthalmic artery occlusion is usually more marked than that seen with acute CRAO. In some eyes, the whitening is so severe that there is ischemic opacification of the retinal pigment epithelium and choroid. Approximately 30% of cases lack a cherry-red spot, in 40% it is questionable, and in the remaining 30% it is present as the choroid reperfuses.[27]

Fluorescein angiography often reveals choroidal perfusion defects in addition to delayed arteriovenous transit time. In the later phases, there may be focal or generalized staining of the retinal pigment epithelium (▸ Fig. 8.14).[27] Electroretinography discloses reduction of both the a-wave and the b-wave.[27]

Because of the choroidal ischemia, there are often long-term RPE changes after acute ophthalmic artery occlusion. They can occur in both the posterior pole and the peripheral fundus. RPE changes are not typically present from CRAO alone.[27]

The causes of acute ophthalmic artery occlusion are generally similar to those for acute CRAO.[27] In particular, giant cell arteritis should be considered in patients older than 55 years with acute ophthalmic artery occlusion. Orbital mucormycosis, in the clinical setting of periorbital infection, has been repeatedly observed to cause acute ophthalmic artery occlusion due to vasculitis.[27]

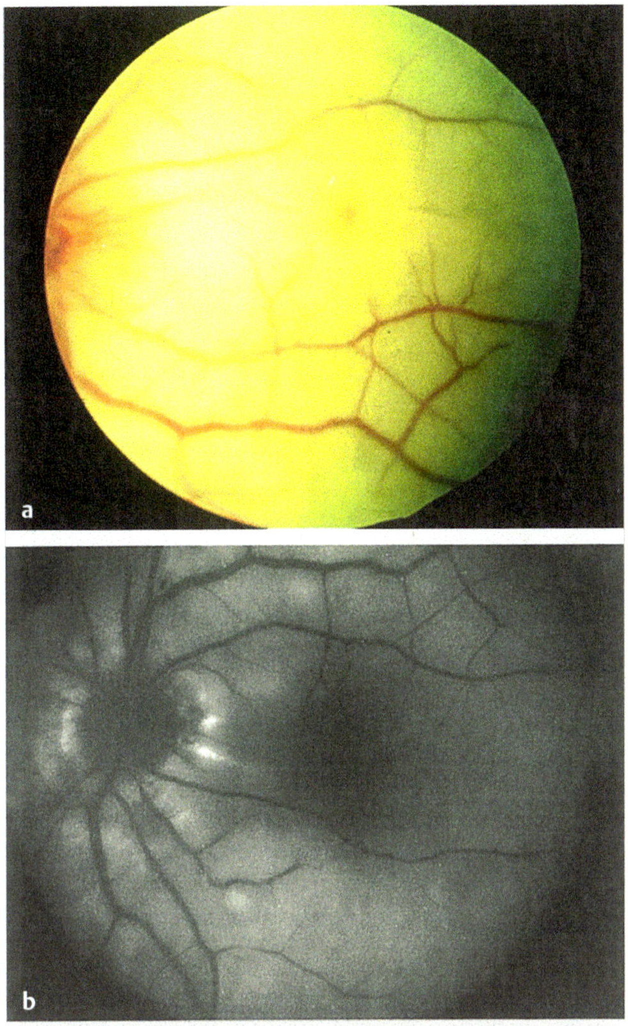

Fig. 8.13 (a) Acute ophthalmic artery occlusion. Marked retinal opacification, caused by inner and outer retinal layer ischemia, is present, and no cherry-red spot can be seen. (b) Fluorescein angiogram corresponding to (a) at 23 seconds after injection reveals lack of dye in the retinal arteries and only minimal peripapillary filling of the choroid. There is diffuse autofluorescence resulting from the yellow color of the fundus.

Treatment of acute ophthalmic artery occlusion is generally unsatisfactory.

8.4 Central Retinal Artery Occlusion

In 1859, von Graefe[29] reported the case of a patient who experienced an acute Central Retinal Artery Occlusion (CRAO). By the beginning of the 20th century, more than two dozen cases of retinal arterial occlusion had appeared in the literature. The mechanisms responsible for CRAO include embolization, intraluminal thrombus, atherosclerotic plaque, hemorrhage under an atherosclerotic plaque, dissecting aneurysm, hypertensive arterial necrosis, vasospasm, circulatory collapse, and vascular inflammation with thickening of arterial walls.[30,31,32,33,34,35,36,37,38,39,40,41,42,43,44,45,46,47,48,49,50]

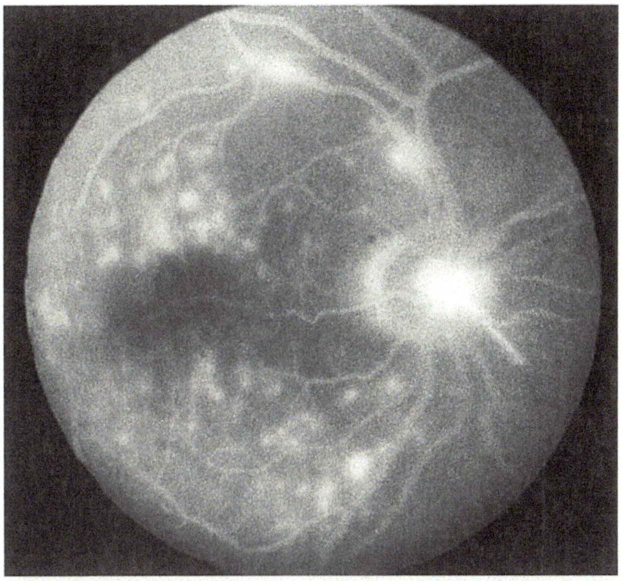

Fig. 8.14 Areas of focal staining at the level of the retinal pigment epithelium in an eye with an acute ophthalmic artery occlusion.

8.4.1 Clinical Features

Demographics

Data from the Retina Vascular Unit at Wills Eye Hospital suggest that CRAO occurs in approximately 1/10,000 outpatient ophthalmologic visits.[28] The mean age at the time of presentation is about 65 years, and men are affected more frequently than women.[28] There appears to be no predilection for one eye over the other. Approximately 1 to 2% of cases are bilateral.[28] When both eyes are affected simultaneously by retinal arterial occlusion, the index of suspicion for cardiac embolic disease, giant cell arteritis, and other vascular inflammations should be heightened. A history of headache, jaw claudication, or recent joint aching should alert the clinician of possible giant cell arteritis as a cause. Since occlusions due to giant cell arteritis have a tendency to be more severe, and because we have seen the fellow eye involved by CRAO within hours after the first, prompt treatment with high-dose corticosteroids should be considered, more so to protect the second eye than to help the first. Nevertheless, anecdotal cases suggest that high-dose corticosteroids can be of benefit in reversing some cases of incomplete occlusion as well.

History

Patients with acute CRAO typically relate a history of abrupt, painless, unilateral visual loss occurring over a period of seconds. Some may have a previous history of amaurosis before the episode of severe visual loss, no matter the cause.

Vision

The visual acuity in eyes with CRAO is usually in the counting fingers to hand-motion range.[28] In most instances, at least a temporal island of vision remains. An afferent pupillary defect appears within seconds after the development of the occlusion.

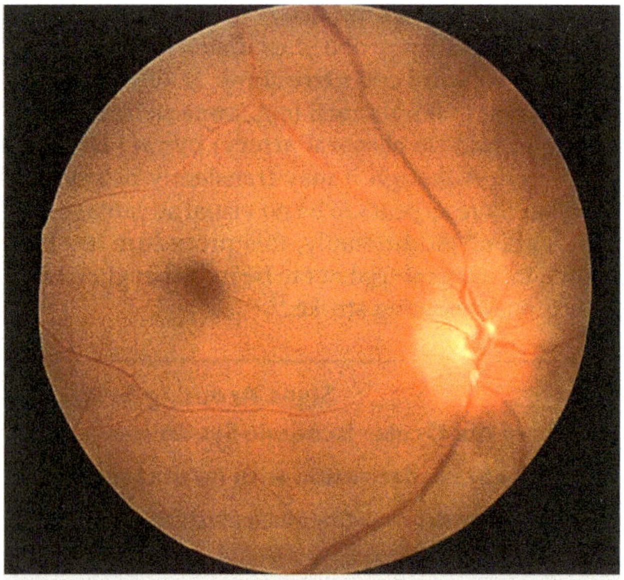

Fig. 8.15 Acute central retinal artery occlusion (CRAO). Superficial retinal opacification is present, and a cherry-red spot can be seen in the foveola. Two large white calcific emboli are present on the optic disc.

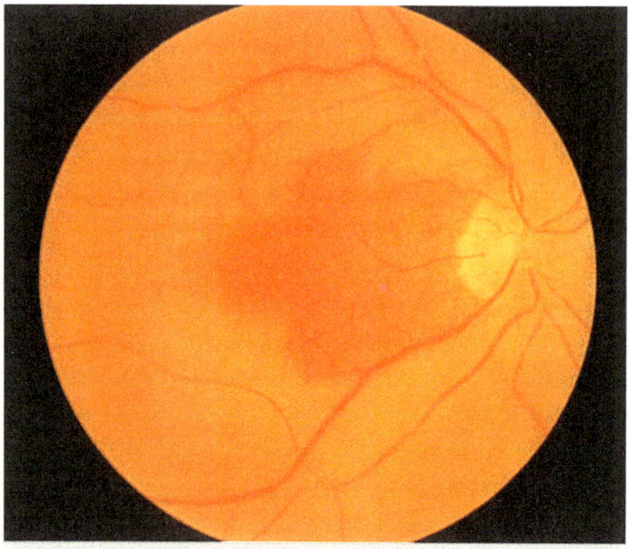

Fig. 8.16 Central retinal artery occlusion (CRAO) with a bifurcating cilioretinal artery emerging temporally on the optic disc and separately from the central retinal arterial system. The patent cilioretinal artery spares the foveolar retina. The visual acuity was 20/50 immediately after the event, improving to 20/20 over several weeks.

Ophthalmoscopy

Fundus examination discloses superficial whitening of the retina, which is most pronounced in the macular region (▸ Fig. 8.15). The whitening typically develops within hours, although in the primate model we have seen it develop within minutes after complete occlusion. In the foveola, where the retina is only 0.1 mm in thickness, a cherry-red spot can be seen. In comparison with the ischemic and opacified perifoveolar retina (approximately 0.5 mm in thickness), the thin foveolar retina still allows visualization of the underlying retinal pigment epithelium and choroid, thus accounting for the cherry-red spot. In mild cases, the whitening can resolve over a period of days. In severe cases, it may take 4 to 10 weeks to disappear. Segmentation of the blood column, or "boxcarring," is present in both the retinal arteries and veins in eyes with severe CRAO.

Cilioretinal Sparing

In approximately 10% of eyes, a patent cilioretinal artery derived from the posterior ciliary arteries, the choroid, or the circle of Zinn–Haller supplies the foveola (▸ Fig. 8.16).[24] These cilioretinal arteries typically originate separately from the central retinal arteries on the optic nerve head or in the temporal peripapillary retina. In these instances, the visual acuity improves to 20/50 or better in 80% of eyes over a period of weeks. The remaining visual field in such cases is variable, but with severe occlusion only a central island of vision may remain. If a patent cilioretinal artery does not reach the foveola, the contribution to visual improvement is minimal.

Emboli

Emboli are seen within the retinal arterial system in approximately 20 to 40% of eyes with CRAO and likely more commonly with branch retinal artery occlusion.[28] Calcific emboli from cardiac valves are usually large and white (▸ Fig. 8.15 and ▸ Fig. 8.17a). They have a greater tendency to cause occlusion than the smaller yellow, glistening cholesterol emboli (Hollenhorst plaques) (▸ Fig. 8.17b). Cholesterol emboli tend to originate from the carotid arteries and/or the aortic arch. In some incidences, they are asymptomatic and are seen in the fundus as incidental findings. Other forms of emboli reported include platelet–fibrin thrombi,[28] atrial myxoma particles,[41,42] corticosteroids,[43,44] talc,[45,46] parasites,[47] contrast media,[48,49] and white blood cell aggregates (leukoemboli).[50]

Ocular Sequelae

Ocular complications of acute CRAO, in addition to visual loss, include neovascularization of the iris and neovascularization of the optic disc.[51,52] Neovascularization of the iris occurs in approximately 18% of eyes, at a mean time of 4 to 5 weeks after the occlusion, with a range of 1 to 15 weeks.[51,52] Laser panretinal photocoagulation has been shown to be effective in causing regression of the new iris vessels in approximately 65% of eyes.[53] NVD has been observed to develop in 2 to 3% of eyes.[54]

8.4.2 Ancillary Studies

Fluorescein Angiography

Intravenous fluorescein angiography often reveals a delay in retinal arterial filling, but the most consistent sign seen with acute CRAO is a delayed arteriovenous transit time. Normally, the arteriovenous transit time (time elapsed from the first appearance of dye within the retinal arteries of the temporal vascular arcade until the corresponding retinal veins are completely filled) is 11 seconds or less. Late staining of the optic disc is variable, but the retinal vessels usually do not stain. Complete lack of filling of the retinal arteries is distinctly unusual and

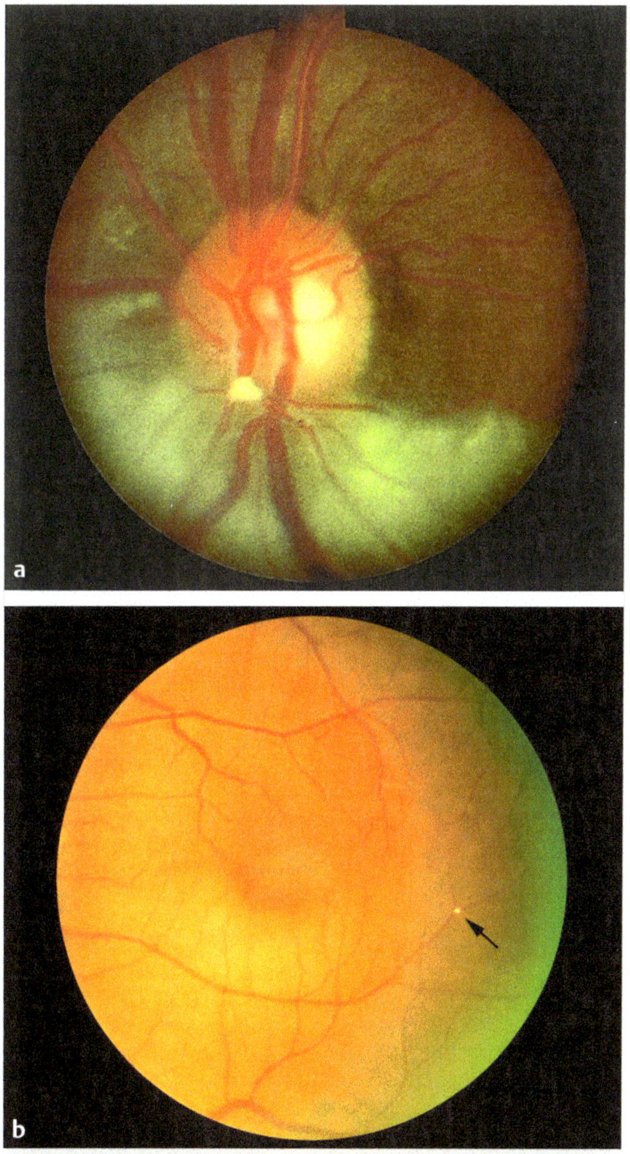

Fig. 8.17 (a) Calcific embolus on the optic disc in the eye of a patient with an inferior papillary branch retinal artery occlusion. (b) Inferior branch retinal artery occlusion in an eye with a cholesterol embolus (Hollenhorst plaque) (arrow) located at a retinal arterial bifurcation where the branching distal vessels narrow. Cholesterol emboli often originate from the carotid arteries and/or aorta and are typically smaller than calcific emboli. Arruga and Sanders (Ophthalmologic findings in 70 patients with evidence of retinal embolism. Ophthalmology 1982;89:1336–1347) noted that 74% of retinal emboli were cholesterol, 10.5% were calcific, and 15.5% were platelet–fibrin.

probably occurs in fewer than 2% of cases.[28] The retinal circulation has a remarkable propensity to become reestablished after CRAO at periods varying from hours to weeks.[55] Thus, although the visual loss may persist, the flow can revert to normal in later fluorescein angiograms.

Electroretinography

Electroretinography (ERG) typically shows a diminution of the amplitude of the b-wave (which corresponds to function of the Müller's and/or bipolar cells), whereas the a-wave (corresponding to photoreceptor function) is usually unaffected.[28] This is in contrast to an ophthalmic artery occlusion, in which there is loss of both a- and b-waves. ERG is particularly useful in confirming a suspected old CRAO. Months after the event, the only fundus abnormality that may be evident is optic nerve pallor. The characteristic electroretinographic finding of b-wave diminution will differentiate an old CRAO from an old optic neuropathy, which would be expected to have normal findings on electroretinography.[56]

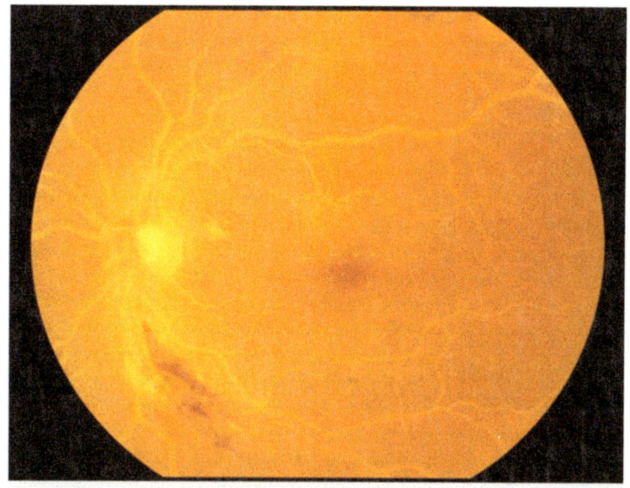

Fig. 8.18 Lipemia retinalis with an appearance somewhat similar to that of a central retinal artery occlusion in a patient with background diabetic retinopathy and a serum triglyceride level of 2,600 mg%. The visual acuity was 20/60, improving to 20/30 when the triglyceride level was brought down to the normal range.

8.4.3 Differential Diagnosis

Tay–Sachs disease typically presents with a cherry-red spot in infancy due to the deposition of gangliosides, a form of sphingolipid, within the retina. Death usually occurs by the age of 4 years; thus, the clinical scenario is vastly different than that seen with CRAO. Lipemia retinalis can also present with a fundus appearance that can be confused with CRAO (▸ Fig. 8.18). In these instances, the serum triglyceride level is typically greater than 2,500 mg% and the vision is mildly to moderately decreased.

8.4.4 Systemic Associations

An evaluation should be undertaken to ascertain the cause of the CRAO. Among the more common underlying associated abnormalities are embolic carotid artery obstructive disease, cardiac valvular disease, atrial fibrillation, collagen vascular diseases, and coagulopathies.[28,36,37,57] Causative systemic abnormalities can be found in about 90% of cases. Systemic arterial hypertension is encountered in about two-thirds of cases, and diabetes mellitus is present in approximately 25%.[28] Both are risk factors for the development of atherosclerosis. Cardiac valvular disease is present in about one-fourth as well,[28] and carotid atherosclerosis in the form of an ipsilateral plaque or stenosis is seen in about 45%.[35] In 20% of cases, the stenosis is 60% or greater.[35]

A more complete list of abnormalities associated with retinal artery occlusion is shown in the following text box. A similar workup should be considered for patients with ophthalmic artery occlusion, branch retinal artery occlusion, cilioretinal artery occlusion, and patients with cotton-wool spots in which no obvious underlying cause is present. The following text box lists numerous disease entities, although the correlation with select abnormalities is much stronger than with entities such as case reports in which the pathophysiologic mechanism may be less clear.[58,61,70,91,92,99,130,142]

Disease Entities Associated with Retinal Arteiral Occlusive Disease

Basic mechanisms of arterial flow diminution:

- Embolus[28]
- Intraluminal thrombus[58]
- Hemorrhage under an atherosclerotic plaque[2]
- Inflammation and thickening of arterial walls[37]
- Immunological[62]
- Atherosclerosis[3,28,35,94]
- Spasm[37,60,137]
- Trauma[59]
- External compression[61]
- Systemic arterial hypotension[143,144]

Clinical entities:

- Abnormalities and situations contributing to embolus formation
  - Systemic arterial hypertension (via atherosclerotic plaque formation; can also cause hypertensive necrosis)[1,2,3,28]
  - Carotid artery atherosclerosis (only 10% of carotid emboli reach the retinal arterial circulation)[1,2,3,28,36,74,75]
  - Aortic arch, ophthalmic artery, central retinal artery atherosclerosis[28,36,74]
  - Cardiac valvular disease
    1. Rheumatic[37]
    2. Mitral valve prolapse[37]
    3. Thrombotic eembolus[132]
  - Atrial fibrillation[67]
  - Cardiac myxoma[4,37,41]
  - Metastatic tumors[50]
  - Intravenous drug abuse[45,46]
  - Lipid emboli (also possible leukoembolization)
    1. Pancreatitis[78]
    2. Purtscher's retinopathy[8,10,90]
  - Loiasis[47]
  - Radiologic studies
    1. Carotid arteriography[97]
    2. Lymphangiography[48]
    3. Hysterosalpingography[49]
  - Head and neck corticosteroid injection[43]
  - Retrobulbar corticosteroids[44]
  - Nasal corticosteroid injection[120]
  - Deep vein thrombosis (via paradoxical embolus and patent foramen ovale)[93]
  - Coil embolization of paraclinoid aneurysm[64]
  - Patent foramen ovale with venous thromboembolism[143]
- Primary retinal arterial damage
  - Intussusception (dissecting aneurysm) of central retinal artery[32]
  - Systemic arterial hypertension[28,143,144]
  - Diabetes mellitus[28,74]
  - Atherosclerosis[28,74]
  - Hemorrhage under an atherosclerotic plaque[29,36]
  - Prepapillary arterial loops[37,72,134]
  - Retinal arterial macroaneurysm (spontaneous arteriolar occlusion in 8%, 16% after laser photocoagulation of macroaneurysm)[128]
  - IRVAN (idiopathic retinitis, vasculitis, aneurysms, and neuroretinitis syndrome)[140]
  - See "Collagen vascular (autoimmune) diseases" and "Other vasculitides"
- Carotid artery disease
  - Emboli[1,2,3,28,36,74,75]
  - Fibromuscular dysplasia[68,118,119]
  - Moyamoya disease[95]
  - Atherosclerotic blockage[3,35,94]
  - Carotid artery dissection[97]
  - Carotid angiography.[100]
  - Takayasu's arteritis[60]
- Trauma
  - Retrobulbar injection[59]
  - Orbital surgery[81]
  - Anesthesia with ocular compression[109,110]
  - Retrobulbar knife injury[27]
  - Drug-induced and/or alcohol-induced stupor with external pressure on the globe[27]
  - External pressure during anesthesia[109,110]
  - Nasal corticosteroid injection[120]
  - Nasal surgery[121,122,123]
  - Photodynamic therapy[63]
  - Laser photocoagulation[128]
  - Coil embolization of paraclinoid aneurysm[64]
  - Avulsion of the optic disc[131]
  - Cosmetic facial filler[66]
  - Cardiopulmonary resuscitation[80]
  - Orbital cavernous hemangioma removal[81]
  - Chiropractic manipulation[99]
  - Radiation retinopathy[88]
  - Purtscher's retinopathy[8,10,89]
  - Intravitreal injection of bevacizumab[139]
- Coagulopathies and other blood abnormalities
  - Sickle hemoglobinopathies (hemoglobins SS, SC, S thalassemia)[37,106]
  - Sickle cell trait with increased intraocular pressure[133]
  - Homocysteinemia[96,97]
  - Oral contraceptives[37]
  - Pregnancy[90]
  - Platelet and/or factor abnormalities[37]
  - Lupus anticoagulant syndrome[38]
  - Protein C deficiency[65,101,102,103,105]
  - Protein S deficiency[101,104]
  - Antithrombin III deficiency[102]
  - Polycythemia vera[69]

- Iron deficiency anemia[130]
- Essential thrombocythemia[98]
- Thrombotic thrombocytopenic purpura[111]

- Ocular conditions associated with retinal arterial occlusion
  - Optic disc drusen[129]
  - Optic disc edema (with ulcerative colitis)[127]
  - Increased intraocular pressure (with sickling hemoglobinopathy)[133]
  - Optic neuropathy.[136]
- Collagen vascular (autoimmune) diseases
  - Systemic lupus erythematosis[37]
  - Polyarteritis nodosa
  - Giant cell arteritis[27,39]
  - Wegener's granulomatosis
  - Churg–Strauss syndrome (allergic granulomatous angiitis)[112]
  - Susac's syndrome (occlusion of arterioles of retina, brain, and inner ear)[83]
  - Antiphospholipid syndrome[113]
- Other vasculitides
  - Radiation retinopathy[87]
  - Behçet's disease[114,115]
  - Crohn's disease[126]
  - Ulcerative colitis[127]
  - Central retinal vein occlusion with cilioretinal artery occlusion[136,138]
- Infection
  - Dengue fever[79]
  - Orbital mucormycosis[27]
  - Toxoplasmosis[107,108]
  - Human immunodeficiency virus (HIV)[82]
  - Lyme disease[91]
  - Cat scratch disease[116]
  - West Nile virus[117]
  - Rocky Mountain spotted fever[125]
- Tumors
  - Non-Hodgkin's large cell lymphoma[92]
  - Central nervous system lymphoma in HIV patient[124]
  - Orbital cavernous hemangioma removal[81]
  - Metastatic tumors[50]
- Drugs
  - Nasal oxymetazoline use[141]
  - Cocaine and methamphetamine abuse[137]
  - Intravenous drug (heroin) abuse[46]
- Miscellaneous associations
  - Sydenham's chorea[77]
  - Migraine[34,37]
  - Systemic arterial hypotension[143]
  - Orbital sarcoid[61]
  - Parry–Romberg syndrome[70]
  - Glabellar injection of hyaluronic acid[73]
  - Childbirth[89]
  - Osteogenesis imperfecta[142]
  - Autosomal dominant polycystic kidney disease[58]

In people under the age of 30 years, carotid artery occlusive disease from atherosclerosis is rare, although entities such as fibromuscular dysplasia[118,119] and Moyamoya disease[95] can precipitate carotid occlusion. The leading systemic associations in this younger group include coagulopathies, migraine, and collagen vascular diseases.[37]

Overall, the mortality in patients with retinal arterial occlusion appears to be increased. Lorentzen[57] found a mean survival time of 5.5 years in people with CRAO versus 15.4 years in an age-matched population. The most common cause of death is cardiovascular disease.[57] With improved therapies for underlying causes of retinal arterial occlusion, such as atherosclerosis, systemic arterial hypertension, collagen vascular diseases, cardiac disease, and so forth, it is likely that this difference has decreased since Lorentzen's report in 1969. In particular, however, the association of cardiovascular disease should be considered, especially since aggressive treatment with HMG-CoA reductase inhibitors (statins) has been demonstrated to reverse coronary atherosclerosis.[144]

Special Considerations

- The clinician should be aware of the high incidence of cardiovascular disease associated with ophthalmic arterial occlusive disease, especially since HMG-CoA reductase inhibitors (statins) have been demonstrated to reverse coronary atherosclerosis.

8.4.5 Management and Course

No treatment has been shown to be consistently effective for improving vision in eyes with acute CRAO. Ocular massage, anterior chamber paracentesis, inhalation treatment with a combination of oxygen and carbon dioxide, administration of antithrombolytic agents via the carotid system and intravenously, and oral vasodilators have all been tried without convincing success.[145,146,147,148,149,150]

Central retinal artery occlusion in association with sickle cell disease has been treated with success with hyperbaric oxygen and exchange transfusion.[151] Nonetheless, limited information is reported on this subject.

An interesting therapy, however, is YAG (yttrium–aluminum–garnet) laser therapy to expel a visible embolus from the central retinal artery or a branch retinal artery. Opremcak and colleagues[152] treated 19 such eyes with central or branch retinal artery occlusion. Transluminal embolysis or embolectomy (expelling the embolus from the artery) was achieved in all 19 eyes. The mean improvement in vision in 17 of 19 (89%) patients was 4.7 lines, suggestive of a better course than the natural history. Vitreous hemorrhage occurred in 7 of 21 (36%) and vitrectomy was required in 5 of 21 (26%). The long-term outcome remains to be seen.

The upper time limit for any treatment modality is uncertain. Animal studies have suggested that the window of opportunity is less than 2 hours for complete occlusion of the central retinal artery.[143,144,153] Nevertheless, in the clinical situation, in which there is often some limited flow through the obstructed artery, visual improvement has been seen clinically as late as 3 days after occlusion.[154] Some advocate performing ocular massage and anterior chamber paracentesis if the occlusion is less than 24 hours in duration. Unfortunately, in a long-term follow-up study of treatment with anterior chamber paracentesis in conjunction with carbogen (95% oxygen, 5% carbon dioxide), it was demonstrated that the treatment group fared only one-fourth line better than the untreated control group.[146]

As mentioned, approximately 18% of eyes with CRAO will progress to develop iris neovascularization, usually within 4 months after the occlusion, with a mean time of 5 weeks after the occlusion.[51,52] Thus, for the first 2 months, these eyes should be followed relatively frequently. If iris neovascularization develops, laser panretinal photocoagulation is successful in causing regression in about 65% of cases, likely reducing progression to neovascular glaucoma.[53] When iris neovascularization is present at the time of the acute CRAO, carotid artery obstructive disease and the OIS should be suspected. In these instances, severe carotid artery occlusion probably leads to neovascular glaucoma and an intraocular pressure that exceeds the perfusion pressure in the central retinal artery.

Pearls

- Close follow-up is needed for patients with an acute CRAO because approximately 18% eyes will develop iris neovascularization. This usually occurs within several weeks after the occlusion.

8.5 Central Retinal Artery/Central Retinal Vein Occlusion

8.5.1 Symptoms

Patients with combined central retinal artery/central retinal vein occlusion typically relate a history of abrupt visual loss and present with the clinical features of both entities.[71,155,156,157,158]

8.5.2 Clinical Features

The visual acuity is usually in the counting fingers to hand-motion range, although in occasional cases it can be surprisingly good. The fundus examination is characterized by the superficial retinal whitening and cherry-red spot seen with CRAO, as well as the dilated and tortuous retinal veins, retinal hemorrhages, and retinal edema encountered with central retinal vein occlusion (▶ Fig. 8.19). The prognosis for visual recovery is generally poor, and effective treatment for the improvement of visual acuity is lacking. Nevertheless, there are rare cases of visual improvement.[156,157]

The pathophysiologic mechanisms that lead to this entity are unclear. One acute case has been reported in which there was histopathologic occlusion in both the central retinal artery and vein.[158] We have seen the artery occlusion can occur before that of the vein, the vein occlusion before that of the artery, and both present simultaneously.

Systemic associations encountered with acute central retinal artery/vein are similar to those seen with acute CRAO (see "Disease Entities Associated with Posterior Segment Arterial (Ophthalmic, Central, Branch, Cilioretinal) Occlusion and/or Cotton-Wool Spots" text box). Nonetheless, almost one-fourth of reported cases occur secondary to complications of retrobulbar injection at the time of ocular surgery.[157]

8.5.3 Ancillary Studies

Fluorescein angiography most commonly reveals severe retinal capillary nonperfusion (▶ Fig. 8.20).[157] The macular retina is often markedly thickened clinically, although in many instances there does not appear to be substantial leakage of dye, probably because of shutdown of much of the retinal vascular bed. Theoretically, the marked extravasation of plasma occurs from the damaged retinal vessels before they undergo complete necrosis and shutdown, although leakage from the remaining viable retinal vessels at the borders of the nonperfused areas may also contribute to the retinal thickening.

8.5.4 Differential Diagnosis

One important entity in the differential diagnosis of combined central retinal artery/central retinal vein occlusion is aminoglycoside toxicity to the retina. This was originally described by McDonald and colleagues[159] after intraocular gentamicin injection, and was demonstrated in the subhuman primate model by Brown et al.[160] Within minutes after intraocular aminoglycoside injection, the retina acquires the appearance of ischemic whitening similar to that in a CRAO. The electroretinogram demonstrates rapid damage to the inner retinal layers followed by damage to the outer layers. By the second day after the insult, a hemorrhagic component typically develops as well. Features that help to differentiate combined central retinal artery/central retinal vein occlusion from aminoglycoside toxicity are shown in ▶ Table 8.3.

Pearls

- Iris neovascularization will develop in approximately 80% of eyes with combined central retinal artery/central retinal vein occlusion.

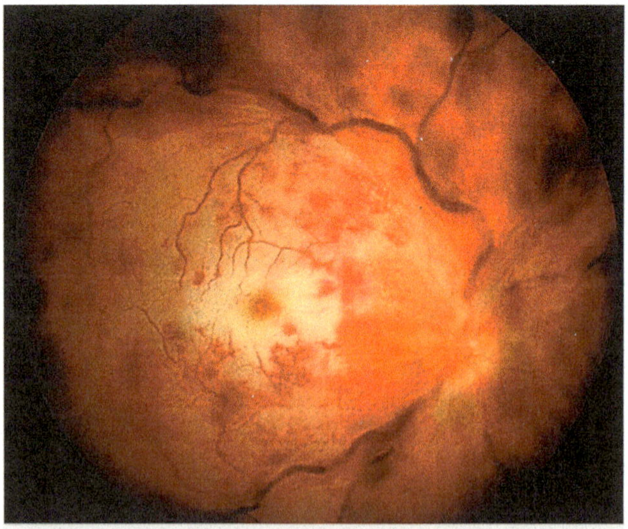

Fig. 8.19 Central retinal artery/vein occlusion in the eye of a 20-year-old woman with systemic lupus erythematosus.

8.5.5 Management and Course

Unfortunately, no treatment has been demonstrated for reversing the visual loss associated with combined central retinal artery/central retinal vein occlusion. In approximately 80% of eyes with combined central retinal artery/central retinal vein occlusion, rubeosis iridis will develop that typically progresses to neovascular glaucoma.[157] This complication can arise as early as 1 to 2 weeks, or as late as 1 year, after occlusion, with a median time of about 6 weeks. The patients should be followed closely during the first 2 months, and laser panretinal photocoagulation should be considered if iris neovascularization begins to develop.

8.6 Branch Retinal Artery Occlusion

Branch retinal artery occlusion causes acute visual field loss in the distribution corresponding to the impaired retina. Although the central visual acuity is often decreased, approximately 80% of eyes improve to 20/40 or better as the zone of hypoxia at the border of the occlusion improves.[37,74] Nevertheless, visual field defects usually remain. Among all retinal artery occlusions, CRAO accounts for 57% of cases, branch retinal artery occlusion for 38%, and cilioretinal artery occlusion for 5%.[41]

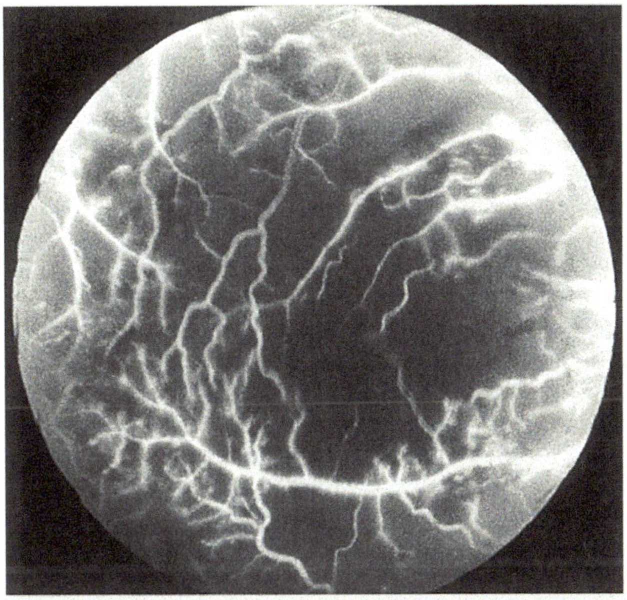

Fig. 8.20 Severe retinal capillary nonperfusion in an eye with a central retinal artery/vein occlusion.

Fundus examination in eyes with acute branch retinal artery occlusion reveals superficial retinal opacification in the affected area (▶ Fig. 8.21a). More intense whitening may be seen at the borders of the ischemic areas since there is axoplasmic damming in addition to the ischemic necrosis. Neovascularization of the iris is extremely unusual after branch retinal artery occlusion, but neovascularization of the retina and/or optic disc, with subsequent preretinal bleeding can rarely occur.[161,162]Arterial-to-arterial collaterals can develop, and are virtually pathognomonic for previous branch retinal artery occlusion.

8.6.1 Optical Coherence Tomography (OCT)

Acutely, there is thickening of ischemic retina, although the typical cystic macular edema present with branch retinal vein occlusion is absent. Over a period of weeks to months, the inner half of the retina is absent due to retinal necrosis and reabsorption (▶ Fig. 8.21b).

8.6.2 Management and Course

Ocular treatment is generally not undertaken because of the relatively favorable visual prognosis, although YAG laser photocoagulation has been suggested as a mechanism of obliterating emboli.[152] Nonetheless, the long-term efficacy for this treatment modality for improving vision remains to be seen.

The systemic workup is essentially similar to that for eyes with CRAO. It should be noted, however, that in cases where the occlusion occurs at an arterial bifurcation the cause is more likely to be embolic than inflammatory.

Recurrent branch retinal artery occlusions can be seen with Susac's syndrome,[83,163] described as a triad of (1) encephalopathy, (2) branch retinal artery occlusions, and (3) hearing loss. It is believed to occur secondary to antibodies to small vessel endothelial cells. The encephalopathy is typically characterized by headaches and white matter lesions that involve the corpus callous. Psychiatric, cognitive, and memory loss changes may progress to dementia. The branch artery occlusions tend to be consecutive over time. Focal staining with fluorescein angiography indicates the vasculitis is still active. Yellow, nonrefractile Gass plaques in the branch retinal arteries are pathognomonic for the disease (▶ Fig. 8.22). The hearing loss is typically in the low-frequency range and pronounced tinnitus may be present. The entity usually resolves within 5 years, but may cause severe damage prior to that time. Oral corticosteroids generally reverse the inflammation relatively quickly, but high-dose intravenous immunoglobulin and drugs such as mycophenolate and azathioprine may be required on a longer-term basis. In

Table 8.3 Features differentiating combined central retinal artery/central retinal vein occlusion from aminoglycoside toxicity

	Combined occlusion	Aminoglycoside toxicity
Scleral perforation and/or intraocular aminoglycoside injection	No	Yes
Cataract formation	No	Yes
Electroretinogram	Reduced b-wave	Extinguished
Late serous retinal detachment	No	Sometimes

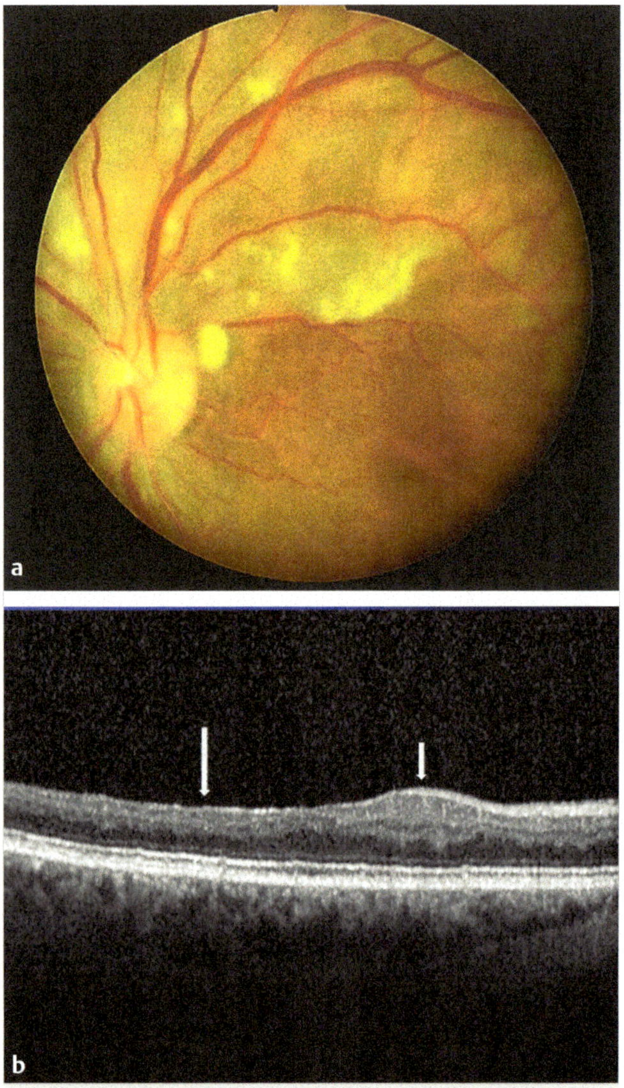

Fig. 8.21 (a) Branch retinal artery occlusion. The retinal whitening is more pronounced at the inferotemporal border of the ischemic retina because of axoplasmic damming in this region. (b) Optical coherence tomography (OCT) from an eye with a branch retinal artery occlusion years before. Loss of the inner retina can be seen (larger arrow). The smaller arrow points to the perifoveal retina that remains normal in thickness.

some instances, we have observed the ocular and aural changes may be present without the encephalopathy or corpus callosum white matter lesions.

8.7 Cilioretinal Artery Occlusion

Cilioretinal arteries are derived from the short posterior ciliary arteries, either directly or via the choroid or the circle of Zinn–Haller. Most commonly, a cilioretinal artery enters the fundus on the optic disc separately from the central retinal artery or its branches. In some instances, it originates from the temporal peripapillary retina. Since it is posterior ciliary in origin, it often fills with fluorescein angiography before the central retinal artery. Three variants of cilioretinal artery occlusion have been described:

- Isolated cilioretinal artery occlusion[127,136]
- Cilioretinal artery occlusion in conjunction with central retinal vein occlusion[136,138,164]
- Cilioretinal artery occlusion in conjunction with anterior ischemic optic neuropathy[136]

Eyes with isolated cilioretinal artery occlusion demonstrate superficial retinal opacification in the distribution of the occluded vessel (▶ Fig. 8.23). The central visual acuity returns to 20/40 or better in 90% of cases. This variant comprises approximately 40% of cilioretinal artery occlusions.[136]

In eyes with cilioretinal occlusion and central retinal vein occlusion, there is superficial retinal opacification in the distribution of the occluded artery in conjunction with features of central retinal vein occlusion, including retinal hemorrhage, dilated retinal veins, and retinal edema (▶ Fig. 8.24). This variant also comprises about 40% of all cilioretinal artery occlusions.[136] Approximately 70% of these eyes eventually improve to a vision of 20/40 or better. Fong and colleagues[165] have noted that approximately 5% of eyes with central retinal vein occlusion also have an associated cilioretinal artery occlusion. The reasons for this association are not clear, but reduced hydrostatic pressure within a cilioretinal artery, in comparison with the central retinal artery, may predispose to stasis and thrombus formation in the situation of central retinal vein occlusion and increased hydrostatic pressure within the central retinal vein. Additionally, swelling of the optic disc may compromise the cross-sectional area of the cilioretinal artery and lead to reduced flow. According to Poiseuille's law, the flow within a blood vessel is proportional to the fourth power of the radius of the vessel, so that a reduction in the radius by 50% will lead to a reduction in flow volume of approximately 94%.

It is not surprising that anterior ischemic optic neuropathy can be associated with cilioretinal artery occlusion, as both abnormalities occur secondary to occlusion of vessels derived from the posterior ciliary circulation. Ophthalmoscopically, there is superficial retinal opacification in association with optic disc swelling (▶ Fig. 8.25). The visual acuity in these eyes, which account for about 15% of cilioretinal artery occlusions, typically remains in the 20/400 range or worse due to the optic neuropathy. In these instances, the possibility of giant cell arteritis should be considered as an underlying cause.

No treatment is indicated for cilioretinal artery occlusion, and the systemic workup is similar to that for other retinal arterial obstructive events. Nonetheless, we typically do not undertake as extensive a systemic arterial workup in the face of a cilioretinal artery occlusion associated with a central retinal vein occlusion since the vein occlusion itself likely predisposes to the cilioretinal artery occlusion by diminishing flow within the cilioretinal artery.

8.8 Cotton-Wool Spots

8.8.1 Ophthalmoscopy

A cotton-wool spot appears clinically as an area of superficial retinal whitening less than one-fourth the disc area in size

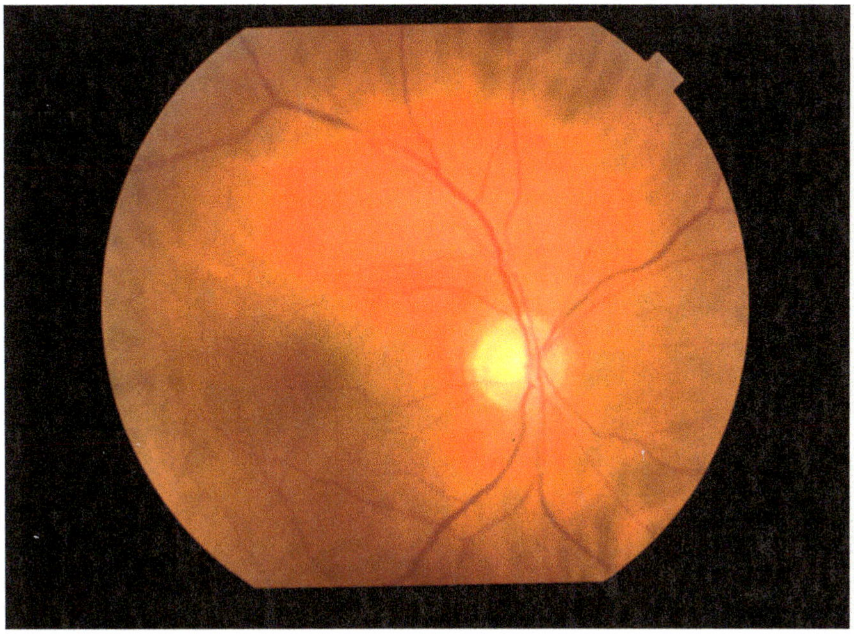

Fig. 8.22 Yellow, focal Gass plaque located one disc diameter inferior to the optic nerve head and presenting as a yellow ring surrounding two branch retinal arteries. This patient with the Susac's syndrome had previous consecutive branch retinal artery occlusions. Residual optic pallor is present due to the prior arterial occlusions.

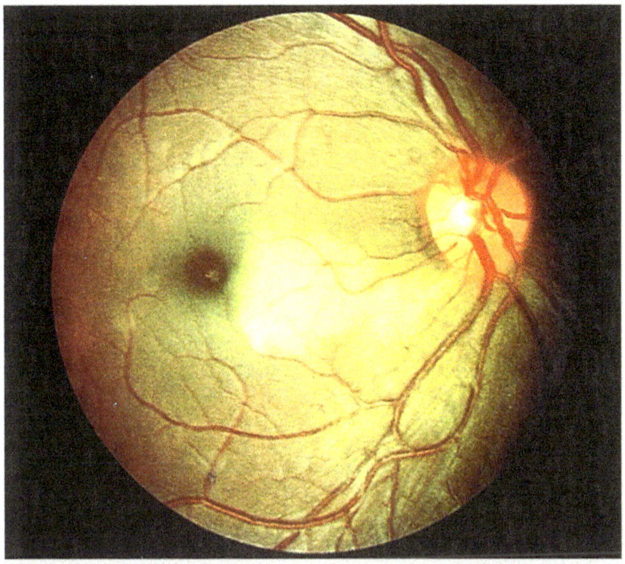

Fig. 8.23 Isolated cilioretinal artery occlusion.

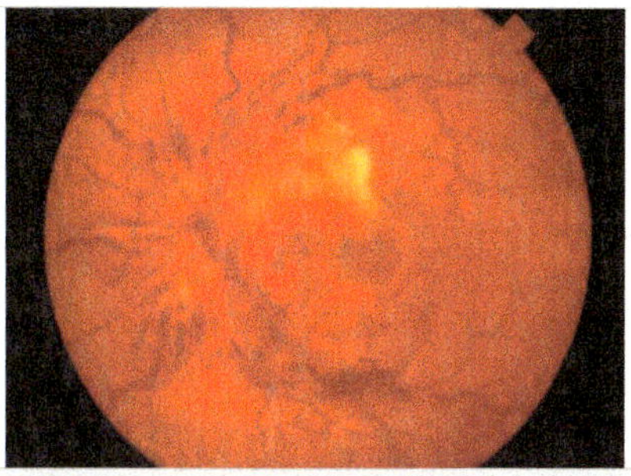

Fig. 8.24 Cilioretinal artery occlusion; in association with central retinal vein occlusion; the latter characterized by a swollen optic disc, dilated and tortuous retinal veins, and retinal hemorrhages.

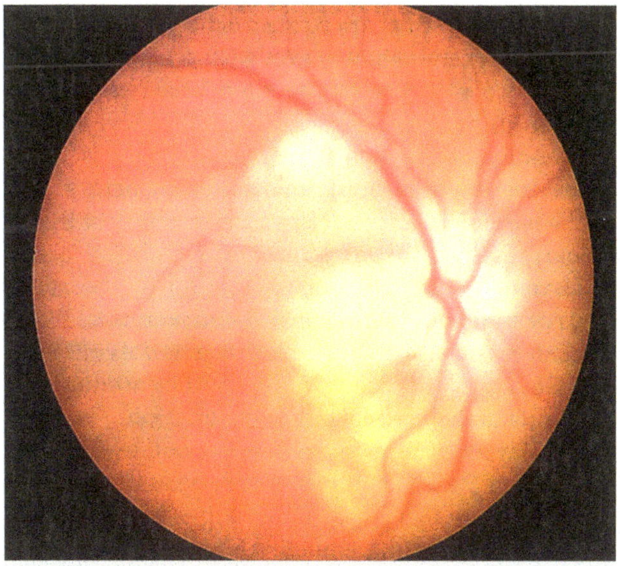

Fig. 8.25 Cilioretinal artery occlusion associated with anterior ischemic optic neuropathy in a patient with giant cell arteritis.

(▶ Fig. 8.26). Cotton-wool spots are typically located in the peripapillary region, along the temporal retinal vascular arcades, or in the macula, and often are multiple (▶ Fig. 8.27). They occur secondary to shutdown of a terminal retinal arteriole, which causes axoplasmic damming and a whitened appearance in the retinal nerve fiber layer.[166] Most cotton-wool spots disappear within 5 to 7 weeks after they develop, although those seen with diabetic retinopathy may take longer to resolve.[166,167]

8.8.2 Differential Diagnosis

Diabetic retinopathy is the leading cause of cotton-wool spots, and approximately 32 to 44% of patients with diabetic retinopathy have cotton-wool spots.[167] When known diabetics are excluded, eyes with a fundus appearance characterized by the

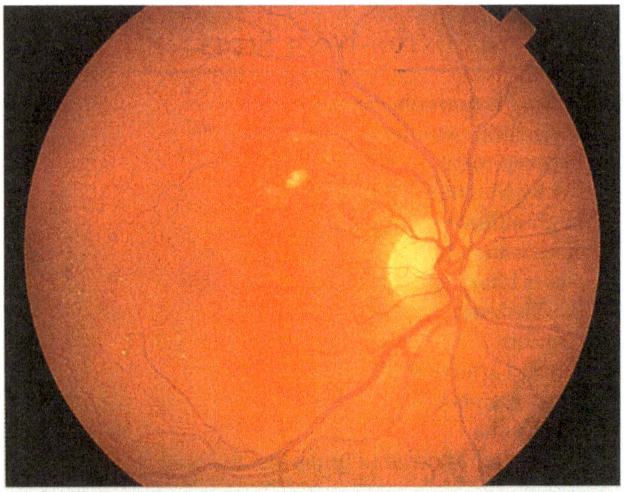

Fig. 8.26 Cotton-wool spot superotemporal to the optic disc in the eye of a patient with diabetic retinopathy.

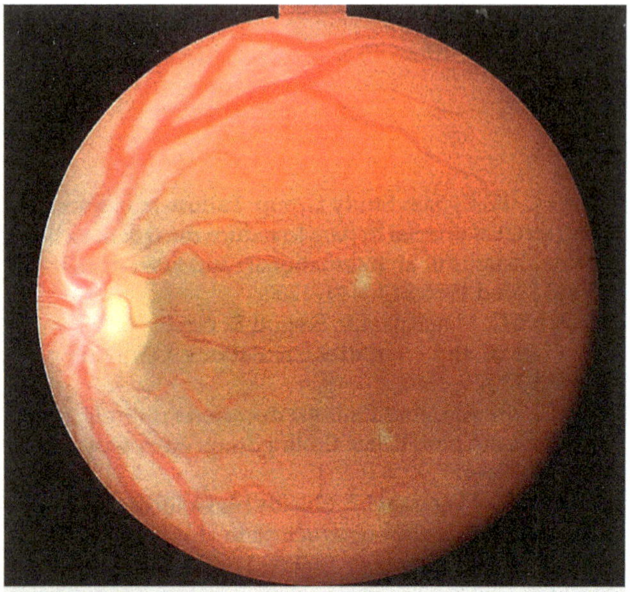

Fig. 8.27 Multiple cotton-wool spots in the eye of a patient with acute undifferentiated leukemia.

presence of at least one cotton-wool spot or a predominance of cotton-wool spots have an associated underlying systemic disease in about 95% of cases.[168] Undiagnosed diabetes mellitus accounts for about 20% of such cases. In these instances, a glucose tolerance test may be necessary to demonstrate the underlying cause. Systemic arterial hypertension accounts for another 20%, and collagen vascular disease comprises a third quintile.

With cases of systemic arterial hypertension, the diastolic blood pressure in adults is usually at least in the range of 110 to 115 mm Hg. (in children, the diastolic pressure may be lower) In these instances, the autoregulatory capacity of the retinal arteries is exceeded and the terminal retinal arterioles downstream are exposed to a level of pressure they cannot effectively tolerate. Subsequent fibrinoid necrosis develops, leading to shutdown of the arteriole.[169] Thus, if someone has cotton-wool spots and the clinician suspects systemic arterial hypertension as the cause, if the diastolic blood pressure is 90 mm Hg, it is very likely that it is rising to 110 to 115 mm Hg at some point.

Pearls

- When cotton-wool spots occur secondary to systemic arterial hypertension in adults, the diastolic blood pressure is usually a minimum of 110 to 115 mm Hg.

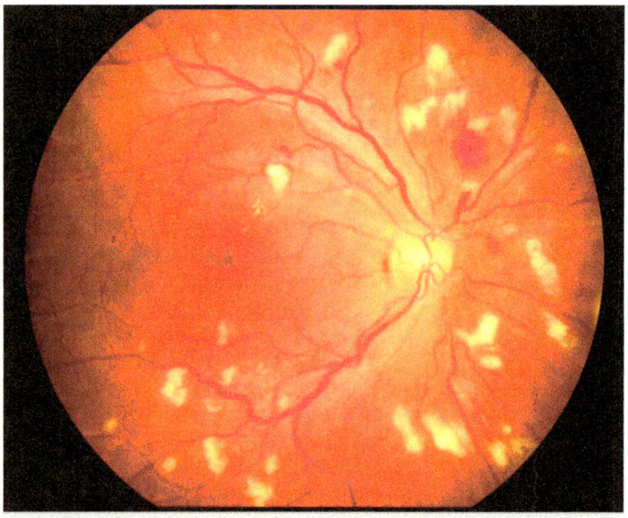

Fig. 8.28 Many cotton-wool spots in the eye of a patient with the acquired immunodeficiency syndrome (AIDS). It has been suggested that immune complexes within the terminal retinal arteriolar walls may predispose to occlusion of these vessels and the development of cotton-wool spots with axoplasmic damming in the subsequent area of focal retinal ischemia.

Another cause of cotton-wool spots is AIDS (acquired immune deficiency syndrome) retinopathy (▶ Fig. 8.28). Cotton-wool spots have been observed clinically in up to 50% of patients with AIDS,[169] with the incidence rising to more than 70% in an autopsy group.[170] It has been suggested that the deposition of immune complexes within retinal blood vessel walls is responsible for the cotton-wool spots seen in the eyes of AIDS patients.[171]

While diabetic retinopathy is the most common cause of cotton-wool spots, other common causes include cardiac valvular disease, radiation retinopathy, Purtscher's traumatic retinopathy, and carotid artery obstructive disease. A more complete list of the more common entities causing cotton-wool spots is shown in text box "Disease entities more commonly associated with cotton-wool spots". Theoretically, any etiologic abnormality associated with retinal arterial occlusion can also be encountered with cotton-wool spots.

These disease entities are more commonly associated with cotton-wool spots:

- Diabetes mellitus
  - Systemic arterial hypertension
  - Collagen vascular diseases
  - Systemic lupus erythematosus
  - Wegener's granulomatosis

  - Polyarteritis nodosa
  - Scleroderma
  - Giant cell arteritis
  - Cardiac valvular disease
  - Mitral valve prolapse
  - Rheumatic heart disease
  - Endocarditis
  - Acquired immunodeficiency syndrome (AIDS)
  - Leukemia
  - Trauma
  - Radiation retinopathy
  - Central retinal artery occlusion (partial)
- Retinal venous occlusion
  - Metastatic carcinoma
  - Leptospirosis
  - Rocky Mountain spotted fever
  - High-altitude retinopathy
  - Severe anemia
  - Acute blood loss
  - Papilledema
  - Papillitis
  - Carotid artery occlusion
  - Dysproteinemias
  - Septicemia
  - Aortic arch syndrome (pulseless disease)
  - Intravenous drug abuse
  - Acute pancreatitis
  - Onchocerciasis

The finding of just one cotton-wool spot in a nondiabetic patient with an otherwise normal fundus necessitates a systemic workup for possible etiologies. The blood pressure should be measured at the time of the initial finding because, as mentioned, cotton-wool spots from systemic arterial hypertension occur only when the autoregulatory capacity of the retinal artery system has been exceeded. In this instance, it is likely that the autoregulatory capacity in other organs, such as kidney and brain, is also exceeded.

Pegylated interferon therapy for chronic hepatitis is associated with cotton-wool spots in approximately 25% of treated patients.[172,173,174] It has also been noted with interferon-beta therapy for multiple sclerosis.[145] While the cotton-wool spots usually do not affect the central vision in these cases, in some instances the retinopathy associated with pegylated interferon can be severe with near confluent cotton-wool spots. In these instances, a discussion with the patient and the patient's treating physician can be considered to decide whether to continue with therapy.

8.8.3 Management and Course

No local ocular treatment is generally necessary for cotton-wool spots, although the underlying systemic entity frequently requires therapy. While a patient may notice small scotomata with coot-wool spots, which are associated with retinal nonperfusion in the area of the lesion, these scotomata generally do not cause long-term symptoms or interfere with central vision.

8.9 Conclusion

Arterial occlusive disease can manifest in the eye as (1) carotid or ophthalmic artery occlusion producing the OIS with subacute vision loss, (2) acute ophthalmic, central, or branch retinal arterial occlusion resulting in sudden vision loss with retinal whitening, and (3) blockage of terminal retinal arterioles causing cotton-wool spots. Each variant is treated differently. Of critical importance for each, however, is the workup for the underlying systemic etiology for the occlusive event(s).

References

[1] Kearns TP, Hollenhorst RW. Venous-stasis retinopathy of occlusive disease of the carotid artery. Proc Staff Meet Mayo Clin. 1963; 38:304–312

[2] Brown GC. The ocular ischemic syndrome. In: Ryan S, ed. Retina. Vol 2. Baltimore, MD: CV Mosby; 1994:1515–1527

[3] Brown GC, Magargal LE. The ocular ischemic syndrome. Clinical, fluorescein angiographic and carotid angiographic features. Int Ophthalmol. 1988; 11 (4):239–251

[4] Sturrock GD, Mueller HR. Chronic ocular ischaemia. Br J Ophthalmol. 1984; 68(10):716–723

[5] Furlan AJ, Whisnant JP, Kearns TP. Unilateral visual loss in bright light. An unusual symptom of carotid artery occlusive disease. Arch Neurol. 1979; 36 (11):675–676

[6] Brown GC, Magargal LE, Schachat A, Shah H. Neovascular glaucoma. Etiologic considerations. Ophthalmology. 1984; 91(4):315–320

[7] Brown GC. Macular edema in association with severe carotid artery obstruction. Am J Ophthalmol. 1986; 102(4):442–448

[8] Brown GC. Anterior ischemic optic neuropathy occurring in association with carotid artery obstruction. J Clin Neuroophthalmol. 1986; 6(1):39–42

[9] Higashide T, Murotani E, Saito Y, Ohkubo S, Sugiyama K. Adverse events associated with intraocular injections of bevacizumab in eyes with neovascular glaucoma. Graefes Arch Clin Exp Ophthalmol. 2012; 250(4):603–610

[10] Jahromi AS, Cinà CS, Liu Y, Clase CM. Sensitivity and specificity of color duplex ultrasound measurement in the estimation of internal carotid artery stenosis: a systematic review and meta-analysis. J Vasc Surg. 2005; 41 (6):962–972

[11] Duker JS, Colt C, Brown GC, Bosley TM, Colt CA, Reber R. Asymmetric proliferative diabetic retinopathy and carotid artery obstructive disease. Ophthalmology. 1990; 97(7):869–874

[12] Sivalingam A, Brown GC, Magargal LE, Menduke H. The ocular ischemic syndrome. II. Mortality and systemic morbidity. Int Ophthalmol. 1989; 13 (3):187–191

[13] Sivalingam A, Brown GC, Magargal LE. The ocular ischemic syndrome. III. Visual prognosis and the effect of treatment. Int Ophthalmol. 1991; 15 (1):15–20

[14] North American Symptomatic Carotid Endarterectomy Trial Collaborators. Beneficial effect of carotid endarterectomy in symptomatic patients with high-grade carotid stenosis. N Engl J Med. 1991; 325(7):445–453

[15] Rerkasem K, Rothwell PM. Carotid endarterectomy for symptomatic carotid stenosis. Cochrane Database Syst Rev. 2011(4):CD001081

[16] Halliday A, Mansfield A, Marro J, et al. MRC Asymptomatic Carotid Surgery Trial (ACST) Collaborative Group. Prevention of disabling and fatal strokes by successful carotid endarterectomy in patients without recent neurological symptoms: randomised controlled trial. Lancet. 2004; 363(9420):1491–1502

[17] Sidawy AN, Zwolak RM, White RA, Siami FS, Schermerhorn ML, Sicard GA, Outcomes Committee for the Society for Vascular Surgery. Risk-adjusted 30-day outcomes of carotid stenting and endarterectomy: results from the SVS Vascular Registry. J Vasc Surg. 2009; 49(1):71–79

[18] Jim J, Rubin BG, Ricotta JJ, II, Kenwood CT, Siami FS, Sicard GA, SVS Outcomes Committee. Society for Vascular Surgery (SVS) Vascular Registry evaluation of comparative effectiveness of carotid revascularization procedures stratified by Medicare age. J Vasc Surg. 2012; 55(5):1313–1320, discussion 1321

[19] Brott TG, Halperin JL, Abbara S, et al. American College of Cardiology, American Stroke Association, American Association of Neurological Surgeons, American College of Radiology, Society of NeuroInterventional Surgery, Society for Vascular Medicine, Society for Vascular Surgery. 2011 ASA/ACCF/AHA/AANN/AANS/ACR/ASNR/CNS/SAIP/SCAI/SIR/SNIS/SVM/SVS guideline on the management of patients with extracranial carotid and vertebral artery disease. A report of the American College of Cardiology Foundation/American Heart Association Task Force on Practice Guidelines, and the American Stroke Association, American Association of Neuroscience Nurses, American Association of Neurological Surgeons, American College of Radiology, American Society of Neuroradiology, Congress of Neurological Surgeons, Society of Atherosclerosis Imaging and Prevention, Society for Cardiovascular Angiography and Interventions, Society of Interventional Radiology, Society of NeuroInterventional Surgery, Society for Vascular Medicine, and Society for Vascular Surgery. Circulation. 2011; 124(4):e54–e130
[20] Beckman JA, Beckman MD. Management of asymptomatic internal carotid artery stenosis. JAMA. 2013; 310(15):1612–1618
[21] Heart Protection Study Collaborative Group. MRC/BHF Heart Protection Study of cholesterol lowering with simvastatin in 20,536 high-risk individuals: a randomised placebo-controlled trial. Lancet. 2002; 360(9326):7–22
[22] Raman G, Moorthy D, Hadar N, et al. Management strategies for asymptomatic carotid stenosis: a systematic review and meta-analysis. Ann Intern Med. 2013; 158(9):676–685
[23] Nicholls SJ, Ballantyne CM, Barter PJ, et al. Effect of two intensive statin regimens on progression of coronary disease. N Engl J Med. 2011; 365 (22):2078–2087
[24] The EC/IC Bypass Study Group. Failure of extracranial-intracranial arterial bypass to reduce the risk of ischemic stroke. Results of an international randomized trial. N Engl J Med. 1985; 313(19):1191–1200
[25] Grubb RL, Jr, Powers WJ, Clarke WR, Videen TO, Adams HP, Jr, Derdeyn CP, Carotid Occlusion Surgery Study Investigators. Surgical results of the Carotid Occlusion Surgery Study. J Neurosurg. 2013; 118(1):25–33
[26] Marshall RS, Festa JR, Cheung YK, et al. RECON Investigators. Randomized Evaluation of Carotid Occlusion and Neurocognition (RECON) trial: main results. Neurology. 2014; 82(9):744–751
[27] Brown GC, Magargal LE, Sergott R. Acute obstruction of the retinal and choroidal circulations. Ophthalmology. 1986; 93(11):1373–1382
[28] Brown GC, Magargal LE. Central retinal artery obstruction and visual acuity. Ophthalmology. 1982; 89(1):14–19
[29] von Graefe A. Ueber Embolie der arteria centralis retinae als Urscahc plotzlicher Erblingdung. Arch Ophthalmol. 1859; 5:136–157
[30] Appen RE, Wray SH, Cogan DG. Central retinal artery occlusion. Am J Ophthalmol. 1975; 79(3):374–381
[31] Dahrling BE, II. The histopathology of early central retinal artery occlusion. Arch Ophthalmol. 1965; 73:506–510
[32] Wolter JR, Hansen KD. Intimo-intimal intussusception of the central retinal artery. Am J Ophthalmol. 1981; 92(4):486–491
[33] Leishman R. The eye in general vascular disease: hypertension and arteriosclerosis. Br J Ophthalmol. 1957; 41(11):641–701
[34] Graveson GS. Retinal arterial occlusion in migraine. BMJ. 1949; 2 (4632):838–840
[35] Shah HG, Brown GC, Goldberg RE. Digital subtraction carotid angiography and retinal arterial obstruction. Ophthalmology. 1985; 92(1):68–72
[36] Gold D. Retinal arterial occlusion. Trans Sect Ophthalmol Am Acad Ophthalmol Otolaryngol. 1977; 83(3, Pt 1):OP392–OP408
[37] Brown GC, Magargal LE, Shields JA, Goldberg RE, Walsh PN. Retinal arterial obstruction in children and young adults. Ophthalmology. 1981; 88(1):18–25
[38] Kleiner RC, Najarian LV, Schatten S, Jabs DA, Patz A, Kaplan HJ. Vaso-occlusive retinopathy associated with antiphospholipid antibodies (lupus anticoagulant retinopathy). Ophthalmology. 1989; 96(6):896–904
[39] Connolly BP, Krishnan A, Shah GK, et al. Characteristics of patients presenting with central retinal artery occlusion with and without giant cell arteritis. Can J Ophthalmol. 2000; 35(7):379–384
[40] Brown GC, Shields JA. Cilioretinal arteries and retinal arterial occlusion. Arch Ophthalmol. 1979; 97(1):84–92
[41] Jampol LM, Wong AS, Albert DM. Atrial myxoma and central retinal artery occlusion. Am J Ophthalmol. 1973; 75(2):242–249
[42] Cogan DG, Wray SH. Vascular occlusions in the eye from cardiac myxomas. Am J Ophthalmol. 1975; 80(3, Pt 1):396–403
[43] Wilson RS, Havener WH, McGrew RN. Bilateral retinal artery and choriocapillaris occlusion following the injection of long-acting corticosteroid suspensions in combination with other drugs: I. Clinical studies. Ophthalmology. 1978; 85(9):967–973
[44] Ellis PP. Occlusion of the central retinal artery after retrobulbar corticosteroid injection. Am J Ophthalmol. 1978; 85(3):352–356
[45] AtLee WE, Jr. Talc and cornstarch emboli in eyes of drug abusers. JAMA. 1972; 219(1):49–51
[46] Siepser SB, Magargal LE, Augsburger JJ. Acute bilateral retinal microembolization in a heroin addict. Ann Ophthalmol. 1981; 13(6):699–702
[47] Corrigan MJ, Hill DW. Retinal artery occlusion in loiasis. Br J Ophthalmol. 1968; 52(6):477–480
[48] Rasmussen KE. Retinal and cerebral fat emboli following lymphography with oily contrast media. Acta Radiol Diagn (Stockh). 1970; 10(3):199–202
[49] Charawanamuttu AM, Hughes-Nurse J, Hamlett JD. Retinal embolism after hysterosalpingography. Br J Ophthalmol. 1973; 57(3):166–169
[50] Tarkkanen A, Merenmies L, Mäkinen J. Embolism of the central retinal artery secondary to metastatic carcinoma. Acta Ophthalmol (Copenh). 1973; 51 (1):25–33
[51] Duker JS, Brown GC. Iris neovascularization associated with obstruction of the central retinal artery. Ophthalmology. 1988; 95(9):1244–1250
[52] Duker JS, Sivalingam A, Brown GC, Reber R. A prospective study of acute central retinal artery obstruction. The incidence of secondary ocular neovascularization. Arch Ophthalmol. 1991; 109(3):339–342
[53] Duker JS, Brown GC. The efficacy of panretinal photocoagulation for neovascularization of the iris after central retinal artery obstruction. Ophthalmology. 1989; 96(1):92–95
[54] Duker JS, Brown GC. Neovascularization of the optic disc associated with obstruction of the central retinal artery. Ophthalmology. 1989; 96(1):87–91
[55] Montzka D, Regillo CD, Brown GC, et al. Color Doppler imaging and central retinal artery obstructions. Invest Ophthalmol Vis Sci. 1994; 35:1635
[56] Chuman H, Maekubo T, Osako T, Kodama Y, Ishiai M, Nao-I N. Rodent model of nonarteritic ischemic optic neuropathy and its electrophysiological evaluation. Jpn J Ophthalmol. 2012; 56(5):518–527
[57] Lorentzen SE. Occlusion of the central retinal artery. A follow-up. Acta Ophthalmol (Copenh). 1969; 47(3):690–703
[58] Qian Q, Younge BR, Torres VE. Retinal arterial and venous occlusions in patients with ADPKD. Nephrol Dial Transplant. 2007; 22(6):1769–1771
[59] Sullivan KL, Brown GC, Forman AR, Sergott RC, Flanagan JC. Retrobulbar anesthesia and retinal vascular obstruction. Ophthalmology. 1983; 90 (4):373–377
[60] Balaskas K, Potamitou D, Spastri A. Branch retinal artery occlusion as the sole ocular manifestation of Takayasu arteritis [in French]. J Fr Ophtalmol. 2010; 33(1):50.e1–50.e3
[61] Kim DS, Korgavkar K, Zahid S, et al. Vision loss after central retinal artery occlusion secondary to orbital sarcoid mass. Ophthal Plast Reconstr Surg. 2016; 32(2):e37–e40
[62] Jarius S, Kleffner I, Dörr JM, et al. Clinical, paraclinical and serological findings in Susac syndrome: an international multicenter study. J Neuroinflammation. 2014; 11:46
[63] Xiao Y, Guo X, Ouyang P. Branch retinal artery occlusion associated with photodynamic therapy in a circumscribed choroidal haemangioma. Photodiagn Photodyn Ther. 2013; 10(4):644–646
[64] Choudhry N, Brucker AJ. Branch retinal artery occlusion after coil embolization of a paraclinoid aneurysm. Ophthalmic Surg Lasers Imaging Retina. 2014; 45 Online:e26–e28
[65] Desai S, Rai N, Kulkarni P, Natarajan S. Combined CRVO with CRAO in a patient with protein C deficiency. Retin Cases Brief Rep. 2014; 8(2):145–149
[66] Park KH, Kim YK, Woo SJ, et al. Korean Retina Society. Iatrogenic occlusion of the ophthalmic artery after cosmetic facial filler injections: a national survey by the Korean Retina Society. JAMA Ophthalmol. 2014; 132(6):714–723
[67] Plunkett O, Lip PL, Lip GY. Atrial fibrillation and retinal vein or artery occlusion: looking beyond the eye. Br J Ophthalmol. 2014; 98(9):1141–1143
[68] Choi JH, Jung J, Park KP, et al. Intracranial fibromuscular dysplasia presenting as various ocular manifestations. J Neurol Sci. 2014; 337(1–2):232–234
[69] Dhrami-Gavazi E, Lee W, Horowitz JD, et al. Jak2 mutation-positive polycythemia vera presenting as central retinal artery occlusion. Retin Cases Brief Rep. 2015; 9(2):127–130
[70] Ehmann D, Riyaz R, Greve M. Central retinal artery occlusion in a child with Parry-Romberg syndrome. Can J Ophthalmol. 2014; 49(1):e9–e10
[71] Brown GC, Lehman R, Magargal LE. Combined retinal artery-vein obstructions. Trans Pa Acad Ophthalmol Otolaryngol. 1988; 40:697–700
[72] Degenhart W, Brown GC, Augsburger JJ, Magargal L. Prepapillary vascular loops. Ophthalmology. 1981; 88(11):1126–1131

[73] Nonomura S, Oshitari T, Miura G, Chiba A, Yamamoto S. A case of ophthalmic artery occlusion following injection of hyaluronic acid into the glabellar area [in Japanese]. Nippon Ganka Gakkai Zasshi. 2014; 118(9):783–787

[74] Karjalainen K. Occlusion of the central retinal artery and retinal branch arterioles. A clinical, tonographic and fluorescein angiographic study of 175 patients. Acta Ophthalmol Suppl. 1971; 109:1–95

[75] Savino PJ, Glaser JS, Cassady J. Retinal stroke. Is the patient at risk? Arch Ophthalmol. 1977; 95(7):1185–1189

[76] Fledelius HC, Sandfeld L, Rasmussen AK, Madsen CV, Feldt-Rasmussen U. Ophthalmic experience over 10 years in an observational nationwide Danish cohort of Fabry patients with access to enzyme replacement. Acta Ophthalmol (Copenh). 2015; 93(3):258–264

[77] Ling W, Oftedal G, Simon T. Central retinal artery occlusion in Sydenham's chorea. Am J Dis Child. 1969; 118(3):525–527

[78] Timoney PJ, Pate JC, Pearson PA, Crandall J. Bilateral central retinal artery occlusion in a patient with acute pancreatitis. Retin Cases Brief Rep. 2009; 3 (3):308–309

[79] Sadiq N, Naqaish T, Arif A, Mohammad K, Jalis M. Central retinal artery occlusion secondary to dengue fever. J Ayub Med Coll Abbottabad. 2014; 26 (1):98–99

[80] Yolcu Ü, Kaldirim Ü, Ilhan A. Valsalva retinopathy and branch retinal artery occlusion after cardiopulmonary cerebral resuscitation. Am J Emerg Med. 2014; 32(10):1293

[81] Sacconi R, Giordano Resti A, Lattanzio R, et al. A case of branch retinal artery occlusion following orbital cavernous hemangioma excision. Eur J Ophthalmol. 2014; 24(6):972–975

[82] Dunn JP, Yamashita A, Kempen JH, Jabs DA. Retinal vascular occlusion in patients infected with human immunodeficiency virus. Retina. 2005; 25 (6):759–766

[83] Susac JO, Egan RA, Rennebohm RM, Lubow M. Susac's syndrome: 1975–2005 microangiopathy/autoimmune endotheliopathy. J Neurol Sci. 2007; 257(1–2):270–272

[84] Jarius S, Neumayer B, Wandinger KP, Hartmann M, Wildemann B. Anti-endothelial serum antibodies in a patient with Susac's syndrome. J Neurol Sci. 2009; 285(1–2):259–261

[85] Dörr J, Krautwald S, Wildemann B, et al. Characteristics of Susac syndrome: a review of all reported cases. Nat Rev Neurol. 2013; 9(6):307–316

[86] Buelens T, Herode L, Nubourgh I, Caspers L, Willermain F, Postelmans L. Central retinal artery occlusion and Susac syndrome: a case report. Retin Cases Brief Rep. 2014; 8(3):187–192

[87] Feresiadou A, Eriksson U, Larsen HC, Raininko R, Nygren I, Melberg A. Recurrence of Susac Syndrome following 23 Years of Remission. Case Rep Neurol. 2014; 6(2):171–175

[88] Noble KG. Central retinal artery occlusion: the presenting sign in radiation retinopathy. Arch Ophthalmol. 1994; 112(11):1409–1410

[89] Kurimoto T, Okamoto N, Oku H, et al. Central retinal artery occlusion resembling Purtscher-like retinopathy. Clin Ophthalmol. 2011; 5:1083–1088

[90] Ayaki M, Yokoyama N, Furukawa Y. Postpartum central retinal artery occlusion simulating Purtscher's retinopathy. Ophthalmologica. 1995; 209(1):37–39

[91] Lightman DA, Brod RD. Branch retinal artery occlusion associated with Lyme disease. Arch Ophthalmol. 1991; 109(9):1198–1199

[92] Gass JD, Trattler HL. Retinal artery obstruction and atheromas associated with non-Hodgkin's large cell lymphoma (reticulum cell sarcoma). Arch Ophthalmol. 1991; 109(8):1134–1139

[93] Hayashi K, Iguchi Y, Kimura K, Shibazaki K, Kobayashi K, Inoue T. Paradoxical brain embolism as a cause of central retinal artery occlusion: a case report. J Neuroimaging. 2007; 17(3):255–257

[94] Leisser C, Kaufmann TA, Feltgen N, Schumacher M, Schmoor C, Meckel S. Distribution of internal carotid artery plaque locations among patients with central retinal artery occlusion in the Eagle study population. Graefes Arch Clin Exp Ophthalmol. 2015; 253(8):1227–1230

[95] Kumar M A, Ganesh B A. CRAO in Moyamoya disease. J Clin Diagn Res. 2013; 7(3):545–547

[96] Berkani Z, Kitouni Y, Belhadj A, et al. Cilioretinal artery occlusion and central retinal vein occlusion complicating hyperhomocysteinemia: a case report [in French]. J Fr Ophtalmol. 2013; 36(7):e119–e127

[97] Patel M, Shah G, Davies JB, Mittra RA, Eliott D. Re-evaluating our perspective on retinal artery occlusion from carotid dissection: a report of three cases and review of the literature. Ophthalmic Surg Lasers Imaging Retina. 2013; 44(6):555–560

[98] Strassman I, Silverstone BZ, Seelenfreund MH, Sheer A, Berson D. Essential thrombocythemia: a rare case of central retinal artery occlusion. Metab Pediatr Syst Ophthalmol (1985). 1991; 14(1):18–20

[99] Jang YJ, Chun JW, Lee SW, Kim HC. A case of central retinal artery occlusion after chiropractic manipulation of the neck. Korean J Ophthalmol. 2012; 26 (2):132–134

[100] Cotineau J, Sorato M, Le Guelec M. Retinal artery occlusions following carotid angiography [author's transl; in French]. J Fr Ophtalmol. 1978; 1(2):119–123

[101] Vignes S, Wechsler B, Elmaleh C, Cassoux N, Horellou MH, Godeau P. Retinal arterial occlusion associated with resistance to activated protein C. Br J Ophthalmol. 1996; 80(12):1111

[102] Bertram B, Remky A, Arend O, Wolf S, Reim M. Protein C, protein S, and antithrombin III in acute ocular occlusive diseases. Ger J Ophthalmol. 1995; 4(6):332–335

[103] Greven CM, Wall AB. Peripheral retinal neovascularization and retinal vascular occlusion associated with activated protein C resistance. Am J Ophthalmol. 1997; 124(5):687–689

[104] Loh BK, Lee SY, Goh KY. Protein S deficiency manifesting simultaneously as central retinal artery occlusion, oculomotor nerve palsy, and systemic arterial occlusive diseases. Eye (Lond). 2007; 21(5):684–686

[105] Glueck CJ, Ping Wang, Hutchins R, Petersen MR, Golnik K. Ocular vascular thrombotic events: central retinal vein and central retinal artery occlusions. Clin Appl Thromb Hemost. 2008; 14(3):286–294

[106] Liem RI, Calamaras DM, Chhabra MS, Files B, Minniti CP, Thompson AA. Sudden-onset blindness in sickle cell disease due to retinal artery occlusion. Pediatr Blood Cancer. 2008; 50(3):624–627

[107] Kianersi F, Ghanbari H, Beni AN, Beni ZN, Fesharaki H, Ahmadi M. Macular branch retinal artery occlusion as the first manifestation of ocular toxoplasmosis. Retin Cases Brief Rep. 2013; 7(4):391–394

[108] Arai H, Sakai T, Okano K, et al. Presumed toxoplasmic central retinal artery occlusion and multifocal retinitis with perivascular sheathing. Clin Ophthalmol. 2014; 8:789–792

[109] Myers MA, Hamilton SR, Bogosian AJ, Smith CH, Wagner TA. Visual loss as a complication of spine surgery. A review of 37 cases. Spine. 1997; 22 (12):1325–1329

[110] Bekar A, Türeyen K, Aksoy K. Unilateral blindness due to patient positioning during cervical syringomyelia surgery: unilateral blindness after prone position. J Neurosurg Anesthesiol. 1996; 8(3):227–229

[111] Schwartz SG, Hickey M, Puliafito CA. Bilateral CRAO and CRVO from thrombotic thrombocytopenic purpura: OCT findings and treatment with triamcinolone acetonide and bevacizumab. Ophthalmic Surg Lasers Imaging. 2006; 37(5):420–422

[112] De Salvo G, Li Calzi C, Anastasi M, Lodato G. Branch retinal vein occlusion followed by central retinal artery occlusion in Churg-Strauss syndrome: unusual ocular manifestations in allergic granulomatous angiitis. Eur J Ophthalmol. 2009; 19(2):314–317

[113] Cobo-Soriano R, Sánchez-Ramón S, Aparicio MJ, et al. Antiphospholipid antibodies and retinal thrombosis in patients without risk factors: a prospective case-control study. Am J Ophthalmol. 1999; 128(6):725–732

[114] Esen E, Sizmaz S, Sariyeva A, Demircan N. Bilateral central retinal artery occlusion in Behçet disease. Ocul Immunol Inflamm. 2015; 23(5):416–419

[115] Ozdal PC, Ortaç S, Taskintuna I, Teke MY, Firat E. Central retinal artery occlusion associated with ocular Behçet's disease. Eur J Ophthalmol. 2002; 12 (4):328–330

[116] Chi SL, Stinnett S, Eggenberger E, et al. Clinical characteristics in 53 patients with cat scratch optic neuropathy. Ophthalmology. 2012; 119(1):183–187

[117] Kaiser PK, Lee MS, Martin DA. Occlusive vasculitis in a patient with concomitant West Nile virus infection. Am J Ophthalmol. 2003; 136(5):928–930

[118] Matonti F, Prost Magnin O, Galland F, et al. [Internal carotid artery dissection on arterial fibromuscular dysplasia causing a central retinal artery occlusion: a case report]. J Fr Ophtalmol. 2006; 29(7):e15

[119] Altun A, Altun G, Olcaysu OO, Kurna SA, Aki SF. Central retinal artery occlusion in association with fibromuscular dysplasia. Clin Ophthalmol. 2013; 7:2253–2255

[120] Whiteman DW, Rosen DA, Pinkerton RM. Retinal and choroidal microvascular embolism after intranasal corticosteroid injection. Am J Ophthalmol. 1980; 89(6):851–853

[121] Cheney ML, Blair PA. Blindness as a complication of rhinoplasty. Arch Otolaryngol Head Neck Surg. 1987; 113(7):768–769

[122] Ramezani A, Haghighatkhah H, Moghadasi H, Taheri MS, Parsafar H. A case of central retinal artery occlusion following embolization procedure for juvenile nasopharyngeal angiofibroma. Indian J Ophthalmol. 2010; 58 (5):419–421

[123] Xing L, Almeida DR, Belliveau MJ, et al. Ophthalmic artery occlusion secondary to fat emboli after cosmetic nasal injection of autologous fat. Retina. 2012; 32(10):2175–2176

[124] Bachman DM, Green WR, Holman R. Bilateral ophthalmic artery occlusion in a patient with acquired immunodeficiency syndrome and central nervous system lymphoma. Ophthalmology. 2002; 109(6):1142–1147
[125] Smith TW, Burton TC. The retinal manifestations of Rocky Mountain spotted fever. Am J Ophthalmol. 1977; 84(2):259–262
[126] Saatci OA, Koçak N, Durak I, Ergin MH. Unilateral retinal vasculitis, branch retinal artery occlusion and subsequent retinal neovascularization in Crohn's disease. Int Ophthalmol. 2001; 24(2):89–92
[127] Rouleau J, Longmuir R, Lee AG. Optic disc edema with adjacent cilioretinal artery occlusion in a male with ulcerative colitis. Semin Ophthalmol. 2007; 22(1):25–28
[128] Panton RW, Goldberg MF, Farber MD. Retinal arterial macroaneurysms: risk factors and natural history. Br J Ophthalmol. 1990; 74(10):595–600
[129] Newsom RS, Trew DR, Leonard TJ. Bilateral buried optic nerve drusen presenting with central retinal artery occlusion at high altitude. Eye (Lond). 1995; 9(Pt 6):806–808
[130] Imai E, Kunikata H, Udono T, Nakagawa Y, Abe T, Tamai M. Branch retinal artery occlusion: a complication of iron-deficiency anemia in a young adult with a rectal carcinoid. Tohoku J Exp Med. 2004; 203(2):141–144
[131] Chong CC, Chang AA. Traumatic optic nerve avulsion and central retinal artery occlusion following rugby injury. Clin Experiment Ophthalmol. 2006; 34(1):88–89
[132] Ayati M, Gori T, Münzel T. Lesions of the mitral valve as a cause of central retinal artery occlusion: presentation and discussion of two cases. Echocardiography. 2010; 27(1):E1–E3
[133] Wolf A, Shalem M, Horowitz J, Geyer O. Retinal vascular occlusion following traumatic hyphema and glaucoma, as a presenting sign of sickle cell trait. Isr Med Assoc J. 2005; 7(7):476–477
[134] Brown GC, Magargal L, Augsburger JJ, Shields JA. Preretinal arterial loops and retinal arterial occlusion. Am J Ophthalmol. 1979; 87(5):646–651
[135] Brown GC, Shields JA, Sanborn G, Augsburger JJ, Savino PJ, Schatz NJ. Radiation retinopathy. Ophthalmology. 1982; 89(12):1494–1501
[136] Brown GC, Moffat K, Cruess A, Magargal LE, Goldberg RE. Cilioretinal artery obstruction. Retina. 1983; 3(3):182–187
[137] Wallace RT, Brown GC, Benson W, Sivalingham A. Sudden retinal manifestations of intranasal cocaine and methamphetamine abuse. Am J Ophthalmol. 1992; 114(2):158–160
[138] Schatz H, Fong AC, McDonald HR, et al. Cilioretinal artery occlusion in young adults with central retinal vein occlusion. Ophthalmology. 1991; 98(5):594–601
[139] Kaur S, Sachdev N. Unilateral branch retinal arterial occlusion following administration of bevacizumab for branch retinal vein occlusion. Int Ophthalmol. 2013; 33(5):549–552
[140] Terrada C, Dethorey G, Ducos G, Lehoang P, Bodaghi B, Souied EH. Spontaneous branch artery occlusion in idiopathic retinitis, vasculitis, aneurysms, and neuroretinitis syndrome despite panretinal laser photocoagulation of widespread retina nonperfusion. Acta Ophthalmol (Copenh). 2011; 89(6): e542–e543
[141] Magargal LE, Sanborn GE, Donoso LA, Gonder JR. Branch retinal artery occlusion after excessive use of nasal spray. Ann Ophthalmol. 1985; 17(8):500–501
[142] Bradish CF, Flowers M. Central retinal artery occlusion in association with osteogenesis imperfecta. Spine. 1987; 12(2):193–194
[143] Hayreh SS. Acute retinal arterial occlusive disorders. Prog Retin Eye Res. 2011; 30(5):359–394
[144] Ferrières J. Effects on coronary atherosclerosis by targeting low-density lipoprotein cholesterol with statins. Am J Cardiovasc Drugs. 2009; 9(2):109–115
[145] Brown MM, Brown GC, Sharma S. Cost-effective analysis. The value component of evidence-based medicine. Cost-utility of treatment for acute, nonarteritic central retinal artery obstruction. Evidence-Based Eye. 2000; 1:243–247
[146] Atebara NH, Brown GC, Cater J. Efficacy of anterior chamber paracentesis and Carbogen in treating acute nonarteritic central retinal artery occlusion. Ophthalmology. 1995; 102(12):2029–2034, discussion 2034–2035
[147] Lim JY, Lee JY, Chung HW, Yoon YH, Kim JG. Treatment of branch retinal artery occlusion with transluminal Nd:YAG laser embolysis. Korean J Ophthalmol. 2009; 23(4):315–317
[148] Ffytche TJ. A rationalization of treatment of central retinal artery occlusion. Trans Ophthalmol Soc U K. 1974; 94(2):468–479
[149] Watson PG. The treatment of acute central retinal artery occlusion. In: Cant JS, ed. The Ocular Circulation in Health and Disease. St. Louis, MO: CV Mosby; 1969:234–245
[150] Kuritzky S. Nitroglycerin to treat acute loss of vision. N Engl J Med. 1990; 323(20):1428
[151] Schmidt D, Schumacher M, Wakhloo AK. Microcatheter urokinase infusion in central retinal artery occlusion. Am J Ophthalmol. 1992; 113(4):429–434
[152] Opremcak E, Rehmar AJ, Ridenour CD, Borkowski LM, Kelley JK. Restoration of retinal blood flow via transluminal Nd:YAG embolysis/embolectomy (TYL/E) for central and branch retinal artery occlusion. Retina. 2008; 28 (2):226–235
[153] Canan H, Ulas B, Altan-Yaycioglu R. Hyperbaric oxygen therapy in combination with systemic treatment of sickle cell disease presenting as central retinal artery occlusion: a case report. J Med Case Reports. 2014; 8:370
[154] Duker JS, Brown GC. Recovery following acute obstruction of the retinal and choroidal circulations. A case history. Retina. 1988; 8(4):257–260
[155] Hayreh SS, Kolder HE, Weingeist TA. Central retinal artery occlusion and retinal tolerance time. Ophthalmology. 1980; 87(1):75–78
[156] Richards RD. Simultaneous occlusion of the central retinal artery and vein. Trans Am Ophthalmol Soc. 1979; 77:191–209
[157] Jorizzo PA, Klein ML, Shults WT, Linn ML. Visual recovery in combined central retinal artery and central retinal vein occlusion. Am J Ophthalmol. 1987; 104(4):358–363
[158] Duker SJ, Brown GC, Sergott R, McNamara JA. Combined arterial and venous disease of the retina. Retina. 1990; 10:105–112
[159] McDonald HR, Schatz H, Allen AW, et al. Retinal toxicity secondary to intraocular gentamicin injection. Ophthalmology. 1986; 93(7):871–877
[160] Brown GC, Duker JS, Lehman R, Eagle RC, Jr. Combined central retinal artery-central vein obstruction. Int Ophthalmol. 1993; 17(1):9–17
[161] Brown GC, Eagle RC, Jr, Shakin EP, Gruber M, Arbizio VV. Retinal toxicity of intravitreal gentamicin. Arch Ophthalmol. 1990; 108(12):1740–1744
[162] Brown GC, Reber R. An unusual presentation of branch retinal artery obstruction in association with ocular neovascularization. Can J Ophthalmol. 1986; 21(3):103–106
[163] Kraushar MF, Brown GC. Retinal neovascularization after branch retinal arterial obstruction. Am J Ophthalmol. 1987; 104(3):294–296
[164] Mateen FJ, Zubkov AY, Muralidharan R, et al. Susac syndrome: clinical characteristics and treatment in 29 new cases. Eur J Neurol. 2012; 19(6):800–811
[165] Fong ACO, Schatz H, McDonald HR, et al. Cilioretinal artery occlusion in young adults with central retinal vein occlusion. Retina. 1992; 12:3–11
[166] McLeod D, Marshall J, Kohner EM, Bird AC. The role of axoplasmic transport in the pathogenesis of retinal cotton-wool spots. Br J Ophthalmol. 1977; 61 (3):177–191
[167] Kohner EM, Dollery CT, Bulpitt CJ. Cotton-wool spots in diabetic retinopathy. Diabetes. 1969; 18(10):691–704
[168] Brown GC, Brown MM, Hiller T, Fischer D, Benson WE, Magargal LE. Cotton-wool spots. Retina. 1985; 5(4):206–214
[169] Robinson F, Riva CE, Grunwald JE, Petrig BL, Sinclair SH. Retinal blood flow autoregulation in response to an acute increase in blood pressure. Invest Ophthalmol Vis Sci. 1986; 27(5):722–726
[170] Freeman WR, Lerner CW, Mines JA, et al. A prospective study of the ophthalmologic findings in the acquired immune deficiency syndrome. Am J Ophthalmol. 1984; 97(2):133–142
[171] Pepose JS, Nestro MS, Holland GN, Cochran AJ, Foos RY. An analysis of retinal cotton-wool spots in the acquired immunodeficiency syndrome. Am J Ophthalmol. 1983; 95:118–120
[172] Seligmann M, Chess L, Fahey JL, et al. AIDS—an immunologic reevaluation. N Engl J Med. 1984; 311(20):1286–1292
[173] Lim JW, Shin MC. Pegylated-interferon-associated retinopathy in chronic hepatitis patients. Ophthalmologica. 2010; 224(4):224–229
[174] Ohira M, Ito D, Shimizu T, Shibata M, Ohde H, Suzuki N. Retinopathy: an overlooked adverse effect of interferon-beta treatment of multiple sclerosis. Keio J Med. 2009; 58(1):54–56

9 Retinal Venous Occlusive Disease

Amol D. Kulkarni, Michael S. Ip, and Ingrid U. Scott

9.1 Introduction

Retinal venous occlusive disease is the second most common retinal vascular disease following diabetic retinopathy.[1] There are three distinct types of retinal vein occlusion (RVO) based on the site of obstruction: branch retinal vein occlusion (BRVO), central retinal vein occlusion (CRVO), and hemiretinal vein occlusion.[2] Population-based studies report a prevalence rate of 0.5 to 2.0% for BRVO and 0.1 to 0.2% for CRVO.[3] The 15-year incidence rate is estimated to be 1.8% for BRVO and 0.5% for CRVO.[4] The most common cause of vision loss in RVO is macular edema (ME); other causes of vision loss include macular ischemia, intraretinal hemorrhage, and neovascularization (NV) with secondary vitreous hemorrhage, tractional retinal detachment, and/or neovascular glaucoma (NVG).[5,6] Many systemic diseases are risk factors for RVO.[7,8] The various treatment options for RVO can be categorized broadly into pharmacotherapy, laser treatment, surgical treatment, and combination therapy.[9] This chapter reviews the pathophysiology, clinical features and various treatment modalities for, RVO.

9.2 Branch Retinal Vein Occlusion

BRVO is four to six times more common than CRVO.[3] Advanced age is an important risk factor, with the prevalence of BRVO in persons older than 80 years being seven times higher than the prevalence of BRVO in people between 40 and 49 years of age.[3] Systemic vascular diseases such as hypertension (HTN), hyperlipidemia (HLD) and peripheral arterial disease (PAD), and metabolic diseases such as diabetes mellitus (DM) have been associated with BRVO.[7] A meta-analysis of risk factors in patients with BRVO reveals that the odds ratio is 3.0 (95% CI: 2.0–4.4) for HTN, 2.3 (95% CI: 1.5–3.5) for HLD, and 1.1 (95% CI: 0.8–1.5) for DM.[10]

Special Considerations

- RVO risk factors
  - Cardiovascular risk profile of patients is more important than thrombophilic risk factors.

The role of thrombophilia in the pathogenesis of BRVO is not clear. A review of the literature reveals a lack of consensus regarding the role in RVO of currently known thrombophilic risk factors such as hyperhomocysteinemia, factor V Leiden mutation, deficiency in protein C and/or S, antithrombin III deficiency, prothrombin gene mutation, anticardiolipin antibodies, lupus anticoagulant, increased packed cell volume, hematocrit, and fibrinogen.[11] Some authors have concluded that, with respect to RVO, cardiovascular risk profile is more important than thrombophilic risk factors.[11] BRVO can also occur secondary to local or systemic vasculitis.[12] Further, BRVO can be a result of direct infiltration leading to venous obstruction such as in sarcoidosis, ocular tuberculosis, or neoplastic diseases.[12] Glaucoma and ocular HTN may predispose to RVO because increased intraocular pressure (IOP) may lead to venous stasis; these conditions are not considered as important risk factors for BRVO as compared to CRVO.[12] Moreover, medications such as oral contraceptives and anabolic steroids have been reported as risk factors for BRVO due to hypercoagulability associated with the use of these medications.[12]

9.2.1 Pathophysiology

BRVO usually develops at arteriovenous (AV) crossing sites where the artery is situated superficially over the vein. Histological examinations have shown that arteriosclerotic changes in the retinal artery may cause compression of the underlying vein, leading to thrombus formation and vein occlusion.[13,14] Other theories include hemodynamic variations due to venous contouring at AV crossing sites as the inciting cause of BRVO. Diseases of the vein wall, such as vasculitis, can also cause BRVO and may not involve AV crossing sites.[15] BRVO leads to localized retinal ischemia which is associated with secretion of vasopermeability factors such as vascular endothelial growth factor (VEGF) and interleukin-6 (IL-6). These factors lead to breakdown of the blood–retinal barrier and development of ME. Release of VEGF and IL-6 at the border between perfused and nonperfused retina is also associated with formation of retinal NV, which may lead to vitreous hemorrhage and abnormal vitreoretinal adhesions.

9.2.2 Clinical Features and Diagnosis

BRVO is typically characterized by clinical findings in a segmental distribution distal to the involved AV crossing site, with the most common location being the superotemporal quadrant of the retina.[16] BRVOs are classified according to their anatomical location either as major, when one of the major branch veins draining one of the retinal quadrants is involved, or as macular, when one of the smaller venules within the macula is occluded.[12] BRVOs can also be classified according to their duration either as acute, when present for less than 6 months, or as chronic, when present for more than 6 months.[9] In an acute BRVO, the involved area is usually wedge-shaped with dilated and tortuous veins surrounded by deep and superficial retinal hemorrhages, cotton-wool spots, and retinal edema (▸ Fig. 9.1). Visual acuity (VA) may be reduced due to retinal hemorrhage, edema, or ischemia involving the central macular region. If the venous blockage is peripheral to branches draining the macula or involves a branch in the nasal retina, VA may be unaffected unless other complications arise. Approximately 50 to 60% of untreated patients will have a final VA of 20/40 or better. However, severe vision loss is not uncommon, with 20 to 25% of patients having a VA of 20/200 or worse.[17] In a chronic BRVO, intraretinal hemorrhages have usually resolved and subtle retinal vascular changes such as capillary abnormalities (telangiectasia and microaneurysms) and collateral vessel formation may be observed. Intravenous fluorescein angiography (FA) may aid in the diagnosis in these cases by better demonstrating the

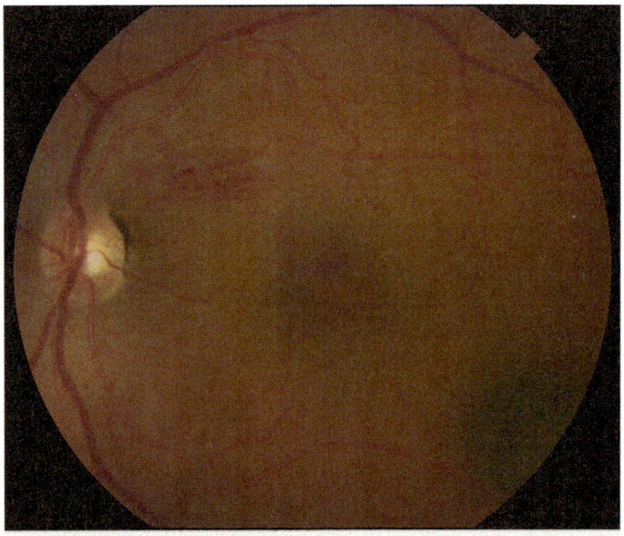

Fig. 9.1 Acute branch retinal vein occlusion. Note the segmental distribution of intraretinal hemorrhages.

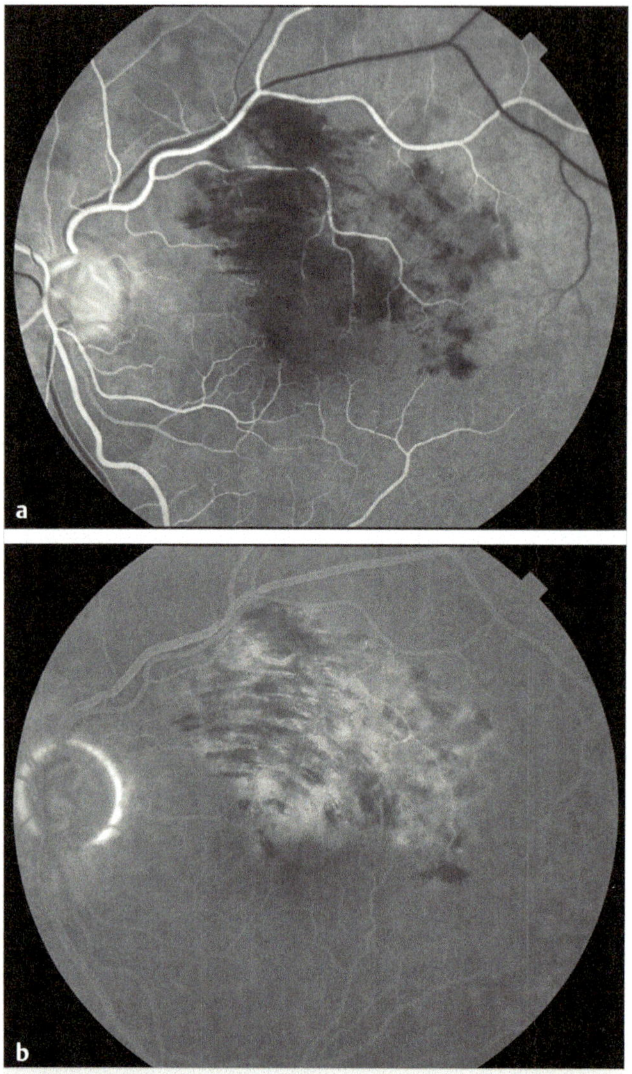

Fig. 9.2 Macular edema associated with a perfused branch retinal vein occlusion. **(a)** Fluorescein angiography demonstrates an intact parafoveal retinal capillary network during the transit phase of the fluorescein angiogram. **(b)** Late accumulation of fluorescein dye is present both parafoveally and in the foveal center.

segmental retinal vascular alterations. Angiographic findings reflect changes in vessel permeability, caliber, and patency, and may assist in identifying areas of ME, NV, and nonperfusion. If the area of retinal capillary nonperfusion is smaller than 5 disc diameters in size on fluorescein angiography, the occlusion is defined as perfused.[18] If the area of nonperfusion is larger than 5 disc diameters in size, the occlusion is defined as nonperfused.[18] Of eyes with a BRVO affecting at least one quadrant of the retina, approximately 50% are nonperfused.[18] It is important to recognize that perfused BRVO may progress to the nonperfused type during ensuing weeks, months, and even years.[19] Visually significant complications associated with BRVO include ME (most common) and intraocular NV, which may result in vitreous hemorrhage or tractional retinal detachment.[19]

9.2.3 Macular Edema

In eyes with a BRVO, ME can be classified angiographically as perfused, nonperfused (ischemic), or mixed (perfused and nonperfused).[17,20] ME is perfused (▶ Fig. 9.2) when fluorescein angiography shows a completely intact parafoveal retinal capillary network during the transit phase of the angiogram followed by the late accumulation of fluorescein dye in and around the foveal center.[20] ME is nonperfused (▶ Fig. 9.3) when fluorescein angiography reveals an irregular parafoveal vascular network with parafoveal and perifoveal retinal capillary nonperfusion and no late accumulation of fluorescein dye in the foveal center.[20] ME is mixed when fluorescein angiography demonstrates a combination of parafoveal retinal capillary dilation with leakage and areas of capillary nonperfusion.[20] In patients with perfused ME, approximately one-third will regain some vision spontaneously.[19] However, this becomes less likely the longer the edema persists. Early in the course of BRVO, macular nonperfusion can result in permanent vision loss.[19] The presence of a significant amount of intraretinal hemorrhage in the central macula may interfere with the angiographic interpretation, and optical coherence tomography (OCT) may be useful in these cases. In fact, OCT has become a mainstay for the detection of ME and for monitoring of treatment efficacy in patients with ME due to RVO.[21] The findings from the Standard Care versus COrticosteroid for REtinal Vein Occlusion (SCORE) Study revealed a modest correlation between OCT-measured center point thickness and VA in patients with BRVO or CRVO.[21]

9.2.4 Intraocular Neovascularization

In the Branch Vein Occlusion Study (BVOS), retinal or disc NV developed in 36% of eyes with 5 disc diameters or more of retinal nonperfusion,[18] and 60% of these eyes developed vitreous hemorrhage if untreated.[18] The NV usually develops within the first 6 to 12 months after the onset of the occlusion but may develop anytime within the first 3 years.[19] Neovascular vessels may be confused with collateral vessels on ophthalmoscopic examination. Fluorescein angiography is useful to differentiate collateral vessels from NV as dye leakage is more prominent

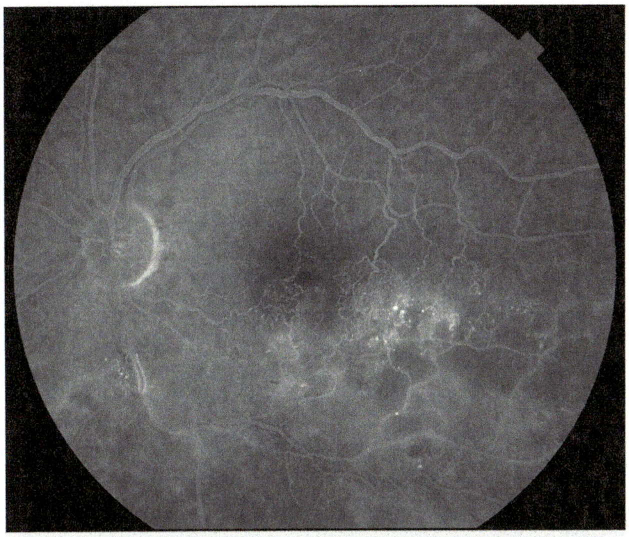

Fig. 9.3 Macular edema associated with a nonperfused branch retinal vein occlusion. The fluorescein angiogram demonstrates an irregular parafoveal vascular network with parafoveal and perifoveal areas of retinal capillary nonperfusion and no late accumulation of fluorescein dye in the foveal center.

from the NV than from the collateral vessels (in contrast to NV, collateral vessels are associated with no or only minimal leakage on FA).[18] Iris NV and NVG are infrequent complications in eyes with BRVO.[19]

Pearls

- Macular edema in RVO
  - OCT has become a mainstay for the detection of ME and for monitoring of treatment efficacy in patients with ME due to RVO.

9.2.5 Management and Course

In addition to a thorough eye examination, initial evaluation of patients with BRVO may include medical assessment to identify any underlying systemic causes. It is important to look for cardiovascular risk factors, and baseline laboratory testing may include fasting blood glucose level, complete blood count with differential and platelets, renal function tests, and lipid profile.[11]

Pearls

- BVOS
  - Retinal or disc NV developed in 36% of eyes with 5 disc diameters or more of retinal nonperfusion.

Further testing may be indicated in patients younger than 50 years with or without suspicion for coagulopathy (see the following list).[11]

Tests for coagulopathy in the assessment of selected patients with RVO[11]:

- Functional protein C and protein S levels
- Antithrombin III levels
- Antiphospholipid antibodies: lupus anticoagulant and anticardiolipin antibodies
- Activated protein C resistance (factor V Leiden mutation [R506Q] polymerase chain reaction assay)
- Factor XII (Hageman factor)
- Prothrombin gene mutation (G20210A)

Various treatments for BRVO are aimed at minimizing visual loss from complications such as ME and NV.[9] Treatment options for ME include pharmacotherapy and laser.[9] Surgical treatments such as AV sheathotomies have been attempted with varied success, but they are not generally considered standard of care due to the associated risk of complications, unpredictable efficacy, and inability to alter the chronic effects from ischemia.[22]

Pharmacotherapy

Intravitreal Pharmacotherapy

Intravitreal injection of pharmacological agents reduces the breakdown of the blood–retinal barrier by inhibiting factors such as VEGF, IL-6, prostaglandins, and protein kinase C. The various pharmacological preparations currently available for intraocular delivery include anti-VEGF agents and corticosteroids.[23]

Intravitreal Anti-VEGF Therapy

Anti-VEGF therapy is typically the first-line treatment in patients with ME associated with BRVO. Anti-VEGF agents currently available for the treatment of ME associated with BRVO by intravitreal injection include ranibizumab (Lucentis), bevacizumab (Avastin), and aflibercept (Eylea).

Ranibizumab

Ranibizumab (Lucentis, Genentech) is a humanized Fab fragment that binds and neutralizes all isoforms of VEGF-A. Ranibizumab was the first anti-VEGF agent to receive Food and Drug Administration (FDA) approval (in June 2010) for the treatment of ME secondary to BRVO.

Pearls

- Intravitreal pharmacotherapy for ME associated with BRVO
  - Anti-VEGF therapy is typically the first-line treatment in patients with ME associated with BRVO.

In the BRanch Retinal Vein Occlusion (BRAVO) study[24] (a phase III, multicenter, prospective clinical trial comparing the efficacy and safety of intravitreal injections of ranibizumab 0.3 mg, intravitreal injections of ranibizumab 0.5 mg, and sham injections), 397 patients with center-involved ME from a BRVO occurring within 12 months of study entry were randomized to receive monthly intraocular injections of 0.3 mg (n =134) or

0.5 mg (n =131) of ranibizumab or sham injections (n = 132). A gain of =15 Early Treatment Diabetic Retinopathy Study (ETDRS letters in best-corrected visual acuity (BCVA) at 6 months compared to baseline (the primary study endpoint) was achieved in 55.2% (0.3 mg) and 61.1% (0.5 mg) of patients in the ranibizumab groups and 28.8% in the sham group ($p < 0.0001$ for each ranibizumab group versus sham). There was greater resolution of ME in the ranibizumab groups compared to the sham group; central subfield thickness (CST) was reduced by 337.3 µm in the 0.3 mg group; 345.2 µm in the 0.5 mg group; and 157.7 µm in the sham group ($p < 0.0001$ for each ranibizumab group versus sham). Rescue grid laser therapy was performed in 18.7% of patients in the 0.3 mg ranibizumab group, 19.8% of patients in the 0.5 mg ranibizumab group, and 54.5% of patients in the sham group. After 6 months, all the patients were evaluated monthly and, if study eye Snellen equivalent BCVA was =20/40 or mean CST was =250 µm, patients received intravitreal ranibizumab; patients in the ranibizumab groups received their assigned dose and patients in the sham group received 0.5 mg of ranibizumab. Between 6 and 12 months, the vision was maintained in the ranibizumab groups, and there was substantial improvement in the sham group (an improvement in VA letter score of =15 compared to baseline was achieved in 28.8% of patients in the sham group at month 6 and in 43.9% of patients in the sham group at month 12).[25] In the BRAVO study, patients in the sham group showed a substantial improvement in vision after receiving ranibizumab as needed, but their vision at month 12 was not as good as that in patients in the ranibizumab groups.[25] This indicates that a delay in instituting treatment may affect the final visual gain.[25]

Bevacizumab

Bevacizumab (Avastin, Genentech) is a full-length humanized monoclonal antibody to VEGF-A. Although bevacizumab is not FDA approved for intravitreal use, numerous case reports and case series have reported that intravitreal bevacizumab is associated with improvement in VA and retinal thickening in eyes with ME due to BRVO.[26,27,28] Fung et al concluded that physician reporting of adverse events after intravitreal bevacizumab injections did not show an increased rate of drug-related ocular or systemic events.[29] There are concerns about tolerance and tachyphylaxis with intravitreal bevacizumab therapy, which may be addressed by switching to other anti-VEGF agents.[30]

Aflibercept

Aflibercept (Eylea, Regeneron) is a small soluble VEGF receptor that acts as a decoy receptor binding free-VEGF. Aflibercept was approved by the FDA for treatment of ME secondary to BRVO in October 2014.[31] In the VIBRANT study[31] (a phase III, multicenter, prospective clinical trial comparing the efficacy and safety of intravitreal aflibercept with macular grid laser for treatment of ME after BRVO), 183 treatment-naive eyes with ME after BRVO of less than 12 months' duration and BCVA between 20/40 and 20/320 Snellen equivalent were randomized to receive either intravitreal aflibercept 2 mg every 4 weeks (n = 91) from baseline to week 20 or grid laser (n = 92) at baseline with a single grid laser rescue treatment, if needed, from weeks 12 through 20. Rescue treatment criteria included (a) a > 50-µm increase in central retinal thickness (CRT) compared with the lowest previous measurement; (b) presence of new or persistent cystic retinal changes, subretinal fluid, or persistent diffuse edema in the central OCT subfield; or (c) loss of =5 ETDRS letters compared with the best previous measurement because of BRVO in conjunction with any increase in CRT. If =1 rescue treatment criterion was met, eyes in the intravitreal aflibercept group received sham laser at either week 12, 16, or 20. Eyes in the laser group eligible for rescue treatment before week 24 received one additional laser treatment from week 12 to 20. A gain of =15 ETDRS letters in BCVA at 24 weeks compared to baseline (the primary study endpoint) was achieved in 52.7% of eyes in the aflibercept group compared to 26.7% in the laser group (p = 0.0003). The mean reduction in CRT at week 24 compared to baseline was 280.5 µm in the aflibercept group and 128.0 µm in the laser group ($p < 0.0001$). There were no cases of intraocular inflammation or endophthalmitis.

Intravitreal Corticosteroids

Intravitreal corticosteroids reduce the breakdown of the blood–retinal barrier by inhibiting factors such as VEGF, IL-6, prostaglandins, and protein kinase C.[32] Several case studies have shown favorable anatomical response to intravitreal injection of triamcinolone acetonide (TA) in eyes with ME associated with RVO.[33,34,35,36,37] Corticosteroid preparations currently available for intraocular use include TA and dexamethasone. Fluocinolone acetonide is a glucocorticoid that can be delivered by polymer-based non-biodegradable platforms to the posterior segment; there is currently no fluocinolone implant approved by the FDA for use in RVO.[9]

Triamcinolone Acetonide (TA)

According to a pharmacokinetics study of human nonvitrectomized eyes, a single 4 mg intravitreal injection of TA has a mean half-life of 18.6 days with measurable concentrations expected to last approximately 3 months.[38] Reported side effects include cataract, increased IOP, and injection-related complications including noninfectious and infectious endophthalmitis, retinal detachment, vitreous hemorrhage, and lens injury.[33,34,35,36,37] The SCORE Study, a multicenter, randomized, phase III National Eye Institute–sponsored study, investigated the efficacy and safety of standard care versus intravitreal injection(s) of TA for ME secondary to BRVO and CRVO.[39,40] Individuals with BRVO or CRVO with associated ME of up to 24 months' duration and BCVA between 19 and 73 ETDRS letters (corresponding to a Snellen VA equivalent of approximately 20/40–20/400) were eligible for participation in the SCORE Study.[39,40,41] The two primary study objectives of the SCORE-BRVO trial were (1) to determine whether intravitreal TA at 1 and 4 mg doses produces greater visual benefit, with an acceptable safety profile, than grid laser (standard care), when appropriate, for the treatment of vision loss associated with ME secondary to BRVO; and (2) to compare the efficacy and safety of the 1- and 4-mg TA doses.[40] The results of the SCORE-BRVO trial demonstrated no significant differences among the three treatment groups for a gain in VA letter score of =15 at 12 months (29, 26, and 27% in the standard care, and 1- and 4-mg TA groups, respectively).[40] An early positive treatment response of a gain in VA letter score of =15 was observed at month 4 in the 4-mg TA group compared with the 1-mg TA and standard care groups. After month 12 and through month 36, the mean improvement from baseline VA letter score was greatest in the standard care group compared with the two TA groups. With respect to OCT-measured center point thickness, all three groups showed a decrease from baseline to month 12. Analogous to the VA results, only at month 4 did the 4-mg TA group demonstrate a greater treatment effect on center point thickness than the 1-mg TA and standard care groups; at all other times investigated (months 8–36), the standard care group demonstrated the greatest overall median decrease in center point thickness from baseline. The rates of adverse events were higher in the 4-mg TA group compared with the 1-mg and standard care groups. There was a dose-dependent higher frequency of initiating IOP-lowering medications in the TA groups (41% in 4 mg and 8% in 1 mg) compared with the standard care group (2%). The proportion of phakic eyes that had new-onset lens opacity or progression of an existing opacity through 12 months based on assessment at the clinical center was greater in the two TA groups (35% in 4 mg and 25% in 1 mg) compared with the standard care group (13%). Most cataract surgeries were performed during the second year of the study and occurred with the highest frequency in the 4-mg TA group (n = 35). The rates of adverse events with respect to cataract surgery and elevated IOP were similar between the standard care and 1 mg TA groups. Thus, the SCORE Study results, at the time of publication, supported grid laser as the standard of care for patients with decreased VA attributable to ME secondary to BRVO.[40]

Dexamethasone Implant

Dexamethasone is a glucocorticoid which is three times more potent than TA.[41] However, it is cleared rapidly from the vitreous cavity (half-life of 5.5 h) in humans. Ozurdex (Allergan) is an extended delivery bioerodable dexamethasone polylactic acid polyglycolic acid (PLGA) copolymer complex.[41] A specially designed proprietary instrument is used for the intravitreal injection of the Ozurdex dexamethasone implant, thus obviating the need for surgery. The Ozurdex dexamethasone implant is approved by the FDA for ME associated with BRVO or CRVO.[42] Two identical, randomized, prospective, multicenter, masked, sham-controlled, phase 3 clinical trials investigated the efficacy of the dexamethasone implant compared with sham treatment for ME associated with BRVO or CRVO.[42] The trials enrolled 1,267 patients aged =18 years with a BCVA between 20/50 and 20/200 secondary to ME of =300 µm in the central 1-mm macular subfield associated with either BRVO or CRVO. The study consisted of a 6-month primary phase followed by a 6-month, open-label, follow-up phase.[43]

> **Special Considerations**
>
> - SCORE BRVO trial
>   - Grid photocoagulation recommended over intravitreal triamcinolone acetonide for patients with decreased VA associated with ME secondary to BRVO.

In the primary phase, enrolled patients were randomized 1:1:1 to receive either a 700-µg dexamethasone implant ($n = 427$), a 350-µg dexamethasone implant ($n = 412$), or a sham injection ($n = 423$). Ninety-four percent of patients completed the study through day 180, and 997 patients continued in the open-label phase. One-third of patients in each group had a diagnosis of CRVO, whereas the remaining two-thirds had a diagnosis of BRVO. The duration of ME was similar among groups. Patients did not receive grid laser in the control arm. All patients were examined at baseline, and at 1, 7, 30, 60, 90, and 180 days after treatment. The primary outcome for the first 6 months was the proportion of eyes achieving at least a 15-letter VA improvement from baseline. The FDA later changed the primary outcome for the second study to be the time to reach a 15-letter improvement from baseline. Following completion of the first portion of the study, patients were eligible to have open-label retreatment with the 700-µg dexamethasone implant regardless of which initial treatment group they were in (sham, 350 µg, or 700 µg), provided that they demonstrated evidence of ME > 250 µm on OCT examination and VA was worse than 20/20 at 6 months.

Both dexamethasone implant groups showed significantly greater improvement in vision than the sham treatment. The cumulative response rate was 41% in the 700-µg group, 40% in the 350-µg group, and 23% in the sham group ($p < 0.001$). Although the proportion of eyes achieving at least a 15-letter improvement from baseline BCVA was greater in the treatment groups at month 1 (21% in the 700-µg group vs. 18% in the 350-µg group vs. 8% in the sham group; $p < 0.001$) and month 3 (22% in the 700-µg group vs. 23% in the 350-µg group versus 13% in the sham group; $p < 0.001$), this effect was not statistically significant at month 6. The reduction in mean OCT central subfield retinal thickness was greater in the 700-µg (208 ± 201 µm) and 350-µg (177 ± 197 µm) groups than in the sham group (85 ± 173 µm) at month 3 ($p < 0.001$), but not statistically significant at month 6. It should be noted that 21% of BRVO and 17% of CRVO eyes required only a single treatment through 12 months. The dexamethasone implant was well tolerated and most eyes had no significant increase in IOP at the 6-month follow-up. Only 0.2% of eyes in either dexamethasone group had an IOP > 35 mm Hg and 1.2% had an IOP > 25 at 6 months. Overall, 29.7% of eyes were treated with IOP-lowering medication at day 90 and the IOP returned to baseline by day 180 in all groups. Five eyes (0.7%) underwent surgical intervention for IOP control, and three of these were for NVG secondary to RVO. Rates of cataract progression up to 1 year did not differ significantly among the groups. The side effect profile was similar during the 6-month open-label extension, during which all eyes received a first (in the case of sham-treated eyes) or second dexamethasone implant. In the extended follow-up, 32.8% of retreated dexamethasone 700-µg/700-µg group patients had at least a 10-mm Hg increase in IOP from baseline at some point over the 12-month period. In this retreatment group, 14 eyes underwent laser or surgery to reduce IOP. Cataracts were reported in 29.8% of phakic study eyes in the retreated dexamethasone 700-µg/700-µg group, 19.8% of the dexamethasone 350-µg/700-µg group, and 10.5% of the delayed treatment (sham/700-µg) group ($p = 0.001$). A total of 11 patients underwent cataract surgery. The results from these two "phase 3" trials have important clinical implications. Earlier treatment was associated with a better VA outcome across subgroups. A three-line VA gain following treatment with the 700-µg implant was seen in 48% of eyes with BRVO =90 days and in 67% of eyes with baseline BCVA worse than 55 letters in the =90-day subset. In addition, there was up to a twofold greater risk of three-line VA loss in sham-treated eyes compared with the 700-µg implant group. Risk of vision loss persisted at 12 months even after the sham group was treated with a 700-µg implant at the 6-month visit.[43]

Laser Photocoagulation

Before the advent of intravitreal anti-VEGF therapy, the standard of care for decreased vision due to BRVO-associated ME was grid laser potocoagulation.[40] The treatment technique consists of applying laser to the macula in a “grid” pattern, targeted to the areas of vascular leakage on fluorescein angiography.[17] The laser spots are applied outside the foveal avascular zone and farther into the periphery inside the major vascular arcade (▶ Fig. 9.4). Thick patches of intraretinal blood are avoided, as laser uptake by the blood within the retina can cause preretinal gliosis. The recommended laser settings are 0.1-second duration, 50- to 100-µm-diameter spot size, and a power setting sufficient to produce a light to medium light burn. A heavy burn should not be used, as this can lead to immediate and delayed complications, such as subretinal hemorrhage and choroidal NV, respectively.[44] The laser uptake occurs at the level of the retinal pigment epithelium (RPE) and is associated with a gradual decrease retinal vascular leakage during the ensuing 2 to 3 months.[45] The response to a laser treatment session is assessed in about 3 months, and repeat laser is performed if the VA is still believed to be reduced due to ME secondary to BRVO and residual areas of leakage on FA are present.[17] Due to the reported efficacy of intravitreal anti-VEGF therapy for ME associated with BRVO, as well as risks of laser therapy such as enlargement of laser scars resulting in scotomas[46] and choroidal NV, monotherapy with grid laser has become less relevant in treating ME secondary to BRVO. Grid laser may be used in combination with anti-VEGF therapy following incomplete response to anti-VEGF agents or in an attempt to reduce the frequency of intravitreal anti-VEGF injections.[47] Published studies with combination therapy have reported mixed results with respect to achieving better visual outcomes[47,48]; however, combination therapy has been associated with a reduced frequency of anti-VEGF injections.[46]

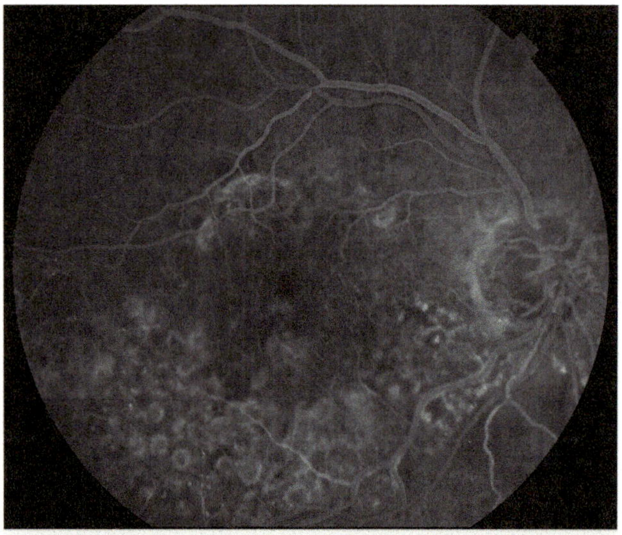

Fig. 9.4 Laser treatment for decreased vision due to macular edema associated with a perfused branch retinal vein occlusion is applied in a “grid” pattern throughout the area of fluorescein angiographic leakage. Treatment should not extend any closer to the fovea than the edge of the capillary-free zone or any farther into the periphery than the major vascular arcade.

Peripheral scatter laser treatment is still the standard of care for retinal or disc NV in eyes with nonperfused BRVO.[18] The treatment technique consists of applying 200- to 500-µm, medium-intensity laser spots spaced about one spot-width apart to the area of ischemic retina, outside 2 disc diameters from the fovea. Laser spots should not be placed over thick intraretinal hemorrhage or elevated neovascular fronds. Supplementation is occasionally needed for persistent neovascular activity. Peripheral scatter laser applied when NV first develops can decrease the chance of vitreous hemorrhage significantly. Analysis of the BVOS data indicates that laser delivered after the development of NV is as effective in preventing vitreous hemorrhage as laser applied before the development of NV.[18] Hence, prophylactic scatter laser is not recommended. A wide-field FA may be useful to determine the perfusion status of the BRVO and to search for the development of any retinal or disc NV.[49]

Pearls

- Treatment of retinal or disc NV associated with BRVO
  - Peripheral scatter laser photocoagulation is the standard of care for retinal or disc NV in eyes with nonperfused BRVO.

Surgery

Vitreous hemorrhage in eyes with BRVO develops either from intraretinal hemorrhage breaking through the internal limiting membrane into the vitreous cavity or from retinal or disc NV. The course and long-term visual consequences of vitreous hemorrhage are variable. In most eyes, the vitreous hemorrhage is mild and may clear spontaneously. Some patients with dense nonclearing vitreous hemorrhage are treated with pars plana vitrectomy and sectoral scatter endolaser.[22] Patients who develop macula-involving or macula-threatening tractional retinal detachment may be treated with pars plana vitrectomy and membrane peeling, with or without sectoral endolaser.

Systemic Therapies

Systemic Anticoagulation

Systemic anticoagulation including oral acetylsalicylic acid, subcutaneous heparin, or intravenous thrombolysis has not been shown to be of ocular benefit in patients with BRVO and may potentially worsen concurrent or future intraretinal hemorrhage.[50] Troxerutin, which inhibits erythrocyte and platelet aggregation and improves erythrocyte deformability, and thereby retinal microcirculation,[50] was studied in a double-masked randomized study of 26 patients with BRVO of less than

5 months' duration. Baseline visual acuities were well matched in the two study arms, and at the end of 4 months follow-up, the troxerutin-treated group, as compared with the placebo group, showed significant improvement in VA ($p = 0.03$), macular threshold ($p = 0.01$), retinal circulation times ($p = 0.04$), and ME ($p = 0.05$). Furthermore, eyes in the troxerutin-treated group demonstrated diminished progression of ischemia ($p = 0.05$) and decreased red blood cell aggregability ($p = 0.006$) when compared with the control eyes. This study was limited by a small sample size and a short follow-up duration (4 months). Ticlopidine is an inhibitor of platelet aggregation and was compared with placebo in treating 54 patients within 3 weeks of the onset of symptoms of BRVO.[50] This study reported a significant difference between the ticlopidine treatment and placebo groups for VA ($p = 0.01$). In the treated group, 69% (20/29) experienced an improvement in VA compared to 52% (13/25) in the placebo group. However, ticlopidine was associated with a higher risk of gastrointestinal symptoms and skin reactions.[50]

Isovolemic Hemodilution

BRVO has been reported to be associated with hyperviscosity due to higher hematocrit and plasma viscosity. It has been reported that hypervolemic or isovolemic hemodilution treatment (IHT), commenced within 3 months of the onset of symptoms of BRVO, accelerates the rate of visual recovery and also has a positive effect on the final VA at 1 year.[51] In this study, patients were randomized to isovolemic hemodilution (IHT) ($n = 18$) or no treatment ($n = 16$). Patients randomized to treatment received IHT for 6 weeks with venesection and volume replacement using hydroxyethyl starch in an outpatient setting, with a target hematocrit of 35%. At the end of the active treatment period, the IHT group showed significant mean improvement in VA of approximately two lines (0.2 logarithm of the minimum angle of resolution [logMAR] units) when compared with a less than one-line improvement (0.01 logMAR units) in the control group ($p = 0.003$). At the end of the follow-up period of 1 year, the difference between the treatment and control group was still significant ($p = 0.03$), with a mean improvement from baseline of approximately four lines (0.43 logMAR units) in the treatment group compared with only a one-line improvement in the control group. Patients with persistent ME were treated with macular grid laser therapy after the 3-month visit; 28% of those in the IHT group and 44% in the control group received laser therapy. Reported complications of hemodilution include deep vein thrombosis and hypotension.[51]

9.3 Central Retinal Vein Occlusion

Major risk factors for CRVO include increasing age, HTN, DM, arteriosclerotic vascular risk factors, and primary open angle glaucoma.[8] The use of anticoagulants in patients at risk of CRVO does not appear to offer any significant protective benefit.[52,53] There appears to be a significant association between whole blood viscosity and erythrocyte deformability index with RVO, indicating that hemorheologic factors may play some role in the pathogenesis.[54] This may explain the occurrence of CRVO in younger patients due to dehydration.[55] The role of thrombophilia in the pathogenesis of CRVO remains controversial because of conflicting results in the literature.[56,57]

Special Considerations

- CRVO and coagulation disorders:
  - The value of widespread screening of patients with CRVO for coagulation disorders is unclear. It is important to consider a work-up for thrombophilic risk factors in patients with personal or family history of venous thromboembolism, venous thrombosis at multiple sites, bilateral or sequential RVO, and young age.

Several small retrospective studies show an association of CRVO with factor V Leiden, hyperhomocysteinemia, protein C and S deficiency, antiphospholipid antibody syndrome, and factor XII deficiency.[58,59,60,61] The value of widespread screening of patients with CRVO for these coagulation disorders is unclear.[57] It is important to consider a work-up for thrombophilic risk factors in patients with a personal or family history of venous thromboembolism, venous thromboses at multiple sites, bilateral or sequential RVO, and young age.

9.3.1 Pathophysiology

The pathogenesis and treatment of CRVO is controversial. Hayreh has suggested that perfused CRVO occurs after occlusion of retinal venous flow, while nonperfused CRVO develops after occlusion of venous and arterial flow at or posterior to the lamina cribrosa.[62] The obstruction to central retinal venous outflow is thought to occur in the region of, and just posterior to, the lamina cribrosa. A histopathologic study noted fresh or a recanalized thrombus in enucleated eyes with chronic, nonperfused CRVO, and NVG.[63] A combination of factors including local anatomical susceptibility, vessel wall changes, and hemorheologic and thrombotic tendencies may all contribute to the development of CRVO. The central retinal vein in the region of the lamina cribrosa shares a common adventitial sheath with the central retinal artery, and compression of the vein by the more rigid arterial wall, especially in individuals with arteriosclerotic vascular disease, may occur.[64] Postmortem studies have demonstrated a natural constriction in the central retinal vein in this region in healthy eyes, and more pronounced changes are seen with increasing age.[64] These changes could then lead to greater shear stresses causing endothelial cell damage, which, in turn, could lead to endothelial cell proliferation and possible thrombus formation.[65] The variation in the clinical picture is most probably related to the location of the blockage in the central retinal vein.[66] An occlusion of the central retinal vein in the lamina cribrosa region may produce a more severe or ischemic-type clinical picture, whereas an occlusion further posterior to the lamina cribrosa may produce a less severe or nonischemic clinical condition.[66] Hypoxia secondary to ischemia induces upregulation of VEGF and appears to play an important role in the development of ME and NV secondary to CRVO.[67] Inhibition of VEGF in a nonhuman primate model of CRVO can prevent the development of iris and angle NV.[68] VEGF induces expression of thromboplastin, a potent procoagulant tissue factor that may aggravate the retinal ischemia induced by the CRVO.[69] Furthermore, VEGF induces retinal endothelial swelling, which may lead to further capillary nonperfusion.[70]

9.3.2 Clinical Features and Diagnosis

Classically, a CRVO presents with marked dilation and tortuosity of the retinal veins, extensive retinal edema, pronounced superficial and deep retinal hemorrhages radiating outward from the optic disc in all quadrants, cotton-wool spots, and optic disc swelling. Approximately two-thirds of CRVOs are perfused (▶ Fig. 9.5), while the remaining one-third are nonperfused.[71] Nonperfused CRVO is often more dramatic in its presentation and is frequently associated with a relative afferent pupillary defect and VA worse than 20/400 (▶ Fig. 9.6). Overlying retinal hemorrhage may impede the ability to evaluate the underlying capillary perfusion status. One-third of perfused CRVOs progress to nonperfused over the course of the disease.[72] Risk factors for progression include worse presenting VA, severe ME, and progressive intraretinal hemorrhage.

The clinical course after a CRVO is highly variable.[71] The retinal hemorrhages may resolve over weeks or may persist for years. The venous dilatation and tortuosity typically resolve with time, and marked fibrous sheathing of the retinal veins and arteries may develop. The disc swelling resolves slowly and may develop disc pallor in nonperfused cases. Optociliary shunt vessels develop commonly following CRVO (▶ Fig. 9.7), and may be associated with a decreased risk of developing anterior segment NV.[71] Microaneurysms are a frequent finding following CRVO, whereas macroaneurysms and hard exudates are less common. ME is common following CRVO, and may resolve quickly, persist chronically, vary intermittently, or develop late in the course of the disease. If NV occurs following a CRVO, it typically develops within the first 7 months of the CRVO and usually forms on the iris (▶ Fig. 9.8); less frequently, NV may develop on the disc or retina.[72] The rate of iris NV is 10% in perfused eyes, and is 45 to 80% in nonperfused eyes. Of the eyes that develop iris NV, approximately two-thirds will develop NVG without treatment.[72]

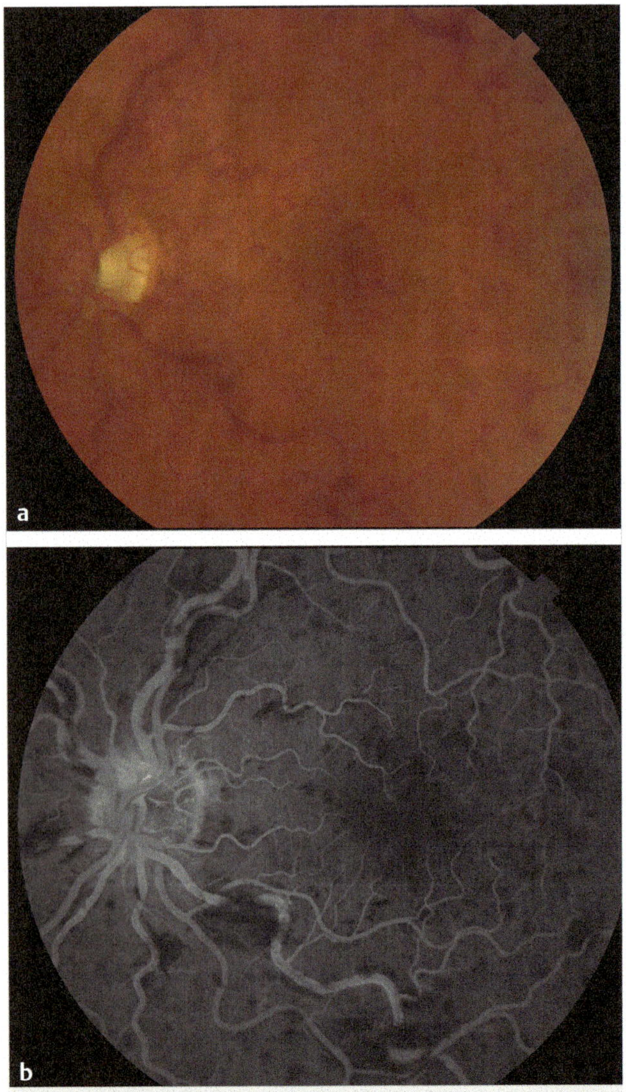

Fig. 9.5 Perfused central retinal vein occlusion. (a) Note the relatively few intraretinal hemorrhages and only mildly dilated and tortuous retinal venous system. (b) Fluorescein angiography demonstrates fewer than 10 disc areas of capillary nonperfusion.

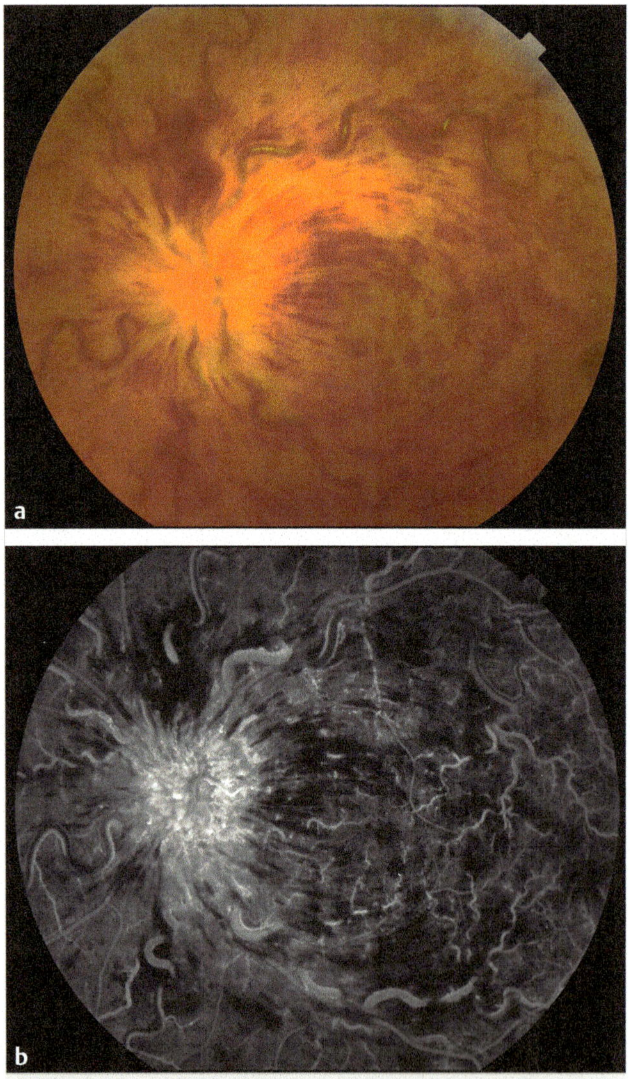

Fig. 9.6 Nonperfused central retinal vein occlusion. (a) Numerous, almost confluent intraretinal hemorrhages and markedly dilated and tortuous retinal veins are evident. (b) Fluorescein angiography reveals 10 or more disc areas of retinal capillary nonperfusion.

Perfusion status is determined most commonly by clinical examination combined with FA.[71] The Central Vein Occlusion Study (CVOS) used 10 disc areas of nonperfusion as its cutoff for predicting risk of developing 2 clock hours of iris NV or any angle NV.[73] In patients with CRVO-associated ME, FA shows parafoveal and paramacular capillary leakage that appears as hyperfluorescence that increases in size and intensity with time, often in a petaloid-type pattern. Nonperfusion near the fovea is associated with worse visual prognosis. Electrophysiologic testing may be helpful when FA cannot demonstrate the extent of nonperfusion (e.g., in cases with extensive intraretinal hemorrhage). ERG b/a-wave amplitude ratios, photopic and scotopic b-wave amplitudes, and flicker amplitudes were significantly smaller in eyes with extensive capillary nonperfusion than in perfused eyes.[74] OCT can aid the clinician in evaluating and monitoring such complications of CRVO as ME and epiretinal membrane formation.

9.3.3 Management and Course

A complete ocular examination, including IOP measurement, slit-lamp biomicroscopy, gonioscopy to rule out NV of the iris or angle, and a dilated fundus examination, is recommended at presentation and at follow-up examinations. Until relatively recently, treatment for CRVO was typically limited to panretinal laser for the neovascular complications of retinal ischemia. Recently, a number of randomized-controlled clinical trials have evaluated the role of various new treatment options. These treatment options can be classified broadly into therapies aimed at relieving the obstruction to venous outflow and those aimed at the sequelae of the venous occlusion (including both ME and the consequences of retinal ischemia).

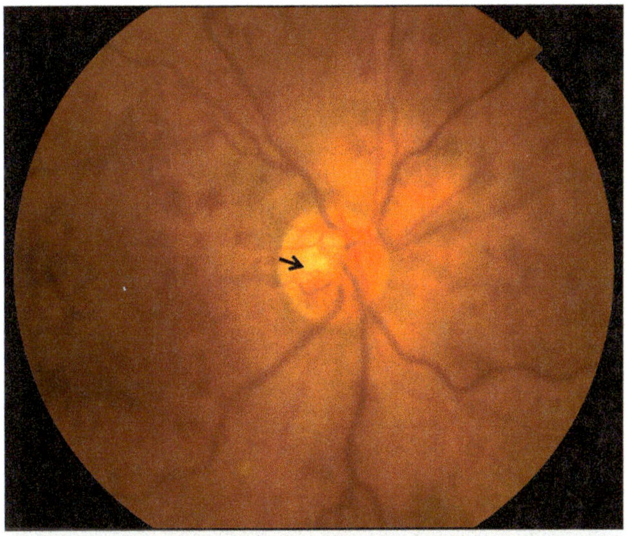

Fig. 9.7 Disc collaterals. These channels appear as tortuous vascular loops on or adjacent to the optic nerve head (arrow). They form between the obstructed disc capillaries and the unobstructed choroidal or pial capillaries.

Therapies for Relieving Venous Occlusion

Anticoagulation

The role of systemic anticoagulation in CRVO is unclear. There is no evidence that agents such as aspirin, heparin, or warfarin alter the natural history of CRVO. Patients taking warfarin have been reported to develop CRVO despite maintaining therapeutic levels of anticoagulation.[52,53] Antiplatelet drugs such as ticlopidine have been noted to have a potentially beneficial effect; however, this has not been studied in prospective, randomized, controlled phase III clinical trials.[50] Thrombolytic agents have been used both systemically and intraocularly in an attempt to lyse the presumed thrombus causing the obstruction to venous outflow.[75] There have been small nonrandomized case series of intravitreal tissue plasminogen activator and direct injection of tissue plasminogen activator into a retinal vein.[9] However, due to significant hemorrhagic side effects associated with systemic thrombolytics, they are no longer used.

Radial Optic Neurotomy

The use of radial optic neurotomy (RON) is based on the hypothesis that a CRVO is similar to a compartment syndrome resulting from increased pressure within the confined space of the scleral outlet affecting the central retinal vein.[76] This procedure involves a pars plana vitrectomy following which a radial incision into the nasal scleral ring of the optic nerve is made to release pressure around the central retinal vein. The initial nonrandomized study[76] showed an average of 2.5 lines of vision gained in up to 71% of eyes; however, another study did not confirm a similar degree of improvement.[77] Chorioretinal anastomoses have been found to occur in up to 47% of eyes treated with a RON, and this may account for the beneficial effect on VA

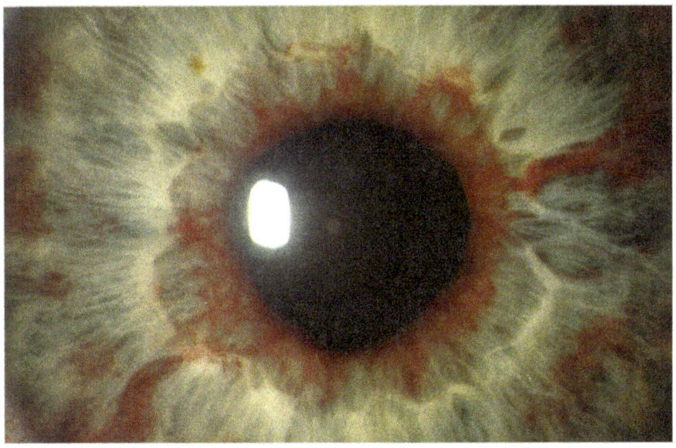

Fig. 9.8 Florid iris neovascularization. Iris neovascularization and consequent neovascular glaucoma occur much more commonly in eyes with central retinal vein occlusion than in eyes with branch retinal vein occlusion.

from this procedure in some eyes.[78] Because of the unclear VA benefit of RON, and the complications associated with this procedure (e.g., vitreous hemorrhage, hemorrhagic retinal detachment, retinal detachment, visual field defects, central retinal artery occlusion, and NV),[79] RON is not generally considered standard of care in the management of CRVO.

Laser-Induced Chorioretinal Anastomosis

The goal of laser-induced chorioretinal anastomosis (L-CRA) is to create a bypass of the occluded central retinal vein by inducing an anastomosis between a retinal vein and the choroidal venous circulation.[80] The procedure involves the use of a high-power argon laser, sometimes combined with an Nd:YAG laser, to rupture both Bruch's membrane and the overlying retinal vein to create a chorioretinal anastomosis.[80] The Central Retinal Vein Bypass Study (CVBS) evaluated L-CRA in 113 consecutive patients with a nonischemic CRVO of > 3 months' duration and VA of =20/50.[81] Patients were randomized to L-CRA (58 patients) or conventional care (55 patients) and followed for 18 months. 53 control patients and 55 treated patients completed the 18-month follow-up. A successful L-CRA was created in 42 (76.4%) eyes in the treatment group. During the 18-month follow-up period, control eyes had a progressive decrease in mean BCVA (–8.9 letters at 18 months compared to baseline). In contrast, the mean change in BCVA in treated eyes at 18 months compared to baseline was + 1.3 letters; among the 42 eyes with a functioning L-CRA, the mean change in BCVA at 18 months compared to baseline was + 3.6 letters. The creation of an L-CRA was also associated with a protective benefit with respect to progressive retinal ischemia. In this study, all eyes were initially nonischemic, and conversion to the ischemic category occurred in 4.9% of eyes in the L-CRA group compared to 20.8% of eyes in the control group ($p = 0.03$).[81] Complications with L-CRA included retinal NV in 18% of eyes (the NV was treated with sectorial laser); vitrectomy was performed in 9% of L-CRA eyes because of either nonresolving vitreous hemorrhage or macular traction. Younger age, better baseline VA, and early evidence of chorioretinal anastomosis occurring at the site of the L-CRA are associated with increased success of the procedure.[82] The definitive role of L-CRA in the management of CRVO is unclear.

Optic Nerve Sheath Decompression

This procedure involves sectioning the posterior scleral ring via an orbital approach.[83] Due to the significant risks associated with this procedure (e.g., ocular motility disorders, pupillary dysfunction, and central retinal artery occlusion), optic nerve sheath decompression is no longer used in the management of eyes with CRVO.[83]

9.4 Therapies for ME

In the CVOS, macular grid laser treatment was associated with reduced angiographic evidence of ME, but there was no visual benefit from grid laser for CRVO-associated ME.[84] Until recently, there were no definitive therapies for ME associated with CRVO.[23] However, with the advent of intravitreal pharmacotherapies, there are various pharmacologic agents that are currently used for management of decreased vision due to CRVO-associated ME.[23]

9.4.1 Intravitreal Anti-VEGF Therapy

Anti-VEGF therapy is typically the first-line treatment in patients with ME associated with CRVO.[85] Currently available intravitreal anti-VEGF agents include ranibizumab, bevacizumab, and aflibercept.

Pearls

- Treatment for ME associated with CRVO
  - Anti-VEGF therapy is typically the first-line treatment in patients with ME associated with CRVO

Ranibizumab

Ranibizumab was the first anti-VEGF agent to receive FDA approval (in June 2010) for the treatment of ME secondary to CRVO. In the Central Retinal Vein OcclUsIon (CRUISE) Study[86] (a phase III, multicenter, prospective clinical trial comparing the efficacy and safety of intravitreal injections of ranibizumab 0.3 mg, intravitreal injections of ranibizumab 0.5 mg, and sham injections), 392 patients with ME secondary to nonischemic CRVO were randomized to receive monthly intravitreal injections of 0.3 mg (n =132) or 0.5 mg (n =130) of ranibizumab or sham injections (n =130). Patients were eligible if they had center-involved ME from a CRVO occurring within 12 months of study entry, BCVA of 20/40 to 20/320, and CST =250 µm. At 6 months, the proportion of patients who gained =15 letters in BCVA was 46.2% (0.3 mg) and 47.7% (0.5 mg) in the ranibizumab groups and 16.9% in the sham group ($p < 0.0001$). There was greater resolution of ME in the ranibizumab groups compared with the sham group (CST was reduced by 433.7 µm in 0.3-mg ranibizumab group and 452.3 µm in 0.5-mg ranibizumab group compared to a 167.7-µm reduction in the sham group). This study demonstrated that monthly injections of ranibizumab 0.3 or 0.5 mg over the course of 6 months reduced ME and provided substantial visual benefit in patients with CRVO-associated ME. After the primary endpoint in the CRUISE Study, all the patients were evaluated monthly, and if study eye Snellen equivalent BCVA was =20/40 or mean CST was =250 µm, patients received intravitreal ranibizumab; patients in the ranibizumab groups received their assigned dose and patients in the sham group received 0.5 mg of ranibizumab. In patients with CRVO, the mean number of ranibizumab injections during the observation period was 3.9, 3.6, and 4.2 in the 0.3-, 0.5-, and sham/0.5-mg groups.[25] At month 12, in the ranibizumab groups, vision was maintained and in the sham group there was substantial vision improvement after receiving ranibizumab (33.1% of patients in the sham group improved from baseline =15 in letter score at month 12 compared to 16.9% at month 6).[25] However, the vision at month 12 in the sham group was not as good as that in patients in the ranibizumab groups.[25] During the second year of ranibizumab treatment, there was a decline in vision, likely due to reduced follow-up and fewer ranibizumab injections.[25] Thus, follow-up and injections should be individualized and patients with CRVO may require more frequent follow-up than every 3 months.[25]

Pearls

- CRUISE study: results in year 2
  - During the second year of ranibizumab treatment, there was a decline in vision, likely due to reduced follow-up and fewer ranibizumab injections.
  - Thus, follow-up and injections should be individualized and CRVO patients may require more frequent follow-up than every 3 months.

Bevacizumab

Although bevacizumab is not FDA-approved for intravitreal use, numerous case reports and series have reported improvement in CRVO-associated ME following treatment with intravitreal bevacizumab.[87,88,89] However, there have been concerns including short-term efficacy and high ME recurrence rate[90] (▶ Fig. 9.9). The Pan-American Collaborative Retina Study group concluded that there was no difference in 2.5- versus 1.25-mg dose of intravitreal bevacizumab at 24 months, although the 2.5-mg dose was associated with more VA improvement and a greater reduction in ME at 6 months compared to the 1.25-mg dose.[27] Ach et al found that CRVO patients who benefited from intravitreal bevacizumab therapy were significantly younger and had lower CRT at baseline than patients who did not demonstrate improvement with intravitreal bevacizumab therapy.[28] Multiple consecutive treatments may be required, and ischemic damage may preclude VA improvement in some cases even if the ME responds to intravitreal bevacizumab.[85]

Aflibercept

Aflibercept was approved by the FDA for treatment of ME secondary to CRVO in September 2012 based on the results of the GALILEO and COPERNICUS Studies.[91,92] In the COPERNICUS Study,[91] 189 eyes with ME secondary to CRVO were randomized 3:2 to receive intravitreal aflibercept 2 mg or sham injection monthly for 6 months. An improvement in BCVA of =15 letters at 6 months compared to baseline was achieved in 56.1% of aflibercept-treated eyes compared to 12.3% of sham-treated eyes ($p < 0.001$).[91] CRT decreased by 457.2 µm in eyes treated with aflibercept versus 144.8 µm in sham-treated eyes ($p < 0.001$), and progression to any NV occurred in 0 and 5 (6.8%) aflibercept- and sham-treated eyes, respectively ($p = 0.006$). In the GALILEO Study (a double-masked phase III trial conducted at 62 centers in Europe and Asia),[92] 177 patients were assigned randomly, in a 3:2 allocation ratio, to receive intravitreal aflibercept 2 mg or sham every 4 weeks until week 24. Between weeks 24 and 52, patients continued monthly monitoring, but the aflibercept eyes received treatment as needed, while the sham group continued to receive sham treatment every 4 weeks. From weeks 52 to 76, the intervisit interval was extended to 8 weeks and sham patients were eligible for aflibercept. During the first 6 months of GALILEO, monthly aflibercept treatment was associated with a mean gain of 18.0 letters compared with 3.3 letters with sham injections ($p < 0.0001$). Mean CRT decreased by 448.6 and 169.3 µm in the aflibercept and sham groups, respectively ($p < 0.0001$). The improvement was largely maintained through week 52, but declined between weeks 52 and 76. After becoming eligible for aflibercept, eyes in the sham group gained vision and had decreased CRT. However, outcomes at week 76 were superior in the eyes that had been treated with aflibercept since the beginning. Results from follow-up to 76 weeks in the phase III GALILEO Study show that intravitreal injection of aflibercept provides substantial improvement in VA in treatment-naive eyes with ME secondary to CRVO. However, the data also suggest the value of close monitoring and early treatment to optimize VA.[92]

Study of Comparative Treatments for Retinal Vein Occlusion 2 (SCORE2)

The Study of Comparative Treatments for Retinal Vein Occlusion 2 (SCORE2) is a multicenter randomized clinical trial which investigated whether intravitreal bevacizumab is noninferior to intravitreal aflibercept for the treatment of ME secondary to

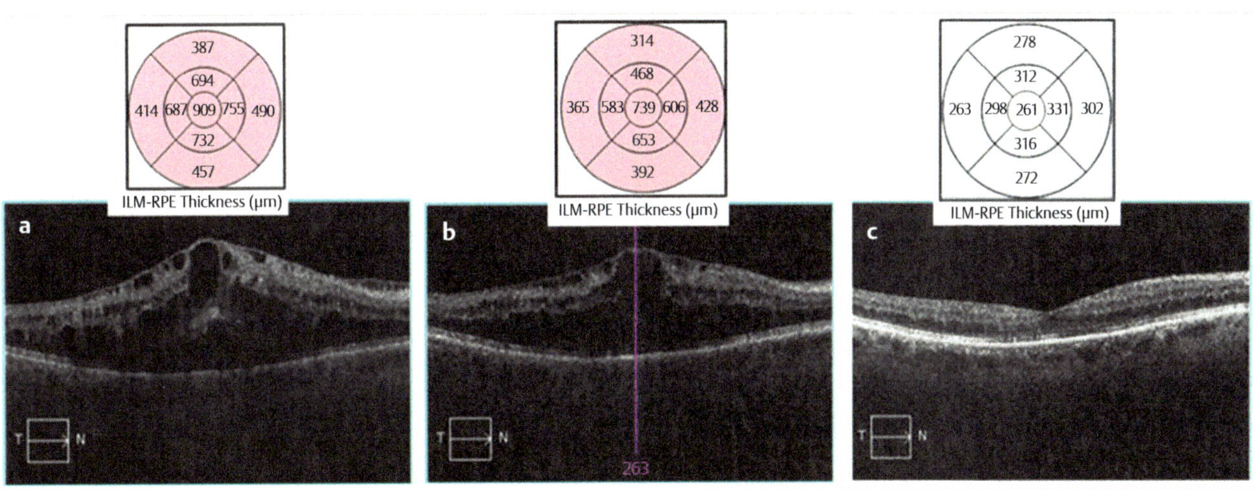

Fig. 9.9 (a) OCT scan of a patient with macular edema secondary to central retinal vein occlusion at baseline. The patient was treated with a series of three intravitreal injections of bevacizumab 1.25 mg 1 month apart. (b) There was minimal resolution of macular edema observed on OCT at 1 month after the third bevacizumab injection. The patient was then treated with a series of three intravitreal injections of aflibercept 2 mg 1 month apart. (c) The macular edema was resolved at 1 month following the third aflibercept injection as noted on OCT.

CRVO or hemiretinal vein occlusion.[93] The study included 362 patients who were randomized 1:1 to receive aflibercept (2.0 mg; n = 180) or bevacizumab (1.25 mg; n = 182) every 4 weeks for 6 months. Following primary outcome assessment at month 6, participants were followed through month 12 according to a protocol-defined treatment strategy based on response at month 6. Eyes with a protocol-defined good response at month 6 were randomized to continue treatment with the originally assigned drug on either a monthly or treat-and-extend schedule. Eyes with a protocol-defined poor response at month 6 were switched to an alternative treatment; eyes in the bevacizumab group with a poor response at month 6 were to receive aflibercept treatment, and eyes in the aflibercept group with a poor response at month 6 were to receive intravitreal dexamethasone implant treatment. To date, 6-month results have been published.[93] The primary outcome was mean change in visual acuity and the non-inferiority margin was 5 letters. At month 6, the mean visual acuity letter score increase from baseline was 18.6 in the bevacizumab group and 18.9 in the aflibercept group. Intravitreal bevacizumab was noninferior to aflibercept with respect to visual acuity after 6 months of treatment. Post hoc analyses at month 6 showed that complete resolution of macular edema occurred in a higher percentage of eyes in the aflibercept group (54.4%) than in the bevacizumab group (28.5%). However, the lower proportion of eyes that had resolution of macular edema in the bevacizumab group did not translate into poorer visual acuity outcomes in that group at 6 months.

9.4.2 Intravitreal Steroids

Triamcinolone Acetonide (TA)

The SCORE Study compared 1- and 4-mg doses of intravitreal TA with standard care (observation) for treatment of vision loss associated with ME secondary to perfused CRVO, and evaluated the efficacy and safety of the 1- and 4-mg TA doses.[94] The primary outcome of the SCORE-CRVO trial, the percentage of participants with a gain in VA letter score of 15 or more from baseline to month 12, was 6.8, 26.5, and 25.6% for the observation, 1-mg TA, and 4-mg TA groups, respectively. More eyes in the 4-mg TA group (35%) initiated IOP-lowering medication through 12 months compared with the 1-mg TA (20%) and observation groups (8%). During the first 12 months of the

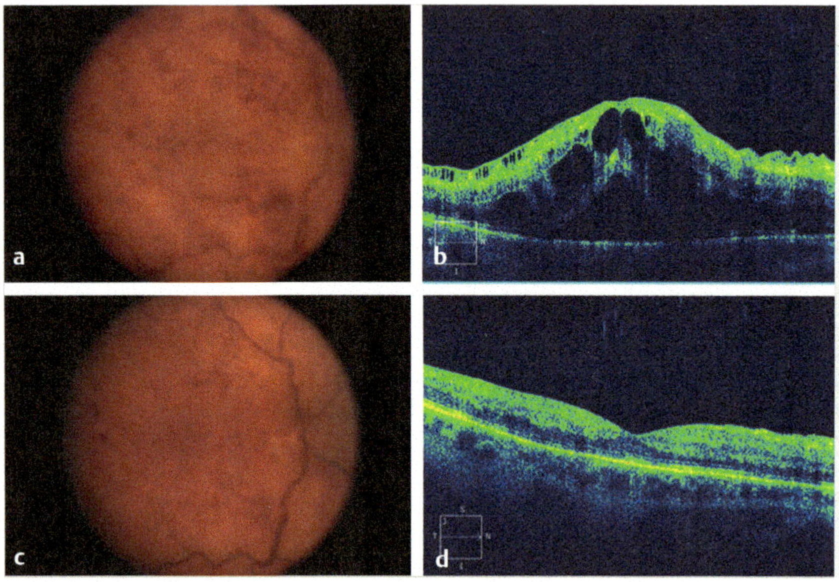

Fig. 9.10 (**a**) Fundus photograph and (**b**) OCT scan of a patient with persistent macular edema secondary to central retinal vein occlusion treated with two intravitreal injections of bevacizumab 1.25 mg 1 month apart. The patient was then treated with an intravitreal injection of triamcinolone acetonide 4 mg and there was resolution of macular edema at 3 months' follow-up as noted on (**c**) fundus photography and (**d**) OCT.

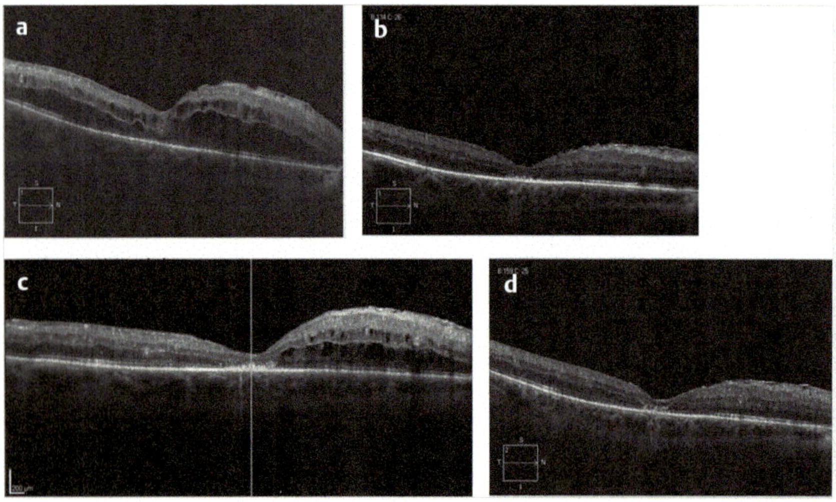

Fig. 9.11 (**a**) OCT scan of a patient with persistent macular edema secondary to central retinal vein occlusion treated with two intravitreal injections of bevacizumab 1.25 mg, one intravitreal injection of triamcinolone acetonide 4 mg, and two intravitreal injections of ranibizumab 0.5 mg. (**b**) The patient was then treated with a dexamethasone implant 700 µg and there was resolution of the macular edema at 1-month follow-up as noted on OCT. (**c**) The macular edema recurred at 3.5 months following injection of the dexamethasone implant 700 µg as noted on OCT. (**d**) The patient was treated with a second injection of a dexamethasone implant 700 µg and has no macular edema at 2 months as noted on OCT.

study, two participants in the 1-mg TA group received tube shunt surgery and between 12 and 24 months, two participants in the 4-mg TA group received tube shunt surgery; the surgery in all participants was deemed by the investigator to be necessary because of NVG rather than steroid-related IOP elevation. Among eyes that were phakic at baseline, the estimate through month 12 of new-onset lens opacity or progression of an existing opacity in the observation group, based on assessment at the clinical center, was 18% compared with 26% and 33% for the 1- and 4-mg TA groups, respectively. While no eyes in the observation or 1-mg TA groups had cataract surgery through month 12, four eyes in the 4-mg TA group received cataract surgery. Similarly, cataract surgery was more frequent between months 12 and 24 in the 4-mg TA group, with 21 eyes receiving cataract surgery compared with three in the 1-mg group and 0 in the observation group. Through month 12, there were no reports of infectious or noninfectious endophthalmitis or retinal detachment in any of the three study groups. In summary, intravitreal TA in both a 1- and 4-mg dose had better VA outcomes over 1 year, and possibly 2 years, than the untreated natural history of ME secondary to perfused CRVO[94] (▶ Fig. 9.10). The superior safety profile of the 1-mg TA dose compared with the 4-mg TA dose, particularly with respect to glaucoma and cataract, makes it the preferred TA dose.

Dexamethasone Implant

The Ozurdex dexamethasone implant, as discussed in the section on BRVO, in a dose of 700 µg was demonstrated to be an effective therapy for ME secondary to RVO (the Ozurdex dexamethasone implant was studied among patients with BRVO or CRVO; separate clinical trials for each of these two disease entities were not performed for the evaluation of the Ozurdex dexamethasone implant)[42,43] (▶ Fig. 9.11).

9.5 Treatment of Ischemic Complications

The CVOS recommended prompt application of panretinal photocoagulation (PRP) after the development of 2 clock hours of iris or any angle NV in eyes with CRVO.[73] Numerous reports describe successful short-term treatment of CRVO-induced NVG with regression of neovascular vessels and improvement in IOP as early as 48 hours after the administration of intravitreal bevacizumab.[95,96,97,98] However, the standard treatment for NVG remains PRP with IOP-lowering medications as needed. Intravitreal bevacizumab may be useful in patients who are unable to undergo PRP, or as bridge therapy until PRP can be performed (e.g., in patients with media opacities).[98] In patients with marked IOP elevation despite maximally tolerated medical therapy, intravitreal bevacizumab may be administered in conjunction with PRP in an attempt to achieve rapid regression of NV, thereby preventing permanent angle synechiae and achieving better IOP control more quickly.[98]

9.6 Hemiretinal Vein Occlusion

Hemiretinal vein occlusion is a term that has been used interchangeably to describe hemicentral retinal vein occlusion (HCRVO) or hemispheric retinal vein occlusion.[99] However, it is important to understand that HCRVO and hemispheric retinal vein occlusion are two different entities.[99] HCRVO occurs due to the occlusion of one of the two trunks of a congenitally abnormal central retinal vein.[100] On the other hand, a hemispheric retinal vein occlusion is believed to be a BRVO which involves either the superior or inferior half of the retina.[101] HCRVO is an anatomical variant of CRVO and may be ischemic or nonischemic. In nonischemic HCRVO, there is typically a good prognosis with respect to the natural history of visual outcome.[99] In ischemic HCRVO, the most prevalent type of NV is retinal NV (29%), with iris NV occurring in 12%, disc NV in 12%, and angle NV in 10%.[99] NVG has been reported to occur in 5% within 6 months of onset.[100]

9.7 Conclusion

RVO is the second most common retinal vascular disease following diabetic retinopathy, and may be associated with significant ocular morbidity. ME represents the most common cause of vision loss due to RVO. There have been recent significant advances in the treatment of RVO-associated ME and ischemic complications. Intravitreal anti-VEGF therapy is currently considered the first-line treatment of decreased vision due to RVO-associated ME. Patients with a partial response or no response to anti-VEGF therapy may benefit from intravitreal injection of TA or the dexamethasone extended release steroid delivery system. Macular grid laser has not been demonstrated to be of visual benefit for patients with CRVO-associated ME, but is a treatment option for patients with BRVO-associated ME without dense macular hemorrhage. When used in combination with intravitreal pharmacotherapy, grid laser may be associated with a decrease in the frequency of anti-VEGF injections in patients with BRVO-associated ME. In the CVBS, laser-induced chorioretinal venous anastomosis was shown to be associated with vision improvement in eyes with CRVO-associated ME, but the improvement in VA was not as much or as rapid as that seen in the CRUISE Study. Treatments in the future may include a combination approach, addressing both the ME and the ischemic consequences of the obstruction to venous outflow.

References

[1] Rogers SL, McIntosh RL, Lim L, et al. Natural history of branch retinal vein occlusion: an evidence-based systematic review. Ophthalmology. 2010; 117 (6):1094–1101.e5

[2] Hayreh SS, Zimmerman MB, Podhajsky P. Incidence of various types of retinal vein occlusion and their recurrence and demographic characteristics. Am J Ophthalmol. 1994; 117(4):429–441

[3] Rogers S, McIntosh RL, Cheung N, et al. International Eye Disease Consortium. The prevalence of retinal vein occlusion: pooled data from population studies from the United States, Europe, Asia, and Australia. Ophthalmology. 2010; 117(2):313–9.e1

[4] Klein R, Moss SE, Meuer SM, Klein BE. The 15-year cumulative incidence of retinal vein occlusion: the Beaver Dam Eye Study. Arch Ophthalmol. 2008; 126(4):513–518

[5] Chatziralli IP, Jaulim A, Peponis VG, Mitropoulos PG, Moschos MM. Branch retinal vein occlusion: treatment modalities: an update of the literature. Semin Ophthalmol. 2014; 29(2):85–107

[6] McIntosh RL, Rogers SL, Lim L, et al. Natural history of central retinal vein occlusion: an evidence-based systematic review. Ophthalmology. 2010; 117 (6):1113–1123.e15

[7] The Eye Disease Case-control Study Group. Risk factors for branch retinal vein occlusion. Am J Ophthalmol. 1993; 116(3):286–296

[8] The Eye Disease Case-Control Study Group. Risk factors for central retinal vein occlusion. Arch Ophthalmol. 1996; 114(5):545–554

[9] Querques G, Triolo G, Casalino G, et al. Retinal venous occlusions: diagnosis and choice of treatments. Ophthalmic Res. 2013; 49(4):215–222

[10] O'Mahoney PR, Wong DT, Ray JG. Retinal vein occlusion and traditional risk factors for atherosclerosis. Arch Ophthalmol. 2008; 126(5):692–699

[11] Yau JW, Lee P, Wong TY, Best J, Jenkins A. Retinal vein occlusion: an approach to diagnosis, systemic risk factors and management. Intern Med J. 2008; 38 (12):904–910

[12] Jaulim A, Ahmed B, Khanam T, Chatziralli IP. Branch retinal vein occlusion: epidemiology, pathogenesis, risk factors, clinical features, diagnosis, and complications. An update of the literature. Retina. 2013; 33(5):901–910

[13] Bowers DK, Finkelstein D, Wolff SM, Green WR. Branch retinal vein occlusion. A clinicopathologic case report. Retina. 1987; 7(4):252–259

[14] Jefferies P, Clemett R, Day T. An anatomical study of retinal arteriovenous crossings and their role in the pathogenesis of retinal branch vein occlusions. Aust N Z J Ophthalmol. 1993; 21(4):213–217

[15] Hoang QV, Freund KB, Klancnik JM, Jr, Sorenson JA, Cunningham ET, Jr, Yannuzzi LA. Focal retinal phlebitis. Retina. 2012; 32(1):120–126

[16] Parodi MB, Bandello F. Branch retinal vein occlusion: classification and treatment. Ophthalmologica. 2009; 223(5):298–305

[17] The Branch Vein Occlusion Study Group. Argon laser photocoagulation for macular edema in branch vein occlusion. Am J Ophthalmol. 1984; 98(3):271–282

[18] Branch Vein Occlusion Study Group. Argon laser scatter photocoagulation for prevention of neovascularization and vitreous hemorrhage in branch vein occlusion. A randomized clinical trial. Arch Ophthalmol. 1986; 104(1):34–41

[19] Rehak J, Rehak M. Branch retinal vein occlusion: pathogenesis, visual prognosis, and treatment modalities. Curr Eye Res. 2008; 33(2):111–131

[20] Finkelstein D. Ischemic macular edema. Recognition and favorable natural history in branch vein occlusion. Arch Ophthalmol. 1992; 110(10):1427–1434

[21] Scott IU, VanVeldhuisen PC, Oden NL, et al. SCORE Study Investigator Group. SCORE Study report 1: baseline associations between central retinal thickness and visual acuity in patients with retinal vein occlusion. Ophthalmology. 2009; 116(3):504–512

[22] Shahid H, Hossain P, Amoaku WM. The management of retinal vein occlusion: is interventional ophthalmology the way forward? Br J Ophthalmol. 2006; 90(5):627–639

[23] Kulkarni A, Gunther J, Ip MS. Pharmacotherapy of retinal vein occlusions. In: Das A, Friberg T, eds. Ocular Angiogenesis Therapy: Principles and Practice. Philadelphia, PA: Lippincott, Williams & Wilkins; 2010:220–234

[24] Campochiaro PA, Heier JS, Feiner L, et al. BRAVO Investigators. Ranibizumab for macular edema following branch retinal vein occlusion: six-month primary end point results of a phase III study. Ophthalmology. 2010; 117 (6):1102–1112.e1

[25] Thach AB, Yau L, Hoang C, Tuomi L. Time to clinically significant visual acuity gains after ranibizumab treatment for retinal vein occlusion: BRAVO and CRUISE trials. Ophthalmology. 2014; 121(5):1059–1066

[26] Badalà F. The treatment of branch retinal vein occlusion with bevacizumab. Curr Opin Ophthalmol. 2008; 19(3):234–238

[27] Wu L, Arevalo JF, Roca JA, et al. Pan-American Collaborative Retina Study Group (PACORES). . Comparison of two doses of intravitreal bevacizumab (Avastin) for treatment of macular edema secondary to branch retinal vein occlusion: results from the Pan-American Collaborative Retina Study Group at 6 months of follow-up. Retina. 2008; 28(2):212–219

[28] Ach T, Hoeh AE, Schaal KB, Scheuerle AF, Dithmar S. Predictive factors for changes in macular edema in intravitreal bevacizumab therapy of retinal vein occlusion. Graefes Arch Clin Exp Ophthalmol. 2010; 248 (2):155–159

[29] Fung AE, Rosenfeld PJ, Reichel E. The International Intravitreal Bevacizumab Safety Survey: using the internet to assess drug safety worldwide. Br J Ophthalmol. 2006; 90(11):1344–1349

[30] De Niro JE, Fu AD, Johnson RN, et al. Intravitreous ranibizumab for persistent macular edema in retinal vein occlusion unresponsive to bevacizumab. Retin Cases Brief Rep. 2013; 7(3):220–224

[31] Campochiaro PA, Clark WL, Boyer DS, et al. Intravitreal aflibercept for macular edema following branch retinal vein occlusion: the 24-week results of the VIBRANT study. Ophthalmology. 2015; 122(3):538–544

[32] Wolfensberger TJ, Gregor ZJ. Macular edema—rationale for therapy. Dev Ophthalmol. 2010; 47:49–58

[33] Lee H, Shah GK. Intravitreal triamcinolone as primary treatment of cystoid macular edema secondary to branch retinal vein occlusion. Retina. 2005; 25 (5):551–555

[34] Yepremyan M, Wertz FD, Tivnan T, Eversman L, Marx JL. Early treatment of cystoid macular edema secondary to branch retinal vein occlusion with intravitreal triamcinolone acetonide. Ophthalmic Surg Lasers Imaging. 2005; 36(1):30–36

[35] Ozkiris A, Evereklioglu C, Erkiliç K, Ilhan O. The efficacy of intravitreal triamcinolone acetonide on macular edema in branch retinal vein occlusion. Eur J Ophthalmol. 2005; 15(1):96–101

[36] Jonas JB, Akkoyun I, Kamppeter B, Kreissig I, Degenring RF. Branch retinal vein occlusion treated by intravitreal triamcinolone acetonide. Eye (Lond). 2005; 19(1):65–71

[37] Chen SD, Sundaram V, Lochhead J, Patel CK. Intravitreal triamcinolone for the treatment of ischemic macular edema associated with branch retinal vein occlusion. Am J Ophthalmol. 2006; 141(5):876–883

[38] Beer PM, Bakri SJ, Singh RJ, Liu W, Peters GB, III, Miller M. Intraocular concentration and pharmacokinetics of triamcinolone acetonide after a single intravitreal injection. Ophthalmology. 2003; 110(4):681–686

[39] Scott IU, Ip MS. It's time for a clinical trial to investigate intravitreal triamcinolone for macular edema due to retinal vein occlusion: the SCORE study. Arch Ophthalmol. 2005; 123(4):581–582

[40] Scott IU, Ip MS, VanVeldhuisen PC, et al. SCORE Study Research Group. A randomized trial comparing the efficacy and safety of intravitreal triamcinolone with standard care to treat vision loss associated with macular Edema secondary to branch retinal vein occlusion: the Standard Care vs Corticosteroid for Retinal Vein Occlusion (SCORE) study report 6. Arch Ophthalmol. 2009; 127(9):1115–1128

[41] London NJ, Chiang A, Haller JA. The dexamethasone drug delivery system: indications and evidence. Adv Ther. 2011; 28(5):351–366

[42] Haller JA, Bandello F, Belfort R, Jr, et al. OZURDEX GENEVA Study Group. Randomized, sham-controlled trial of dexamethasone intravitreal implant in patients with macular edema due to retinal vein occlusion. Ophthalmology. 2010; 117(6):1134–1146.e3

[43] Haller JA, Bandello F, Belfort R, Jr, et al. Ozurdex GENEVA Study Group. Dexamethasone intravitreal implant in patients with macular edema related to branch or central retinal vein occlusion twelve-month study results. Ophthalmology. 2011; 118(12):2453–2460

[44] Han DP, Mieler WF, Burton TC. Submacular fibrosis after photocoagulation for diabetic macular edema. Am J Ophthalmol. 1992; 113(5):513–521

[45] Wilson DJ, Finkelstein D, Quigley HA, Green WR. Macular grid photocoagulation. An experimental study on the primate retina. Arch Ophthalmol. 1988; 106(1):100–105

[46] Schatz H, Madeira D, McDonald HR, Johnson RN. Progressive enlargement of laser scars following grid laser photocoagulation for diffuse diabetic macular edema. Arch Ophthalmol. 1991; 109(11):1549–1551

[47] Leitritz MA, Gelisken F, Ziemssen F, Szurman P, Bartz-Schmidt KU, Jaissle GB. Grid laser photocoagulation for macular oedema due to branch retinal vein occlusion in the age of bevacizumab? Results of a prospective study with crossover design. Br J Ophthalmol. 2013; 97(2):215–219

[48] Donati S, Barosi P, Bianchi M, Al Oum M, Azzolini C. Combined intravitreal bevacizumab and grid laser photocoagulation for macular edema secondary to branch retinal vein occlusion. Eur J Ophthalmol. 2012; 22(4):607–614

[49] Prasad PS, Oliver SC, Coffee RE, Hubschman JP, Schwartz SD. Ultra wide-field angiographic characteristics of branch retinal and hemicentral retinal vein occlusion. Ophthalmology. 2010; 117(4):780–784

[50] McIntosh RL, Mohamed Q, Saw SM, Wong TY. Interventions for branch retinal vein occlusion: an evidence-based systematic review. Ophthalmology. 2007; 114(5):835–854

[51] Chen HC, Wiek J, Gupta A, Luckie A, Kohner EM. Effect of isovolaemic haemodilution on visual outcome in branch retinal vein occlusion. Br J Ophthalmol. 1998; 82(2):162–167

[52] Browning DJ, Fraser CM. Retinal vein occlusions in patients taking warfarin. Ophthalmology. 2004; 111(6):1196–1200

[53] Mruthyunjaya P, Wirostko WJ, Chandrashekhar R, et al. Central retinal vein occlusion in patients treated with long-term warfarin sodium (Coumadin) for anticoagulation. Retina. 2006; 26(3):285–291

[54] Sofi F, Mannini L, Marcucci R, et al. Role of haemorheological factors in patients with retinal vein occlusion. Thromb Haemost. 2007; 98(6):1215–1219

[55] Francis PJ, Stanford MR, Graham EM. Dehydration is a risk factor for central retinal vein occlusion in young patients. Acta Ophthalmol Scand. 2003; 81 (4):415–416

[56] Janssen MC, den Heijer M, Cruysberg JR, Wollersheim H, Bredie SJ. Retinal vein occlusion: a form of venous thrombosis or a complication of atherosclerosis? A meta-analysis of thrombophilic factors. Thromb Haemost. 2005; 93 (6):1021–1026

[57] Fegan CD. Central retinal vein occlusion and thrombophilia. Eye (Lond). 2002; 16(1):98–106

[58] Chua B, Kifley A, Wong TY, Mitchell P. Homocysteine and retinal vein occlusion: a population-based study. Am J Ophthalmol. 2005; 139(1):181–182

[59] Vine AK. Hyperhomocysteinemia: a risk factor for central retinal vein occlusion. Am J Ophthalmol. 2000; 129(5):640–644

[60] Cobo-Soriano R, Sánchez-Ramón S, Aparicio MJ, et al. Antiphospholipid antibodies and retinal thrombosis in patients without risk factors: a prospective case-control study. Am J Ophthalmol. 1999; 128(6):725–732

[61] Bashshur ZF, Taher A, Masri AF, Najjar D, Arayssi TK, Noureddin BN. Anticardiolipin antibodies in patients with retinal vein occlusion and no risk factors: a prospective study. Retina. 2003; 23(4):486–490

[62] Hayreh SS. Prevalent misconceptions about acute retinal vascular occlusive disorders. Prog Retin Eye Res. 2005; 24(4):493–519

[63] Green WR, Chan CC, Hutchins GM, Terry JM. Central retinal vein occlusion: a prospective histopathologic study of 29 eyes in 28 cases. Trans Am Ophthalmol Soc. 1981; 79:371–422

[64] Taylor AW, Sehu W, Williamson TH, Lee WR. Morphometric assessment of the central retinal artery and vein in the optic nerve head. Can J Ophthalmol. 1993; 28(7):320–324

[65] Williamson THA. A "throttle" mechanism in the central retinal vein in the region of the lamina cribrosa. Br J Ophthalmol. 2007; 91(9):1190–1193

[66] Beaumont PE, Kang HK. Pattern of vascular nonperfusion in retinal venous occlusions occurring within the optic nerve with and without optic nerve head swelling. Arch Ophthalmol. 2000; 118(10):1357–1363

[67] Boyd SR, Zachary I, Chakravarthy U, et al. Correlation of increased vascular endothelial growth factor with neovascularization and permeability in ischemic central vein occlusion. Arch Ophthalmol. 2002; 120(12):1644–1650

[68] Adamis AP, Shima DT, Tolentino MJ, et al. Inhibition of vascular endothelial growth factor prevents retinal ischemia-associated iris neovascularization in a nonhuman primate. Arch Ophthalmol. 1996; 114(1):66–71

[69] Sassa Y, Hata Y, Murata T, et al. Functional role of Egr-1 mediating VEGF-induced tissue factor expression in the retinal capillary endothelium. Graefes Arch Clin Exp Ophthalmol. 2002; 240(12):1003–1010

[70] Hofman P, van Blijswijk BC, Gaillard PJ, Vrensen GF, Schlingemann RO. Endothelial cell hypertrophy induced by vascular endothelial growth factor in the retina: new insights into the pathogenesis of capillary nonperfusion. Arch Ophthalmol. 2001; 119(6):861–866

[71] Quinlan PM, Elman MJ, Bhatt AK, Mardesich P, Enger C. The natural course of central retinal vein occlusion. Am J Ophthalmol. 1990; 110(2):118–123

[72] Magargal LE, Donoso LA, Sanborn GE. Retinal ischemia and risk of neovascularization following central retinal vein obstruction. Ophthalmology. 1982; 89(11):1241–1245

[73] Central Vein Occlusion Study Group. A randomized clinical trial of early panretinal photocoagulation for ischemic central vein occlusion. The Central Vein Occlusion Study Group N report. Ophthalmology. 1995; 102(10):1434–1444

[74] Matsui Y, Katsumi O, Mehta MC, Hirose T. Correlation of electroretinographic and fluorescein angiographic findings in unilateral central retinal vein obstruction. Graefes Arch Clin Exp Ophthalmol. 1994; 232 (8):449–457

[75] Elman MJ. Thrombolytic therapy for central retinal vein occlusion: results of a pilot study. Trans Am Ophthalmol Soc. 1996; 94:471–504

[76] Opremcak EM, Rehmar AJ, Ridenour CD, Kurz DE. Radial optic neurotomy for central retinal vein occlusion: 117 consecutive cases. Retina. 2006; 26 (3):297–305

[77] Weizer JS, Stinnett SS, Fekrat S. Radial optic neurotomy as treatment for central retinal vein occlusion. Am J Ophthalmol. 2003; 136(5):814–819

[78] García-Arumíi J, Boixadera A, Martinez-Castillo V, Castillo R, Dou A, Corcostegui B. Chorioretinal anastomosis after radial optic neurotomy for central retinal vein occlusion. Arch Ophthalmol. 2003; 121(10):1385–1391

[79] Williamson TH, Poon W, Whitefield L, Strothidis N, Jaycock P. A pilot study of pars plana vitrectomy, intraocular gas, and radial neurotomy in ischaemic central retinal vein occlusion. Br J Ophthalmol. 2003; 87 (9):1126–1129

[80] McAllister IL, Douglas JP, Constable IJ, Yu DY. Laser-induced chorioretinal venous anastomosis for nonischemic central retinal vein occlusion: evaluation of the complications and their risk factors. Am J Ophthalmol. 1998; 126 (2):219–229

[81] McAllister IL, Gillies ME, Smithies LA, et al. The Central Retinal Vein Bypass Study: a trial of laser-induced chorioretinal venous anastomosis for central retinal vein occlusion. Ophthalmology. 2010; 117(5):954–965

[82] McAllister IL, Gillies ME, Smithies LA, et al. Factors promoting success and influencing complications in laser-induced central vein bypass. Ophthalmology. 2012; 119(12):2579–2586

[83] Dev S, Buckley EG. Optic nerve sheath decompression for progressive central retinal vein occlusion. Ophthalmic Surg Lasers. 1999; 30(3):181–184

[84] Evaluation of grid pattern photocoagulation for macular edema in central vein occlusion. The Central Vein Occlusion Study Group M report. Ophthalmology. 1995; 102(10):1425–1433

[85] Braithwaite T, Nanji AA, Lindsley K, Greenberg PB. Anti-vascular endothelial growth factor for macular oedema secondary to central retinal vein occlusion. Cochrane Database Syst Rev. 2014; 5:CD007325

[86] Brown DM, Campochiaro PA, Singh RP, et al. CRUISE Investigators. Ranibizumab for macular edema following central retinal vein occlusion: six-month primary end point results of a phase III study. Ophthalmology. 2010; 117 (6):1124–1133.e1

[87] Iturralde D, Spaide RF, Meyerle CB, et al. Intravitreal bevacizumab (Avastin) treatment of macular edema in central retinal vein occlusion: a short-term study. Retina. 2006; 26(3):279–284

[88] Costa RA, Jorge R, Calucci D, Melo LA, Jr, Cardillo JA, Scott IU. Intravitreal bevacizumab (Avastin) for central and hemicentral retinal vein occlusions: IBeVO study. Retina. 2007; 27(2):141–149

[89] Axer-Siegel R, Dotan A, Mimouni K, Bor E, Weinberger D, Bourla DH. Intravitreous bevacizumab treatment for macular edema due to central retinal vein occlusion. Curr Eye Res. 2012; 37(9):818–822

[90] Epstein DL, Algvere PV, von Wendt G, Seregard S, Kvanta A. Benefit from bevacizumab for macular edema in central retinal vein occlusion: twelve-month results of a prospective, randomized study. Ophthalmology. 2012; 119(12):2587–2591

[91] Boyer D, Heier J, Brown DM, et al. Vascular endothelial growth factor Trap-Eye for macular edema secondary to central retinal vein occlusion: six-month results of the phase 3 COPERNICUS study. Ophthalmology. 2012; 119 (5):1024–1032

[92] Korobelnik JF, Holz FG, Roider J, et al. GALILEO Study Group. Intravitreal aflibercept injection for macular edema resulting from central retinal vein occlusion: one-year results of the Phase 3 GALILEO Study. Ophthalmology. 2014; 121(1):202–208

[93] Scott IU, VanVeldhuisen PC, Ip MS, et al. Effect of bevacizumab vs aflibercept on visual acuity among patients with macular edema due to central retinal vein occlusion. The SCORE2 randomized clinical trial. JAMA. 2017; 317 (20):2072–2087

[94] Ip MS, Scott IU, VanVeldhuisen PC, et al. SCORE Study Research Group. A randomized trial comparing the efficacy and safety of intravitreal triamcinolone with observation to treat vision loss associated with macular edema secondary to central retinal vein occlusion: the Standard Care vs Corticosteroid for Retinal Vein Occlusion (SCORE) study report 5. Arch Ophthalmol. 2009; 127(9):1101–1114

[95] Ehlers JP, Spirn MJ, Lam A, Sivalingam A, Samuel MA, Tasman W. Combination intravitreal bevacizumab/panretinal photocoagulation versus panretinal photocoagulation alone in the treatment of neovascular glaucoma. Retina. 2008; 28(5):696–702

[96] Batioglu F, Astam N, Ozmert E. Rapid improvement of retinal and iris neovascularization after a single intravitreal bevacizumab injection in a patient with central retinal vein occlusion and neovascular glaucoma. Int Ophthalmol. 2008; 28(1):59–61

[97] Kahook MY, Schuman JS, Noecker RJ. Intravitreal bevacizumab in a patient with neovascular glaucoma. Ophthalmic Surg Lasers Imaging. 2006; 37 (2):144–146

[98] Iliev ME, Domig D, Wolf-Schnurrbursch U, Wolf S, Sarra GM. Intravitreal bevacizumab (Avastin) in the treatment of neovascular glaucoma. Am J Ophthalmol. 2006; 142(6):1054–1056

[99] Hayreh SS. Ocular vascular occlusive disorders: natural history of visual outcome. Prog Retin Eye Res. 2014; 41:1–25

[100] Hayreh SS, Hayreh MS. Hemi-central retinal vein occlusion. Pathogenesis, clinical features, and natural history. Arch Ophthalmol. 1980; 98(9):1600–1609

[101] Sanborn GE, Magargal LE. Characteristics of the hemispheric retinal vein occlusion. Ophthalmology. 1984; 91(12):1616–1626

10 Diabetic Retinopathy

Jennifer K. Sun and Lloyd Paul Aiello

10.1 Introduction

Due largely to numerous well-designed landmark clinical trials performed over the past half century, the methods by which diabetic retinopathy is diagnosed, classified, and treated have evolved enormously since Jaegar first described direct evidence of alterations in the macula of patients with glycosuria in 1856.[1] Although diabetic retinopathy is still the leading cause of vision loss in the working age population of many developed countries such as the United States, visual outcomes in diabetic patients continue to improve with substantial advancements in systemic diabetes control and more effective retinopathy therapy.

In 1952, Luft and associates[2] performed a hypophysectomy in the hope of ameliorating the vascular complications of diabetes, and in 1960, photocoagulation for the treatment of diabetic retinopathy was first reported by Meyer-Schwickerath,[3] who used a xenon arc photocoagulator to directly treat new vessels on the surface of the retina. Despite these efforts, by 1967 there were still no effective treatments available, prompting Duke-Elder to describe the visual complications of diabetes mellitus as "not preventable" and "relatively untreatable."

Treatments developed in the early 1970s, such as argon laser photocoagulation as proposed by Beetham et al[4] and pars plana vitrectomy, were put to the test during the ensuing years in several landmark clinical trials that ultimately proved their remarkable effectiveness in preserving vision in patients with diabetes mellitus. The first of such trials was the Diabetic Retinopathy Study (DRS) of 1976, which showed that the rate of severe visual loss (SVL) in high-risk proliferative diabetic retinopathy (PDR) could be reduced by as much as 60% following the timely application of panretinal photocoagulation (PRP).[5] In the mid-1980s, results from the Early Treatment Diabetic Retinopathy Study (ETDRS) and the Diabetic Retinopathy Vitrectomy Study (DRVS) become available. The ETDRS demonstrated that providing PRP at or as an eye-approached high-risk PDR could reduce the risk of SVL by 96%. The ETDRS also demonstrated that focal laser photocoagulation treatment to the macula could substantially reduce the risk of moderate visual acuity loss in patients with diabetic macular edema.[6] The Diabetic Retinopathy Vitrectomy Study (DRVS) showed that in eyes with severe vitreous hemorrhage, early intervention with pars plana vitrectomy resulted in better visual outcomes than deferral of surgery in patients with type I diabetes mellitus.[7]

The past decade has witnessed the advent of anti-vascular endothelial growth factor (anti-VEGF) agents for diabetic eye disease. Major phase 3 clinical trials including the Diabetic Retinopathy Clinical Research Network (DRCR.net) Protocol I,[8] RIDE/RISE,[9] and VISTA/VIVID[10] studies have demonstrated that these medications are highly effective and superior to macular laser photocoagulation in improving visual acuity outcomes in eyes with diabetic macular edema. The formation of the National Institutes of Health–sponsored DRCR.net, the nation's largest collaborative network of academic and community sites dedicated to research in diabetic retinopathy, was another recent landmark in the field of clinical research for diabetic retinopathy. Since its inception in 2002, the DRCR.net has designed, implemented, and reported on more than 20 clinical studies that have informed the current standard of care for diabetic eye disease on diverse topics including imaging of the diabetic retina, optimal protocols for macular laser photocoagulation, and the safety and efficacy of intravitreal anti-VEGF and steroid treatment for diabetic macular edema.

Clinical trials have better defined those eyes at greatest risk, the appropriate times to intervene, and the therapeutic modalities that are most effective in preserving vision in patients with diabetes. This chapter reviews the clinical manifestations and pathophysiologic mechanisms underlying the visual complications of diabetes mellitus, as well as the current appropriate management of diabetic retinopathy based on the results of major clinical studies.

10.2 Epidemiology

Despite treatment advances, and overall improvements in glycemic and hypertensive control over the past few decades, diabetic retinopathy remains a leading cause of new-onset blindness in working age adults in the United States. It is estimated that approximately 7.7 million Americans had diabetic retinopathy in 2010, but this number will nearly double to 14.6 million by the year 2050.[11] The strongest risk factors for development of diabetic retinopathy are longer duration of diabetes and worse glycemic control. The prevalence of all types of retinopathy increases with the duration of diabetes, probably reflecting the consequences of prolonged hyperglycemia. Early reports suggested that, after 15 years of diabetes duration, nearly all patients (98%) with type 1 diabetes and more than 78% of patients with type 2 diabetes have some degree of retinopathy.[12,13] Uncontrolled hypertension and cholesterol have also been related to worse outcomes in diabetic retinopathy. Young persons with type 1 diabetes are more likely to suffer severe visual complications from PDR during their lifetime, whereas a greater total number of older patients with type 2 diabetes mellitus experience visual loss from macular edema.

The projected rapid rise in diabetes over the next few decades will place approximately 592 million individuals at risk for vision complications from diabetes worldwide by the year 2035.[14] Major challenges will be the timely evaluation and triage of these patients in order to provide access to expert care across potential socioeconomic and geographic barriers. In this era, a critical role for the ophthalmologist is to identify accurately the stages of retinopathy at which patients are most amenable to treatment, as ocular interventions such as intravitreal anti-VEGF injections, laser photocoagulation, and surgery are most effective in preserving vision when initiated before vision is lost from macular edema or the complications of proliferative retinopathy.

10.3 Preclinical Molecular and Pathophysiologic Changes in the Diabetic Retina

Diverse molecular pathways have been implicated in the mechanisms that underlie the development of diabetic retinopathy. Eyes with active neovascularization from diabetes or with diabetic macular edema have been shown to have increased levels of VEGF,[15] which is a potent enhancer of both ocular angiogenesis and retinal vascular permeability. Currently, the most effective clinical interventions for diabetic macular edema target the VEGF molecule to block its activity. Such approaches are currently being studied to determine their efficacy in the treatment of PDR. Multiple earlier stage pathways may play key roles in the onset or worsening of diabetic eye disease, including increased oxidative stress, activation of protein kinase C, and the presence of advanced glycation end products. The sorbitol pathway has also been a subject of investigation because under hyperglycemic conditions, aldose reductase reduces many aldose sugars (glucose, galactose) to their respective sugar alcohols (sorbitol, galactitol), which can subsequently accumulate to high levels in cells. Animal studies have demonstrated increased pericyte dropout, formation of microaneurysms, and capillary acellularity in nondiabetic dogs fed a diet enriched with galactose.[16] However, the role of aldose reductase inhibitors (sorbinil) in preventing these microvascular changes in animal models has been controversial, and their efficacy in slowing down the progression of diabetic retinopathy in humans has not been demonstrated.[17]

Although there is increasing evidence that abnormalities of the neural retina such as thinning of the inner retinal layers are present in early diabetes,[18] the fundus changes observed in diabetic retinopathy are primarily the result of pathologic changes within the retinal blood vessels. One of the earliest findings in the diabetic retina is loss of pericytes, the supporting mural cells of the retinal capillaries. In the normal retinal vasculature, endothelial cells and intramural pericytes are distributed in equal numbers in a ratio of approximately 1:1. Trypsin-digest preparations have shown that eyes with diabetic retinopathy demonstrate a preferential loss of microvascular pericytes.[19] Diabetic retinal capillaries can also become acellular, and studies correlating fluorescein angiograms with trypsin-digest preparations provide direct evidence that acellular ghost capillaries are usually nonperfused.[20] Perhaps as a response to retinal hypoxia, the adjacent capillary bed becomes dilated and hypercellular. Intraluminal factors that contribute to abnormalities in the retinal vasculature even before clinically observable signs of retinal vasculopathy include slowing of retinal blood flow and blood viscosity abnormalities due to elevated plasma fibrinogen, increased platelet adhesiveness, and abnormal aggregation properties of erythrocytes. Thickening of endothelial basement membranes also occurs, which can cause luminal narrowing and potentially lead to retinal capillary closure.

The endothelial cell is the principal site of breakdown in the inner blood–retinal barrier that leads to abnormal vascular permeability in the diabetic eye. Defects in the tight junctions between endothelial cells may arise secondary to obstruction of adjacent vessels, or from the well-documented dropout of capillary pericytes.[21] Even before any retinopathy is demonstrable clinically, evidence of abnormal vascular permeability may be seen on fluorescein angiography as focal staining of the arteriole wall. As the leakage becomes more widespread, accumulation of fluid and plasma constituents in the surrounding retina can lead to marked retinal thickening, cystoid changes in the fovea, and the formation of hard exudates (composed of plasma lipoprotein).

10.4 Clinical Features

Diabetic retinopathy is broadly classified as either nonproliferative diabetic retinopathy (NPDR) or PDR. The microvascular changes that occur in NPDR are limited to the confines of the retina and do not include the growth of new vessels from the existing retinal vasculature. In contrast, PDR is characterized by the growth and possible extension of retinal neovascularization beyond the internal limiting membrane. Diabetic macular edema, the most common cause of decreased central vision in patients with diabetes, can occur in either NPDR or PDR. Each of these manifestations of diabetic retinal vascular pathology is associated with hallmark lesions that are described in this section.

Pearls

- Macular edema is the most common cause of decreased visual acuity in patients with diabetes mellitus. Although more common with more advanced disease, it can be present at any stage of diabetic retinopathy.

One of the earliest and most common clinically observable lesions in diabetic retinopathy is the microaneurysm, a saccular outpouching of the retinal capillary (▶ Fig. 10.1). Initially detectable only on fluorescein angiography as small hyperfluorescent foci that may or may not leak fluorescein in the late phase of the angiogram, they subsequently enlarge and appear as scattered, red dots on ophthalmoscopic examination. Two hypotheses that have been proposed for microaneurysm

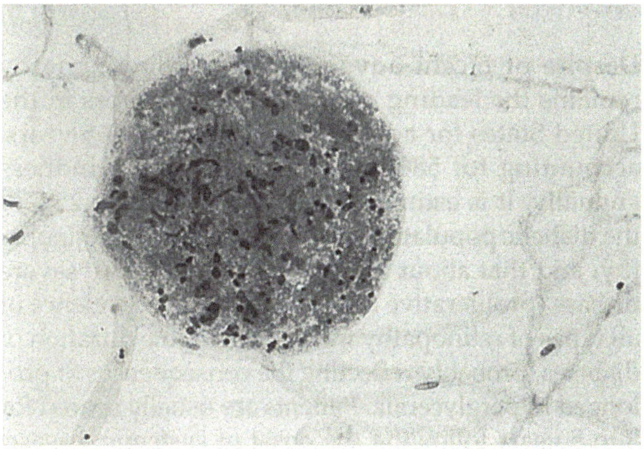

Fig. 10.1 Microaneurysm formation represents the first clinically visible manifestation of diabetic retinopathy and occurs adjacent to areas of capillary closure. (Image courtesy of George H. Bresnick, MD.)

formation are as follows: (1) saccular outpouchings occur at the sites of pericyte degeneration and (2) microaneurysm formation involves a proliferative cellular response to focal retinal hypoxia. Microaneurysms tend to cluster at the margins of capillary nonperfusion and follow a typical life cycle of gradual enlargement, thickening, and hyalinization of the wall, and eventual auto-occlusion by encroachment of the thickened wall into the lumen. It has been suggested that the rate of formation and turnover appears to be correlated with the level and severity of diabetic retinopathy.[22]

With progression of NPDR, intraretinal hemorrhages resulting from ruptured microaneurysms and decompensated capillaries become visible, with superficial flame-shaped hemorrhages being located in the nerve fiber layer and dot-shaped hemorrhages within the deeper retina (▶ Fig. 10.2). Occasionally, retinal hemorrhages in diabetes may demonstrate a white center, reflecting either their fibrin component or their origin from a hyalinized microaneurysm.

Another important fundus sign of retinal ischemia is the development of intraretinal microvascular abnormalities (IRMAs), a descriptive term for irregular, segmental dilations and vascular looping of the retinal capillary bed (▶ Fig. 10.3b). IRMAs are thought to represent either a compensatory dilation of preexisting vascular channels (shunt vessels) or a form of intraretinal neovascularization. In longitudinal fluorescein angiographic studies, IRMAs have been shown to develop slowly within the focal areas of arteriolar nonperfusion over the course of months.[23] The network of dilated capillaries appears to originate from the venous side of the circulation and also drains into the retinal veins, with a direct connection to a retinal arteriole being a rare finding. IRMAs are distinguishable from preretinal neovascularization in that they remain within the confines of the retina and do not leak fluorescein. An additional hallmark finding in diabetic retinopathy is venous caliber abnormalities, or venous beading, consisting of alternating areas of dilation and constriction of the retinal venules (▶ Fig. 10.3a). “Reduplication” of venous segments and abnormal venous “loop” formation are also common in the diabetic retina.

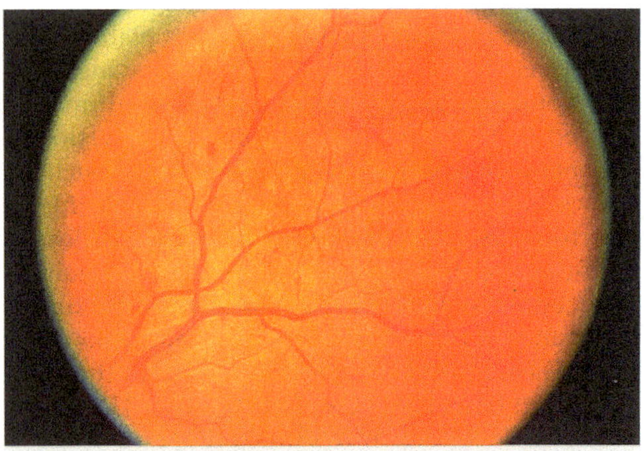

Fig. 10.2 Moderate nonproliferative diabetic retinopathy: Standard photograph 2A demonstrating a moderate degree of intraretinal hemorrhages and microaneurysms. (Image courtesy of the Early Treatment Diabetic Retinopathy Study Group.)

Increased vascular permeability of the diabetic retina is manifested by the exudation of fluid, lipoproteins, and various other plasma constituents into the retinal neural tissue. The leakage stems from microaneurysms and defective small retinal vessels and can result in the formation of intraretinal cysts and/or accumulation of subretinal fluid (▶ Fig. 10.4). Hard exudates are commonly seen along the borders of zones of current or previous retinal thickening and consist of intraretinal yellow cholesterol deposits that are hyperreflective on imaging with optical coherence tomography (OCT).

Retinal capillary abnormalities can affect adjacent arterioles, resulting in arteriolar closure and discrete areas of capillary dropout or nonperfusion. Clinically, the most obvious manifestation of such arteriolar ischemia is the cotton-wool spot (▶ Fig. 10.5), a localized infarct of the nerve fiber layer that results from occlusion of the terminal arteriole (precapillary arteriole). Cotton-wool spots in diabetic eyes tend to persist for extended periods; their mean half-life is approximately 8 months in diabetic patients younger than 40 years and 17 months in those older than 40 years, compared with about 6 weeks in hypertensive retinopathy.[24] Once the cotton-wool spot resolves, the inner retina layers may become atrophic, with the site becoming ophthalmoscopically visible as a focal, depressed area. Data from the ETDRS suggest that isolated cotton-wool spots represent a common but nonprognostic sign of diabetic retinopathy and do not necessarily correlate with either the angiographic evidence of retinal ischemia or a high likelihood of progression to proliferative retinopathy.[25]

In performing fundus examinations, it is important to keep in mind that the characteristic intraretinal lesions of diabetic retinopathy may be absent in the severely ischemic stages of NPDR. Cotton-wool spots and retinal exudates tend to resolve with time, and blot hemorrhages and IRMAs may also disappear following extensive capillary nonperfusion. With a reduction in the normal vascularity of the retina, fewer hemorrhages and microaneurysms may be apparent and some arterioles may become thin, white threads, producing a fundus appearance

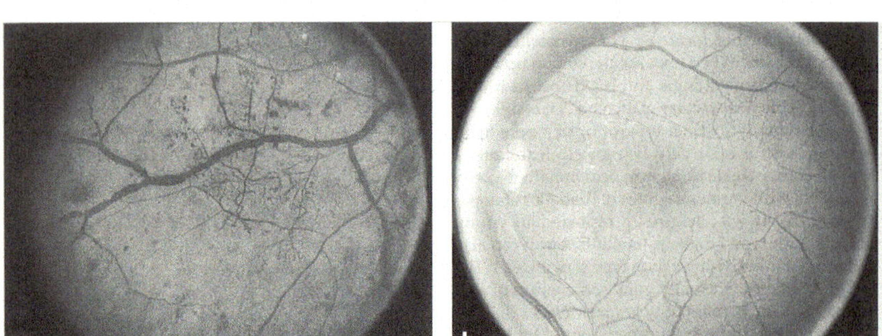

Fig. 10.3 Severe nonproliferative diabetic retinopathy: (**a**) Severe venous beading. (**b**) Prominent intraretinal microvascular abnormalities (IRMA) superotemporal to the macular center. (Image courtesy of the Early Treatment Diabetic Retinopathy Study Group.)

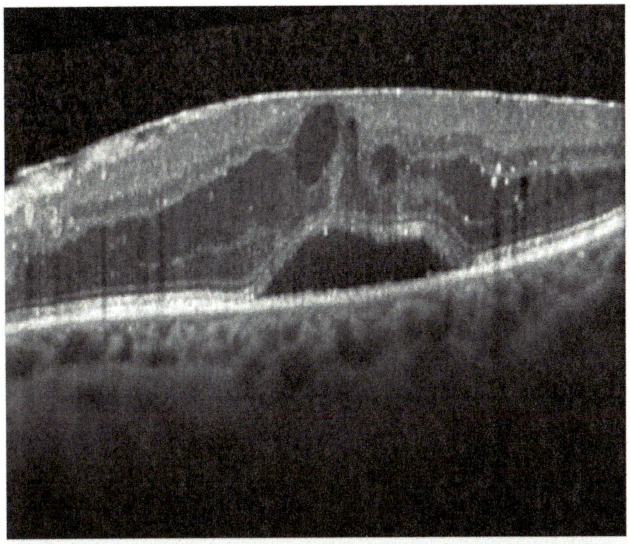

Fig. 10.4 Optical coherence tomography B-scan demonstrating a cross-section of a retina with diabetic macular edema. Findings include intraretinal cysts, subretinal fluid, and hard exudates. There is an epiretinal membrane across the surface of the retina as well.

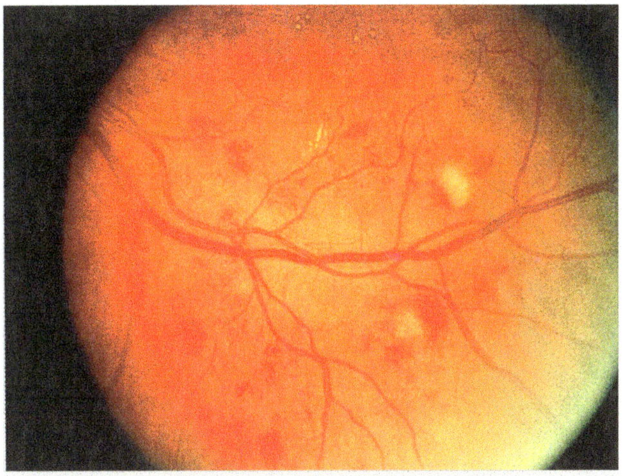

Fig. 10.5 Severe nonproliferative diabetic retinopathy: Numerous intraretinal hemorrhages and scattered cotton-wool spots are evident in this fundus photograph.

that has been described as "featureless" retina. On a cursory inspection, such an absence of lesions can mislead the examiner into substantially underestimating the severity of the retinopathy.

Pearls

- In some cases, as the NPDR progresses and the retina becomes severely ischemic, the usual characteristics of nonproliferative retinopathy may actually become *less* apparent. This presentation is often referred to as a "featureless" fundus, and with a cursory retinal examination, the severity of the retinopathy may be underestimated.

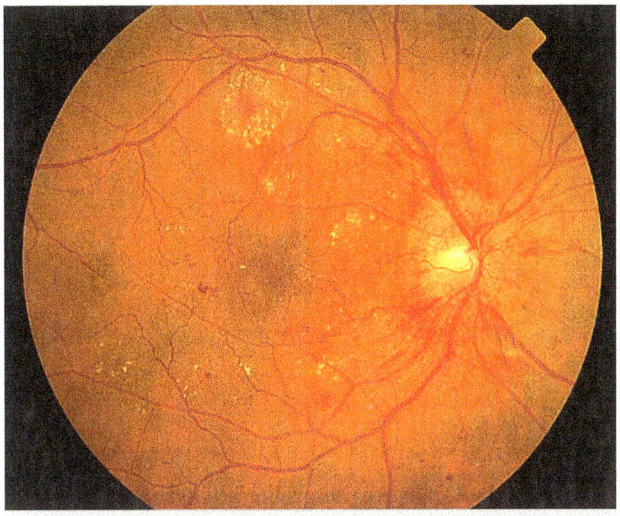

Fig. 10.6 Diabetic papillopathy: Hyperemic, diffuse disc swelling is evident in this eye with moderate nonproliferative diabetic retinopathy. (Image courtesy of Carl D. Regillo, MD)

In response to retinal ischemia resulting from retinal capillary nonperfusion, vasoproliferative factors such as VEGF are released from the retina and induce the development of neovascularization on the retina, optic nerve head, and/or iris. Preretinal neovascular networks have a propensity to bleed into the vitreous cavity and obscure vision. They also retain the potential for differentiation into fibroblasts, and this fibrous component contributes to the formation of firm adhesions at the interface between the retina and vitreous body. As the fibrovascular tissue contracts, these vitreoretinal adhesions may lead to complications involving the underlying retina, such as traction retinal detachment, focal areas of retinoschisis, and retinal breaks. When neovascularization occurs in the anterior chamber angle and iris (rubeosis iridis), increased intraocular pressure from neovascular glaucoma can result.

A presumably distinct type of optic nerve head swelling with a relatively benign clinical course, termed *diabetic papillopathy*, is occasionally seen in patients with various degrees of diabetic retinopathy (▶ Fig. 10.6). This entity was originally reported in young patients with type 1 diabetes mellitus, but it can also occur in older individuals with type 2 diabetes.[26] It is more likely to occur in patients with worse glycemic control. The visual prognosis is usually good and the optic disc edema is often self-limited. As a cause of disc edema, diabetic papillopathy is considered a diagnosis of exclusion but can be differentiated by the following constellation of features: common bilateral (simultaneous or sequential) presentation, minimal or no signs or symptoms of significant optic nerve dysfunction, hyperemic disc swelling (with prominent, telangiectatic disc vessels), and resolution occurring during a period of months without the appearance of optic atrophy. Clinically, it is important to distinguish the radially oriented, telangiectatic vessels of diabetic papillopathy from disc neovascularization, which is more randomly oriented and typically elevated above the plane of the disc and retina. An association between diabetic papillopathy and widespread retinal capillary disease has been found in a large series, supporting the suspicion that diabetes-related microangiopathy is related pathogenetically to the disc swelling in some way.[26]

Controversial Points

- Diabetic papillopathy is a transient swelling of the optic nerve head in the setting of diabetic retinopathy. Clinically, it is differentiated from an ischemic optic neuropathy by the lack of significant, permanent optic nerve dysfunction. Whether these cases represent mild ischemic events or vascular incompetence of the optic nerve head remains controversial.

Although a history of systemic hyperglycemia and the bilateral, generally rather symmetric presentation of diabetic retinopathy makes the diagnosis obvious in most cases, other entities that may present with similar microangiopathic changes in the posterior pole should be considered in the differential diagnosis for diabetic retinopathy. The most common ocular diseases that may mimic diabetic retinopathy are other retinal vascular disorders, including central and branch retinal vein occlusion (CRVO, BRVO), hypertensive retinopathy, ocular ischemic syndrome (OIS), radiation retinopathy, human immunodeficiency virus (HIV) retinopathy, and idiopathic juxtafoveal telangiectasis. The fundus appearance, accompanying systemic history, and asymmetry of presentation are useful in ruling out the majority of these conditions. A recent CRVO may closely resemble the fundus findings of diabetic retinopathy, and typically presents with venous dilation, cotton-wool spots, and a distribution of retinal hemorrhages involving all four quadrants. These two conditions also affect similar populations, and CRVOs are thought to occur with a higher frequency in diabetic patients, particularly in the younger age groups. However, the symptoms associated with a CRVO tend to be more acute, and there is typically more asymmetry between the eyes. Finally, it should be kept in mind that patients sometimes present with two different retinal diseases simultaneously (i.e., BRVO or HIV retinopathy and NPDR).

10.5 Nonproliferative Diabetic Retinopathy

10.5.1 Diagnosis and Staging

The ETDRS validated a classification system for diabetic retinopathy severity grading that has been utilized thereafter in numerous epidemiologic and interventional clinical studies that have set the current gold standards for the diagnosis and management of diabetic retinopathy. This system relies on grading of diabetic retinopathy findings in comparison to standard photographs. NPDR is divided into severity levels (▶ Table 10.1) that predict the risk for retinopathy progression over time. The risk of diabetic retinopathy progression for an individual eye is strongly related to the presence and extent of the following clinical findings: increasing severity of intraretinal hemorrhages and microaneurysms, venous beading, and IRMAs. Conversely, hard exudate deposits have not been found to be a significant risk factor for diabetic retinopathy progression (although they are associated with visual loss from diabetic macular edema), and the presence of cotton-wool spots is only weakly correlated with subsequent progression to PDR. With stratification into three general groups based on these intraretinal findings, the ETDRS found a substantial difference in the

Table 10.1 Levels of diabetic retinopathy and recommended management

Diabetes type/retinopathy levels	First fundus exam/fundus findings	Follow-up (minimum)	Treatment[a]
Type 1 diabetes	Within 5 y of diagnosis	Yearly	N/A
Type 2 diabetes	At diagnosis	Yearly	N/A
Before pregnancy	Before conception or first trimester	3 mo	N/A
A. Mild NPDR	At least one MA, mild HE, CWS, H (criteria not met for *B*)	1 y	N/A
B. Moderate NPDR	H/Ma (> photograph 2A), CWS, VB, IRMA present (criteria not met for C)	6 mo	N/A
C. Severe NPDR	Any one or more of the following criteria: 1. H/Ma (= photograph 2A) in all four quadrants 2. VB in two or more quadrants 3. IRMA (= photograph 8A) in one or more quadrants	3–4 mo	Consider PRP in select cases (e.g., patients with type 2 diabetes)
D. Early PDR	New vessels present (criteria not met for *E*)	2–3 mo	Consider PRP or anti-VEGF
E. PDR with high-risk characteristics	Any one or more of the following criteria: 1. NVD *with* VH 2. NVD = 1/4–1/3 DD (= photograph 10A) *without* VH 3. NVE = 1/2 DD *with* VH	2–3 mo	Immediate PRP or anti-VEGF

Abbreviations: COM, center of macula; CWS, cotton-wool spots; DD, disc diameter; H, retinal hemorrhages; HE, hard exudates; IRMA, intraretinal microvascular abnormalities; MA, microaneurysms; NPDR, nonproliferative diabetic retinopathy; NVD, neovascularization within 1 DD of disc; NVE, neovascularization elsewhere (on the retina); PRP, panretinal (scatter) photocoagulation; VB, venous beading; VEGF, vascular endothelial growth factor. VH, vitreous (or preretinal) hemorrhage;

[a]At all levels of retinopathy, diabetic macular edema may be present and should be treated if it involves the retinal center and especially if there is accompanying visual impairment.

1-year risk for development of proliferative retinopathy between the mildest and most severe levels of NPDR.[27]

Mild NPDR is defined as the presence of at least one retinal microaneurysm and a minimal number of intraretinal hemorrhages. Patients with mild NPDR have a 4% risk for progression to PDR within 1 year and a 15% risk for progression to high-risk PDR within 5 years. *Moderate* NPDR is characterized by more extensive hemorrhages and microaneurysms (more than on standard photograph 2A, ▶ Fig. 10.2). Cotton-wool spots and a limited amount of venous beading can also be seen in this stage. With moderate NPDR, the risk for progression to PDR within 1 year is 8 to 18%, and the risk for progression to high-risk PDR within 5 years is 24 to 39%.

Severe NPDR (formerly known as *preproliferative retinopathy*) is characterized by any one of the following ("four-two-one rule"):

1. Numerous hemorrhages and microaneurysms (greater than or equal to standard photograph 2A) in *four* quadrants
2. Definite venous beading in *two* or more quadrants
3. IRMA (greater than or equal to standard photograph 8A) in *one* or more quadrants

The intraretinal findings of severe NPDR reflect widespread arteriolar closure, and angiographic studies of patients with severe NPDR demonstrate extensive zones of capillary nonperfusion (▶ Fig. 10.7). Eyes with severe NPDR have a 33% risk for development of PDR within 1 year and a 58% risk for development of high-risk PDR within 5 years. In certain situations, patients with severe NPDR may be candidates for scatter (panretinal) laser photocoagulation. Because progression to proliferative stages of retinopathy is often rapid in eyes with severe NPDR, frequent surveillance is important, and evaluation at 2- to 4-month intervals is recommended (▶ Table 10.1).

Pearls

- Eyes meeting the criteria for severe NPDR must be followed up closely, as the risk for progression to PDR is high. If close follow-up is not possible, scatter (panretinal) laser treatment should be considered to reduce the risk of vision loss from progression to PDR and PDR-related complications.

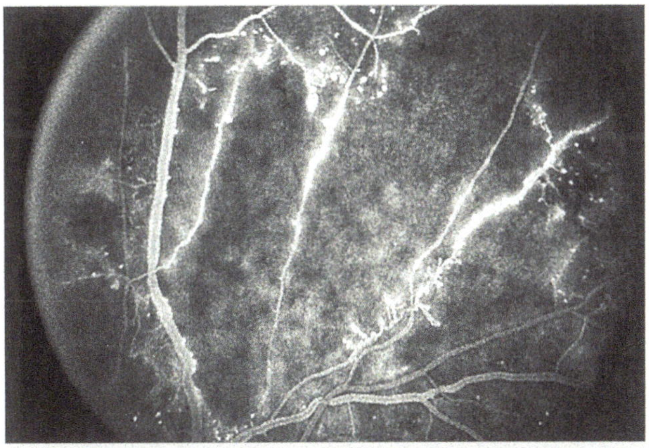

Fig. 10.7 Capillary nonperfusion: Fluorescein angiography photograph showing widespread capillary dropout or nonperfusion in the midperipheral fundus. This is a significant risk factor for progression to proliferative diabetic retinopathy.

Analysis of angiographic characteristics from the ETDRS untreated (deferred) eyes indicates that fluorescein leakage, capillary loss and dilation, and various other arteriolar abnormalities are associated with the likelihood of progression to PDR.[28] Widespread capillary nonperfusion is a particularly significant risk factor for progression to PDR (▶ Fig. 10.7); the extent of capillary closure seen on angiography appears to be correlated with the severity of new vessels involving the retina, optic disc, and anterior chamber angle.[29] Despite this correlation and the additional risk factors provided by fluorescein angiography, clinical examinations and/or color fundus photographs appear to give the same prognostic information. Therefore, the increase in power to predict progression to PDR provided by fluorescein angiography is not of enough clinical importance to warrant routine ordering of angiograms for patients with NPDR.[28] Ophthalmoscopic examination supplemented by color photography remains the mainstay of staging diabetic retinopathy severity levels, and periodic follow-up of all patients with diabetic retinopathy continues to be of fundamental importance to document progression.

The recent availability of instruments that can provide ultrawide field imaging of the retina, obtaining fields of up to 200 degrees with a single image, has sparked renewed interest in whether careful documentation of the retinal periphery outside the standard ETDRS 7 fields allows the detection of more retinal pathology and a more accurate assessment of risk for future worsening in eyes with diabetic retinopathy. Multiple studies have demonstrated that peripheral pathology is common in eyes of patients with diabetes and that this pathology suggests a more severe level of diabetic retinopathy than that documented within the ETDRS fields approximately 9 to 10% of the time (▶ Fig. 10.8).[30] Studies have also found that eyes in which diabetic lesions are greater in extent or severity in the periphery as compared to within the ETDRS fields at baseline have a threefold higher risk of diabetic retinopathy worsening and a nearly fivefold higher risk of new-onset PDR over the subsequent 4 years.[31] If these results are confirmed in currently ongoing large, multicenter studies, these findings may

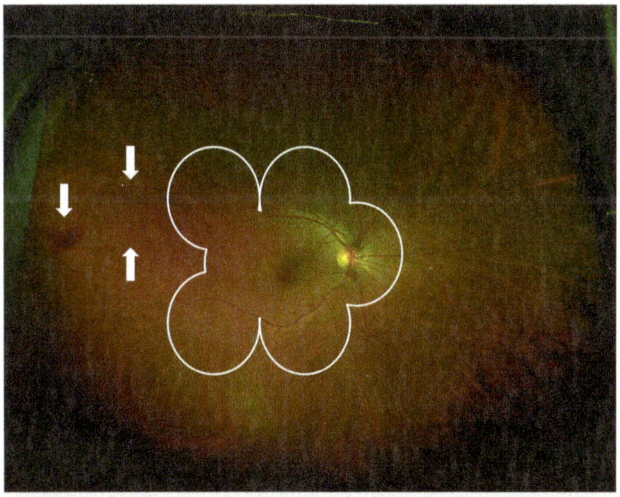

Fig. 10.8 Photograph of a 200-degree ultrawide field fundus demonstrating peripheral retinal neovascularization (*arrows*) in an eye with only nonproliferative lesions present within the area covered by the standard 7 ETDRS fields (white outline).

substantively impact the manner in which we determine diabetic retinopathy severity and necessitate revision of the current standard severity grading guidelines.

10.5.2 Management and Course

The management of NPDR is based on the optimal medical control of diabetes, as patients with NPDR generally do not require PRP, nor are they treated with anti-VEGF therapy in the absence of diabetic macular edema. These eyes can be followed up safely at 2- to 12-month intervals as determined by the severity of retinopathy (▶ Table 10.1). The most important systemic factor affecting the course of retinopathy appears to be blood glucose levels, although blood pressure and lipids play a role as well.

The Diabetes Control and Complications Trial (DCCT) evaluated the role of intensive diabetic management on the course of retinopathy in patients with insulin-dependent diabetes mellitus (IDDM). The DCCT showed that intensive glucose control with three or more daily injections of insulin delayed the onset and decreased the progression of all levels of retinopathy (beginning after 3 years of therapy) in comparison with treatment with conventional insulin dosing in the control group.[32] Intensive control also reduced the likelihood of requiring laser treatment (for proliferative retinopathy) by almost 60%. Careful monitoring is recommended for patients with significant eye disease who are starting on intensive control regimens, as a minority of patients may experience an initial worsening of retinopathy. However, long-term, intensive therapy still results in better outcomes. Although all levels of retinopathy included in the DCCT appeared to benefit from intensive glucose control, intensive therapy was more effective in preventing progression when initiated early in the course of IDDM. Additionally, the Epidemiology of Diabetes Interventions and Complications (EDIC) study conclusively showed that the benefits of early glycemic control in the DCCT intensive control group as compared to the conventional control group persisted for decades even after subsequent glycemic control in these two groups became equivalent.[33] All microvascular complications and the need for retinopathy treatment were dramatically reduced in the intensive versus conventional control group for nearly two decades after the DCCT ended. The rate of ocular surgery was reduced in the intensive control group as compared to the conventional control group by approximately 50% over a median follow-up of 23 years.[34] Therefore, the importance of early optimal control of blood glucose levels should be reinforced to patients as highly significant in reducing the risk for visual complications. Other systemic factors, such as hypertension, hyperlipidemia, and renal failure, can also contribute to the further progression of retinopathy and should be managed appropriately.

One of the aims of the ETDRS was to test the efficacy of systemic *aspirin therapy* in influencing the course of diabetic retinopathy.[35] In patients with NPDR or early PDR, taking two aspirin tablets a day (650 mg/d) did not produce any demonstrable effects on the progression of NPDR, rates of development of PDR, or visual acuity outcomes. Aspirin therapy also did not increase the risk for vitreous hemorrhage. Although these data do not support a therapeutic role for aspirin to affect diabetic retinopathy favorably, the results indicate that there are no ocular contraindications to aspirin at this dose if required for other medical issues.

Special Considerations

- Although the regular use of aspirin does not favorably affect the course of diabetic retinopathy, its use for other indications, such as to reduce the risk of cardiovascular or cerebrovascular mortality, does not have adverse ocular effects in patients with any degree of diabetic retinopathy.

The potential accelerating effects of pregnancy on the natural course of diabetic retinopathy have long been acknowledged, and prospective studies have confirmed a strong association between the onset of pregnancy and worsening of retinopathy severity.[36,37] Those pregnant patients at highest risk for progression typically have had diabetes for an extended period and possess significant degrees of retinopathy at conception, whereas women who begin pregnancy with no retinopathy or mild background retinopathy, are unlikely to develop vision-threatening complications during pregnancy.[37] In the counseling of diabetic women who are pregnant or considering pregnancy, their baseline severity of retinopathy should be considered the most important prognostic factor for possible visual complications. Frequent retinal examinations are currently recommended for all pregnant women with diabetes (at least once per trimester), and earlier laser photocoagulation may be prudent in eyes with severe NPDR or early PDR in the setting of pregnancy.

10.5.3 Regression of NPDR with Intravitreal Anti-VEGF Therapy

The widespread use of anti-VEGF therapy as first-line treatment for center-involved diabetic macular edema has provided additional insight into the response of nonproliferative diabetic pathology to anti-VEGF. Clinical trials of the anti-VEGF agents, aflibercept and ranibizumab which are used to treat diabetic macular edema, have consistently demonstrated significantly reduced rates of two- and three-step worsening and increasing rates of two- and three-step improvement on the ETDRS diabetic retinopathy severity scale in eyes that are treated with these agents as compared with eyes that receive macular laser photocoagulation alone.[10,38] Substantial improvements in diabetic retinopathy severity level have been documented in eyes receiving treatment on an as needed basis for diabetic macular edema as well as in eyes receiving monthly anti-VEGF therapy.[39] These improvements can occur early in the course of therapy. Two-step and even three-step improvement in diabetic retinopathy severity was documented by 3-month follow-up in some eyes treated with monthly ranibizumab in the RIDE/RISE trials. A substantial proportion of eyes receiving anti-VEGF will eventually experience improvement. By 36 months of follow-up, 39 and 15% of the cohort of eyes that had received continuous monthly therapy with 0.3 mg ranibizumab in the RIDE/RISE studies had two- and three-step improvements, respectively.[38]

Although these results are promising, treatment with anti-VEGF agents for NPDR in the absence of center-involved macular edema is not currently considered standard care. Phase 3 clinical trials of anti-VEGF for this indication are still pending. One consideration that may limit the use of current formulations of anti-VEGF for NPDR alone is that it is yet unclear how durable the effects of anti-VEGF are on retinopathy regression. In the RIDE/RISE open-label extension phase, eyes that initially received 36 months of continuous, monthly anti-VEGF treatment were transitioned to as needed dosing based solely on macular edema status. Although many of these eyes remained stable or improved in retinopathy severity level as compared to the start of the open-label extension, there were some eyes that worsened over time with this reduced frequency of anti-VEGF dosing.[40] Fortunately, there did not appear to be dramatic rebound rates of diabetic retinopathy worsening even in eyes receiving no anti-VEGF during the open-label extension. The majority of eyes remained stable or improved as compared to the start of the RIDE/RISE trials.

10.6 Proliferative Diabetic Retinopathy

The proliferative stage of diabetic retinopathy (PDR) is characterized by extraretinal neovascular proliferation that is thought to result from a compensatory response to widespread retinal ischemia. In addition to worse glycemic control, the factor most closely related to increased risk of PDR is longer duration of diabetes. In population-based studies, the prevalence of PDR in patients with diabetes onset at age younger than 30 years is near zero when diabetes has been present for less than 10 years, but then it rises rapidly to about 50% when the duration of diabetes reaches 20 years or longer.[12,13]

10.6.1 Diagnosis

The diagnosis of PDR involves the observation of preretinal new vessels and/or fibrous tissue arising from the optic disc or elsewhere on the retina. These proliferative, immature vessels extend along the inner surface of the retina or into the vitreous cavity and are abnormal in their propensity to bleed into the vitreous cavity, thus obscuring vision. Furthermore, they can result in firm adhesions between the retina and vitreous body, and with contracture or attempted separation of the vitreous gel, they may give rise to the development of traction retinal detachments. Vitreous hemorrhage and traction retinal detachments involving the macula are two of the most common causes of SVL in eyes with PDR (▶ Fig. 10.9).

Although new vessels may arise anywhere in the retina, they are most frequently observed in the posterior aspect of the fundus (within 45 degrees of the optic nerve), and are particularly common on the disc itself (▶ Fig. 10.10 and ▶ Fig. 10.11). Among 1,377 control group eyes in the DRS with new vessels present in baseline photographs, 60% demonstrated neovascularization within 1 disc diameter of the optic disc (NVD).[41] NVD is usually readily identified as fine loops of vessels lying on the surface of the disc or bridging across the physiologic cup. New vessels arising from elsewhere on the retina (neovascularization of the retina elsewhere [NVE]) often form wheel-like networks, with vessels radiating like spokes from the center of the patch and a circumferential vessel bounding the periphery. NVE complexes may also be irregular in shape without a distinct radial pattern, or lie over retinal veins and appear to drain into them. A review of DRS baseline photographs demonstrated that 59% of eyes with NVE had their most advanced lesions in the temporal quadrants, suggesting that this is a common area for nonperfusion.[42]

It is often difficult to distinguish between IRMAs and nonelevated NVE. A magnified stereoscopic view, obtained with either contact lens biomicroscopy or stereoscopic 30-degree photographs, may aid in the differentiation of early neovascularization by demonstrating its extraretinal nature and more superficial location. OCT can also aid in determining the preretinal location of retinal neovascularization. Preretinal new vessels can also be distinguished by their unique ability to cross both arterioles and veins in the underlying retina. In particularly difficult cases, fluorescein angiography can be used to demonstrate the profuse dye leakage, characteristic of true neovascularization. Routine examination for early NVE should

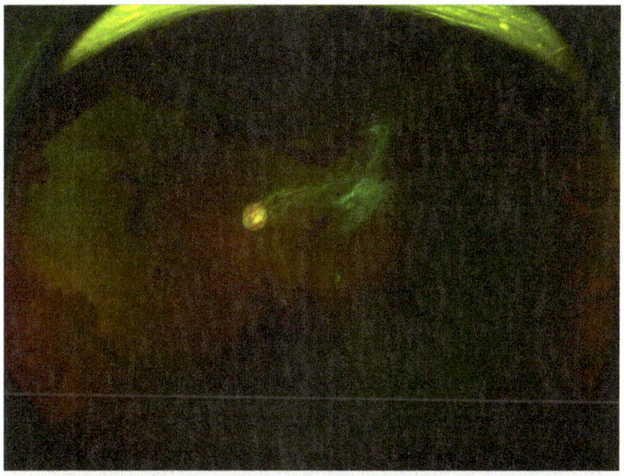

Fig. 10.9 Eye with retinal neovascularization from proliferative diabetic retinopathy that has resulted in a traction retinal detachment extending across the temporal arcades and central macula. Preretinal hemorrhage is present in the superior and nasal retinal periphery with vitreous hemorrhage obscuring much of the fundus.

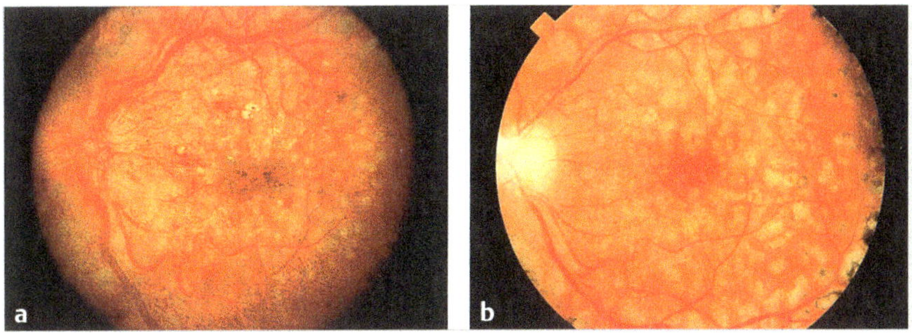

Fig. 10.10 (a) Extensive disc neovascularization that regressed (b) after panretinal laser therapy. Note that this eye also had (a) diffuse macular edema immediately following grid laser photocoagulation that was resolved (b) 2 years after laser treatment.

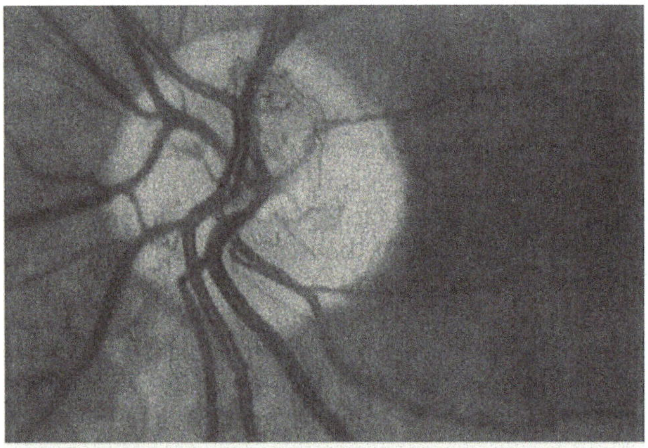

Fig. 10.11 Standard photograph 10A: The minimal amount of disc neovascularization (*without hemorrhage*) that would classify an eye as having high-risk characteristics and proliferative disease. (Image courtesy of the Diabetic Retinopathy Study Group.)

include both slit-lamp biomicroscopy of the posterior pole and examination for preretinal or vitreous hemorrhages in the periphery with indirect ophthalmoscopy.

When a patient presents with a fresh vitreous hemorrhage in the absence of any detectable neovascularization, examination of the more peripheral retina with the Goldmann three-mirror lens or fluorescein angioscopy using the indirect ophthalmoscope may be helpful. When new vessels still cannot be found, one should remember that a vitreous hemorrhage may also arise from a peripheral retinal tear, a partially avulsed retinal vessel, or the complete avulsion of a small neovascular patch from its connections to the disc or retina.

10.6.2 Pathophysiology

A generally accepted explanation for the pathogenesis of endothelial cell proliferation and new vessel formation is ischemia of the inner retinal layers leading to the release of "vasoproliferative factors" from the ischemic retina, such as VEGF. Such vessel-stimulating growth factors act locally and also diffuse through the vitreous to other areas of the retina, the optic disc, and the anterior chamber, causing neovascularization at these sites. Preretinal new vessels characteristically evolve through a cycle of proliferation followed by partial or complete regression. Their initial appearance is that of fine new vessels accompanied by minimal fibrous tissue that grow along the anterior surface of the retina. As the abnormal vessels increase in size and extent, the accompanying fibrous component, composed of both fibrocytes and glial cells, also undergoes a comparable rate of growth. A period of regression ensues, characterized by a decrease in the number and caliber of the vessels at the center of the patch, followed by their partial replacement with fibrous tissue. Fresh, active vessels are commonly seen emerging from the edges of partially regressed patches, and patches of neovascularization at different stages of development may be seen in the same eye.

Neovascular complexes may cycle through all these stages without causing any visual sequelae. Most of the visual complications of PDR can be attributed to the contraction of fibrovascular tissue growing along the posterior hyaloid face, which leads to the onset of posterior vitreous detachment (PVD). Like the age-related PVD that occurs secondary to vitreous syneresis, vitreous detachment in diabetic eyes usually begins in the posterior pole, most frequently near the superotemporal vessels, temporal to the macula, and above or below the disc.[43] However, PVD in diabetic eyes with PDR is not a smoothly progressive process and often spreads in an asymmetric, abrupt fashion, its advancing edge impeded by vitreoretinal adhesions associated with patches of neovascularization. The posterior vitreous surface also tends to vary in thickness, with alternating thin and thicker areas imparting a "Swiss cheese" appearance, but without actual hole formation.[43] Traction exerted by the shrinking vitreous body on fragile fibrovascular proliferations contributes to the recurrent vitreous hemorrhages that coincide with the progression of a PVD, and symptomatic vitreous hemorrhages are typically accompanied by some clinical evidence of localized PVD.

In addition to vitreous hemorrhage, vitreous contraction can also lead to complications involving the underlying retina, such as avulsion of retinal vessels, distortion or dragging of the macula, formation of retinal breaks, and traction retinal detachments. Tractional detachments in the setting of PDR are usually confined to the posterior fundus, most commonly along the temporal arcades, with possible extension into the macula. Continued vitreoretinal traction can also lead to the formation of retinal breaks and the development of a combined traction–rhegmatogenous retinal detachment. Retinal breaks in PDR are typically small, difficult to identify, and located adjacent to areas of fibrovascular proliferations. Traction on the retina can also cause focal areas of retinoschisis that may be difficult to distinguish from full-thickness retinal detachment.

When a PVD has reached completion or is no longer progressing, proliferative retinopathy tends to enter the burned-out or "involutional" stage. Vitreous hemorrhages decrease in frequency as well as severity, although many months may elapse before there is substantial vitreous clearing from previous hemorrhages. A marked reduction in the caliber and number of retinal vessels is also characteristic. Loss of central vision experienced at this quiescent stage is best explained by severe macular ischemia, central vitreous hemorrhage, or involvement of the macula by traction retinal detachment.

10.6.3 Management and Course

The main therapeutic goal in PDR is to preserve vision by promoting regression of existing neovascular tissue and preventing future proliferations or PDR-related complications of vitreous hemorrhage and retinal traction. Direct laser treatment to close neovascular fronds was the aim of early investigators, but it soon became evident that this was difficult to achieve and not particularly effective. However, there were subsequent observations of apparent neovascular regression at some distance from the directly treated areas, as well as reports of decreased retinopathy in diabetic patients with unilateral chorioretinal scarring, a high degree of myopia, and optic atrophy. These clinical observations led to the first studies demonstrating success with laser burns scattered across the peripheral retina. Since then, the efficacy of PRP for PDR has been well documented in numerous randomized clinical trials.

PRP, or "scatter" laser, currently remains the mainstay of treatment for active PDR. Its mechanism of action has only become reasonably certain recently with the understanding that PRP improves retinal oxygenation by allowing oxygen diffusion from the choroid through the laser burns to the retina. In addition, there is decreased expression of VEGF due to PRP-related destruction of ischemic VEGF producing cells and a relative increase in perfusion to viable retina after the procedure.

The DRS demonstrated that the timely application of PRP was effective in inhibiting the progression of retinopathy and reducing the risk of SVL from PDR. The DRS randomized patients to either argon or xenon laser treatment groups, with one eye of each patient being randomly assigned to immediate photocoagulation treatment and the other eye to indefinite deferral of treatment.[5] Both the argon and xenon laser techniques consisted of applying laser spots in the peripheral retina for 360 degrees (see Technique). The primary outcome was *SVL*, defined as visual acuity of less than 5/200 on two consecutive follow-up examinations, 4 months apart. The DRS demonstrated an overall reduction in the rate of SVL from 15.9% in untreated eyes to 6.4% in treated eyes, a reduction of 60% at the 2-year mark.

By analyzing various risk factors for SVL, the DRS identified the specific proliferative features that benefited most from PRP.[44,45] These are known as *high-risk characteristics (HRC)*, and by definition, an eye has PDR with HRC when one or more of the following is present:

1. Any neovascularization located on or within 1 disc diameter of the disc (NVD) associated *with* preretinal or vitreous hemorrhage
2. Moderate to severe degree of NVD (greater than or equal to one-fourth to one-third disc diameter, standard photograph 10A) *without* associated preretinal or vitreous hemorrhage (▶ Fig. 10.11)
3. NVE (greater than or equal to one-half disc area) associated *with* preretinal or vitreous hemorrhage

In the DRS, increasingly severe levels of retinopathy were associated with correspondingly higher rates of SVL.[46] For untreated eyes, the 2-year risk for SVL increased from 3.2% in eyes with NPDR to 7.0% in eyes with PDR without HRC and 26.2% in eyes with HRC.[47] Treatment reduced the risk for SVL by 50 to 65% in all groups, but the percentage of treated eyes that benefited was smaller as retinopathy levels decreased. This visual benefit of overall improvement in SVL risk had to be weighed against the potential increased risk of visual loss in individual eyes. The study found a 3 to 11% permanent reduction in visual acuity (two lines or more) associated with PRP. Taking all these into consideration, the *DRS investigators concluded that PRP should be performed promptly for eyes reaching HRC, as the benefits of treatment clearly outweighed its risks in this subgroup.* Clear conclusions regarding treatment strategies for eyes with severe NPDR or early PDR (i.e., without HRC), however, could not be drawn from DRS data alone.

The ETDRS subsequently attempted to determine whether the benefits of *early* PRP (i.e., before the development of HRC) justified the risks or side effects of laser treatment.[48] Like the DRS, the ETDRS found that early scatter treatment reduced the risk for SVL (or progression to a stage requiring vitrectomy) to about one-half that in the deferral group. However, because the 5-year incidence of SVL was low for both treatment and deferral groups, only 2 to 4% of patients with NPDR or early PDR ended up benefiting from early PRP. Based on these data, the ETDRS concluded that for mild to moderate NPDR, it is best to defer scatter laser treatment until the retinopathy reaches more advanced stages, provided that careful follow-up can be maintained. When retinopathy is more severe (i.e., severe NPDR and early PDR), PRP can be considered, especially for patients with type 2 diabetes who may have significantly reduced rates of vision loss with early PRP.[49]

Detection of neovascularization on the iris (rubeosis iridis) or anterior chamber angle is an indication for prompt scatter photocoagulation, whether or not PDR meeting high-risk criteria is present. Rubeosis iridis is a sign of severe retinal ischemia, and such eyes can progress rapidly to total synechial closure of the anterior chamber angle with the onset of typically difficult-to-control neovascular glaucoma. Even in eyes with significant portions of the angle already closed by synechiae, remarkable regression of these new vessels can be achieved with complete PRP. In severe cases, use of anti-VEGF agents can provide a remarkable but transient response, allowing time for PRP to be applied for longstanding effect. If neovascular glaucoma has already developed, PRP is still recommended, as regression of anterior chamber vessels may improve the success of subsequent filtration surgery.

Technique of Scatter (Panretinal) Laser Photocoagulation

The amount of therapy necessary to achieve the goals of PRP is determined by the clinical response. Additional laser treatment is applied until regression of neovascular vessels is achieved, until vitreous hemorrhage precludes further therapy, or until there is no remaining area appropriately treatable with laser. Currently, a variety of wavelengths are available when commercial ophthalmic lasers are used for PRP. Numerous studies have suggested that the benefits of panretinal treatment are attained with similar burns regardless of the wavelength used to obtain them and primarily depend on the absorption of laser energy by the pigment epithelium. This layer absorbs all wavelengths so well that PRP can probably be performed with equal efficacy when any currently available wavelength is used. Some wavelengths may have some benefits in reaching the retina given different media conditions, but the main goal is to produce an appropriately placed, correct intensity burn. The DRS used argon blue–green laser (a mixture of 488-nm blue and 515-nm green wavelengths). However, blue light may be harmful for the patient and for the surgeon administering the treatment because of possible absorption by macular xanthophyll pigment. For this reason, the green wavelength is preferred to blue–green for retinal laser photocoagulation. Patients treated with xenon light in the DRS for PDR- although showing benefit-experienced greater losses of visual field and central visual acuity than did patients treated with the argon laser, and its use is no longer recommended.

Commercial dye lasers offer yellow (577-nm), orange (610-nm), and red (630-nm) wavelengths. Yellow probably has effects on the pigment epithelium similar to those of green wavelengths and is presumed to be of equal efficacy. Orange should be avoided, as some studies have suggested the presence of a poorly defined chromophore in human retinas that may absorb orange wavelengths, thereby causing retinal damage. Both dye red and krypton red (647 ran) have nearly identical absorption spectra in the human eye and can be used interchangeably. The advantage of red wavelengths lies in their ability to penetrate through media opacities, such as vitreous hemorrhage or cataract. Unfortunately, red wavelengths also penetrate through the pigment epithelium more deeply than shorter wavelengths and have the potential to cause more choroidal damage and, possibly, choroidal-retinal vascular anastomoses. Red wavelengths also induce significantly more ocular pain, and their use more often requires retrobulbar anesthesia to complete treatment. The availability of the pattern scan diode laser has provided an alternative laser treatment option that allows clinicians to place multiple spots at a time in preset patterns, providing faster treatment times and more exact burn spacing.

A standard, "full-scatter" PRP using the argon laser consists of the application of 1,200 to 1,600 spots approximately 500 µm in size on the retina, with an exposure time of 0.1 second (▶ Table 10.2). The number of spots is increased when the pattern scan laser is used with up to 1,800 to 2,400 spots typically delivered with an exposure time of 0.02 seconds. The power is adjusted to obtain moderately intense white burns spaced approximately one burn width apart for argon lasers and one-half burn width apart for pattern scan lasers (▶ Fig. 10.10). The power level required to achieve burns of this strength depends on the clarity of the media and the pigmentation of the fundus, even if spot size settings and duration are kept constant. The size of the burn is determined mainly by the spot size but is also influenced by the power and duration settings and by the type of contact lens used. This "full-scatter" protocol used in the ETDRS was found to be preferable to "mild-scatter" treatments utilizing greater spacing between burns. Some eyes may require more than 1,600 laser spots, and treatment should be tailored to the individual case. In particular, eyes with marked ischemia and rapidly progressive neovascularization often require aggressive treatment to achieve regression.

In the ETDRS, the initial (complete) PRP treatment was divided into two or more sessions, separated by at least 2 weeks for two sessions and 4 days or so for three or more sessions. Among the techniques currently performed by most retinal surgeons, the number of episodes in which scatter treatment is carried out varies from one to four or more. Although some reports have

Table 10.2 Recommended techniques for laser treatment of diabetic retinopathy

	Laser type	Spot size on retina (µm)	Duration (s)	Intensity[a]	Number	Placement
Argon Laser Technique	Focal-direct	50	0.05–0.1	Mild burn under MA	Sufficient to target all leaking MA	500–3,000 µm from COM, 300–500 µm if < 20/40 and retreatment
	Focal-grid	50	0.05–0.1	Mild, light burns	Cover areas of diffuse edema and capillary nonperfusion	Spaced 2 burn widths apart, 500–3,000 µm from COM, 500 µm from disc
	Scatter (PRP)	400–500	0.05–0.2 (0.1 recommended)	Moderately intense burns	1,200–1,600	Spaced 1 burn width apart, > 2 DD from COM to equator, 500 µm from disc
	Local (direct)	200–500	0.05–0.2	Moderately intense	Overlapping, confluent treatment, 500 µm around margins	> 2 DD from COM scar < 2 DD in diameter
Patter Scan Laser Technique	Focal-direct	50[b]	0.01	Mild burn under MA	Sufficient to target all leaking MA	500–3,000 µm from COM, 300–500 µm if < 20/40 and retreatment
	Focal-grid	50[b]	0.01	Mild, light burns	Cover areas of diffuse edema and capillary nonperfusion	Spaced 2 burn widths apart, 500–3,000 µm from COM, 500 µm from disc
	Scatter (PRP)	400	0.02	Moderately intense burns	1,800–2,400	Spaced 1/2 burn width apart, > 2 DD from COM to equator, 500 µm from disc
	Local (direct)	200–400	0.02	Moderately intense	Overlapping, confluent treatment, 500 µm around margins	> 2 DD from COM scar < 2 DD in diameter

Abbreviations: COM, center of macula; DD, disc diameter; MA, microaneurysm; PRP, panretinal (scatter) photocoagulation.

[a]No specific settings are given for power, as power should be started at a low setting (usually 50–100 mW and titrated upward as needed to achieve the burn intensity described in this column).

[b]Usually set as a 60-µm spot on the machine itself.

suggested that initial associated complications, including serous detachment of the peripheral choroid and ciliary body, are more frequent when PRP is carried out in a single episode, a DRCR.net randomized trial comparing single-session treatment versus PRP delivered over four sessions did not find any clinically meaningful differences in OCT-measured central retinal thickness or visual acuity over the course of 34 weeks of follow-up.[50]

Controversial Points

- Advantages of dividing PRP into multiple sessions may include better patient tolerance and therefore a reduced need for retrobulbar anesthesia. There has been no conclusive evidence that a single-session administration of PRP results in a greater rate of diabetic macular edema or permanent vision loss than a multiple-session approach.

The posterior margin of the treatment should be placed no closer than 2 disc diameters above, temporal to, and below the center of the macula and 500 µm from the nasal margin of the disc (▶ Fig. 10.12). Placement of a single row of spots inside the temporal vascular arcades is acceptable. Anteriorly, laser burns are extended peripherally to or beyond the equator, avoiding direct treatment of major retinal vessels as well as areas of fibrosis, chorioretinal scarring, and large patches of intraretinal hemorrhage. Eyes that have met high-risk PDR criteria are probably more at risk for visual disability from the complications of PDR than from the side effects of panretinal treatment, and the ETDRS protocol should be followed in most cases.

Direct Treatment of Neovascularization of the Retina Elsewhere

Direct (local) treatment of NVE can be effective in destroying new vessels on the surface of the retina. It is primarily used after standard scatter treatment as outlined in the ETDRS treatment protocol has already been performed and directed only at recurrent, relatively small, flat NVE. The technique consists of applying overlapping (confluent) burns to the patch of NVE, with extension of the treatment beyond the margin of the NVE by about 500 µm. To start, laser parameters of 500-µm spot size and 0.1-second duration are used and the power adjusted for a moderately intense tissue uptake. Stronger burns can then be applied using a smaller spot size (200 µm) and longer duration (0.2–0.5 second) to optimize direct destruction of the neovascular focus (▶ Table 10.2). Direct treatment of NVE is discouraged within 2 disc diameters of the center of the macula and whenever local treatment would produce a scar larger than 2 disc diameters. Treatment is also not recommended over major retinal veins, preretinal hemorrhages, or darkly pigmented chorioretinal scars.

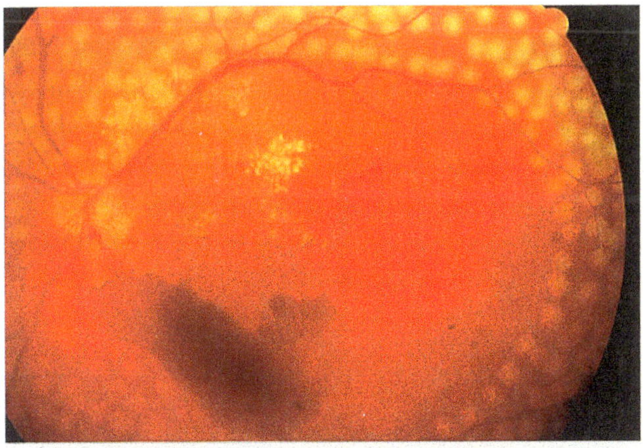

Fig. 10.12 "Full-scatter" panretinal photocoagulation therapy immediately following treatment in an eye with proliferative diabetic retinopathy and high-risk characteristics: Laser spots are of moderate intensity and spaced approximately one-half spot width apart. The posterior margin of the treatment is about 2 disc diameters above, temporal to, and below the center of the macula.

Follow-up for Recurrent Neovascularization

Follow-up at 2- to 4-month intervals is recommended following the initial application of PRP therapy. Careful examinations are necessary, as it may be difficult to identify areas of recurrent or persistent retinal neovascularization against the background of extensive laser scars. Indirect ophthalmoscopy or ultrawide field imaging to visualize the far periphery should also be performed to identify small, visually asymptomatic vitreous or preretinal hemorrhages. Such a finding should prompt the examiner to look more closely for patches of recurrent neovascularization and to consider performing fluorescein angiography or angioscopy in certain cases. Various strategies to consider in the follow-up treatment of persistent or recurrent neovascularization include additional scatter laser treatment, direct (local) laser to NVE, pars plana vitrectomy for uncontrollable fibrovascular proliferation and retinal traction, or perhaps simply continued observation.

Many observers have noted that in some eyes, new vessels continue to grow despite full-scatter treatment or, more commonly, recur after showing evidence of partial or complete regression (▶ Fig. 10.13). When eyes with widespread capillary nonperfusion or severe levels of proliferative retinopathy (NVD and/or vitreous hemorrhage) are treated, regression from high-risk stages may be difficult to achieve despite multiple treatment sessions and an extensive number of laser spots. On the basis of various studies, it appears that additional treatment is justified in at least 25% of eyes following completion of initial scatter photocoagulation, and multiple treatment sessions requiring close follow-up should be anticipated in patients with severe retinal ischemia and advanced stages of PDR, particularly in juvenile-onset type 1 diabetes.

Pearls

- On follow-up examinations after PRP, indirect ophthalmoscopy should be routinely performed to identify small, visually asymptomatic vitreous or preretinal hemorrhages, which can be a sign of persistent (active) neovascularization or new foci of neovascularization. Eyes with such findings that progress or threaten the macula will typically require supplemental PRP.

In follow-up, if new vessels appear to be active and significant vitreous or preretinal hemorrhage occurs, additional

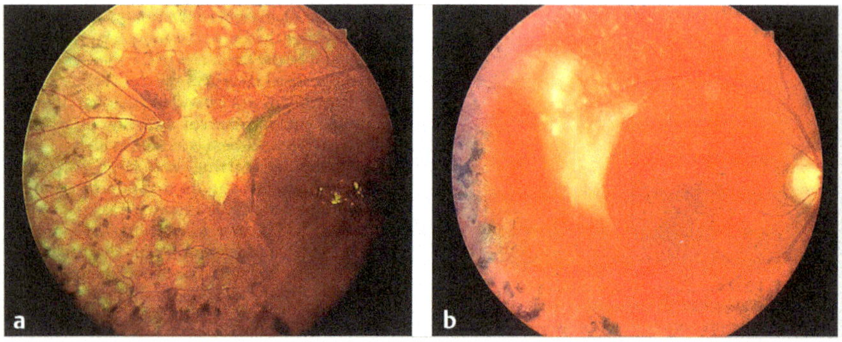

Fig. 10.13 (a) Partially regressed but still active retinal neovascularization along the temporal border of the macula: Recent, supplemental scatter laser spots are seen in the adjacent peripheral retina. (b) Complete regression of the neovascularization with residual fibrosis is evident in this photograph taken 3 months after treatment.

photocoagulation is strongly considered (▶ Fig. 10.13). The case for retreatment is especially convincing if the extent of new vessels is substantially greater than that demonstrated at the time of initial scatter treatment, or if new vessels show continued growth in comparison with previous visits. If the original scatter burns appear widely spaced, or if there are areas where treatment was omitted, additional "fill-in" photocoagulation spots are placed in these areas. The laser indirect ophthalmoscope delivery system is particularly useful to "fill in" the far periphery in cases of continued neovascular activity and good posterior scatter.

Adverse Effects of Panretinal Laser Photocoagulation

A temporary decrease in central visual acuity is frequently observed following scatter photocoagulation, with recovery to the pretreatment level occurring in most cases within several weeks. In the DRS, 21% of argon-treated eyes and 46% of the xenon-treated group showed a decrease in visual acuity of two or more lines at 6 weeks, compared with 9% of untreated eyes.[47] Permanent losses of two or more lines of vision were attributed to scatter treatment in 3% of the argon-treated and 11% of the xenon-treated eyes. In the ETDRS, similar harmful effects of PRP were observed, with 9.7% of the full-scatter group experiencing a three-line or greater loss of vision at the 4-month visit, compared with 3.8% of eyes in the deferral group.[51] Although this figure was reduced to 2.3% in eyes that received focal treatment before scatter treatment, the initial detrimental effect of scatter photocoagulation on central vision appeared to be persistent, as delayed focal treatment applied 4 months later did not reduce the rate of visual loss. Because both the DRS and ETDRS support the clinical impression that eyes with macular edema may worsen following scatter photocoagulation, patients should routinely undergo treatment for center-involved diabetic macular edema (now typically with an anti-VEGF agent) in preparation for scatter treatment.

In the xenon laser-treated group of the DRS, 18% of the eyes with either severe fibrous proliferations or localized traction retinal detachments demonstrated a decrease in visual acuity of five lines or more.[52] In such eyes, progressive contraction of fibrous proliferation sometimes occurred following the PRP, resulting in extension of traction detachment into the center of the macula. A subgroup analysis, however, indicated that even in these eyes, the benefits of scatter treatment outweighed its potential complications. Thus, when high-risk PDR is present in eyes at risk for tractional complications, PRP should still be carried out, with precautions taken to avoid areas of fibrous proliferation, while using mild to moderate laser settings, and treatments divided among several sessions.

Controversial Points

- In eyes with extensive fibrovascular proliferations and localized traction retinal detachments, PRP may promote extension of the traction detachment in some cases. These eyes still benefit from PRP; however, in hopes of minimizing this potential side effect, heavy laser burns close to areas of traction should be avoided and PRP can be divided into several sessions.

Other side effects associated with PRP include decreased night vision, color vision, and peripheral vision, as well as photopsia and a temporary loss of accommodation. Some individuals may experience significant postoperative pain, particularly when extensive treatments are performed in younger patients. Foveal photocoagulation is a rare complication that can be avoided by maintaining proper orientation in the fundus at all times. Ciliochoroidal effusions are more likely to occur with heavy treatments applied in a single episode, with treatments covering large surface areas of the retina, and in eyes with shorter axial lengths.[53,54,55] Fortunately, in the vast majority of cases, they are asymptomatic and resolve without sequelae. (See the following list for a complete list of potential side effects or complications of PRP.) In eyes with diabetic macular edema and concomitant high-risk proliferative retinopathy, the initiation of scatter or PRP may exacerbate the macular edema. These patients are best served if therapy with anti-VEGF medication is performed first for the macular edema in preparation for possible impending scatter treatment.

- Panretinal Laser Photocoagulation: Side Effects and Complications
  - Decreased visual acuity
  - Increased macular edema
  - Decreased night vision
  - Decreased (constricted) peripheral vision
  - Decreased hue discrimination
  - Loss of accommodation and pupillary changes
  - Transient pain
  - Exudative retinal detachment
  - Ciliochoroidal effusions
  - Secondary angle closure and increased intraocular pressure

- Inadvertent foveolar burns
- Exacerbation of traction retinal detachments (controversial)

Anti-VEGF Treatment for PDR

VEGF is a key driver of ocular angiogenesis in PDR, and the retinal neovascularization of PDR is highly sensitive to anti-VEGF therapy. An early report demonstrated that intravitreal treatment with bevacizumab at even 100th the dose typically used for intravitreal injection to treat posterior segment disease can achieve transient regression of NVD and NVE from diabetes.[56] The response of retinal neovascularization to intravitreal anti-VEGF therapy is usually rapid, with visible decreases in perfusion, vascular caliber, and fluorescein leakage often apparent within the first week after treatment (▶ Fig. 10.14).

Phase 3 clinical trials that have evaluated the efficacy of anti-VEGF treatment for diabetic macular edema have reported substantially decreased rates of PDR-related outcomes in these eyes, including less new onset of PDR, vitreous hemorrhage, and need for PRP or vitrectomy.[39] Primary results from the DRCR.net Protocol S, a multicenter trial of prompt PRP versus anti-VEGF treatment with deferred PRP for treatment of PDR, demonstrate that treatment with as needed ranibizumab (0.5 mg) results in visual acuity at 2 years that is noninferior to that in eyes that receive baseline PRP. Advantages of ranibizumab treatment over PRP included greater average visual acuity, decreased loss of peripheral visual field, decreased rates of DME development, and reductions in need for vitrectomy over 2 years. One eye in the ranibizumab-treated group developed endophthalmitis, but no substantial differences were seen between the groups in systemic safety events, including thromboembolic adverse events.

Although the Protocol S results are promising for the use of anti-VEGF as a first-line therapy alternative to PRP, and many eyes with PDR experience rapid and marked regression of neovascularization in response to anti-VEGF therapy, clinical experience reveals that both NVD and NVE can recur once anti-VEGF treatment is withheld. Thus, PRP which has a lasting and durable effect may be a better choice in the eyes of patients who have difficulty with monthly follow-up due to travel or health concerns or who are otherwise noncompliant. Monthly injections of anti-VEGF also expose the patient to the ongoing risk of endophthalmitis and other potential associated adverse events with each injection. Finally, increasing fibrous proliferation can cause progressive traction of the retina in eyes treated with anti-VEGF, putting these eyes at risk for traction detachments that may adversely and severely affect vision if left untreated. Recent studies, however, have suggested this occurs only infrequently. A DRCR.net study comparing ranibizumab versus saline intravitreal injection in eyes with vitreous hemorrhage from PDR found that after injections at baseline, 4 and 8 weeks, traction retinal detachments were present at 16-week follow-up in 6% of eyes in the ranibizumab group as compared to 7% in the saline group.[51] Nevertheless, surgery either alone or in combination with anti-VEGF may be a better first-line treatment in eyes with macula-threatening traction.

Despite these concerns, anti-VEGF treatment for PDR is a promising alternative to PRP in many eyes. In eyes with active PDR that will already be initiating anti-VEGF therapy for center-involved diabetic macular edema, scatter laser photocoagulation can often be delayed, as it may be expected that the PDR will regress substantially in response to the anti-VEGF therapy. These eyes can be reevaluated for need for PDR treatment once anti-VEGF treatment is no longer needed for the macular edema. Furthermore, intravitreal anti-VEGF treatment is useful prior to surgery in eyes for which vitrectomy is planned for active PDR and its complications. The preoperative administration of anti-VEGF in these eyes causes regression of new vessels and thereby reduces intraoperative bleeding. Anti-VEGF in these cases should generally be given no longer than 1 week prior to surgery in order to minimize chances of worsening macular traction.

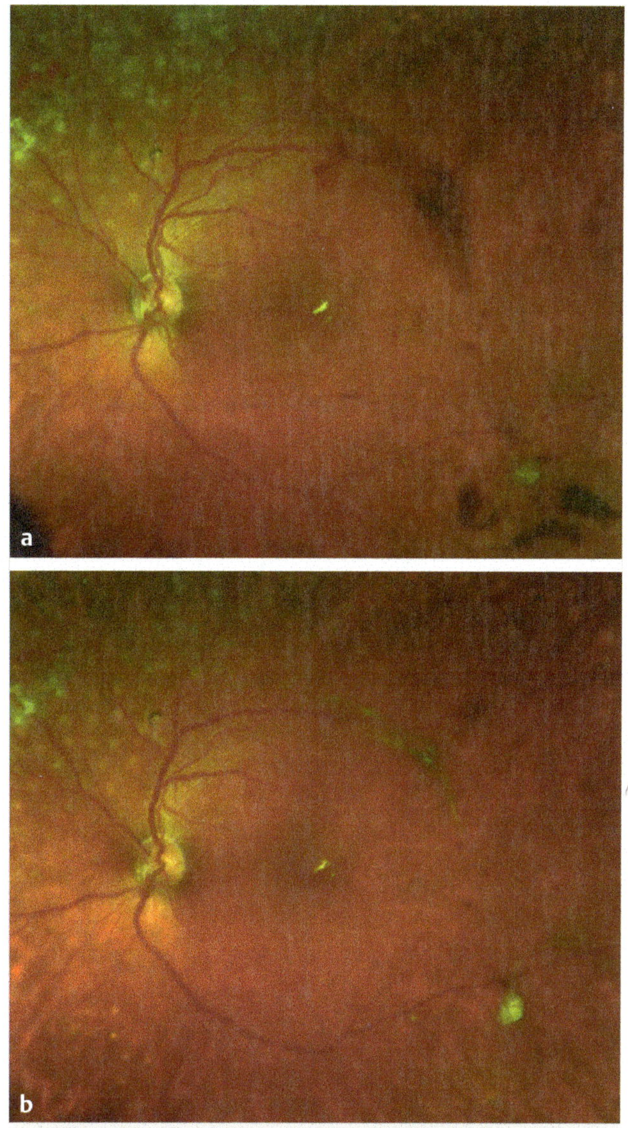

Fig. 10.14 Response of proliferative diabetic retinopathy to intravitreal anti-vascular endothelial growth factor (anti-VEGF) therapy: (**a**) Baseline ultrawide field fundus photograph demonstrating large, active areas of neovascularization of the retina elsewhere (NVE) along the supero- and inferotemporal arcades. (**b**) One month after anti-VEGF treatment, the areas of NVE are regressed and fibrotic.

10.7 Diabetic Macular Edema

Diabetic macular edema may be present at any level of retinopathy and occurs in approximately 10% of all patients with diabetes mellitus.[17] As might be expected, the prevalence of macular edema is directly related to the overall severity of the retinopathy and its duration, ranging from 3% among eyes with mild NPDR to 38% among eyes with moderate to severe NPDR and 71% among eyes with PDR.[57] Macular edema may occur earlier in the course of diabetes for older patients (higher incidence in the first 5 years after diagnosis), likely in part because many patients with type 2 diabetes may have had subclinical diabetes for an indeterminate period of time prior to their diagnosis. The subset of older-onset patients requiring insulin has the highest prevalence of macular edema among all groups.[57]

10.7.1 Clinical Features

Diabetic macular edema results from abnormal increased vascular permeability leading to accumulations of intraretinal or subretinal fluid. Vitreomacular traction can also play a role in the retinal thickening from diabetic macular edema. The cellular distortion and impairment that results from macular edema is initially reversible. However, chronic leakage affecting the central macula can lead to a permanent loss of vision, either from extensive hard exudate deposition or degenerative changes in the fovea. Intraretinal hard exudates are composed of plasma lipoproteins derived from leaking microaneurysms, and they are deposited predominantly in the outer and inner plexiform layers. Occasionally, this exudate may be deposited beneath the sensory retina and evolve into an organized plaque, leading to photoreceptor degeneration, SVL, and fibrous metaplasia of the retinal pigment epithelium (RPE).[58] A dysfunction in the barrier and transport functions of the RPE may also contribute to the development of diffuse macular edema.[59] Some patients with diffuse patterns of edema manifest signs of systemic fluid retention from concurrent heart failure, renal disease, or systemic hypertension, and appropriate treatment of these systemic abnormalities may induce some resolution of the visual impairment.

In the current era in which intravitreal anti-VEGF therapy is considered first-line treatment for most eyes with center-involved diabetic macular edema, the most relevant characteristic that helps determine management recommendations is whether or not the retinal thickening involves the 1 mm in diameter central zone of the macula. If the central 1 mm zone is thickened, the eye is considered to have *center* (or *central) involved diabetic macular edema.* If the central 1 mm zone is not affected, but there is retinal thickening within the macula, the eye has *non–center-involved diabetic macular edema.* Currently, eyes with non-center-involved diabetic macular edema are generally observed for progression to central involvement before anti-VEGF therapy is initiated, as the risk of vision loss is low in these cases.

Prior to the time when intravitreal anti-VEGF treatment was available, the ETDRS defined the presence of *clinically significant macular edema (CSME)* as the threshold for instituting focal/grid macular laser photocoagulation. CSME was defined as the presence of any one of the following criteria (▶ Fig. 10.15):

1. Retinal thickening at or within 500 µm of the center of the macula
2. Hard exudates at or within 500 µm of the center of the macula, if associated with thickening of adjacent retina (which may be outside the 500-µm limit)
3. Zone or zones of retinal thickening 1 disc area in size, at least part of which is within 1 disc diameter of the center of the macula

Diabetic macular edema may also be described as either localized or diffuse retinal thickening, with or without deposits of intraretinal hard exudates. *Localized (or focal) edema* refers to a circumscribed area of retinal thickening resulting from discrete foci of leaking microaneurysms. The characteristic appearance is a circular area of edema demarcated by a ring of hard exudate in a circinate pattern, with clusters of leaking microaneurysms at its center (▶ Fig. 10.16). *Diffuse edema* is more widespread retinal thickening caused by generalized leakage from

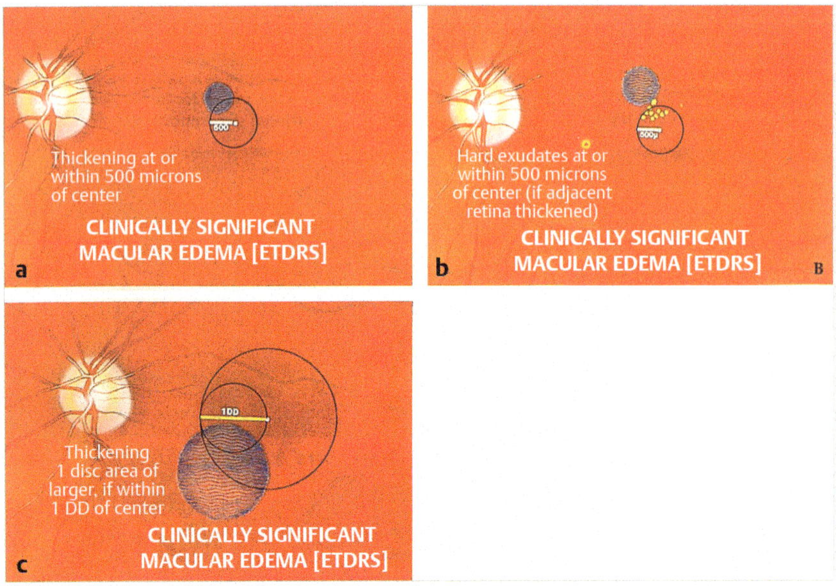

Fig. 10.15 Three subtypes of clinically significant macular edema (CSME) as defined in the Early Treatment Diabetic Retinopathy Study (ETDRS)

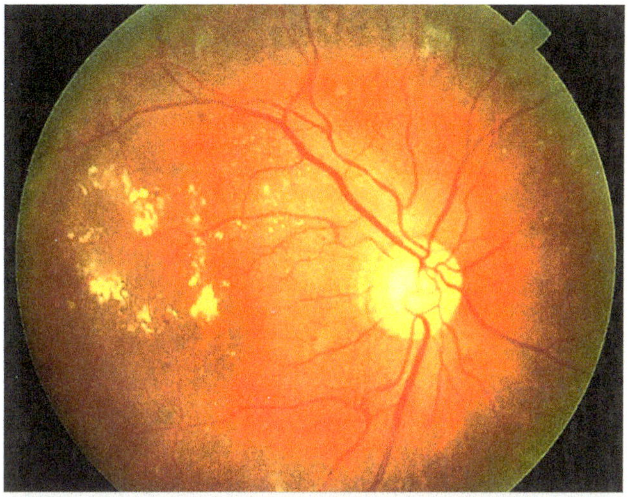

Fig. 10.16 Focal macular edema: A discrete area of retinal thickening with a typical circinate ring of hard exudate formation.

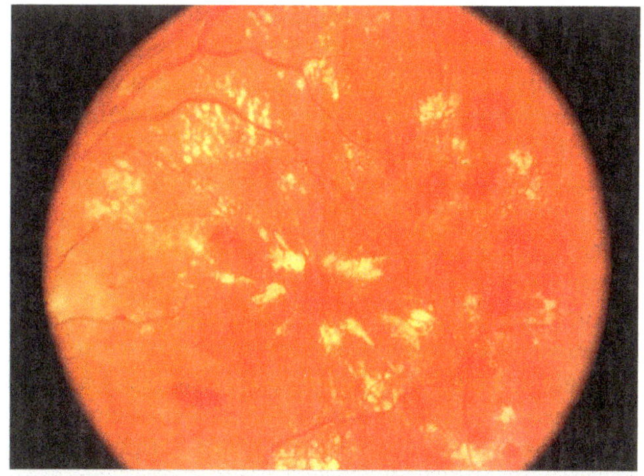

Fig. 10.17 Diffuse macular edema: Retinal thickening and scattered hard exudates are present throughout the macula.

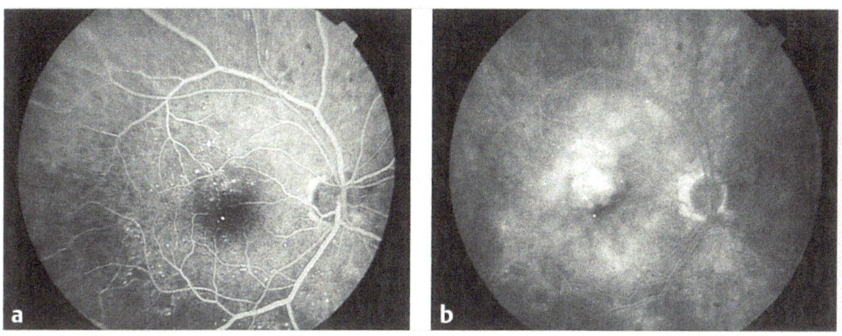

Fig. 10.18 Mixed focal and diffuse diabetic macular edema: Early (**a**) and late (**b**) frame fluorescein angiogram photographs showing a cluster of leaking microaneurysms and more widespread intraretinal dye leakage evident only later in the study.

abnormally permeable and dilated capillaries throughout the posterior pole (▶ Fig. 10.17 and ▶ Fig. 10.18), often associated with areas of retinal nonperfusion.

Ischemic maculopathy, either with or without macular edema, is another source of central vision loss in patients with diabetic retinopathy. It represents closure or nonperfusion of perifoveal capillaries (▶ Fig. 10.19).[57] Despite the considerable overlap in the dimensions of the foveal avascular zone (FAZ) between normal and diabetic patients, there does appear to be a correlation between FAZ size and advancing levels of retinopathy, with enlargement greater than 1,000 µm being seen almost exclusively in eyes with severe PDR.[60] More specific signs of diabetes-related FAZ abnormalities include irregularities of the avascular zone margins, capillary "budding" into zones of capillary closure, and widening of the intercapillary spaces in the perifoveal capillary bed.[60]

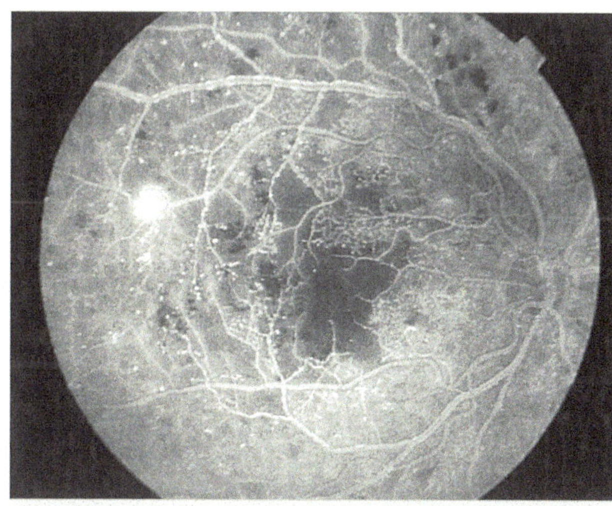

Fig. 10.19 Macular ischemia: Fluorescein angiogram photograph showing extensive perifoveal capillary dropout resulting in an abnormally enlarged and irregular foveal avascular zone. (The patient had markedly reduced visual acuity but no significant macular thickening)

10.7.2 Management and Course

Anti-VEGF Therapy

Multiple, large-scale clinical trials have clearly established intravitreously administered anti-VEGF therapy as the current first-line treatment for eyes with visual impairment from center-involved diabetic macular edema. The DRCR.net Protocol I study ("Randomized Trial Evaluating Ranibizumab Plus Prompt or Deferred Laser or Triamcinolone Plus Prompt Laser for Diabetic Macular Edema") was the first major phase 3 study to demonstrate the substantial increased efficacy of anti-VEGF treatment over macular focal/grid laser photocoagulation in improving visual acuity outcomes in eyes with center-involved diabetic macular edema.[56] At the primary outcome time point of 1 year, the two ranibizumab-treated groups (one treated with prompt laser starting at baseline and the other treated with deferred laser starting at 6 months if there was persistent edema despite anti-VEGF treatment) gained eight and nine letters in visual acuity as compared to the laser-treated group which gained only three letters of vision. This difference in visual outcome was maintained throughout 2 years, with mean differences of nearly four and six letters in the ranibizumab plus prompt and deferred laser groups, respectively, as compared with the sham plus laser group. The anatomic results reflected the visual outcomes, with greater reduction in retinal thickening in the anti-VEGF arms than in the laser control arm of this study. Similar results demonstrating a clear benefit of anti-VEGF over macular laser treatment alone have been reported in additional phase 3 studies utilizing monthly ranibizumab and trials of aflibercept for diabetic macular edema.

Commercially available anti-VEGF agents include aflibercept, bevacizumab, pegaptanib, and ranibizumab. Of these, only aflibercept and ranibizumab are currently approved by the United States Food and Drug Administration for the treatment of diabetic macular edema. Despite its off-label status, however, bevacizumab has also been used widely for diabetic macular edema because it provides an alternative that is of substantially lower cost and yet roughly comparable efficacy. In 2015, the DRCR.net reported results from a comparative effectiveness study (Protocol T) that enrolled eyes with center-involved diabetic macular edema with vision of 20/32 to 20/320 and randomized these eyes to treatment with aflibercept, bevacizumab, or ranibizumab.[61] Six hundred and sixty participants, each with a single study eye, were enrolled in this study. This study demonstrated substantial visual acuity improvement in all three treatment arms. However, in the overall cohort, aflibercept treatment led to significantly better visual outcomes at the primary outcome 1 year time point. Aflibercept-treated eyes gained 13 letters of vision as compared to 11 and 10 letters of visual improvement in the ranibizumab and bevacizumab-treated groups, respectively. It is important to recognize that this difference in treatment effect was driven by outcomes from the eyes with worse baseline visual acuity (20/50 or worse). In this group, which represented approximately 50% of the total cohort, aflibercept-treated eyes gained 19 letters of vision as compared to 14 and 12 letters gained by the ranibizumab and bevacizumab groups, respectively. The rate of 10 or more letters vision gain in this subset with worse baseline visual acuity was correspondingly much higher in the aflibercept arm than in either the ranibizumab or bevacizumab arms (77, 69, and 60%, respectively). In contrast, there was no significant difference between 1 year vision outcomes in eyes with vision of 20/32 or 20/40 at baseline. On average, each of the groups gained 8 letters of vision over the first year of treatment, and rates of 10-letter improvement were similar between the three treatment arms (aflibercept 50%, bevacizumab 45%, and ranibizumab 50%). In all groups, rates of 10 or more letters of vision loss were low at 4% or less. The retinal thickness outcomes were generally consistent with the visual outcomes, but revealed that bevacizumab-treated eyes had the least improvement in central retinal edema regardless of baseline visual acuity status.

The optimal dosing schedule and retreatment algorithm for eyes with diabetic macular edema may not be fully established, but given the excellent visual results obtained in both the DRCR.net Protocol I and T studies, many clinicians utilize the protocols outlined in these studies for anti-VEGF retreatment guidelines. Eyes enrolled in Protocol T were treated at the baseline visit and reinjected at each subsequent visit if there was improvement or worsening (defined by thresholds of five or more letters visual acuity change or a 10% or more change in the central subfield thickness on OCT). Injections were deferred only if an eye had been stable over the last two injections. In eyes in which treatment was deferred for stability, injections were resumed if there was any worsening by either the vision or OCT criteria. Visits occurred monthly over the first year, but the follow-up intervals were extended in the second year of treatment to a maximum of 16 weeks if treatment continued to be deferred. On average, following these treatment guidelines, eyes received 8 to 10 injections over the first year of Protocol T. In Protocol I, using similar guidelines, the need for treatment declined after the first year to only two to three injections in the second year, one to two injections in the third year, and zero to one injections in the fourth and fifth years of the study.

Data from both Protocol I and the RIDE/RISE studies suggest that visual gains obtained during an initial period of monthly administration of anti-VEGF can be maintained as eyes are transitioned to less frequent as-needed treatment as long as sufficient early therapy has been given. However, a delay of 2 years or more in initiating anti-VEGF therapy may lead to worse visual outcomes as evidenced by the fact that the RIDE/RISE group initially treated with sham injections did not achieve the same visual gains after 1 year of continuous monthly therapy as did the groups that had started monthly ranibizumab 2 years before.[9]

Additional data suggest that intravitreal anti-VEGF therapy may be similarly effective in eyes that have previously undergone vitrectomy as in eyes that have not been vitrectomized. Initial reports of decreased half-lives for bevacizumab and ranibizumab in rabbit eyes after vitrectomy implied that effectiveness of anti-VEGF agents might be limited in eyes with diabetic macular edema that had previously been vitrectomized due to faster clearance of the drugs.[62] However, a review of eyes enrolled in the DRCR.net Protocol I that were randomized to ranibizumab treatment revealed that the visual acuity and retinal thickness outcomes did not differ substantially between vitrectomized eyes and the nonvitrectomized cohort through 3 years.[63] Thus, the use of intravitreal anti-VEGF therapy appears warranted for the treatment of center-involved diabetic macular edema regardless of an eye's prior history of vitrectomy.

Much scrutiny has been given to the safety profile of intravitreal anti-VEGF treatments because of the increased risk for thromboembolic events when anti-VEGF medications are given systemically in much higher doses (several hundred-fold the doses used for ocular treatments) as chemotherapeutic agents for cancer. Fortunately, intravitreal anti-VEGF appears to be safe and well tolerated in eyes treated for diabetic macular edema. The most common associated serious adverse events, such as endophthalmitis, are related to the intravitreal injection procedure rather than the medication. Studies have not found any consistent association between intravitreal anti-VEGF therapy and increased rates of thromboembolic events such as those included in the combination endpoint defined by the Antiplatelet Trialists' Collaboration of non–fatal myocardial infarction, non–fatal stroke, or vascular death.

Although the majority of eyes demonstrate at least a partially favorable response to anti-VEGF treatment for diabetic macular edema, approximately 40 to 50% of eyes treated with anti-VEGF therapy will not have a complete response resulting in 20/20 or better vision or complete resolution of macular edema. Given the high potency and excellent selectivity of the available anti-VEGF medications, this suboptimal response in the face of frequent and sustained treatment suggests that diabetic macular edema is a multifactorial process and that pathways other than those related to VEGF may be active in eyes with incomplete response.

Pearls

- Intravitreal anti-VEGF treatment should be considered first-line therapy for most eyes with center-involved diabetic macular edema and associated visual impairment. Although optimal therapy requires frequent, monthly injections over the first year of treatment, it is usually possible to substantially reduce the number and frequency of injections in the following years while maintaining excellent visual results.

Steroid Therapy

Initial reports of intravitreal steroid treatment in eyes with diabetic macular edema were highly encouraging, in that rapid reductions in retinal thickening and associated improvements in visual acuity were seen within the first few months after steroid administration.[64] However, longer-term studies over the course of a year and more revealed that these short-term gains were not sustained over longer durations. The DRCR.net Protocol B compared safety and efficacy of intravitreal triamcinolone monotherapy with macular laser photocoagulation for diabetic macular edema.[65] Although visual acuity and retinal thickness were better in the steroid-treated eyes at 4 months, there were no significant differences in visual outcomes between the steroid and laser groups at 1 year and by 16 months, and mean visual acuity was better in the laser group than in the steroid groups. Similar results were seen in Protocol I in which early gains in the steroid with prompt laser group had disappeared by the 1-year visit. At the 1-year primary outcome time point, this group had visual outcomes that were equivalent to the laser control arm and inferior to either of the anti-VEGF–treated arms.

Steroid-related ocular adverse events are common and include cataract development, and intraocular pressure rises that can lead to glaucoma. Indeed, much of the decline in vision in the Protocol I steroid group was likely related to cataract development in the phakic eyes, as steroid-treated eyes that were pseudophakic at baseline in this trial had very similar visual outcomes to those treated with anti-VEGF medication. By month 24 of this study, more than 70% of steroid-treated eyes underwent cataract surgery as compared to approximately 20% of the anti-VEGF and laser-treated eyes.[66] Rates of elevated intraocular pressure were also more common in the steroid arm.

Although intravitreal steroid is generally not considered first-line treatment for eyes with diabetic macular edema, steroids do have a role, particularly as second-line treatment in eyes that have not previously responded well to anti-VEGF therapy. As currently available steroid formulations have duration of action ranging from approximately 3 months to 3 years, and phase 3 studies have demonstrated some efficacy for diabetic macular edema,[67,68] steroids may also be a viable alternative for some patients who cannot comply with the monthly follow-up visits necessary during the first year of anti-VEGF treatment, especially if they are pseudophakic.

Intravitreal Injection Technique

Both anti-VEGF and steroid agents are delivered via intravitreal injection. Repeated experience over tens of thousands of intravitreal injections in eyes of patients with diabetes strongly suggests that these injections are generally safe and well tolerated with either topical or subconjunctival anesthesia. Over the course of the first 8,027 intravitreal injections performed within DRCR.net studies, there were only seven cases of endophthalmitis.[69] Six of these cases occurred with the use of topical antibiotics and one case occurred without the use of topical antibiotics. Other associated serious ocular complications are rare, including retinal tears or detachment, vitreous hemorrhage, or traumatic cataract. Common, mild adverse events may be associated with intravitreal injection and the eye preparation procedure can include conjunctival injection, subconjunctival hemorrhage, superficial punctate keratitis, corneal abrasion, and transient, self-limited floaters.

Intravitreal injections are performed 3.5 to 4 mm posterior to the limbus. The DRCR.net protocol for intravitreal injection required the use of topical povidone iodine and a sterile lid speculum, but did not mandate the use of pre- or postinjection antibiotics, sterile gloves, or a sterile drape. The use of a lid speculum reduces lid movement during the injection and therefore theoretically may decrease the chance of contamination of the conjunctival surface. However, use of a lid speculum does not appear to have an effect on the rate of postinjection infection based on other studies. Although intraocular pressure rises immediately postinjection due to the increased volume in the eye, this elevation is typically mild and self-limited and usually does not require either topical ocular antihypertensives or aqueous paracentesis. Nonetheless, it is important to check for the restoration of optic nerve perfusion and return of vision to the eye before allowing the patient to leave the clinic.

Pearls

- When performing an intravitreal injection, the use of topical povidone iodine is essential to minimize the risk for subsequent endophthalmitis.

Focal/Grid Macular Laser Treatment

Although macular laser treatment is no longer considered first-line therapy for most eyes with center-involved diabetic macular edema, laser photocoagulation still has an important role as adjunctive therapy in eyes that have persistent edema despite anti-VEGF treatment. In addition, laser is an excellent option for patients who either cannot tolerate invasive procedures or who cannot comply with the monthly visits required for the optimal initiation of anti-VEGF therapy. Some eyes with easily identifiable focal leakage from specific microaneurysms may also benefit from laser procedures that target these microaneurysms and ameliorate the retinal edema over a limited number of treatment sessions. Eyes with DME that is not center involved can often be observed rather than treated, as rates of progression to center involvement are generally low, and outcomes with anti-VEGF treatment once DME affects the central retina are excellent. Nonetheless, specific cases of non–center-involved DME (such as those threatening the center with circinate rings indicating highly focal leakage) may benefit from focal laser treatment that targets the leaking microaneurysms, thereby resolving the DME and obviating the need for future anti-VEGF therapy.

The ETDRS demonstrated that eyes with CSME benefited from immediate focal argon laser photocoagulation, which significantly reduces the risk for moderate visual loss (MVL) (▶ Fig. 10.20). (In the ETDRS, MVL was defined as loss of 15 or more letters on a standardized visual acuity chart, which was equivalent to a doubling of the visual angle, e.g., from 20/25 to 20/50.) Further analysis showed that focal laser treatment was most beneficial for eyes meeting criteria for CSME, decreasing the incidence of visual loss by approximately 50% at the 3-year mark (30% risk for MVL reduced to 15%).[6] The subgroup of eyes with CSME involving the center of the macula experienced an even more profound visual acuity benefit with treatment (33% risk for MVL reduced to 13%). Eyes in which macular edema was not clinically significant at baseline had low rates of visual loss, and differences between the treatment and deferral groups were small, particularly in the first 2 years of follow-up. Focal laser treatment also increased the likelihood of visual improvement, with 16% of patients gaining more than one line of acuity (▶ Fig. 10.21). Major adverse side effects were not noted with focal treatment, except for minor losses of visual field and occasional paracentral scotomas. With a large benefit-to-risk ratio, the ETDRS recommended that focal photocoagulation should be considered for all eyes with CSME.

Visual prognosis after macular laser for diabetic macular edema tends to be most favorable when areas of leakage are primarily focal in nature and less favorable when leakage is diffuse. Other factors that predict a poor response to focal photocoagulation include ischemic maculopathy with extensive perifoveal capillary nonperfusion, cystoid changes resulting from chronic edema, and hard exudate deposits in the foveola. Patients of increased age and on treatment for systemic hypertension have been identified on retrospective reviews not to respond as well to focal laser therapy.[70,71]

Controversial Points

- Although macular laser treatment is no longer considered first-line therapy for most eyes with center-involved diabetic macular edema, laser still has an important role as adjunctive therapy in eyes that have not responded completely to anti-VEGF therapy and also for eyes that may not be candidates for repeated anti-VEGF injections. Some eyes with purely focal leakage from microaneurysms may be good candidates for primary laser treatment that can resolve retinal thickening in only one or two therapeutic sessions that may obviate the need for further treatment.

Technique

As described in the ETDRS, *direct treatment* involves the application of laser photocoagulation spots to all leaking microaneurysms between 500 and 3,000 µm (2 disc diameters) from the center of the macula. Treatment of focal leaks between 300 and 500 µm from the center may be performed if (1) previous treatment has been applied and CSME persists, (2) vision is less than 20/40, and (3) treatment is not likely to destroy the remaining perifoveal capillary network. Treatment of microaneurysms or other focal points of leakage farther than 2 disc diameters from the center of the macula is optional but can be

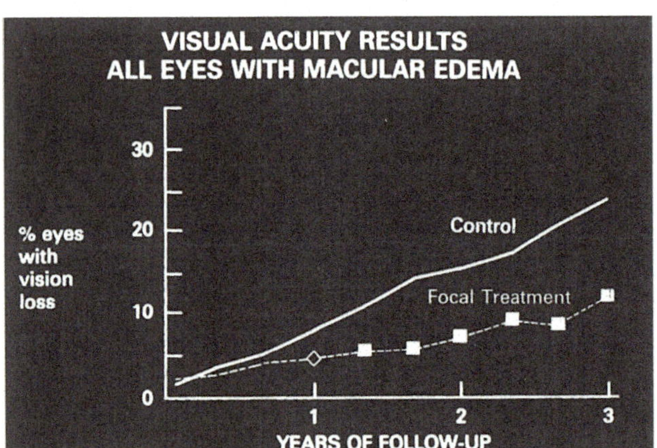

Fig. 10.20 Visual acuity results of the Early Treatment Diabetic Retinopathy Study Group demonstrating that immediate focal photocoagulation for macular edema reduces the risk for moderate visual loss (doubling of the visual angle) by 50%.

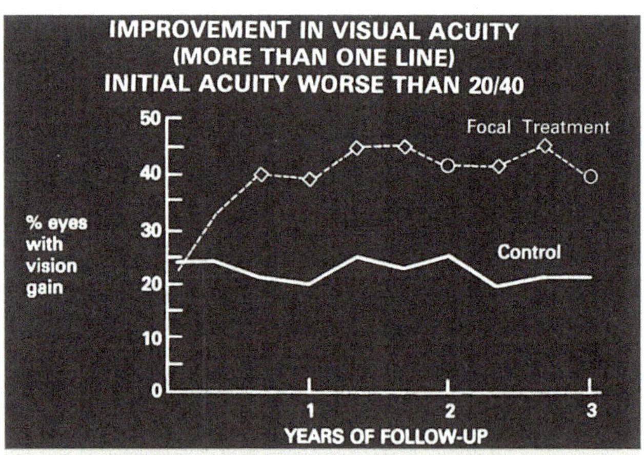

Fig. 10.21 Results of the Early Treatment Diabetic Retinopathy Study Group showing percentage of patients with improvement in visual acuity (six letters or more) assigned to either immediate focal photocoagulation or deferral of treatment: Focal laser treatment for clinically significant macular edema increases the chances for visual improvement.

considered if they leak prominently and are associated with retinal thickening or hard exudate rings that extend into the macula (▶ Table 10.2). Power is initially set at 50 mW and increased slowly to obtain a burn under the microaneurysm. Originally whitening or darkening of the microaneurysm at the minimum power settings (▶ Fig. 10.22) was considered an endpoint, as a color change usually indicates that sufficient heat has been generated to coagulate the wall of the microaneurysm. This is rarely achieved with microaneurysms smaller than 40 µm and currently the expected endpoint is simply mild to moderate whitening of the underlying retina, with care being taken to avoid rupturing Bruch's membrane.

Grid treatment is the primary mode of laser therapy for eyes with diffuse macular edema. Grid treatment consists of placing light burns, 50 to 200 µm in size, at the level of the RPE in areas of leakage that are more than 500 µm from the center of the macula and 500 µm from the temporal margin of the optic nerve. Exposure time is 0.1 second or less, and power settings are started at 10 mW and increased slowly to obtain a light gray-white lesion in the outer retina (▶ Table 10.2). In general, the spot should be significantly less intense than a PRP burn and just light enough so that it can be barely visualized, a minimum criterion to ensure proper spacing between burns. Overtreatment should be avoided to minimize paracentral scotomas, keeping in mind that future enlargement of laser spots can lead to coalescence of the chorioretinal scars in the macula (▶ Fig. 10.23).

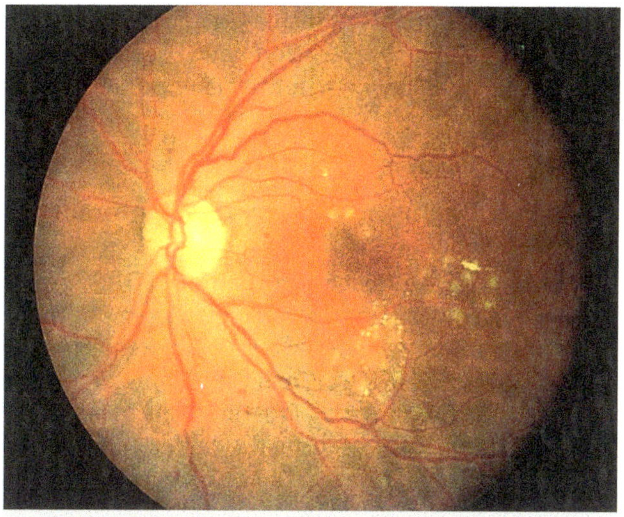

Fig. 10.22 Focal laser photocoagulation: Laser spots (immediately after treatment) directed at microaneurysms within the discrete areas of macular thickening.

Pearls

To avoid complications of focal/grid laser photocoagulation treatment of DME:

- Treat only areas of the macula that are thickened.
- Treat lightly by starting with low-power settings and titrating in small increments.
- Do not treat within 500 µm of the foveal center with the first treatment session.
- Do not space laser spots less than one spot width apart.
- Avoid placing laser spots in intraretinal hemorrhage or at the edge of an enlarged FAZ

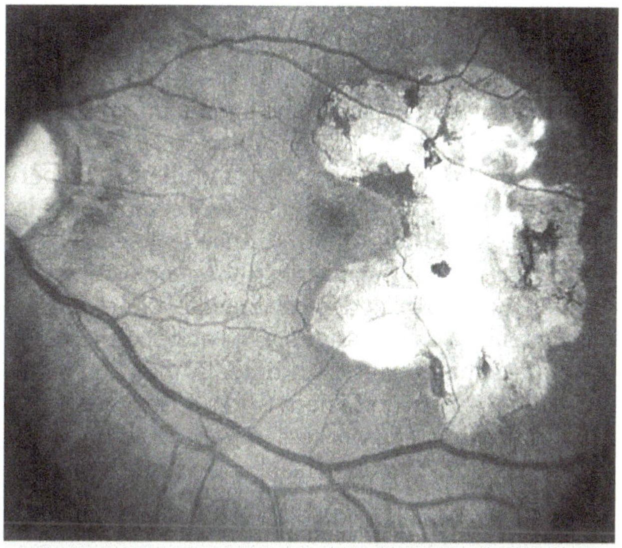

Fig. 10.23 Focal photocoagulation spots that were too high in intensity resulted in a large, confluent, symptomatic chorioretinal scar.

The majority of cases are best treated with a combination of direct and grid treatment, with the proper sequence being the administration of direct treatment first, followed by subsequent grid laser therapy. The exact mechanism responsible for the efficacy of focal laser treatment for DME is not known, although treatment effects presumably are based on stimulation of RPE, changes in VEGF expression, and direct closure of leaking microaneurysms.

When focal laser treatment in the macula is performed, care must be taken to avoid rupturing Bruch's membrane, which can result in the subsequent development of choroidal neovascularization (CNV). This rare but serious complication has been reported to originate from previous photocoagulation scars in the macula, with the postulated mechanism being high-intensity, often small (50-µm) burns (mean power used, 256 mW) causing iatrogenic breaks in Bruch's membrane.[72] Cases of avascular submacular fibrosis have also been reported following macular laser therapy.[73] Although specific predisposing factors for this scarring could not be identified, such cases emphasize the need to avoid excessive energy delivery to the macula. (See the following list for a complete list of potential side effects or complications of focal laser treatment.)

- Focal Laser Photocoagulation: Side Effects and Complications
  - Paracentral scotomas
  - Transient increased edema/decreased vision
  - Choroidal neovascularization
  - Subretinal fibrosis
  - Photocoagulation scar expansion
  - Inadvertent foveolar burns

Follow-up

Patients should be aware that it usually takes at least 1 to 4 months for the maximum effect of edema resorption to be seen after a session of focal laser treatment, and follow-up intervals of 3 to 4 months are recommended for most patients. A temporary increase in the amount of exudate immediately following laser therapy is not unusual and should not be considered an indication for retreatment. In fact, this can represent rapid resorption of the edema with deposition of the lipid components, which generally resolves some time later. If there is residual CSME at 4 months, the fluorescein angiogram may be repeated and retreatment performed if treatable lesions are present. These consist of persistent leaking microaneurysms more than 500 µm from the center of the macula or 300 µm from the center if vision is less than 20/40 and there is no perifoveal capillary dropout. Grid laser therapy can also be administered to areas of diffuse leakage 500 µm from the center of the macula if these areas have not been treated previously; retreatment over areas treated previously is not recommended, as excessive spread and coalescence of laser scars may result with time. In many patients, multiple treatment sessions spread through many months are necessary to stabilize vision.

10.8 Surgery in the Diabetic Eye

10.8.1 Pars Plana Vitrectomy

When pars plana vitrectomy was introduced in 1971, its initial indications in diabetic patients included longstanding vitreous hemorrhage and traction retinal detachment involving the posterior pole (▶ Fig. 10.24).[74] As vitrectomy surgery came into more widespread use, it was recognized that earlier intervention might be of value in eyes with severe PDR. The DRVS was a clinical trial designed to evaluate the efficacy of early vitrectomy for eyes with visually debilitating vitreous hemorrhage.[7,75,76] In the DRVS, eyes with recent vitreous hemorrhage and visual acuity of less than 5/200 for at least 1 month were assigned randomly to either early vitrectomy (1–6 months) or conventional management (follow-up unless retinal detachment involved the center of the macula or the hemorrhage failed to clear during a 1-year waiting period). After 2 years of follow-up, recovery of good levels of vision (visual acuity of 10/20 or better) was observed more frequently in the early vitrectomy group (25 vs. 15% in the conventional management group).

The DRVS classified patients as having type 1 diabetes mellitus if the diagnosis was made at or before 20 years of age and if the patients were receiving insulin at the time of entrance into the study. Patients aged 40 or older at the time of diagnosis (regardless of insulin use) were classified as having type 2 diabetes mellitus, as were patients with diabetes diagnosed at a younger age if they were not receiving insulin at the time of entering the study. Further analysis from the DRVS showed that early vitrectomy was clearly advantageous only for the type 1 group, in which good vision (visual acuity of 10/20 or better) was attained by 36% of patients undergoing early vitrectomy versus 12% of those in the conventional management group. The greatest advantage for early vitrectomy was shown for the subgroup of patients with type 1 disease of less than 20 years' duration (34 vs. 2% in the conventional management group).

A possible explanation for the disparate advantage of early vitrectomy in patients with type 1 diabetes mellitus is that younger patients typically have more severe proliferative disease and are at higher risk for the development of new vessels and vitreoretinal traction complications while they are waiting for the vitreous hemorrhage to clear. Older patients, on the other hand, more often have milder proliferative disease at the time of vitreous hemorrhage presentation, and waiting for the hemorrhage to clear may not be as detrimental. One should, however, not interpret the DRVS data to conclude that it is safe to wait many months for *all* patients with type 2 disease and dense vitreous hemorrhage. Early vitrectomy should be considered in these patients if the neovascular proliferation is known to be (or suspected of being) extensive or rapidly progressive.[76]

A number of other diabetic retinopathy complications can benefit from surgical intervention. Most, but not all, of these complications arise during the more advanced, proliferative stages of the disease. Overall, the main indications for vitrectomy in the setting of diabetic retinopathy are summarized as follows:

- Visually significant, nonclearing vitreous hemorrhage.
- Traction retinal detachment involving or threatening the macula.
- Combined traction–rhegmatogenous retinal detachment.
- Miscellaneous:
  - Progressive fibrovascular proliferation (despite extensive PRP).
  - Refractory macular edema with an attached posterior hyaloid.
  - Traction on the macula (without detachment) causing decreased visual acuity.
  - Eyes with rubeosis and media opacities precluding PRP.
  - Opacified premacular membrane or posterior hyaloid face.

It is important to note that surgical advances over the last decade, including smaller gauge instrumentation, laser endocoagulation, bimanual techniques, and improved widefield viewing systems, have enabled faster surgical times and markedly reduced complication rates, probably making the specific results of the DRVS no longer reflective of current surgical

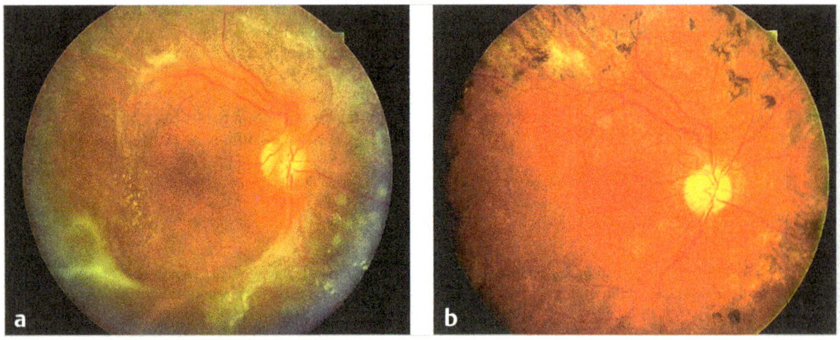

Fig. 10.24 Proliferative diabetic retinopathy with traction retinal detachments: **(a)** Extensive, confluent fibrovascular proliferation along the disc and temporal arcades with early macula-involving traction detachment and decreased visual acuity. **(b)** Six months after pars plana vitrectomy, membrane peeling, and panretinal laser, an attached retina is completely free of traction and there is no active proliferative retinopathy. (Image courtesy of Carl D. Regillo, MD)

intervention results. Additional information regarding vitrectomy surgical techniques and indications can be found in Chapter 40.

10.8.2 Cataract Surgery and Diabetic Retinopathy

Cataract extraction in diabetic patients is commonly indicated, both for visual rehabilitation and for improved visualization of the fundus. In the current era of small incision techniques, visual results are usually excellent. However, the visual prognosis for diabetic patients undergoing cataract surgery can be suboptimal, mainly because of the risk of worsening retinopathy severity or macular edema. Almost all cases demonstrate progression within the first 6 months after surgery, manifested most commonly as worsening of NPDR and exacerbation of macular edema, although a minority of eyes progress to PDR, vitreous hemorrhage, and iris neovascularization.[77]

When extracapsular cataract extraction (ECCE) with posterior chamber lens implantation is performed in diabetic eyes, the overall rate of retinopathy progression is approximately 30 to 39%.[77,78] Patients undergoing intracapsular cataract extraction (ICCE) experience a much higher rate of retinopathy progression when compared with groups undergoing extracapsular surgery. It is speculated that an intact posterior lens capsule acts as a semipermeable barrier to the diffusion of various factors between the anterior and posterior chambers, reducing both the neovascular and inflammatory complications postoperatively. In eyes with PDR that have undergone ICCE, the rate of anterior segment neovascularization can be as high as 40%.[79] Similar risks apply to ECCE cases complicated by vitreous loss and a ruptured posterior capsule, although subsequent posterior capsulotomy does not appear to increase the rate of visual deterioration.[80] Eyes with active PDR at the time of surgery have the highest risk for retinopathy progression and the worst prognosis for visual improvement. Conversely, eyes that have no maculopathy and have reached a quiescent stage of proliferative retinopathy (either through prior photocoagulation or vitrectomy) usually demonstrate a favorable course, with approximately 50% attaining a visual acuity of 20/40 or better.[80]

Current cataract surgeons predominantly utilize phacoemulsification or other advanced techniques. These techniques result in shorter operative time, less tissue damage, faster recovery, and fewer complications than ICCE and ECCE. Rates of diabetic retinopathy progression do not appear to be substantially higher after an uncomplicated phacoemulsification than those that occur with the natural history of the disease.[81] However, it is clear that more severe preoperative diabetic retinopathy as well as worse glycemic control and longer diabetes duration are risk factors for increased chance of retinopathy worsening after phacoemulsification.[82,83]

An important determinant of the visual outcome in cataract surgery is the severity of the preoperative retinopathy. The visual prognosis for patients without any diabetic retinopathy approximates that of nondiabetic individuals, with almost 90% of patients attaining a visual acuity of 20/40.[84] For patients demonstrating preexisting retinopathy, the postoperative vision can be affected by the development of a diffuse, exudative form of macular edema, particularly in women and older individuals.[80,85] Cystoid macular edema (CME) is another common cause of poor vision in the postoperative period, and approximately 50% of patients with preexisting retinopathy show evidence of persistent CME at 1 year.[84,86] Eyes that present with non–center-involved macular edema at the time of cataract surgery that have undergone prior treatment for diabetic macular edema have a rate of postsurgical progression to center involvement between 13 and 28%. Fortunately, when there is no baseline center-involved diabetic macular edema present and no history of treatment for diabetic macular edema, the risk of subsequent development of center-involved macular edema is low, between 1 and 8%.[87]

Ideally, proliferative retinopathy and macular edema should be stabilized by treatment with appropriate anti-VEGF therapy and/or laser photocoagulation *before* cataract removal and, if possible, before the density of the cataract precludes such treatment. When the cataract surgery is planned, the necessity of a good fundus view and the possibility of future posterior segment laser treatments should always be kept in mind; thus, wider pupillary apertures should be maintained and posterior chamber intraocular lenses with large optics are preferred. The use of silicone intraocular lenses should be avoided due to an increased tendency for condensation on these lenses during any subsequently necessary vitrectomy with intraoperative fluid–gas exchange. Limbal or corneal incisions should be sutured more frequently in diabetic patients who have a tendency toward poorer wound healing. Because of the significant risk for CME and fibrinoid uveitis in the postoperative period, prophylactic use of anti-inflammatory agents is recommended. Close follow-up for progression of retinopathy is essential, particularly in the first 6 months after surgery, with early initiation of focal or scatter photocoagulation treatment as indicated. With proper counseling, careful surgical planning, and appropriate follow-up, cataract extraction can lead to gratifying visual results for patients with diabetes mellitus, as well as an improved fundus view that facilitates early diagnosis and treatment of any clinically significant diabetic retinopathy that may develop subsequently.

Special Considerations

- Measures that can optimize the visual results of cataract surgery in diabetic patients include proper timing of surgery before the cataract becomes highly dense, performance of appropriate preoperative treatment to stabilize retinopathy and macular edema, and intraoperative maintenance of an intact posterior lens capsule.

10.9 Conclusion

Over the coming decades, the worldwide epidemic of diabetes will place a staggering number of patients at risk for vision loss from diabetic eye disease. Fortunately, advances in treatments including the development of laser photocoagulation and medical therapies such as intravitreal anti-VEGF medications and steroids have dramatically improved visual outcomes related to diabetic retinopathy. First-line treatment for diabetic macular edema has evolved from macular focal/grid laser photocoagulation to anti-VEGF therapy for most eyes. Laser and occasionally steroids can be used in cases that are not candidates for anti-VEGF or as adjunctive treatment as needed for incomplete response to anti-VEGF therapy. Standard care treatment for PDR remains panretinal PRP, but evidence now demonstrates that anti-VEGF therapies are no worse than and have potential benefits as compared to PRP over 1 year, and large-scale clinical trials that may shed light on the potential efficacy of anti-VEGF therapy for long-term treatment of retinal neovascularization are ongoing. Continued clinical research efforts are assessing alternative ways to identify and triage patients at risk for vision threatening complications of diabetic retinopathy and exploring more effective treatments for earlier stage disease in order to best preserve vision. Thus, for patients with diabetic retinopathy, the efficacy of currently available therapeutic options is exceptional, and the promise of additional future advances remains strong.

References

[1] Wolfensberger TJ, Hamilton AM. Diabetic retinopathy—an historical review. Semin Ophthalmol. 2001; 16(1):2–7

[2] Luft R, Olivecrona H, Sjögren B. [Hypophysectomy in man]. Nord Med. 1952; 47(11):351–354

[3] Meyer-Schwickerath G. Light coagulation [Drance SM, transl.]. St. Louis: Mosby Year Book, 1960

[4] Beetham WP, Aiello LM, Balodimos MC, Koncz L. Ruby-laser photocoagulation of early diabetic neovascular retinopathy: preliminary report of a long-term controlled study. Trans Am Ophthalmol Soc. 1969; 67:39–67

[5] The Diabetic Retinopathy Study Research Group. Preliminary report on effects of photocoagulation therapy. Am J Ophthalmol. 1976; 81(4):383–396

[6] Early Treatment Diabetic Retinopathy Study Research Group. Photocoagulation for diabetic macular edema: ETDRS report number 1. Arch Ophthalmol. 1985; 103:1796–1806

[7] The Diabetic Retinopathy Vitrectomy Study Research Group. Early vitrectomy for severe vitreous hemorrhage in diabetic retinopathy. Two-year results of a randomized trial. Diabetic Retinopathy Vitrectomy Study report 2. Arch Ophthalmol. 1985; 103(11):1644–1652

[8] Elman MJ, Aiello LP, Beck RW, et al. Diabetic Retinopathy Clinical Research Network. Randomized trial evaluating ranibizumab plus prompt or deferred laser or triamcinolone plus prompt laser for diabetic macular edema. Ophthalmology. 2010; 117(6):1064–1077.e35

[9] Brown DM, Nguyen QD, Marcus DM, et al. RIDE and RISE Research Group. Long-term outcomes of ranibizumab therapy for diabetic macular edema: the 36-month results from two phase III trials: RISE and RIDE. Ophthalmology. 2013; 120(10):2013–2022

[10] Brown DM, Schmidt-Erfurth U, Do DV, et al. Intravitreal Aflibercept for Diabetic Macular Edema: 100-Week Results From the VISTA and VIVID Studies. Ophthalmology. 2015; 122(10):2044–2052

[11] National Eye Institute. Diabetic Retinopathy. Available at: https://nei.nih.gov/eyedata/diabetic; Accessed October 7, 2015

[12] Klein R, Klein BE, Moss SE, Davis MD, DeMets DL. The Wisconsin epidemiologic study of diabetic retinopathy. III. Prevalence and risk of diabetic retinopathy when age at diagnosis is 30 or more years. Arch Ophthalmol. 1984; 102(4):527–532

[13] Klein R, Klein BE, Moss SE, Davis MD, DeMets DL. The Wisconsin epidemiologic study of diabetic retinopathy. II. Prevalence and risk of diabetic retinopathy when age at diagnosis is less than 30 years. Arch Ophthalmol. 1984; 102(4):520–526

[14] International Diabetes Federation. IDF Diabetes Atlas: Sixth Edition, 2014 Update. Available at: http://www.idf.org/diabetesatlas/update-2014; Accessed October 7, 2015

[15] Aiello LP, Avery RL, Arrigg PG, et al. Vascular endothelial growth factor in ocular fluid of patients with diabetic retinopathy and other retinal disorders. N Engl J Med. 1994; 331(22):1480–1487

[16] Engerman RL, Kern TS. Experimental galactosemia produces diabetic-like retinopathy. Diabetes. 1984; 33(1):97–100

[17] Sorbinil Retinopathy Trial Research Group. A randomized trial of sorbinil, an aldose reductase inhibitor, in diabetic retinopathy. Arch Ophthalmol. 1990; 108(9):1234–1244

[18] Stem MS, Gardner TW. Neurodegeneration in the pathogenesis of diabetic retinopathy: molecular mechanisms and therapeutic implications. Curr Med Chem. 2013; 20(26):3241–3250

[19] Cogan DG, Toussaint D, Kuwabara T. Retinal vascular patterns. IV. Diabetic retinopathy. Arch Ophthalmol. 1961; 66:366–378

[20] De Venecia G, Davis M, Engerman R. Clinicopathologic correlations in diabetic retinopathy. I. Histology and fluorescein angiography of microaneurysms. Arch Ophthalmol. 1976; 94(10):1766–1773

[21] Antonetti DA, Klein R, Gardner TW. Diabetic retinopathy. N Engl J Med. 2012; 366(13):1227–1239

[22] Kohner EM, Sleightholm M. Does microaneurysm count reflect severity of early diabetic retinopathy? Ophthalmology. 1986; 93(5):586–589

[23] Muraoka K, Shimizu K. Intraretinal neovascularization in diabetic retinopathy. Ophthalmology. 1984; 91(12):1440–1446

[24] Kohner EM, Dollery CT, Bulpitt CJ. Cotton-wool spots in diabetic retinopathy. Diabetes. 1969; 18(10):691–704

[25] Roy MS, Rick ME, Higgins KE, McCulloch JC. Retinal cotton-wool spots: an early finding in diabetic retinopathy? Br J Ophthalmol. 1986; 70(10):772–778

[26] Regillo CD, Brown GC, Savino PJ, et al. Diabetic papillopathy. Patient characteristics and fundus findings. Arch Ophthalmol. 1995; 113(7):889–895

[27] Early Treatment Diabetic Retinopathy Study Research Group. Fundus photographic risk factors for progression of diabetic retinopathy. ETDRS report number 12. Ophthalmology. 1991; 98(5) Suppl:823–833

[28] Early Treatment Diabetic Retinopathy Study Research Group. Classification of diabetic retinopathy from fluorescein angiograms. ETDRS report number 11. Ophthalmology. 1991; 98(5) Suppl:807–822

[29] Shimizu K, Kobayashi Y, Muraoka K. Midperipheral fundus involvement in diabetic retinopathy. Ophthalmology. 1981; 88(7):601–612

[30] Silva PS, Cavallerano JD, Sun JK, Soliman AZ, Aiello LM, Aiello LP. Peripheral lesions identified by mydriatic ultrawide field imaging: distribution and potential impact on diabetic retinopathy severity. Ophthalmology. 2013; 120(12):2587–2595

[31] Silva PS, Cavallerano JD, Haddad NM, et al. Peripheral lesions identified on ultrawide field imaging predict increased risk of diabetic retinopathy progression over 4 years. Ophthalmology. 2015; 122(5):949–956

[32] Diabetes Control and Complications Trial Research Group. Progression of retinopathy with intensive versus conventional treatment in the Diabetes Control and Complications Trial. Ophthalmology. 1995; 102(4):647–661

[33] Aiello LP, DCCT/EDIC Research Group. Diabetic retinopathy and other ocular findings in the Diabetes Control and Complications Trial/Epidemiology of Diabetes Interventions and Complications study. Diabetes Care. 2014; 37(1):17–23

[34] Aiello LP, Sun W, Das A, et al. DCCT/EDIC Research Group. Intensive diabetes therapy and ocular surgery in type 1 diabetes. N Engl J Med. 2015; 372(18):1722–1733

[35] Early Treatment Diabetic Retinopathy Study Research Group. Effects of aspirin treatment on diabetic retinopathy. ETDRS report number 8. Ophthalmology. 1991; 98(5) Suppl:757–765

[36] Klein BEK, Moss SE, Klein R. Effect of pregnancy on progression of diabetic retinopathy. Diabetes Care. 1990; 13(1):34–40

[37] Axer-Siegel R, Hod M, Fink-Cohen S, et al. Diabetic retinopathy during pregnancy. Ophthalmology. 1996; 103(11):1815–1819

[38] Ip MS, Domalpally A, Sun JK, Ehrlich JS. Long-term effects of therapy with ranibizumab on diabetic retinopathy severity and baseline risk factors for worsening retinopathy. Ophthalmology. 2015; 122(2):367–374

[39] Bressler SB, Qin H, Melia M, et al. Diabetic Retinopathy Clinical Research Network. Exploratory analysis of the effect of intravitreal ranibizumab or triamcinolone on worsening of diabetic retinopathy in a randomized clinical trial. JAMA Ophthalmol. 2013; 131(8):1033–1040

[40] Sun JK, Wang P, Fung A. Impact of treatment delay and durability of diabetic retinopathy (DR) improvement with PRN ranibizumab (RBZ) during the RIDE/RISE Open-Label Extension (OLE). 2015 Macula Society Abstract

[41] Diabetic Retinopathy Study Research Group. Design, methods, and baseline results: DRS report number 6. Invest Ophthalmol Vis Sci. 1981; 21:149–209

[42] Prud'homme GJ, Rand L, The Diabetic Retinopathy Study Research Group. Distribution of maximum grade of lesions in proliferative diabetic retinopathy. Invest Ophthalmol Vis Sci. 1981; 20:59

[43] Davis MD. Vitreous contraction in proliferative diabetic retinopathy. Arch Ophthalmol. 1965; 74(6):741–751

[44] The Diabetic Retinopathy Study Research Group. Four risk factors for severe visual loss in diabetic retinopathy. The third report from the Diabetic Retinopathy Study. Arch Ophthalmol. 1979; 97(4):654–655

[45] Photocoagulation treatment of proliferative diabetic retinopathy. Clinical application of Diabetic Retinopathy Study (DRS) findings, DRS Report Number 8. The Diabetic Retinopathy Study Research Group. Ophthalmology. 1981 Jul;88(7):583-600.

[46] The Diabetic Retinopathy Study Research Group. Factors influencing the development of visual loss in advanced diabetic retinopathy: DRS report number 10. Invest Ophthalmol Vis Sci. 1985; 26:983–991

[47] The Diabetic Retinopathy Study Research Group. Indications for photocoagulation treatment of diabetic retinopathy: DRS report number 14. Int Ophthalmol Clin. 1987; 27:239–253

[48] Early Treatment Diabetic Retinopathy Study Research Group. Early photocoagulation for diabetic retinopathy. ETDRS report number 9. Ophthalmology. 1991; 98(5) Suppl:766–785

[49] Ferris F. Early photocoagulation in patients with either type I or type II diabetes. Trans Am Ophthalmol Soc. 1996; 94:505–537

[50] Brucker AJ, Qin H, Antoszyk AN, et al. Diabetic Retinopathy Clinical Research Network. Observational study of the development of diabetic macular edema following panretinal (scatter) photocoagulation given in 1 or 4 sittings. Arch Ophthalmol. 2009; 127(2):132–140

[51] Diabetic Retinopathy Clinical Research Network*. Randomized clinical trial evaluating intravitreal ranibizumab or saline for vitreous hemorrhage from proliferative diabetic retinopathy. JAMA Ophthalmol. 2013; 131(3):283–293

[52] Diabetic Retinopathy Study Research Group. Photocoagulation treatment of proliferative diabetic retinopathy: relationship of adverse treatment effects to retinopathy severity: DRS report number 5. Dev Ophthalmol. 1981; 2:248–261

[53] Doft BH, Blankenship GW. Single versus multiple treatment sessions of argon laser panretinal photocoagulation for proliferative diabetic retinopathy. Ophthalmology. 1982; 89(7):772–779

[54] Blankenship GW. A clinical comparison of central and peripheral argon laser panretinal photocoagulation for proliferative diabetic retinopathy. Ophthalmology. 1988; 95(2):170–177

[55] Gentile RC, Stegman Z, Liebmann JM, et al. Risk factors for ciliochoroidal effusion after panretinal photocoagulation. Ophthalmology. 1996; 103(5):827–832

[56] Avery RL, Pearlman J, Pieramici DJ, et al. Intravitreal bevacizumab (Avastin) in the treatment of proliferative diabetic retinopathy. Ophthalmology. 2006; 113(10):1695.e1–1695.e15

[57] Klein R, Klein BE, Moss SE, Davis MD, DeMets DL. The Wisconsin epidemiologic study of diabetic retinopathy. IV. Diabetic macular edema. Ophthalmology. 1984; 91(12):1464–1474

[58] Sigurdsson R, Begg IS. Organised macular plaques in exudative diabetic maculopathy. Br J Ophthalmol. 1980; 64(6):392–397

[59] Bresnick GH. Diabetic maculopathy. A critical review highlighting diffuse macular edema. Ophthalmology. 1983; 90(11):1301–1317

[60] Bresnick GH, Condit R, Syrjala S, Palta M, Groo A, Korth K. Abnormalities of the foveal avascular zone in diabetic retinopathy. Arch Ophthalmol. 1984; 102(9):1286–1293

[61] Wells JA, Glassman AR, Ayala AR, et al. Diabetic Retinopathy Clinical Research Network. Aflibercept, bevacizumab, or ranibizumab for diabetic macular edema. N Engl J Med. 2015; 372(13):1193–1203

[62] Christoforidis JB, Williams MM, Wang J, et al. Anatomic and pharmacokinetic properties of intravitreal bevacizumab and ranibizumab after vitrectomy and lensectomy. Retina. 2013; 33(5):946–952

[63] Bressler SB, Melia M, Glassman AR, et al. Diabetic Retinopathy Clinical Research Network. Ranibizumab plus prompt or deferred laser for diabetic macular edema in eyes with vitrectomy before anti-vascular endothelial growth factor therapy. Retina. 2015; 35(12):2516–2528

[64] Martidis A, Duker JS, Greenberg PB, et al. Intravitreal triamcinolone for refractory diabetic macular edema. Ophthalmology. 2002; 109(5):920–927

[65] Diabetic Retinopathy Clinical Research Network. A randomized trial comparing intravitreal triamcinolone acetonide and focal/grid photocoagulation for diabetic macular edema. Ophthalmology. 2008; 115(9):1447–1449, 1449.e1–1449.e10

[66] Elman MJ, Bressler NM, Qin H, et al. Diabetic Retinopathy Clinical Research Network. Expanded 2-year follow-up of ranibizumab plus prompt or deferred laser or triamcinolone plus prompt laser for diabetic macular edema. Ophthalmology. 2011; 118(4):609–614

[67] Boyer DS, Yoon YH, Belfort R, Jr, et al. Ozurdex MEAD Study Group. Three-year, randomized, sham-controlled trial of dexamethasone intravitreal implant in patients with diabetic macular edema. Ophthalmology. 2014; 121(10):1904–1914

[68] Campochiaro PA, Brown DM, Pearson A, et al. FAME Study Group. Sustained delivery fluocinolone acetonide vitreous inserts provide benefit for at least 3 years in patients with diabetic macular edema. Ophthalmology. 2012; 119(10):2125–2132

[69] Bhavsar AR, Stockdale CR, Ferris FL, III, Brucker AJ, Bressler NM, Glassman AR, Diabetic Retinopathy Clinical Research Network. Update on risk of endophthalmitis after intravitreal drug injections and potential impact of elimination of topical antibiotics. Arch Ophthalmol. 2012; 130(6):809–810

[70] McDonald HR, Schatz H. Grid photocoagulation for diffuse macular edema. Retina. 1985; 5(2):65–72

[71] Browning DJ, Zhang Z, Benfield JM, Scott AQ. The effect of patient characteristics on response to focal laser treatment for diabetic macular edema. Ophthalmology. 1997; 104(3):466–472

[72] Lewis H, Schachat AP, Haimann MH, et al. Choroidal neovascularization after laser photocoagulation for diabetic macular edema. Ophthalmology. 1990; 97(4):503–510, discussion 510–511

[73] Han DP, Mieler WF, Burton TC. Submacular fibrosis after photocoagulation for diabetic macular edema. Am J Ophthalmol. 1992; 113(5):513–521

[74] Machemer R, Buettner H, Norton EW, Parel JM. Vitrectomy: a pars plana approach. Trans Am Acad Ophthalmol Otolaryngol. 1971; 75(4):813–820

[75] The Diabetic Retinopathy Vitrectomy Study Research Group. Early vitrectomy for severe proliferative diabetic retinopathy in eyes with useful vision. Results of a randomized trial—Diabetic Retinopathy Vitrectomy Study Report 3. Ophthalmology. 1988; 95(10):1307–1320

[76] Diabetic Retinopathy Vitrectomy Study Research Group. Early vitrectomy for severe vitreous hemorrhage. Four-year results of a randomized trial: Diabetic Retinopathy Study report 5. Arch Ophthalmol. 1990; 108:958–964

[77] Pollack A, Dotan S, Oliver M. Progression of diabetic retinopathy after cataract extraction. Br J Ophthalmol. 1991; 75(9):547–551

[78] Pollack A, Leiba H, Bukelman A, Abrahami S, Oliver M. The course of diabetic retinopathy following cataract surgery in eyes previously treated by laser photocoagulation. Br J Ophthalmol. 1992; 76(4):228–231

[79] Aiello LM, Wand M, Liang G. Neovascular glaucoma and vitreous hemorrhage following cataract surgery in patients with diabetes mellitus. Ophthalmology. 1983; 90(7):814–820

[80] Hykin PG, Gregson RM, Stevens JD, Hamilton PA. Extracapsular cataract extraction in proliferative diabetic retinopathy. Ophthalmology. 1993; 100(3):394–399

[81] Haddad NM, Sun JK, Abujaber S, Schlossman DK, Silva PS. Cataract surgery and its complications in diabetic patients. Semin Ophthalmol. 2014; 29(5–6):329–337

[82] Mittra RA, Borrillo JL, Dev S, Mieler WF, Koenig SB. Retinopathy progression and visual outcomes after phacoemulsification in patients with diabetes mellitus. Arch Ophthalmol. 2000; 118(7):912–917

[83] Kato S, Fukada Y, Hori S, Tanaka Y, Oshika T. Influence of phacoemulsification and intraocular lens implantation on the course of diabetic retinopathy. J Cataract Refract Surg. 1999; 25(6):788–793

[84] Cheng H, Franklin SL. Treatment of cataract in diabetics with and without retinopathy. Eye (Lond). 1988; 2(Pt 6):607–614

[85] Jaffe GJ, Burton TC. Progression of nonproliferative diabetic retinopathy following cataract extraction. Arch Ophthalmol. 1988; 106(6):745–749

[86] Pollack A, Leiba H, Bukelman A, Oliver M. Cystoid macular oedema following cataract extraction in patients with diabetes. Br J Ophthalmol. 1992; 76(4):221–224

[87] Baker CW, Almukhtar T, Bressler NM, et al. Diabetic Retinopathy Clinical Research Network Authors/Writing Committee. Macular edema after cataract surgery in eyes without preoperative central-involved diabetic macular edema. JAMA Ophthalmol. 2013; 131(7):870–879

11 Cystoid Macular Edema

Stephen J. Kim and Ingrid U. Scott

11.1 Introduction

Cystoid macular edema (CME) can be broadly defined as the accumulation of excess fluid in the extracellular space of the neurosensory retina presenting clinically with cyst-like (cystic) spaces and abnormal thickening of the macula. It was first described by Irvine in 1953,[1] but Gass and Norton[2] provided the first detailed microscopic and angiographic description of this condition in 1966, and the condition later became known as Irvine–Gass syndrome. Although intracellular edema of Müller's cells has been observed, the classic pathology of CME consists of large cystic spaces in the outer plexiform layer of Henle.[3] With modern imaging, fluid-filled spaces can often be seen in multiple layers of the retina, including the subretinal space. Although the definitive cause of CME cannot be precisely determined in most cases, several basic pathophysiologic processes contribute to the development of CME, depending on the underlying etiology and clinical context. As a final common complication of many retinal conditions, CME can be considered a leading cause of central vision loss and is, therefore, of enormous socioeconomic importance.

Therapeutic approaches to CME have evolved over the past two decades as research has led to greater understanding of underlying etiology and pathophysiologic mechanisms. The recent availability of drugs to inhibit vascular endothelial growth factor (VEGF) has been a remarkable advance in the treatment of CME due to underlying retinal vascular disease. Recent advances in drug delivery, particularly enhanced bioavailability of topically applied and intravitreally delivered anti-inflammatory drugs, have also improved treatment options.

11.2 Classification and Diagnosis

CME can be classified as clinical (retinal thickening observed on biomicroscopic examination in combination with vision impairment), angiographic (leakage detected on fluorescein angiography [FA]), and, more recently, in terms of the presence of intraretinal (with or without subretinal) fluid on optical coherence tomography (OCT). Although moderate and severe cases of CME can be observed reliably by direct biomicroscopy, mild cases may be missed. FA has been the traditional method to detect CME and can reveal a petaloid-like pattern of hyperfluorescence in the macula during the late phase due to dye leakage from perifoveal capillaries and dye accumulation within cystic spaces in the outer plexiform layer (▶ Fig. 11.1). OCT is a relatively newer technology and provides high-resolution cross-sectional imaging that directly measures macular thickness. It has several advantages over angiography, including faster speed, noninvasiveness, and reproducibility. In addition, its measurements are quantifiable and, therefore, OCT lends itself well to clinical trials.[4] Consequently, OCT has been used increasingly to grade and assess CME in clinical practice. Despite these inherent advantages, mild diffuse cases of CME with minimal thickening may be missed on OCT but observed more readily on angiography, which shows direct leakage from retina blood vessels (▶ Fig. 11.2).

CME is not a specific disease but rather a clinical finding of intraretinal fluid in the macula (macular edema [ME]) typically (but not always) with cystic changes that is a common complication of many diseases. Because of its historical description by Gass and Norton[2] after cataract surgery (Irvine–Gass syndrome) and its presumed relationship with inflammation,[5] CME is often used in the literature to describe ME in the setting of cataract surgery, uveitis, and other conditions (e.g., retinitis pigmentosa [RP]) where inflammation is thought to be primarily involved. In contrast, ME is more commonly used in the literature to describe similar clinical findings in the setting of retinal vein occlusions (RVOs), radiation retinopathy, and other

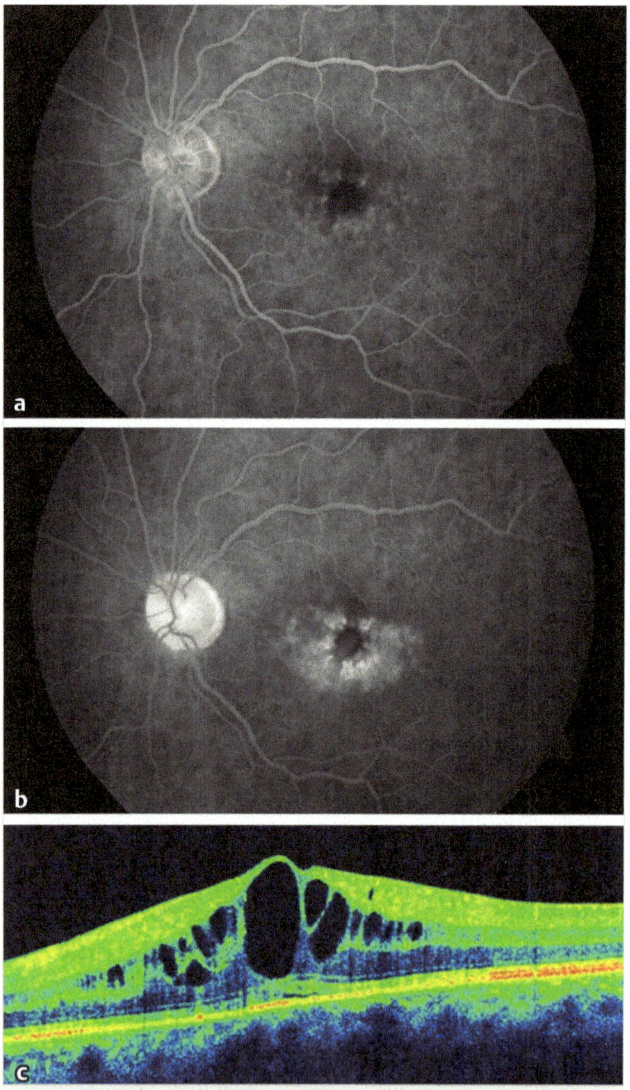

Fig. 11.1 (**a**) Early and (**b**) late fluorescein angiography images demonstrate typical petaloid-like pattern of hyperfluorescence in the macula during the late phase due to dye leakage from perifoveal capillaries. (**c**) Corresponding optical coherence tomography (OCT) image demonstrates cystic spaces predominately in the outer plexiform layer.

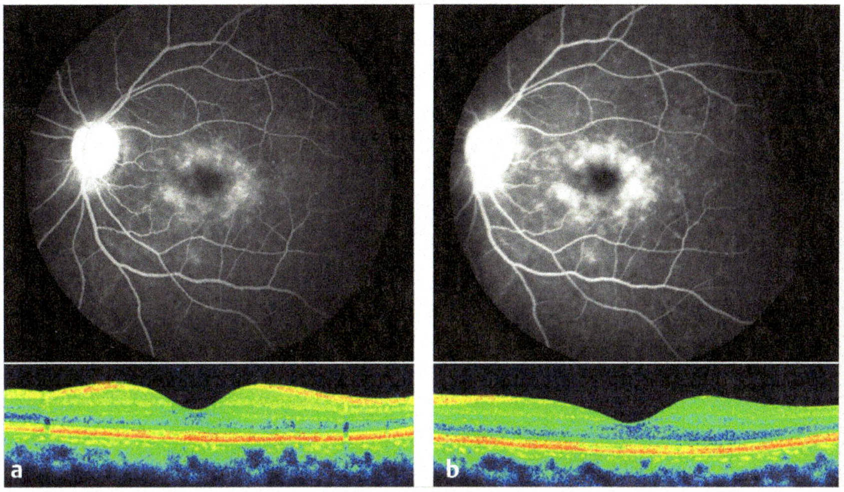

Fig. 11.2 (a) Early and (b) late fluorescein angiography images with corresponding OCT images below demonstrate definite angiographic leakage without obvious cystoid changes on OCT.

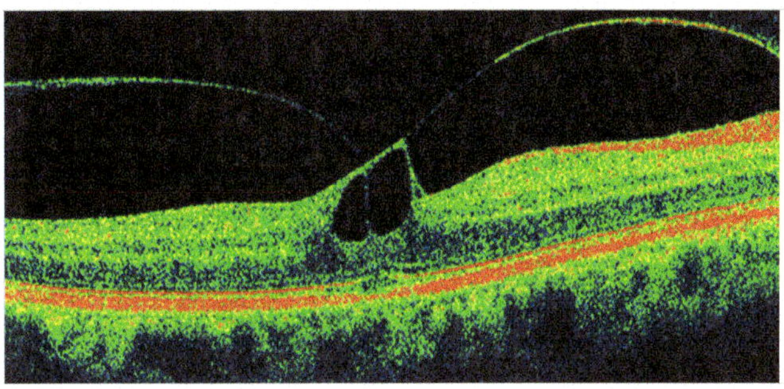

Fig. 11.3 Vitreomacular traction with cystoid spaces in the inner retina.

retinovascular diseases. Furthermore, when observed in the setting of diabetes, the descriptive term *diabetic macular edema* (DME) is used routinely. It is now generally accepted that chronic inflammation plays a more prominent role in the pathogenesis of ME in retinal vascular diseases than recognized previously, obscuring the boundaries of this traditional classification.[6,7] Therefore, throughout this chapter, CME and ME are intended to be viewed as overlapping rather than distinctive terms,[8] but where appropriate the more cited term will be used for historical consistency.

Pearls

- CME is not a specific disease but a clinical finding which complicates many diseases. As such, its application can overlap with ME and DME. Consequently, distinguishing CME from ME or DME is not always clinically possible or even important as treatment approaches are often similar.

11.3 Pathophysiology

The volume and composition of the extracellular compartment of the neurosensory retina is tightly regulated under normal circumstances by the inner (retinal capillary endothelial cell tight junctions) and outer (retinal pigment epithelium [RPE] cell tight junctions) blood–retinal barriers and by the active pumping function of the RPE cells.[3,9] Consequently, cellular (endothelial or RPE) impairment/death, loss of tight junction integrity, and increased intraluminal pressure can disrupt and/or overwhelm these barriers/RPE pump capacity and result in accumulation of intraretinal fluid (see text box).[10,11] While vitreomacular traction also results in cystic spaces on OCT (▶ Fig. 11.3) and in some circumstances traction-induced macular capillary leakage on FA, its pathophysiology is distinct and primarily due to mechanical traction and separation of intraretinal layers.

Main Pathophysiologic Mechanisms in Cystoid Macular Edema

- Increased vascular permeability
  - Inflammation
  - Loss of pericytes and endothelial cells
  - Vascular incompetence (e.g., Coats' disease)
  - Vasopermeability factors (e.g., VEGF)
  - Leukocyte stasis
- Increased intraluminal pressure
  - Increased blood flow
  - Vasodilation
  - Increased blood volume
  - Vascular occlusion (e.g., vein occlusion)
- Dysfunction of RPE barrier/pump
- Drug toxicity

Despite its multiple mechanisms, ME occurs most commonly due to pathologic hyperpermeability of retinal capillaries, which can occur as a result of endothelial cell damage/impairment (e.g., diabetes, Coats' disease) or increased vascular permeability from inflammation (e.g., postsurgical, uveitis; ▶ Table 11.1).[3] Adherence of leukocytes to vessel walls

Table 11.1 Pathologic conditions causing cystoid macular edema

Inflammatory disorders	Intraocular surgery
	Intraocular inflammation (uveitis)
	Laser procedures
Retinal vascular diseases	Diabetic retinopathy
	Radiation retinopathy
	Retinal venous occlusion
	Hypertensive retinopathy
Drug induced	Prostaglandin analogs
	Epinephrine
	Nicotinic acid
	Taxanes (docetaxel, paclitaxel)
	Tamoxifen
	Thiazolidinediones (glitazones)
	Interferons
	Fingolimod
Inherited retinal dystrophies	Retinitis pigmentosa
	Autosomal dominant cystoid macular edema
Others	Choroidal tumors
	Retinal vascular tumors (e.g., capillary angioma)
	Choroidal neovascularization
	Vitreomacular traction syndrome
	Exudative retinal detachment
	Optic nerve head abnormalities (coloboma, pit)

Source: Reused with permission by Elsevier from Johnson.[3]

(leukostasis), an early finding in diabetic retinopathy (DR) and mediated by intercellular adhesion molecule-1 (ICAM-1),[12] results in progressive endothelial damage from nitric oxide and inflammatory mediators. These mediators include prostaglandins, leukotrienes, protein kinase C (PKC), VEGF, nitric oxide, and various cytokines which result in increased retinal vascular permeability by directly or indirectly causing vasodilation and disruption of endothelial tight junctions.[13,14,15] Subsequent increased vascular permeability results in extravasation of proteins, fluid, and other macromolecules into the extracellular space and retinal interstitium. This causes a shift in the balance of hydrostatic and oncotic pressure, favoring the accumulation of fluid within the extracellular space and the development of ME. The majority of cases of ME demonstrate fluid in the outer layers of the retina, but severe occurrences can result in secondary fluid migration into the subretinal space.

Extravasation and accumulation of fluid into the retina can also be caused by disruption of the RPE barrier and/or pump function which may occur in conditions such as central serous retinopathy, retinitis pigmentosa (RP), and drug-induced toxicity and which may result in serous macular detachment and secondary ME. Retinal permeability can be increased by conditions that increase blood volume, flow, and intraluminal pressure (e.g., central retinal vein occlusion [CRVO]) or by factors that promote vasodilation.

Independent of the mechanism(s) of CME, visual acuity depends on a number of factors, including duration and severity of edema, underlying health of the RPE and photoreceptors, and macular perfusion. With the notable exception of postsurgical ME occurring in healthy retinas preoperatively,[8] many studies report poor correlation between macular thickness and visual acuity in eyes with recurrent or longstanding ME.[16]

11.4 Major Pathologic Conditions

11.4.1 Intraocular Surgery

More than 2 million cataract surgeries are performed annually in the United States, and development of CME remains the most common cause of postoperative vision loss. Incidence rates of CME vary substantially throughout the literature depending on which definition is used and the type of patients included in the study. It is clear that CME occurs at a higher frequency in patients with uveitis or diabetes.[17,18] Recent studies have reported incidences following modern, small-incision, uncomplicated cataract surgery in healthy individuals (without diabetes or uveitis) as high as 9 to 19% using FA, but visually important CME is reported at much lower rates (in the range of 1–4%).[4] Although CME can be treated, its development increases the cost of cataract surgery by approximately 50% (additional cost in 2014: $1,092) and chronic disease can result in permanent visual impairment.[19]

Although the exact pathogenesis of CME after cataract surgery remains unknown, disruption of the blood–retinal barrier due to inflammation may play a prominent role. It has been hypothesized that release of prostaglandins and other inflammatory mediators presumably from anterior uveal tissue increases permeability of perifoveal capillaries, resulting in accumulation of fluid and cystic changes in the retinal layers.[5] In agreement with this, a higher incidence of CME is seen in complicated cataract surgeries with vitreous loss, adhesions to the cataract wound, and retained lens material where inflammation would likely be more pronounced and prolonged.[20] Recent studies have confirmed higher rates of ME in diabetic eyes after cataract surgery, particularly in those eyes with a previous history of DME and, therefore, likely to have existing retinal vasculature hyperpermeability and compromise.[21] While it is virtually impossible to distinguish postsurgical CME (Irvine–Gass) versus exacerbation of DME in diabetic eyes after cataract surgery, such a distinction is mostly academic, as treatment goals and strategies for each entity are similar. Instead, emphasis should be focused on preventive measures in eyes with preexisting DME undergoing cataract surgery.

Pearls

- History of previous DME is significantly associated with development of ME after cataract surgery.[21] Such at-risk eyes should receive appropriate preventive measures which may consist of preoperative topical corticosteroid and/or nonsteroidal anti-inflammatory drops and periocular or intraocular corticosteroids.

Similarly, measures should be taken to ensure that inflammation is controlled for at least 3 months in eyes with uveitis before elective cataract surgery. A recent prospective trial demonstrated that administration of perioperative systemic prednisone starting 2 days before surgery with rapid taper after surgery reduced the risk of CME at 4 weeks by sevenfold.[18]

Pearls

- Perioperative systemic prednisone significantly reduced the incidence of CME at 4 weeks after cataract surgery by sevenfold in eyes with uveitis.[18]

Although much attention has focused on CME after cataract surgery, CME has also been reported after other types of intraocular surgery[22,23] and laser therapy.[24,25,26] New or exacerbation of CME is well known to occur following panretinal photocoagulation in diabetic eyes.[24] CME has also been reported to occur after neodymium-doped yttrium aluminum garnet (Nd:YAG) posterior capsulotomy[25] and selective laser trabeculoplasty.[26]

Although there is no Food and Drug Administration (FDA)-approved therapy for CME, both prophylaxis and treatment are directed toward blocking inflammatory mediators (mainly prostaglandins) produced in the anterior uvea through the use of topical corticosteroids and nonsteroidal anti-inflammatory drugs (NSAIDs). An extensive meta-analysis of the world literature in 1998 concluded that NSAIDs are beneficial for the treatment and prevention of CME following cataract surgery.[27] A subsequent major review of the literature on this topic in 2010 reported similar findings but emphasized the paucity of well-designed studies and the lack of evidence of long-term benefit.[28] In particular, as many cases of CME are mild and resolve spontaneously, it remains unknown whether prophylactic treatment improves long-term visual outcomes.

Despite markedly increasing intraocular pressure in a small percentage of patients, corticosteroids should continue to be a mainstay of prevention and treatment of postsurgical CME, given their long track record of use and potent anti-inflammatory properties. A step-wise approach should be taken, with initial efforts focused on prevention usually with topical corticosteroids. If CME develops and is mild, increased dosing and/or prolonged use of a topical corticosteroid can be attempted. In more severe cases, local or intravitreal injection may be necessary.[29] Carbonic anhydrase inhibitors have been reported to be useful in some cases.[30] Both bevacizumab and ranibizumab have been used to treat refractory CME after surgery in uncontrolled case series with inconsistent results.[31,32]

Controversial Points

- Despite widespread use, the benefit of topical NSAIDs in combination with topical corticosteroids in the prevention and treatment of postsurgical CME remains unknown.

11.4.2 Uveitis

Uveitis is responsible for approximately 10% of all cases of legal blindness in the United States.[33] CME is the primary cause of vision loss associated with uveitis and complicates a wide variety of uveitic syndromes, particularly posterior uveitis and panuveitis.[34] While the pathogenesis of CME is not entirely understood, resolution of CME in response to anti-inflammatory treatment strongly implicates inflammatory mediators such as prostaglandins, leukotrienes, and cytokines, with resulting compromise of the inner blood–retinal barrier. Over time, RPE barrier and/or pump function may permanently decline and contribute to persistent fluid accumulation despite adequate control of inflammation. This later occurrence is supported by the observed therapeutic benefit for uveitic CME of carbonic anhydrase inhibitors, which function primarily by facilitating fluid transport across the RPE.[35,36] Over the past two decades, greater emphasis has been focused on sustained suppression of chronic inflammation to prevent CME and permanent vision loss.[37] Therapeutic strategies employed rely on topical corticosteroids; adjuvant, systemic, low-dose prednisone (= 10 mg/d); and steroid-sparing immunosuppressive drugs.[38] Typically, control of ocular inflammation requires much higher doses of steroid-sparing drugs than needed to treat systemic autoimmune disease. Administration of systemic treatment with prednisone and/or a steroid-sparing agent is particularly advantageous in patients with bilateral disease and, unlike local therapy, downgrades activation and proliferation of leukocytes in peripheral lymph nodes.

Similar to postsurgical CME, treatment of more refractory or chronic cases requires a step-wise approach. There are two sustained delivery devices that are FDA approved for the treatment of uveitis.[39,40] A 0.7-mg dexamethasone implant (Ozurdex; Allergan, Inc.) can be injected in the office and provides sustained release of the drug for up to 6 months. Its efficacy in reducing inflammation was proven in a large randomized trial with acceptable rates of cataract formation and elevated intraocular pressure.[39,41] The dexamethasone implant may be particularly advantageous in vitrectomized eyes where the half-life of intravitreally injected triamcinolone acetonide is markedly reduced. A surgically implantable device containing 0.59-mg fluocinolone acetonide provides sustained release of the drug for over 2 years and was comparable to chronic systemic immunosuppression in a large randomized clinical trial.[42] Although the implant was associated with a much higher rate of ocular side effects, mainly cataract formation and intraocular pressure elevation, it controlled inflammation slightly better than systemic immunosuppression and was associated with higher quality-of-life scores. It therefore remains a viable option to control recalcitrant uveitis and CME particularly in patients intolerant of systemic immunosuppression. Treatment of uveitic CME with anti-VEGF therapy has also been reported to be beneficial in small and uncontrolled case series.[14]

11.4.3 Diabetic Retinopathy

Nearly 300 million individuals have diabetes worldwide, and diabetic retinopathy (DR) is the leading cause of blindness among working-age adults. Approximately 35% of diabetic patients will have some form of DR, and 5 to 10% of these individuals will suffer from vision loss due to diabetic macular edema (DME).[43] Although diabetes may cause vision loss by several means, including cataract formation and proliferative retinopathy, DME is the most common cause (▶ Fig. 11.4). Early histological findings in DR include capillary basement membrane thickening, loss of pericytes, and loss of endothelial cells. Subsequent formation of microaneurysms, breakdown of the inner blood–retinal barrier, and consequent vascular leakage may result in ME.

The pathophysiology of DME is multifactorial, incompletely understood, and complex. Chronic hyperglycemia is a major initiator of microvascular complications and results in a series of metabolic events with the accumulation of polyols through the aldose reductase pathway, overproduction of reactive oxygen intermediates, increased formation of advanced glycation end products (AGEs), and pathologic activation of PKC.[3,6] In particular, some of the earliest changes seen histologically in DR involve the accumulation of AGEs, which bind to Receptor for Advanced Glycation End-Products (RAGE) and result in expression of VEGF, ICAM-1, tumor necrosis factor-a, and a number of other inflammatory mediators.[44] PKC is a family of serine threonine kinases that are activated by growth hormones.[45] At least 13 isoforms exist and the PKC-$ß_2$ isoforms appear to play an important role in increased vascular permeability due to VEGF. In animal models, administration of ruboxistaurin (RBX), a PKC-ß–specific inhibitor, has been shown to block more than 95% of VEGF's effect on increased vascular permeability.[46] The PKC-ß–specific inhibitor RBX has been evaluated in several large, multicenter, randomized control trials with regard to its effect on DR, but was not approved by the FDA for DME due to lack of efficacy.[47,48]

A growing body of scientific evidence indicates that inflammation contributes to the pathogenesis of DME.[7,49,50] The retinal vasculature of patients with diabetes contains increased numbers of adherent leukocytes, and breakdown of the inner blood–retinal barrier develops early in the course of DR.[50,51] Both phenomena presumably lead to progressive dysfunction and death of endothelial cells and pericytes which are pathophysiological hallmarks of DR.[52,53] In support of this, a number of proinflammatory cytokines are consistently elevated in the aqueous and vitreous of patients with advanced stages of DR

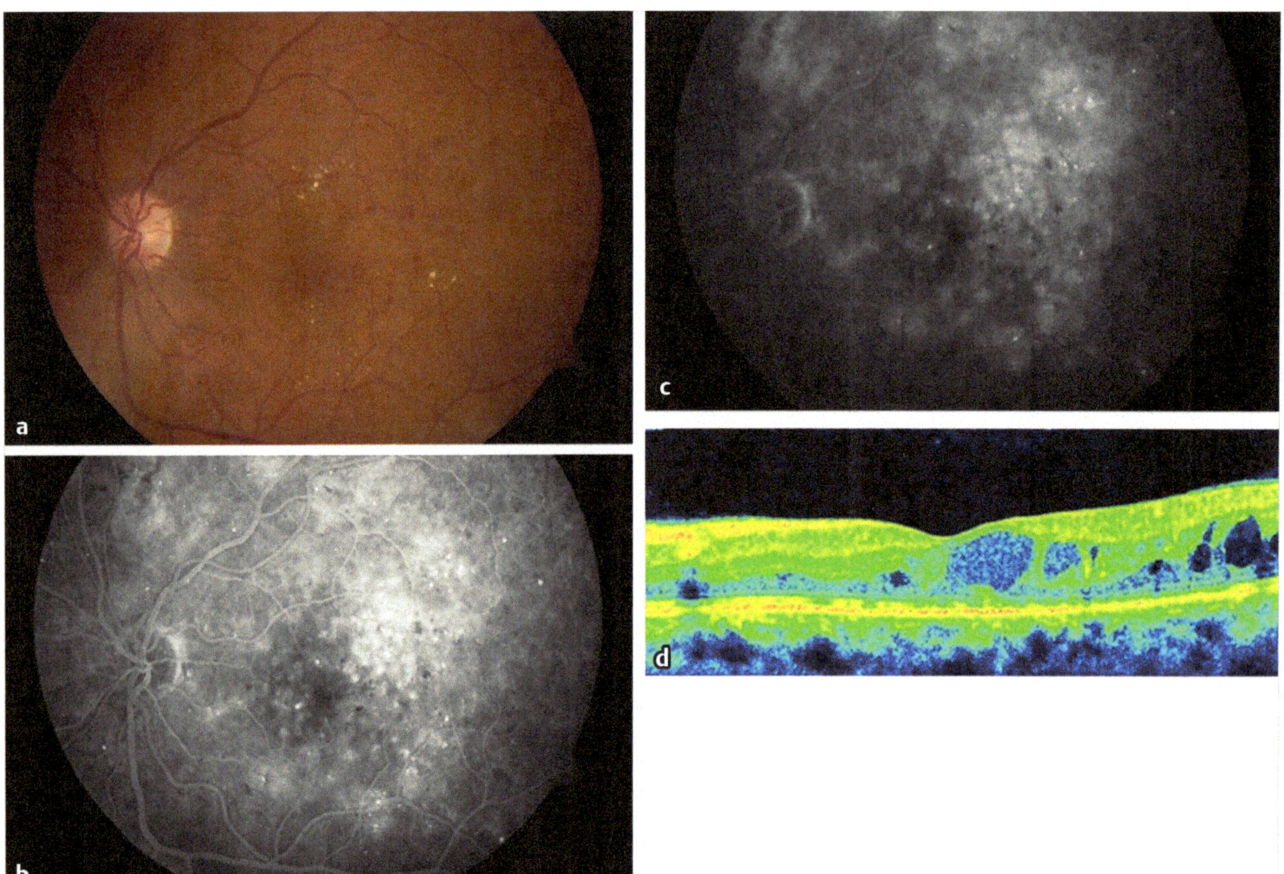

Fig. 11.4 **(a)** Color fundus photograph and **(b)** early and **(c)** late fluorescein angiography (FA) images demonstrate diabetic retinopathy. There are microaneurysms and lipid exudate visible on the color photograph with early hyperfluorescence and late staining and leakage visible on FA. Note the presence of prior focal laser scars. **(d)** Corresponding OCT demonstrates diffuse DME.

and DME.[54,55,56,57,58] Chronic inflammation-mediated vascular disease then may result in subsequent capillary nonperfusion, retinal ischemia, and vascular leakage that are key clinical features of advanced DR and DME and result in irreversible vision loss. Progressive ischemia from altered blood flow may further promote upregulation of VEGF and other inflammatory mediators, which could then self-perpetuate this process.[50,59]

The Early Treatment of Diabetic Retinopathy Study (ETDRS) Group established level I guidelines for treating patients with DME with macular laser photocoagulation.[60] When delivered appropriately in patients with a focal pattern of leakage, laser treatment is safe, effective, and has long-term benefits. In contrast, laser photocoagulation is less effective for diffuse patterns of DME. These clinical laser treatment guidelines were established before the use of adjunctive pharmacologic agents. VEGF, a highly potent vasopermeability factor, has been shown to play a central role in DME.[61]

At the time of this writing, there are two major anti-VEGF agents that have been evaluated in large, prospective, randomized, multicenter trials and are FDA approved for the treatment of DME: ranibizumab (Lucentis, Genentech, Inc.)[62,63] and aflibercept (Eylea, Regeneron Pharmaceuticals, Inc.).[64,65] Off-label use of a third agent, bevacizumab (Avastin, Genentech, Inc.), is common.[66] Ranibizumab is a recombinant humanized immunoglobulin G1 kappa isotype therapeutic antibody fragment which binds to and inhibits the biologic activity of all isoforms of human VEGF-A. It was approved by the FDA in August 2012 for the treatment of DME. Aflibercept, approved by the FDA in August 2014 for the treatment of DME, is a 115-kDa recombinant fusion protein consisting of the VEGF-binding domains of the human VEGF receptors 1 and 2 fused to the Fc domain of human immunoglobulin G1. Aflibercept competitively inhibits VEGF and also binds placental growth factors 1 and 2. Bevacizumab is a full-length monoclonal antibody that also binds all isoforms of VEGF-A. It is approved by the FDA for intravenous use in the treatment of metastatic colorectal cancer, non–small cell lung cancer, metastatic renal cell carcinoma, and glioblastoma.

Pearls

- Delay in treatment of DME with intraocular anti-VEGF drugs may negatively affect long-term visual outcomes. Early treatment may, therefore, be considered even in eyes with mild center-involved DME and relatively good vision.

While anti-VEGF agents have been a remarkable advance for the treatment of DME, clinical responses are generally transient and require repeat and serial injections. Long-term benefits beyond 3 years also remain unproven which is particularly germane, as DME occurs in younger patients and serial intravitreal injections are burdensome for working-age patients.[61]

Prior to the availability of anti-VEGF agents, intravitreal corticosteroids were commonly used to treat DME.[67,68] Rationale for their use was based on their broad suppression of inflammatory mediators including VEGF which were presumed to be directly involved in leukostasis and disruption of the blood–retinal barrier.[50,69] The Diabetic Retinopathy Clinical Research Network (DRCR) performed a prospective, randomized trial comparing focal/grid laser photocoagulation versus 1- and 4-mg intravitreal triamcinolone acetonide for the treatment of DME.[70] While there was an early benefit at 4 months in the 4-mg group compared to focal/grid laser, by 2 years focal/grid laser was more effective with fewer side effects. Another DRCR trial reported that intravitreal triamcinolone combined with focal/grid laser did not result in superior visual acuity outcomes compared with laser alone, but did appear to have a visual acuity benefit similar to ranibizumab in pseudophakic eyes.[71,72] Consequently, use of intravitreal triamcinolone should continue to play an important role in the treatment of DME in some patients. In June 2014, a 0.7-mg dexamethasone intravitreal implant (Ozurdex) was approved for the treatment of DME in eyes which had already undergone cataract surgery or were undergoing cataract surgery.[73] This Ozurdex implant may be particularly beneficial in eyes that have undergone vitrectomy due to the markedly shortened half-life of intravitreally injected drugs.[74] A global clinical study, known as *FAME (Fluocinolone Acetonide in Diabetic Macular Edema)*, consisted of two prospective, randomized, multicenter trials which evaluated the safety and efficacy of a fluocinolone acetonide (0.19 mg) intravitreal implant (ILUVIEN, Alimera Sciences, Inc) that releases drug for up to 36 months.[75] In September 2014, ILUVIEN was approved by the FDA for the treatment of DME in patients treated previously with a course of corticosteroids and did not have a clinically significant rise in intraocular pressure.

Pearls

- Intravitreal corticosteroids should continue to play an important role in the treatment of DME in some eyes, particularly those with pseudophakia.

While there is little debate regarding the benefits of vitrectomy surgery for DME with an obvious tractional component, the role of the vitrectomy in the treatment of DME without evident traction is controversial.[76,77] It has been argued that removal of the vitreous may improve oxygenation and allow greater diffusion of inflammatory mediators which may be concentrated near the retinal surface in the setting of an intact posterior hyaloid.[78] No compelling trials have demonstrated a long-term benefit of vitrectomy for DME without a tractional component. Furthermore, any potential benefit of vitrectomy needs to be balanced against the prospect of a shortened half-life of intravitreally injected anti-VEGF drugs.

Controversial Points

- The potential benefits of vitrectomy surgery for DME should be weighed carefully against the negative consequences of reduced duration of intravitreally injected drugs, which may negatively impact long-term management of DME.

11.4.4 Radiation Retinopathy

ME is an early complication of radiation retinopathy and is a leading cause of vision loss in patients with this condition. Histologic findings are similar to DR and include loss of pericytes and retinal endothelial cells, microaneurysms, capillary dropout and occlusion, increased vasopermeability, and neovascularization (▶ Fig. 11.5).[79] Radiation-induced ME is a predictable complication that follows external beam radiation as well as plaque brachytherapy. Radiation maculopathy has been reported to occur in 10 to 63% of eyes treated with plaque brachytherapy for choroidal melanoma.[80,81] Approaches for treating radiation-induced ME have included intravitreal bevacizumab, intravitreal triamcinolone acetonide, and laser photocoagulation, with a few case reports describing other methods. However, no effective treatment for this condition has been established. Studies have reported that concurrent administration of corticosteroids and intravitreal anti-VEGF agents may be helpful,[82] and a recent report suggests that concurrent vitrectomy with placement of 1,000 centistokes silicone oil may reduce the incidence of radiation retinopathy.[83]

11.4.5 Retinal Venous Occlusion

ME as a complication of branch retinal vein occlusion (BRVO) and CRVO is a leading cause of decreased central visual acuity secondary to RVO. Clinical features of RVO include retinal hemorrhages, dilated and tortuous retinal vessels, cotton-wool spots, optic disc edema with splinter hemorrhages, and ME. In addition, subretinal fluid and serous macular detachment can complicate BRVO and CRVO. Immediate elevation of intravascular pressure in retinal veins distal to the occlusion site results in greater transudation of fluid into the extracellular space due to increased transmural hydrostatic pressure.[3] Vascular stasis causing ischemia and resulting in upregulation of VEGF and other inflammatory mediators increases vasopermeability and further promotes extravasation of fluid.

Visual acuity loss following RVOs occurs commonly due to ME, but also may result from macular ischemia or neovascular complications (e.g., vitreous hemorrhage, neovascular glaucoma). Macular grid-pattern laser photocoagulation was evaluated and shown in a randomized trial to have modest benefit in perfused ME due to BRVO but not in eyes with ME due to CRVO.[84,85] Corticosteroid-based pharmacotherapies are thought to decrease edema by stabilizing vascular permeability, downregulating inflammatory mediators, and indirectly inhibiting the actions of VEGF.[86] The dexamethasone intravitreal implant (Ozurdex) is FDA approved for the treatment of ME associated with RVO, and several formulations of triamcinolone acetonide are used off-label for this indication.[87,88] The SCORE Study,

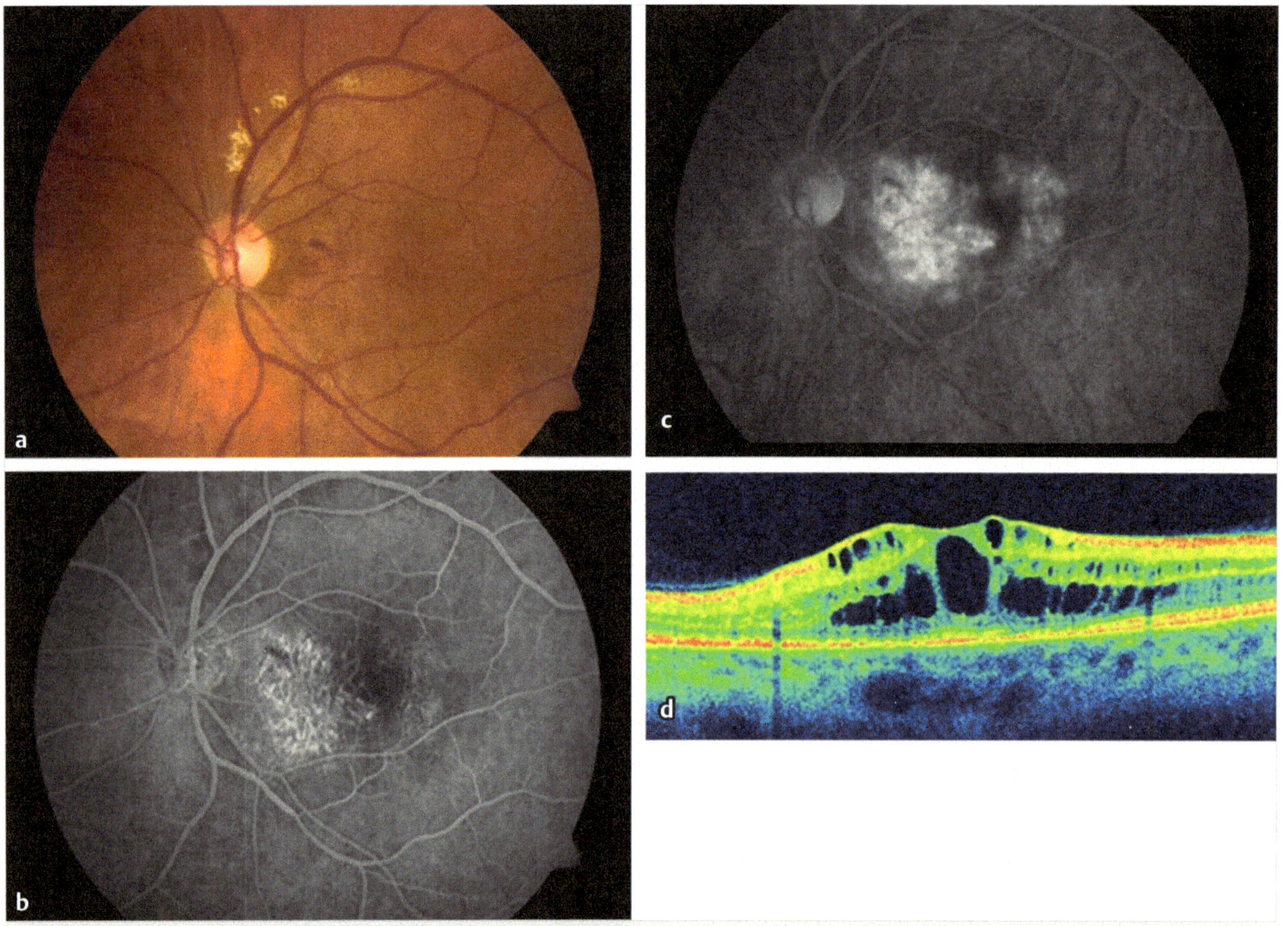

Fig. 11.5 (**a**) Color fundus photograph and (**b**) early and late (**c**) fluorescein angiography images demonstrate microaneurysms and lipid exudates with diffuse hyperfluorescence and leakage in a patient with radiation retinopathy secondary to treatment of a pituitary tumor. (**d**) Corresponding OCT demonstrates diffuse edema. Macular edema resolved completely with monthly injections of bevacizumab, and visual acuity has been maintained at 20/40 for over 3 years with continued maintenance injections every 6 weeks.

funded by the National Eye Institute, demonstrated a modest benefit of a noncommercially available preservative-free formulation of triamcinolone acetonide over standard care at the time of the study (observation for CRVO, grid laser for BRVO) for ME due to CRVO but not for ME due to BRVO.[89,90] At the time of this writing, pharmacotherapy with anti-VEGF drugs has become the predominant means to treat ME due to RVO. Both ranibizumab[91,92,93] and aflibercept[94,95] are FDA approved for the treatment of ME associated with RVO, and off-label use of bevacizumab is common.[96,97] While several other potential treatments for ME associated with RVO have been reported, including pars plana vitrectomy,[98] radial optic neurotomy,[99] intravitreal or retinal intravascular tissue plasminogen activator, and laser-induced chorioretinal anastomosis,[100] these treatments are less proven and/or are not associated with a similar magnitude of visual improvement as demonstrated with anti-VEGF drugs. Several large, prospective, crossover studies have also shown that delay in treatment with anti-VEGF drugs deleteriously affects long-term visual acuity outcomes in eyes with ME due to RVO.[92,95]

Pearls

- Delay in treatment of ME due to RVO with intraocular anti-VEGF drugs deleteriously affects long-term visual outcomes. Early treatment of ME should be encouraged.

11.5 Other Localized Retinal Vascular Disorders

There are several retinal vascular diseases that cause ME, including type 1 macular telangiectasia and Coats' disease. These conditions are usually limited to localized segments of retinal blood vessels and typically result in progressive vascular permeability and accumulation of ME.

11.5.1 Retinal Dystrophies

CME develops in approximately 10% of patients with retinitis pigmentosa (RP) and is usually accompanied by vitreous inflammation (▶ Fig. 11.6). It is generally believed that dysfunction of the RPE pumping mechanism is the predominant cause of CME, but disruption of the outer blood–retinal barrier may also contribute.[101] Consequently, carbonic anhydrase inhibitors, particularly oral acetazolamide, have been reported to be effective in treating CME due to RP because they facilitate fluid transport across the RPE.[102,103] CME unresponsive to acetazolamide may respond to intravitreal corticosteroids, but anatomic benefit is usually temporary and recurrences are common. FA will demonstrate a variable amount of slow leakage, and OCT typically shows cystoid changes over time, often in the setting of a thin retina. Autosomal dominant CME is a rare bilateral disease characterized by hyperopia, subnormal electro-oculogram, and fluorescein leakage. This is in contrast to foveal schisis

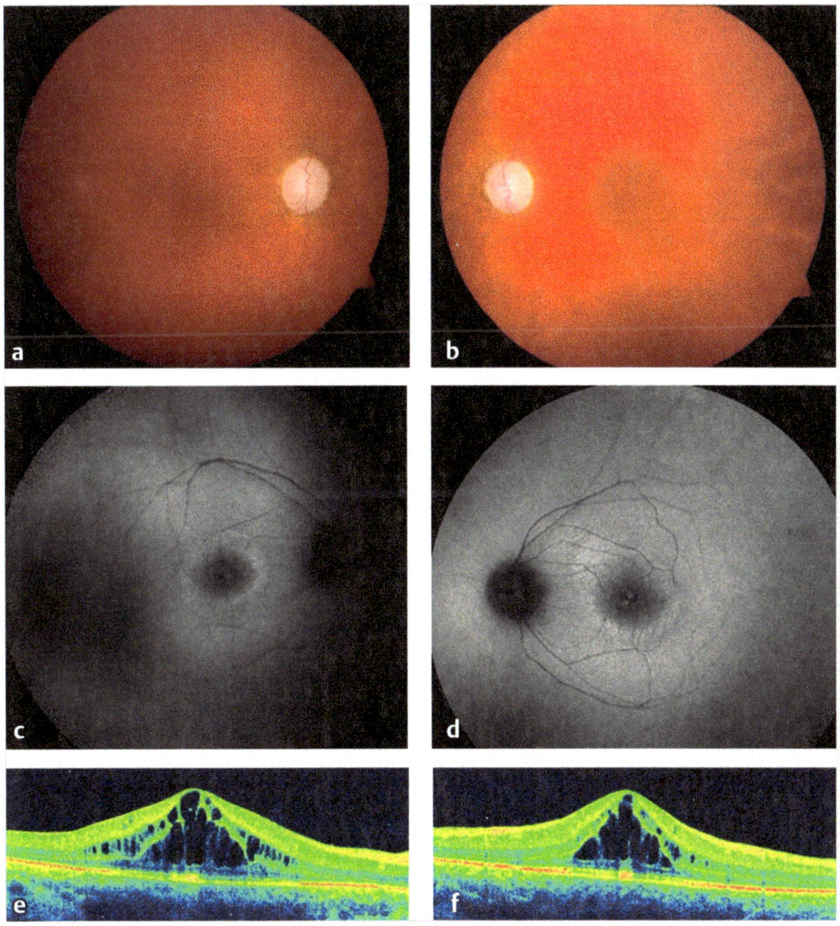

Fig. 11.6 (**a, b**) Color fundus photographs, (**c, d**) fundus autofluorescence, and (**e, f**) OCT images of a patient with retinitis pigmentosa with chronic CME. Note the classic waxy pallor of the optic disc and arteriole attenuation. The CME responded to treatment with oral acetazolamide.

which does not leak on FA and can be associated with conditions such as X-linked juvenile retinoschisis and Goldmann–Favre syndrome.[3]

11.5.2 Drug Toxicity

Several medications have been implicated in the development of ME.[104] Topical prostaglandin analogs such as latanoprost have been reported to cause CME, particularly in eyes with intraocular inflammation.[105] Topical epinephrine was first reported to cause CME (characterized by FA findings identical to Irvine–Gass syndrome) in aphakic eyes.[106] A prospective study of eyes undergoing vitrectomy surgery demonstrated that the addition of epinephrine to the infusion solution increased postoperative intraocular inflammation, which supports an inflammatory mechanism.[107] Thiazolidinediones (TZDs) such as rosiglitazone and pioglitazone were reported to cause peripheral edema and fluid retention in 5 to 15% of diabetic patients.[104] Subsequently, TZDs were associated with the development and exacerbation of DME in patients, but this association remains tenuous.[108] Fingolimod is FDA approved for relapsing forms of multiple sclerosis and was associated with a dose-dependent risk of ME in patients.[109] According to FDA recommendations, patients should undergo a baseline ophthalmic examination prior to starting fingolimod therapy and a second examination 3 to 4 months after starting treatment. High oral doses of nicotinic acid (= 3 g/d) for the treatment of hypercholesterolemia may cause CME (which is typically bilateral) in a small percentage of patients. Although the biomicroscopic appearance of nicotinic acid–induced CME is indistinguishable from that of inflammatory CME, FA shows no evidence of retinal capillary leakage in eyes with nicotinic acid–induced CME.[110] ME without fluorescein leakage can also develop in patients taking taxanes (docetaxel and paclitaxel) which are widely used chemotherapy agents, but the pathophysiologic mechanism is unknown.[111,112] Tamoxifen is an oral nonsteroidal antiestrogen primarily used as prophylaxis in woman regarded as high risk for developing breast cancer or as therapy against estrogen receptor–positive breast cancer. There have been several reports of tamoxifen-induced retinopathy and ME, but mostly from isolated case reports reflecting the rarity of this condition.[113] Interferon (INF)-a, INF-ß, and INF-? are naturally occurring cytokines that modulate the activity of the immune system. INF-ß is used for treating multiple sclerosis and INF-a is used to treat several cancers and hepatitis C. The most frequent ocular complication of INF therapy is retinopathy characterized by retinal hemorrhages and cotton-wool spots, but ME has rarely been reported.[114]

References

[1] Irvine SR. A newly defined vitreous syndrome following cataract surgery. Am J Ophthalmol. 1953; 36(5):599–619

[2] Gass JD, Norton EW. Cystoid macular edema and papilledema following cataract extraction. A fluorescein fundoscopic and angiographic study. Arch Ophthalmol. 1966; 76(5):646–661

[3] Johnson MW. Etiology and treatment of macular edema. Am J Ophthalmol. 2009; 147(1):11–21.e1

[4] Kim SJ, Bressler NM. Optical coherence tomography and cataract surgery. Curr Opin Ophthalmol. 2009; 20(1):46–51

[5] Miyake K, Ibaraki N. Prostaglandins and cystoid macular edema. Surv Ophthalmol. 2002; 47 Suppl 1:S203–S218

[6] Bhagat N, Grigorian RA, Tutela A, Zarbin MA. Diabetic macular edema: pathogenesis and treatment. Surv Ophthalmol. 2009; 54(1):1–32

[7] Schoenberger SD, Kim SJ. Nonsteroidal anti-inflammatory drugs for retinal disease. Int J Inflamm. 2013; 2013:281981

[8] Kim SJ, Belair ML, Bressler NM, et al. A method of reporting macular edema after cataract surgery using optical coherence tomography. Retina. 2008; 28 (6):870–876

[9] Cunha-Vaz JG, Travassos A. Breakdown of the blood-retinal barriers and cystoid macular edema. Surv Ophthalmol. 1984; 28 Suppl:485–492

[10] Scholl S, Kirchhof J, Augustin AJ. Pathophysiology of macular edema. Ophthalmologica. 2010; 224:8–15

[11] Singh A, Stewart JM. Pathophysiology of diabetic macular edema. Int Ophthalmol Clin. 2009; 49(2):1–11

[12] Miyamoto K, Khosrof S, Bursell SE, et al. Prevention of leukostasis and vascular leakage in streptozotocin-induced diabetic retinopathy via intercellular adhesion molecule-1 inhibition. Proc Natl Acad Sci U S A. 1999; 96 (19):10836–10841

[13] Saishin Y, Saishin Y, Takahashi K, Melia M, Vinores SA, Campochiaro PA. Inhibition of protein kinase C decreases prostaglandin-induced breakdown of the blood-retinal barrier. J Cell Physiol. 2003; 195(2):210–219

[14] Cordero Coma M, Sobrin L, Onal S, Christen W, Foster CS. Intravitreal bevacizumab for treatment of uveitic macular edema. Ophthalmology. 2007; 114 (8):1574–1579.e1

[15] Leal EC, Manivannan A, Hosoya K, et al. Inducible nitric oxide synthase isoform is a key mediator of leukostasis and blood-retinal barrier breakdown in diabetic retinopathy. Invest Ophthalmol Vis Sci. 2007; 48 (11):5257–5265

[16] Catier A, Tadayoni R, Paques M, et al. Characterization of macular edema from various etiologies by optical coherence tomography. Am J Ophthalmol. 2005; 140(2):200–206

[17] Kim SJ, Equi R, Bressler NM. Analysis of macular edema after cataract surgery in patients with diabetes using optical coherence tomography. Ophthalmology. 2007; 114(5):881–889

[18] Bélair ML, Kim SJ, Thorne JE, et al. Incidence of cystoid macular edema after cataract surgery in patients with and without uveitis using optical coherence tomography. Am J Ophthalmol. 2009; 148(1):128–35.e2

[19] Schmier JK, Halpern MT, Covert DW, Matthews GP. Evaluation of costs for cystoid macular edema among patients after cataract surgery. Retina. 2007; 27(5):621–628

[20] Konstantopoulos A, Yadegarfar G, Madhusudhana K, et al. Prognostic factors that determine visual outcome following cataract surgery complicated by vitreous loss. Eur J Ophthalmol. 2009; 19(2):247–253

[21] Baker CW, Almukhtar T, Bressler NM, et al. Diabetic Retinopathy Clinical Research Network Authors/Writing Committee. Macular edema after cataract surgery in eyes without preoperative central-involved diabetic macular edema. JAMA Ophthalmol. 2013; 131(7):870–879

[22] Kramer SG. Cystoid macular edema after aphakic penetrating keratoplasty. Ophthalmology. 1981; 88(8):782–787

[23] Benson SE, Ratclliffe S, Van Raders P, et al. A randomized comparison of parecoxib/valdecoxib and placebo for the prevention of cystoid macular edema after scleral buckling surgery. Retina. 2009; 29(3):387–394

[24] Falavarjani KG, Modarres M, Nazari H, Naseripour M, Parvaresh MM. Diabetic macular edema following panretinal photocoagulation. Arch Ophthalmol. 2010; 128(2):262–, author reply 262

[25] Steinert RF, Puliafito CA, Kumar SR, Dudak SD, Patel S. Cystoid macular edema, retinal detachment, and glaucoma after Nd:YAG laser posterior capsulotomy. Am J Ophthalmol. 1991; 112(4):373–380

[26] Wechsler DZ, Wechsler IB. Cystoid macular oedema after selective laser trabeculoplasty. Eye (Lond). 2010; 24(6):1113

[27] Rossetti L, Chaudhuri J, Dickersin K. Medical prophylaxis and treatment of cystoid macular edema after cataract surgery. The results of a meta-analysis. Ophthalmology. 1998; 105(3):397–405

[28] Kim SJ, Flach AJ, Jampol LM. Nonsteroidal anti-inflammatory drugs in ophthalmology. Surv Ophthalmol. 2010; 55(2):108–133

[29] Kiernan DF, Mieler WF. Intraocular corticosteroids for posterior segment disease: 2012 update. Expert Opin Pharmacother. 2012; 13(12):1679–1694

[30] Ismail RA, Sallam A, Zambarakji HJ. Pseudophakic macular edema and oral acetazolamide: an optical coherence tomography measurable, dose-related response. Eur J Ophthalmol. 2008; 18(6):1011–1013

[31] Spitzer MS, Ziemssen F, Yoeruek E, Petermeier K, Aisenbrey S, Szurman P. Efficacy of intravitreal bevacizumab in treating postoperative pseudophakic cystoid macular edema. J Cataract Refract Surg. 2008; 34(1):70–75

[32] Demirel S, Batioglu F, Özmert E. Intravitreal ranibizumab for the treatment of cystoid macular edema in Irvine-Gass syndrome. J Ocul Pharmacol Ther. 2012; 28(6):636–639

[33] Nussenblatt RB. The natural history of uveitis. Int Ophthalmol. 1990; 14(5–6):303–308

[34] Rothova A, Suttorp-van Schulten MS, Frits Treffers W, Kijlstra A. Causes and frequency of blindness in patients with intraocular inflammatory disease. Br J Ophthalmol. 1996; 80(4):332–336

[35] Rho D. Acetazolamide treatment of CME in patients with uveitis. Ophthalmology. 1996; 103(11):1717–, author reply 1717–1718

[36] Zierhut M, Thiel HJ, Schlote T. Treatment of uveitic macular edema with acetazolamide. Doc Ophthalmol. 1999; 97(3–4):409–413

[37] Nguyen QD, Callanan D, Dugel P, et al. Treating chronic noninfectious posterior segment uveitis: the impact of cumulative damage. Proceedings of an expert panel roundtable discussion. Retina. 2006(Suppl):1–16

[38] Jabs DA, Rosenbaum JT, Foster CS, et al. Guidelines for the use of immunosuppressive drugs in patients with ocular inflammatory disorders: recommendations of an expert panel. Am J Ophthalmol. 2000; 130(4):492–513

[39] Lowder C, Belfort R, Jr, Lightman S, et al. Ozurdex HURON Study Group. Dexamethasone intravitreal implant for noninfectious intermediate or posterior uveitis. Arch Ophthalmol. 2011; 129(5):545–553

[40] Callanan DG, Jaffe GJ, Martin DF, Pearson PA, Comstock TL. Treatment of posterior uveitis with a fluocinolone acetonide implant: three-year clinical trial results. Arch Ophthalmol. 2008; 126(9):1191–1201

[41] Williams GA, Haller JA, Kuppermann BD, et al. Dexamethasone DDS Phase II Study Group. Dexamethasone posterior-segment drug delivery system in the treatment of macular edema resulting from uveitis or Irvine-Gass syndrome. Am J Ophthalmol. 2009; 147(6):1048–1054, 1054.e1–1054.e2

[42] Kempen JH, Altaweel MM, Holbrook JT, et al. Multicenter Uveitis Steroid Treatment (MUST) Trial Research Group. Randomized comparison of systemic anti-inflammatory therapy versus fluocinolone acetonide implant for intermediate, posterior, and panuveitis: the multicenter uveitis steroid treatment trial. Ophthalmology. 2011; 118(10):1916–1926

[43] Antonetti DA, Klein R, Gardner TW. Diabetic retinopathy. N Engl J Med. 2012; 366(13):1227–1239

[44] Wenick AS, Bressler NM. Diabetic macular edema: current and emerging therapies. Middle East Afr J Ophthalmol. 2012; 19(1):4–12

[45] Danis RP, Sheetz MJ. Ruboxistaurin: PKC-beta inhibition for complications of diabetes. Expert Opin Pharmacother. 2009; 10(17):2913–2925

[46] Aiello LP, Bursell SE, Clermont A, et al. Vascular endothelial growth factor-induced retinal permeability is mediated by protein kinase C in vivo and suppressed by an orally effective beta-isoform-selective inhibitor. Diabetes. 1997; 46(9):1473–1480

[47] PKC-DMES Study Group. Effect of ruboxistaurin in patients with diabetic macular edema: thirty-month results of the randomized PKC-DMES clinical trial. Arch Ophthalmol. 2007; 125(3):318–324

[48] Aiello LP, Davis MD, Girach A, et al. PKC-DRS2 Group. Effect of ruboxistaurin on visual loss in patients with diabetic retinopathy. Ophthalmology. 2006; 113(12):2221–2230

[49] Adamis AP, Berman AJ. Immunological mechanisms in the pathogenesis of diabetic retinopathy. Semin Immunopathol. 2008; 30(2):65–84

[50] Tang J, Kern TS. Inflammation in diabetic retinopathy. Prog Retin Eye Res. 2011; 30(5):343–358

[51] Joussen AM, Poulaki V, Le ML, et al. A central role for inflammation in the pathogenesis of diabetic retinopathy. FASEB J. 2004; 18(12):1450–1452

[52] Tu Z, Li Y, Smith DS, et al. Retinal pericytes inhibit activated T cell proliferation. Invest Ophthalmol Vis Sci. 2011; 52(12):9005–9010

[53] Li Y, Smith D, Li Q, et al. Antibody-mediated retinal pericyte injury: implications for diabetic retinopathy. Invest Ophthalmol Vis Sci. 2012; 53(9):5520–5526

[54] Schoenberger SD, Kim SJ, Sheng J, Rezaei KA, Lalezary M, Cherney E. Increased prostaglandin E2 (PGE2) levels in proliferative diabetic retinopathy, and correlation with VEGF and inflammatory cytokines. Invest Ophthalmol Vis Sci. 2012; 53(9):5906–5911

[55] Sohn HJ, Han DH, Kim IT, et al. Changes in aqueous concentrations of various cytokines after intravitreal triamcinolone versus bevacizumab for diabetic macular edema. Am J Ophthalmol. 2011; 152(4):686–694

[56] Funk M, Schmidinger G, Maar N, et al. Angiogenic and inflammatory markers in the intraocular fluid of eyes with diabetic macular edema and influence of therapy with bevacizumab. Retina. 2010; 30(9):1412–1419

[57] Lange CA, Stavrakas P, Luhmann UF, et al. Intraocular oxygen distribution in advanced proliferative diabetic retinopathy. Am J Ophthalmol. 2011; 152 (3):406–412.e3

[58] Zhou J, Wang S, Xia X. Role of intravitreal inflammatory cytokines and angiogenic factors in proliferative diabetic retinopathy. Curr Eye Res. 2012; 37(5):416–420

[59] Spijkerman AM, Gall MA, Tarnow L, et al. Endothelial dysfunction and low-grade inflammation and the progression of retinopathy in Type 2 diabetes. Diabet Med. 2007; 24(9):969–976

[60] Early Treatment Diabetic Retinopathy Study research group. Photocoagulation for diabetic macular edema. Early Treatment Diabetic Retinopathy Study report number 1. Early Treatment Diabetic Retinopathy Study research group. Arch Ophthalmol. 1985; 103(12):1796–1806

[61] Ho AC, Scott IU, Kim SJ, et al. Anti-vascular endothelial growth factor pharmacotherapy for diabetic macular edema: a report by the American Academy of Ophthalmology. Ophthalmology. 2012; 119(10):2179–2188

[62] Mitchell P, Bandello F, Schmidt-Erfurth U, et al. RESTORE study group. The RESTORE study: ranibizumab monotherapy or combined with laser versus laser monotherapy for diabetic macular edema. Ophthalmology. 2011; 118 (4):615–625

[63] Nguyen QD, Brown DM, Marcus DM, et al. RISE and RIDE Research Group. Ranibizumab for diabetic macular edema: results from 2 phase III randomized trials: RISE and RIDE. Ophthalmology. 2012; 119(4):789–801

[64] Do DV, Schmidt-Erfurth U, Gonzalez VH, et al. The DA VINCI Study: phase 2 primary results of VEGF Trap-Eye in patients with diabetic macular edema. Ophthalmology. 2011; 118(9):1819–1826

[65] Do DV, Nguyen QD, Boyer D, et al. da Vinci Study Group.. One-year outcomes of the da Vinci Study of VEGF Trap-Eye in eyes with diabetic macular edema. Ophthalmology. 2012; 119:1658–1665

[66] Rajendram R, Fraser-Bell S, Kaines A, et al. A 2-year prospective randomized controlled trial of intravitreal bevacizumab or laser therapy (BOLT) in the management of diabetic macular edema: 24-month data: report 3. Arch Ophthalmol. 2012; 130(8):972–979

[67] Qi HP, Bi S, Wei SQ, Cui H, Zhao JB. Intravitreal versus subtenon triamcinolone acetonide injection for diabetic macular edema: a systematic review and meta-analysis. Curr Eye Res. 2012; 37(12):1136–1147

[68] Stewart MW. Corticosteroid use for diabetic macular edema: old fad or new trend? Curr Diab Rep. 2012; 12(4):364–375

[69] Schröder S, Palinski W, Schmid-Schönbein GW. Activated monocytes and granulocytes, capillary nonperfusion, and neovascularization in diabetic retinopathy. Am J Pathol. 1991; 139(1):81–100

[70] Beck RW, Edwards AR, Aiello LP, et al. Diabetic Retinopathy Clinical Research Network (DRCR.net). Three-year follow-up of a randomized trial comparing focal/grid photocoagulation and intravitreal triamcinolone for diabetic macular edema. Arch Ophthalmol. 2009; 127(3):245–251

[71] Elman MJ, Aiello LP, Beck RW, et al. Diabetic Retinopathy Clinical Research Network. Randomized trial evaluating ranibizumab plus prompt or deferred laser or triamcinolone plus prompt laser for diabetic macular edema. Ophthalmology. 2010; 117(6):1064–1077.e35

[72] Elman MJ, Bressler NM, Qin H, et al. Diabetic Retinopathy Clinical Research Network. Expanded 2-year follow-up of ranibizumab plus prompt or deferred laser or triamcinolone plus prompt laser for diabetic macular edema. Ophthalmology. 2011; 118(4):609–614

[73] Haller JA, Kuppermann BD, Blumenkranz MS, et al. Dexamethasone DDS Phase II Study Group. Randomized controlled trial of an intravitreous dexamethasone drug delivery system in patients with diabetic macular edema. Arch Ophthalmol. 2010; 128(3):289–296

[74] Boyer DS, Faber D, Gupta S, et al. Ozurdex CHAMPLAIN Study Group. Dexamethasone intravitreal implant for treatment of diabetic macular edema in vitrectomized patients. Retina. 2011; 31(5):915–923

[75] Campochiaro PA, Brown DM, Pearson A, et al. FAME Study Group. Sustained delivery fluocinolone acetonide vitreous inserts provide benefit for at least 3 years in patients with diabetic macular edema. Ophthalmology. 2012; 119 (10):2125–2132

[76] Haller JA, Qin H, Apte RS, et al. Diabetic Retinopathy Clinical Research Network Writing Committee. Vitrectomy outcomes in eyes with diabetic macular edema and vitreomacular traction. Ophthalmology. 2010; 117(6):1087–1093.e3

[77] Doi N, Sakamoto T, Sonoda Y, et al. Comparative study of vitrectomy versus intravitreous triamcinolone for diabetic macular edema on randomized paired-eyes. Graefes Arch Clin Exp Ophthalmol. 2012; 250(1):71–78

[78] Jiramongkolchai K, Lalezary M, Kim SJ. Influence of previous vitrectomy on incidence of macular oedema after cataract surgery in diabetic eyes. Br J Ophthalmol. 2011; 95(4):524–529

[79] Archer DB, Amoaku WM, Gardiner TA. Radiation retinopathy—clinical, histopathological, ultrastructural and experimental correlations. Eye (Lond). 1991; 5(Pt 2):239–251

[80] Wen JC, Oliver SC, McCannel TA. Ocular complications following I-125 brachytherapy for choroidal melanoma. Eye (Lond). 2009; 23(6):1254–1268

[81] Wen JC, McCannel TA. Treatment of radiation retinopathy following plaque brachytherapy for choroidal melanoma. Curr Opin Ophthalmol. 2009; 20 (3):200–204

[82] Shah NV, Houston SK, Markoe A, Murray TG. Combination therapy with triamcinolone acetonide and bevacizumab for the treatment of severe radiation maculopathy in patients with posterior uveal melanoma. Clin Ophthalmol. 2013; 7:1877–1882

[83] McCannel TA, McCannel CA. Iodine 125 brachytherapy with vitrectomy and silicone oil in the treatment of uveal melanoma: 1-to-1 matched case-control series. Int J Radiat Oncol Biol Phys. 2014; 89(2):347–352

[84] The Branch Vein Occlusion Study Group. Argon laser photocoagulation for macular edema in branch vein occlusion. Am J Ophthalmol. 1984; 98 (3):271–282

[85] Central Vein Occlusion Study Group. Evaluation of grid pattern photocoagulation for macular edema in central vein occlusion. The Central Vein Occlusion Study Group M report. Ophthalmology. 1995; 102(10):1425–1433

[86] Park SP, Ahn JK. Changes of aqueous vascular endothelial growth factor and interleukin-6 after intravitreal triamcinolone for branch retinal vein occlusion. Clin Experiment Ophthalmol. 2008; 36(9):831–835

[87] Haller JA, Bandello F, Belfort R, Jr, et al. OZURDEX GENEVA Study Group. Randomized, sham-controlled trial of dexamethasone intravitreal implant in patients with macular edema due to retinal vein occlusion. Ophthalmology. 2010; 117(6):1134–1146.e3

[88] Haller JA, Bandello F, Belfort R, Jr, et al. Ozurdex GENEVA Study Group. Dexamethasone intravitreal implant in patients with macular edema related to branch or central retinal vein occlusion twelve-month study results. Ophthalmology. 2011; 118(12):2453–2460

[89] Ip MS, Scott IU, VanVeldhuisen PC, et al. SCORE Study Research Group. A randomized trial comparing the efficacy and safety of intravitreal triamcinolone with observation to treat vision loss associated with macular edema secondary to central retinal vein occlusion: the Standard Care vs Corticosteroid for Retinal Vein Occlusion (SCORE) study report 5. Arch Ophthalmol. 2009; 127(9):1101–1114

[90] Scott IU, Ip MS, VanVeldhuisen PC, et al. SCORE Study Research Group. A randomized trial comparing the efficacy and safety of intravitreal triamcinolone with standard care to treat vision loss associated with macular Edema secondary to branch retinal vein occlusion: the Standard Care vs Corticosteroid for Retinal Vein Occlusion (SCORE) study report 6. Arch Ophthalmol. 2009; 127(9):1115–1128

[91] Brown DM, Campochiaro PA, Singh RP, et al. CRUISE Investigators. Ranibizumab for macular edema following central retinal vein occlusion: six-month primary end point results of a phase III study. Ophthalmology. 2010; 117 (6):1124–1133.e1

[92] Campochiaro PA, Brown DM, Awh CC, et al. Sustained benefits from ranibizumab for macular edema following central retinal vein occlusion: twelve-month outcomes of a phase III study. Ophthalmology. 2011; 118(10):2041–2049

[93] Heier JS, Campochiaro PA, Yau L, et al. Ranibizumab for macular edema due to retinal vein occlusions: long-term follow-up in the HORIZON trial. Ophthalmology. 2012; 119(4):802–809

[94] Boyer D, Heier J, Brown DM, et al. Vascular endothelial growth factor Trap-Eye for macular edema secondary to central retinal vein occlusion: six-month results of the phase 3 COPERNICUS study. Ophthalmology. 2012; 119 (5):1024–1032

[95] Brown DM, Heier JS, Clark WL, et al. Intravitreal aflibercept injection for macular edema secondary to central retinal vein occlusion: 1-year results from the phase 3 COPERNICUS study. Am J Ophthalmol. 2013; 155(3):429–437.e7

[96] Epstein DL, Algvere PV, von Wendt G, Seregard S, Kvanta A. Bevacizumab for macular edema in central retinal vein occlusion: a prospective, randomized, double-masked clinical study. Ophthalmology. 2012; 119(6):1184–1189

[97] Epstein DL, Algvere PV, von Wendt G, Seregard S, Kvanta A. Benefit from bevacizumab for macular edema in central retinal vein occlusion: twelve-month results of a prospective, randomized study. Ophthalmology. 2012; 119(12):2587–2591

[98] Raszewska-Steglinska M, Gozdek P, Cisiecki S, Michalewska Z, Michalewski J, Nawrocki J. Pars plana vitrectomy with ILM peeling for macular edema secondary to retinal vein occlusion. Eur J Ophthalmol. 2009; 19(6):1055–1062

[99] Opremcak EM, Rehmar AJ, Ridenour CD, Kurz DE, Borkowski LM. Radial optic neurotomy with adjunctive intraocular triamcinolone for central retinal vein occlusion: 63 consecutive cases. Retina. 2006; 26(3):306–313

[100] McAllister IL, Gillies ME, Smithies LA, et al. The Central Retinal Vein Bypass Study: a trial of laser-induced chorioretinal venous anastomosis for central retinal vein occlusion. Ophthalmology. 2010; 117(5):954–965

[101] Scorolli L, Morara M, Meduri A, et al. Treatment of cystoid macular edema in retinitis pigmentosa with intravitreal triamcinolone. Arch Ophthalmol. 2007; 125(6):759–764

[102] Cox SN, Hay E, Bird AC. Treatment of chronic macular edema with acetazolamide. Arch Ophthalmol. 1988; 106(9):1190–1195

[103] Fishman GA, Gilbert LD, Fiscella RG, Kimura AE, Jampol LM. Acetazolamide for treatment of chronic macular edema in retinitis pigmentosa. Arch Ophthalmol. 1989; 107(10):1445–1452

[104] Makri OE, Georgalas I, Georgakopoulos CD. Drug-induced macular edema. Drugs. 2013; 73(8):789–802

[105] Rowe JA, Hattenhauer MG, Herman DC. Adverse side effects associated with latanoprost. Am J Ophthalmol. 1997; 124(5):683–685

[106] Kolker AE, Becker B. Epinephrine maculopathy. Arch Ophthalmol. 1968; 79 (5):552–562

[107] Kim SJ, Martin DF, Hubbard GB, III, et al. Incidence of postvitrectomy macular edema using optical coherence tomography. Ophthalmology. 2009; 116 (8):1531–1537

[108] Ryan EH, Jr, Han DP, Ramsay RC, et al. Diabetic macular edema associated with glitazone use. Retina. 2006; 26(5):562–570

[109] Minuk A, Belliveau MJ, Almeida DR, Dorrepaal SJ, Gale JS. Fingolimod-associated macular edema: resolution by sub-tenon injection of triamcinolone with continued fingolimod use. JAMA Ophthalmol. 2013; 131(6):802–804

[110] Gass JDM. Nicotinic acid maculopathy. Am J Ophthalmol. 1973; 76(4):500–510

[111] Telander DG, Sarraf D. Cystoid macular edema with docetaxel chemotherapy and the fluid retention syndrome. Semin Ophthalmol. 2007; 22(3):151–153

[112] Joshi MM, Garretson BR. Paclitaxel maculopathy. Arch Ophthalmol. 2007; 125(5):709–710

[113] Griffiths MF. Tamoxifen retinopathy at low dosage. Am J Ophthalmol. 1987; 104(2):185–186

[114] Tokai R, Ikeda T, Miyaura T, Sato K. Interferon-associated retinopathy and cystoid macular edema. Arch Ophthalmol. 2001; 119(7):1077–1079

12 Retinopathy of Prematurity

Yoshihiro Yonekawa and R. V. Paul Chan

First edition chapter originally authored by J. Arch McNamara and Brian P. Connolly

12.1 Introduction

Retinopathy of prematurity (ROP) is a potentially blinding retinal vascular disorder that affects the retina of premature infants. ROP has become more frequent, as advances in neonatal medicine have allowed increased survival of premature infants. Well over half of infants with a birth weight of 700 g[1] and those born at 24 weeks of gestational age (GA)[2] are now able to survive. Neonates who are born very premature and with an extremely low birth weight are at greatest risk for the development of ROP. For example, in the Early Treatment for ROP (ETROP) study, 6,998 infants with birth weight < 1,251 g were screened from 2000 to 2002, and any degree of ROP was found in 68% of these babies.[3] However, ROP developed in 93% of patients with birth weight < 750 g compared to 44% of those with birth weights 1,000 to 1,250 g and in 89% of patients = 27 weeks of GA compared to 14% of those = 32 weeks of GA.[3]

12.2 Initial Findings and the Role of Oxygen

The first description of ROP as a disease entity related to prematurity was made by Terry in 1942, and he coined the term *retrolental fibroplasia* to refer to the late presentation of total retinal detachment with overlying fibrovascular membranes behind the lens.[4,5] Within a decade of his initial reports, ROP was the leading reported cause of childhood blindness in industrialized nations.[6] Oxygen exposure was noted as an association with ROP in the early 1950s,[7] and subsequent studies illustrated the role of supplemental oxygen treatment in the development of ROP.[8] Health care providers in neonatal nurseries were encouraged to curtail oxygen therapy, and the incidence of ROP rapidly declined. However, in the 1960s, oxygen deprivation was reported to be associated with increased neonatal mortality from neurological and pulmonary disorders, and this led to more liberal use of oxygen and the resurgence of ROP.[9] The advent of continuous transcutaneous oxygen monitoring allowed health care providers to set goals for oxygenation saturation in an attempt to balance the risks of ROP and mortality, but the target range for oxygenation saturation remains controversial.[10,11,12] Furthermore, it is now recognized that ROP is a complex and multifactorial disease, rather than a retinopathy due solely to supplemental oxygen exposure.

12.3 Prevalence

The overall prevalence of ROP in a given nation is related to socioeconomic status and neonatal intensive care unit (NICU) capacities. Low-income nations have low rates of ROP because the mortality rates for premature infants are high. More severe forms of ROP are seen in high-income nations due to advances in neonatal care that allow the youngest and sickest infants to survive, but often with worse ocular and systemic sequelae. The ETROP study took place in the United States in the 2000s,[3] and while the overall incidence of ROP was similar to the Cryotherapy for Retinopathy of Prematurity (CRYO-ROP) study from the 1980s, there were more patients with posterior disease in the ETROP study, which occurred most often in the youngest and sickest infants.

Middle-income nations are currently experiencing a "third epidemic" of ROP due to increased numbers of NICUs, but many such NICUs lack sophisticated oxygen-monitoring devices.[13] Based on 1993 epidemiological data, the World Health Organization estimated that more than 50,000 children were blinded by ROP throughout the world.[14] Most of these children lived in Latin America and former socialist economies.

12.4 Clinical Features

It is fortunate that the natural history of acute ROP favors spontaneous regression in the majority of cases. Among infants whose ROP regressed spontaneously, Flynn et al[15] reported that ROP lasted for an average of 15 weeks. The earliest sign of regression is vascularization of the retina beyond the fibrovascular ridge. As the arterioles and venules extend into the avascular retina, the caliber and tortuosity of the vessels posterior to the shunt and in the posterior pole diminish.

Those infants who progress to advanced stages of ROP represent a small minority. The most important risk factors are low birth weight and young GA. In the CRYO-ROP study, of 4,099 infants who were screened, 291 (7%) reached threshold disease that required randomization.[16] The mean birth weight of these infants was 800 ± 165 g and the mean GA was 26.3 ± 1.8 weeks.

Pearls

- In the United States, 83% of infants with birth weights less than 1,000 g are at greatest risk for the development of ROP.[3]

12.5 Pathogenesis

Retinal vessels normally reach the nasal ora serrata by 36 weeks of gestation and temporally by 40 weeks, although complete remodeled vascularization is achieved 2 to 3 months after term birth.[17] Premature infants are born prior to full vascularization of the retina, and the relatively hyperoxic extrauterine environment and supplemental oxygen cause downregulation of growth factors such as vascular endothelial growth factor (VEGF), which slows down vascular development.[18] Existing vasculature becomes attenuated and may undergo apoptosis.[19] The vaso-obliteration and the increasing metabolic demands of the maturing peripheral retina make the retina hypoxic, resulting in upregulation of growth factors. This leads to pathologic

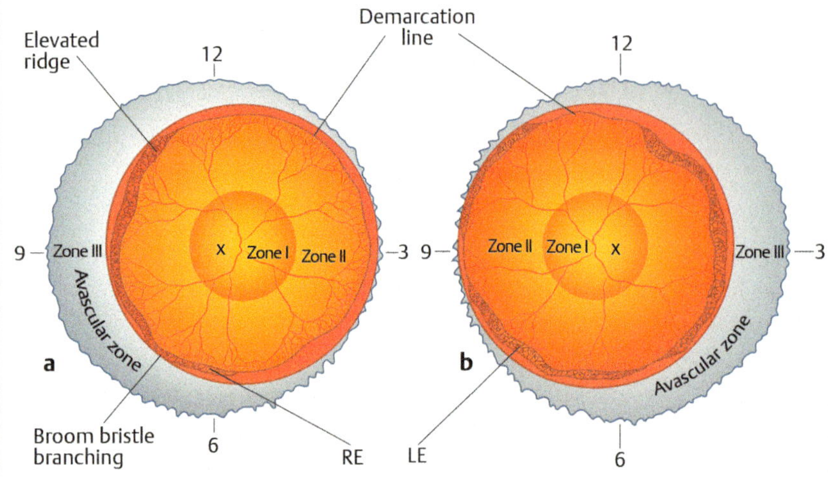

Fig. 12.1 Two schematic eyes that have reached threshold criteria for retinopathy of prematurity in one of two ways: (**a**) 5 contiguous clock hours of stage 3 disease; (**b**) 8 cumulative clock hours of stage 3 disease. Plus disease (not shown here) is also required for the classification of threshold disease.

fibrovascular proliferation. The attenuated vessels merge with surrounding mesenchymal cells to form arteriovenous shunts, represented as the demarcation line in stage 1 ROP as described in the next section.[20] The shunt regresses in most cases and peripheral retinal vascularization occurs. However, the neovascular drive may persist in high-risk infants, causing the primitive endothelial cells of the shunt to proliferate through the internal limiting membrane and into the vitreous.[21] This fibrovascular tissue exerts vitreoretinal contractile forces, which can lead to tractional retinal detachment.

12.6 Diagnosis and Classification

In 1984, a classification system for acute ROP, devised by 23 ophthalmologists from 11 countries, was published and widely accepted.[22] The International Classification for Retinopathy of Prematurity (ICROP) systematically defined the location of the disease in the retina as well as the extent of the developing vasculature that was involved. Moreover, this classification system laid the groundwork for controlled randomized clinical trials. Three parameters are used to characterize the amount of disease that is present: zone, stage, and (the presence or absence of) "plus" disease. The extent of disease is further specified as number of clock hours (▶ Fig. 12.1).

To define the anatomic location of disease in the retina, the retina is divided into three zones centered around the optic disc. Zone I is a circle with a radius defined as twice the distance between the center of the optic nerve and the foveal center. Zone II extends from the anterior edge of zone I to a circle whose radius is equal to the distance between the center of the optic disc and the nasal ora serrata. Finally, zone III represents the temporal crescent of the retina anterior to zone II.

Pearls

- Fortunately, acute ROP regresses in most eyes without treatment.

When an abnormal vascular response is present, it is the basis for the second parameter, the stage of disease. When there is no demarcation line between vascularized and nonvascularized retina, immature vasculature (but not acute ROP) is said to be present (▶ Fig. 12.2a). Four stages were included in the original classification, and they are described as follows. Stage 1 (demarcation line) is defined by the presence of a thin but definite structure that separates the avascular retina anteriorly from vascularized retina posteriorly (▶ Fig. 12.2b). Abnormal branching or arcading of vessels is seen leading up to the line. The line is flat and white and is in the plane of the retina. Stage 2 (ridge) is present when the line of stage 1 has grown, has height and width, and extends out of the plane of the retina (▶ Fig. 12.2c). The ridge may be either pink or white in color. Vessels may leave the plane of the retina to enter the ridge. Small tufts of new vessels may be noted on the surface of the retina posterior to the ridge. These vessels do not constitute fibrovascular growth, which is a necessary condition for stage 3 ROP. Stage 3 (ridge with extraretinal fibrovascular proliferation) exists when extraretinal neovascularization is added to the ridge of stage 2 ROP (▶ Fig. 12.2d). Stage 4 (retinal detachment) is the addition of (partial) tractional retinal detachment to stage 3 findings (▶ Fig. 12.3a,b), and stage 5 is total retinal detachment, often with retrolenticular tissue (▶ Fig. 12.4). Stage 5 retinal detachments are total. Stage 5 is subdivided based on the shape of the funnel. The funnel is divided into anterior and posterior parts, allowing for four subdivisions depending on whether the funnel is open or narrow in both its parts.

Progressive vascular incompetence, occurring in association with changes at the edge of the abnormally developing retinal vasculature, is confirmed by increasing dilation and tortuosity of the peripheral retinal vessels, iris vascular engorgement, pupillary rigidity, and vitreous haze. When vascular changes are so marked that the posterior veins are enlarged and the arterioles are tortuous, a plus sign is added to the ROP stage number ("plus" disease) (▶ Fig. 12.5a). At least two quadrants of plus disease are required for the diagnosis of plus disease. Although it is not part of the classification, the committee recognized that regression is the most common outcome of ROP. The myriad patterns of regression were thought to be too numerous to classify, but they were listed as shown in ▶ Table 12.1.

In 2005, the ICROP report was updated using wide-angle digital fundus photographs, and included the following revisions[23]: (1) The classification of "preplus" disease was introduced. It

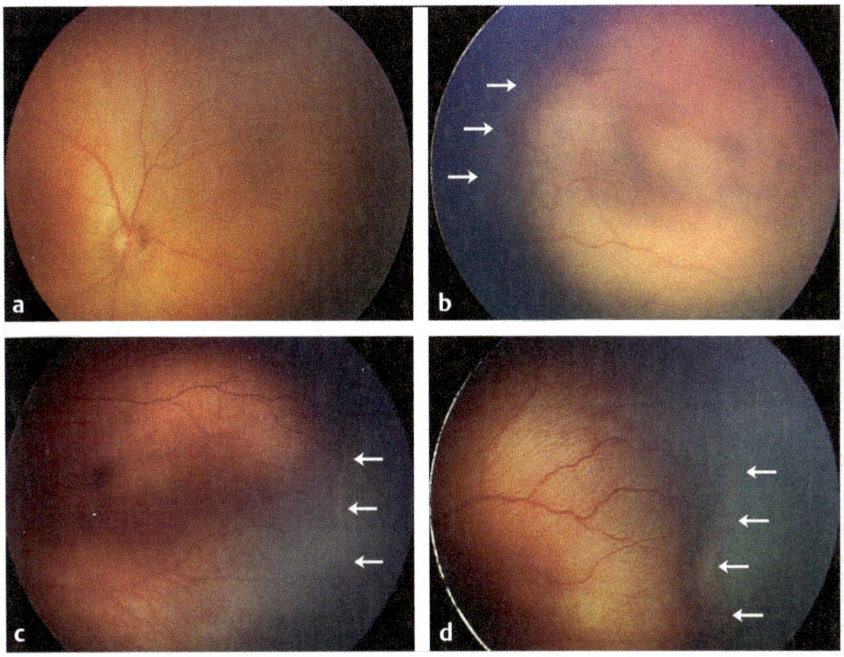

Fig. 12.2 The stages of retinopathy of prematurity. (**a**) Immature vascularization: No distinct border between vascular and avascular retina, and vascularization extends to zone II. (**b**) Stage 1: White demarcation line (arrows) dividing vascularized and avascular retina. (**c**) Stage 2: Elevated ridge (arrows) dividing vascularized and avascular retina. (**d**) Stage 3: Extraretinal fibrovascular proliferation (arrows).

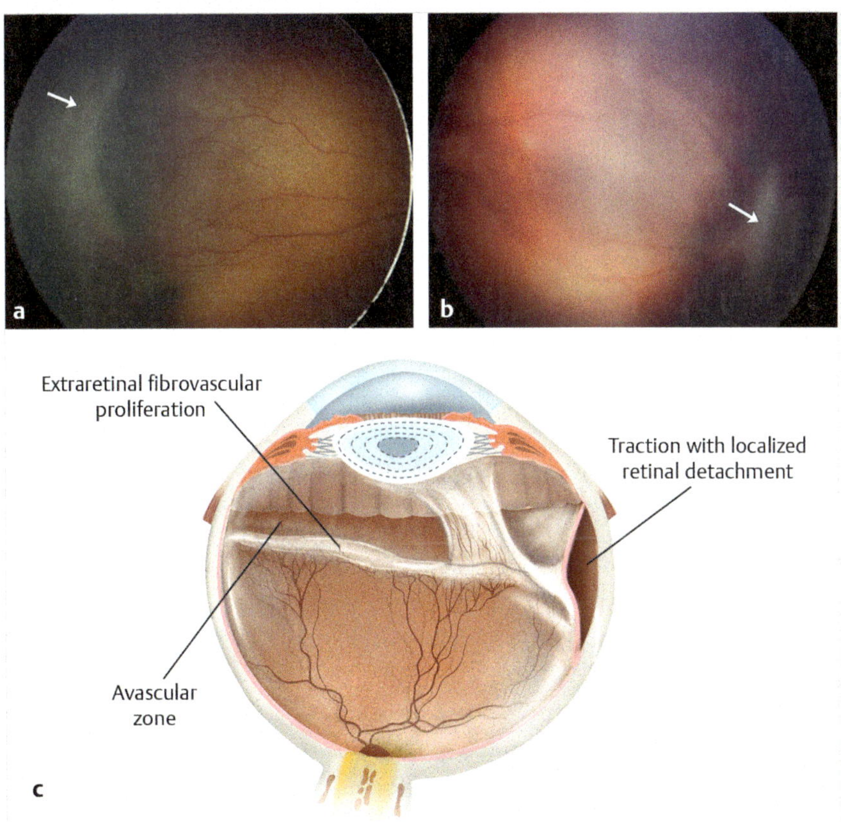

Fig. 12.3 Stage 4 retinopathy of prematurity. (**a**) Stage 4A is a retinal detachment caused by tractional membranes (arrow) that spares the fovea. (**b**) Stage 4B is a tractional (arrow) retinal detachment that involves the fovea. (**c**) Schematic of a partial retinal detachment with vitreoretinal traction directed anteriorly and centrally.

represents posterior pole vascular changes that do not meet criteria for plus disease (▶ Fig. 12.5b). (2) A severe form of ROP called “aggressive posterior ROP” (AP-ROP) was also recognized (▶ Fig. 12.5c). This occurs in the youngest infants, and is characterized by posterior plus disease, often with flat neovascularization and rapid progression that may skip the classic ROP stages.

Pearls

- AP-ROP is a rapidly progressive form of ROP found in zone I or posterior zone II of very premature infants, and may skip the traditional ROP stages. AP-ROP needs to be treated immediately.

12.6.1 Flourescein Angiography and Optical Coherence Tomography

Wide-field fluorescein angiography (FA) can be accomplished in patients with ROP using digital imaging systems, for example, RetCam (Clarity Medical Systems).[25,26,27,28,29,30] It allows precise delineation of the vascular–avascular junction, clear visualization of the fibrovascular proliferation, and identification of areas of capillary nonperfusion. Flat stage 3 disease often seen in posterior ROP, and popcorn lesions (small isolated tufts of regressing stage 3), may also be more easily appreciated on angiography, compared to clinical or digital fundus images alone. Other features such as focal capillary dilatations, arteriovenous shunting, and irregular branching of peripheral vessels are also observed on angiography. Finally, FA can be used to image areas of residual avascularity after treatment to determine appropriate re-retreatments or timing of follow-up (▶ Fig. 12.6). It may be useful but at this time is not considered essential in routine ROP management.

Optical coherence tomography (OCT) has provided new insights into ROP pathophysiology and foveal development (▶ Fig. 12.7a).[31] Initial techniques required prone positioning of neonates under general anesthesia to set the infants' chins onto the OCT interfaces,[32,33] but hand-held systems have been developed to allow easier and safer scanning in the supine position.[34,35,36] With OCT imaging, it was observed that approximately half of premature infants develop cystoid macular changes (▶ Fig. 12.7b).[37,38] This appears to be independent of clinical ROP staging.[38,39] Many patients with a history of ROP may have poor visual outcomes despite good anatomic results. Previously, the poor vision was commonly attributed to cerebral dysfunction, but the maculopathy appreciated on OCT may also be contributory.[33] Furthermore, OCT is being investigated as a method for analysis of choroidal[40] and optic nerve[41] development.

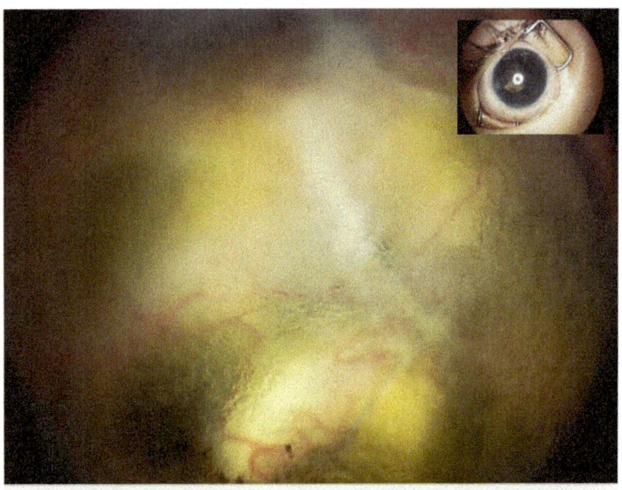

Fig. 12.4 Stage 5 retinopathy of prematurity is a total retinal detachment that often presents with retrolental tissue.

12.6.2 Screening Examination Schedule

The key elements of the recently updated recommendations for the initial ophthalmologic examination of premature infants are as follows[44]:

- All infants with a birth weight = 1,500 g or GA of 30 weeks or less should be examined. Additionally, infants with a birth weight 1,500 to 2,000 g or GA > 30 weeks who have experienced an unstable clinical course may also be screened at the discretion of the treating neonatologist or pediatrician.
- The first examination should take place either at 31 weeks of postmenstrual age (PMA) or 4 weeks after delivery.

After the initial examination, follow-up is determined by the following guideline, but will be determined by the practitioner:

- 1 week or less: zone I stage 1 or 2, zone II stage 3, or suspicion for AP-ROP
- 1 to 2 weeks: posterior zone II immature, or zone II stage 2
- 2 weeks: zone II immature, stage 1, or regressing.
- 2 to 3 weeks: zone III stage 1, 2, or regressing.

Criteria to help the clinician decide to conclude acute ROP screenings include the following:

- Vascularization to zone III in eyes with no previous ROP.
- Full vascularization to the ora serrata for.
- PMA 50 weeks with no prethreshold disease or worse.
- Regression of ROP, with no abnormal vascular tissues that may reactivate.

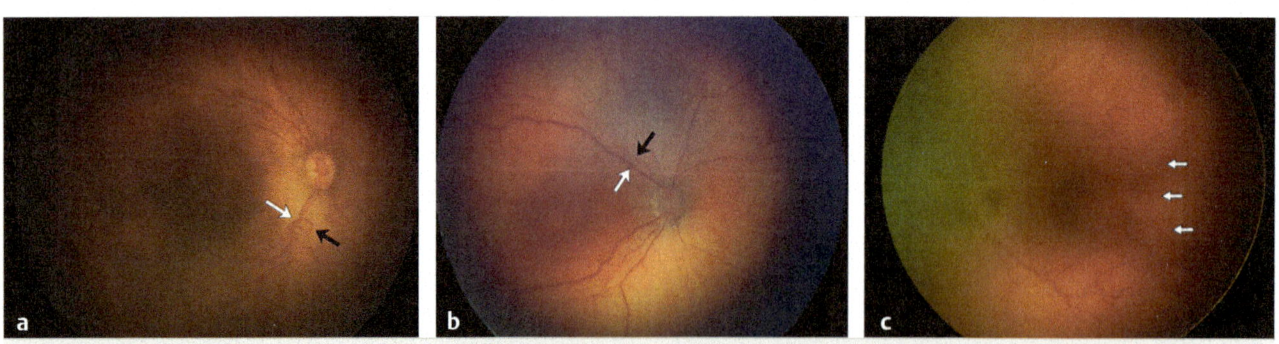

Fig. 12.5 Plus disease. (a) Plus disease is characterized by dilated venules (white arrow) and tortuous arterioles (black arrow). At least two quadrants of vascular changes are required to meet criteria for plus disease. (b) Preplus disease describes posterior pole vascular changes with mild venous dilation (white arrow) and arterial tortuosity (black arrow) that do not meet criteria for plus disease. (c) Aggressive posterior retinopathy of prematurity (AP-ROP) is rapidly progressive, with hallmarks of posterior stage 3 disease and substantial plus disease. This photograph of AP-ROP illustrates prominent plus disease with flat neovascularization (arrow) in zone I.

Table 12.1 Sequelae and signs of previous history of retinopathy of prematurity[22,24]

	Peripheral	Posterior
Vascular	• Failure to vascularize peripheral retina • Abnormal nondichotomous branching of retinal vessels • Vascular arcades with circumferential interconnection • Telangiectatic vessels	• Vascular tortuosity • Straightening of blood vessels in temporal arcade • Decrease in angle of insertion of major temporal arcade
Retinal	• Pigmentary changes • Vitreoretinal interface changes • Thin retina • Peripheral folds • Vitreous membranes with or without attachment to retina • Lattice-like degeneration • Retinal breaks • Traction or rhegmatogenous retinal detachment	• Pigmentary changes • Distortion and ectopia of macula • Stretching and folding of macula • Vitreoretinal interface changes • Vitreous membranes • Dragging of retina over disc • Traction or rhegmatogenous retinal detachment

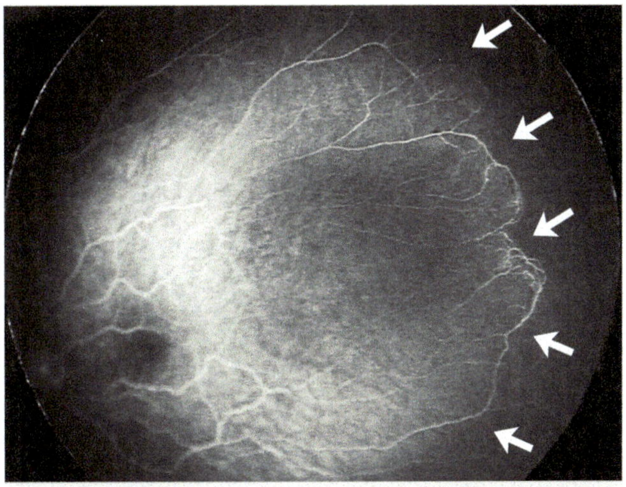

Fig. 12.6 Wide-field fluorescein angiography in an eye with retinopathy of prematurity shows incomplete peripheral vascularization after treatment with intravitreal bevacizumab.

In eyes treated with intravitreal bevacizumab, follow-up examinations are recommended until there is full vascularization of the retina.

Pearls

It is recommended that infants with high-risk prethreshold, or *Type 1* ROP (which has a > 15% risk of retinal detachment), be treated with laser within 72 hours. Waiting until threshold disease is no longer recommended. *Type 1* ROP includes the following:

- Zone I: any stage with plus.
- Zone I: stage 3 without plus.
- Zone II: stage 2 or 3 with plus.

It is recommended that infants with *Type 2* ROP (which has a < 15% risk of retinal detachment) be followed closely. *Type 2* ROP includes the following:

- Zone I: stage 1 or 2 without plus.
- Zone II: stage 3 without plus.

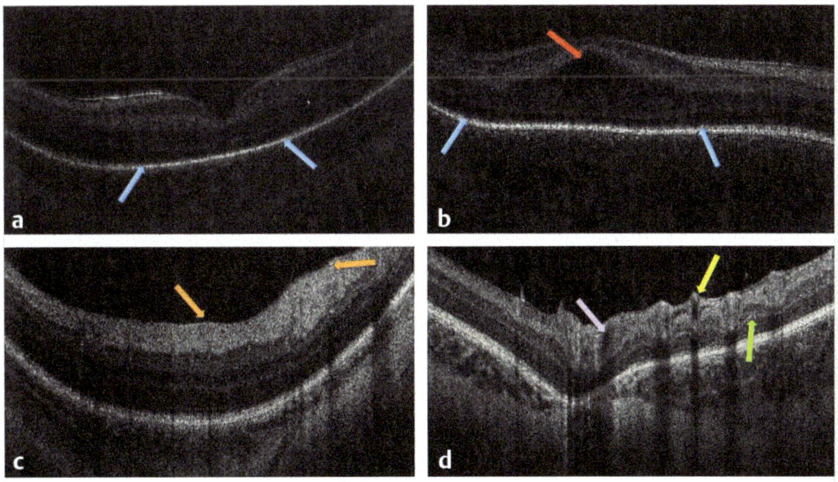

Fig. 12.7 Spectral domain optical coherence tomography (SD-OCT) of retinopathy of prematurity. (**a**) SD-OCT of a premature infant at 34 weeks' PMA with no cystoid macular edema. However, the photoreceptors are underdeveloped as the end of the ellipsoid zone (blue arrows) has not migrated out to the foveal center. (**b**) SD-OCT of a premature infant at 34 weeks' PMA with cystoid macular edema in the inner nuclear layer, causing the fovea to bulge upward (red arrow). The photoreceptors are also underdeveloped (blue arrows). (**c**) SD-OCT of a premature infant at 41 weeks' PMA with no plus disease. This infant had normal vascular features (orange arrows). (**d**) SD-OCT of a premature infant at 42 weeks' PMA with plus disease. This infant had vascular abnormalities including elevated vessels (yellow arrow), scalloped inner retinal layers (green arrow), and hyporeflective vessels (purple arrow).[42,43] (Images courtesy of Cynthia A. Toth, MD.)

Examinations usually take place in the intensive care nursery with monitoring of the infant by the nursery staff. To decrease the risks of emesis and aspiration, examinations should take place no sooner than 1 hour after feeding. Although various other regimens of mydriatic agents can be used, we use three drops of a combination of cyclopentolate 0.2% and phenylephrine 1% (Cyclomydril, Alcon). Topical anesthesia with 0.5% proparacaine or 0.5% tetracaine is administered, and a lid speculum is inserted. Anterior segment examination followed by binocular indirect ophthalmoscopy with a 28-diopter lens is then performed.

The degree of pupillary dilation should be noted on anterior segment examination. Poor dilation may reflect iris vascular engorgement, implying very active ROP. This is often mistaken for iris neovascularization. The presence or absence of "plus" disease should be noted before scleral depression. Scleral depression can modify the amount of vascular engorgement that is apparent. On indirect ophthalmoscopy, the zone should be graded and the stage noted for each clock hour.

If vitreous hemorrhage or stage 5 ROP is present, B-scan ultrasonography may be needed. Ultrasonography can help determine whether a retinal detachment exists behind vitreous hemorrhage that precludes adequate visualization of the retina. In advanced stage 5 ROP, the configuration of the entire funnel-shaped retinal detachment can be evaluated. The anterior and posterior parts of the funnel can be graded as open or closed. This is helpful for providing prognosis and in planning surgery.

12.6.3 Telemedical ROP Screening

The incidence of severe ROP is on the rise,[45,46] and it is becoming increasingly difficult for ophthalmologists to keep up with the demand for ROP screening services.[47] To improve access to care, telemedical ROP screening may provide a viable alternative or adjunct to conventional bedside screening. Currently, the telemedicine model that appears to be best suited for ROP screening is for trained personnel to acquire bedside fundus images using wide-field digital fundus cameras. The images are then uploaded for remote review by expert readers in a "store-and-forward" manner.[48,49] The concepts of "referral-warranted"[50] and "clinically significant"[51] ROP were introduced to identify patients who would benefit from bedside examinations with indirect ophthalmoscopy by the treating ophthalmologist. Studies have shown that remote digital fundus imaging has high sensitivity and specificity,[52,53,54] especially in older infants.[54,55] Telemedical screening programs have demonstrated the reliability of identifying patients who require treatment.[56,57]

In 2012, the American Academy of Ophthalmology published an Ophthalmic Technology Assessment of detecting clinically significant ROP with wide-angle digital photography, and classified seven studies with Level I evidence.[58] Benefits of the technology included objective documentation, being able to compare photographs longitudinally and send them for outside consultations, and the opportunities for education and research. Challenges included personnel training, medicolegal issues, HIPAA compliance, coordination with the NICU, and clear designation of responsibilities.

12.7 Cryotherapy and the CRYO-ROP Study

For infants with progressive ROP, various interventions can stabilize or cause regression of the disease. As early as 1967, Nagata et al[59] noted regression of ROP after xenon arc photocoagulation. Nonetheless, this method was cumbersome and was supplanted by cryotherapy, which was first reported to induce regression by Yamashita[60] in 1972. Several pilot studies of cryotherapy paved the way for the landmark multicenter trial of CRYO-ROP.[16,61,62] This study demonstrated the effectiveness of cryotherapy for reducing the likelihood of an "unfavorable outcome" in infants with *threshold* disease. In the CRYO-ROP study, an unfavorable outcome was defined as the presence of retinal folds involving the macula, retinal detachment involving zone I, or retrolental tissue or "mass." *Threshold* disease was defined as 5 contiguous or 8 cumulative clock hours of stage 3 ROP with plus disease.[22] Treating threshold ROP resulted in reduction in unfavorable outcomes from 51% in the observation group to 31% in the cryotherapy treatment group (a risk reduction of about 40%).[62] This translated into a lower risk of blindness in the treatment group.[63]

An infant's systemic status may preclude treatment. In the CRYO-ROP study,[62] 9% of infants suffered bradycardia, arrhythmia, or significant apnea during administration of anesthesia and cryotherapy. Brown et al reported three instances of respiratory arrest and one of cardiopulmonary arrest in 80 consecutive infants treated with cryotherapy for ROP.[64] These severe systemic complications underscore the need to have infants monitored carefully by a neonatologist or anesthesiologist during treatment. If the neonatologist believes that cryotherapy may be too stressful for the infant, then treatment should be deferred.

12.8 Laser Photocoagulation and the ETROP Study

In the late 1980s, indirect ophthalmoscopic delivery systems for laser photocoagulation became available. Building on the foundation provided by the CRYO-ROP study, McNamara et al[65] and Iverson et al[66] compared argon laser photocoagulation with cryotherapy in prospective randomized clinical trials. Landers et al[67] also reported the use of argon laser for threshold ROP. Subsequently, portable diode and argon indirect lasers were manufactured and have been shown to be effective in treating infants with ROP.[68] Portable lasers have the advantage that they can be brought directly into nurseries. Capone et al showed that laser treatment was particularly beneficial for posterior disease.[69] In a randomized comparison of cryotherapy and laser photocoagulation for threshold ROP, White and Repka noted a trend in which laser-treated eyes tended to have better visual acuity and less myopia than cryotherapy-treated eyes.[70] Earlier laser treatment of prethreshold ROP was piloted in a small controlled trial by Vander et al, whose study resulted in similar rates of unfavorable outcomes between infants treated at threshold and prethreshold.[71]

Such pilot studies led to the organization of the ETROP study. Mathematical algorithms were developed from CRYO-ROP data and converted into a risk analysis program known as Risk Model (RM)-ROP.[72,73] *Threshold* disease confers a 50% risk for unfavorable functional and structural outcomes. *Prethreshold* eyes calculated to have a risks of 15% or higher for unfavorable functional and structural outcomes were considered to be *high-risk prethreshold* (also known as *Type 1 ROP*: zone I any stage with plus, zone I stage 3 with or without plus, or zone II stage 2 or 3 with plus). *Prethreshold* eyes calculated to have a risk of less than 15% for unfavorable functional and structural outcomes were *low-risk prethreshold* (*Type 2 ROP*: zone I stage 1 or 2 without plus, or zone II stage 3 without plus). In ETROP, eyes were randomized to treatment at either threshold or high-risk prethreshold. Most infants received laser treatment, but cryotherapy was also allowed. Unlike the 72-hour treatment window in the CRYO-ROP study, treatment was provided within 48 hours. ETROP showed that earlier treatment at Type 1 ROP resulted in reduction in both unfavorable visual (from 19.5 to 14.5%) and structural (from 15.6 to 9.1%) outcomes at 9 months.[74] Similar trends were seen at 6 years.[75] These data lead to the current standard of care: treatment of Type 1 ROP and close monitoring of Type 2 ROP.

Despite treatment, ROP may progress to stage 4 or stage 5. Retinal detachment occurred in 89 of 718 randomized eyes (12%) in ETROP.[76] Partial or complete ROP-related retinal detachments were treated with surgery (e.g., vitrectomy, scleral buckle)

12.9 Anti-VEGF Treatment

There is growing interest in the off-label use of intravitreal anti-VEGF therapy to target the hypoxia-induced upregulation of VEGF during the second phase of ROP's pathologic neovascularization. The current literature regarding the use of anti-VEGF therapy (typically bevacizumab [Avastin, Genentech]) for the treatment of ROP consists primarily of case reports and small case series, and provides evidence that anti-VEGF treatment promotes regression of neovascularization in patients with acute ROP.[77,78,79] However, anti-VEGF therapy for ROP remains controversial.

There are several theoretical advantages to anti-VEGF therapy compared to laser photocoagulation for the treatment of ROP.[80] (1) Laser ablation of the peripheral retina causes visual field loss, while anti-VEGF agents may allow better preservation of the peripheral retina. (2) Vascular regression is usually faster after anti-VEGF therapy than after laser treatment. (3) Intravitreal injections can be performed under topical anesthesia, and is a much quicker procedure. (4) Resource-poor nations may have easier access to bevacizumab than portable laser systems. (5) Refractive errors may be less common than with laser therapy.[81,82] (6) Anti-VEGF therapy may allow longer treatment windows due to its rapid onset of action, which may decrease the number of infants who ultimately receive treatment.

The BEAT-ROP trial was the first published prospective, controlled, multicenter trial that evaluated intravitreal bevacizumab for the treatment of ROP.[83] A total of 150 infants with zone I or posterior zone II stage 3+disease were enrolled, and randomized to either treatment with bilateral 0.625 mg of bevacizumab or bilateral laser therapy. Overall, 6 of 140 eyes in the bevacizumab group experienced recurrence, compared to 32 of 146 eyes treated with laser ($p = 0.002$). In the subset of eyes with zone I disease, 2 recurred in the bevacizumab group, compared to 23 in the laser group ($p = 0.003$). Benefit of bevacizumab was not observed in zone II eyes. The trial was not powered to assess safety, but there were four deaths related to pulmonary complications in the bevacizumab group, compared to one in the laser group.

One of the main concerns with intravitreal anti-VEGF treatment is its systemic safety in the premature infant. It is known that bevacizumab administered intravitreally in infants with ROP is absorbed systemically and leads to reduced systemic VEGF.[84,85,86] The impact of transiently decreased systemic VEGF levels on the development of other organ systems is unknown. Pulmonary distress is a major cause of morbidity and death in premature infants, and VEGF likely plays an important role in lung development.[87] There are many reports of arteriothrombotic and hemorrhagic events in adults that have been linked with anti-VEGF treatment.[88,89] Intravenous administration of bevacizumab as a chemotherapeutic agent is known to cause such complications as hypertension, stroke, and gastrointestinal bleeding.[90] There are also concerns of potential local adverse events. Eyes with tractional components of ROP pretreatment may develop an increase in traction after anti-VEGF therapy due to rapid involution of the fibrovascular membranes, leading to retinal detachment.[91] There are also reports in the ROP literature of vitreous and retinal hemorrhage,[92] cataract,[93] vascular attenuation with exudation and optic atrophy,[94] and choroidal ischemia.[95] RetCam wide-field angiography has also shown that approximately half of eyes with ROP treated with intravitreal bevacizumab can remain with incomplete peripheral vascularization.[96]

Unlike age-related macular degeneration and diabetic retinopathy, conditions in which VEGF is upregulated continuously and, thus, multiple injections of anti-VEGF therapy may be required, a single intravitreal injection of an anti-VEGF agent may theoretically be able to suppress the neovascular drive in active ROP. Unlike laser treatment, which prevents additional VEGF release from the avascular retina, anti-VEGF therapy allows quenching of the existing VEGF. Anti-VEGF treatment, however, should not be viewed as a one-time treatment without need for follow-up. Recurrence of ROP has been noted to occur after anti-VEGF treatment much later than one would expect after laser treatment.[97,98,99,100] Consensus on a recommended follow-up schedule has not yet been achieved, but infants who were treated with an anti-VEGF agent will often need to be continued to be examined longer than those who were treated with laser, due to delayed full peripheral vascularization and late reactivation of ROP.

The use of anti-VEGF therapy to treat ROP remains controversial, especially in industrialized nations with easy access to portable laser systems, as photocoagulation has proven effective with long-term follow-up. Regression of neovascular disease in ROP has been demonstrated for anti-VEGF agents, but patients must be selected carefully, and the informed consent process with parents should be performed meticulously. In resource-limited nations with poor access to laser systems and well-trained pediatric ophthalmologists or retina specialists, anti-VEGF treatment may be a much-needed option. Further studies will allow better definition of the indications, timing, and follow-up for anti-VEGF treatment of ROP.

12.10 Treatment Techniques

12.10.1 Cryotherapy

Cryotherapy currently has limited indications in the treatment for ROP due to the superior outcomes demonstrated with laser photocoagulation. However, cryotherapy may be required in eyes in which poor pupillary dilation or vitreous hemorrhage do not allow indirect laser application, or if laser systems are not available. Cryotherapy can be applied with topical, subconjunctival, or general anesthesia. If topical or local anesthesia is chosen, intravenous sedation should be administered. Conjunctival swelling from injection of a local anesthetic adds to the edema that occurs during cryotherapy and may obscure the cornea, necessitating termination of the procedure. For topical anesthesia, 0.5% proparacaine or tetracaine can be applied to the cornea every 20 minutes during treatment. Subconjunctival 1% lidocaine can also be provided. To avoid possible cardiopulmonary complications, no more than 0.5 mL should be injected.[64]

A standard retinal or neonatal cryoprobe is used. It is best to start treatment nasally, as pressure from the cryoprobe softens the globe and thus facilitates treatment temporally, where the avascular zone is usually more posterior. Contiguous spots of cryotherapy should be applied throughout the avascular retina anterior to the ridge (▶ Fig. 12.5). Typically, 30 to 50 applications of cryotherapy are necessary, depending on the extent of avascular retina. Care should be taken to avoid prolonged scleral depression, which increases the intraocular pressure and risk for central retinal artery occlusion. A small conjunctival peritomy to fit the cryoprobe may be required to treat posterior disease.

Occasionally, corneal clouding obscures the view during treatment. Removing the lid speculum and waiting several minutes often results in clearing. If waiting fails, the epithelium may be removed with a cotton-tipped swab dipped in 4% lidocaine. Vitreous hemorrhage may also occur during treatment, necessitating termination of the procedure. This is usually a consequence of bleeding from an area of florid extraretinal fibrovascular proliferation and may be precipitated by pressure on the globe from the cryoprobe. Treatment should be completed when the vitreous hemorrhage clears. In the CRYO-ROP study, retinal, preretinal, or vitreous hemorrhage occurred in 22% of treated eyes.[62]

If the view of the fundus is obscured by anterior segment changes or vitreous hemorrhage, cryotherapy should not be applied, and ultrasonography should be performed. If, during the active stage of ROP, there is vitreous hemorrhage obscuring the view posteriorly, vitrectomy should be considered to clear the view for treatment. If anterior segment changes, such as corneal opacity or cataract, are present in both eyes or in a fellow eye when the other eye is blind, and if retinal detachment is seen on ultrasound, combined anterior segment and vitreous surgery should be considered.

12.10.2 Laser Photocoagulation

Clear media are essential for successful laser photocoagulation. Anterior segment changes, such as cataract, corneal clouding, and vitreous hemorrhage may hinder laser treatment in eyes in which cryotherapy or intravitreal injections may be performed.

Although laser photocoagulation delivered by the indirect ophthalmoscope can be performed under general anesthesia, topical anesthesia allows treatment in the nursery (for safety reasons, treatment should be performed in an isolated treatment room if possible). Gentle manipulation is performed with a scleral depressor to position the globe for viewing of the peripheral retina.

Spots should be placed in a near-confluent pattern with a dull white laser photocoagulation mark as the end point.[101,102] We prefer to use the diode laser. If, however, argon laser is used, the initial power can be set to 200 mW at a 0.1-second duration. The power can then be increased gradually to achieve the appropriate desired end point. With the diode laser, we set the initial power setting slightly lower (150 mW) with a longer duration (0.2 second) to avoid rupture of Bruch's membrane and choroidal hemorrhage. The entire anterior avascular retina should be treated (▶ Fig. 12.8). If the infant's movement under topical anesthesia hampers adequate focusing of the laser, the neonatologist or anesthesiologist may administer intravenous sedation. Infants should be monitored by a neonatologist and/or anesthesiologist during treatment.

Potential ocular complications from photocoagulation include anterior segment burns to the cornea, iris, or lens (see the following list). The risk of anterior segment burns may be diminished by limiting infant movement with sedation. Ensuring a clearly focused aiming beam on the retina is critical. Diode laser has the theoretical advantage of lessening the likelihood of lens burns in premature infants with persistent tunica vasculosa lentis. The diode laser, emitting at 810 nm, is not absorbed by the hemoglobin in those vessels, whereas argon green, emitting at 514 nm, is absorbed by hemoglobin.

Ocular Complications of Laser Photocoagulation for Retinopathy of Prematurity

- Stray burns in the retina or anterior segment
- Cataract

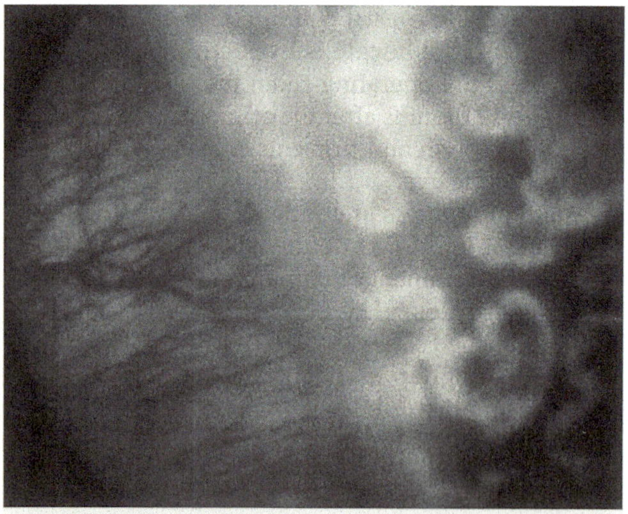

Fig. 12.8 Laser photocoagulation for threshold retinopathy of prematurity. Two weeks after treatment, the laser spots show early pigmentation, and there is good regression of the extraretinal fibrovascular tissue.

- Vitreous hemorrhage
- Late retinal detachment

12.10.3 Intravitreal Anti-VEGF Injection

The unique anatomy of the neonatal eye must be considered when administering intravitreal injections. Most importantly, the lens occupies a relatively larger volume of a smaller globe. Topical anesthesia usually suffices for premature infants, and 5% povidone iodine is used to scrub the lids, and a lid speculum is inserted. The injection is administered with a 30-gauge needle inserted approximately 0.5-1.0 mm posterior to the limbus, which corresponds to the location of the pars plicata. The optimal dose or intravitreal bevacizumab for the treatment of ROP has not been determined. The BEAT-ROP study used 0.625 mg in 0.025 mL of solution, which is half the dose used for adults,[83] but doses as low as 0.25 mg have been reported to be effective.[84]

12.10.4 Scleral Buckle

Retinal detachment in ROP is typically tractional in nature, with or without an exudative component. Tractional detachment of the retina can occur due to progressive fibrous proliferation. This tractional force is often circumferential, and the retina may detach as if a purse string were being tightened. Exuberant extraretinal fibrovascular proliferation may lead to subretinal serous fluid accumulation. Rhegmatogenous retinal detachments are rare but may present years later as a delayed complication of ROP. Retinal detachments often occur at the border between treated and untreated retina.[103] In ETROP, 16% (63 of 401) of infants developed retinal detachment despite laser treatment.[76] Macular reattachment was achieved in 36% (25 of 70) of eyes overall, 34% (17 of 50) after vitrectomy with or without scleral buckling, 67% (6 of 9) after scleral buckling alone, and 18% (2 of 11) with observation. Stage 4A ROP may regress spontaneously or as a result of ablative or anti-VEGF therapy; thus, these detachments should be followed closely and repaired only if they appear to be progressing. When involvement of the fovea is present (stage 4B) or imminent, treatment should be considered.

Scleral buckling was the standard of care for ROP detachments for many years, but in the current era of microincisional vitrectomy surgery and wide-angle viewing systems, it has been largely replaced by lens-sparing vitrectomy (LSV). Scleral buckling is still an effective treatment option in resource-limited nations, and may be a useful adjunct to vitrectomy when the fibrovascular ridge is anterior to the equator and for rhegmatogenous components.

Vitreous hemorrhage is a relative contraindication to scleral buckling surgery. If the hemorrhage is mild and the view of the fundus is adequate to permit staging and appreciation of the amount of fibrous proliferation, then scleral buckling may be performed. If the hemorrhage is too dense or there is any concern that a funnel-shaped retinal detachment is present, vitrectomy is the superior option.

In general, the principle of scleral buckling in ROP is to indent the sclera over the area of vitreoretinal traction just enough to allow the retina to settle and become reapposed to the retinal pigment epithelium and choroid. The globe is typically encircled, and subretinal fluid may or may not be drained externally. Drainage of the subretinal fluid is at the discretion of the surgeon. The neonatal sclera is thin, and the surgeon must keep this in mind when depressing the globe and passing sutures.

Because these eyes are often very small at the time of treatment, the buckle is frequently transected or removed in the operating room under general anesthesia 3 to 6 months after the original operation. This facilitates growth of the globe and prevents erosion of the scleral buckle into the eye. Encircling bands also induce significant myopic anisometropia, which can be reduced by dividing the buckle. Although not a complication of buckle division per se, nonattachment of the retina is an undesired result if it occurs. This may be a result of the disease process itself (persistent or progressive tractional detachment) and also of a loose buckle. If the height of the buckle seems inadequate, the scleral buckle should be revised.

Anatomic success after scleral buckling for retinal detachment in ROP is defined as macular reattachment (full attachment of retina between the temporal vascular arcades). The reported success rate varies between 46 and 75%.[104,105,106,107,108,109,110,111] Higher reattachment rates have been achieved when additional vitreous or scleral buckling surgery was performed. Although the anatomic success rates in these studies are encouraging, the visual results are disappointing.

12.10.5 Vitrectomy

With progressive severity of ROP, the surgical techniques for attempted repair become more complicated and the visual outcomes are generally worse. Vitreous surgery techniques are used to treat stage 4 and 5 retinal detachments. In infants with regression of ROP and good potential for vision in one eye, but with severe stage 4B or 5 disease in the fellow eye, one may consider conservative management, especially if the general anesthesia risk is high.

As with other forms of surgery, the infant's systemic condition should be considered before proceeding with vitrectomy. Vitreous surgery is performed under general anesthesia, and contraindications to this form of anesthesia may necessitate delaying the surgery. Vitreous surgery for ROP continues to evolve. A few dedicated surgeons, notably Machemer, Schepens, Charles, Trese, Hirose, Tasman, and de Juan,[112,113,114,115,116,117] have contributed greatly to our understanding of the surgical pathologic anatomy and the development of surgical techniques for advanced ROP. Lensectomy was a routine component of vitrectomy for ROP detachments until the mid-1900s. In 1992, Maguire and Trese introduced LSV.[118] In this technique, pars plicata vitrectomy is performed using a two-port system with an infusion light pipe, vitreous cutter, and membrane peeler cutter scissors. The sclerotomies are created parallel to the visual axis, but may need to be modified[119] to make the entry in the plane between the lens and retina. Traction is released by removing the organized vitreous ridge-to-ridge, ridge-to-periphery, ridge-to-lens, and ridge-to-disc. Subsequent series, some with modifications to the technique, reported relatively favorable outcomes in eyes with stage 4A and 4B ROP.[120,121,122,123,124,125,126,127,128,129] Surgical adjuncts, such as enzymatic vitreolysis to facilitate vitreous manipulation[130,131,132] and endoscopic-assisted vitrectomy,[133,134] are under investigation. The details of ROP vitrectomy have been described extensively.[135,136]

The timing of surgery is important. It is best for ROP to be quiescent before vitreous surgery is undertaken, but this is not a contraindication. If there is persistent plus disease, with engorgement of the iris vasculature and tortuosity and dilation of the retinal vessels, the risk for intraoperative hemorrhage can be higher. Because of the widespread knowledge of the CRYO-ROP and ETROP results, most patients have already received ablative therapy before presenting with advanced retinal detachment. The detachment occurs because of failure of the ablation to arrest the progression of tractional retinal detachment. Nonetheless, ablative therapy usually induces regression of severe plus disease, making subsequent vitreous surgery safer. Some surgeons have advocated for early vitrectomy in patients with AP-ROP to prevent progression of disease.[137,138]

If there is persistent and severe plus disease, Trese[139] recommends a two-step approach. Patients are treated initially with peripheral avascular retinal ablation, and this area of treated retina usually does not detach; the configuration of retinal detachments in treated patients is typically such that a peripheral trough forms, with the more anterior avascular retina remaining attached. In approximately 3 weeks, plus disease has generally regressed to the point where vitreous surgery can be performed.

The goals of retinal detachment surgery in infants with ROP are different from those in adults undergoing vitreoretinal surgery. As preretinal tissue in infants with ROP is attached firmly and, at times, is integrated into the retina, it is dangerous to attempt to remove all membranes. The tissues can be segmented and left in place if the vitreoretinal tractional forces have been relieved. In addition to massive hemorrhage and infection, another significant potential complication in eyes undergoing vitrectomy for far-advanced ROP is retinal break formation. Retinal breaks occur most often anteriorly in the region of the pars plana during dissection of very adherent epiretinal membranes. When a retinal break occurs, flattening of the retina to permit adequate cryotherapy or laser around the break and on the retina in the area of the scleral buckle is difficult. In none of the cases reported by Zilis et al[116] in which a retinal break was noted during surgery did reattachment occur. When a retinal break is not seen but schlieren (small masses or streaks occurring when two clear fluids of different optical densities mix) is observed, a retinal break should be assumed to be present—although pockets of denser fluid can reside within areas enclosed by membranes or folds and may present with schlieren-like appearances when liberated.

The goals for LSV in stage 4A ROP are to minimize posterior pole distortion, achieve retinal reattachment, and maintain a clear visual axis. If successful, LSV should halt the progression to stage 4B/5. For stage 4B, posterior pole distortion should be minimized as much as possible, but macular dragging will be common, total retinal reattachment may not be possible in most cases, and the lens may have to be sacrificed in some cases. Ambulatory vision is the functional goal. For stage 5 ROP, attempts should be made to reattach as much of the retina as possible, without causing iatrogenic breaks. LSV may be possible in some open-funnel detachments, but lensectomy is usually performed for stage 5 detachments and certainly if extensive fibrovascular proliferation is displacing the lens anteriorly. Staged approaches can be taken by performing a lensectomy and external drainage on the first surgery and returning several weeks later to work on membrane dissection. Determining the configuration of the retinal detachment is the first essential step in surgical planning. Form vision is still possible after stage 5 ROP surgery.[140,141,142]

Although now performed uncommonly, open-sky vitrectomy is another method of ROP surgery that requires lensectomy.[113,114,140] The main advantages of open-sky vitrectomy (vitreous surgery through a trephined opening in the cornea) are easy access to, and visualization of, the anterior retina and epiretinal membranes. Disadvantages of open-sky vitrectomy include lack of control of intraocular pressure and difficulty in posterior manipulation. Currently, open-sky vitrectomy may be appropriate for eyes with cloudy corneas that prevent closed vitrectomy or for eyes with very narrow-funnel stage 5 retinal detachments. The basic steps include trephining the cornea, extracting the lens with a cryoprobe, and then dissecting the epiretinal fibrous proliferation stepwise in an anterior-to-posterior direction.

12.11 Conclusion

The increased survival rate of premature infants has led to an increased incidence of advanced ROP, a new epidemic in middle-income nations. Great strides in ROP management have been made with three seminal efforts to combat the disease: CRYO-ROP and ETROP to guide treatment protocols, and ICROP to promote international clinical research efforts by standardizing nomenclature. New developments in the past decade that are being assessed carefully include anti-VEGF therapy, telemedical screening, and new imaging technologies. Caring for neonates with ROP is a multidimensional effort that requires optimization of access to care, risk factor assessment, screening, imaging, and surgical and nonsurgical treatment, as well as consideration of complicated socioeconomic and medicolegal issues.

References

[1] Wilcox A, Skjaerven R, Buekens P, Kiely J. Birth weight and perinatal mortality. A comparison of the United States and Norway. JAMA. 1995; 273 (9):709–711

[2] Stoll BJ, Hansen NI, Bell EF, et al. Eunice Kennedy Shriver National Institute of Child Health and Human Development Neonatal Research Network. Neonatal outcomes of extremely preterm infants from the NICHD Neonatal Research Network. Pediatrics. 2010; 126(3):443–456

[3] Good WV, Hardy RJ, Dobson V, et al. Early Treatment for Retinopathy of Prematurity Cooperative Group. The incidence and course of retinopathy of prematurity: findings from the early treatment for retinopathy of prematurity study. Pediatrics. 2005; 116(1):15–23

[4] Terry TL. Extreme prematurity and fibroblastic overgrowth of persistent vascular sheath behind each crystalline lens. I. Preliminary report. Am J Ophthalmol. 1942; 25:203–204

[5] Terry TL. Retrolental fibroplasia in the premature infant: V. Further studies on fibroplastic overgrowth of the persistent tunica vasculosa lentis. Trans Am Ophthalmol Soc. 1944; 42:383–396

[6] Patz A. The role of oxygen in retrolental fibroplasia. Trans Am Ophthalmol Soc. 1968; 66:940–985

[7] Campbell K. Intensive oxygen therapy as a possible cause of retrolental fibroplasia; a clinical approach. Med J Aust. 1951; 2(2):48–50

[8] Patz A, Hoeck LE, De La Cruz E. Studies on the effect of high oxygen administration in retrolental fibroplasia. I. Nursery observations. Am J Ophthalmol. 1952; 35(9):1248–1253

[9] Cross KW. Cost of preventing retrolental fibroplasia? Lancet. 1973; 2 (7835):954–956
[10] Carlo WA, Finer NN, Walsh MC, et al. SUPPORT Study Group of the Eunice Kennedy Shriver NICHD Neonatal Research Network. Target ranges of oxygen saturation in extremely preterm infants. N Engl J Med. 2010; 362 (21):1959–1969
[11] Schmidt B, Whyte RK, Asztalos EV, et al. Canadian Oxygen Trial (COT) Group. Effects of targeting higher vs lower arterial oxygen saturations on death or disability in extremely preterm infants: a randomized clinical trial. JAMA. 2013; 309(20):2111–2120
[12] Stenson BJ, Tarnow-Mordi WO, Darlow BA, et al. BOOST II United Kingdom Collaborative Group, BOOST II Australia Collaborative Group, BOOST II New Zealand Collaborative Group. Oxygen saturation and outcomes in preterm infants. N Engl J Med. 2013; 368(22):2094–2104
[13] Gilbert C, Rahi J, Eckstein M, O'Sullivan J, Foster A. Retinopathy of prematurity in middle-income countries. Lancet. 1997; 350(9070):12–14
[14] Gilbert C, Fielder A, Gordillo L, et al. International NO-ROP Group. Characteristics of infants with severe retinopathy of prematurity in countries with low, moderate, and high levels of development: implications for screening programs. Pediatrics. 2005; 115(5):e518–e525
[15] Flynn JT, Bancalari E, Bachynski BN, et al. Retinopathy of prematurity. Diagnosis, severity, and natural history. Ophthalmology. 1987; 94(6):620–629
[16] Cryotherapy for Retinopathy of Prematurity Cooperative Group. Multicenter trial of cryotherapy for retinopathy of prematurity. One-year outcome—structure and function. Arch Ophthalmol. 1990; 108(10):1408–1416
[17] Cogan DG. Development and senescence of the human retinal vasculature. Trans Ophthalmol Soc U K. 1963; 83:465–489
[18] Pierce EA, Foley ED, Smith LE. Regulation of vascular endothelial growth factor by oxygen in a model of retinopathy of prematurity. Arch Ophthalmol. 1996; 114(10):1219–1228
[19] Ashton N. Oxygen and the growth and development of retinal vessels. In vivo and in vitro studies. The XX Francis I. Proctor Lecture. Am J Ophthalmol. 1966; 62(3):412–435
[20] Flynn JT. Retinopathy of prematurity. Pediatr Clin North Am. 1987; 34 (6):1487–1516
[21] Foos RY. Retinopathy of prematurity. Pathologic correlation of clinical stages. Retina. 1987; 7(4):260–276
[22] The Committee for the Classification of Retinopathy of Prematurity. An international classification of retinopathy of prematurity. Arch Ophthalmol. 1984; 102(8):1130–1134
[23] International Committee for the Classification of Retinopathy of Prematurity. The International Classification of Retinopathy of Prematurity revisited. Arch Ophthalmol. 2005; 123(7):991–999
[24] The International Committee for the Classification of the Late Stages of Retinopathy of Prematurity. An international classification of retinopathy of prematurity. II. The classification of retinal detachment. Arch Ophthalmol. 1987; 105(7):906–912
[25] Yokoi T, Hiraoka M, Miyamoto M, et al. Vascular abnormalities in aggressive posterior retinopathy of prematurity detected by fluorescein angiography. Ophthalmology. 2009; 116(7):1377–1382
[26] Hoang QV, Kiernan DF, Chau FY, Shapiro MJ, Blair MP. Fluorescein angiography of recurrent retinopathy of prematurity after initial intravitreous bevacizumab treatment. Arch Ophthalmol. 2010; 128(8):1080–1081
[27] Lepore D, Molle F, Pagliara MM, et al. Atlas of fluorescein angiographic findings in eyes undergoing laser for retinopathy of prematurity. Ophthalmology. 2011; 118(1):168–175
[28] Kang KB, Wessel MM, Tong J, D'Amico DJ, Chan RVP. Ultra-widefield imaging for the management of pediatric retinal diseases. J Pediatr Ophthalmol Strabismus. 2013; 50(5):282–288
[29] Tsui I, Franco-Cardenas V, Hubschman J-P, Schwartz SD. Pediatric retinal conditions imaged by ultra wide field fluorescein angiography. Ophthalmic Surg Lasers Imaging Retina. 2013; 44(1):59–67
[30] Yonekawa Y, Chan RVP. Widefield imaging-guided treatment of pediatric vitreoretinal diseases. Retina Today. 2014:54–57
[31] Maldonado RS, O'Connell RV, Sarin N, et al. Dynamics of human foveal development after premature birth. Ophthalmology. 2011; 118(12):2315–2325
[32] Patel CK. Optical coherence tomography in the management of acute retinopathy of prematurity. Am J Ophthalmol. 2006; 141(3):582–584
[33] Joshi MM, Trese MT, Capone A, Jr. Optical coherence tomography findings in stage 4A retinopathy of prematurity: a theory for visual variability. Ophthalmology. 2006; 113(4):657–660
[34] Chavala SH, Farsiu S, Maldonado R, Wallace DK, Freedman SF, Toth CA. Insights into advanced retinopathy of prematurity using handheld spectral domain optical coherence tomography imaging. Ophthalmology. 2009; 116 (12):2448–2456
[35] Muni RH, Kohly RP, Charonis AC, Lee TC. Retinoschisis detected with handheld spectral-domain optical coherence tomography in neonates with advanced retinopathy of prematurity. Arch Ophthalmol. 2010; 128(1):57–62
[36] Vinekar A, Sivakumar M, Shetty R, et al. A novel technique using spectral-domain optical coherence tomography (Spectralis, SD-OCT+HRA) to image supine non-anaesthetized infants: utility demonstrated in aggressive posterior retinopathy of prematurity. Eye (Lond). 2010; 24(2):379–382
[37] Vinekar A, Avadhani K, Sivakumar M, et al. Understanding clinically undetected macular changes in early retinopathy of prematurity on spectral domain optical coherence tomography. Invest Ophthalmol Vis Sci. 2011; 52 (8):5183–5188
[38] Maldonado RS, O'Connell R, Ascher SB, et al. Spectral-domain optical coherence tomographic assessment of severity of cystoid macular edema in retinopathy of prematurity. Arch Ophthalmol. 2012; 130(5):569–578
[39] Dubis AM, Subramaniam CD, Godara P, Carroll J, Costakos DM. Subclinical macular findings in infants screened for retinopathy of prematurity with spectral-domain optical coherence tomography. Ophthalmology. 2013; 120 (8):1665–1671
[40] Moreno TA, O'Connell RV, Chiu SJ, et al. Choroid development and feasibility of choroidal imaging in the preterm and term infants utilizing SD-OCT. Invest Ophthalmol Vis Sci. 2013; 54(6):4140–4147
[41] Tong AY, El-Dairi M, Maldonado RS, et al. Evaluation of optic nerve development in preterm and term infants using handheld spectral-domain optical coherence tomography. Ophthalmology. 2014; 121(9):1818–1826
[42] Rothman AL, Tran-Viet D, Gustafson KE, et al. Poorer neurodevelopmental outcomes associated with cystoid macular edema identified in preterm infants in the intensive care nursery. Ophthalmology. 2015; 122(3):610–619
[43] Maldonado RS, Yuan E, Tran-Viet D, et al. Three-dimensional assessment of vascular and perivascular characteristics in subjects with retinopathy of prematurity. Ophthalmology. 2014; 121(6):1289–1296
[44] Fierson WM, American Academy of Pediatrics Section on Ophthalmology, American Academy of Ophthalmology, American Association for Pediatric Ophthalmology and Strabismus, American Association of Certified Orthoptists. Screening examination of premature infants for retinopathy of prematurity. Pediatrics. 2013; 131(1):189–195
[45] Lad EM, Hernandez-Boussard T, Morton JM, Moshfeghi DM. Incidence of retinopathy of prematurity in the United States: 1997 through 2005. Am J Ophthalmol. 2009; 148(3):451–458
[46] Lad EM, Nguyen TC, Morton JM, Moshfeghi DM. Retinopathy of prematurity in the United States. Br J Ophthalmol. 2008; 92(3):320–325
[47] Roach L. ROP crisis near, survey says. EyeNet July 2006
[48] Lorenz B, Bock M, Müller HM, Massie NA. Telemedicine based screening of infants at risk for retinopathy of prematurity. Stud Health Technol Inform. 1999; 64:155–163
[49] Schwartz SD, Harrison SA, Ferrone PJ, Trese MT. Telemedical evaluation and management of retinopathy of prematurity using a fiberoptic digital fundus camera. Ophthalmology. 2000; 107(1):25–28
[50] Ells AL, Holmes JM, Astle WF, et al. Telemedicine approach to screening for severe retinopathy of prematurity: a pilot study. Ophthalmology. 2003; 110 (11):2113–2117
[51] Photographic Screening for Retinopathy of Prematurity (Photo-ROP) Cooperative Group. The photographic screening for retinopathy of prematurity study (photo-ROP). Primary outcomes. Retina. 2008; 28(3) Suppl:S47–S54
[52] Chiang MF, Keenan JD, Starren J, et al. Accuracy and reliability of remote retinopathy of prematurity diagnosis. Arch Ophthalmol. 2006; 124(3):322–327
[53] Chiang MF, Starren J, Du YE, et al. Remote image based retinopathy of prematurity diagnosis: a receiver operating characteristic analysis of accuracy. Br J Ophthalmol. 2006; 90(10):1292–1296
[54] Chiang MF, Wang L, Busuioc M, et al. Telemedical retinopathy of prematurity diagnosis: accuracy, reliability, and image quality. Arch Ophthalmol. 2007; 125(11):1531–1538
[55] Yen KG, Hess D, Burke B, Johnson RA, Feuer WJ, Flynn JT. Telephotoscreening to detect retinopathy of prematurity: preliminary study of the optimum time to employ digital fundus camera imaging to detect ROP. J AAPOS. 2002; 6(2):64–70
[56] Lorenz B, Spasovska K, Elflein H, Schneider N. Wide-field digital imaging based telemedicine for screening for acute retinopathy of prematurity (ROP). Six-year results of a multicentre field study. Graefes Arch Clin Exp Ophthalmol. 2009; 247(9):1251–1262
[57] Fijalkowski N, Zheng LL, Henderson MT, et al. Stanford University Network for Diagnosis of Retinopathy of Prematurity (SUNDROP): five years of

screening with telemedicine. Ophthalmic Surg Lasers Imaging Retina. 2014; 45(2):106–113

[58] Chiang MF, Melia M, Buffenn AN, et al. Detection of clinically significant retinopathy of prematurity using wide-angle digital retinal photography: a report by the American Academy of Ophthalmology. Ophthalmology. 2012; 119(6):1272–1280

[59] Nagata M, Kobayashi Y, Fukuda H, Suekane K. Photocoagulation for the treatment of retinopathy of prematurity. Jpn J Clin Ophthalmol. 1968; 22:419–427

[60] Yamashita Y. Studies on retinopathy of prematurity. III. Cryocautery for retinopathy of prematurity. Jpn J Clin Ophthalmol. 1972; 26:385–393

[61] Cryotherapy for Retinopathy of Prematurity Cooperative Group. Multicenter trial of cryotherapy for retinopathy of prematurity. Preliminary results. Arch Ophthalmol. 1988; 106(4):471–479

[62] Cryotherapy for Retinopathy of Prematurity Cooperative Group. Multicenter trial of cryotherapy for retinopathy of prematurity. Three-month outcome. Arch Ophthalmol. 1990; 108(2):195–204

[63] Cryotherapy for Retinopathy of Prematurity Cooperative Group. Multicenter trial of cryotherapy for retinopathy of prematurity. Snellen visual acuity and structural outcome at 5 1/2 years after randomization. Arch Ophthalmol. 1996; 114(4):417–424

[64] Brown GC, Tasman WS, Naidoff M, Schaffer DB, Quinn G, Bhutani VK. Systemic complications associated with retinal cryoablation for retinopathy of prematurity. Ophthalmology. 1990; 97(7):855–858

[65] McNamara JA, Tasman W, Brown GC, Federman JL. Laser photocoagulation for stage 3 + retinopathy of prematurity. Ophthalmology. 1991; 98(5):576–580

[66] Iverson DA, Trese MT, Orgel IK, Williams GA. Laser photocoagulation for threshold retinopathy of prematurity. Arch Ophthalmol. 1991; 109 (10):1342–1343

[67] Landers MB, III, Toth CA, Semple HC, Morse LS. Treatment of retinopathy of prematurity with argon laser photocoagulation. Arch Ophthalmol. 1992; 110(1):44–47

[68] McNamara JA, Tasman W, Vander JF, Brown GC. Diode laser photocoagulation for retinopathy of prematurity. Preliminary results. Arch Ophthalmol. 1992; 110(12):1714–1716

[69] Capone A, Jr, Diaz-Rohena R, Sternberg P, Jr, Mandell B, Lambert HM, Lopez PF. Diode-laser photocoagulation for zone 1 threshold retinopathy of prematurity. Am J Ophthalmol. 1993; 116(4):444–450

[70] White JE, Repka MX. Randomized comparison of diode laser photocoagulation versus cryotherapy for threshold retinopathy of prematurity: 3-year outcome. J Pediatr Ophthalmol Strabismus. 1997; 34(2):83–87, quiz 121–122

[71] Vander JF, Handa J, McNamara JA, et al. Early treatment of posterior retinopathy of prematurity: a controlled trial. Ophthalmology. 1997; 104 (11):1731–1735, discussion 1735–1736

[72] Hardy RJ, Palmer EA, Schaffer DB, Phelps DL, Davis BR, Cooper CJ. Outcome-based management of retinopathy of prematurity. Multicenter Trial of Cryotherapy for Retinopathy of prematurity Cooperative Group. J AAPOS. 1997; 1 (1):46–54

[73] Hardy RJ, Palmer EA, Dobson V, et al. Cryotherapy for Retinopathy of Prematurity Cooperative Group. Risk analysis of prethreshold retinopathy of prematurity. Arch Ophthalmol. 2003; 121(12):1697–1701

[74] Early Treatment For Retinopathy Of Prematurity Cooperative Group. Revised indications for the treatment of retinopathy of prematurity: results of the early treatment for retinopathy of prematurity randomized trial. Arch Ophthalmol. 2003; 121(12):1684–1694

[75] Good WV, Hardy RJ, Dobson V, et al. Early Treatment for Retinopathy of Prematurity Cooperative Group. Final visual acuity results in the early treatment for retinopathy of prematurity study. Arch Ophthalmol. 2010; 128 (6):663–671

[76] Repka MX, Tung B, Good WV, et al. Outcome of eyes developing retinal detachment during the Early Treatment for Retinopathy of Prematurity Study (ETROP). Arch Ophthalmol. 2006; 124(1):24–30

[77] Wykoff CC, Houston SK, Berrocal AM. Anti-vascular endothelial growth factor agents for pediatric retinal diseases. Int Ophthalmol Clin. 2011; 51 (1):185–199

[78] Micieli JA, Surkont M, Smith AF. A systematic analysis of the off-label use of bevacizumab for severe retinopathy of prematurity. Am J Ophthalmol. 2009; 148(4):536–543.e2

[79] Mititelu M, Chaudhary KM, Lieberman RM. An evidence-based meta-analysis of vascular endothelial growth factor inhibition in pediatric retinal diseases: part 1. Retinopathy of prematurity. J Pediatr Ophthalmol Strabismus. 2012; 49(6):332–340

[80] Mintz-Hittner HA. Treatment of retinopathy of prematurity with vascular endothelial growth factor inhibitors. Early Hum Dev. 2012; 88(12):937–941

[81] Harder BC, von Baltz S, Schlichtenbrede FC, Jonas JB. Early refractive outcome after intravitreous bevacizumab for retinopathy of prematurity. Arch Ophthalmol. 2012; 130(6):800–801

[82] Harder BC, Schlichtenbrede FC, von Baltz S, Jendritza W, Jendritza B, Jonas JB. Intravitreal bevacizumab for retinopathy of prematurity: refractive error results. Am J Ophthalmol. 2013; 155(6):1119–1124.e1

[83] Mintz-Hittner HA, Kennedy KA, Chuang AZ, BEAT-ROP Cooperative Group. Efficacy of intravitreal bevacizumab for stage 3 + retinopathy of prematurity. N Engl J Med. 2011; 364(7):603–615

[84] Sato T, Wada K, Arahori H, et al. Serum concentrations of bevacizumab (avastin) and vascular endothelial growth factor in infants with retinopathy of prematurity. Am J Ophthalmol. 2012; 153(2):327–333.e1

[85] Matsuyama K, Ogata N, Matsuoka M, Wada M, Takahashi K, Nishimura T. Plasma levels of vascular endothelial growth factor and pigment epithelium-derived factor before and after intravitreal injection of bevacizumab. Br J Ophthalmol. 2010; 94(9):1215–1218

[86] Karaca C, Oner AO, Mirza E, Polat OA, Sahiner M. Bilateral effect of unilateral bevacizumab injection in retinopathy of prematurity. JAMA Ophthalmol. 2013; 131(8):1099–1101

[87] Meller S, Bhandari V. VEGF levels in humans and animal models with RDS and BPD: temporal relationships. Exp Lung Res. 2012; 38(4):192–203

[88] Curtis LH, Hammill BG, Schulman KA, Cousins SW. Risks of mortality, myocardial infarction, bleeding, and stroke associated with therapies for age-related macular degeneration. Arch Ophthalmol. 2010; 128(10):1273–1279

[89] Ueta T, Yanagi Y, Tamaki Y, Yamaguchi T. Cerebrovascular accidents in ranibizumab. Ophthalmology. 2009; 116(2):362–362

[90] Hapani S, Sher A, Chu D, Wu S. Increased risk of serious hemorrhage with bevacizumab in cancer patients: a meta-analysis. Oncology. 2010; 79(1–2):27–38

[91] Mintz-Hittner HA, Best LM. Antivascular endothelial growth factor for retinopathy of prematurity. Curr Opin Pediatr. 2009; 21(2):182–187

[92] Wu W-C, Yeh P-T, Chen S-N, Yang C-M, Lai C-C, Kuo H-K. Effects and complications of bevacizumab use in patients with retinopathy of prematurity: a multicenter study in Taiwan. Ophthalmology. 2011; 118(1):176–183

[93] Wu W-C, Kuo H-K, Yeh P-T, Yang C-M, Lai C-C, Chen S-N. An updated study of the use of bevacizumab in the treatment of patients with prethreshold retinopathy of prematurity in Taiwan. Am J Ophthalmol. 2013; 155(1):150–158.e1

[94] Jalali S, Balakrishnan D, Zeynalova Z, Padhi TR, Rani PK. Serious adverse events and visual outcomes of rescue therapy using adjunct bevacizumab to laser and surgery for retinopathy of prematurity. The Indian Twin Cities Retinopathy of Prematurity Screening database Report number 5. Arch Dis Child Fetal Neonatal Ed. 2013; 98(4):F327–F333

[95] Chhablani J, Rani PK, Balakrishnan D, Jalali S. Unusual adverse choroidal reaction to intravitreal bevacizumab in aggressive posterior retinopathy of prematurity: the Indian Twin Cities ROP screening (ITCROPS) data base report number 7. Semin Ophthalmol. 201 4; 29(4):222–225

[96] Tahija SG, Hersetyati R, Lam GC, Kusaka S, McMenamin PG. Fluorescein angiographic observations of peripheral retinal vessel growth in infants after intravitreal injection of bevacizumab as sole therapy for zone I and posterior zone II retinopathy of prematurity. Br J Ophthalmol. 2014; 98(4):507–512

[97] Blair M, Shapiro MJ. Bevacizumab for ROP. Ophthalmology. 2012; 119 (2):431–432, author reply 432

[98] Moshfeghi DM, Berrocal AM. Retinopathy of prematurity in the time of bevacizumab: incorporating the BEAT-ROP results into clinical practice. Ophthalmology. 2011; 118(7):1227–1228

[99] Hu J, Blair MP, Shapiro MJ, Lichtenstein SJ, Galasso JM, Kapur R. Reactivation of retinopathy of prematurity after bevacizumab injection. Arch Ophthalmol. 2012; 130(8):1000–1006

[100] Ittiara S, Blair MP, Shapiro MJ, Lichtenstein SJ. Exudative retinopathy and detachment: a late reactivation of retinopathy of prematurity after intravitreal bevacizumab. J AAPOS. 2013; 17(3):323–325

[101] Banach MJ, Ferrone PJ, Trese MT. A comparison of dense versus less dense diode laser photocoagulation patterns for threshold retinopathy of prematurity. Ophthalmology. 2000; 107(2):324–327, discussion 328

[102] Rezai KA, Eliott D, Ferrone PJ, Kim RW. Near confluent laser photocoagulation for the treatment of threshold retinopathy of prematurity. Arch Ophthalmol. 2005; 123(5):621–626

[103] Greven CM, Tasman W. Rhegmatogenous retinal detachment following cryotherapy in retinopathy of prematurity. Arch Ophthalmol. 1989; 107 (7):1017–1018
[104] McPherson AR, Hittner HM, Lemos R. Retinal detachment in young premature infants with acute retrolental fibroplasia. Thirty-two new cases. Ophthalmology. 1982; 89(10):1160–1169
[105] Topilow HW, Ackerman AL, Wang FM. The treatment of advanced retinopathy of prematurity by cryotherapy and scleral buckling surgery. Ophthalmology. 1985; 92(3):379–387
[106] Greven C, Tasman W. Scleral buckling in stages 4B and 5 retinopathy of prematurity. Ophthalmology. 1990; 97(6):817–820
[107] Noorily SW, Small K, de Juan E, Jr, Machemer R. Scleral buckling surgery for stage 4B retinopathy of prematurity. Ophthalmology. 1992; 99(2):263–268
[108] Trese MT. Scleral buckling for retinopathy of prematurity. Ophthalmology. 1994; 101(1):23–26
[109] Ricci B, Santo A, Ricci F, Minicucci G, Molle F. Scleral buckling surgery in stage 4 retinopathy of prematurity. Graefes Arch Clin Exp Ophthalmol. 1996; 234 Suppl 1:S38–S41
[110] Chuang YC, Yang CM. Scleral buckling for stage 4 retinopathy of prematurity. Ophthalmic Surg Lasers. 2000; 31(5):374–379
[111] Hinz BJ, de Juan E, Jr, Repka MX. Scleral buckling surgery for active stage 4A retinopathy of prematurity. Ophthalmology. 1998; 105(10):1827–1830
[112] Treister G, Machemer R. Results of vitrectomy for rare proliferative and hemorrhagic diseases. Am J Ophthalmol. 1977; 84(3):394–412
[113] Schepens CL. Clinical and research aspects of subtotal open-sky vitrectomy. XXXVII Edward Jackson Memorial Lecture. Am J Ophthalmol. 1981; 91 (2):143–171
[114] Hirose T, Schepens CL, Lopansri C. Subtotal open-sky vitrectomy for severe retinal detachment occurring as a late complication of ocular trauma. Ophthalmology. 1981; 88(1):1–9
[115] Tasman W, Borrone RN, Bolling J. Open sky vitrectomy for total retinal detachment in retinopathy of prematurity. Ophthalmology. 1987; 94 (4):449–452
[116] Zilis JD, deJuan E, Machemer R. Advanced retinopathy of prematurity. The anatomic and visual results of vitreous surgery. Ophthalmology. 1990; 97 (6):821–826
[117] de Juan E, Jr, Machemer R, Charles ST, Hirose T, Tasman WS, Trese MT. Surgery for stage 5 retinopathy of prematurity. Arch Ophthalmol. 1987; 105 (1):21
[118] Maguire AM, Trese MT. Lens-sparing vitreoretinal surgery in infants. Arch Ophthalmol. 1992 Feb; 110(2):284:6
[119] Ho LY, Ranchod TM, Drenser KA, Capone A, Jr, Trese MT. Ab interno incision for pediatric vitreoretinal surgery. Retina. 2010; 30(9):1542–1543
[120] Capone A, Jr, Trese MT. Lens-sparing vitreous surgery for tractional stage 4A retinopathy of prematurity retinal detachments. Ophthalmology. 2001; 108 (11):2068–2070
[121] Hubbard GB, III, Cherwick DH, Burian G. Lens-sparing vitrectomy for stage 4 retinopathy of prematurity. Ophthalmology. 2004; 111(12):2274–2277
[122] Moshfeghi AA, Banach MJ, Salam GA, Ferrone PJ. Lens-sparing vitrectomy for progressive tractional retinal detachments associated with stage 4A retinopathy of prematurity. Arch Ophthalmol. 2004; 122(12):1816–1818
[123] Chan-Kai BT, Lauer AK. Transconjunctival, sutureless 25-gauge lens sparing vitrectomy for stage 4 retinopathy of prematurity-related retinal detachments. Retina. 2009; 29(6):854–859
[124] Kychenthal A, Dorta P. 25-gauge lens-sparing vitrectomy for stage 4A retinopathy of prematurity. Retina. 2008; 28(3) Suppl:S65–S68
[125] Lakhanpal RR, Davis GH, Sun RL, Albini TA, Holz ER. Lens clarity after 3-port lens-sparing vitrectomy in stage 4A and 4B retinal detachments secondary to retinopathy of prematurity. Arch Ophthalmol. 2006; 124(1):20–23
[126] Gonzales CR, Boshra J, Schwartz SD. 25-Gauge pars plicata vitrectomy for stage 4 and 5 retinopathy of prematurity. Retina. 2006; 26(7) Suppl:S42–S46
[127] Luna JD, Caribaux LJ, Reviglio VE, Juarez CP. Lens-sparing surgery for retinopathy of prematurity. Ophthalmology. 2003; 110(8):1669
[128] Singh R, Reddy DM, Barkmeier AJ, Holz ER, Ram R, Carvounis PE. Long-term visual outcomes following lens-sparing vitrectomy for retinopathy of prematurity. Br J Ophthalmol. 2012; 96(11):1395–1398
[129] Wu W-C, Lai C-C, Lin R-I, et al. Modified 23 gauge vitrectomy system for stage 4 retinopathy of prematurity. Arch Ophthalmol. 2011; 129(10):1326–1331
[130] Wong SC, Capone A, Jr. Microplasmin (ocriplasmin) in pediatric vitreoretinal surgery: update and review. Retina. 2013; 33(2):339–348
[131] Wu W-C, Drenser KA, Lai M, Capone A, Trese MT. Plasmin enzyme-assisted vitrectomy for primary and reoperated eyes with stage 5 retinopathy of prematurity. Retina. 2008; 28(3) Suppl:S75–S80
[132] Tsukahara Y, Honda S, Imai H, et al. Autologous plasmin-assisted vitrectomy for stage 5 retinopathy of prematurity: a preliminary trial. Am J Ophthalmol. 2007; 144(1):139–141
[133] Yonekawa Y, Papakostas TD, Marra KV, Arroyo JG. Endoscopic pars plana vitrectomy for the management of severe ocular trauma. Int Ophthalmol Clin. 2013; 53(4):139–148
[134] Wong SC, Lee TC, Heier JS, Ho AC. Endoscopic vitrectomy. Curr Opin Ophthalmol. 2014; 25(3):195–206
[135] Faia LJ, Trese MT. Retinopathy of prematurity. In: Ryan SJ, Wilkinson CP, Wiedemann P, eds. Retina. Vol. 3, 5 ed. Philadelphia, PA: Elsevier; 2013:1920–1932
[136] Capone AJ, Trese MT, Hartnett ME. Treatment of stages 4 and 5 retinopathy of prematurity. In: Hartnett ME, Trese MT, Capone AJ, Keats B, Caputo G, eds. Pediatric Retina. 2nd ed. New York, NY: Lippincott Williams & Wilkins; 2014:597–603
[137] Micelli Ferrari T, Furino C, Lorusso VV, et al. Three-port lens-sparing vitrectomy for aggressive posterior retinopathy of prematurity: early surgery before tractional retinal detachment appearance. Eur J Ophthalmol. 2007; 17(5):785–789
[138] Nishina S, Yokoi T, Yokoi T, Kobayashi Y, Hiraoka M, Azuma N. Effect of early vitreous surgery for aggressive posterior retinopathy of prematurity detected by fundus fluorescein angiography. Ophthalmology. 2009; 116 (12):2442–2447
[139] Trese MT. Surgical therapy for stage V retinopathy of prematurity. A two-step approach. Graefes Arch Clin Exp Ophthalmol. 1987; 225(4):266–268
[140] Hirose T, Katsumi O, Mehta MC, Schepens CL. Vision in stage 5 retinopathy of prematurity after retinal reattachment by open-sky vitrectomy. Arch Ophthalmol. 1993; 111(3):345–349
[141] Mintz-Hittner HA, O'Malley RE, Kretzer FL. Long-term form identification vision after early, closed, lensectomy-vitrectomy for stage 5 retinopathy of prematurity. Ophthalmology. 1997; 104(3):454–459
[142] Trese MT, Droste PJ. Long-term postoperative results of a consecutive series of stages 4 and 5 retinopathy of prematurity. Ophthalmology. 1998; 105 (6):992–997

13 Miscellaneous Retinal Vascular Conditions

Frank S. Siringo, Ingrid U. Scott, Naresh Mandava, and Lawrence A. Yannuzzi

13.1 Hypertensive Retinopathy

- Grade 0: No changes
- Grade 1: Barely detectable arteriolar narrowing
- Grade 2: Obvious arteriolar narrowing with focal irregularities
- Grade 3: Grade 2 plus retinal hemorrhages and/or exudate
- Grade 4: Grade 3 plus disc swelling

Systemic arterial hypertension can accelerate the progression of diabetic retinopathy and is associated with an increased risk for retinal arterial and venous occlusive disease. *Hypertensive retinopathy* refers to any retinal vascular change related directly to the systemic hypertension.

13.1.1 Clinical Features

Retinal vascular changes secondary to hypertension most commonly do not cause visual loss or other ocular symptoms. In typical primary, chronic hypertension, the most common fundus sign is focal narrowing of the major retinal arterial branches.[1] There can also be generalized retinal arteriolar narrowing, with the vessels taking on a "copper wire" or "silver wire" appearance, reflecting moderate and severe arteriolosclerosis, respectively.[2] These color changes of the vessels are the result of diffusion of the normal light reflex secondary to the diminution of the size of the vascular lumen. Finally, arteriovenous "nicking" is sometimes seen in chronic hypertension. It refers to the focal narrowing of a retinal vein at an arteriovenous crossing. Because there is a common adventitial sheath at the crossings, enlargement of the retinal arteriolar wall by arteriolosclerosis will cause some degree of venous compression or narrowing at that point.[3]

When the hypertension is severe or acute, a variety of other fundus changes can be seen. In the retina, there can be pronounced focal arteriolar narrowing or closure, intraretinal hemorrhages, cotton-wool spots, or lipid exudates (▶ Fig. 13.1). Complications include hemorrhagic detachment of the internal limiting membrane as well as epiretinal membrane formation in the perimacular area.[1] Hemorrhages, cotton-wool spots, and lipid exudate eventually disappear once the blood pressure is brought under reasonable control (see "Management and Course"). However, subtle microvascular abnormalities or focal areas of retinal depression corresponding to previous cotton-wool spots may persist.[4]

With very high blood pressure, optic nerve head swelling may occur. This is, by definition, malignant hypertension (or grade 4 hypertensive retinopathy according to the modified Scheie's classification).[5] Optic nerve head swelling in this setting could represent papilledema from intracranial hypertension, especially if bilateral, or it could be a result of optic nerve head ischemia from local vascular compromise (see later). A macular star pattern of lipid exudate associated with optic nerve head swelling is a classic but not specific finding of severe systemic hypertension.

In summary, the modified Scheie's classification allows the clinician to stratify hypertensive retinopathy as such: it can be absent (grade 0), minor with mild focal narrowing of arterioles (grade 1), moderate with widespread arteriolar narrowing (grade 2), maked as when retinal hemorrhage is present in concert with widespread arteriolar narrowing (grade 3), or severe when optic disc edema is present (grade 4).[5]

Hypertensive choroidopathy may accompany the retinal vascular disease. Clinically evident choroidal involvement is indicative of acute hypertensive disease, which leads to focal choroidal hypoperfusion. Ophthalmoscopically, hypertensive choroidopathy may manifest as Elschnig's spots with or without exudative retinal detachment (▶ Fig. 13.2).[6] The spots represent foci of retinal pigment epithelial (RPE) infarction from underlying choriocapillaris fibrinoid necrosis.[6,7] In the acute phase, these RPE changes appear as deep, gray-yellow spots; with time, they become hyperpigmented. The overlying exudative retinal detachment resolves as the blood pressure comes under better control. Similar foci of ischemia and resultant fibrinoid necrosis along choroidal arterioles leads to the clinical development of linear, pigmented lesions known as Siegrist's streaks.[6,7]

Women whose pregnancies are complicated by preeclampsia are at risk for the acute manifestations of hypertensive retinopathy and choroidopathy. Rapid vision loss may be due to macula-involving, serous retinal detachment overlying areas of choroidal hypoperfusion.[8] More insidious evidence of choroidal hypoperfusion has been demonstrated in such patients with the recent advent of enhanced depth imaging of spectral-domain optical coherence tomography (EDI-SDOCT). While pregnancy is associated with an increase in subfoveal choroidal thickness, it is significantly decreased in preeclamptic women compared with healthy pregnant controls, matching that of a third group of age-matched nongravid healthy women.[9,10,11] In a study of retinal macular volume and choroidal thickness in *postpartum* preeclamptic women, healthy postpartum women, and age-matched nongravid controls, increased choroidal thickness and retinal macular volume were noted in preeclamptic postpartum women compared with both normal postpartum and nonpregnant controls, who were similar with respect to choroidal thickness and retinal macular volume.[12] Taken together, these studies suggest dysfunction in choroidal vascular autoregulation in women with preeclampsia both during and after delivery, with increased susceptibility to hypertensive choroidopathy.

Pearls

- Young patients with rapidly accelerating hypertension are most likely to manifest signs of hypertensive choroidopathy.

Visual loss resulting directly from hypertensive retinopathy can be caused by exudation of lipid or serous material into the foveal area from incompetent paramacular capillaries. In the setting of grade 4 disease, ischemic damage to the optic nerve head may be the source of vision loss. Finally, significant

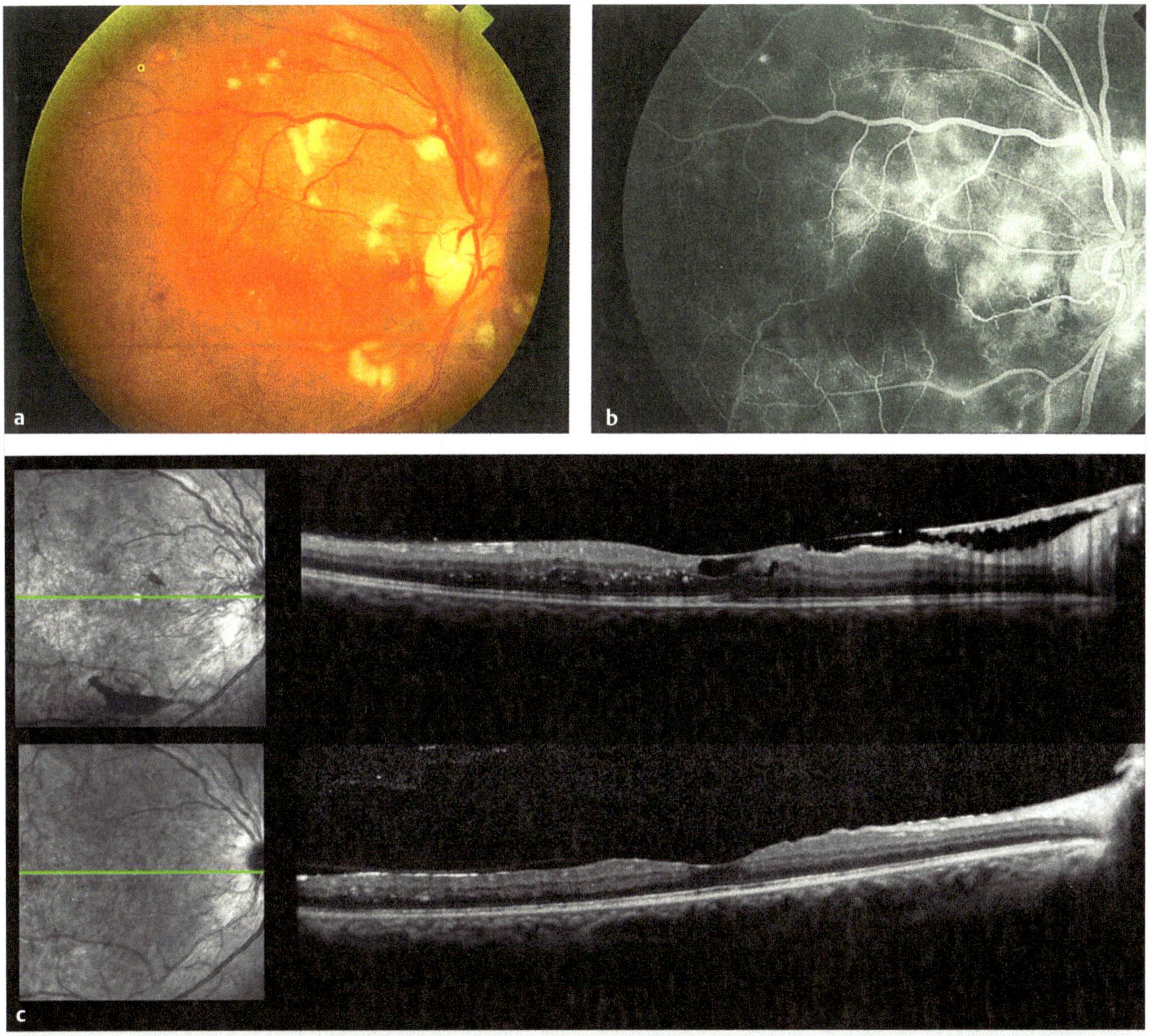

Fig. 13.1 Acute hypertensive retinopathy. **(a)** Multiple cotton-wool spots and intraretinal hemorrhages are present in the posterior pole. There is also some punctate lipid exudate in the central macula. **(b)** Corresponding midphase fluorescein angiogram shows scattered microaneurysms, capillary nonperfusion, and intraretinal leakage of dye. **(c)** Upper image: Acute hypertensive retinopathy in a 24 year old pregnant woman with preeclampsia demonstrating optic disc edema, intraretinal lipid exudate, preretinal and intraretinal hemorrhage, and intrafoveal cystic changes on scanning laser ophthalmoscopy (SLO) and spectral domain optical coherence tomography (SD-OCT). Lower image: Same patient six months later, after sustained improvement in blood pressure.

choroidal involvement can also contribute to vision loss, particularly if there is an exudative retinal detachment that involves the macula.

Fluorescein angiographic findings in hypertensive retinopathy include microaneurysmal dilation of capillaries, telangiectasis, capillary nonperfusion, and leakage from retinal vessels or the optic nerve head (▸ Fig. 13.1). Following hypertensive control, these small-vessel alterations may persist to some degree, being mainly evident in the peripapillary area and the posterior pole. Angiographic findings in hypertensive choroidopathy include focal hyperfluorescence and leakage at the level of the RPE corresponding to the location of the "acute" Elschnig's spots (▸ Fig. 13.2)[13] (see also Chapter 30).

Common ophthalmic diseases associated with systemic hypertension include retinal vein occlusions, arterial macroaneurysm, and ischemic optic neuropathy. Eyes with these conditions may or may not have fundus findings of hypertensive retinopathy.

13.1.2 Differential Diagnosis

The differential diagnosis of hypertensive retinopathy is extensive because of the wide spectrum of acute and chronic manifestations. Patients with evidence of capillary abnormalities, such as capillary nonperfusion or microaneurysms, may have diabetic retinopathy, radiation retinopathy, venous occlusive disease, perifoveal telangiectasis, or systemic illness, such as a

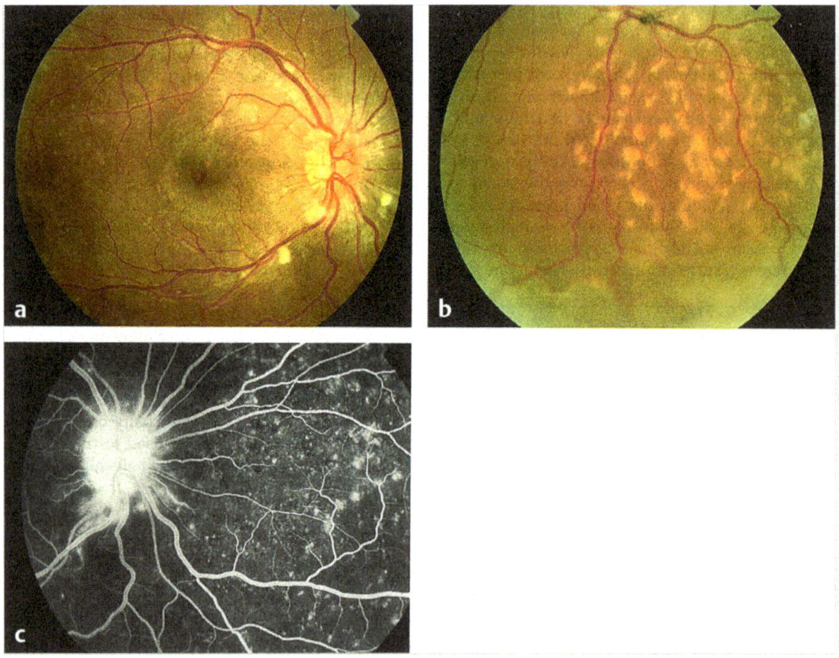

Fig. 13.2 Acute hypertensive choroidopathy: Fundus photographs of the macula (**a**) and inferonasal retina (**b**) reveal multiple gray-yellow spots at the level of the retinal pigment epithelium. Note also the inferior (exudative) retinal detachment and peripapillary cotton-wool spots. (**c**) Corresponding midphase fluorescein angiogram shows multiple, deep hyperfluorescent foci and leakage from the optic disc.

collagen vascular disease. Not uncommonly, two disease entities may be at play (e.g., systemic lupus erythematosus [SLE] and secondary hypertension). Patients with optic nerve head swelling and macular star (lipid) must have blood pressure checked immediately. With this clinical presentation, the differential diagnosis includes neuroretinitis (cat-scratch disease, toxoplasmosis), diabetic papillopathy, and optic neuritis of infectious (sarcoidosis, syphilis, Lyme disease) or inflammatory etiology. Often, headache is present in patients with malignant hypertension; nevertheless, papilledema secondary to intracranial disease also presents with headache and must be ruled out.

13.1.3 Pathogenesis

Arteriolosclerosis refers to the alteration of the arteriolar wall secondary to long-standing hypertension. Early changes result from an increase in the elastic tissue in the intima. Gradually, the intima is replaced by hyaline and the muscular wall becomes fibrotic.[2,14] In acute cases, damage to blood vessel walls can also result from leakage of blood components into the arteriolar wall. This results in narrowing or closure of the vascular lumen. In addition, focal areas of capillary nonperfusion to the nerve fiber layer result in ischemic zones, which appear as cotton-wool spots. Cotton-wool spots appear white because of axoplasmic stasis in the area of retinal ischemia.[4,13] Remodeling of the retinal microcirculation results in microaneurysmal formation and telangiectasis, and it can also result in intraretinal exudation secondary to increased vascular permeability.[1] Macular star formation results from damage to optic nerve head capillaries and parafoveal capillaries, with passage of lipid-rich material along a plane in the outer plexiform layer into the macula to form a starlike pattern.[1] Experimental evidence in an animal model suggests that optic nerve head swelling may result from the accumulation of axoplasmic components secondary to axoplasmic stasis, as shown by Tso and Jampol.[7]

13.1.4 Management and Course

Fundus changes from chronic hypertensive retinopathy, such as retinal arterial narrowing and arteriovenous nicking, tell little about recent blood pressure control. Because these features represent permanent changes in the vessel walls, they persist long after blood pressure has normalized.

In contrast, the acute manifestations indicate poor blood pressure control at the time of the ocular examination. Retinal hemorrhages and cotton-wool spots would be expected when the autoregulatory mechanisms of the retinal arterioles are overwhelmed. In normal individuals, this occurs when the mean arterial blood pressure rises suddenly above 115 mm Hg.[14] In individuals with preexisting hypertension, still higher levels of blood pressure are probably needed to produce the acute retinal changes.

Management consists of controlling the blood pressure; appropriate systemic therapy leads to resolution of the acute, potentially sight-threatening manifestations. Some degree of permanent visual loss may be encountered if there is significant macular or optic nerve involvement. When there are signs of severe hypertensive retinopathy, choroidopathy, or any optic nerve head swelling, the blood pressure must be checked in the office immediately. Very high systemic blood pressure is a medical emergency and necessitates prompt referral to a comprehensive health care facility.

Pearls

- Optic nerve head swelling in the setting of hypertensive retinopathy is presumed to represent malignant hypertension and, therefore, a potential medical emergency. Blood pressure should be checked immediately in the office and the patient referred promptly if uncontrolled hypertension is confirmed.

13.2 Coats' Disease

Coats' disease is an idiopathic condition that was first characterized by George Coats in 1908.[15] Coats described this entity as abnormal telangiectatic or aneurysmal retinal vessels associated with intraretinal and massive subretinal exudates. He classified patients having the disease into three groups with varying degrees of vascular abnormality, but all with massive subretinal exudates. Group 3 patients had arteriovenous malformation and exudation, which von Hippel later characterized as a distinct entity, angiomatosis retinae, leading Coats to remove it from his classification. Later, Leber[16] described a disease, Leber's multiple miliary aneurysms, characterized by the same vascular abnormalities as Coats' disease but lacking the massive subretinal exudates. The possibility that these entities were part of a spectrum of disease was confirmed when Reese[17] documented a case of presumptive multiple miliary aneurysms in which massive subretinal exudation typical of Coats' disease developed. He was also the first to use the term *retinal telangiectasis*, which many authors feel better describes the disease and its wide spectrum of presentations and varying degrees of severity.

13.2.1 Clinical Features

Congenital retinal telangiectasis, or Coats' disease, is predominantly a disease of childhood; however, a less severe form of the disease may develop in adults.[18,19,20,21,22,23,24] The majority of cases are diagnosed by 20 years of age, with a peak incidence at the end of the first decade.[18,19] Male patients are affected up to four times as frequently as female patients and there is no racial or ethnic predisposition.[13] It is classically thought of as an exclusively unilateral process.[21,23,25,26] Recent reports, however, have shown a high incidence of subtle retinal vascular abnormalities in the fellow eyes of patients with Coats' disease; these abnormalities include peripheral nonperfusion, telangiectasias, and microaneurysms observed with fluorescein angiography.[27]

Traditionally, the term *Coats' disease* is used to describe the most severe end of the disease spectrum, characterized by massive yellow subretinal lipid exudation and secondary retinal detachment in children.[26] Infants and young children can present with leukocoria secondary to subretinal lipid deposition and exudative retinal detachment or strabismus from the poor vision that results. Because of the common presentation of leukocoria and strabismus in other childhood diseases, other diagnoses must be investigated (▶ Table 13.1).[27,28]

Table 13.1 Perifoveal retinal telangiectasis (Gass's classification)

Group 1A	Unilateral, congenital parafoveolar telangiectasis
Group 1B	Unilateral, idiopathic, focal juxtafoveolar telangiectasis
Group 2A	Bilateral, idiopathic, acquired perifoveolar telangiectasis
Group 3A	Occlusive, idiopathic, juxtafoveolar retinal telangiectasis
Group 3B	Occlusive, idiopathic, juxtafoveolar, retinal telangiectasis associated with central nervous system vasculopathy

Reprinted with permission from Gass JDM, Oyakawa RT. Idiopathic juxtafoveolar retinal telangiectasis. Arch Ophthalmol. 1982; 100(5): 769–780.

The diagnosis is typically made by ophthalmoscopy alone. The term *retinal telangiectasis* is appropriate, as this is a disease principally of the retinal capillaries. Telangiectasis, increased tortuosity, and exudation from incompetence of small-caliber vessels are typical features (▶ Fig. 13.3). However, larger vessels, including large arteries and veins, can be affected with sheathing, aneurysmal dilations, and exudation. Interestingly, retinal neovascularization is rare despite the presence of capillary nonperfusion and adjacent, relatively normal blood vessels. Vitreous hemorrhage and neovascularization are seen only when larger zones of capillary nonperfusion or retinal detachment are present. Despite the low incidence of neovascularization, it has been demonstrated that in vivo vascular endothelial growth factor (VEGF) levels rise in accordance with the stage of Coats' disease compared to controls.[28] In addition, elevated levels of VEGF and VEGF-receptor 2 were demonstrated in enucleated eyes of patients with Coats' disease.[29] This has led researchers to investigate new treatment modalities, namely, the adjunctive use of antiangiogenic agents such as bevacizumab and ranibizumab.

In contrast to the often aggressive childhood presentation and course, adult-onset disease—known as idiopathic macular telangiectasia (IMT) type 1, discussed later—is typically less severe, with telangiectasis and intraretinal exudation often simulating other diseases. Visual loss is secondary to leakage from perifoveal telangiectases, causing cystoid macular edema and often a circinate ring of lipid deposition around the macula (▶ Fig. 13.4). Often, the ophthalmoscopic and angiographic picture in the adult form of disease is difficult to differentiate from that of other perifoveal microvascular abnormalities (▶ Table 13.1). Exudative retinal detachment typical of the childhood form is rarely seen in adults.

The aggressive form of the disease is typically seen in children and infants. Initially, severe retinal vascular leakage causes subretinal deposition of protein and lipid-rich exudate. Massive accumulation of yellow subretinal exudation causes the bullous retinal detachment characteristic of Coats' disease. In time, nonresolving subretinal lipid deposition can lead to fibrovascular tissue formation and even choroidal neovascularization (CNV). Disciform scars can then develop from CNV and these scars are, unfortunately, most common in the macula, where lipid from peripheral exudative lesions tend to track. In fact, disciform scars are most common in children and infants with broader zones of peripheral involvement.[22]

Other than disciform scars, the complications of long-standing exudative retinal detachments are numerous. Cataract, iridocyclitis, neovascular glaucoma, and eventually phthisis bulbi can occur. Rarely, organization of subretinal fluid in long-standing detachments can lead to a clinical picture simulating that of other diseases. Coalescence of intraretinal cystic spaces in unresolved detachments have reportedly led to hemorrhagic retinal macrocysts.[30] There is also a report of orbital cellulitis developing from transscleral leakage of subretinal toxins in a child with advanced Coats' disease.[31]

Although no conclusive evidence of a genetic transmission of Coats' disease has been demonstrated, multiple associations with systemic and ocular diseases have been reported. Alport's disease, tuberous sclerosis, Turner's syndrome, Senior–Løken syndrome, and the ichthyosis hystrix variant of epidermal nevus syndrome have all anecdotally been reported to be

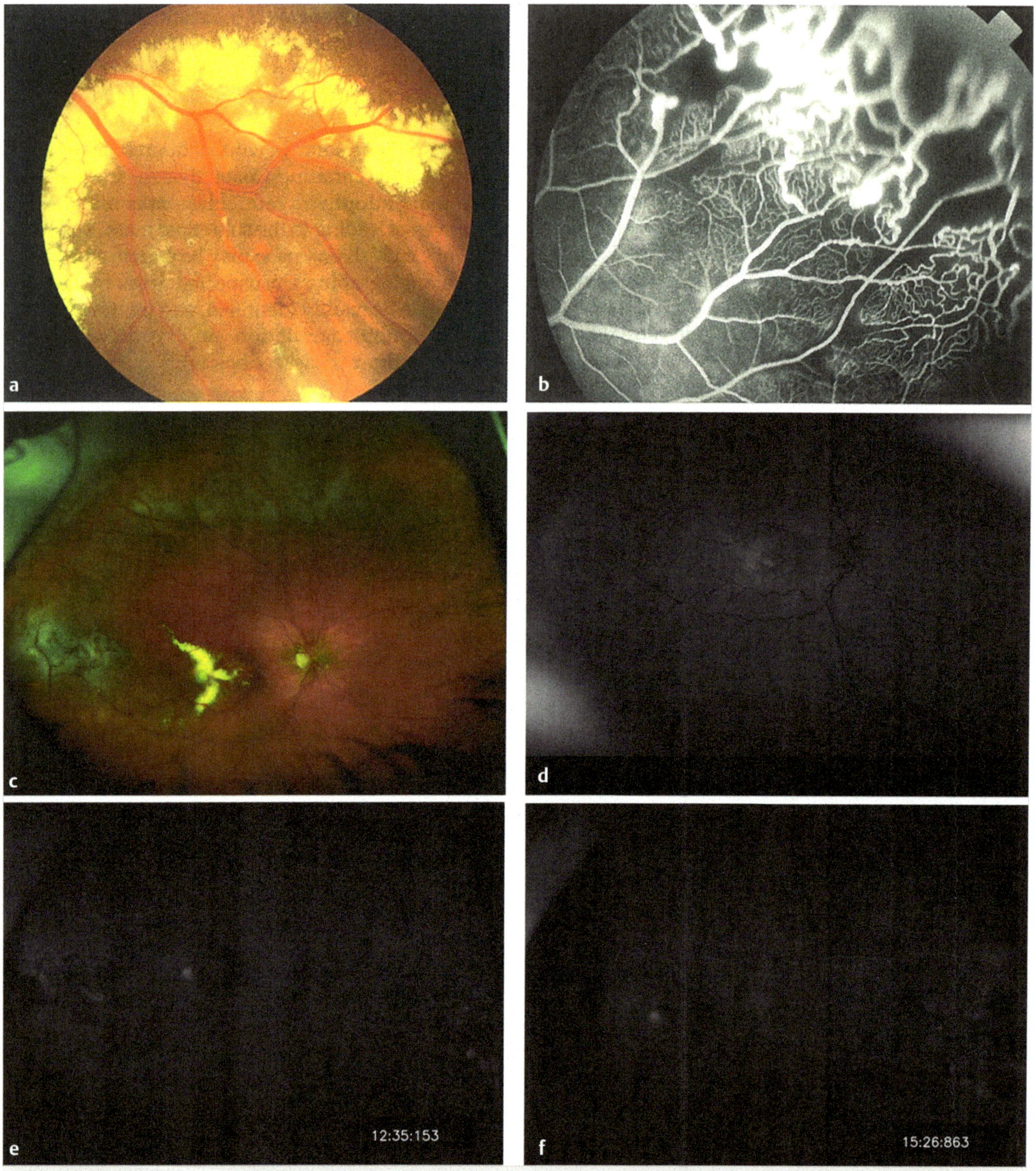

Fig. 13.3 Coats' disease. (**a**) Fundus photograph showing peripheral retinal telangiectasis, aneurysm-like abnormalities, and lipid exudate. (**b**) Fluorescein angiogram of a different eye with Coats' disease shows the typical peripheral retinal vascular abnormalities and adjacent capillary nonperfusion. (**c, d**) Ultra-widefield and autofluorescence images demonstrating temporal telangiectasias, aneurysms, shallow inferotemporal exudative detachment, and marked macular lipid deposition. (**e, f**) Same patient, recirculation phase oral fluorescein images demonstrating aneurysms and peripheral nonperfusion nasally and temporally. Delayed time shots represent increased time for gastrointestinal absorption of fluorescein.

associated with a Coats'-like response. Multiple reports of an association with muscular dystrophy, and more recently with facioscapulohumeral dystrophy, exist. In 1956, Zamorani[32] was the first to report an association of retinitis pigmentosa with Coats' disease. Morgan and Crawford[33] have since described multiple cases of Coats'-like findings in patients with retinitis pigmentosa. In a literature review, Khan et al[34] reported 46 cases of retinitis pigmentosa associated with Coats'-like

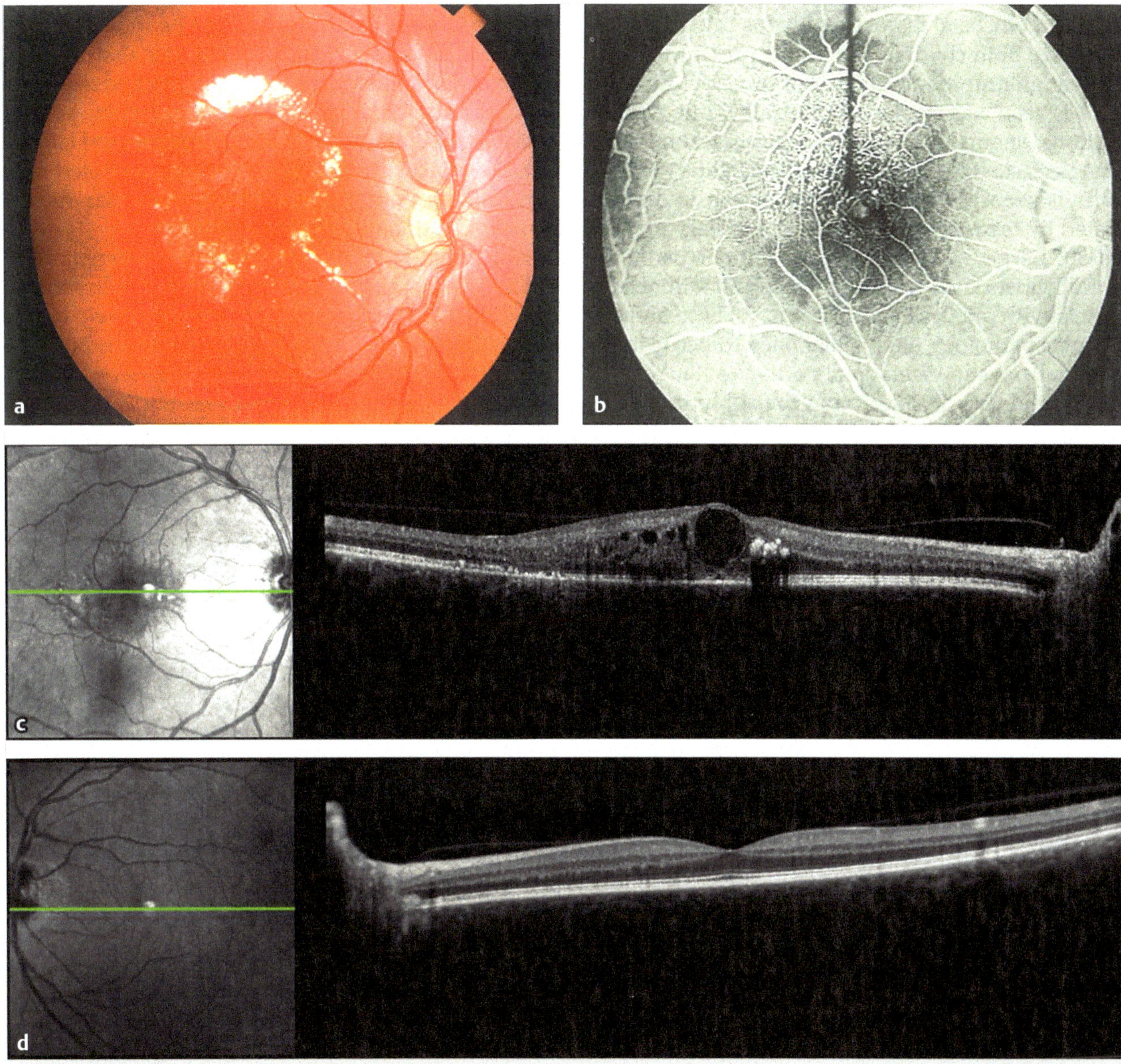

Fig. 13.4 Coats' disease. (a) Localized area of microaneurysms and telangiectatic change in the macula. Note the circinate ring of lipid exudate tracking through the fovea. (b) Fluorescein angiogram better depicts the microaneurysms and related vascular abnormalities. (c, d) Upper image: SLO and SDOCT images of a 45-year-old man with idiopathic macular telangiectasia (IMT) type 1, demonstrating intraretinal hyperreflective deposits consistent with lipid, and intrafoveal cystic edema. Lower image: normal fellow eye.

findings, or 1.2 to 3.6% of retinitis pigmentosa patients affected among the sites reporting data. Pruett differentiated Coats'-like findings in patients with retinitis pigmentosa from traditional Coats' disease, noting that the aneurysmal telangiectasias and exudative detachments in patients with retinitis pigmentosa are more often bilateral, without gender predilection, and found in the inferior fundus.[35] The adult form of Coats' disease has also been associated with hypercholesterolemia.

Fluorescein angiography demonstrates the vascular origin of Coats' disease and helps confirm the diagnosis. Both children and adults present with the same angiographic findings. Large-vessel involvement is seen as saccular ("light bulb") aneurysmal dilations, anomalous vascular communications, and telangiectasia (▶ Fig. 13.3). Occasionally, beading of vessel walls is seen.[16] Capillary involvement is demonstrated by telangiectasia as well as capillary nonperfusion. Large areas of capillary nonperfusion are typically associated with neighboring abnormal large vessels with aneurysmal dilations.[21] These areas of vascular pathology have a tendency to occur in the temporal and superotemporal portions of the retina.[20] Fluorescein dye does leak into the subretinal space but stains only minimally. Large zones of exudative retinal detachment distal to the telangiectasias do not stain. However, fluorescein dye does fill intraretinal cystic spaces, often showing a pattern characteristic of cystoid macular edema.[21] Interestingly, many cases with exudation originally reported as not having a frankly visible vascular origin have since been shown to have associated vascular anomalies by fluorescein angiography. Most recently, ultrawide-field color fundus and fluorescein imaging has contributed to a greater understanding of this spectrum of peripheral retinal vascular disease, particularly in the realm of pediatric retina. Single-shot images of the posterior pole and retinal periphery are obtained quickly without the need for examination under anesthesia. Fluorescein angiograms may be obtained with oral intake of sodium fluorescein. While precise choroidal fills are difficult to time with this modality, useful angiographic images are nonetheless obtainable with a modicum of cooperation (see ▶ Fig. 13.3e–f). This is helpful both to document novel findings in known conditions—such as the previously mentioned subtle fellow-eye vasculopathy in patients with Coats' disease—as well as for diagnostic purposes in new or challenging cases.[36]

There may be some benefit to fluorescein angiography in differentiating Coats' disease from retinoblastoma. Endophytic retinoblastomas may have a feeder vessel leading to the subretinal mass. The treatment of Coats' disease also may be enhanced by fluorescein angiography. Unsuspected areas of vascular leakage can be readily identified, and treatment in the form of photocoagulation or cryotherapy then directed to those areas (see Management and Course).[15]

13.2.2 Differential Diagnosis

The differential diagnosis in the childhood form of Coats' disease presenting with leukocoria or exudative retinal detachment is extensive (see text box Differential Diagnosis of Coats' Disease).[37] Most importantly, retinoblastoma must be ruled out, as it is life threatening. In a large series by Howard and Ellsworth,[38] 3.9% of children initially thought to have retinoblastoma were found to have Coats' disease. A thorough history and clinical examination are most important for an accurate diagnosis; unlike retinoblastoma, Coats' disease occurs primarily in males and has no genetic predisposition.[37] Furthermore, Coats' disease presents with more lipid exudation than retinoblastoma, and the characteristic vascular anomalies are usually recognizable in patients with Coats' disease.

Angiomatosis retinae (retinal capillary hemangioma, or von Hippel's lesion) and the peripheral, acquired retinal angioma can present with significant lipid exudation. In angiomatosis retinae, the rate of bilaterality is high, and the lesions are often associated with dilated feeder and draining vessels, unlike the lesions of Coats' disease.[37] The acquired peripheral capillary angioma, however, can be more difficult to differentiate from Coats' disease, as it also does not have very prominent feeder and drainer vessels and can present with heavy lipid exudation, serous detachment, epiretinal membrane, and telangiectatic vascular change. Despite these associated similarities, a discrete, peripheral retinal vascular mass is usually identifiable (see Chapter 28).

Ancillary tests may be pivotal in the differentiation of Coats' disease from retinoblastoma. Ultrasound and computed tomographic (CT) imaging help detect intraocular calcification, which would support the diagnosis of retinoblastoma.[39] Also, thin sections with contrast CT imaging can detect vascularization of the subretinal space, sometimes found in retinoblastoma lesions. Fluorescein angiography may also be useful in evaluating the vasculature of an endophytic mass, as described earlier.[16] Retinoblastomas can present with a feeder vascular stalk seen by angiography. Aqueous lactate dehydrogenase and isoenzyme levels have not assisted in the diagnosis. However, the presence of cholesterol-laden macrophages in the subretinal fluid is unique to Coats' disease but is of little help clinically when one is trying to establish the diagnosis noninvasively.[38,40]

Localized telangiectasis and leakage are seen in the adult form of Coats' disease. Gass[21] referred to these cases as *unilateral congenital parafoveolar retinal telangiectasis* (group 1A of his classification of idiopathic perifoveal retinal telangiectasis, see later) and is termed *IMT type 1* in the updated Yannuzzi's classification (▶ Table 13.1). The differential diagnosis includes all perifoveal retinal microvascular abnormalities that can present with or without leakage (see text box). Certainly, diabetic retinopathy and venous occlusive disease present more commonly in this manner than does Coats' disease. Idiopathic, acquired perifoveal retinal telangiectasis (group 2 by Gass' classification) can have minimal intraretinal serous exudation but, by definition, does not have lipid exudation.[41] It is also typically a bilateral disease and has no gender predilection. (Other features unique to this form of perifoveal telangiectasis are discussed in the next section.) Capillary nonperfusion and perifoveal microvascular disease seen in the adult form of Coats' disease are also seen in radiation retinopathy and sickle-cell retinopathy. Cavernous hemangioma is a relatively discrete retinal vascular anomaly that can be likened to a cluster of grapes. There is no clinical or angiographic evidence for vascular incompetence, as there is in Coats' disease. Acquired arterial macroaneurysms have a zone of leakage typically surrounding a single lesion by angiography. Idiopathic retinal vasculitis, aneurysms, and neuroretinitis (IRVAN) presents with a constellation of findings not typical of Coats' disease.

Differential Diagnosis of Coats' Disease

- Childhood disease (leukocoria or exudative retinal detachment)
  - Retinoblastoma
  - Persistent hyperplastic primary vitreous
  - Retinopathy of prematurity
  - Familial exudative vitreoretinopathy
  - Norrie's disease
  - Toxocariasis
  - von Hippel–Lindau disease (angiomatosis retinae)
  - Peripheral acquired retinal angioma
  - Incontinentia pigmenti
  - Pars planitis
  - Retinitis pigmentosa with Coats'-like retinal telangiectasias and exudates
- Parafoveal telangiectasis with or without lipid exudation
  - Diabetic retinopathy
  - Branch retinal vein occlusion
  - Idiopathic perifoveal retinal telangiectasis
  - Epiretinal membrane with secondary vascular leakage
  - Sickle-cell retinopathy
  - Radiation retinopathy
  - Acquired inflammatory diseases
- Localized telangiectasis with arterial or venous aneurysms
  - Cavernous hemangioma of retina
  - • IRVAN
  - Acquired retinal arterial macroaneurysm

13.2.3 Pathogenesis and Histopathology

Historically, infectious and inflammatory processes were implicated in Coats' disease. A vascular etiology has also been described; this is supported by the presence of material that stains with periodic acid–Schiff (PAS) and thickening of endothelial basement membrane.[42] However, these histopathologic changes may be nonspecific and seen with other etiologies. For example, an endocrine disturbance for Coats' disease has been suggested based on the similarity in basement membrane disease to diabetes and pregnancy-related vascular diseases. Other systemic abnormalities have been investigated. A defect in cholesterol transport has been proposed.[43] The known association between hypercholesterolemia and the adult form of Coats' disease may be further evidence of a serum lipid abnormality.[44]

Because of improvements in diagnostic testing, enucleation of eyes with Coats' disease is now very rare. Most histopathologic reports of Coats' disease are from earlier studies. By light microscopy, all reports describe abnormal telangiectatic vessels that leak plasma and exudate into retinal tissues as well as subretinally.[42,45,46] Lipid-engorged macrophages are found in the subretinal space. Green[46] reported that it is uncertain whether these macrophages originate from retinal vessels and migrate subretinally or travel from the choroidal circulation to phagocytose lipid in the subretinal space.

Electron microscopy confirms abnormalities at the level of the retinal vascular endothelium in eyes with Coats' disease.[47] In addition, Egbert et al[42] demonstrated retinal vascular aneurysms and deposition of PAS-positive material in retinal vascular walls after trypsin digestion in 10 eyes. Trypsin digestion studies demonstrate diffuse capillary involvement, even in the peripheral retina.[45]

Chronic lipid deposition leads to the growth of fibrovascular tissue and, eventually, a disciform scar clinically. Histopathologically, RPE hyperplasia is often seen overlying this organized subretinal fibrovascular tissue.[46] Fibrous metaplasia of the RPE has been reported, with the occasional presence of calcium and even bone in these organized fibrous nodules.[45]

13.2.4 Management and Course

An understanding of the spectrum of disease severity and the remitting and exacerbating nature of the disease is crucial. Although rare, complete remissions have been reported.[48,49] The rare patient with bilateral disease typically presents with only mild involvement of the second eye, often to a clinically insignificant level.[20]

Multiple treatment strategies have been proposed for the management of Coats' disease. Early treatments for the disease with corticotropin (adrenocorticotropic hormone), steroids, and antibiotics were unsuccessful. Although some authors reported an occasional benefit to transscleral diathermy and radiotherapy, it was not until Meyer-Schwickerath[50] applied his new laser techniques to eyes with Coats' disease that significant cure rates were established.

In the 1970s, treatments of vascular lesions in Coats' disease by xenon arc, argon laser photocoagulation, or cryotherapy were minimally successful. The major prognostic factor despite the most aggressive treatment was the area of involvement of disease.[20,22,51] Egerer and colleagues[20] reported visual improvement only in eyes with two or fewer quadrants of pathology. The previous report of Harris[22] echoed this finding. Harris also concluded that lipid deposition in the macula was irreversible. Later, Spitznas[52] reported several cases of Coats' disease with resolution of lipid deposition in the macula after treatment. However, he surmised that early treatment was preferred, as more severe lipid deposition did not resolve and often led to permanent visual loss. Most investigators deduced that early treatment of vascular lesions, before lipid accumulation in the macula, was beneficial.[20,22,51,52]

Pearls

- Early treatment of vascular abnormalities in Coats' disease provides the best control of leakage and appears to minimize the chances of vision loss. Multiple treatment sessions are often necessary to arrest the leakage.

In 1982, in a retrospective review of 41 patients, Ridley et al[23] reported more severe disease in Coats' disease patients younger than 4 years. Their report suggested that aggressive treatment with photocoagulation, cryotherapy, and repair of retinal detachments was beneficial. In fact, among children older than 4 years, only 25% of untreated patients maintained at least their previous visual acuity, whereas more than 70% of children who underwent aggressive treatment maintained their previous acuity. The visual outcomes were worse for children younger than 4 years; however, aggressive treatment still carried a better prognosis. When there is significant retinal elevation from exudation, external or internal drainage of subretinal fluid may be necessary for adequate uptake of laser photocoagulation or cryotherapy and ultimate control of the leaking retinal vessels.[20,23,52] Machemer and Williams[53] reported two patients with traction retinal detachments secondary to Coats' disease in whom spontaneous retinal reattachment and resolution of exudates occurred after vitrectomy. Adequate treatment of leaking vessels prevented further exudation and membrane formation.

Complications of laser photocoagulation of these aneurysmal lesions include vitreous hemorrhage secondary to destruction of vascular walls and macular pucker secondary to vitreous contraction.[20,22,23] Rarely, progressive fibrosis and traction retinal detachments can develop. Therefore, laser energy should be used sparingly to avoid these complications. We use laser whenever possible, as it minimizes epiretinal membrane formation in comparison with cryotherapy. Treatment of the aneurysms directly or scatter treatment in the distribution of the telangiectasia works. Our preference is to treat the aneurysms in the course of scatter treatment. Multiple sessions of laser are often necessary to treat residual leaking vessels, which may become visible when exudates clear. In addition, recurrences have been reported up to 5 years after complete resolution of the Coats' process.[20] This necessitates close observation of all patients with Coats' disease, even after stabilization of the disease process.

In the modern era of anti-angiogenic therapy, intravitreal bevacizumab and ranibizumab have been employed either as monotherapy or in combination with laser, cryotherapy, or local steroids to treat patients with Coats' disease. Some studies report promising results with improvement or stabilization of visual acuity and resolution of exudates and telangiectasias.[54,55] Other investigators are more sanguine about the role of these agents in Coats' disease, urging caution and noting the risk of traction retinal detachment from vitreoretinal fibrosis, which can approach 50%.[56] Some investigators question whether anti-angiogenic agents truly alter the natural history of Coats' disease, which may involve fibrosis and vitreoretinal traction, given the small sample sizes and lack of randomized controlled studies noted by those urging restraint.[57] In the absence of definitive data, it may be reasonable to use anti-angiogenic medications in an adjunctive or monotherapeutic role, particularly in advanced cases with widespread exudative detachment, where conventional laser or cryotherapy is likely to fail and the visual prognosis is poor.

13.3 Idiopathic Macular Telangiectasia

Idiopathic macular telangiectasia, an updated terminology and classification of the term *perifoveal or juxtafoveal telangiectasis* described by Gass, is a unique entity associated with dilation and incompetence of retinal capillaries solely in the perifoveal area of one or both eyes. Here, we discuss the bilateral variant, type 2 IMT, previously known as *idiopathic perifoveal telangiectasis (IPT)* or group 2A of the Gass's classification of perifoveal telangiectasis (▶ Table 13.1).[58] The other entities are rare except for group 1A, or the "Coats' variant," which has already been discussed. The changes of type 2 IMT are likely acquired, but by definition, no associated retinal vascular diseases should be present.

13.3.1 Clinical Features

Type 2 IMT is a bilateral condition most commonly presenting in patients 50 to 60 years of age, with a mean age of 55 years.[41,59] It has no gender predilection and, as mentioned earlier, no association with systemic diseases, although a link with diabetes mellitus has been suggested.[60]

Patients typically present with decreased visual acuity to the level of 20/30 or better.[41,59] Most commonly, patients have an area of occult telangiectasis, smaller than one disc diameter, confined to the temporal macula, although larger zones of capillary abnormality may be present. There is only minimal intraretinal serous exudation and no lipid exudation, as opposed to type 1 macular telangiectasis, also known as *aneurysmatic telangiectasia*.

Clinical features are best understood by staging of the severity of disease.[58] Stage 1 shows mild staining in the outer retina of the temporal macula on fluorescein angiography, with no biomicroscopic or angiographic evidence of telangiectasis. In stage 2 disease, some graying of the involved area develops, and fluorescein angiography shows formation of mild telangiectasis with more prominent late leakage of fluorescein dye. In stage 3 disease, severely blunted, dilated, right-angle venules are seen "diving" deep into the outer retinal plexus. The hallmark of stage 4 disease is the formation of stellate RPE plaques along the right-angle venules secondary to an RPE hyperplastic response (▶ Fig. 13.5). These intraretinal stellate pigment plaques are characteristic of this disease. These first four stages are classified by Yannuzzi as nonproliferative, whereas in stage 5, CNV develops. In addition, peculiar retinochoroidal anastomoses unique to the disease occur in the vicinity of the pigment plaques.

Other clinical findings can include small, refractile, golden crystalline deposits, seen in approximately one half of patients with stage 2 through 5 diseases (▶ Fig. 13.6).[61] In 5% of affected patients, a yellow foveal lesion develops in one or both eyes. This may appear as a lamellar macular hole secondary to progressive atrophy of the outer retina.[62] The advent of SDOCT has provided greater insight into the microarchitectural retinal changes in this group of disorders, confirming the clinical observations made by Gass, Blodi, and Yannuzzi (▶ Fig. 13.5c–h).[63,64]

Importantly, severe complications, such as subretinal neovascularization, subretinal hemorrhage, and disciform scar formation (i.e., stage 5 proliferative disease), with vision worse than 20/50, develop in fewer than 5% of patients. Patients with significant perifoveal capillary nonperfusion do not have classic IMT; in fact, they may be diagnosed with Gass's group 3 disease after a proper workup to rule out malignancy or other systemic illness.[58,65]

13.3.2 Differential Diagnosis

The diagnosis of IMT is often elusive because its principal features are seen in other disease processes. Telangiectatic vascular change is seen in diabetic retinopathy, venous occlusive disease, radiation retinopathy, Coats' disease, cystoid macular edema secondary to uveitis or the Irvine–Gass variant, and even in Eales' disease. The most important distinguishing feature of IMT in comparison with these other diseases is the limitation of the disease process to the perifoveal macular region (first temporally). This is not typical of the other conditions, although all of them may present in this manner.

Patients with IMT may be initially diagnosed with diabetic retinopathy or central serous chorioretinopathy, until it is realized that the clinical findings have either not progressed or have resolved. In elderly patients, IMT may resemble age-related macular degeneration, especially when pigmentary change and fibrovascular scarring is present. Importantly, Coats' disease may be confused with IMT; however, the presence of microvascular abnormalities outside the immediate perifoveal region, unilaterality, and the presence of lipid are key features of Coats' disease and not of IMT. The presence of retinal crystals may mimic other crystalline retinopathies. Finally, progressive outer retinal atrophy may simulate a lamellar macular hole. Often, the fellow eye has pathology more typical of IMT, making the diagnosis more straightforward.

Pearls

- Lipid is not seen in IPT, but it can be seen in central serous chorioretinopathy, CNV, diabetic retinopathy, and Coats' disease.

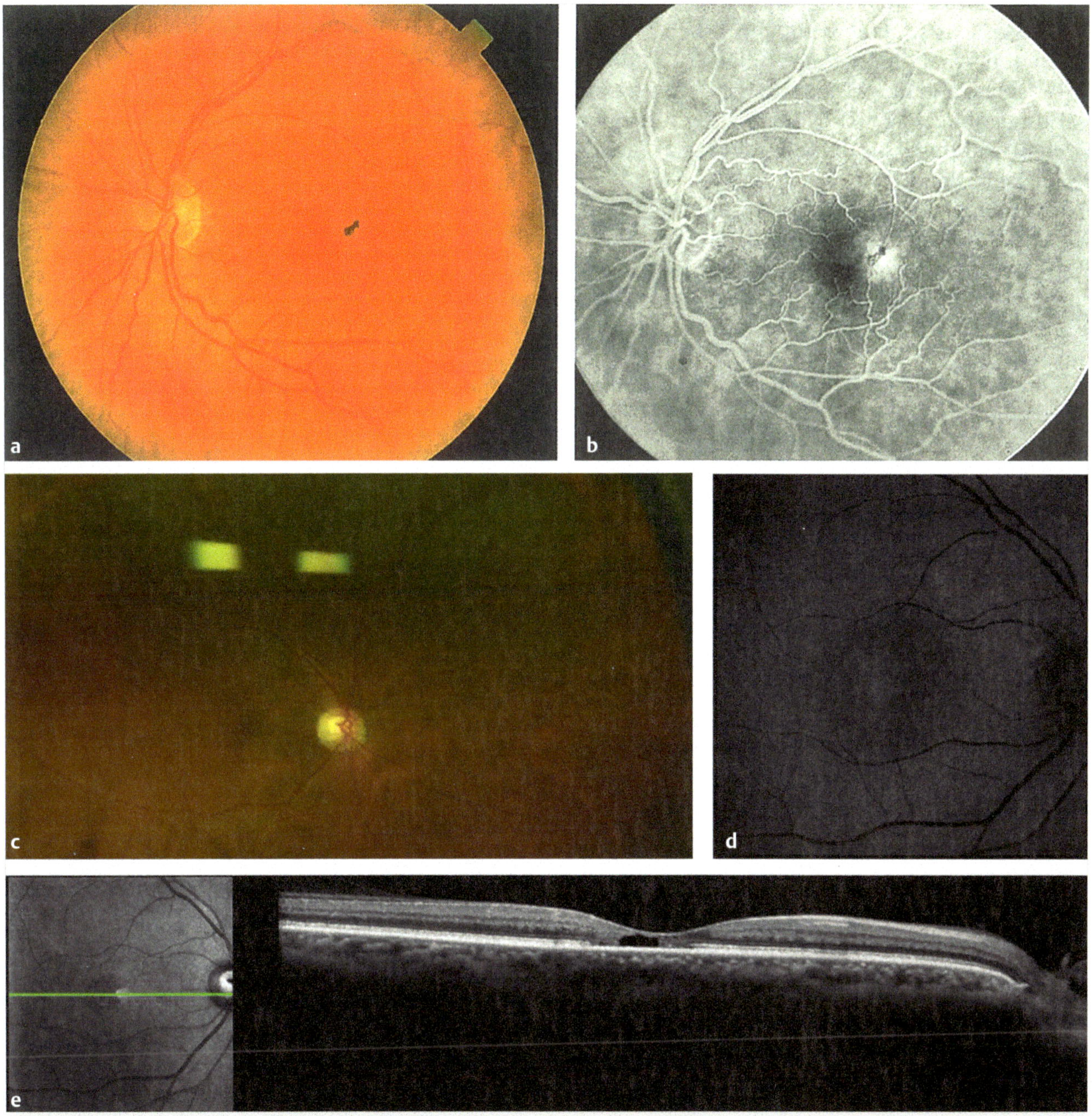

Fig. 13.5 Idiopathic perifoveal telangiectasis. (a) Mild retinal thickening with a blunted foveal reflex and an adjacent intraretinal pigment clump in the temporal foveal area. (b) Corresponding late-phase fluorescein angiogram shows intraretinal leakage of dye around the pigment clump. (c, d) Ultra-widefield color and short-wave fundus autofluorescence (FAF) imaging of a 59-year-old man with IMT type 2, demonstrating decreased macular pigment and corresponding attenuation of normal foveal hypoautofluorescence. Best-corrected vision was 20/200 (eccentric). (e) SLO and SDOCT image of same patient demonstrating foveal pseudohole and outer retinal atrophy. (continued)

13.3.3 Pathogenesis and Histopathology

The pathogenesis of IMT is unknown. Although 15% of patients have hypertension, mild diabetes, or atherosclerotic disease, no significant correlation with other diseases exists.[41] One study did find a correlation with abnormal glucose metabolism in patients with IMT.[66] Gass and Blodi[59] reported one family with two siblings affected by IMT, suggesting a genetic component, although similar environmental factors may have been causative.

Histopathologic examination revealed thickening of the capillary endothelial wall of affected vessels in a patient with IMT; however, no evidence of capillary telangiectasis was observed.[67] Gass[58] contended that retinal capillary invasion of the retinal receptor layer and accumulation of extracellular fluid within the retina are seen in IMT. In addition, the angiographic staining pattern typical of IMT is secondary to

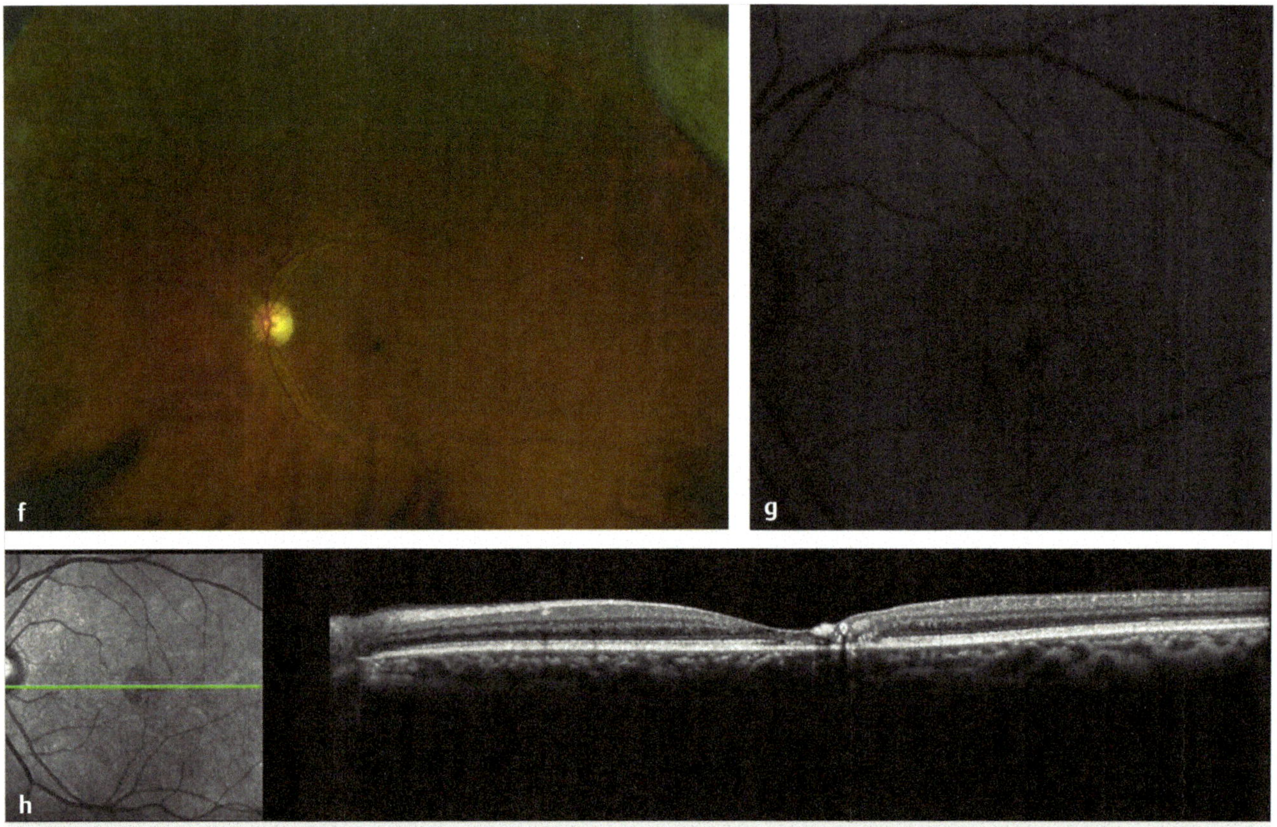

Fig. 13.5 (continued) **(f–h)** Upper image: ultra-widefield color and FAF images of the fellow eye of the same patient, demonstrating abnormal petaloid hypoautofluorescence in the fovea corresponding to intraretinal pigment migration seen on color imaging. Lower image: SLO and SDOCT images of the same patient, demonstrating intraretinal hyperreflectivity consistent with pigment migration and outer retinal atrophy. Best-corrected vision was 20/50.

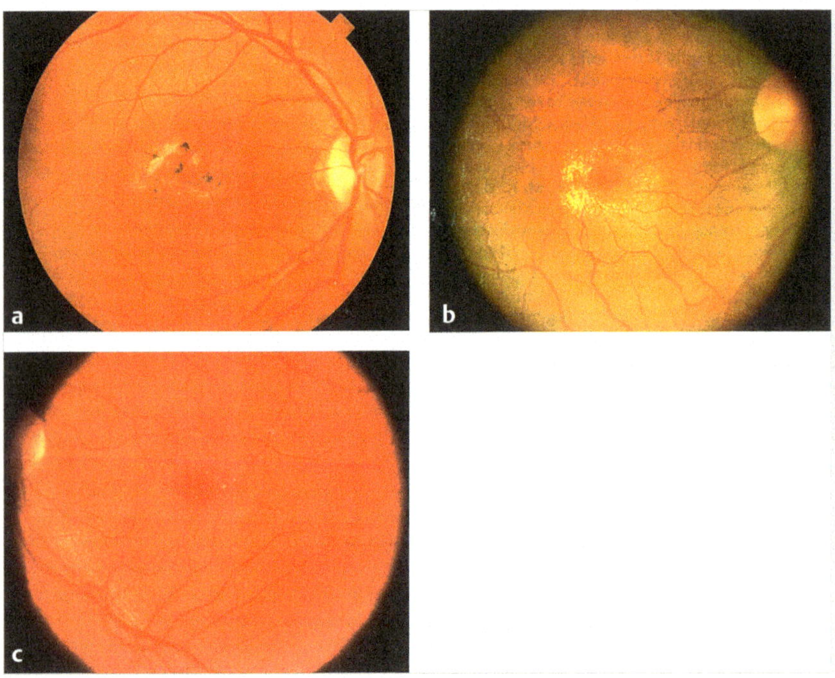

Fig. 13.6 Other findings of idiopathic perifoveal telangiectasis. **(a)** Late disease with extensive pigment epithelial hyperplasia and fibrous metaplasia. **(b)** Crystals on the retinal surface, principally in temporal portion of macula, associated with telangiectasis. **(c)** Early grayish discoloration surrounding fovea and the appearance of a lamellar macular hole, indicative of outer retinal atrophy.

nutritional deprivation of the middle retina, which leads to cellular damage. Eventually, degeneration of outer retinal cell layers leads to outer retinal atrophy. Vasoproliferative changes begin in the deep retinal venous plexus and extend into the subsensory retinal space in advanced disease. RPE hyperplasia and migration occur along right-angle venules. The reason for vasoproliferation and pigment migration in this disease is not understood. The etiology of the inner retinal crystals is unknown; however, degenerative products of cellular metabolism in the internal limiting membrane may be causative.

13.3.4 Management and Course

The use of laser in IMT is considered in only those patients with persistent, advanced nonproliferative disease.[66] The disease is typically self-limited and visual acuity stabilizes at the 20/30 level in most patients. As visual loss is usually secondary to atrophy of retinal tissue rather than accumulation of serous exudation secondary to incompetent vasculature, laser has little therapeutic rationale. Although nonproliferative disease is typically observed, macular edema has been treated with anti-angiogenic agents.

Unfortunately, this offers short-term anatomic improvement, but little to no visual benefit. Patients with secondary CNV —in decades past treated with laser or photodynamic therapy—are now routinely offered intravitreal anti-angiogenic therapy with more promising results, as decreased vascular permeability and resolution of subretinal neovascular complexes often preserves or restores vision.[69]

Controversial Points

- Laser to the area of abnormal retinal vessels in idiopathic macular telangiectasia may decrease the amount of intraretinal leakage, but it is not thought to affect the final visual outcome favorably in most cases. Anti-angiogenic therapy may be useful in proliferative IMT.

13.4 Eales' Disease

In 1880, Henry Eales first described a disease associated with abnormal retinal veins and hemorrhages. The disease he originally described most likely included several different diseases in its spectrum. Nonetheless, the disease entity presenting with idiopathic obliterative vasculopathy, retinal perivasculitis, peripheral nonperfusion, and bilateral recurrent vitreous hemorrhages has been termed *Eales' disease.* Most importantly, this remains a diagnosis of exclusion. Interestingly, the disease is more common in the Middle East and India.

13.4.1 Clinical Features

Eales' disease most commonly affects young adults 20 to 30 years of age and may have a male predominance, although some have reported an equal distribution among male and female patients.[70,71] In approximately 80 to 90% of patients, bilateral disease develops.[72]

The inflammatory component of the disease presents with retinal vascular sheathing, ranging from minimal white sheathing of vessels to heavier focal areas of exudation. The veins may be affected more than arteries, although some have reported equal involvement.[68,69] Cell and flare and keratic precipitates are seen in the anterior chamber, whereas vitritis and macular edema are seen posteriorly.

The vascular component of the disease can vary from mild microvascular abnormalities at the margin of perfused and nonperfused retina to frank neovascularization, which is present in approximately 80% of patients. The area of nonperfusion is typically in the peripheral retina and may have white sclerotic vessels. The junctional area may have microaneurysms, arteriovenous shunts, venous beading, or collaterals.[71,73] In addition, cotton-wool spots and hard exudates are more prominent in this region. Neovascularization most commonly occurs at the border of perfused and nonperfused retina (▶ Fig. 13.7) and can lead to vitreous hemorrhage and complicated retinal detachment (which may at first be fractional but later develop a rhegmatogenous component).

Visual loss occurs secondary to vitreous hemorrhage, retinal vasculitis, and macular edema associated with uveitis. Visual outcomes can be excellent, as the macula is often spared; however, in the setting of macular involvement, the visual outcome can be poor. Concomitant branch retinal vein occlusion has been reported in patients with Eales' disease, and this can also lead to visual loss. Rubeosis and neovascular glaucoma are late complications of severe nonperfusion or chronic retinal detachment. Rarely, focal central nervous system involvement with strokes has been reported in some patients with Eales' disease.[74,75] In particular, hearing loss, possibly secondary to cochlear ischemia, has been reported in up to 50% of patients.[75]

13.4.2 Differential Diagnosis

Because Eales' disease is a diagnosis of exclusion, many ocular and systemic diseases, particularly posterior segment inflammatory diseases and entities causing peripheral neovascularization, must be ruled out. Peripheral neovascularization without concomitant inflammation is seen in sickle-cell diseases, diabetic retinopathy, incontinentia pigmenti, retinopathy of prematurity, and familial exudative vitreoretinopathy. Inflammation associated with similar retinal vascular abnormalities can be seen in sarcoidosis, pars planitis, and collagen vascular diseases, such as lupus erythematosus. Rarely, systemic diseases such as ulcerative colitis can present with similar findings. A fractional retinal detachment in a patient with Eales' disease must be distinguished from bullous retinal detachments seen in diseases such as central serous chorioretinopathy.[76]

Pearls

- Eales' disease is a bilateral, obliterative retinal vasculopathy of young adults that may result in extensive peripheral nonperfusion, retinal neovascularization, and recurrent vitreous hemorrhage. It is a diagnosis of exclusion, as many known infectious and noninfectious conditions can produce a similar ocular picture.

13.4.3 Pathogenesis and Histopathology

The etiology of Eales' disease is unknown. The most common reported association is prior exposure to tuberculin protein; however, an association with active tuberculosis has not been

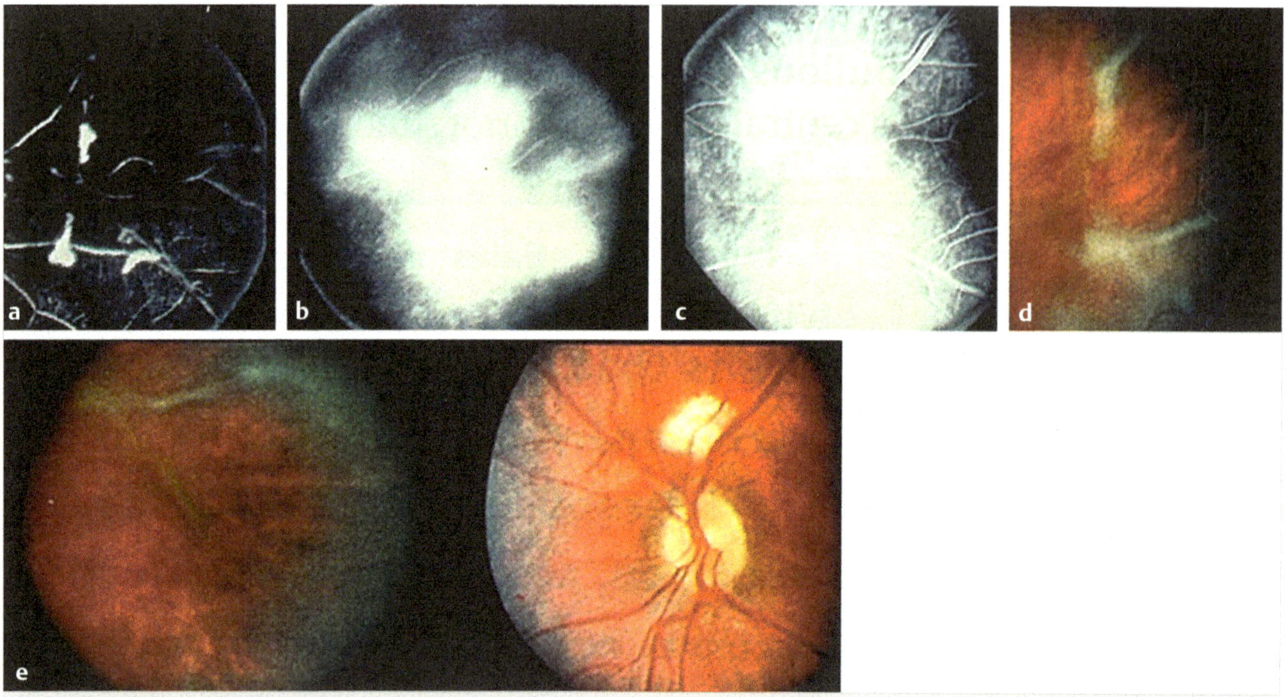

Fig. 13.7 Eales disease. **(a–c)** Fluorescein angiogram photographs show peripheral nonperfusion with neovascularization at the margin of severe capillary nonperfusion. Late leakage of fluorescein dye is typical of neovascularization. **(d, e)** Fundus photographs reveal fibrous proliferation at the margin of capillary nonperfusion, a precursor of traction retinal detachment. *(continued)*

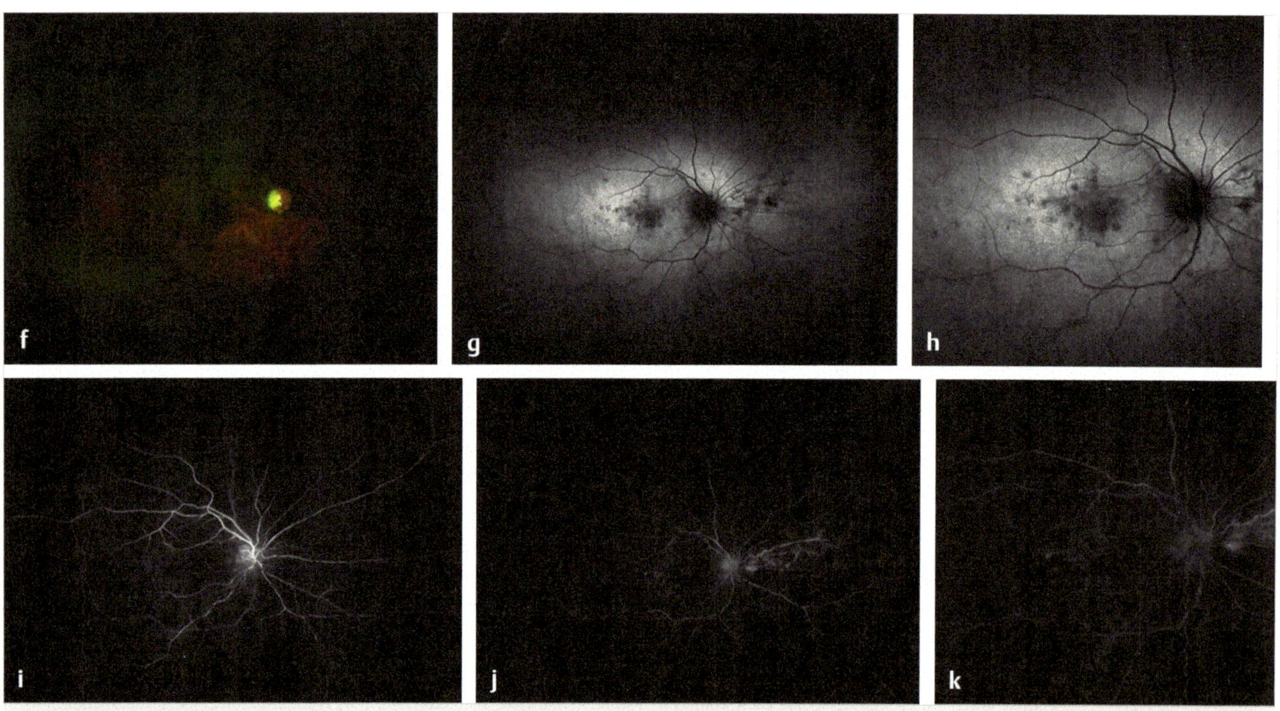

Fig. 13.7 *(continued)* **(f–h)** Ultra-widefield color and FAF photographs demonstrating nasal intraretinal hemorrhage and speckled macular hypoautofluorescence consistent with retinal pigment epithelium (RPE) dysfunction. **(i–k)** Upper images: early (left) and late (right and lower) phase fundus fluorescein angiography demonstrating blocking hypofluorescence corresponding to nasal hemorrhage with adjacent hypoperfusion and retinal vasculitis. The macula demonstrates hyperfluorescent RPE window defects in areas of hypoautofluorescence.

established. Gass[41] reported elevated levels of alpha-1 acid glycoprotein and other serum proteins, although these may be nonspecific findings in patients with acute inflammation.

13.4.4 Management and Course

There appears to be no effective treatment to reduce the inflammatory component of the disease. To date, steroids have been relatively ineffective. The treatment is limited to stimulating regression of neovascularization by applying laser to the nonperfused retina.[77] Some have also advocated treatment of the junctional area of perfused retina.[70] Murphy et al[71] have reported better than 20/40 vision in 67% of patients. Severe vision loss was reported in approximately 10% of patients and was caused most frequently by vitreous hemorrhage, retinal detachment, and neovascular glaucoma. Vitrectomy is indicated for nonclearing vitreous hemorrhage, epiretinal membrane, and traction or combined traction and rhegmatogenous retinal detachment.

13.5 Acquired Retinal Macroaneurysm

Acquired retinal arterial macroaneurysms are typically solitary, fusiform dilations of retinal arterioles occurring in 50- to 60-year-old individuals, more commonly in women than in men. The vascular abnormality is usually in the posterior pole and often occurs near an arterial bifurcation or arteriovenous crossing. Visual loss occurs secondary to hemorrhage or exudate tracking into the central macula area and, as such, the most common presentation is the superotemporal arterial macroaneurysm. Approximately two-thirds of affected individuals have systemic hypertension and other risk factors for stroke and coronary artery disease.[78] Robertson[79] first used the term *retinal macroaneurysm* to describe these vascular abnormalities because they are larger than the microaneurysms seen in diabetic retinopathy and venous occlusive disease.

13.5.1 Clinical Features

As described earlier, the most common presentation of retinal arterial macroaneurysm is visual loss from a lesion along the superotemporal arcade that has resulted in lipid exudation or hemorrhage into the fovea. It is uncommon to see more than one macroaneurysm; however, multiple macroaneurysms can affect the same vessel or occur independently in another region of the fundus. Multiple macroaneurysms should alert the clinician to other entities with similar presentation (see "Differential Diagnosis"). Approximately 10% of patients with acquired retinal macroaneurysm have bilateral involvement. Macroaneurysms involving the cilioretinal artery and the optic nerve head vessels have been reported.[80]

The macroaneurysm is often readily identified ophthalmoscopically when an area of circinate lipid surrounds the lesion; however, not uncommonly, the presentation is less obvious when hemorrhage obscures the lesion. The most distinctive feature of an acquired macroaneurysm is the potential presence of hemorrhage in every possible anatomic compartment—subretinal, intraretinal, subinternal limiting membrane, immediately preretinal, and vitreous (▶ Fig. 13.8). The hourglass hemorrhage is virtually pathognomonic for a retinal macroaneurysm. The severity of lipid exudation can vary from mild to exuberant and may increase after laser treatment (▶ Fig. 13.9).[81] The presence of focal arterial yellow plaques in 10% of patients previously was thought to indicate embolic foci but most likely represents areas of atheroma formation on damaged vessel walls. Gass[80] has seen these foci develop into macroaneurysms.

Pearls

- The most distinctive feature of acquired macroaneurysm is the potential presence of hemorrhage in every possible anatomic compartment—subretinal, intraretinal, subinternal limiting membrane, immediately preretinal, and vitreous. The hourglass hemorrhage is virtually pathognomonic for retinal macroaneurysm.

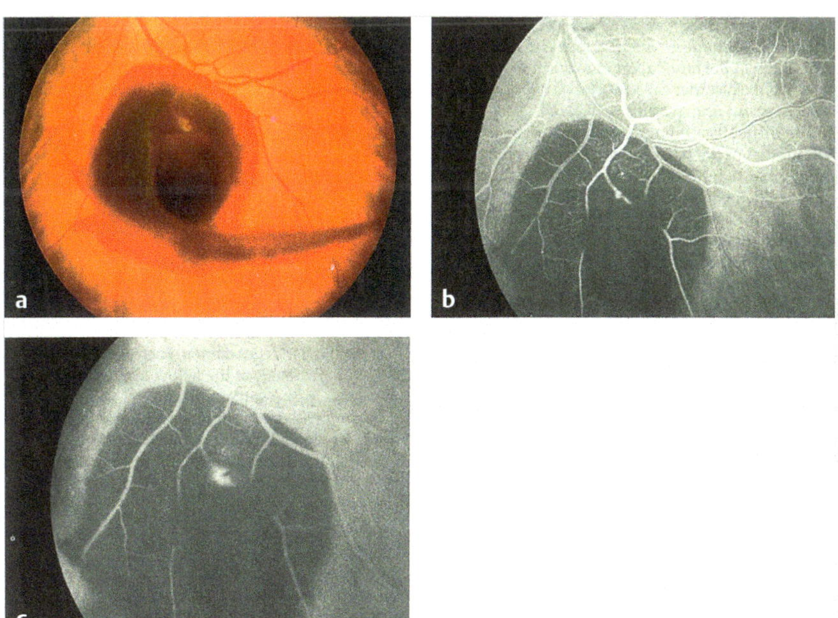

Fig. 13.8 Acquired retinal macroaneurysm. **(a)** Preretinal, intraretinal, and subretinal hemorrhage is present. Early-phase **(b)** and late-phase **(c)** fluorescein angiogram photographs show the macroaneurysm as a leaking focus along the course of a retinal arteriole.

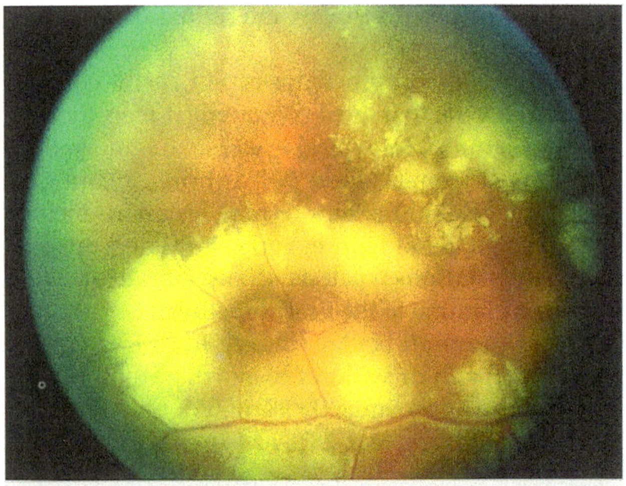

Fig. 13.9 Acquired retinal macroaneurysm. Lipid exudate rather than hemorrhage predominates in this affected eye. Laser has been applied directly to the macroaneurysm.

Fluorescein angiography is useful for confirming the diagnosis and quantitating the perfusion of the involved retinal artery as well as the leakage of the macroaneurysm. A macroaneurysm typically fills early and the damaged vascular wall stains later in the angiogram (▶ Fig. 13.8). Leakage of fluorescein dye into the extravascular area coincides with the degree of lipid exudation seen clinically. Often, a significant area of capillary nonperfusion is seen surrounding the lesion, and the neighboring vasculature may exhibit microaneurysms and intra-arterial collateral formation. The distal portion of the involved vessel may fill with fluorescein dye slowly, indicating a partial occlusion of the artery. The artery most commonly remains completely patent, but a classic branch retinal artery occlusion with complete distal occlusion is not uncommon.[80] Indocyanine green angiography (ICGA) shows similar findings, with the aneurysm being hyperfluorescent and exhibiting late leakage. The hyperfluorescent focus on ICGA, but not on fluorescein angiography, may still be visible under a moderately thick layer of blood.

13.5.2 Differential Diagnosis

Large fusiform dilations of retinal arterioles (macroaneurysms) can be seen in other disease processes, such as angiomatosis retinae, Eales' disease, Leber's multiple miliary aneurysms, Coats' disease, and branch retinal vein occlusions. The clinical features of these diseases help distinguish them from the solitary, acquired macroaneurysm. The presence of multiple, bilateral, "Y-shaped" macroaneurysms occurring principally at the bifurcation of major retinal arteries is seen in the disorder called *IRVAN*.[82]

The difficulty in diagnosis often arises from the obscuration of the retinal lesion by hemorrhage. The differential diagnosis in the setting of hemorrhage includes diabetic retinopathy, retinal telangiectasis, retinal capillary angioma, and cavernous hemangioma of the retina. A dark-colored region deep to the RPE often seen in acquired macroaneurysm can also be seen with sub-RPE hemorrhage in age-related macular degeneration or, importantly, in malignant melanoma of the choroid.[83] The presence of other features of macular degeneration, such as drusen formation or involvement of the fellow eye, will aid in the diagnosis. In the setting of malignant melanoma, ultrasound will demonstrate low internal reflectivity. When the blood is not very thick, ICGA may aid in detecting the macroaneurysm or rule out other causes, such as CNV, as described earlier.

13.5.3 Pathogenesis and Histopathology

There is a strong association between systemic arterial hypertension and macroaneurysm formation. Breaks in the arterial wall resulting in focal dilation of the involved vessel are presumed to result from long-standing hypertension. Similar manifestations of hypertension are known to occur in the cerebral arteries. Others have reported an association with lipid and lipoprotein abnormalities. Histopathology reveals fibrin–platelet clot formation; extravasated blood, exudate, hemosiderin, and lipid-laden macrophages; and fibroglial proliferation within and around the involved vessel.[80,83,84,85] The natural course of untreated macroaneurysm involves thrombosis, involution, and resolution of exudation. Typically, the involved artery remains patent.

13.5.4 Management and Course

The natural course of retinal macroaneurysm is resolution of the hemorrhagic and exudative manifestations. As such, treatment is usually considered only in the setting of persistent visual loss secondary to chronic exudation or hemorrhage into the macula. We use the argon green or dye yellow laser and apply a large spot size (500 µm) with a long duration of 0.5 second and low energy. The aneurysm is treated directly, and the neighboring area of nonperfusion and other microvascular changes is not treated. Complications of laser include occlusion of the distal retinal artery and hemorrhage, both of which may be seen during the treatment session. Hemorrhage may be controlled by manual compression of the lens to the globe, which raises the intraocular pressure and closes the retinal arterial circulation. Intravitreal bevacizumab has been reported to be an effective treatment in patients with central macular edema due to retinal macroaneurysms as evidenced by decreased leakage on posttreatment compared with pretreatment fluorescein angiography, reduced central retinal thickness, and improved visual acuity.[86] However, one case–control study demonstrated only a quicker improvement of these metrics but similar final outcomes between treated and observed groups.[87]

Controversial Points

- The visual prognosis after a retinal arterial macroaneurysm has caused exudation or hemorrhage is generally good. However, treatment may be considered if there is persistent or progressive visual loss from chronic exudation into the macula.

Visual outcomes after surgical drainage of subretinal blood or preretinal hemorrhage are typically no better than the natural course. Recently, some investigators have reported better visual outcomes with the use of tissue plasminogen activator (tPA) to facilitate removal of subfoveal hemorrhage.[88,89] The use of Nd:YAG (neodymium:yttrium-aluminum-garnet) laser may expedite visual recovery in patients with subinternal limiting membrane hemorrhage.[90] Generally, patients with chronic lipid exudation into the macula or subfoveal hemorrhage have limited, if any, visual recovery.

13.6 Collagen Vascular Diseases

Many ocular problems can result from the various collagen vascular diseases (see text box). The scope of this section is limited to those conditions that have been reported to affect the retinal or choroidal vasculature.

Etiologies of Retinal Vasculitis

Systemic conditions

Noninfectious

- Behçet's disease
- Wegener's granulomatosis
- SLE
- Polyarteritis nodosa
- Whipple's disease
- Crohn's disease
- Sarcoidosis
- Multiple sclerosis
- After vaccination
- Buerger's disease
- Takayasu's disease
- Sjögren's syndrome
- Churg–Strauss syndrome

Infectious

- Syphilis
- Lyme disease
- Toxoplasmosis
- *Toxocara canis* infection
- Coccidioidomycosis
- Tuberculosis
- Cytomegalovirus (CMV) infection
- Herpes simplex or zoster virus infection
- Candidiasis
- Brucellosis
- Leptospirosis
- Rickettsial infection
- Amebiasis
- Epstein–Barr virus infection (mononucleosis)

Ocular conditions

- Birdshot chorioretinopathy
- Pars planitis (intermediate uveitis)
- Eales' disease
- IRVAN
- Frosted branch angiitis (postviral, CMV, other)
- Multifocal choroiditis and panuveitis

Source: Information presented in this text box was obtained in personal oral communication with Thomas E. Flynn, MD, 1998 (Columbia University and St. Luke's Roosevelt Medical Center, New York).

SLE is the collagen vascular disease that most commonly affects the retinal vasculature. The typical systemic manifestations of SLE include malar rash, polyarthritis, arthralgias, fever, and weight loss. Serious manifestations include hypertension, renal failure, and central nervous system manifestations, such as seizures or stroke. The eye is not immune to the vasculopathy of SLE. In fact, the most common ocular finding in SLE is cotton-wool spots with or without hemorrhages. Retinopathy is seen in approximately 3% of SLE patients in the ambulatory setting and 28% of patients in the inpatient setting.[91,92]

Vascular occlusive diseases such as central or branch retinal artery occlusion and central or branch retinal vein occlusion have been reported in patients with SLE. In fact, the risk seems to be greater than one would expect from hypertension alone. In some patients, a severe vasculitic response develops, with nonperfusion of the retinal capillaries, which may be localized or widespread, and sometimes permanent vision loss (▶ Fig. 13.10 and ▶ Fig. 13.11). Large zones of capillary nonperfusion may lead to neovascularization, vitreous hemorrhage, and other complications similar to those seen in diabetic retinopathy. Vasculitis may improve with appropriate immunosuppression, particularly if begun early (▶ Fig. 13.11).

Lupus choroidopathy results from ischemia of the choroidal circulation. The typical fundus appearance consists of multifocal exudative neurosensory retinal detachments with acute Elschnig's spots or Siegrist's streaks.[93] These findings are identical to those seen in hypertensive choroidopathy and exudative retinal detachment secondary to organ transplantation.

The differential diagnosis of retinopathy in SLE includes diabetic retinopathy, hypertension retinopathy, radiation retinopathy, and other collagen vascular diseases or systemic vasculitides such as scleroderma, dermatomyositis, relapsing polychondritis, polyarteritis nodosa, Wegener's granulomatosis, and Behçet's disease. Certain systemic vasculitic syndromes such as the hemoglobinopathies and infectious causes such as AIDS and Lyme disease can present with cotton-wool spots and retinal vasculopathy as well.

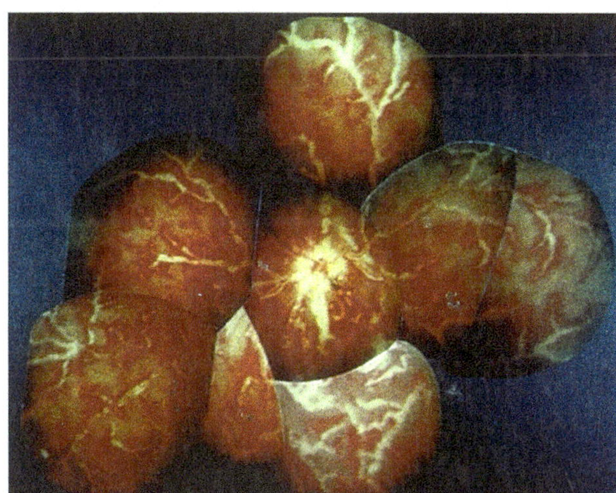

Fig. 13.10 Lupus retinopathy. There is widespread involvement of both retinal arteries and veins. Note the frosted branch angiitis-like picture and prominent intraretinal hemorrhages, indicative of venous occlusive disease.

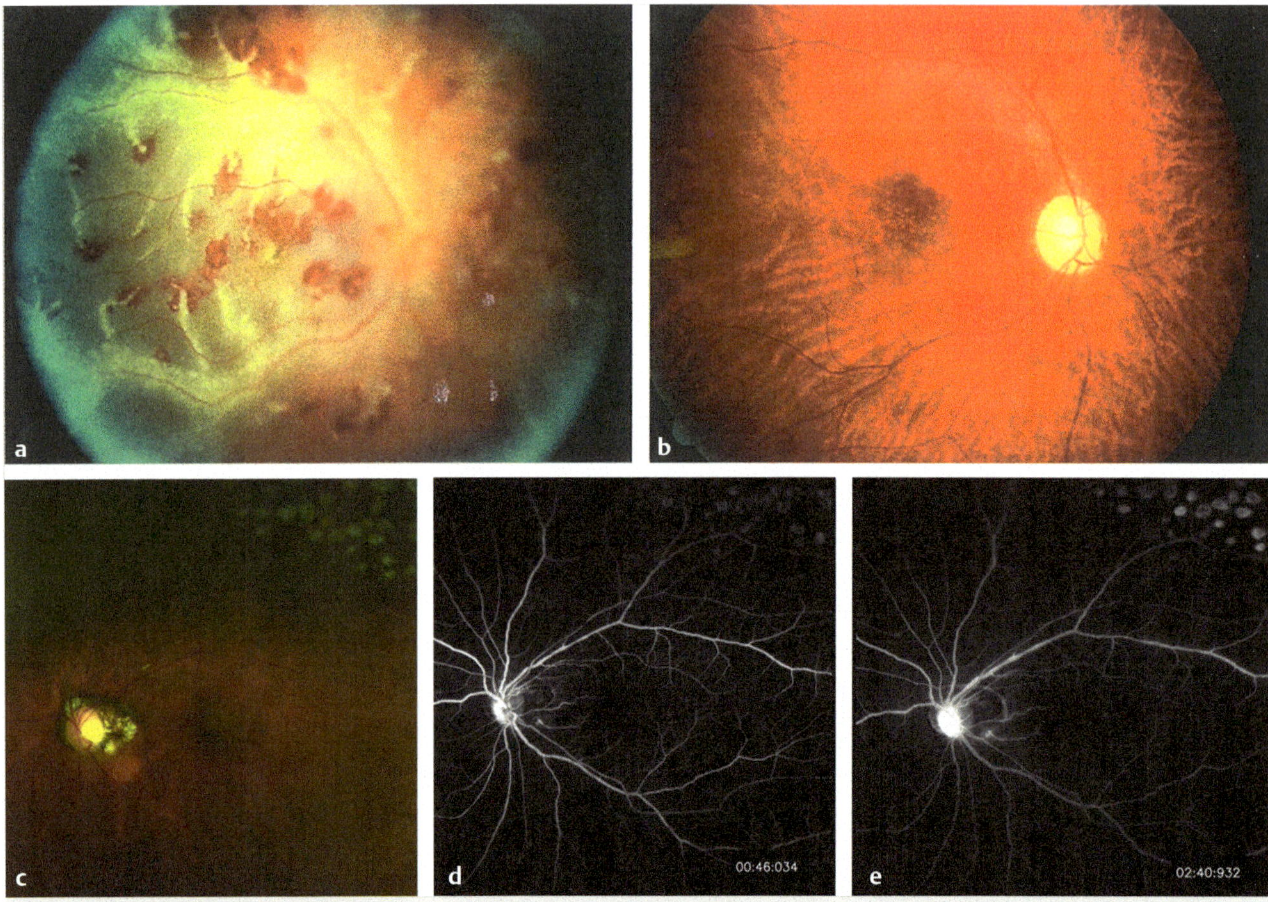

Fig. 13.11 Lupus retinopathy. (**a**) Acute presentation with severe vasculitis. (**b**) After treatment with systemic corticosteroids, the vasculitic manifestations completely resolved, but optic disc pallor was evident. (**c–e**) Patient with old retinal vascular occlusions and active systemic lupus vasculitis. Fluorescein angiogram demonstrates progressive retinal vascular staining along the superior arcade and nonperfusion in the distribution of the cilioretinal arteriole.

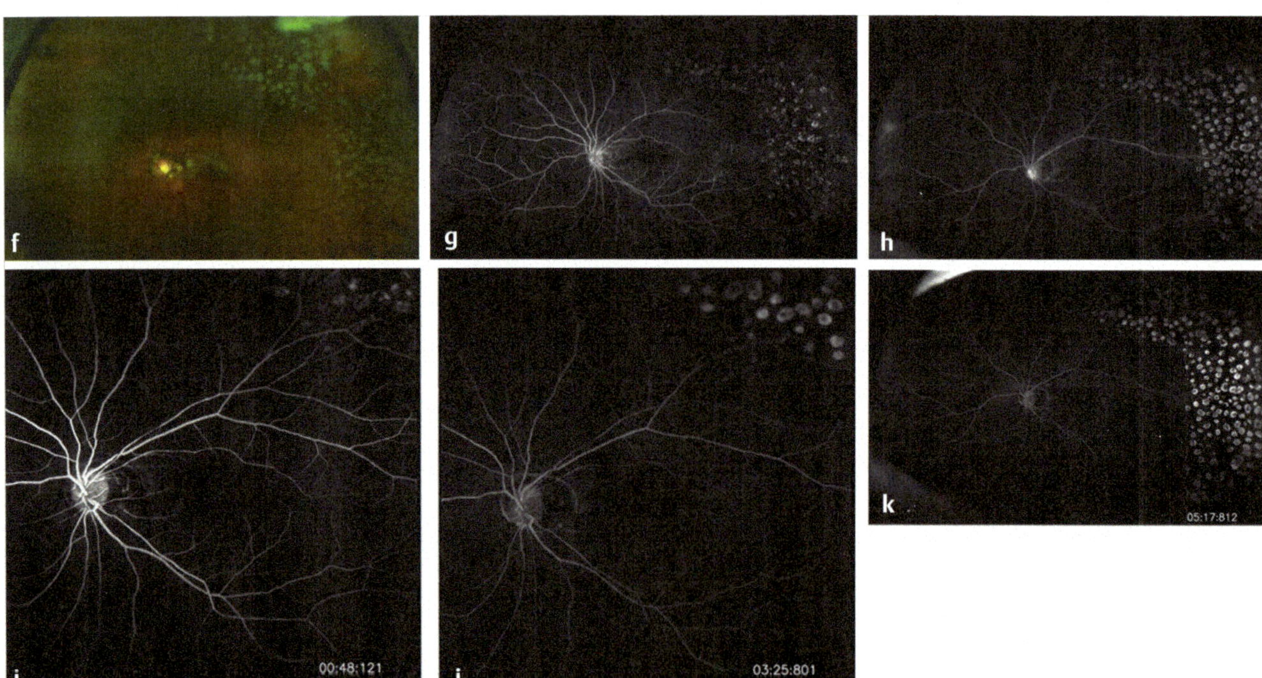

Fig. 13.11 (**f–h**) Ultra-widefield images of the same patient reveal peripheral retinal vasculitis. (**i–k**) Resolved retinal vasculitis in the same patient two months after beginning immunosuppressive therapy with oral steroids and methotrexate.

The pathogenesis of SLE vasculopathy may not be inflammatory, as many patients with SLE have a circulating antiphospholipid antibody or anticardiolipin antibody, which causes a hypercoagulable state.[94] Interestingly, the histopathology of central nervous system lupus microangiopathy is very similar to that of the retinopathy.

Treatment of SLE-related retinopathy is aimed at controlling the hypertensive manifestations of the primary disease and treating the autoimmune disease with steroids or other immunosuppressive medications if necessary. Often, treatment with oral steroids and control of blood pressure are adequate (▶ Fig. 13.11). Laser to the area of capillary nonperfusion may be necessary in the setting of severe nonperfusion and retinal neovascularization. Laser may be useful in the rare setting of persistent lupus choroidopathy.[93]

Other collagen vascular diseases may present with retinal vascular involvement as a primary manifestation or as a result of secondary hypertension. Rheumatoid arthritis is rarely associated with cotton-wool spots in the fundus. Although the primary ocular manifestations of scleroderma are dry eye and anterior segment disease, sometimes cotton-wool spots, retinal hemorrhages, and even optic disc edema may develop. These changes, however, seem primarily attributable to hypertension associated with the disease. The identical histopathology in scleroderma and hypertensive retinopathy, as well as the resolution of retinopathy with hypertensive control, supports this hypothesis.[95] Cotton-wool spots alone have been reported in dermatomyositis, and a few vaso-occlusive episodes have been reported in relapsing polychondritis.

Both polyarteritis nodosa and Wegener's granulomatosis have been reported to be associated with cotton-wool spots, hemorrhages, and vascular occlusion, although ischemic optic neuropathy is a more common manifestation.[96] In addition to the typical central retinal artery occlusion or ischemic optic neuropathy presentation, the clinician should also consider giant cell arteritis with an otherwise unexplained, nonspecific occlusive retinopathy consisting of just cotton-wool spots and hemorrhages. Expeditious diagnosis and treatment are always necessary in giant cell arteritis to avoid bilateral vision loss. Behçet's disease classically presents with oral ulcers, genital ulcers, and a hypopyon uveitis. The characteristic retinal vasculitis, when present, involves both the artery and vein and is associated with severe arteriolar occlusion and retinal necrosis (see Chapter 25).

13.7 Systemic Vasculitic Syndromes

Retinal vascular involvement is seen in many diseases affecting the entire systemic vasculature, including the hemoglobinopathies, disseminated intravascular coagulation syndrome, and some hypercoagulable syndromes, such as protein C or protein S deficiencies, resistance to activated protein C, and antiphospholipid antibody syndrome (▶ Fig. 13.12). It is often difficult to discern whether retinal vascular occlusive disease is related to a vasculitic process, a hypercoagulable process, or a combination of both, as in disseminated intravascular coagulation. Systemic causes of true vasculitis include infectious and inflammatory disorders (see text box in section "Collagen Vascular Diseases"). Infectious diseases, such as syphilis, cat scratch disease, AIDS, *T. canis* infection, toxoplasmosis, and Lyme disease are commonly associated with retinal vasculitis. A detailed discussion of these diseases can be found in Chapter 24.

Systemic causes of vasculitis, including the collagen vascular diseases discussed previously, must be ruled out. Sarcoidosis, an autoimmune disorder, is associated with retinal vasculitis and is discussed in Chapter 25. Finally, multiple sclerosis has been associated with uveitis and retinal vasculitis, particularly periphlebitis (▶ Fig. 13.13).[97]

Crohn's disease and other inflammatory bowel diseases are typically associated with anterior segment findings alone; however, retinal vasculitis and systemic thrombotic diatheses leading to branch retinal artery occlusion have been reported. In addition, Whipple's disease presents with uveitis and retinal vasculitis. In general, inflammatory and infectious diseases with retinal vasculitis involve the veins preferentially or to the same degree as the arteries. Behçet's disease and syphilis are notable exceptions in that there is a preferential involvement of the arteries. The vasculitic component of these diseases may manifest as sheathing of vessels, which refers to the fundus appearance of white-outlined vessels, either segmental or continuous in configuration.

Pearls

- In general, inflammatory and infectious diseases with retinal vasculitis tend to involve the veins more than or to the same degree as the arteries. Notable exceptions include Behçet's disease and syphilis.

13.8 Valsalva Retinopathy

At the annual meeting of the American Ophthalmological Society in 1972, Dr. Thomas Duane described a series of patients with fundus findings in the wake of distant trauma to the circulation.[98] Perhaps the most striking case was of the patient who

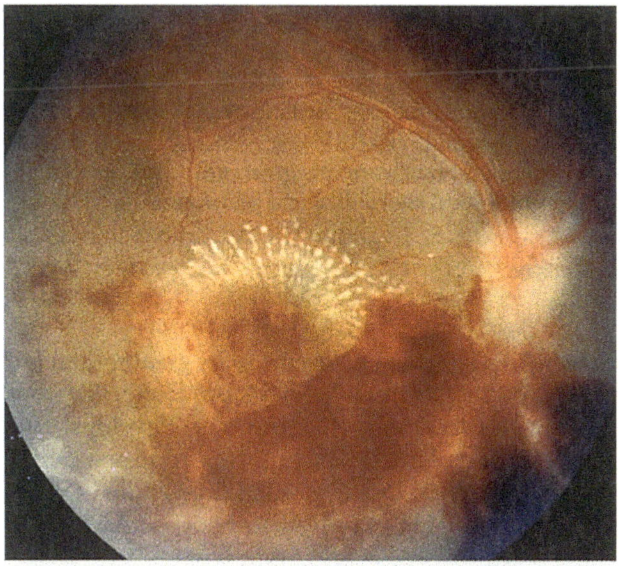

Fig. 13.12 Hypercoagulable syndrome with protein C deficiency manifesting as a branch retinal vein occlusion. A vasculitic component is also evident.

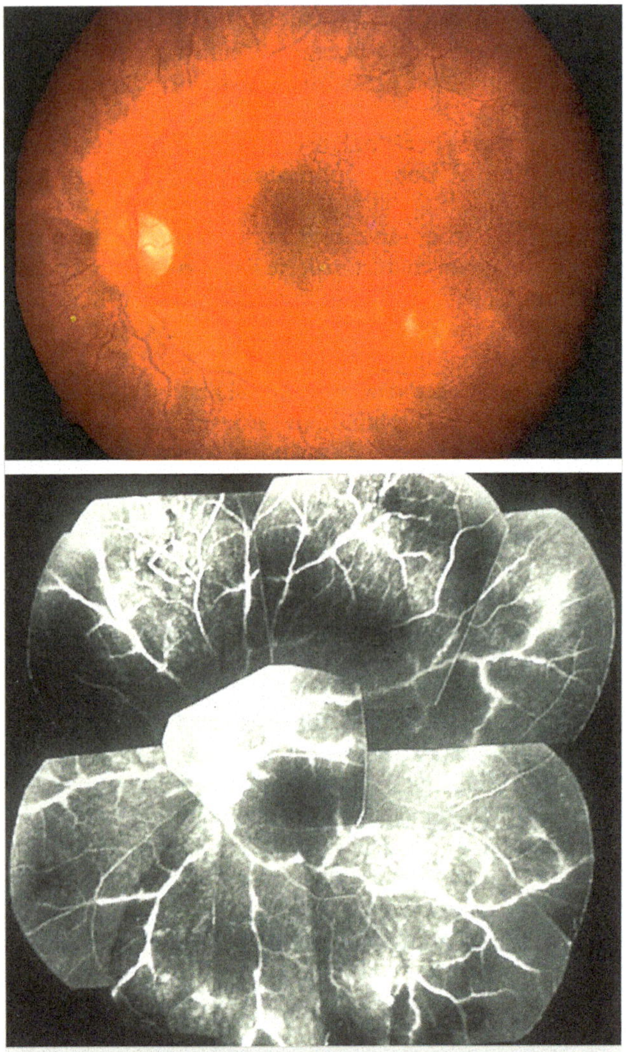

Fig. 13.13 Multiple sclerosis-related vasculitis. Fundus photograph reveals segmental retinal vascular sheathing and deep retinal white lesions scattered in the temporal midperiphery. Fluorescein angiogram composite shows widespread vasculitis with staining primarily of retinal veins. There is also extensive peripheral retinal capillary nonperfusion.

had "reflex spasm of the trachea and bronchial tree" during sodium pentothal anesthesia for an orthopedic procedure, which necessitated a "rather heroic form of tracheal intubation." The patient awoke "with many complaints, but a sore throat and greatly disturbed vision in each eye were predominant."[98] Dilated fundus exam revealed bilateral macular preretinal hemorrhages, which resolved over a few months, with no long-term visual consequences. At the same meeting, Dr. Edward Norton presented three patients with identical self-resolving fundus findings after comparatively more mundane episodes: one each with vomiting, coughing, and "a fit of rage."[98]

13.8.1 Clinical Features

Such inciting events and ocular sequelae illustrate the hallmarks of Valsalva hemorrhagic retinopathy: sudden increase in intrathoracic or intra-abdominal pressure, often against a closed glottis, with resultant increase in retinal intravenous pressure, exceeding the autoregulatory mechanisms at the level of the retinal capillaries. As a result, a cascade of extravasation may occur, ranging from intraretinal edema to intraretinal hemorrhage, and the visually consequential subhyaloid or (preretinal) hemorrhage, or even into the vitreous cavity itself.[99,100] Recent investigations with SD-OCT have delineated many of these hemorrhages as in fact occurring in the subinternal limiting membrane space.[101] The amplitude and duration of the force applied, as well as preexisting health of the retinal vasculature, likely interact to determine the level of fundus involvement. Nonetheless, even large pre-retinal macular hemorrhages are reported to self-resolve over time, with full recovery of vision.[99,100] Rare associated complications after Valsalva maneuvers include central retinal vein occlusion and macular hole (▶ Fig. 13.14).[102,103]

Valsalva retinopathy has since been described in a variety of antecedent settings including pregnancy, labor, pushups, sexual intercourse, colonoscopy, esophagogastroduodenoscopy, and even during an oratorical contest.[104,105,106,107,108,109,110] Retinal vascular diseases such as retinal arteriolar macroaneurysm, proliferative diabetic retinopathy, and proliferative sickle-cell retinopathy also can present with similar subretinal or subinternal limiting membrane hemorrhages.[111,112] and can be considered in the differential diagnosis, or possibly as predisposing factors if there is a history of antecedent Valsalva maneuver. While controlled studies are lacking, compromised retinal capillary integrity may increase the risk of clinically significant hemorrhage during Valsalva maneuvers.

13.8.2 Management and Course

As the natural history of Valsalva hemorrhagic retinopathy is favorable,[99,100] observation is usually the treatment of choice. Yet as visual recovery may take months, patients and physicians alike may seek intervention. The most well-studied treatment is Nd:YAG membrane puncture, initially reported by Raymond for the treatment of premacular hemorrhage in proliferative diabetic retinopathy and retinal arterial macroaneurysm,[111] and since utilized for Valsalva retinopathy.[113,114,115,116] The goal of treatment is laser perforation of the posterior hyaloid or internal limiting membrane and hence drainage of hemorrhage into the vitreous.

Nd:YAG membrane puncture has been shown to be a safe and relatively rapid method to restore vision,[116] with precise lysis of the posterior hyaloid or internal limiting membrane demonstrated via pre- and post-laser SD-OCT.[113,115] Pars plana vitrectomy with elevation of the posterior hyaloid with or without internal limiting membrane peeling has also been employed with favorable results.[117] However, the benign natural history of Valsalva retinopathy should give pause to the clinician when considering laser or surgical intervention.

Pearls

- Acute monocular or binocular loss of vision after Valsalva maneuver is caused by macular subhyaloid or subinternal limiting membrane hemorrhage. The natural history is very favorable, though restoration of vision may take months. Nd:YAG laser membrane puncture or pars plana vitrectomy may be employed in select cases.

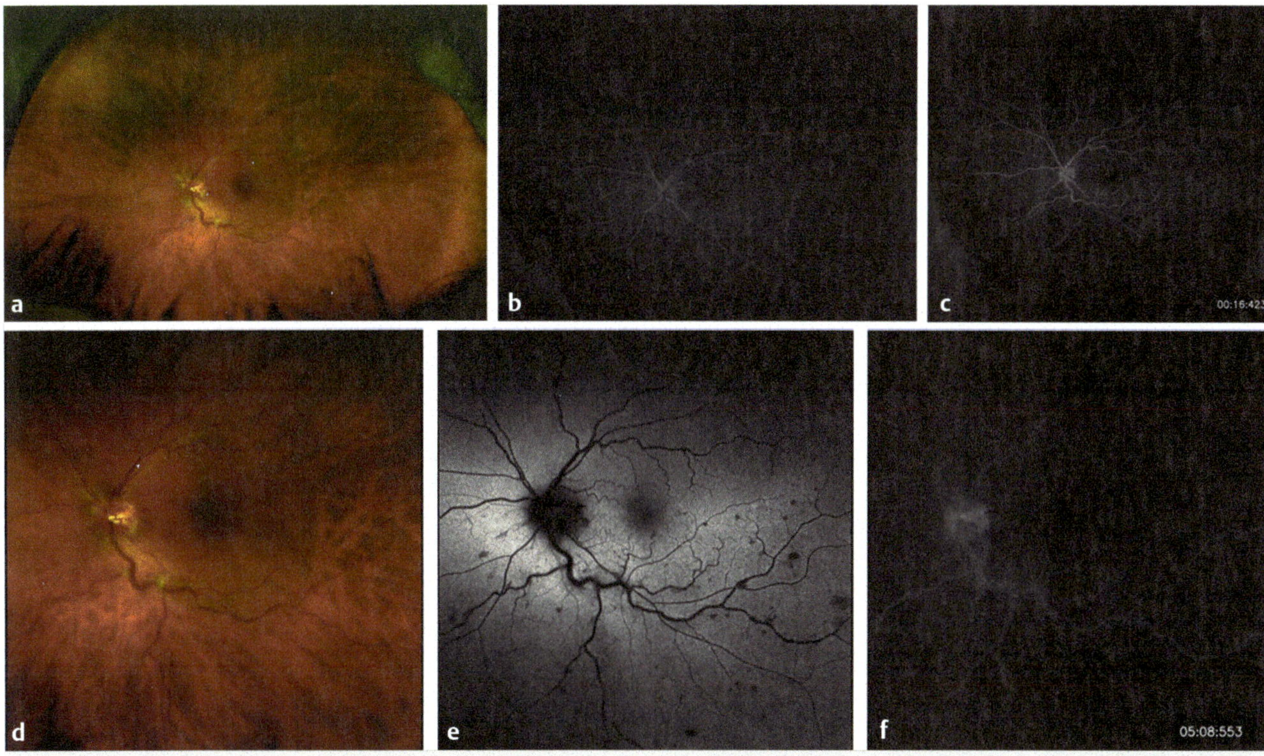

Fig. 13.14 (a–c) A 42-year-old man with perfused central retinal vein occlusion and antiphospholipid antibody syndrome. Best-corrected vision was 20/30. **(d–f)** Same patient with color, FAF, and late-phase fluorescein images demonstrating marked retinal vascular tortuosity, cotton-wool spots, and intraretinal hemorrhages with no neovascularization or nonperfusion.

References

[1] Gass JDM. Stereoscopic Atlas of Macular Diseases: Diagnosis and Treatment, 4th ed. St. Louis, MO: Mosby-Year Book; 1997:467–471

[2] Murphy RP, Chew EY. Hypertension. In: Ryan SJ, ed. Retina. 2nd ed. St Louis, MO: Mosby-Year Book; 1994:1413–1419

[3] Green WR. Systemic diseases with retinal involvement. In: Spencer WH, ed. Ophthalmic Pathology: An Atlas and Textbook. Philadelphia, PA: WB Saunders; 1985:1034–1047

[4] Goldbaum MH. Retinal depression sign indicating a small retinal infarct. Am J Ophthalmol. 1978; 86(1):45–55

[5] Scheie HG. Evaluation of ophthalmoscopic changes of hypertension and arteriolar sclerosis. AMA Arch Opthalmol. 1953; 49(2):117–138

[6] de Venecia G, Wallow I, Houser D, Wahlstrom M. The eye in accelerated hypertension. I. Elschnig's spots in nonhuman primates. Arch Ophthalmol. 1980; 98(5):913–918

[7] Tso MOM, Jampol LM. Pathophysiology of hypertensive retinopathy. Ophthalmology. 1982; 89(10):1132–1145

[8] Dewilde E, Huygens M, Cools G, Van Calster J. Hypertensive choroidopathy in pre-eclampsia: two consecutive cases. Ophthalmic Surg Lasers Imaging Retina. 2014; 45(4):343–346

[9] Sayin N, Kara N, Pirhan D, et al. Subfoveal choroidal thickness in preeclampsia: comparison with normal pregnant and nonpregnant women. Semin Ophthalmol. 2014; 29(1):11–17

[10] Kara N, Sayin N, Pirhan D, et al. Evaluation of subfoveal choroidal thickness in pregnant women using enhanced depth imaging optical coherence tomography. Curr Eye Res. 2014; 39(6):642–647

[11] Atas M, Açmaz G, Aksoy H, et al. Evaluation of the macula, retinal nerve fiber layer and choroid in preeclampsia, healthy pregnant and healthy non-pregnant women using spectral-domain optical coherence tomography. Hypertens Pregnancy. 2014; 33(3):299–310

[12] Garg A, Wapner RJ, Ananth CV, et al. Choroidal and retinal thickening in severe preeclampsia. Invest Ophthalmol Vis Sci. 2014; 55(9):5723–5729

[13] Ashton N, Harry J. The pathology of cotton wool spots and cytoid bodies in hypertensive retinopathy and other diseases. Trans Ophthalmol Soc U K. 1963; 83:91–114

[14] Robinson F, Riva CE, Grunwald JE, Petrig BL, Sinclair SH. Retinal blood flow autoregulation in response to an acute increase in blood pressure. Invest Ophthalmol Vis Sci. 1986; 27(5):722–726

[15] Coats G. Forms of retinal disease with massive subretinal exudation. R Lond Ophthalmic Hosp Rep. 1908; 17:440–525

[16] Leber TH. Verber ein durch Yorkommen miltipler Miliaraneurisimen characterisierte Form von Retinal degeneration. Graefes Arch Clin Exp Ophthalmol. 1912; 81:1–14

[17] Reese AB. Telangiectasis of the retina and Coats' disease. Am J Ophthalmol. 1956; 42(1):1–8

[18] Gomez Morales A. Coats' disease. Natural history and results of treatment. Am J Ophthalmol. 1965; 60(5):855–865

[19] Spitznas M, Joussen F, Wessing A, Meyer-Schwickerath G. Coat's disease. An epidemiologic and Fluorescein angiographic study. Albrecht Von Graefes Arch Klin Exp Ophthalmol. 1975; 195(4):241–250

[20] Egerer I, Tasman W, Tomer TT. Coats disease. Arch Ophthalmol. 1974; 92 (2):109–112

[21] Gass JDM. Stereoscopic Atlas of Macular Diseases: Diagnosis and Treatment. 4th ed. St. Louis, MO: Mosby-Year Book; 1997:494–502

[22] Harris GS. Coats' disease, diagnosis and treatment. Can J Ophthalmol. 1970; 5(4):311–320

[23] Ridley ME, Shields JA, Brown GC, Tasman W. Coats' disease. Evaluation of management. Ophthalmology. 1982; 89(12):1381–1387

[24] Pauleikhoff D, Kruger K, Heinrich T, Wessing A. Epidemiologic features and therapeutic results in Coats' disease. Invest Ophthalmol. 1988; 29:335

[25] Green WR. Bilateral Coats' disease. Massive gliosis of the retina. Arch Ophthalmol. 1967; 77(3):378–383

[26] McGettrick PM, Loeffler KU. Bilateral Coats' disease in an infant (a clinical, angiographic, light and electron microscopic study). Eye (Lond). 1987; 1(Pt 1):136–145

[27] Blair MP, Ulrich JN, Elizabeth Hartnett M, Shapiro MJ. Peripheral retinal nonperfusion in fellow eyes in coats disease. Retina. 2013; 33(8):1694–1699

[28] Zhao Q, Peng XY, Chen FH, et al. Vascular endothelial growth factor in Coats' disease. Acta Ophthalmol (Copenh). 2014; 92(3):e225–e228

[29] Kase S, Rao NA, Yoshikawa H, et al. Expression of vascular endothelial growth factor in eyes with Coats' disease. Invest Ophthalmol Vis Sci. 2013; 54(1):57–62

[30] Goel SD, Augsburger JJ. Hemorrhagic retinal macrocysts in advanced Coats disease. Retina. 1991; 11(4):437–440
[31] Judisch GF, Apple DJ. Orbital cellulitis in an infant secondary to Coats' disease. Arch Ophthalmol. 1980; 98(11):2004–2006
[32] Zamorani G. A rare association of Coats' and retinitis pigmentosa. G Ital Oftalmol. 1956; 9:429–443
[33] Morgan WE, III, Crawford JB. Retinitis pigmentosa and Coats' disease. Arch Ophthalmol. 1968; 79(2):146–149
[34] Khan JA, Ide CH, Strickland MP. Coats'-type retinitis pigmentosa. Surv Ophthalmol. 1988; 32(5):317–332
[35] Pruett RC. Retinitis pigmentosa: clinical observations and correlations. Trans Am Ophthalmol Soc. 1983; 81:693–735
[36] Kang KB, Wessel MM, Tong J, D'Amico DJ, Chan RV. Ultra-widefield imaging for the management of pediatric retinal diseases. J Pediatr Ophthalmol Strabismus. 2013; 50(5):282–288
[37] Shields JA, Shields CL. Intraocular Tumors. A Text and Atlas. Philadelphia, PA: WB Saunders; 1992:356–358
[38] Howard GM, Ellsworth RM. Differential diagnosis of retinoblastoma. A statistical survey of 500 children. I. Relative frequency of the lesions which simulate retinoblastoma. Am J Ophthalmol. 1965; 60(4):610–618
[39] Tasman WS. Coats' disease. In: Tasman WS, ed. Clinical Decisions in Medical Retinal Disease. St. Louis, MO: Mosby-Year Book; 1994:204–210
[40] Haik BG. Advanced Coats' disease. Trans Am Ophthalmol Soc. 1991; 89:371–476
[41] Gass JDM, Oyakawa RT. Idiopathic juxtafoveolar retinal telangiectasis. Arch Ophthalmol. 1982; 100(5):769–780
[42] Egbert PR, Chan CC, Winter FC. Flat preparations of the retinal vessels in Coats' disease. J Pediatr Ophthalmol. 1976; 13(6):336–339
[43] Yeung J, Harris GS. Coats' disease: a study of cholesterol transport in the eye. Can J Ophthalmol. 1976; 11(1):61–68
[44] Woods AC, Duke JR. Coats' disease. I. Review of the literature, diagnostic criteria, clinical findings, and plasma lipid studies. Br J Ophthalmol. 1963; 47:385–412
[45] Chang MM, McLean IW, Merritt JC. Coats' disease: a study of 62 histologically confirmed cases. J Pediatr Ophthalmol Strabismus. 1984; 21(5):163–168
[46] Green WR. Congenital variations and abnormalities. In: Spencer WH, ed. Ophthalmic Pathology. 3rd ed. Philadelphia, PA: WB Saunders; 1985:624–630
[47] Tripathi R, Ashton N. Electron microscopical study of Coat's disease. Br J Ophthalmol. 1971; 55(5):289–301
[48] Campbell FP. Coats' disease and congenital vascular retinopathy. Trans Am Ophthalmol Soc. 1976; 74:365–424
[49] Deutsch TA, Rabb MF, Jampol LM. Spontaneous regression of retinal lesions in Coats' disease. Can J Ophthalmol. 1982; 17(4):169–172
[50] Meyer-Schwickerath G. Light Coagulation. St. Louis, MO: CV Mosby; 1960:103
[51] McGrand JC. Photocoagulation in Coats' disease. Trans Ophthalmol Soc U K. 1970; 90:47–56
[52] Spitznas M. Coats' disease: an epidemiologic and fluorescein angiographic study. Graefes Arch Clin Exp Ophthalmol. 1976; 199:31
[53] Machemer R, Williams JM, Sr. Pathogenesis and therapy of traction detachment in various retinal vascular diseases. Am J Ophthalmol. 1988; 105(2):170–181
[54] Zheng XX, Jiang YR. The effect of intravitreal bevacizumab injection as the initial treatment for Coats' disease. Graefes Arch Clin Exp Ophthalmol. 2014; 252(1):35–42
[55] Lin CJ, Chen SN, Hwang JF, Yang CM. Combination treatment of pediatric coats' disease: a bicenter study in Taiwan. J Pediatr Ophthalmol Strabismus. 2013; 50(6):356–362
[56] Ramasubramanian A, Shields CL. Bevacizumab for Coats' disease with exudative retinal detachment and risk of vitreoretinal traction. Br J Ophthalmol. 2012; 96(3):356–359
[57] Gaillard MC, Mataftsi A, Balmer A, Houghton S, Munier FL. ranibizumab in the management of advanced Coats disease Stages 3B and 4: long-term outcomes. Retina. 2014; 34(11):2275–2281
[58] Gass JDM. Stereoscopic Atlas of Macular Diseases: Diagnosis and Treatment. 4th ed. St. Louis: Mosby-Year Book; 1997:506–510
[59] Gass JDM, Blodi BA. Idiopathic juxtafoveolar retinal telangiectasis. Update of classification and follow-up study. Ophthalmology. 1993; 100(10):1536–1546
[60] Chew EY, Murphy RP, Newsome DA, Fine SL. Parafoveal telangiectasis and diabetic retinopathy. Arch Ophthalmol. 1986; 104(1):71–75
[61] Moisseiev J, Lewis H, Bartov E, Fine SL, Murphy RP. Superficial retinal refractile deposits in juxtafoveal telangiectasis. Am J Ophthalmol. 1990; 109(5):604–605
[62] Patel B, Duvall J, Tullo AB. Lamellar macular hole associated with idiopathic juxtafoveolar telangiectasia. Br J Ophthalmol. 1988; 72(7):550–551
[63] Wong WT, Forooghian F, Majumdar Z, et al. Fundus autofluorescence in type 2 macular telangiectasia: correlation with optical coherence tomography and microperimetry. Am J Ophthalmol. 2009; 148:573–583
[64] Wolff B, Basdekidou C, Vasseur V, et al. "En Face" optical coherence tomography imaging in type 2 idiopathic macular telangiectasia. Retina. 2014; 34:2072–2078
[65] Minnella AM, Yannuzzi LA, Slakter JS, Rodriquez A. Bilateral perifoveal ischemia associated with chronic granulocytic leukemia. Case report. Arch Ophthalmol. 1988; 106(9):1170–1171
[66] Millay RH, Klein ML, Handelman IL, Watzke RC. Abnormal glucose metabolism and parafoveal telangiectasia. Am J Ophthalmol. 1986; 102(3):363–370
[67] Green WR, Quigley HA, De la Cruz Z, Cohen B. Parafoveal retinal telangiectasis. Light and electron microscopy studies. Trans Ophthalmol Soc U K. 1980; 100(Pt 1):162–170
[68] Chopdar A. Retinal telangiectasis in adults: fluorescein angiographic findings and treatment by argon laser. Br J Ophthalmol. 1978; 62(4):243–250
[69] Kovach JL, Rosenfeld PJ. Bevacizumab (avastin) therapy for idiopathic macular telangiectasia type II. Retina. 2009; 29(1):27–32
[70] Elliot AJ, Harris GS. The present status of the diagnosis and treatment of periphlebitis retinae (Eales' disease). Can J Ophthalmol. 1969; 4(2):117–122
[71] Murphy RP, Renie WA, Proctor LR, et al. A survey of patients with Eales' disease. In: Fine SL, Owens SL, eds. Management of Retinal Vascular and Macular Disorders. Baltimore, MD: Williams & Wilkins; 1983
[72] Elliot AJ. 30-year observation of patients with Eale's disease. Am J Ophthalmol. 1975; 80(3, Pt 1):404–408
[73] Spitznas M, Meyer-Schwickerath G, Stephan B. The clinical picture of Eales' disease. Albrecht Von Graefes Arch Klin Exp Ophthalmol. 1975; 194(2):73–85
[74] Misra UK, Jha S, Kalita J, Sharma K. Stroke—a rare presentation of Eales' disease. A case report. Angiology. 1996; 47(1):73–76
[75] Renie WA, Murphy RP, Anderson KC, et al. The evaluation of patients with Eales' disease. Retina. 1983; 3(4):243–248
[76] Gass JD, Little H. Bilateral bullous exudative retinal detachment complicating idiopathic central serous chorioretinopathy during systemic corticosteroid therapy. Ophthalmology. 1995; 102(5):737–747
[77] Meyer-Schwickerath G. Eales' disease: treatment with light photocoagulation. Mod Probl Ophthalmol. 1966; 4:10–18
[78] Green WR. Retinal ischemia: vascular and circulatory conditions and diseases. In: Spencer WH, ed. Ophthalmic Pathology. Philadelphia, PA: WB Saunders; 1985
[79] Robertson DM. Macroaneurysms of the retinal arteries. Trans Am Acad Ophthalmol Otolaryngol. 1973; 77(1):OP55–OP67
[80] Gass JDM. Stereoscopic Atlas of Macular Diseases: Diagnosis and Treatment. 4th ed. St. Louis, MO: Mosby-Year Book; 1997:472–476
[81] Panton RW, Goldberg MF, Farber MD. Retinal arterial macroaneurysms: risk factors and natural history. Br J Ophthalmol. 1990; 74(10):595–600
[82] Chang TS, Aylward GW, Davis JL, et al. Idiopathic retinal vasculitis, aneurysms, and neuro-retinitis. Retinal Vasculitis Study. Ophthalmology. 1995; 102(7):1089–1097
[83] Perry HD, Zimerman LE, Benson WE. Hemorrhage from isolated aneurysm of a retinal artery: report of two cases simulating malignant melanoma. Arch Ophthalmol. 1977; 95(2):281–283
[84] Fichte C, Streeten BW, Friedman AH. A histopathologic study of retinal arterial aneurysms. Am J Ophthalmol. 1978; 85(4):509–518
[85] Gold DH, La Piana F, Zimmerman LE. Isolated retinal arterial aneurysms. Am J Ophthalmol. 1976; 82(6):848–857
[86] Pichi F, Morara M, Torrazza C, et al. Intravitreal bevacizumab for macular complications from retinal arterial macroaneurysms. Am J Ophthalmol. 2013; 155(2):287–294.e1
[87] Cho HJ, Rhee TK, Kim HS, et al. Intravitreal bevacizumab for symptomatic retinal arterial macroaneurysm. Am J Ophthalmol. 2013; 155(5):898–904
[88] Peyman GA, Nelson NC, Jr, Alturki W, et al. Tissue plasminogen activating factor assisted removal of subretinal hemorrhage. Ophthalmic Surg. 1991; 22(10):575–582
[89] Moriarty AP, McAllister IL, Constable IJ. Initial clinical experience with tissue plasminogen activator (tPA) assisted removal of submacular haemorrhage. Eye (Lond). 1995; 9(Pt 5):582–588

[90] Tassignon MJ, Stempels N, Van Mulders L. Retrohyaloid premacular hemorrhage treated by Q-switched Nd-YAG laser. A case report. Graefes Arch Clin Exp Ophthalmol. 1989; 227(5):440–442
[91] Gold D, Feiner L, Henkind P. Retinal arterial occlusive disease in systemic lupus erythematosus. Arch Ophthalmol. 1977; 95(9):1580–1585
[92] Lanham JG, Barrie T, Kohner EM, Hughes GRV. SLE retinopathy: evaluation by fluorescein angiography. Ann Rheum Dis. 1982; 41(5):473–478
[93] Jabs DA, Hanneken AM, Schachat AP, Fine SL. Choroidopathy in systemic lupus erythematosus. Arch Ophthalmol. 1988; 106(2):230–234
[94] Kleiner RC, Najarian LV, Schatten S, Jabs DA, Patz A, Kaplan HJ. Vaso-occlusive retinopathy associated with antiphospholipid antibodies (lupus anticoagulant retinopathy). Ophthalmology. 1989; 96(6):896–904
[95] Ashton N, Coomes EN, Garner A, Oliver DO. Retinopathy due to progressive systemic sclerosis. J Pathol Bacteriol. 1968; 96(2):259–268
[96] Bullen CL, Liesegang TJ, McDonald TJ, DeRemee RA. Ocular complications of Wegener's granulomatosis. Ophthalmology. 1983; 90(3):279–290
[97] Vine AK. Severe periphlebitis, peripheral retinal ischemia, and preretinal neovascularization in patients with multiple sclerosis. Am J Ophthalmol. 1992; 113(1):28–32
[98] Duane TD. Valsalva hemorrhagic retinopathy. Trans Am Ophthalmol Soc. 1972; 70:298–313
[99] Szelog JT, Lally DR, Heier JS. Natural history of Valsalva-induced subhyaloid hemorrhage. JAMA Ophthalmol. 2015; 133(2):e143268
[100] García Fernández M, Navarro JC, Castaño CG. Long-term evolution of Valsalva retinopathy: a case series. J Med Case Reports. 2012; 6:346
[101] Shukla D, Naresh KB, Kim R. Optical coherence tomography findings in Valsalva retinopathy. Am J Ophthalmol. 2005; 140(1):134–136
[102] Weiss KD, Kuriyan AE, Flynn HW, Jr. Central retinal vein occlusion after prolonged vomiting and repeated valsalva maneuvers associated with gastroenteritis and dehydration. Ophthalmic Surg Lasers Imaging Retina. 2014; 45 Online:e23–e25
[103] Xie ZG, Yu SQ, Chen X, Zhu J, Chen F. Macular hole secondary to Valsalva retinopathy after doing push-up exercise. BMC Ophthalmol. 2014; 14(98):98
[104] Deane JS, Ziakas N. Valsalva retinopathy in pregnancy. Eye (Lond). 1997; 11 (Pt 1):137–138
[105] Ladjimi A, Zaouali S, Messaoud R, et al. Valsalva retinopathy induced by labour. Eur J Ophthalmol. 2002; 12(4):336–338
[106] Hassan M, Tajunisah I. Valsalva haemorrhagic retinopathy after push-ups. Lancet. 2011; 377(9764):504
[107] Al Rubaie K, Arevalo JF. Valsalva retinopathy associated with sexual activity. Case Rep Med. 2014; 2014:524286
[108] Oboh AM, Weilke F, Sheindlin J. Valsalva retinopathy as a complication of colonoscopy. J Clin Gastroenterol. 2004; 38(9):793–794
[109] Park JH, Sagong M, Chang W. Valsalva retinopathy following esophagogastroduodenoscopy under propofol sedation: a case report. World J Gastroenterol. 2014; 20(11):3056–3058
[110] Kim JY, Lee DH, Lee JH, Yoon IeN. Valsalva retinopathy associated with an oratorical contest. Korean J Ophthalmol. 2009; 23(4):318–320
[111] Raymond LA. Neodymium:YAG laser treatment for hemorrhages under the internal limiting membrane and posterior hyaloid face in the macula. Ophthalmology. 1995; 102(3):406–411
[112] Konotey-Ahulu F. Valsalva vitreous haemorrhage and retinopathy in sickle cell haemoglobin C disease. Lancet. 1997; 349(9067):1774
[113] Sabella P, Bottoni F, Staurenghi G. Spectral-domain OCT evaluation of Nd: YAG laser treatment for Valsalva retinopathy. Graefes Arch Clin Exp Ophthalmol. 2010; 248(4):599–601
[114] Bourne RA, Talks SJ, Richards AB. Treatment of preretinal Valsalva haemorrhages with neodymium:YAG laser. Eye (Lond). 1999; 13(Pt 6):791–793
[115] Goel N, Kumar V, Seth A, Raina UK, Ghosh B. Spectral-domain optical coherence tomography following Nd:YAG laser membranotomy in valsalva retinopathy. Ophthalmic Surg Lasers Imaging. 2011; 42(3):222–228
[116] Durukan AH, Kerimoglu H, Erdurman C, Demirel A, Karagul S. Long-term results of Nd:YAG laser treatment for premacular subhyaloid haemorrhage owing to Valsalva retinopathy. Eye (Lond). 2008; 22(2):214–218
[117] De Maeyer K, Van Ginderdeuren R, Postelmans L, Stalmans P, Van Calster J. Sub-inner limiting membrane haemorrhage: causes and treatment with vitrectomy. Br J Ophthalmol. 2007; 91(7):869–872

14 Age-Related Macular Degeneration

Ashleigh L. Levison, Paula E. Pecen, and Peter K. Kaiser

14.1 Introduction

Age-related macular degeneration (AMD) is a chronic, progressive disease of the macula, and it is the leading cause of severe irreversible central vision loss and legal blindness in individuals 65 years of age or older in the United States and in other Western countries.[1,2,3,4,5,6] A meta-analysis reported that, in Caucasians aged 40 years and older, the prevalence of early AMD was 6.8%, and the prevalence of late AMD was 1.5%, with prevalence increasing with patient age.[7] Overall, AMD is estimated to affect more than 8 million people in the United States, with advanced AMD affecting 1.75 million individuals.[6]

Special Considerations

- AMD is the leading cause of irreversible central vision loss in people older than 65 years in the United States.

AMD is classified into two well-defined clinical forms. The more common form is non-neovascular AMD (non-NVAMD), also known as "dry" or "nonexudative" AMD.[8,9] The second form is NVAMD, also referred to as "wet" or "exudative" AMD. Differentiating dry versus wet disease has important implications for both prognosis and treatment. Findings of non-NVAMD include abnormalities of the retinal pigment epithelium (RPE) and drusen. Early dry AMD is associated with minimal visual acuity loss; however, it may progress to late dry AMD, otherwise referred to as geographic atrophy, where there is loss of the RPE. Late dry AMD accounts for nearly 20% of legal blindness related to AMD.[9,10] NVAMD is defined by the appearance of choroidal neovascularization (CNV) and can be associated with severe vision loss with subsequent subretinal fibrosis or disciform scarring if left untreated. While CNV occurs in 10 to 15% of all patients with AMD, it accounts for more than 80% of cases of severe central vision loss associated with AMD.[11]

In the past two decades, significant advancements have been made in the diagnosis of AMD, especially the development of optical coherence tomography (OCT). Historically, clinical biomicroscopy with a contact lens and imaging in the form of fluorescein angiography were used for the evaluation of CNV; however, current OCT scanners are able to provide rapid, noninvasive cross-sectional images of the retina and even choroid, rendering contact lens examinations nearly obsolete. With the evolution of technology from time domain to spectral domain and now swept-source OCT, physicians are able to obtain progressively higher resolution OCT images, which provide detailed information about the pathological changes in AMD.[12]

Prior to 2004, treatment options for exudative AMD included laser photocoagulation, verteporfin (Visudyne, Valeant) in photodynamic therapy (PDT), submacular surgery, and macular translocation. Unfortunately, these therapies had minimal success in maintaining vision, and most patients experienced progressive vision loss. In 2004, the treatment of exudative AMD was revolutionized by the advent of anti–vascular endothelial growth factor (anti-VEGF) therapy. Instead of preventing vision loss, the prognosis of exudative AMD was redefined, with the potential to improve vision, and in most cases preserve vision.[9]

This chapter reviews the current knowledge of AMD, critical to understanding present management and potential future treatment strategies.

14.2 Non-Neovascular Age-Related Macular Degeneration

14.2.1 Clinical Features

The features of non-NVAMD include drusen (singular, "druse"), areas of increased pigmentation or hyperpigmentation in the outer retina associated with drusen, and areas of depigmentation or hypopigmentation of the RPE. The later stages of dry AMD may include geographic and nongeographic areas of RPE atrophy. All of these features are termed "non-neovascular," as they do not involve manifestations associated with the growth of CNV (a feature of the late stage of AMD), discussed in the second section of this chapter.[10]

Drusen

The pathogenesis of early AMD is characterized by thickening of Bruch's membrane due to lipid and protein accumulation, leading to the formation of sub-RPE deposits referred to as "drusen."[10] Drusen appear as yellowish white lesions at the level of the RPE and can appear clinically in various shapes and sizes. The size of drusen can be classified as small (< 63 µm), intermediate (63–125 µm), or large (> 125 µm).[13,14] Drusen are then further described by their appearance as either "hard" or "soft." If a significant number of drusen coalesce, they are described as "confluent."[6,10]

Drusen are composed of lectin binding saccharides, including mannose, glucosamines, galactose, and sialic acid. Lectins are glycoproteins that can bind reversibly to specific saccharide sequences. Multiple proteins are present in drusen including amyloid P component, apolipoprotein E, immunoglobulins, and complement.[15,16] In addition, drusen contain molecules associated with both humoral and cellular immunity.[15,16] Hard drusen are typically small (< 63 µm) and have well-defined borders (▶ Fig. 14.1). The presence of at least one small druse in the macula is nearly ubiquitous and is not believed to be associated with an increased risk of the development of vision loss from geographic atrophy or the neovascular form of AMD.[3,17,18] On fluorescein angiography, hard drusen may show hyperfluorescence during the early transit phase as underlying choroidal fluorescence shows through the tiny "window defects" created by the drusen. This fluorescence fades as the choroidal fluorescence fades in the late-phase frames.

Soft drusen are defined as having a greatest linear dimension of more than 63 µm and borders without sharp edges (▶ Fig. 14.2). Soft drusen are believed to be a hallmark of AMD. Development of CNV and geographic atrophy of the RPE appear to be more frequently associated with soft drusen than with

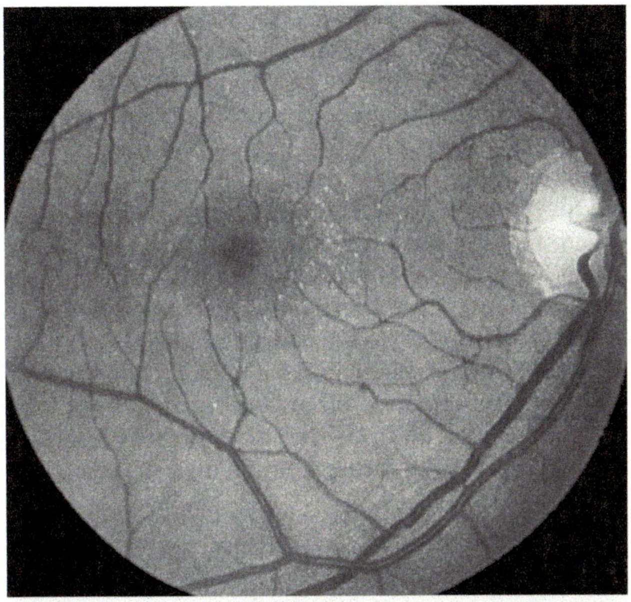

Fig. 14.1 Hard drusen. This fundus photograph demonstrates hard drusen: small, round, discrete yellowish-white deposits. Reproduced with permission by Elsevier from Bressler et al.[61]

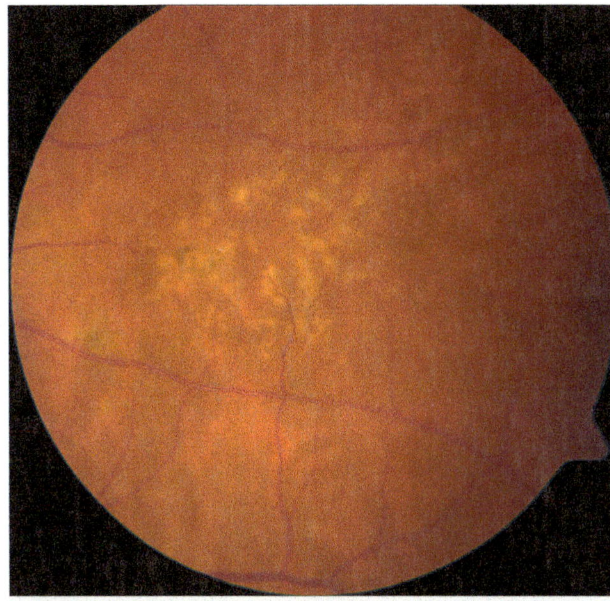

Fig. 14.2 Soft drusen. This fundus photograph demonstrates soft drusen, which are larger than hard drusen and have nondiscrete borders. Soft drusen are more highly associated with development of choroidal neovascularization than hard drusen.

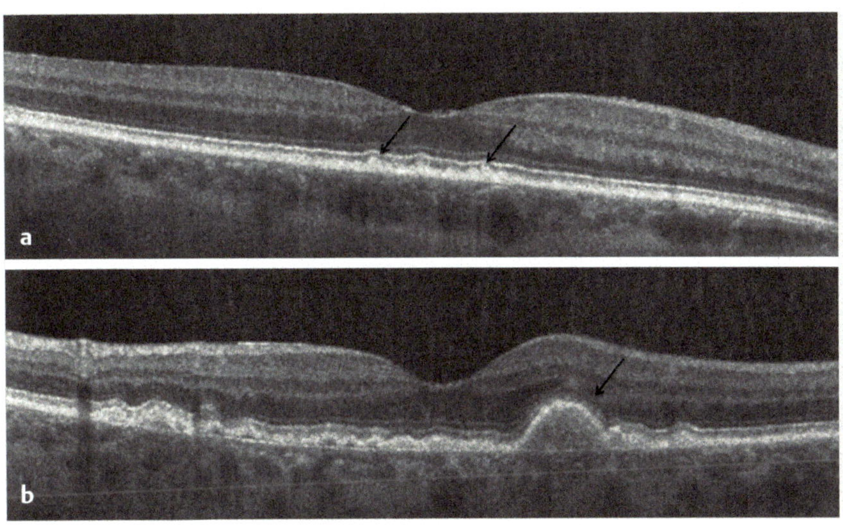

Fig. 14.3 Optical coherence tomography (OCT) images of drusen. (**a**) Small drusen are demonstrated by the arrows. They appear as hyperreflective material under the retinal pigment epithelium. (**b**) The arrow points to a large drusenoid pigment epithelial detachment (PED). Drusenoid PEDs do not indicate the presence of choroidal neovascularization.

hard drusen alone.[14,18,19,20,21,22] Angiographically, soft drusen may exhibit hypo- or hyperfluorescence. Some investigators have suggested that the intensity of staining may be due to variable polarity of the drusen components.[23] Alternatively, the variability in fluorescence may be due to the degree of pigment epithelial detachment (PED), allowing fluorescein to pool or variability in the degree of overlying RPE depigmentation which allows for more or less transmission of underlying fluorescence.

On spectral domain OCT (SD-OCT), small and intermediate drusen can be seen as discrete areas of RPE elevation with variable reflectivity underlying the RPE (▶ Fig. 14.3a). Drusen can be associated with changes in the overlying outer retina, specifically with evidence of disruption of the outer segment (OS) ellipsoid zone (previously known as the inner segment/outer segment junction zone).[12]

Pearls

- CNV appears to be more frequently associated with soft drusen than with hard drusen alone.

Drusen larger than 125 µm have greater clinical significance than smaller drusen and are typically described as soft in appearance. Larger drusen may become confluent and evolve into drusenoid RPE detachments.[6] On OCT, larger drusen or drusenoid pigment epithelium detachments (PEDs) create RPE elevations that are often dome shaped, with a hypo- or medium-reflective material between the RPE and underlying Bruch's membrane (▶ Fig. 14.3b).[12] On fluorescein angiography, a drusenoid PED fluoresces faintly during the early transit

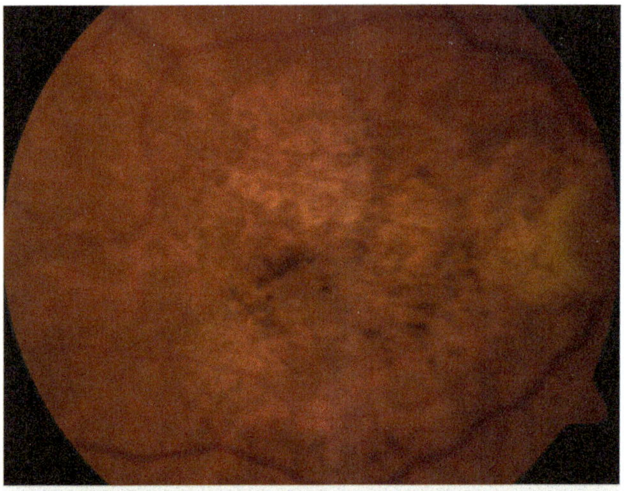

Fig. 14.4 Retinal pigment epithelial (RPE) hyperplasia. The photograph shows multiple areas of RPE hyperplasia as well as areas of RPE atrophy. RPE hyperplasia is a common clinical finding seen in age-related macular degeneration.

phase and does not progress to bright hyperfluorescence in late frames. Reticulated pigment clumping is frequently seen overlying the detachment.

In AMD, there are significant morphological changes at the level of the RPE in addition to the presence of drusen. There are two variations of sub-RPE deposits, also referred to as basal deposits, which are separated by the RPE basement membrane. "Basal laminar deposits" refer to a layer of abnormal basement membrane material on the inner aspect of the RPE basement membrane. "Basal linear deposits" are formed by a layer of membranous debris on the external aspect of the RPE basement membrane and lie within the inner collagenous zone of Bruch's membrane.[6]

Abnormalities of the Retinal Pigment Epithelium

Focal hyperpigmentation seen clinically corresponds to clumps of pigmented cells at the level of the RPE or pigment that has migrated to the level of the photoreceptor nuclei in the outer retina (▸ Fig. 14.4).[20,24] On OCT, pigment clumping and migration can be seen as focal areas of hyperreflectivity. These areas are often seen in the outer nuclear layer or near areas of the RPE overlying drusen.[12] It has been shown that the presence of focal pigment clumping correlates with an increased risk of developing CNV or atrophy of the RPE.[19,25,26]

Pearls

- The presence of focal pigment clumping correlates with an increased risk of developing CNV or geographic atrophy.

Geographic Atrophy

Atrophic abnormalities of the RPE may be another manifestation of AMD. With atrophy of the RPE, the overlying outer layers of the retina and the underlying choriocapillaris may also deteriorate and become atrophic. "Geographic atrophy" is an area of retina that is sharply demarcated with loss of the underlying RPE and is usually initially located extrafoveally. This atrophy allows for increased visualization of the underlying choroidal vessels (▸ Fig. 14.5a).[27] The fovea itself is typically spared until late in the course of the disease. Before geographic atrophy involves the fovea, vision is limited by the size of the functioning fovea so that only a portion of a word or an image may be perceived. As geographic atrophy extends into the fovea, patients will experience severe vision loss.[27] Vision loss in geographic atrophy is usually perceived by the patient to be gradual, even when central fixation is involved.[20]

OCT is able to successfully identify areas of geographic atrophy visualized as loss of the RPE and the overlying photoreceptors, leading to retinal thinning in the region of geographic atrophy (▸ Fig. 14.5b). There is choroidal hyperreflectivity due to thinning of the overlying retina and RPE.[12] At the edges of the geographic atrophy, the external limiting membrane (ELM) and OS ellipsoid zone may be abnormal and taper off. This abnormality at the borders of retinal thinning suggests that there is photoreceptor loss beyond the margins of the geographic atrophy. OCT offers a mechanism to objectively quantify and follow geographic atrophy over time.[12]

Fundus autofluorescence (FAF) is another important imaging modality for identifying and monitoring progression of geographic atrophy. Normally, RPE cells have natural autofluorescence due to the accumulation of lipofuscin. The loss of RPE autofluorescence represents disruption of the RPE–photoreceptor complex, likely due to the death of photoreceptor cells and/or RPE cells. Thus, areas of geographic atrophy appear as discrete hypoautofluorescent lesions. There are various patterns seen on FAF imaging in patients with geographic atrophy, suggesting multiple different phenotypes of geographic atrophy.[28] Comparison of OCT and FAF images in patients with geographic atrophy shows that loss of FAF signal correlates with changes in reflectivity of the choriocapillaris on OCT images (▸ Fig. 14.6).[27] Similar to OCT, FAF can be used to monitor for progression of GA over time.

14.2.2 Differential Diagnosis

Several other maculopathies have features that resemble AMD but have distinctly different etiologies. The need to recognize and differentiate them from AMD is paramount, as prognosis and treatment may vary greatly from that of AMD.

Reticular Pseudodrusen

Reticular pseudodrusen form a yellowish interlacing network about 250 µm in diameter that resembles soft, confluent drusen. These pseudodrusen typically present first in the outer macula, but can then develop more peripherally. They are best identified on red-free imaging and do not fluoresce on fluorescein angiography. Clinically, pseudodrusen can appear similar to soft confluent drusen, but can be easily distinguished from drusen on SD-OCT. On SD-OCT, the deposits are seen above the RPE, which is distinctly different from the sub-RPE space in which drusen are found.[29,30] When evaluated histologically, reticular pseudodrusen have a similar composition to that of

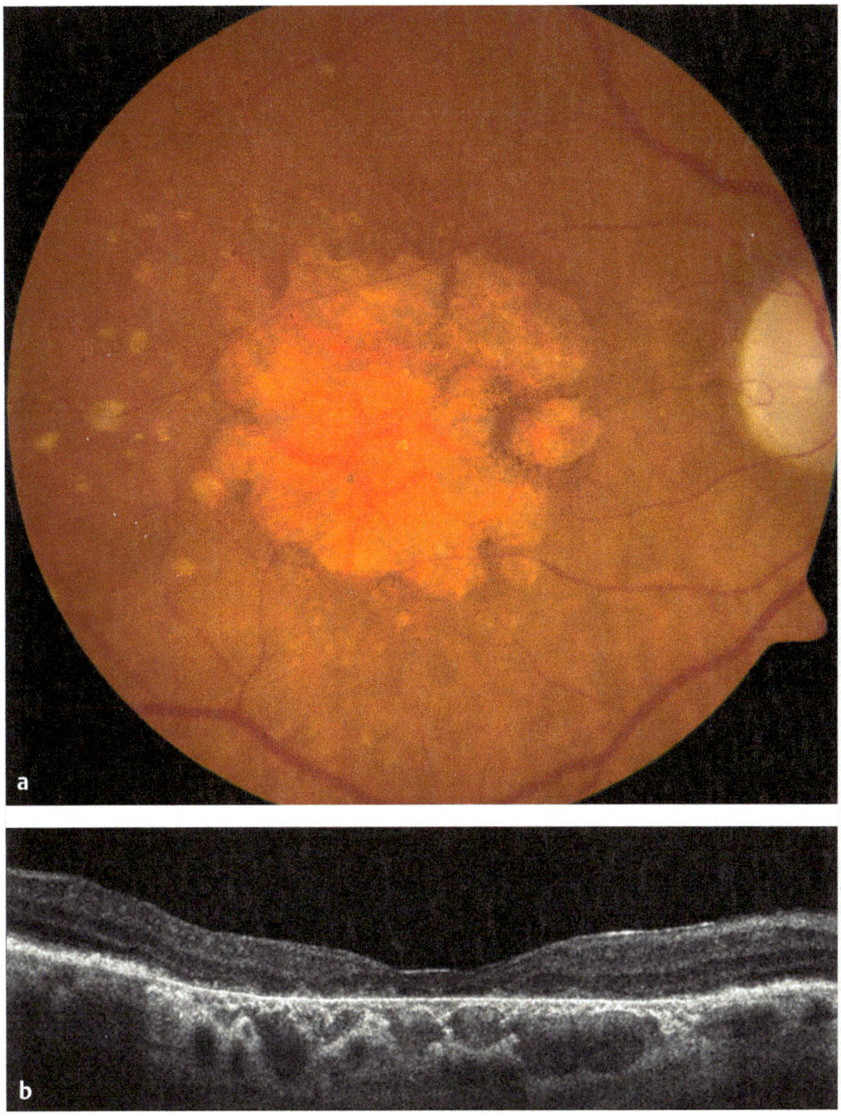

Fig. 14.5 Geographic atrophy. (a) This fundus photograph shows a large area of geographic atrophy. There is loss of the outer retina with RPE atrophy. Corresponding to this atrophy is the increased ability to see the underlying choroidal vessels. (b) This is an OCT image of a different patient with central geographic atrophy. There is atrophy of the outer retina with loss of the ellipsoid zone.

soft drusen.[31] The risk of progression to late AMD is much lower with reticular pseudodrusen than with soft drusen.[6]

Basal Laminar Drusen (Cuticular Drusen)

Basal laminar drusen, also known as "cuticular drusen," are multiple, small, discrete, round, yellow sub-RPE lesions (▶ Fig. 14.7a). The clinical term "basal laminar drusen" should not be confused with the histopathological terms "basal laminar deposits" and "basal linear deposits" (defined in subsection "Drusen").[24] On OCT, cuticular drusen cause a saw-tooth elevation of the RPE with some disruption of the OS ellipsoid zone and ELM. On fluorescein angiography, cuticular drusen demonstrate early hyperfluorescence, creating a "starry night" appearance that fades in the later phase frames (▶ Fig. 14.7b). Historically, basal laminar drusen were thought to be secondary to thickening of the RPE; however, it is now thought that, histopathologically, they are unlikely different from drusen.[12,32] Eyes that have cuticular drusen can form a pseudovitelliform macular detachment. The natural course of these pseudovitelliform lesions may be progressive collapse with the development of marked geographic atrophy or clearing with minimal atrophy. Nevertheless, patients with basal laminar drusen are at risk for developing CNV and any suggestion of CNV on OCT or fluorescein angiography should be considered for treatment.

Pattern Dystrophy

Pattern dystrophies are a heterogenous group of disorders characterized by bilateral, symmetric pigmentary disturbance of the central macula, with an onset in midlife and usually mild reductions in visual acuity. Inheritance of most of these appears to be autosomal dominant and the prognosis for retention of useful vision into late adulthood appears to be good. Clinically, various patterns of yellow-orange lesions that appear at the level of the RPE have been described. They are usually bilateral and located in the central macula (▶ Fig. 14.8). Occasionally, they can be unilateral or eccentric. The best known of these patterns includes adult-onset foveomacular pigment epithelial dystrophy, butterfly-shaped pigment dystrophy, and reticular pigment dystrophy. Differentiation among them may be difficult because the same dystrophy may have variable phenotypic expression within a family.[33,34]

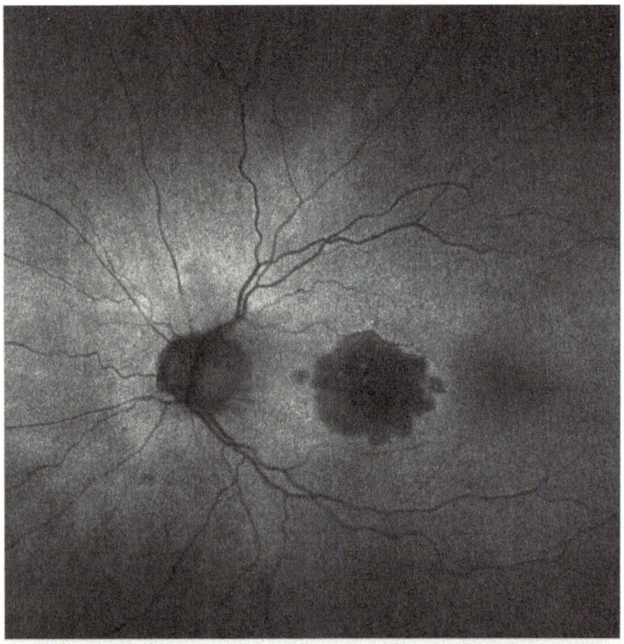

Fig. 14.6 Geographic atrophy on fundus autofluorescence. There is marked hypofluorescence in the area corresponding to geographic atrophy on examination. There is atrophy and, therefore, loss of lipofuscin. The loss of lipofuscin leads to loss of hyperfluorescence in the macula.

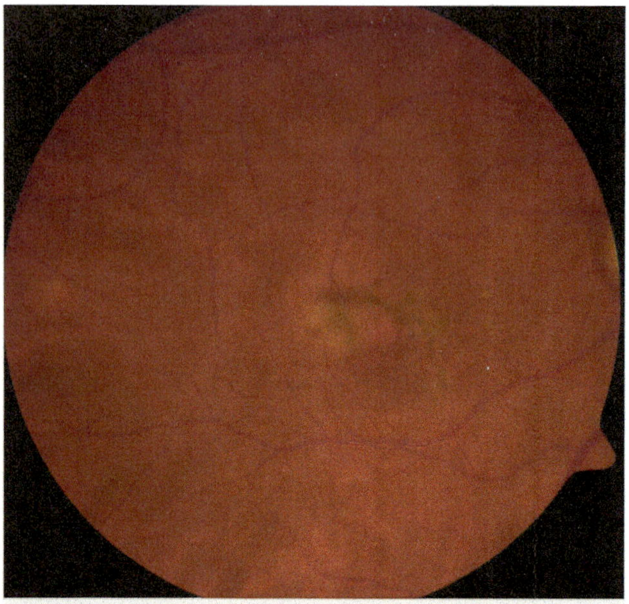

Fig. 14.8 Pattern dystrophy with a vitelliform lesion. In pattern dystrophies, yellow, orange, and gray lesions along with reticulated pigment clumping are present at the level of the retinal pigment epithelium. It is important not to mistake this lesion for age-related macular degeneration as choroidal neovascularization occurs less commonly in association with pattern dystrophies than with age-related macular degeneration.

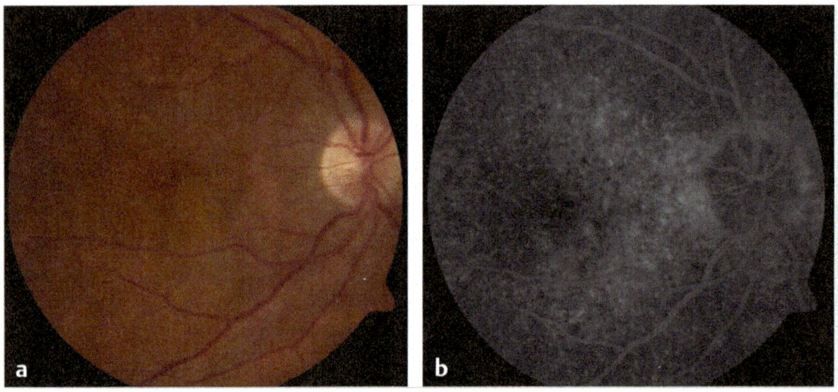

Fig. 14.7 Cuticular drusen. **(a)** The fundus photograph shows many small discrete round yellow basal laminar drusen, also referred to as cuticular drusen. **(b)** On fluorescein angiography, the cuticular drusen have a "starry night" appearance.

Ophthalmoscopic clues that suggest a macular dystrophy rather than AMD are the absence of typical soft drusen as well as a difference in the character of the pigmentation, which is deep to the retina, gray-greenish in appearance, and often reticular with a macular dystrophy. The pigmentation is sometimes best appreciated on transillumination, as direct illumination may reveal only subtle changes. The "pattern" may also be highlighted on fluorescein angiography with blockage of fluorescence by the pigment and hyperfluorescence surrounding the pigment. Clinicopathologic correlation demonstrates a thick layer of periodic acid–Schiff (PAS) positive material between an atrophic RPE and Bruch's membrane, with large pigmented cells filled with lipofuscin and extracellular pigment superficial to Bruch's membrane. Like basal laminar drusen, these disorders may be associated with a vitelliform lesion that mimics CNV in its fluorescent pattern on angiography. Again, it is important to differentiate this vitelliform lesion from CNV, given the former does not need treatment, while CNV generally requires treatment.[35]

14.2.3 Management and Course

Severe vision loss in AMD results from fovea-involving atrophy or complications of CNV. With the development of anti-VEGF agents, severe vision loss associated with CNV has been significantly reduced especially with early intervention. The main predictor of visual acuity outcome following anti-VEGF treatment is the visual acuity at the time of initiation of treatment; therefore, early detection and prompt initiation of treatment are essential.

Given the infrequency of clinical examination, it is important for patients with dry AMD to perform self-monitoring. Ideally, the patient with non-NVAMD should perform monocular checks of vision to detect metamorphopsia or scotomas on a daily basis using an Amsler grid. Upon detecting new visual symptoms, patients should present promptly for examination.

Development of CNV can often be asymptomatic; therefore, it is recommended that patients with non-NVAMD be examined every 6 to 12 months, perhaps even more often for patients at higher risk for conversion from dry to wet AMD. Some retinal specialists monitor dry AMD patients with OCT images to ensure detection of early exudation. If there is evidence of neovascular abnormalities such as intraretinal fluid, subretinal fluid, or hemorrhage on clinical examination or OCT, then fluorescein angiography may be indicated.

Recently, advances have been made in computerized home monitoring systems to detect development and progression of AMD. The Home Monitoring of Eye (HOME) study recruited participants, aged 55 to 90 years, at significant risk of developing NVAMD. The patients had either bilateral large drusen or large drusen in one eye in addition to advanced AMD in the other eye. This was an unmasked, multicenter, randomized trial comparing the ForeseeHome (Notal Vision) device in addition to standard of care alone. Standard[36] care consists of instructions provided specifically from each investigator for self-monitoring, including use of Amsler grids. The ForeseeHome device uses preferential hyperacuity perimetry and telemonitoring to detect changes in visual function associated with development of CNV due to AMD.[36] The study found that participants at risk of development of CNV benefited from the home monitoring strategy for earlier detection. Those patients in the device arm had a 5-day median time of alerts or symptoms to examination, whereas those patients in the standard care arm had a median time to examination of 7.5 days. During the study period, 82 patients progressed to CNV. Of those, 51 were detected in the device arm, while only 31 were detected in the standard care arm. The device arm also had significantly better mean visual acuity at the time of CNV diagnosis compared to the standard care arm. Early detection increases the likelihood of better visual acuity results with intravitreal anti-VEGF therapy.[36]

Pearls

- With the goal of detecting CNV as early as possible, patients with AMD should perform monocular checks of vision for metamorphopsia or scotoma using an Amsler grid on a daily basis.

14.2.4 Risk Factors for Progression to Late Age-Related Macular Degeneration

Several genetic and nongenetic risk factors for AMD have been identified. Some of these risk factors are modifiable, while others are not. Antioxidant and mineral supplementations have been demonstrated to lower the risk of conversion from nonexudative to exudative AMD.

Genetic Risk of Age-Related Macular Degeneration

Several genes have been identified as risk factors for development of AMD. Patients with specific single-nucleotide polymorphisms (SNPs) in the complement factor H region (CFH) and age-related maculopathy susceptibility protein 2 (ARMS2) genes have been shown to have higher association with geographic atrophy and exudative AMD than with early AMD.[37,38] In 2005, a strong association between AMD and CFH was identified.[39] This association has been confirmed in multiple ethnic groups around the world. Complement factor H is a serum glycoprotein that serves as a natural inhibitor of complement factor 3 (C3) convertase and blocks the activation of the alternative complement pathway in normal cells. Identification of susceptibility genes associated with the complement pathway confirms the hypothesis that inflammatory pathways play an important role in the pathogenesis of AMD.[9,39]

In addition to the inflammatory pathway, it is believed that oxidative stress also plays a strong role in AMD progression. Certain genetic mutations that predispose patients to oxidative cellular injury likely have an important role in AMD predisposition. The exact function of ARMS2 is not yet known; however, the protein was originally found in the outer membrane of mitochondria. Mitochondria help control oxidative stress via their role in oxidative phosphorylation in the retina.[9]

The Beaver Dam Eye Study found that the estimated population-attributable risk fraction, when at least one CFH risk allele was present, was 9.6 and 53.2% for early and late AMD, respectively. When at least one ARMS2 risk allele was present, that risk was 5.0 and 43.0%, respectively.[37]

Besides CFH and ARMS2, a meta-analysis evaluating 14 case–control studies regarding the HTRA1 promoter polymorphism identified an important association with AMD. Because the HRTA1 promoter is close to the ARMS2 gene, it is possible that both together influence AMD susceptibility.[9] Multiple other genes have been studied and are being currently investigated for their association with AMD, but their role is not felt to be as strong as CFH and ARMS2.[39]

Genetic testing has now become commercially available for patients with AMD, but it has not been widely adopted into clinical practice. A recent publication has suggested that those patients with certain genetic makeups may have a differential response to AREDS supplementation, and in some cases may in fact have poorer outcomes with standard AREDS formulations.[40,41] However, this is controversial[40,42] and, to date, no other investigators have found a similar link. As more information becomes available, there may be increased interest in genetic testing of AMD.

Nongenetic Risk Factors for Development of Age-Related Macular Degeneration

A meta-analysis was published in 2010 that evaluated 45 studies looking at 16 risk factors that were felt to be associated with development of advanced AMD. Of the 16 risk factors identified in this systematic review and meta-analysis, age, smoking, cataract surgery, and family history were strongly and consistently associated with late AMD.[43] Most studies have shown no difference between male and female genders for risk of development of AMD; however, at the 10-year follow-up from the original AREDS study, female gender was identified as a risk for progression to NVAMD.[44]

The largest modifiable risk factor for AMD is smoking. Jonasson and colleagues showed that of 2,196 patients who smoked and were without evidence of AMD at baseline examination, 14.9% developed AMD. The odds ratio (OR) of developing AMD in a current smoker was 2.07, while it was 1.36 for former smokers.[1] The Beaver Dam Eye Study also confirmed that smoking is associated with an increased risk of progression of minimal to moderate early AMD, as well as from severe early to late AMD.[45] Many other studies have also validated this association.[39,46,47]

Besides smoking, other systemic risk factors including cardiovascular disease, hypertension, and obesity have been associated with increased risk of developing late AMD. Some systemic risk factors have stronger evidence than others.[39,48,49] Pooled data in a meta-analysis showed a statistically significant increased risk for those with cardiovascular disease and hypertension.[43]

There has been a question as to the role of ultraviolet (UV) light exposure in AMD. UV light exposure is thought to possibly contribute to the development of AMD by producing reactive oxygen species and free radicals in the outer retina. The hypothesis of phototoxicity being associated with AMD development is based on experimental and animal studies. Some studies have found an association while others have not. Currently, large epidemiological studies have not shown convincing evidence of the association of UV light and AMD.[39,50,51,52]

Some studies have reported evidence that cataract surgery is associated with progression of AMD. In 2003, a study was published that showed that exudative AMD or geographic atrophy developed in 6 to 7% of pseudophakic patients, but in only 0.7% of phakic patients.[53] The AREDS study, however, did not find any clear association between cataract surgery and the risk of progression of AMD.[5]

Modifying Risk for Progression of Age-Related Macular Degeneration

Various studies from the 1980s and 1990s suggested a role of antioxidant status and zinc levels with the risk of AMD.[10,54,55,56] Since those studies were published, two large, randomized, controlled trials have shown the benefit of vitamin and mineral supplementation in the prevention of progression to advanced AMD. The first was the Age-Related Eye Disease Study (AREDS), which enrolled 4,575 patients into four different categories based on size and extent of drusen, RPE abnormalities in each eye, the presence of advanced AMD in the fellow eye, and visual acuity.[5]

Those with category 1 disease had fewer than 5 small (< 63 µm) drusen and had good visual acuity of 20/32 or better in both eyes. Patients with category 2 disease had multiple small drusen, at least one intermediate druse (63–124 µm), and/or pigment changes with vision of 20/32 or better in both eyes. Category 3 eyes had absence of advanced AMD in both eyes, one eye with at least 20/32 vision, at least one large druse (> 125 µm), significant intermediate drusen, and/or geographic atrophy outside of the center of the macula. The final group, category 4, had visual acuity of 20/32 or better, and no advanced AMD in the study eye, but the fellow eye had advanced AMD or vision less than 20/32 and AMD changes that accounted for the reduced visual acuity.[5]

Patients were randomized to take daily oral tablets with (1) antioxidants (500 mg vitamin C, 400 IU vitamin E, and 15 mg beta carotene), (2) 80 mg zinc oxide and 2 mg cupric oxide, (3) antioxidants plus zinc, or (4) placebo.[5] The AREDS demonstrated that patients with categories 3 and 4 AMD benefited from antioxidant and mineral supplementation. The risk reduction for those patients taking antioxidants and zinc together was 25%.[5] As a result of the study, the AREDS formula was recommended for all patients with category 3 or 4 AMD.

A follow-up study, AREDS2, evaluated the safety and efficacy of removing beta-carotene while adding lutein and zeaxanthin and/or omega-3 long-chain polyunsaturated fatty acid (LCPUFA) supplementation to the original AREDS formulation to reduce the risk of progressing to advanced AMD. For the primary analysis, AREDS2 enrolled 4,203 participants, ages 50 to 85 years, at 82 clinical sites across the United States. Of the 4,203 participants, 3,036 agreed to a secondary randomization, which aimed to evaluate the effect of eliminating beta-carotene and reducing the zinc level from the original AREDS formulation.[57]

Both lutein and zeaxanthin are significant components making up macular pigment; therefore, it was felt that these compounds might be of benefit in reducing risk of progression to advanced AMD. While planning the original AREDS, it was believed that lutein may have a potential benefit in reducing risk of progression; however, at the time of the first study, lutein was not commercially available.[58] The reason for removing beta-carotene from the AREDS formula stemmed from a reported increased risk of lung cancer associated with beta-carotene nutritional supplementation in smokers.[14]

In the primary analysis, the AREDS2 showed no positive or negative effect of adding lutein, zeaxanthin, omega-3 LCPUFAs, or the combination on the progression to advanced AMD compared to the original formulation. Removing beta-carotene also did not have any statistically significant effect on the progression to advanced AMD when lutein and zeaxanthin were added.[57] With regard to the comparison of 80 to 25 mg of zinc, there was not enough evidence to make a recommendation regarding ideal dose. While the primary analysis did not show an independent benefit of lutein and zeaxanthin, some secondary analyses have shown there might be some positive effect. Therefore, given all of these findings and the increased risk of lung cancer in smokers with beta-carotene supplementation, beta-carotene was removed from the AREDS2 formulation and lutein and zeaxanthin were added.

Pearls

The AREDS2 formulation includes:

- 500 mg vitamin C
- 400 IU vitamin E
- 10 mg lutein
- 2 mg zeaxanthin
- 80 mg zinc
- 2 mg cupric oxide/copper

(Note: No beta carotene or omega-3 fatty acids.)

Special Considerations

- The original AREDS formula should not be recommended for patients who smoke.

Grading Risk of Progression of Age-Related Macular Degeneration

As we have gained significant knowledge about risk factors for progression to late AMD, some investigators have tried to create models to help identify individuals at risk for progression. Some of these risk models are more complicated than others. In 2013, a large committee convened to create a new classification system of AMD. They determined risk of progression to late AMD based on two basic characteristics seen on clinical examination: if there was one or more large drusen (> 125 µm) and/or any hyperpigmented or hypopigmented abnormalities associated with drusen. For each risk factor in each eye, a risk score of 1 is associated. There is a maximum total score of 4 for a person, 2 per eye. The 5-year risk of advanced AMD is 100-fold larger between those patients with a score of 0 and those with a score of 4. The risk of progression to advanced AMD with a score of 1 is 12%, 25% for those between 2 and 3, and 50% for those between 3 and 4. These percentages are then further modified based on other systemic and external risk factors for progression of AMD. For example, the risk for progression varies based on smoking status.[44,59,60]

14.3 Neovascular Age-Related Macular Degeneration

Characterized by the growth of fibrovascular tissue from the choroidal circulation, NVAMD is the leading cause of severe vision loss in people older than 65 years in the United States and Western world. Although it accounts for only 8% of patients with late stage of AMD, it is responsible for 85% of the severe visual loss caused by AMD.[4] The vision loss is caused by the resultant subretinal fibrosis from the CNV and is irreversible.

14.3.1 Clinical Features

CNV should be suspected in anyone complaining of metamorphopsia or scotoma, especially if the person is older than 65 years and is known to have non-NVAMD.[61] Slit-lamp biomicroscopy may reveal retinal elevation from underlying fluid or blood, pigment epithelial elevation from sub-RPE fluid, blood or fibrovascular tissue, intraretinal or subretinal lipid, or cystic edema of the sensory retina overlying the CNV membrane (▸ Fig. 14.9a). Other causes of subretinal hemorrhage, such as macroaneurysms, lacquer cracks in pathologic myopia, or choroidal tumors, should be ruled out. The fundus may appear normal in spite of the presence of CNV, especially if the only sign present is subretinal fluid, which may be very subtle by ophthalmoscopy.

Fluorescein angiography is the gold standard in the diagnosis of exudative AMD to identify and characterize CNV. Early-, mid-, and late-phase frames of the macula enable determination of the CNV boundaries (well demarcated or poorly demarcated), pattern (classic or occult), and location (subfoveal or extrafoveal).

CNV may have a variety of appearances on fluorescein angiography. The basic patterns recognized are *classic* and *occult* (▸ Fig. 14.10). While these classifications are no longer used as frequently as they were in the past, prior to the use of anti-VEGF agents, they can provide some important prognostic information. *Classic* CNV is apparent on the early transit-phase frames as a bright, well-demarcated area of hyperfluorescence with significant leakage apparent in the later phase frames as the dye pools in the subretinal space and obscures the boundary of this area of hyperfluorescence. Lacy vessels, sometimes visualized in the early-phase frames, are not required for a lesion to be considered classic. In fact, this appearance is present in only a minority of the classic CNV lesions associated with AMD and may be seen in a lesion judged to have a fluorescent pattern of *occult* CNV, as both classic and occult CNV consist of new blood vessels.

The term *occult* CNV refers to two types of patterns seen in eyes with AMD-related CNV. The first pattern, termed a *fibrovascular pigment epithelial detachment* (FVPED), is best appreciated with stereoscopic views at approximately 1 to 2 minutes after dye injection; it appears as an irregular elevation of the RPE stippled with hyperfluorescent dots. Staining or leakage is evident in the late-phase frames as fluorescein collects within the fibrous tissue or pools in the subretinal space overlying the FVPED. The exact boundaries of FVPEDs can be determined only when fluorescence sharply outlines the elevated RPE. The amount of elevation is dependent on the quality of the stereophotograph and the thickness of the fibrovascular tissue. Unfortunately, the boundary of a FVPED is usually not well demarcated. The second pattern, *late leakage of an undetermined source*, refers to late choroidal-based leakage in which there is no clearly identifiable classic CNV or FVPED in the early or midphase of the angiogram to account for an area of leakage in the late phase. Often, this pattern of occult CNV can appear as speckled hyperfluorescence overlying pooling of dye in the subretinal space.

The terminology of classic and occult CNV is currently less commonly used due to the transition away from laser treatment and toward using intravitreal anti-VEGF therapy. With the increased use of OCT, a new classification scheme has been

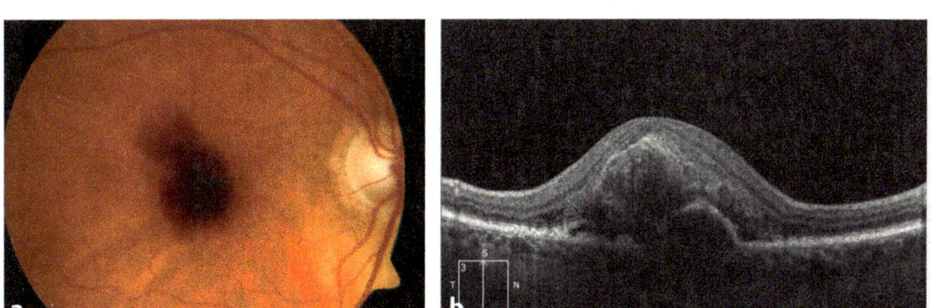

Fig. 14.9 Neovascular age-related macular degeneration. **(a)** Fundus photograph showing both drusen and subretinal hemorrhage. **(b)** OCT of the macula in the same patient showing hyperreflective material under the retina consistent with subretinal hemorrhage.

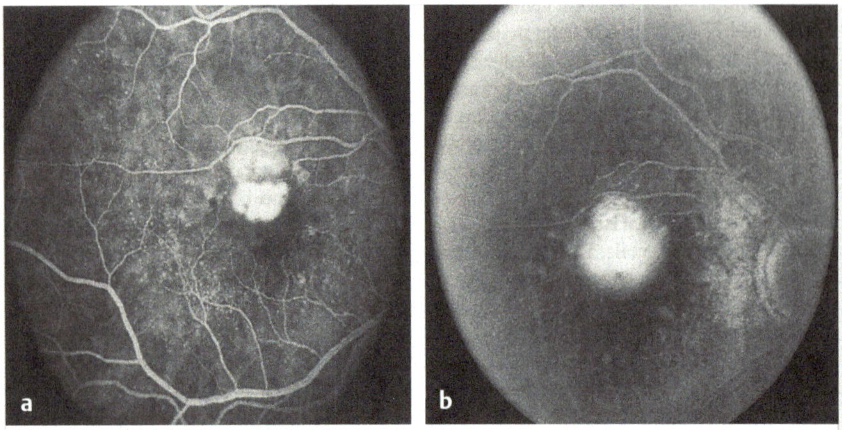

Fig. 14.10 Classic and occult choroidal neovascularization (CNV). **(a)** "Classic" CNV is apparent in the inferior half of this lesion in the early phase of the angiogram as a brightly hyperfluorescent, well-demarcated lesion with the suggestion of lacy or cartwheel features. "Occult" CNV in the form of a fibrovascular pigment epithelial detachment (FVPED) is evident in the superior half of the lesion as an area of less intense, stippled hyperfluorescence; the retinal pigment epithelium is elevated in this region. **(b)** Profuse leakage from the classic CNV is seen in the late-phase frame. The FVPED demonstrates progressive staining in the late phase. (Reproduced with permission by Wolters Kluwer from Bressler SB. The Wilmer Retina Update 1995;1:3–7.)

created. SD-OCT is able to identify CNV and its associated intraretinal fluid, subretinal fluid, and PEDs (▶ Fig. 14.9b).[12] Type 1 CNV originates in the choroid and then breaks through Bruch's membrane and extends under the RPE. If the neovascularization comes from the choroidal circulation and then extends through the RPE and into the subretinal space, then it is referred to as type 2 CNV. Often, CNV is a combination of both type 1 and type 2 disease. If the disease is predominantly type 1, it is referred to as minimally classic. If it is predominantly type 2, then it is predominantly classic.[32,62] Type 3 neovascularization refers to retinal angiomatous proliferation (RAP). This is characterized by retinal neovascularization that emanates from the deep capillary plexus of the retina. There are multiple stages of progression of RAP, with the final stage including choroidal and retinal neovascularization that consolidates to become a retinal–choroidal anastomosis. This is associated with leakage within and below the retina and involves development of a PED.[63,64]

With the increased use of SD-OCT imaging, new features of AMD have been discovered that had not been identified previously. The presence of what have now been named outer retinal tubulations (ORTs) are seen in some patients with many diseases associated with retinal injury and photoreceptor disruption, but most commonly with exudative AMD.[65] ORTs represent photoreceptor rearrangement and degeneration. On SD-OCT, ORTs appear as round, hyporeflective structures that are surrounded by a hyperreflective lining, usually overlying areas of pigment epithelial alteration or subretinal fibrosis. The hyperreflective border of the tubulation is thought to be the inner segment–outer segment junction of the photoreceptors. It is important to distinguish ORTs from cystoid macular edema because of the implications for treatment with anti-VEGF therapy, as ORTs do not represent active exudation.[65,66]

The end stage of exudative AMD is the development of a fibrotic disciform scar (▶ Fig. 14.11). The intraretinal and subretinal fluid, as well as hemorrhage, associated with CNV can lead to disorganization of the retina. There is extensive loss of RPE and photoreceptors with development of a disciform scar. When these scars involve the fovea, there is significant vision loss.[67] Although a disciform scar represents end-stage disease, there can still be reactivation of CNV leading to further hemorrhage; therefore, these patients should be followed up at less frequent but regular intervals.[68]

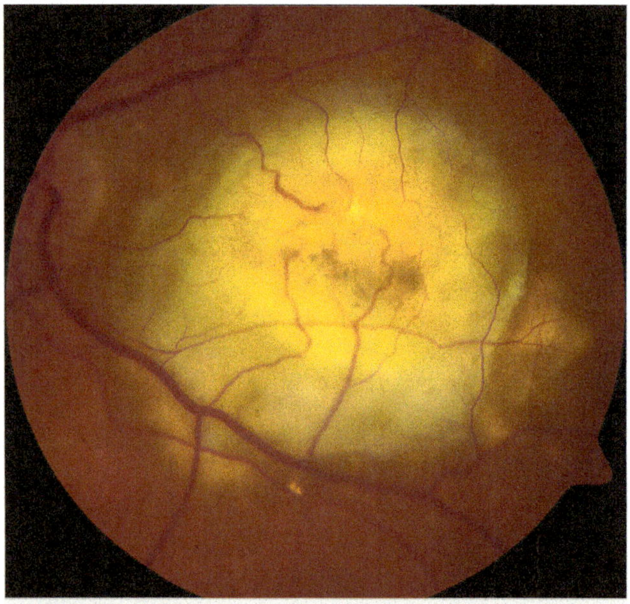

Fig. 14.11 Disciform scar. This is the end stage of exudative age-related macular degeneration with significant subretinal fibrosis and profound vision loss.

Pigment Epithelial Detachments

Various lesions in AMD will result in elevation of the pigment epithelial layer of the retina. A fibrovascular PED is a type of occult CNV described earlier (▶ Fig. 14.12). A serous detachment of the RPE (▶ Fig. 14.13) is distinguishable angiographically from a fibrovascular PED by the appearance of well-circumscribed, bright, uniform hyperfluorescence in the early phase with persistence of bright fluorescence in the later phases, with little, if any, leakage into the subretinal space. Although the clinical course is variable, most of these patients will show evidence of CNV within 1 to 2 years. Some serous PEDs manifest a notch at the edge that is believed to be a sign of occult CNV.[69]

On OCT, PEDs are broad elevations of the RPE above Bruch's membrane. Fibrovascular PEDs are associated with variable amounts of serous exudation and/or hemorrhage. Owing to this

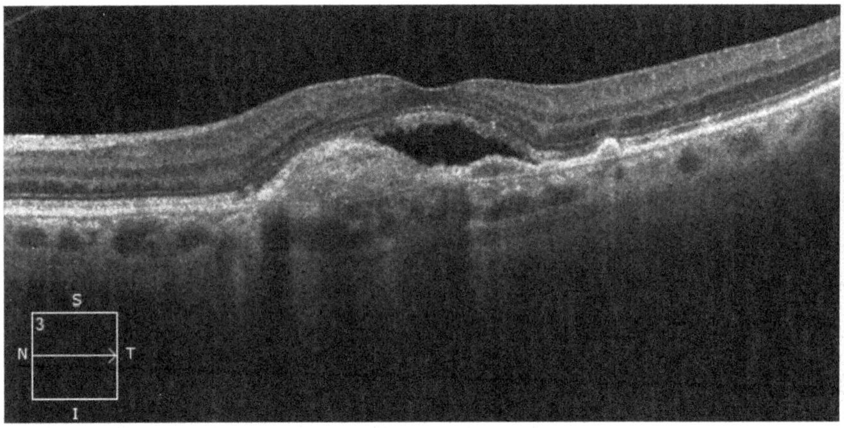

Fig. 14.12 Fibrovascular retinal pigment epithelial detachment (PED). The OCT scan shows an elevation of the retinal pigment epithelium, a PED, with associated subretinal fluid. The PED is associated with hyperreflection under it, consistent with a fibrovascular PED. It represents choroidal neovascularization which has resulted in the presence of subretinal fluid.

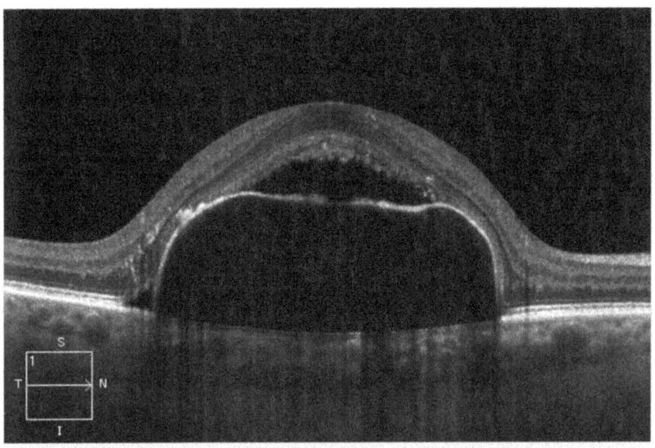

Fig. 14.13 Serous retinal pigment epithelial detachment (PED). The OCT raster scan demonstrates a serous PED with associated subretinal fluid. Unlike the fibrovascular PED above, a serous PED has an underlying homogenous hyporeflective space. The underlying Bruch's membrane can be identified. (Image courtesy of Dr. Justis Ehlers.)

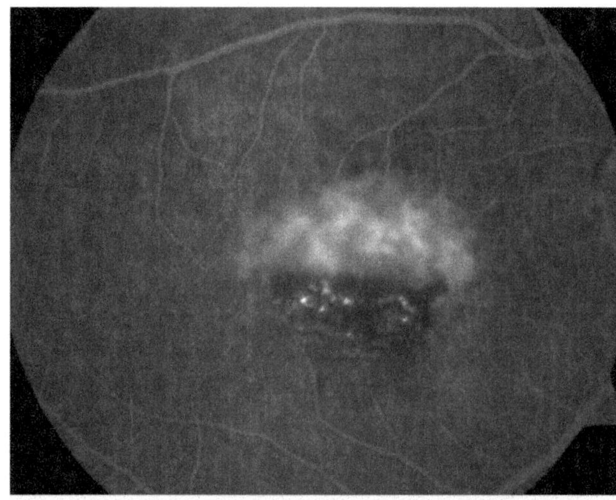

Fig. 14.14 Tear of the retinal pigment epithelium (RPE). Fluorescein angiography demonstrates early hyperfluorescence within the torn region. The bright region corresponds to choroidal fluorescence that is no longer blocked by RPE and the dark region corresponds to fluorescence blocked by the mass of RPE tissue.

exudation, the slope of the PED may vary depending on its fluid content. On OCT, avascular serous PEDs appear as dome-shaped elevations of the RPE. Underlying the RPE is a homogenously hyporeflective space. Vascularized serous PEDs likely occur with growth of a CNV lesion in the sub-RPE space that has significant associated exudation. This exudation creates a serous fluid compartment that looks similar to that of avascular PEDs; however, some have small collections of solid material (fibrovascular proliferation) adherent to the outer surface of the RPE.

Hemorrhagic PEDs form when there is hemorrhage in the sub-RPE space from neovascularization. The hemorrhage obscures the view to Bruch's membrane.[12] A hemorrhagic PED decreases the ability to detect CNV beneath the blood on fluorescein angiography as well. The appearance of a hemorrhagic PED sometimes may mimic a choroidal melanoma; however, the lack of low internal reflectivity on ultrasound examination will assist in this distinction.

A tear of the RPE can occur spontaneously in an eye with a serous PED or following treatment.[70] Studies have shown that the incidence of RPE tears after anti-VEGF therapy is similar to spontaneous RPE tears associated with the natural history of the disease.[71] On OCT, the discontinuity of the RPE can often be seen. If the torn area has no underlying fibrovascular tissue, one will see early bright, sharply demarcated hyperfluorescence on fluorescein angiography in the area denuded of RPE. An adjacent hypofluorescent area will be apparent where the scrolled RPE is now blocking underlying fluorescence (▶ Fig. 14.14). If fibrovascular tissue persists in the area of torn RPE, the fluorescence may not be as bright in the denuded area.

With RPE tears, visual acuity may fall precipitously. Some studies have shown that the majority of patients will have continued vision loss with longer follow-up. The major factor that determines visual prognosis is whether or not there is loss of RPE in the foveal center. Unfortunately, RPE tears are often associated with progressive fibrovascular scarring, which also contributes to vision loss.[71] Thus, when using anti-VEGF agents, if a RPE rip occurs and there is persistent activity of the choroidal neovascular membranes, most still recommend continued treatment with anti-VEGF therapy to help prevent fibrovascular scarring. While there may be concern for enlargement of the RPE tear with further consolidation of the CNV with treatment, studies have shown benefit to treatment.[72] Tears of the RPE where visual acuity was preserved even though subfoveal RPE was absent have been reported, but these cases did not have evidence of associated CNV.[9,33] Coco and colleagues described a series of patients with RPE tears that did not involve the foveal center. They found that continued anti-VEGF therapy led to a statistically significant improvement in vision.[72] Studies have been published that show some patients regain vision with repopulation of the RPE after the tear.[73]

14.3.2 Differential Diagnosis of Exudative Age-Related Macular Degeneration

CNV is associated with disease entities other than AMD. This is important to recognize, as the prognosis of CNV in other conditions may be different from AMD-related CNV. The presence of soft drusen and RPE abnormalities (pigmentation and/or atrophy) in both eyes of an individual older than 50 years will help establish AMD as the underlying diagnosis. Some other conditions associated with CNV include ocular histoplasmosis syndrome (OHS), pathologic myopia, choroidal rupture, angioid streaks, optic nerve drusen, a history of focal laser photocoagulation, and choroidal inflammatory syndromes such as multifocal choroiditis and punctate inner choroidopathy (PIC).

One also must be aware that other conditions can produce the biomicroscopic and OCT findings associated with CNV, that is, subretinal fluid, blood, and lipid exudate. Subretinal and intraretinal blood can develop in association with retinal macroaneurysms, lacquer cracks in pathologic myopia, traumatic choroidal rupture, central serous chorioretinopathy (CSCR), polypoidal vascular chorioretinopathy, and retinal vascular disease such as vein occlusion. Subretinal fluid also may develop in conjunction with choroidal tumors such as melanomas, nevi, osteomas, hemangiomas, and metastases, inflammatory conditions such as Harada's disease or posterior scleritis, and uveal effusion syndrome.

Central Serous Chorioretinopathy

Idiopathic central serous chorioretinopathy (CSCR) is a disease of the macula characterized by serous detachments of the neurosensory retina and RPE. With resolution of the serous detachments, there can be pigmentary mottling that might suggest a pattern of pigment clumping and atrophy of non-NVAMD. When the patient is older than 55 years, it may be difficult to differentiate these two conditions. Absence of soft drusen and the presence of multifocal areas of mottled RPE in both eyes, especially if located outside the macula, suggest the diagnosis of CSCR over AMD. In severe cases of CSCR, "guttering" of subretinal fluid—that is, spread of the fluid by gravity in a pseudopod fashion to the inferior fundus—will leave pigmentary mottling in this distribution. This guttering effect can be seen well on FAF (▶ Fig. 14.15). Although typically affecting men between the ages of 20 and 45 years, it occasionally will present in a patient older than 65 years, suggesting the possibility of AMD-related CNV. Angiographically, the subretinal fluid of CSCR, unlike CNV in AMD, usually extends far beyond the early- and midphase leakage. OCT confirms PEDs and subretinal fluid. With enhanced depth imaging (EDI) and now swept source OCT technology, the thickened choroid associated with patients with CSCR can be identified.[74,75] It is critical to differentiate CSCR from CNV in AMD. CSCR does not generally respond to anti-VEGF therapy but often responds well to PDT.

Polypoidal Choroidal Vasculopathy

Polypoidal choroidal vasculopathy (PCV) presents very similar to AMD and there is still debate as to whether this is a distinct entity or a variant of type 1 CNV in AMD. The disease is associated with polypoidal vascular lesions in the subretinal space that can lead to serous and hemorrhagic PEDs as well as subretinal hemorrhage.[76] Some patients can have episodes with repeated bleeding leading to significant vision loss and scarring. PCV occurs in both men and women, and is seen most commonly in Asian patients; however, it is also seen in African American and Caucasian patients. Fluorescein angiography cannot always reliably distinguish polypoidal choroidal vasculopathy from AMD; thus, PCV is often best characterized on indocyanine green angiography (ICGA) imaging[77] (▶ Fig. 14.16). Distinguishing PCV from AMD is important because the polyps may fail to resolve with anti-VEGF therapy, but have been shown to involute with ocular PDT. The EVEREST study found that verteporfin PDT in addition to ranibizumab (Lucentis Genentech/Roche) or PDT alone, was more effective than ranibizumab in leading to complete regression of polyps on ICGA in patients with PCV.[77]

14.3.3 Management and Course

Over the past 10 years, the treatment of exudative AMD has been revolutionized with the discovery and development of anti-VEGF agents. Historically, conventional laser, PDT, subfoveal surgery, and macular translocation were performed for exudative AMD but were associated with significantly worse visual acuity outcomes as compared to those associated with anti-VEGF therapy.

Treatment of CNV in Age-Related Macular Degeneration

CNV involves the development of new blood vessels growing from the choriocapillaris that break through Bruch's membrane into the subretinal pigment epithelial space or subretinal space,

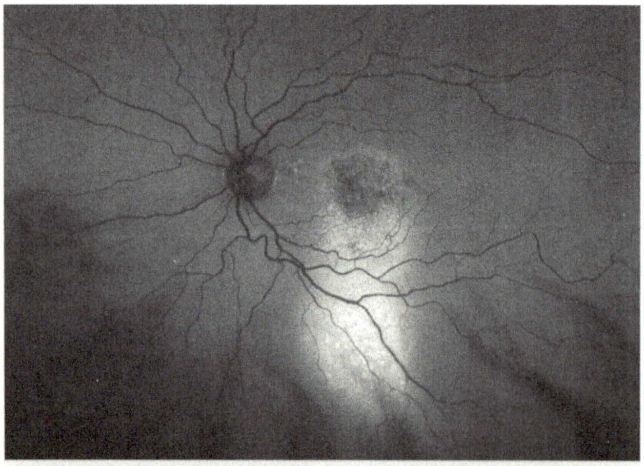

Fig. 14.15 Central serous chorioretinopathy. The fundus autofluorescence photograph shows an area of hyporeflectivity underlying the central macular abnormality which represents evidence of a gutter from central serous chorioretinopathy.

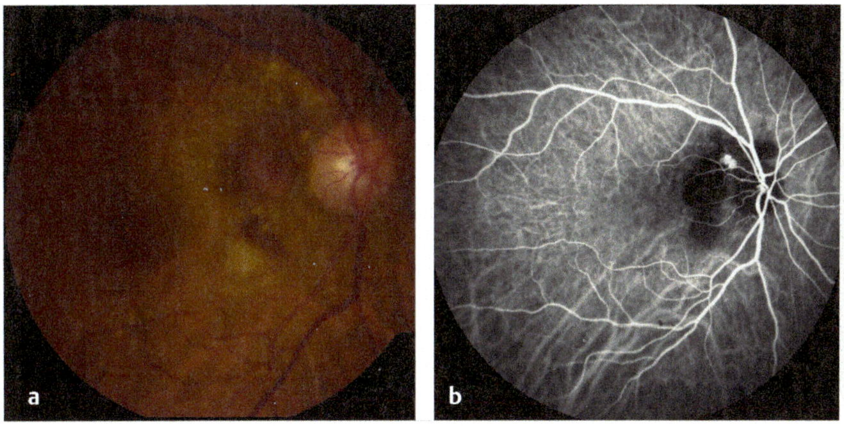

Fig. 14.16 Polypoidal chorioretinopathy. (**a**) The clinical fundus photograph shows evidence of subretinal hemorrhage and exudates. (**b**) The indocyanine angiography image shows evidence of a polyp just temporal to the optic nerve.

which can be associated with leakage of fluid and blood. Several factors are involved in angiogenesis, or development of new blood vessels from preexisting blood vessels. VEGF plays a fundamental role in angiogenesis, but other factors may also be important as well, including fibroblast growth factor (FGF), angiopoietin (Ang), platelet-derived growth factor (PDGF), pigment epithelium-derived factor, nitric oxide, matrix metalloproteinases, and tissue inhibitors of metalloproteinases.[78]

Laser Photocoagulation

Prior to the development of anti-VEGF therapy, the Macular Photocoagulation Study (MPS) showed that there were benefits of laser treatment over observation for several defined types of neovascular presentations. There were three sets of studies: the argon, krypton, and foveal studies. Each compared focal laser photocoagulation to observation.[79,80,81] While laser photocoagulation is typically no longer performed, the studies are important from a historical perspective.

In the first MPS report on new subfoveal lesions, laser-treated eyes, on average, retained better levels of visual acuity, reading speed, and contrast sensitivity compared to untreated eyes. An immediate decrease in vision usually occurred after treatment, but the benefits of treatment were noted 1 to 2 years after treatment as vision continued to decline in the eyes randomized to observation, but not in eyes randomized to laser treatment.[81]

In 1991, the MPS group published the long-term (5-year) results of a randomized prospective trial designed to evaluate the effectiveness of laser photocoagulation for *extrafoveal* CNV (CNV > 200 µm from the foveal center).[80] Untreated eyes lost a mean of 7.1 lines of visual acuity, while laser treated eyes lost 5.2 lines. Unfortunately, persistent or recurrent CNV was observed in 54% of treated eyes. Eyes with CNV persistence or recurrence were associated with significant visual loss.[80]

The 5-year results for *juxtafoveal* CNV (CNV 1–199 µm from the foveal center) in AMD were updated in 1994. As with extrafoveal lesions, there was a statistically significant visual benefit to treating juxtafoveal CNV. Twenty-five percent of the treated eyes compared to 15% of the untreated eyes maintained their baseline level of visual acuity. In addition, more than twice as many treated patients retained a visual acuity of 20/40 or better. Unfortunately, by the 5-year follow-up examination, 78% of those treated had either persistent or recurrent CNV involving the foveal center.[79]

When the original studies demonstrating the benefit of laser photocoagulation for lesions not involving the fovea were initiated, a distinction was not made between occult and classic CNV. A subsequent reanalysis of all fluorescein angiograms from the juxtafoveal AMD MPS trial strengthened the conclusion that treatment of lesions that involved classic CNV with no occult CNV was beneficial compared to observation when treatment covered the entire lesion.[81] Treatment of classic CNV only in lesions that had both classic and occult components was essentially equivalent to no treatment. There were too few eyes with occult CNV only with variable coverage of the lesion to draw conclusions about the benefit of treatment in this subgroup. However, 41% of the eyes with occult CNV only that were not treated lost significant vision by 1 year after study entry, usually following the development of classic CNV.[82]

Submacular Surgery

The Submacular Surgery Trials (SST) Research Group performed multicenter, randomized clinical trials aimed to determine whether surgical removal of subfoveal CNV stabilizes or improves vision more often than observation. The studies showed that vision did not improve for most patients who had submacular surgery for AMD. The conclusion was that submacular surgery was not helpful for most CNV lesions in AMD.[83,84]

Macular Translocation

Prior to the development of anti-VEGF agents for the treatment of exudative AMD, macular translocation was developed for the treatment of subfoveal CNV. Macular translocation with a 360-degree retinectomy moved the macular retina away from the area of subfoveal CNV and diseased RPE to a new location with healthier RPE and choroid. The purpose was to improve visual function.[85,86] This surgery has been abandoned in the era of anti-VEGF medications.

Photodynamic Therapy

PDT with verteporfin (Visudyne; Novartis Pharma AG) is approved for treatment of CNV from AMD.[87] The mechanism of action of verteporfin involves uptake of the photosensitizing dye that, when activated by specific laser energy, selectively closes the choroidal neovascular membrane by thrombosis.[88] The Treatment of Age-Related Macular Degeneration With

Photodynamic Therapy (TAP) trial found that at 24 months, fewer patients treated with PDT compared to placebo had lost less than three lines. Subgroup analysis showed there was more benefit in treatment with PDT in those eyes with larger than a 50% classic component of the CNV. A report of the 5-year outcomes suggested results remain stable in those who remained in follow-up.[87] The Verteporfin in Photodynamic Therapy (VIP) study enrolled patients who were not eligible for the TAP study. The majority of the participants enrolled in the study had occult with no classic CNV.[88] There was less benefit of PDT in these patients.

Given the greater benefit of anti-VEGF agents, PDT is no longer commonly used for the treatment of exudative AMD. It is still used in patients who are poor responders to anti-VEGF and in patients who are unable or unwilling to undergo frequent treatment with anti-VEGF drugs.[89] Poor response to anti-VEGF agents may suggest the possibility of polypoidal choroidopathy which does respond better to PDT in combination with anti-VEGF compared to anti-VEGF alone.[77]

Anti–Vascular Endothelial Growth Therapy

Pegaptanib

Pegaptanib (Macugen; Valeant Ophthalmics) was the first therapy developed to inhibit VEGF in the treatment of NVAMD and was approved by the U.S. Food and Drug Administration (FDA) in 2004 for the treatment of NVAMD. Pegaptanib is an RNA oligonucleotide (or aptamer) that specifically binds and blocks the activity of the extracellular 165-aminoacid isoform of VEGF ($VEGF_{165}$). In 2004, the results of the VEGF Inhibition Study in Ocular Neovascular (VISION) trial were published. VISION consisted of a randomized, prospective, multicenter, double-masked controlled clinical trial involving 1,186 patients and compared various doses of pegaptanib given every 6 weeks over a 48-week period to sham injection. By 54 weeks, pegaptanib was associated with an increase in the proportion of patients who lost fewer than 15 letters of vision (70% of patients treated with pegaptanib compared to 55% of controls). As early as 6 weeks after beginning therapy and at all subsequent time points, the mean visual acuity was better among patients treated with pegaptanib than in those receiving sham injections.[90] This anti-VEGF treatment has now been replaced by bevacizumab, ranibizumab, and aflibercept due to more favorable results than with pegaptanib.[91,92,93]

Bevacizumab

Bevacizumab (Avastin; Genentech/Roche) is a 149-kDa, full-length monoclonal antibody against all isoforms of VEGF-A, and was FDA approved in 2004 as a systemic therapy for the treatment of metastatic colorectal cancer. In 2004, the Systemic Avastin for Neovascular AMD (SANA) trial was initiated and demonstrated that bevacizumab was also effective in the treatment of exudative AMD. In this uncontrolled, open-label, single-central clinical study, 18 patients underwent two to three *intravenous* infusions of bevacizumab (5 mg/kg) at 2-week intervals. Initially, systemic bevacizumab caused mildly elevated systolic blood pressure, which was controlled by antihypertensive medications and was no longer significantly elevated by 12 weeks after treatment. By 24 weeks, systemic bevacizumab therapy was associated with an increased mean visual acuity of 14 letters and decreased mean central retinal thickness of 112 µm as measured with OCT.[94,95]

In 2005, the first reported case of intravitreal injection of bevacizumab was given to a patient with recurrent CNV who was treated previously with verteporfin PDT in combination with triamcinolone acetonide followed by pegaptanib injections. A 1.0-mg intravitreal injection of bevacizumab was associated with decreased central retinal thickness on OCT and improved visual distortion within 1 week, and the improved macular appearance was sustained for at least 4 weeks after injection.[96]

At the time when bevacizumab was being studied as an off-label treatment of NVAMD, clinical trials using pegaptanib and ranibizumab were underway, and there was some concern that the 149-kDa bevacizumab was too large to penetrate the retina to treat CNV effectively compared to the much smaller 48-kDa ranibizumab. However, in 2006 Shahar and colleagues reported that intravitreal injection of bevacizumab could be found in the subretinal space within 24 hours of injection in rabbits.[97] Several small studies were published documenting the improvement in mean visual acuity and reduction in OCT thickness in patients with NVAMD treated with intravitreal bevacizumab. In 2010, results of a randomized, double-masked phase III/IV study of the efficacy and safety of Avastin (Bevacizumab) intravitreal injections compared to standard therapy in subjects with CNV secondary to age-related macular degeneration (ABC) trial were published, which was a prospective, double-masked, multicenter, randomized controlled trial that involved 131 patients with NVAMD at three centers in the United Kingdom, randomized 1:1 to intervention or control. Intervention was intravitreal bevacizumab injection (1.25 mg in 0.05 mL given as three loading doses every 6 weeks, followed by additional injections given every 6 weeks as needed [PRN]). The control therapy was the standard of care, which at the time was verteporfin PDT for predominantly classic CNV, or pegaptanib injection or sham injection for minimally classic or occult CNV. A significantly higher proportion of patients in the bevacizumab group gained 15 or more letters from baseline visual acuity compared to the standard care group (32 vs. 3%), irrespective of lesion type. By the end of the study at 54 weeks, the mean change in vision was + 7.0 letters in the bevacizumab group and -9.4 letters in the standard care group, providing the first level I evidence of efficacy of bevacizumab for the treatment of NVAMD.[98]

Ranibizumab

Ranibizumab (Lucentis; Genentech/Roche) is a humanized anti-VEGF-A recombinant Fab fragment that has been affinity matured to increase its binding affinity to VEGF-A. In 2006, the Minimally Classic/Occult Trial of the Anti-VEGF Antibody Ranibizumab in the Treatment of Neovascular Age-Related Macular Degeneration (MARINA) study was published, which was a multicenter, 2-year, double-masked, sham-controlled study of 716 patients with NVAMD and minimally classic or occult CNV, randomized to receive either 24 monthly, ranibizumab intravitreal injections (0.3 or 0.5 mg) or sham injections. At 24 months, there was a significant increase in the number of patients with visual acuity improvement of at least 15 letters in the 0.5-mg ranibizumab group compared to the sham injection group (33 vs. 4%). About 1% of patients ($n=5$) who received intravitreal ranibizumab developed endophthalmitis. There were no increased systemic vascular complications in the ranibizumab groups compared to the control group, including hypertension, risk of myocardial infarction, stroke, and nonocular hemorrhage, although the study was not powered to detect small differences among groups for these uncommon adverse events.[92]

The Anti-VEGF Antibody for the Treatment of Predominantly Classic Choroidal Neovascularization in the Age-Related Macular Degeneration (ANCHOR) study was published in 2006 and 2009, and was also a multicenter, 2-year, double-masked study of 423 patients with NVAMD and predominantly classic CNV, randomized 1:1:1 to receive either monthly ranibizumab intravitreal injections (0.3 or 0.5 mg) plus sham verteporfin PDT or monthly sham injections plus active verteporfin PDT PRN every 3 months. At 24 months, there was a significant increase in the number of patients with visual acuity improvement of at least 15 letters in the 0.5-mg ranibizumab group compared to the verteporfin PDT group (41 vs. 6%). The mean change in visual acuity was + 10.7 letters in the 0.5-mg ranibizumab group and − 9.8 letters in the verteporfin PDT group. About 1.1% (3 of 277) of patients who received intravitreal ranibizumab developed endophthalmitis (rate per injection = 3/5,921, or 0.05%). There were no increased systemic vascular complications in the ranibizumab groups compared to the control group, including hypertension, risk of myocardial infarction, stroke, and nonocular hemorrhage.[99,100]

As visual acuity improvement seemed to plateau by 4 months in both the MARINA and ANCHOR trials, and monthly injections were considered inconvenient for patients, alternative treatment regimens were evaluated in the phase IIIb, multicenter, randomized, double-masked, sham injection-controlled study of the efficacy and safety of ranibizumab in subjects with subfoveal CNV with or without classic CNV secondary to age-related macular degeneration (PIER) and efficacy and safety of ranibizumab in patients with subfoveal CNV secondary to age-related macular degeneration (EXCITE) studies. In 2008 and 2010, the year 1 and 2 results of the PIER study were published. The PIER study was a multicenter, randomized, double-masked trial of 184 patients with NVAMD and subfoveal CNV, randomized 1:1:1 to 0.3 mg ranibizumab, 0.5 mg ranibizumab, or sham injection, with injections administered every month for 3 months, followed by additional injections every 3 months.[101] During year 2, eligible sham group patients crossed over to the 0.5-mg ranibizumab quarterly injection group. Later in year 2, all eligible randomized patients rolled over to 0.5 mg ranibizumab monthly.[102] At month 3, the mean change in visual acuity was + 4.3 letters in the 0.5 mg ranibizumab group. At year 1, mean change in visual acuity was −0.2 letters in the 0.5-mg ranibizumab group and −16.3 letters in the sham injection group. At year 2, mean change in visual acuity was −2.3 letters in the 0.5-mg ranibizumab group and −21.4 letters in the sham injection group. Visual acuity of sham patients that crossed over to the ranibizumab quarterly group lost 3.5 letters at 10 months after crossover. The 0.3 and 0.5 mg groups that rolled over into the monthly 0.5-mg ranibizumab group during year 2 increased mean visual acuity by 2.2 and 4.1 letters, respectively, 4 months after rollover. Thus, quarterly injections of ranibizumab do not appear to provide the same likelihood of visual improvement as monthly ranibizumab, and monthly ranibizumab injections could provide additional visual benefit to treated patients if patients were rolled over to monthly dosing, but not to patients who began receiving ranibizumab after more than 14 months of sham injections.[101,102] Therefore, early initiation of anti-VEGF treatment is important in NVAMD.

The EXCITE study was published in 2011, and was a 12-month, multicenter, double-masked trial of 293 patients with NVAMD and subfoveal CNV, randomized 1:1:1 to 0.3 mg quarterly, 0.5 mg quarterly, or 0.3 mg monthly doses of ranibizumab after a loading phase of three consecutive monthly injections. By 12 months, visual acuity increased in all groups from baseline by + 4.9, + 3.8, and + 8.3 letters in the 0.3 mg quarterly, 0.5 mg quarterly, and 0.3 mg monthly dosing groups, respectively. At month 12, there was also decreased central retinal thickness on OCT in all groups from baseline: −96.0, −105.6, and −105.3 µm in the 0.3 mg quarterly, 0.5 mg quarterly, and 0.3 mg monthly, respectively. At month 12, the visual acuity gain associated with the monthly regimen was higher than the visual acuity gain associated with the quarterly regimens, and the noninferiority of a quarterly regimen was not achieved with 5.0 letter noninferiority margins.[103]

Thus, data from the MARINA, ANCHOR, PIER, and EXCITE studies showed that, after a loading dose of three monthly injections, subsequent monthly injections of ranibizumab were superior to quarterly injections.

The Prospective OCT Imaging of Patients with Neovascular AMD Treated with Intraocular Lucentis (PrONTO) study, published in 2007 and 2009, was a 2-year study of a variable-dosing regimen of intravitreal ranibizumab in 40 patients with NVAMD and subfoveal CNV and a central retinal thickness of at least 300 µm measured by OCT. Patients initially received three consecutive monthly intravitreal injections of 0.5 mg ranibizumab, and retreatment with ranibizumab was performed if one of the following changes occurred: (1) a loss of 5 letters of vision in conjunction with fluid in the macula detected by OCT, (2) an increase in OCT central retinal thickness of at least 100 µm, (3) new-onset classic CNV, (4) new macular hemorrhage, or (5) persistent macular fluid detected by OCT at least 1 month after the previous injection. Patients were monitored with monthly OCT. At 24 months, mean visual acuity improved by 11.1 letters and the central retinal thickness on OCT decreased by 212 µm, with an average of 9.9 injections. The PrONTO study suggested that OCT-guided variable dosing of intravitreal ranibizumab resulted in comparable visual acuity outcomes to prior monthly injection studies, but with fewer intravitreal injections.[104,105]

The Safety Assessment of Intravitreal Lucentis for AMD (SAILOR) study was a phase IIIb study to evaluate the safety of 0.3 and 0.5 mg ranibizumab in 4,307 patients with NVAMD and subfoveal CNV. Patients were assigned randomly to either dose, and initially given three consecutive monthly injections followed by retreatment every 3 months PRN if vision decreased by greater than 5 letters from the patient's best level of visual acuity, or if there was an increase in central retinal thickness on OCT greater than 100 µm with intraretinal or subretinal fluid. At 1 year, treatment-naive patients had improved mean visual acuity of + 0.5 and + 2.3 letters in the 0.3 and 0.5 mg groups, respectively, while previously treated patients had mean visual acuity improvements of + 1.7 and + 2.3 letters, respectively. There was a higher rate of cerebrovascular stroke associated with 0.5 mg compared to 0.3 mg ranibizumab (1.2 vs. 0.7%), but this was not statistically significant, and a prior history of stroke, arrhythmias, and congestive heart failure were significant risk factors for stroke. The PRN regimen in SAILOR was associated with less favorable visual outcomes compared to monthly therapy in the MARINA and ANCHOR trials, and also compared unfavorably to the PrONTO study treatment regimen, although different retreatment criteria and regimens were utilized.[106]

The Safety and Efficacy of a Flexible Dosing Regimen of Ranibizumab in Neovascular Age-Related Macular Degeneration (SUSTAIN) study, published in 2011, was a multicenter, open-label, single-arm study of 513 patients with NVAMD and subfoveal CNV naive to ranibizumab treatment, and was performed in 10 European countries and Australia. Patients were given three initial monthly injections of 0.3 mg ranibizumab, then PRN retreatment for 9 months (of note, the dose of ranibizumab was switched to 0.5 mg after ranibizumab approval in Europe). Patients were monitored at monthly follow-up visits, and retreatment occurred if vision decreased by greater than 5 letters or if there was an increase in central retinal thickness on OCT of greater than 100 µm. There was an option to not retreat if vision was greater than or equal to 79 letters or if the central retinal thickness was less than or equal to 225 µm. Mean visual acuity peaked at month 3 at + 5.8 letters, and was + 3.6 at month 12. Mean change in central retinal thickness was −101 µm at month 3 and −92 µm at month 12. The average number of retreatments from months 3 to 11 was 2.7.[107]

Thus, PRN treatment regimens in SAILOR and SUSTAIN achieved less favorable visual acuity outcomes compared to the monthly dosing regimens in ANCHOR and MARINA, but the PRN regimen in the PrONTO study had more comparable results to monthly dosing of ranibizumab.

Comparison of Age-related Macular Degeneration Treatments Trials

The efficacy of ranibizumab has been established for the treatment of NVAMD in multiple clinical trials. However, despite the lack of clear level I evidence supporting the off-label use of bevacizumab for the treatment of NVAMD prior to the ABC trial published in 2010, the most commonly used pharmacological treatment of NVAMD in 2008 was bevacizumab. A retrospective review of the Medicare fee-for-service part B claims file in 2008 found that 58% of all intravitreal injections were bevacizumab and 41% were ranibizumab.[108] Thus, the Comparison of Age-related Macular Degeneration Treatments Trials (CATT) study was designed to compare the efficacy of bevacizumab and ranibizumab, administered monthly or PRN, for the treatment of NVAMD. CATT was a multicenter, randomized clinical trial of 1,107 patients with previously untreated subfoveal CNV due to AMD. At the time of enrollment, patients were assigned to one of four treatment groups based on drug (0.5 mg ranibizumab or 1.25 mg bevacizumab) and dosing regimen (monthly or PRN). At 1 year, patients initially in the monthly treatment group were randomly reassigned to monthly or PRN treatment, without changing the drug assignment. Among patients following the same regimen for 2 years, mean gain in visual acuity was not statistically significant and similar for both drugs (bevacizumab–ranibizumab difference, −1.4 letters; 95% confidence interval: −3.7 to + 0.8 letters). The mean gain in visual acuity was slightly significantly higher for the monthly versus PRN treatment (difference, −2.4 letters; 95% confidence interval: −4.8 to −0.1 letters). The proportion of patients without fluid on OCT was greatest at 46% in the ranibizumab monthly group, 30% in the bevacizumab monthly group, 22% in the ranibizumab PRN group, and least at 14% in the bevacizumab PRN group. Switching from monthly to PRN treatment was associated with a greater mean decrease in vision during year 2 (−2.2 letters) and a lower proportion of eyes without fluid (19%). Rates of death and arteriothrombotic events (ATEs) were similar for both drugs. There was a significantly higher proportion of patients with one or more systemic serious adverse events with bevacizumab than with ranibizumab (39.9 vs. 31.7%); however, most of these adverse events have not been previously associated with systemic anti-VEGF therapy. Thus, ranibizumab and bevacizumab were reported to have similar effects on visual acuity over a 2-year period. Treatment PRN was associated with slightly less gain in visual acuity, whether PRN treatment was instituted initially or after 1 year of monthly treatment. There were no significant differences between drugs in rates of deaths or ATEs. The slightly higher rates of serious adverse events associated with bevacizumab warrant further study, given that these conditions lack an association with VEGF inhibition.[91,109] Although cost was not a primary endpoint of CATT, the average annual cost per patient given monthly injections was $595 for bevacizumab and $23,400 for ranibizumab.

Several studies comparing ranibizumab and bevacizumab for NVAMD have been published since the first CATT results were published in 2011. Similar findings to CATT were reported from the Group d'Evaluation Francais Avastin versus Lucentis (GEFAL) study in France in 2013, a randomized controlled trial of alternative treatments to inhibit VEGF in age-related choroidal neovascularization (IVAN) study in the United Kingdom in 2013, a randomized double-masked trial comparing the visual outcome after treatment with ranibizumab or bevacizumab in patients with neovascular age-related macular degeneration (MANTA) study in Austria in 2013, the Lucentis Compared to Avastin Study (LUCAS) in Norway presented in 2013, and the study comparing effectiveness of bevacizumab to ranibizumab in patients with exudative age-related macular degeneration (BRAMD) in the Netherlands in 2014.[110,111,112,113,114]

Controversial Points

- Multiple studies have now reported no significant difference between bevacizumab and ranibizumab for the treatment of exudative AMD. There is a significant cost difference between the two medications.

Aflibercept

Aflibercept (Eylea; Regeneron) is a fusion protein that combines the ligand-binding elements from the extracellular domains of VEGF receptors 1 and 2 fused to the Fc constant portion of human immunoglobulin G. Aflibercept has a much higher binding affinity for VEGF than ranibizumab or bevacizumab and, unlike bevacizumab or ranibizumab (which only inhibit VEGF-A), aflibercept also binds VEGF-B and placental growth factors.[115] The "VEGF Trap-Eye: Investigation of Efficacy and Safety in Wet AMD" studies (VIEW 1 and VIEW 2) were similarly designed prospective, double-masked, multinational, controlled, randomized clinical trials. Patients in VIEW 1 were randomized at 154 sites in the United States and Canada, while patients in VIEW 2 were randomized at 172 sites in Europe, the Middle East, Asia Pacific, and Latin America. Patients with exudative AMD were randomized 1:1:1:1 to 0.5 mg aflibercept monthly (0.5q4), 2 mg aflibercept monthly (2q4), 2 mg aflibercept every 2 months (following three monthly loading doses; 2q8), or 0.5 mg ranibizumab monthly (Rq4), during the first year of study. PRN dosing with both agents, with a dose administered at least every 3 months (but not more often than monthly), was evaluated during year 2. Year 1 results were published in 2012 and year 2 results were published in 2014.[116,117] The mean visual acuity gains were similar across all treatment groups from baseline to 2 years, +6.6, +7.6, +7.6, and+7.9 letters for the 0.5q4, 2q4, 2q8, and Rq4 groups, respectively. The mean number of injections during weeks 52 through 96 was 4.6, 4.1, 4.2, and 4.7 for the 0.5q4, 2q4, 2q8, and Rq4 groups, respectively. There was a statistically significant lower number of injections in the 2q4 and 2q8 groups versus the Rq4 group (differences of -0.64 [95% confidence interval: -0.89 to -0.40] and -0.55 [95% confidence interval: -0.79 to -0.30]). The incidence of arterial thromboembolic events was similar across all groups. Thus, all aflibercept and ranibizumab groups were equally effective in improving visual acuity at 96 weeks. The 2-mg aflibercept every 2 months group was similar to ranibizumab in visual acuity outcomes at 96 weeks, but with an average of five fewer injections (11.2 vs. 16.5 injections).[116,117] See ▶ Table 14.1 for a summary of the VIEW 1/2 results as well as the prior clinical trials involving anti-VEGF therapy.

14.3.4 Current Management of Neovascular Age-Related Macular Degeneration

Presently in clinical practice, many physicians follow a "treat-and-extend" or a "PRN" (PRN) approach to the treatment of NVAMD, instead of following a monthly anti-VEGF injection protocol which has demonstrated efficacy in MARINA, ANCHOR, CATT, and VIEW 1/2, as discussed later. In response to the burden of monthly injections and visits on both the physician and the patient, the "treat-and-extend" as well as the "PRN" treatment protocols were evaluated in recent years. As previously discussed, the PrONTO trial injected ranibizumab monthly for 3 months, followed by PRN treatment based on prespecified criteria. Overall, PRN dosing in PrONTO led to comparable visual outcomes compared to monthly injections, though with fewer injections; however, another PRN regimen in SAILOR was associated with less favorable visual outcomes compared to monthly therapy.[104,105,106] More recently, a treat-and-extend protocol was published in 2014 in patients with CNV due to AMD; treatment consisted of three initial monthly ranibizumab or bevacizumab injections followed by monthly injections until there was no evidence of CNV activity. Once there was no evidence of CNV activity, the interval to the next visit/injection was extended by 2 weeks to a maximum of 12 weeks. Results of the "treat-and-extend" protocol were similar to the results of monthly ranibizumab with a mean improvement in visual acuity from baseline of+9.5 and+8.0 letters at 12 and 24 months, respectively.[118] To date, there has not been a head-to-head trial comparing a "treat-and-extend" regimen to a "PRN" regimen, but as of now there seems to be some evidence supporting the use of both practices. As opposed to the treatment of diabetic macular edema, which seems to have decreasing need for anti-VEGF therapy over time, CNV activity in NVAMD is chronic and persistent, with the majority of patients needing continuous active treatment beyond 2 years.[119]

OCT is crucial to monitoring intraretinal or subretinal fluid associated with CNV activity, as trace amounts of fluid observed on OCT are often subclinical on exam. Fluorescein angiography is important in characterizing the choroidal neovascular membrane, but is used less frequently now with greater use of OCT. Uncommonly, NVAMD responds poorly to anti-VEGF therapy and/or further imaging with indocyanine green may reveal a polypoidal choroidal vasculopathy-like CNV, wherein PDT may be considered as a treatment option. Another variant of CNV, peripapillary CNV, may still be successfully treated with laser photocoagulation, as results from the MPS previously demonstrated decreased risk of vision loss with laser as opposed to observation.[80] However, anti-VEGF intravitreal injections are now the mainstay of the treatment of NVAMD, with PDT and laser photocoagulation uncommonly being utilized.

14.3.5 Future Treatments

Currently under development are other intravitreal agents aimed at reducing VEGF levels with longer durations of action, but also agents against other molecules related to angiogenesis. At present, frequent intravitreal injections create a significant burden on both the patient and the treating physician and, therefore, various mechanisms to reduce this burden are being investigated. As some success has been achieved in improving the outcomes of patients with exudative AMD, attention is now being placed on dry AMD, both with respect to reducing progression of geographic atrophy and reducing the risk of progression from dry to wet disease.

Currently, Fovista (OphthoTech) is undergoing Phase III, multicentered, double-masked randomized control trials for the treatment of exudative AMD. Fovista is designed to target PDGF and, in conjunction with anti-VEGF drugs, acts to impair the formation of CNV. Fovista hinders PDGF from binding to PDGF receptors on pericytes, decreasing pericyte presence in choroidal neovascular membranes. In a Phase IIB study, patients treated with a combination of Fovista and ranibizumab gained a mean of 10.6 ETDRS letters at 24 weeks compared to the 6.5 ETDRS letters that were gained by patients treated with ranibizumab alone. The study also found that those patients who received Fovista combination therapy lost less vision then those with ranibizumab alone.[120]

As mentioned earlier, need for frequent injections of anti-VEGF therapy creates significant treatment burden. Development of drugs with longer durations of action would have a significant positive impact on the treatment of exudative AMD. Currently in trial is ESBA1008 (Alcon), a single-chain antibody fragment, which has shown similar reduction in central subfield thickness and possibly has a longer duration of effect

Table 14.1 Summary of clinical trials involving anti–vascular endothelial growth factor treatment of neovascular age-related macular degeneration

Clinical trial (date published, location, duration of study)	Treatment group (n)	Treatment schedule	Mean change in vision (letters)	Vision gain = 15 letters	Mean number of injections	Mean change in central retinal thickness on OCT (μm)	No fluid on OCT
ABC trial (2010, United Kingdom, 54 wk)	Bevacizumab 1.25 mg injection (n = 66)	q6 wk × 3, then q6 wk PRN	+7.0	32%	7.1	–91	N/A
	Standard of care (PDT for predominantly classic CNV or pegaptanib vs. sham injection for minimally classic/occult CNV) (n = 65)	PDT q3 mo PRN or pegaptanib vs. sham injection q6 wk	–9.4	3%	PDT 3.2 (treatments), pegaptanib 8.9, sham 7.3	–55	N/A
MARINA (2006, United States, 24 mo)	Sham injection (n = 238)	Monthly	–14.9	4%	Not reported	N/A	N/A
	Ranibizumab 0.5 mg injection (n = 240)		+6.6	33%	Not reported	N/A	N/A
ANCHOR (2009, United States, 24 mo)	Sham injection + PDT (n = 110)	Injection monthly, PDT q3 mo	–9.8	6%	PDT 3.8 (treatments)	N/A	N/A
	Ranibizumab 0.5 mg injection + sham PDT (n = 116)		+10.7	41%	21.3	N/A	N/A
PIER (2010, United States, 24 mo)	Sham injection (n = 63)	Monthly × 3, then q3 mo injection	–21.4	4.8%	2.6	N/A	N/A
	Ranibizumab 0.5 mg injection (n = 61)		–2.3	8.2%	2.5	N/A	N/A
PrONTO (2009, United States, 24 mo)	Ranibizumab 0.5 mg injection (n = 40)	Monthly × 3, then PRN injection monthly	+11.1	43%	9.9	–212	N/A
SUSTAIN (2011, Europe and Australia, 12 mo)	Ranibizumab 0.3 (then 0.5) mg (n = 513)	Monthly × 3, then PRN injection monthly	+3.6	19.3%	5.7	–92	N/A
CATT (2012, United States,2 y)	Ranibizumab 0.5 mg injection (n = 134)	Monthly	+8.8	33%	22.4	–190	46%
	Bevacizumab 1.25 mg injection (n = 129)	Monthly	+7.8	32%	23.4	–180	30%
	Ranibizumab 0.5 mg injection (n = 264)	PRN	+6.7	31%	12.6	–166	22%
	Bevacizumab 1.25 mg injection (n = 251)	PRN	+5.0	28%	14.1	–153	14%

Table 14.1 continued

Clinical trial (date published, location, duration of study)	Treatment group (*n*)	Treatment schedule	Mean change in vision (letters)	Vision gain = 15 letters	Mean number of injections	Mean change in central retinal thickness on OCT (µm)	No fluid on OCT
VIEW 1/2 (2014, multinational, 96 wk)	Ranibizumab 0.5 mg injection (*n* = 595)	Monthly	+ 7.9	32%	16.5	Not reported	46%
	Aflibercept 2 mg injection (*n* = 613)	Monthly	+ 7.6	31%	16.0	Not reported	54%
	Aflibercept 2 mg injection (*n* = 607)	q2 mo	+ 7.6	33%	11.2	Not reported	50%

Abbreviations: CNV, choroidal neovascularization; N/A, not available; PDT, photodynamic therapy; PRN, as needed; OCT, optical coherence tomography.

when compared to ranibizumab for treatment of exudative AMD.[121] Besides developing medications that last longer than those currently available, development of drug delivery devices would allow for prolonged controlled release of medications without the need for frequent repeat injections.

Another goal of wet AMD treatment is to replace intravitreal injections with a less invasive method of treatment. Ophthalmic eye drops would offer a noninvasive way of treating AMD. Squalamine Lactate Ophthalmic Solution 0.2% (Ohr Pharmaceutical Inc) is undergoing a Phase II study comparing ranibizumab alone versus Squalamine in combination with ranibizumab. An interim report suggested that the combination therapy may be more effective in improving visual acuity outcomes compared to ranibizumab alone. The Phase II study should be completed in early 2015.[122]

While there have been significant advancements in the treatment of exudative AMD, besides the introduction of AREDS supplementation there has not been much change in the treatment of dry AMD. A promising agent, lampalizumab (Roche), also known as *anti–factor D*, has been introduced as a treatment to prevent progression of geographic atrophy. Lampalizumab is an antigen-binding fragment (Fab) of a humanized, monoclonal antibody directed against complement factor D. Complement factor D is a rate-limiting enzyme that is important for the activation of the alternative complement pathway. Increased activity of this pathway is felt to play a role in development of geographic atrophy.[115] The MAHALO study was a Phase II multicentered, single-masked, controlled study of monthly or every other month injections of lampalizumab or sham. At 20 months, there was a 20.4% reduction in the rate of progression of area of geographic atrophy in patients who underwent monthly injections of lampalizumab compared to controls.[123]

It is an exciting time for research and drug and device development for AMD. Over the next few years, we will likely see release of many new drugs giving patients with AMD continued and greater hope for preservation of vision with improved quality of life.

14.4 Conclusion

The diagnosis and treatment of AMD has been transformed by the development of OCT and anti-VEGF therapy. When a patient with nonexudative AMD experiences symptoms of metamorphopsia or visual change, a prompt examination by an ophthalmologist skilled in the recognition of neovascular complications is paramount. Visual acuity outcomes of exudative AMD are largely dependent on the visual acuity at the time of treatment initiation; therefore, early detection of CNV is important. The future of AMD management will hopefully involve prevention of neovascular complications.

14.5 Financial Disclosures

Peter K. Kaiser is a consultant to Alcon, Bayer, Novartis, Genentech, Regeneron, Ohr Pharmaceutical, Oraya, Digisight, Ophthotech, Thrombogenics, Genzyme, Santen, Aerpio. Dr. Kaiser also receives equity from Ohr Pharmaceuticals. Ashleigh L. Levison and Paula E. Pecen have nothing to declare.

References

[1] Jonasson F, Fisher DE, Eiriksdottir G, et al. Five-year incidence, progression, and risk factors for age-related macular degeneration: the age, gene/environment susceptibility study. Ophthalmology. 2014; 121(9):1766–1772

[2] Klein R, Klein BE, Jensen SC, Meuer SM. The five-year incidence and progression of age-related maculopathy: the Beaver Dam Eye Study. Ophthalmology. 1997; 104(1):7–21

[3] Klein R, Klein BE, Linton KL. Prevalence of age-related maculopathy. The Beaver Dam Eye Study. Ophthalmology. 1992; 99(6):933–943

[4] Vingerling JR, Dielemans I, Hofman A, et al. The prevalence of age-related maculopathy in the Rotterdam Study. Ophthalmology. 1995; 102(2):205–210

[5] Age-Related Eye Disease Study Research Group. A randomized, placebo-controlled, clinical trial of high-dose supplementation with vitamins C and E, beta carotene, and zinc for age-related macular degeneration and vision loss: AREDS report no. 8. Arch Ophthalmol. 2001; 119(10):1417–1436

[6] Ryan SSA, Wilkinson C, Hinton D, Sadda V, Wiedemann P. Retina. Vols. 1-3. 5th ed. Philadelphia, PA: Elsevier; 2012

[7] Lim LS, Mitchell P, Seddon JM, Holz FG, Wong TY. Age-related macular degeneration. Lancet. 2012; 379(9827):1728–1738

[8] Bressler NM, Bressler SB. Preventative ophthalmology. Age-related macular degeneration. Ophthalmology. 1995; 102(8):1206–1211

[9] Velez-Montoya R, Oliver SC, Olson JL, Fine SL, Mandava N, Quiroz-Mercado H. Current knowledge and trends in age-related macular degeneration: today's and future treatments. Retina. 2013; 33(8):1487–1502

[10] Bowes Rickman C, Farsiu S, Toth CA, Klingeborn M. Dry age-related macular degeneration: mechanisms, therapeutic targets, and imaging. Invest Ophthalmol Vis Sci. 2013; 54(14):ORSF68–80

[11] Ferris FL, III, Fine SL, Hyman L. Age-related macular degeneration and blindness due to neovascular maculopathy. Arch Ophthalmol. 1984; 102 (11):1640–1642

[12] Keane PA, Patel PJ, Liakopoulos S, Heussen FM, Sadda SR, Tufail A. Evaluation of age-related macular degeneration with optical coherence tomography. Surv Ophthalmol. 2012; 57(5):389–414

[13] Ferris FL, Davis MD, Clemons TE, et al. Age-Related Eye Disease Study (AREDS) Research Group. A simplified severity scale for age-related macular degeneration: AREDS Report No. 18. Arch Ophthalmol. 2005; 123 (11):1570–1574

[14] Goodman GE, Thornquist MD, Balmes J, et al. The Beta-Carotene and Retinol Efficacy Trial: incidence of lung cancer and cardiovascular disease mortality during 6-year follow-up after stopping beta-carotene and retinol supplements. J Natl Cancer Inst. 2004; 96(23):1743–1750

[15] Russell SR, Mullins RF, Schneider BL, Hageman GS. Location, substructure, and composition of basal laminar drusen compared with drusen associated with aging and age-related macular degeneration. Am J Ophthalmol. 2000; 129(2):205–214

[16] D'souza Y, Jones CJ, Bonshek R. Glycoproteins of drusen and drusen-like lesions. J Mol Histol. 2008; 39(1):77–86

[17] Bressler NM, Bressler SB, West SK, Fine SL, Taylor HR. The grading and prevalence of macular degeneration in Chesapeake Bay watermen. Arch Ophthalmol. 1989; 107(6):847–852

[18] Klein BE, Klein R. Cataracts and macular degeneration in older Americans. Arch Ophthalmol. 1982; 100(4):571–573

[19] Bressler SB, Maguire MG, Bressler NM, Fine SL, The Macular Photocoagulation Study Group. Relationship of drusen and abnormalities of the retinal pigment epithelium to the prognosis of neovascular macular degeneration. Arch Ophthalmol. 1990; 108(10):1442–1447

[20] Sarks JP, Sarks SH, Killingsworth MC. Evolution of geographic atrophy of the retinal pigment epithelium. Eye (Lond). 1988; 2(Pt 5):552–577

[21] Pauleikhoff D, Barondes MJ, Minassian D, Chisholm IH, Bird AC. Drusen as risk factors in age-related macular disease. Am J Ophthalmol. 1990; 109 (1):38–43

[22] Bird AC, Bressler NM, Bressler SB, et al. The International ARM Epidemiological Study Group. An international classification and grading system for age-related maculopathy and age-related macular degeneration. Surv Ophthalmol. 1995; 39(5):367–374

[23] Killingsworth MC. Age-related components of Bruch's membrane in the human eye. Graefes Arch Clin Exp Ophthalmol. 1987; 225(6):406–412

[24] Green WR, Enger C. Age-related macular degeneration histopathologic studies. The 1992 Lorenz E. Zimmerman Lecture. Ophthalmology. 1993; 100 (10):1519–1535

[25] Smiddy WE, Fine SL. Prognosis of patients with bilateral macular drusen. Ophthalmology. 1984; 91(3):271–277

[26] Holz FG, Wolfensberger TJ, Piguet B, et al. Bilateral macular drusen in age-related macular degeneration. Prognosis and risk factors. Ophthalmology. 1994; 101(9):1522–1528

[27] Schmitz-Valckenberg S, Fleckenstein M, Göbel AP, Hohman TC, Holz FG. Optical coherence tomography and autofluorescence findings in areas with geographic atrophy due to age-related macular degeneration. Invest Ophthalmol Vis Sci. 2011; 52(1):1–6

[28] Bindewald A, Schmitz-Valckenberg S, Jorzik JJ, et al. Classification of abnormal fundus autofluorescence patterns in the junctional zone of geographic atrophy in patients with age related macular degeneration. Br J Ophthalmol. 2005; 89(7):874–878

[29] Zweifel SA, Imamura Y, Spaide TC, Fujiwara T, Spaide RF. Prevalence and significance of subretinal drusenoid deposits (reticular pseudodrusen) in age-related macular degeneration. Ophthalmology. 2010; 117(9):1775–1781

[30] Zweifel SA, Spaide RF, Curcio CA, Malek G, Imamura Y. Reticular pseudodrusen are subretinal drusenoid deposits. Ophthalmology. 2010; 117(2):303–12.e1

[31] Rudolf M, Malek G, Messinger JD, Clark ME, Wang L, Curcio CA. Sub-retinal drusenoid deposits in human retina: organization and composition. Exp Eye Res. 2008; 87(5):402–408

[32] Yannuzzi LA. The Retinal Atlas. Philadelphia, PA: Saunders/Elsevier; 2010

[33] Thomann U, Büchi ER, Suppiger M, Kryenbühl C, Schipper I, Spiegel R. Age-dependent phenotypic expression of a pattern dystrophy of the retina. Eur J Ophthalmol. 1995; 5(2):107–112

[34] Zerbib J, Querques G, Massamba N, et al. Reticular pattern dystrophy of the retina: a spectral-domain optical coherence tomography analysis. Am J Ophthalmol. 2013; 156(6):1228–1237

[35] Todd KSH, Crawford JB. Pathological findings in pseudo-vitelliform macular degeneration. Invest Ophthalmol Vis Sci. 1986; 27:198

[36] Chew EY, Clemons TE, Bressler SB, et al. AREDS2-HOME Study Research Group. Randomized trial of a home monitoring system for early detection of choroidal neovascularization home monitoring of the Eye (HOME) study. Ophthalmology. 2014; 121(2):535–544

[37] Klein R, Myers CE, Meuer SM, et al. Risk alleles in CFH and ARMS2 and the long-term natural history of age-related macular degeneration: the Beaver Dam Eye Study. JAMA Ophthalmol. 2013; 131(3):383–392

[38] Horie-Inoue K, Inoue S. Genomic aspects of age-related macular degeneration. Biochem Biophys Res Commun. 2014; 452(2):263–275

[39] Katta S, Kaur I, Chakrabarti S. The molecular genetic basis of age-related macular degeneration: an overview. J Genet. 2009; 88(4):425–449

[40] Chew EY, Klein ML, Clemons TE, et al. No clinically significant association between CFH and ARMS2 genotypes and response to nutritional supplements: AREDS report number 38. Ophthalmology. 2014; 121(11):2173–2180

[41] Awh CC, Lane AM, Hawken S, Zanke B, Kim IK. CFH and ARMS2 genetic polymorphisms predict response to antioxidants and zinc in patients with age-related macular degeneration. Ophthalmology. 2013; 120(11):2317–2323

[42] Wittes J, Musch DC. Should we test for genotype in deciding on age-related eye disease study supplementation? Ophthalmology. 2015; 122(1):3–5

[43] Chakravarthy U, Wong TY, Fletcher A, et al. Clinical risk factors for age-related macular degeneration: a systematic review and meta-analysis. BMC Ophthalmol. 2010; 10:31

[44] Chew EY, Clemons TE, Agrón E, et al. Age-Related Eye Disease Study Research Group. Ten-year follow-up of age-related macular degeneration in the age-related eye disease study: AREDS report no. 36. JAMA Ophthalmol. 2014; 132(3):272–277

[45] Myers CE, Klein BE, Gangnon R, Sivakumaran TA, Iyengar SK, Klein R. Cigarette smoking and the natural history of age-related macular degeneration: the Beaver Dam Eye Study. Ophthalmology. 2014; 121(10):1949–1955

[46] Berendschot TT, Willemse-Assink JJ, Bastiaanse M, de Jong PT, van Norren D. Macular pigment and melanin in age-related maculopathy in a general population. Invest Ophthalmol Vis Sci. 2002; 43(6):1928–1932

[47] Klein R, Klein BE, Moss SE. Relation of smoking to the incidence of age-related maculopathy. The Beaver Dam Eye Study. Am J Epidemiol. 1998; 147 (2):103–110

[48] Johnson EJ. Obesity, lutein metabolism, and age-related macular degeneration: a web of connections. Nutr Rev. 2005; 63(1):9–15

[49] van Leeuwen R, Ikram MK, Vingerling JR, Witteman JC, Hofman A, de Jong PT. Blood pressure, atherosclerosis, and the incidence of age-related maculopathy: the Rotterdam Study. Invest Ophthalmol Vis Sci. 2003; 44(9):3771–3777

[50] Khan JC, Shahid H, Thurlby DA, et al. Genetic Factors in AMD Study. Age related macular degeneration and sun exposure, iris colour, and skin sensitivity to sunlight. Br J Ophthalmol. 2006; 90(1):29–32

[51] Darzins P, Mitchell P, Heller RF. Sun exposure and age-related macular degeneration. An Australian case-control study. Ophthalmology. 1997; 104 (5):770–776

[52] Stryker WS, Kaplan LA, Stein EA, Stampfer MJ, Sober A, Willett WC. The relation of diet, cigarette smoking, and alcohol consumption to plasma beta-carotene and alpha-tocopherol levels. Am J Epidemiol. 1988; 127(2):283–296

[53] Wang JJ, Klein R, Smith W, Klein BE, Tomany S, Mitchell P. Cataract surgery and the 5-year incidence of late stage age-related maculopathy: pooled findings from the Beaver Dam and Blue Mountains eye studies. Ophthalmol ogy. 2003; 110(10):1960–1967

[54] The Eye Disease Case-Control Study Group. Risk factors for neovascular age-related macular degeneration. Arch Ophthalmol. 1992; 110(12):1701–1708

[55] Eye Disease Case-Control Study Group. Antioxidant status and neovascular age-related macular degeneration. Arch Ophthalmol. 1993; 111(1):104–109

[56] Goldberg J, Flowerdew G, Smith E, Brody JA, Tso MO. Factors associated with age-related macular degeneration. An analysis of data from the first National Health and Nutrition Examination Survey. Am J Epidemiol. 1988; 128 (4):700–710

[57] Age-Related Eye Disease Study 2 Research Group. Lutein + zeaxanthin and omega-3 fatty acids for age-related macular degeneration: the Age-Related Eye Disease Study 2 (AREDS2) randomized clinical trial. JAMA. 2013; 309 (19):2005–2015

[58] Aronow ME, Chew EY. Age-related Eye Disease Study 2: perspectives, recommendations, and unanswered questions. Curr Opin Ophthalmol. 2014; 25(3):186–190

[59] Ferris FL, III, Wilkinson CP, Bird A, et al. Beckman Initiative for Macular Research Classification Committee. Clinical classification of age-related macular degeneration. Ophthalmology. 2013; 120(4):844–851

[60] Klein ML, Francis PJ, Ferris FL, III, Hamon SC, Clemons TE. Risk assessment model for development of advanced age-related macular degeneration. Arch Ophthalmol. 2011; 129(12):1543–1550

[61] Bressler NM, Bressler SB, Fine SL. Age-related macular degeneration. Surv Ophthalmol. 1988; 32(6):375–413

[62] Jung JJ, Chen CY, Mrejen S, et al. The incidence of neovascular subtypes in newly diagnosed neovascular age-related macular degeneration. Am J Ophthalmol. 2014; 158(4):769–779.e2

[63] Yannuzzi LA, Freund KB, Takahashi BS. Review of retinal angiomatous proliferation or type 3 neovascularization. Retina. 2008; 28(3):375–384

[64] Freund KB, Ho IV, Barbazetto IA, et al. Type 3 neovascularization: the expanded spectrum of retinal angiomatous proliferation. Retina. 2008; 28 (2):201–211

[65] Jung JJ, Freund KB. Long-term follow-up of outer retinal tubulation documented by eye-tracked and en face spectral-domain optical coherence tomography. Arch Ophthalmol. 2012; 130(12):1618–1619

[66] Wolff B, Matet A, Vasseur V, Sahel JA, Mauget-Faÿsse M. En Face OCT Imaging for the Diagnosis of Outer Retinal Tubulations in Age-Related Macular Degeneration. J Ophthalmol. 2012; 2012:542417

[67] Sarks J, Tang K, Killingsworth M, Arnold J, Sarks S. Development of atrophy of the retinal pigment epithelium around disciform scars. Br J Ophthalmol. 2006; 90(4):442–446

[68] Coco RM, Sala-Puigdollers A. Management of significant reactivation of old disciform scars in wet age-related macular degeneration. BMC Ophthalmol. 2014; 14:82

[69] Gass JD. Serous retinal pigment epithelial detachment with a notch: a sign of occult choroidal neovascularization. 1984. Retina. 2003; 23(6) Suppl:205–220

[70] Bressler NM, Finklestein D, Sunness JS, Maguire AM, Yarian D. Retinal pigment epithelial tears through the fovea with preservation of good visual acuity. Arch Ophthalmol. 1990; 108(12):1694–1697

[71] Gutfleisch M, Heimes B, Schumacher M, et al. Long-term visual outcome of pigment epithelial tears in association with anti-VEGF therapy of pigment epithelial detachment in AMD. Eye (Lond). 2011; 25(9):1181–1186

[72] Coco RM, Sanabria MR, Hernandez AG, Fernández Muñoz M. Retinal pigment epithelium tears in age-related macular degeneration treated with antiangiogenic drugs: a controlled study with long follow-up. Ophthalmologica. 2012; 228(2):78–83

[73] Peiretti E, Iranmanesh R, Lee JJ, Klancnik JM, Jr, Sorenson JA, Yannuzzi LA. Repopulation of the retinal pigment epithelium after pigment epithelial rip. Retina. 2006; 26(9):1097–1099

[74] Ferrara D, Mohler KJ, Waheed N, et al. En face enhanced-depth swept-source optical coherence tomography features of chronic central serous chorioretinopathy. Ophthalmology. 2014; 121(3):719–726

[75] Jirarattanasopa P, Ooto S, Tsujikawa A, et al. Assessment of macular choroidal thickness by optical coherence tomography and angiographic changes in central serous chorioretinopathy. Ophthalmology. 2012; 119(8):1666–1678

[76] Koh AH, Chen LJ, Chen SJ, et al. Expert PCV Panel. Polypoidal choroidal vasculopathy: evidence-based guidelines for clinical diagnosis and treatment. Retina. 2013; 33(4):686–716

[77] Koh A, Lee WK, Chen LJ, et al. EVEREST study: efficacy and safety of verteporfin photodynamic therapy in combination with ranibizumab or alone versus ranibizumab monotherapy in patients with symptomatic macular polypoidal choroidal vasculopathy. Retina. 2012; 32(8):1453–1464

[78] Ambati J, Ambati BK, Yoo SH, Ianchulev S, Adamis AP. Age-related macular degeneration: etiology, pathogenesis, and therapeutic strategies. Surv Ophthalmol. 2003; 48(3):257–293

[79] Macular Photocoagulation Study Group. Krypton laser photocoagulation for idiopathic neovascular lesions. Results of a randomized clinical trial. Arch Ophthalmol. 1990; 108(6):832–837

[80] Macular Photocoagulation Study Group. Argon laser photocoagulation for neovascular maculopathy. Five-year results from randomized clinical trials. Arch Ophthalmol. 1991; 109(8):1109–1114

[81] Macular Photocoagulation Study Group. Laser photocoagulation of subfoveal neovascular lesions of age-related macular degeneration. Updated findings from two clinical trials. Arch Ophthalmol. 1993; 111(9):1200–1209

[82] Macular Photocoagulation Study Group. Occult choroidal neovascularization. Influence on visual outcome in patients with age-related macular degeneration. Arch Ophthalmol. 1996; 114(4):400–412

[83] Hawkins BS, Bressler NM, Miskala PH, et al. Submacular Surgery Trials (SST) Research Group. Surgery for subfoveal choroidal neovascularization in age-related macular degeneration: ophthalmic findings: SST report no. 11. Ophthalmology. 2004; 111(11):1967–1980

[84] Bressler NM, Bressler SB, Childs AL, et al. Submacular Surgery Trials (SST) Research Group. Surgery for hemorrhagic choroidal neovascular lesions of age-related macular degeneration: ophthalmic findings: SST report no. 13. Ophthalmology. 2004; 111(11):1993–2006

[85] Lai JC, Lapolice DJ, Stinnett SS, et al. Visual outcomes following macular translocation with 360-degree peripheral retinectomy. Arch Ophthalmol. 2002; 120(10):1317–1324

[86] Park CH, Toth CA. Macular translocation surgery with 360-degree peripheral retinectomy following ocular photodynamic therapy of choroidal neovascularization. Am J Ophthalmol. 2003; 136(5):830–835

[87] Kaiser PK, Treatment of Age-Related Macular Degeneration with Photodynamic Therapy (TAP) Study Group. Verteporfin therapy of subfoveal choroidal neovascularization in age-related macular degeneration: 5-year results of two randomized clinical trials with an open-label extension: TAP report no. 8. Graefes Arch Clin Exp Ophthalmol. 2006; 244(9):1132–1142

[88] Wormald R, Evans J, Smeeth L, Henshaw K. Photodynamic therapy for neovascular age-related macular degeneration. Cochrane Database Syst Rev. 2007(3):CD002030

[89] Amoaku WM, Chakravarthy U, Gale R, et al. Defining response to anti-VEGF therapies in neovascular AMD. Eye (Lond). 2015; 29(6):721–31

[90] Gragoudas ES, Adamis AP, Cunningham ET, Jr, Feinsod M, Guyer DR, VEGF Inhibition Study in Ocular Neovascularization Clinical Trial Group. Pegaptanib for neovascular age-related macular degeneration. N Engl J Med. 2004; 351 (27):2805–2816

[91] Martin DF, Maguire MG, Ying GS, Grunwald JE, Fine SL, Jaffe GJ, CATT Research Group. Ranibizumab and bevacizumab for neovascular age-related macular degeneration. N Engl J Med. 2011; 364(20):1897–1908

[92] Rosenfeld PJ, Brown DM, Heier JS, et al. MARINA Study Group. Ranibizumab for neovascular age-related macular degeneration. N Engl J Med. 2006; 355 (14):1419–1431

[93] Brown DM, Heier JS, Ciulla T, et al. CLEAR-IT 2 Investigators. Primary endpoint results of a phase II study of vascular endothelial growth factor trap-eye in wet age-related macular degeneration. Ophthalmology. 2011; 118 (6):1089–1097

[94] Michels S, Rosenfeld PJ, Puliafito CA, Marcus EN, Venkatraman AS. Systemic bevacizumab (Avastin) therapy for neovascular age-related macular degeneration twelve-week results of an uncontrolled open-label clinical study. Ophthalmology. 2005; 112(6):1035–1047

[95] Moshfeghi AA, Rosenfeld PJ, Puliafito CA, et al. Systemic bevacizumab (Avastin) therapy for neovascular age-related macular degeneration: twenty-

four-week results of an uncontrolled open-label clinical study. Ophthalmology. 2006; 113(11):2002.e1–12

[96] Rosenfeld PJ, Moshfeghi AA, Puliafito CA. Optical coherence tomography findings after an intravitreal injection of bevacizumab (Avastin) for neovascular age-related macular degeneration. Ophthalmic Surg Lasers Imaging. 2005; 36(4):331–335

[97] Shahar J, Avery RL, Heilweil G, et al. Electrophysiologic and retinal penetration studies following intravitreal injection of bevacizumab (Avastin). Retina. 2006; 26(3):262–269

[98] Tufail A, Patel PJ, Egan C, et al. ABC Trial Investigators. Bevacizumab for neovascular age related macular degeneration (ABC Trial): multicentre randomised double masked study. BMJ. 2010; 340:c2459

[99] Brown DM, Michels M, Kaiser PK, Heier JS, Sy JP, Ianchulev T, ANCHOR Study Group. Ranibizumab versus verteporfin photodynamic therapy for neovascular age-related macular degeneration: two-year results of the ANCHOR study. Ophthalmology. 2009; 116(1):57–65.e5

[100] Brown DM, Kaiser PK, Michels M, et al. ANCHOR Study Group. Ranibizumab versus verteporfin for neovascular age-related macular degeneration. N Engl J Med. 2006; 355(14):1432–1444

[101] Regillo CD, Brown DM, Abraham P, et al. Randomized, double-masked, sham-controlled trial of ranibizumab for neovascular age-related macular degeneration: PIER Study year 1. Am J Ophthalmol. 2008; 145(2):239–248

[102] Abraham P, Yue H, Wilson L. Randomized, double-masked, sham-controlled trial of ranibizumab for neovascular age-related macular degeneration: PIER study year 2. Am J Ophthalmol. 2010; 150(3):315–324.e1

[103] Schmidt-Erfurth U, Eldem B, Guymer R, et al. EXCITE Study Group. Efficacy and safety of monthly versus quarterly ranibizumab treatment in neovascular age-related macular degeneration: the EXCITE study. Ophthalmology. 2011; 118(5):831–839

[104] Lalwani GA, Rosenfeld PJ, Fung AE, et al. A variable-dosing regimen with intravitreal ranibizumab for neovascular age-related macular degeneration: year 2 of the PrONTO Study. Am J Ophthalmol. 2009; 148(1):43–58.e1

[105] Fung AE, Lalwani GA, Rosenfeld PJ, et al. An optical coherence tomography-guided, variable dosing regimen with intravitreal ranibizumab (Lucentis) for neovascular age-related macular degeneration. Am J Ophthalmol. 2007; 143 (4):566–583

[106] Boyer DS, Heier JS, Brown DM, Francom SF, Ianchulev T, Rubio RG. A Phase IIIb study to evaluate the safety of ranibizumab in subjects with neovascular age-related macular degeneration. Ophthalmology. 2009; 116(9):1731–1739

[107] Holz FG, Amoaku W, Donate J, et al. SUSTAIN Study Group. Safety and efficacy of a flexible dosing regimen of ranibizumab in neovascular age-related macular degeneration: the SUSTAIN study. Ophthalmology. 2011; 118 (4):663–671

[108] Brechner RJ, Rosenfeld PJ, Babish JD, Caplan S. Pharmacotherapy for neovascular age-related macular degeneration: an analysis of the 100% 2008 Medicare fee-for-service part B claims file. Am J Ophthalmol. 2011; 151(5):887–895.e1

[109] Martin DF, Maguire MG, Fine SL, et al. Comparison of Age-related Macular Degeneration Treatments Trials (CATT) Research Group. Ranibizumab and bevacizumab for treatment of neovascular age-related macular degeneration: two-year results. Ophthalmology. 2012; 119(7):1388–1398

[110] Kodjikian L, Souied EH, Mimoun G, et al. GEFAL Study Group. Ranibizumab versus Bevacizumab for Neovascular Age-related Macular Degeneration: Results from the GEFAL Noninferiority Randomized Trial. Ophthalmology. 2013; 120(11):2300–2309

[111] Chakravarthy U, Harding SP, Rogers CA, et al. IVAN study investigators. Alternative treatments to inhibit VEGF in age-related choroidal neovascularisation: 2-year findings of the IVAN randomised controlled trial. Lancet. 2013; 382(9900):1258–1267

[112] Berg K. Lucentis Compared to Avastin Study (LUCAS): treating exudative AMD with Lucentis (ranibizumab) versus Avastin (bevacizumab) following an “inject and extend” protocol, 1-year results. Paper presented at: the American Academy of Ophthalmology 2013 Annual Meeting; November 15–19, 2013; New Orleans, LA

[113] Schauwvlieghe AM, Dijkman G, Hooyman JM, et al; Comparing the effectiveness of bevacizumab to ranibizumab in patients with exudative age-related macular degeneration. BRAMD. Paper presented at: Association for Research in Vision and Ophthalmology Annual Meeting; May 3–8, 2014; Orlando, FL

[114] Krebs I, Schmetterer L, Boltz A, et al. MANTA Research Group. A randomised double-masked trial comparing the visual outcome after treatment with ranibizumab or bevacizumab in patients with neovascular age-related macular degeneration. Br J Ophthalmol. 2013; 97(3):266–271

[115] Nguyen QD, Shah SM, Browning DJ, et al. A phase I study of intravitreal vascular endothelial growth factor trap-eye in patients with neovascular age-related macular degeneration. Ophthalmology. 2009; 116(11):2141–8.e1

[116] Heier JS, Brown DM, Chong V, et al. VIEW 1 and VIEW 2 Study Groups. Intravitreal aflibercept (VEGF trap-eye) in wet age-related macular degeneration. Ophthalmology. 2012; 119(12):2537–2548

[117] Schmidt-Erfurth U, Kaiser PK, Korobelnik JF, et al. Intravitreal aflibercept injection for neovascular age-related macular degeneration: ninety-six-week results of the VIEW studies. Ophthalmology. 2014; 121(1):193–201

[118] Abedi F, Wickremasinghe S, Islam AF, Inglis KM, Guymer RH. Anti-VEGF treatment in neovascular age-related macular degeneration: a treat-and-extend protocol over 2 years. Retina. 2014; 34(8):1531–1538

[119] Rasmussen A, Sander B. Long-term longitudinal study of patients treated with ranibizumab for neovascular age-related macular degeneration. Curr Opin Ophthalmol. 2014; 25(3):158–163

[120] Fovista. Available at: http://www.ophthotech.com/product-candidates/fovista. Accessed August 29, 2014

[121] Dugel P. Results of ESBA 1008, a single-chain antibody fragment, for the treatment of neovascular AMD. Paper presented at: American Society of Retina Specialists 2014 Annual Meeting; August 9–13, 2014; San Diego, CA

[122] Slakter J. Interim results from a phase 2 study of squalamine lactate ophthalmic solution 0.2% in the treatment of neovascular age-related macular degeneration. Paper presented at: American Society of Retina Specialists 2014 Annual Meeting; August 9–13, 2014; San Diego, CA

[123] Regillo C. Lampalizumab (anti-factor D) in patients with geographic atrophy: the MAHALO phase 2 results. Paper presented at: the American Academy of Ophthalmology 2013 Annual Meeting; November 15–19, 2013; New Orleans, LA

15 Miscellaneous Macular Degenerations

Samuel K. Steven Houston III and Allen C. Ho

15.1 Pathologic Myopia

Pathologic myopia is one of the leading causes of blindness in the world. In the United States and Europe, it ranks seventh among all the diseases that cause significant, uncorrectable visual loss.[1] Loss of visual acuity is caused by either exudative or progressively atrophic macular degeneration. In general, affected individuals have at least 6 diopters of myopia. Progressive myopia is the hallmark of the condition and is attributed to progressive elongation of the eye.[2] The prevalence of pathologic myopia varies among different races and ethnic groups, and appears to be more common in women than men. In the United States, the condition is found in 2.1% of 17-year-olds.[1] In comparison, the prevalence elsewhere has been reported to be as low as 0.2% in Egypt and as high as 9.6% in Spain.[3]

15.1.1 Clinical Features

The clinical findings in pathologic myopia are believed to be the result of progressive elongation of the eye. Some of these features may be present in patients with low to moderate degrees of myopia (less than 6 diopters of myopia), whereas some patients with high degrees of myopia may demonstrate a relatively normal fundus.

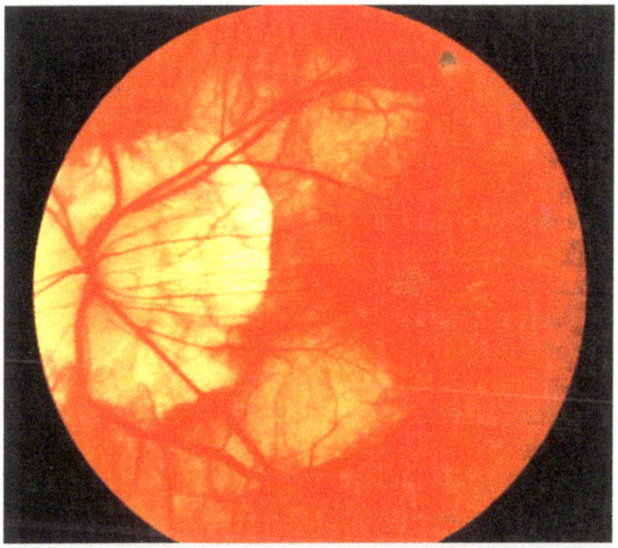

Fig. 15.1 Pathologic myopia: A peripapillary myopic crescent located predominantly on the temporal aspect of the optic disc. A macular hemorrhage adjacent to a lacquer crack is also evident.

The hallmark ophthalmoscopic finding is a peripapillary "myopic" crescent (▶ Fig. 15.1). It usually appears as a hypopigmented, sharply defined area on the temporal aspect of the optic disc, where there is attenuation of the retinal pigment epithelium (RPE), smaller choroidal vessels, and a scleral shell. The borders of the crescent may extend superiorly and nasally and are commonly irregularly delineated by clumps of pigment. Occasionally the myopic crescent extends into the macula and through fixation. Uncommonly, it is located only on the nasal side (myopia inversus). The presence of the crescent correlates with axial length but not with overall total refractive error, as the latter is also influenced by corneal and lenticular factors. Commonly, the optic disc is vertically elongated and may be tilted, with a flattened temporal side. This optic nerve head configuration can make it difficult to assess the degree of cupping when glaucoma is suspected.

Posterior pole staphylomas may also be observed and are characterized by well-circumscribed, nummular areas of chorioretinal atrophy that are white in appearance (▶ Fig. 15.2). When these lesions enlarge and extend into the central macula, loss of vision can follow. The prevalence of staphyloma is also related to increasing axial length.

Less dramatic but important fundus features may be observed in eyes with pathologic myopia. The RPE of the macula may demonstrate varying degrees of mottling. Yellow, linear, subretinal streaks in the macula are known as *lacquer cracks* and are observed in 4% of highly myopic eyes.[4] They correspond to disruptions in Bruch's membrane, and because they herald subsequent widespread chorioretinal degeneration, they are a poor visual prognostic sign (▶ Fig. 15.1).[5] Fuchs' spots are round or oval areas of subretinal hyperpigmentation, which may be found in up to 10% of individuals with pathologic myopia, typically after the age of 30 years (▶ Fig. 15.3). These spots are bilateral in 40% of the patients, with the second eye being involved within 5 years.[5] Fuchs' spots are believed to be the sequelae of previous subretinal hemorrhage or choroidal neovascularization (CNV). They may have a surrounding area of depigmented atrophy and can significantly affect vision if close to the fovea.

Most patients with pathologic myopia slowly lose central vision because of the progressive atrophic, degenerative

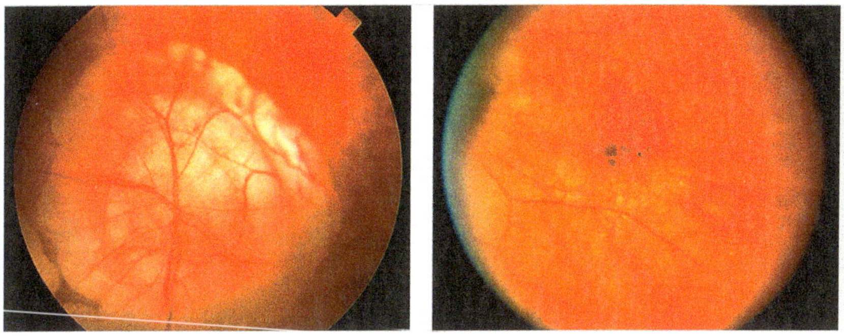

Fig. 15.2 Pathologic myopia: A posterior pole staphyloma encompassing the optic disc and also extending into the macular region. Note the excavated appearance and discrete borders of the lesion. Also note the difference in focus at the optic disc and the adjacent pigmented retina, which reflects the staphylomatous axial elongation.

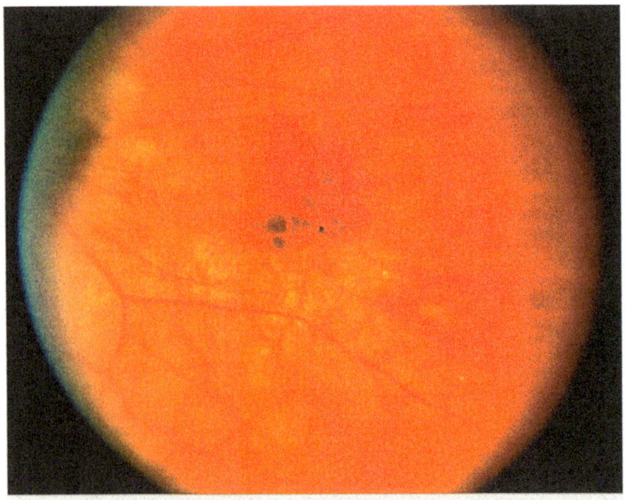

Fig. 15.3 Pathologic myopia: A Fuchs' spot with an adjacent macular hemorrhage. Fuchs' spots are the sequelae of previous subretinal hemorrhage or choroidal neovascularization.

changes described earlier. Sudden and often more severe loss of visual acuity is typically a consequence of superimposed, subretinal exudative changes resulting from CNV (▶ Fig. 15.4).[6] The exudative changes consist primarily of subretinal hemorrhage and fluid. There may be an associated elevation of the RPE that can be seen on spectral-domain optical coherence tomography (SD-OCT). SD-OCT can also identify subretinal and intraretinal hemorrhage or fluid. Fluorescein angiography (FA) usually reveals well-delineated, typically classic CNV lesions located near or beneath the fovea (▶ Fig. 15.5). Overall, the neovascular process tends to be less extensive and less aggressive than that found in age-related macular degeneration (AMD), with much less subretinal fluid or macular edema.

Pearls

- Myopic macular hemorrhage demonstrates a variable visual prognosis. For subfoveal hemorrhage associated with CNV, anti–vascular endothelial growth factor (anti-VEGF) treatment has emerged as the treatment of choice.

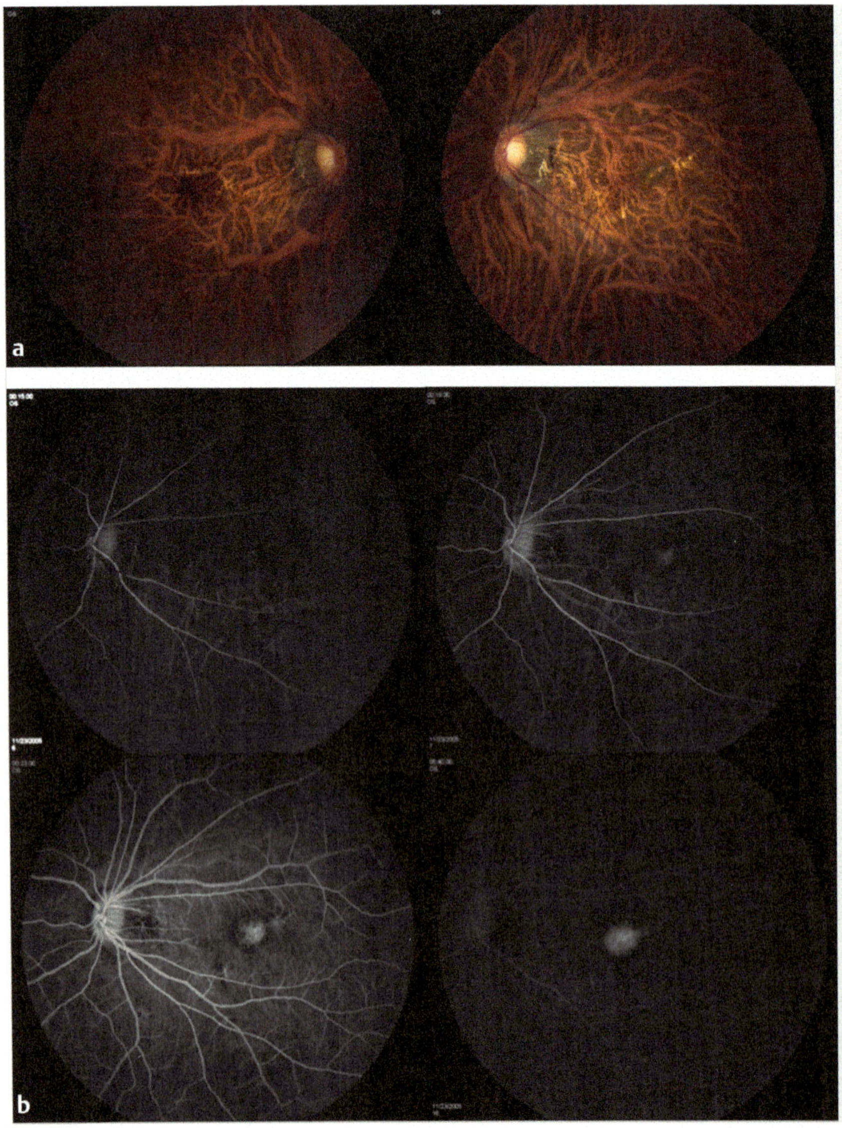

Fig. 15.4 Pathologic myopia: Both eyes show atrophy of the retinal pigment epithelium with visualization of the deep choroidal vessels. The left eye shows a gray-green choroidal neovascularization juxtafoveally, just temporal to the fovea. (**a**) Fluorescein angiography shows a classic lesion in the early phase, (**b**) with progressive leakage through the later phases.

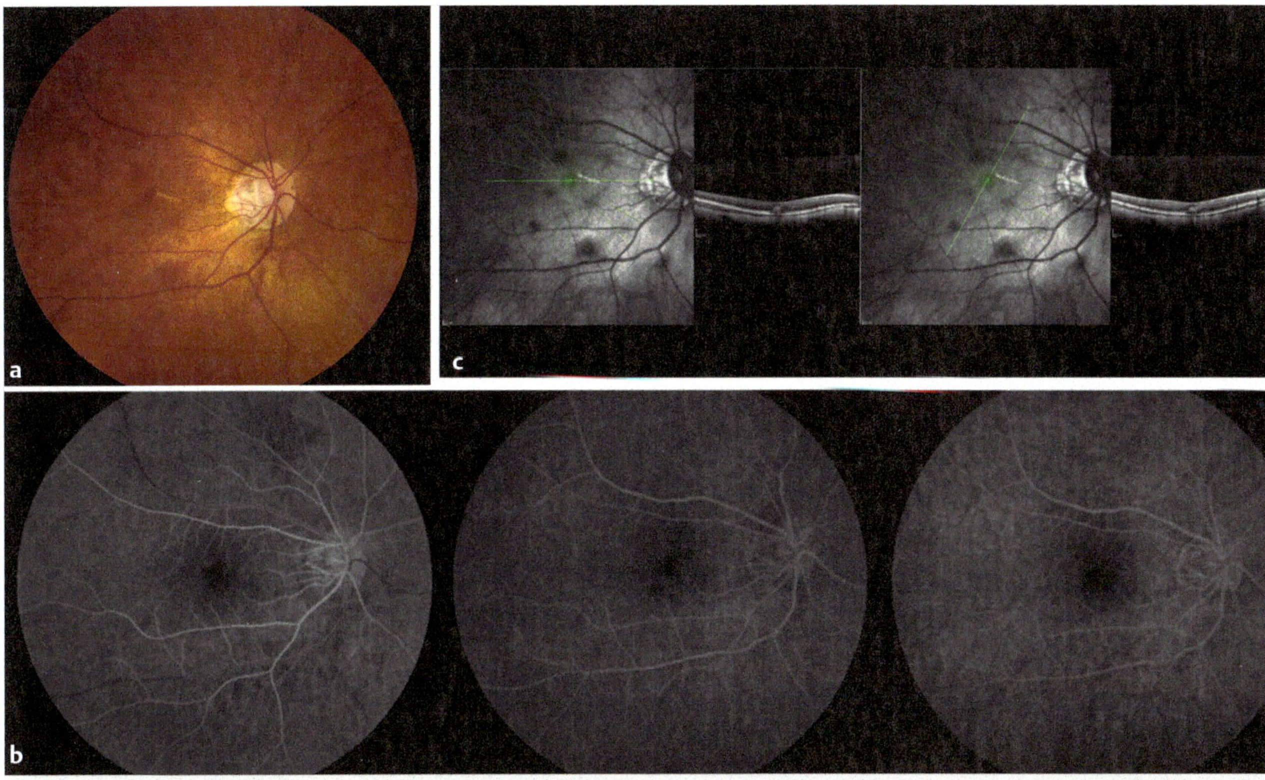

Fig. 15.5 Pathologic myopia. (a) The right eye shows a central foveal retinal hemorrhage. (b) Fluorescein angiography shows hypofluorescence from blockage by the blood. (c) SD-OCT shows subretinal elevation with intraretinal hyperreflectivity.

Of note is that some patients who present with new macular hemorrhages in the setting of pathologic myopia may not have evidence of CNV on FA (▶ Fig. 15.1). In this situation, neovascularization is either occult (obscured by the hemorrhage) or not present. Regardless of the source, submacular hemorrhages in eyes with pathologic myopia are associated with a variable visual prognosis depending on proximity to the fovea, and it is important to realize that many patients with extrafoveal lesions can retain excellent central visual acuity. However, in patients with subfoveal or juxtafoveal lesions, treatment with photodynamic therapy (PDT) and anti-VEGF agents has been investigated.

The peripheral retina of patients with pathologic myopia generally demonstrates diffuse pigmentary alterations and often has a tigroid appearance. Patchy or diffuse areas of atrophy of the retina and choroid are often observed. Patients with pathologic myopia are at increased risk for retinal tears and retinal detachment.

15.1.2 Diagnosis

The diagnosis of pathologic myopia is suggested by the history of requiring correction for high refractive error and, occasionally, by family history. The axial length of the eye is typically greater than 26 mm. The diagnosis is then confirmed by observing the constellation of fundus features described earlier.

The differential diagnosis varies depending on the predominant clinical features. Patients with anomalous, tilted discs usually demonstrate an inferior scleral crescent with an irregular vascular pattern emanating from the optic nerve head and an area of fundus ectasia inferotemporally. The myopic crescent is more commonly located temporally. The presumed ocular histoplasmosis syndrome (POHS) demonstrates peripapillary pigmentary alterations, scattered "punched-out" chorioretinal atrophic lesions, and macular CNV. This syndrome, however, has no predilection for patients with high myopic refractive errors. Macular conditions that manifest serous or serosanguinous exudations, such as AMD or central serous chorioretinopathy, may be confused with myopic macular degeneration when incidental myopia and peripapillary pigmentary changes are present. Gyrate atrophy is an uncommon autosomal recessive condition characterized by multiple, sharply demarcated areas of geographic chorioretinal atrophy beginning in the midperipheral fundus in childhood and then coalescing to involve larger portions of the fundus with increasing age. These patients are often highly myopic, and if this precocious pattern of degeneration is observed, gyrate atrophy should be considered in the differential diagnosis (see Chapter 22).

15.1.3 Pathogenesis and Histopathology

The pathogenesis of the macular degenerative changes in highly myopic eyes is not well understood, although they are believed to be influenced in part by genetic factors. Progressive axial elongation distends the ocular coats and causes the peripapillary, retinal, choroidal, and scleral degenerative changes. Resultant abnormalities at the level of Bruch's membrane probably underlie the predisposition to CNV, as is the case with the other diseases discussed in this chapter.

Histopathologically, the sclera is thin, with areas of corresponding changes in the architecture of its collagen bundles. Degenerative changes involving the choriocapillaris, Bruch's membrane, and the RPE are also observed, with thinning of the choroid and an absence of vasculature in some areas.[7] The RPE cells appear flatter and larger than usual. Bruch's membrane is thinned and areas of dehiscences can be observed. There is also an associated thinning of the neurosensory retina, particularly in areas overlying choroidal atrophy. The thickness of the neurosensory macula is reduced partially because of thinning of the ganglion cell layer.

15.1.4 Management and Course

At this time, there are no proven therapies to prevent progressive elongation of the globe in pathologic myopia. In the hope of slowing down or preventing significant atrophic macular degeneration, scleral resection and reinforcement procedures have been performed. Limited reports indicate achievement of some degree of axial length or staphyloma stabilization.[8,9] However, beneficial effects on the visual outcome have never been demonstrated definitively.

Efforts have concentrated on CNV detection and treatment. Patients who experience sudden loss of vision and who manifest macular exudative or hemorrhagic changes should have a SD-OCT and an FA to identify and determine the extent of the CNV (▶ Fig. 15.4 and ▶ Fig. 15.5). If there is just blocked fluorescence from hemorrhage, indocyanine green angiography (ICG) may help to identify or rule out underlying CNV. Unfortunately, when CNV is identified, it is located under the foveal center in approximately 60 to 75% of cases.[3,5] Although the behavior of CNV is not as aggressive as it is in AMD, it is nonetheless associated with a variable degree of central visual loss.[10]

For nonsubfoveal CNV in eyes with myopic degeneration, laser photocoagulation has been shown to be effective in preventing visual loss.[11,12] However, recurrence rates of CNV can be high, and of particular concern, there can be significant, progressive enlargement of the laser photocoagulation scars with time (▶ Fig. 15.6).[13] As a result, patients with juxtafoveal (within 200 µm from the foveal center) and particularly with subfoveal CNV are not good candidates for laser treatment. Prior to the advent of anti-VEGF agents, PDT was used in the treatment of CNV associated with myopic degeneration. The VIP Study was a randomized, controlled clinical trial investigating the use of verteporfin with PDT versus placebo in the treatment of myopia-associated CNV. The study enrolled 120 patients with subfoveal CNV; approximately 90% had evidence of a classic CNV lesion. The 1-year results showed that PDT with verteporfin was associated with less visual acuity loss compared to placebo. The main outcome measure (proportion of eyes with a

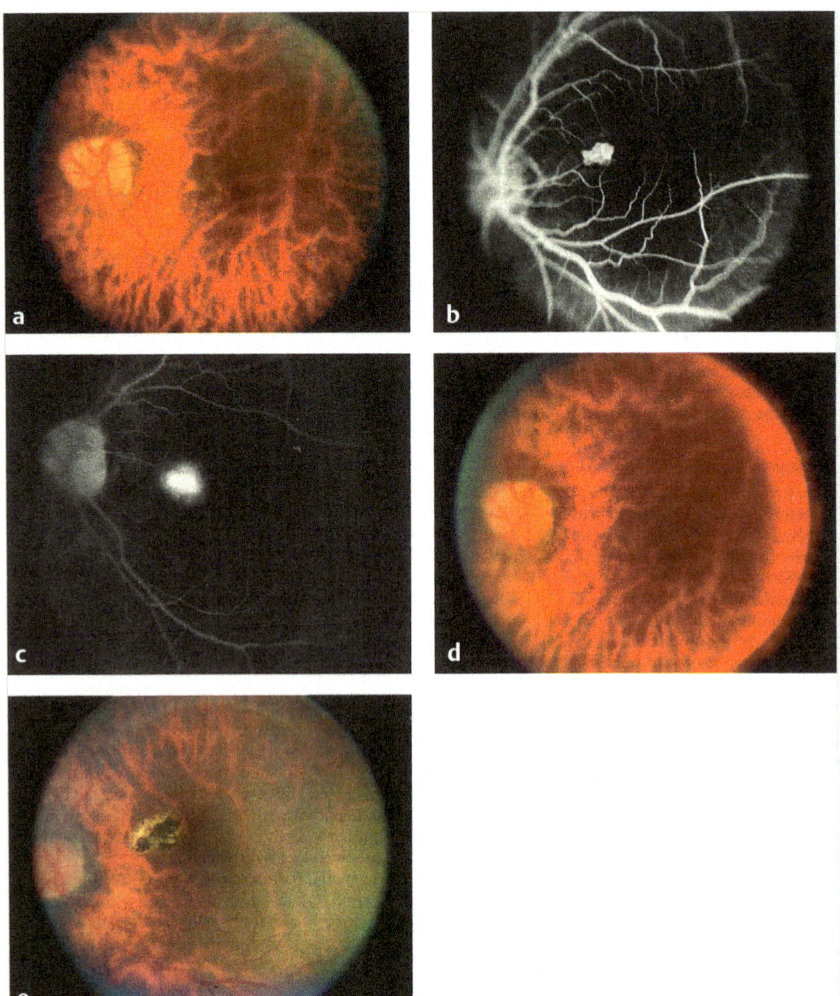

Fig. 15.6 Pathologic myopia. (**a**) A grayish green subretinal lesion is present just nasal to the fovea. There is some associated subretinal hemorrhage and fluid. The vision is 20/25. (**b**) Early-phase fluorescein angiogram demonstrates early hyperfluorescence of the lesion. (**c**) Late-phase fluorescein angiogram frame reveals dye leakage, consistent with choroidal neovascularization. (**d**) The eye was treated with laser photocoagulation because the fellow eye had a poor visual outcome resulting from choroidal neovascularization. Shortly after treatment, there was resolution of the exudative signs. (**e**) By 6 months after treatment, increased pigmentation and expansion of the laser scar were evident. The vision was stable at 20/25.

visual acuity loss of less than 8 Early Treatment Diabetic Retinopathy Study (ETDRS) letters) was statistically significant between the groups (72 vs. 44%; $p < 0.01$). In the PDT group, 86% of patients lost less than 15 ETDRS letters of vision, compared to 67% in the control group. In addition, 32% of patients treated with PDT gained at least 5 ETDRS letters compared to 15% in controls.[14] At the 2-year follow-up, the main outcome measure (loss of less than 8 ETDRS letters) was no longer statistically significant (64 vs. 49%; $p = 0.11$). However, 40% of patients in the PDT group gained 5 or more letters compared to only 13% in the control group.[15] This study led to the adoption of PDT with verteporfin as treatment for subfoveal CNV secondary to myopic degeneration until the use of anti-VEGF agents in 2006.[16,17]

The use of intravitreal bevacizumab led to a paradigm shift in the management of AMD-associated CNV, with the ANCHOR[18] and MARINA[19] trials showing that anti-VEGF therapy with ranibizumab not only prevented severe visual loss in the majority of patients, but also was associated with a mean gain in visual acuity of 8 to 10 ETDRS letters; almost 40% of patients gained three or more lines of vision (=15 ETDRS letters). Early case series demonstrated the efficacy of intravitreal bevacizumab for the treatment of CNV secondary to myopic degeneration.[16,17] A systematic review and meta-analysis demonstrated that anti-VEGF agents were superior to PDT at 2 years in improving visual acuity in eyes with myopia-associated CNV. The pooled data showed that 35% of 513 patients gained three or more lines of visual acuity with an associated decrease in OCT-measured central retinal thickness.[20] Although anti-VEGF therapy has proven efficacy in stabilizing and often improving visual acuity in myopia-associated CNV, optimal treatment protocols have not been determined. Most studies utilize either one injection followed by pro re nata (PRN) treatment based on OCT findings, visual acuity, and clinical examination or three monthly injections followed by PRN treatment. The RADIANCE study[21] was a randomized, double-masked, controlled trial investigating intravitreal ranibizumab versus PDT in the treatment of CNV secondary to pathologic myopia. The study included 277 patients divided into three groups: (1) two initial monthly ranibizumab injections followed by PRN injections based on visual acuity; (2) one initial ranibizumab injection followed by PRN injections based on disease activity; and (3) PDT with verteporfin with rescue ranibizumab after month 3. Intravitreal ranibizumab was found to be superior to PDT with respect to visual acuity outcomes. At month 3, the two ranibizumab groups gained on average 10.5 ETDRS letters compared to 2.2 letters in the PDT group. At month 12, the ranibizumab monotherapy groups gained an average of 13.8 to 14.4 ETDRS letters. The group that received PDT followed by ranibizumab after month 3 gained an average of 9.3 letters compared to baseline but did not catch up to the ranibizumab monotherapy. Both intravitreal ranibizumab treatment protocols were associated with similar visual acuity gains, with group 1 receiving a median of four injections compared to two injections in group 2.

Although studies have used both bevacizumab and ranibizumab in the treatment of CNV secondary to pathologic myopia, small case series show similar efficacy between agents[22] and the CATT and IVAN[23,24] studies reported similar clinical efficacy between ranibizumab and bevacizumab in eyes with exudative AMD. Despite the efficacy of anti-VEGF therapy in the management of myopia-related CNV, patients need close follow-up after cessation of treatment. Monitoring with a home Amsler grid combined with frequent follow-up including SD-OCT and clinical examination may identify disease reactivation that has been shown to occur in up to 25% of patients.[25] Risk factors for CNV recurrence include increasing age, greater myopia, decreased choroidal thickness, larger CNV lesions, and subfoveal hemorrhage. Lacquer cracks extending through the fovea, baseline visual acuity, and peripapillary choroidal atrophy were prognostic factors for visual acuity after treatment.[26]

Intravitreal anti-VEGF therapy has emerged as the standard of care in the treatment of CNV secondary to myopic degeneration. Unlike AMD, myopia-related CNV usually responds to two to four injections with the majority of retina specialists utilizing a PRN treatment approach.

15.2 Presumed Ocular Histoplasmosis Syndrome

Histoplasma capsulatum is a soil mold found predominantly in the central and eastern United States, particularly the Ohio–Mississippi River Valley area.[27] Respiratory tract infections are usually asymptomatic and self-limited. POHS is likely the result of a subclinical systemic infection by this organism many years prior. The clinical syndrome of peripapillary chorioretinal changes, multiple macular and peripheral chorioretinal atrophic lesions, macular CNV, and an absence of inflammation was first described in 1960.[28] It is unusual to have active *H. capsulatum* intraocular infection. Panuveitis has been described in chronically ill and immunocompromised patients but is not a feature of POHS.[29]

15.2.1 Clinical Features

The classic triad of POHS includes peripapillary chorioretinal atrophy, multiple "punched-out" chorioretinal scars, and acute or chronic macular exudative changes from CNV (▶ Fig. 15.7). Patients are often young, usually between 20 and 50 years of age, and have visited or lived in the Ohio–Mississippi River Valley area; the incidence of "histo spots" is estimated to be 2.6% in this endemic area.[30] Prior exposure to pigeons, chickens, or parakeets may be significant.

The peripapillary chorioretinal atrophic changes can vary in degree. A rim of pigment separating the optic disc from the adjacent atrophy may be present.[31] The "punched-out" lesions are scattered throughout the fundus, are typically less than 1 mm in diameter, often have surrounding hyperpigmentation, and do not demonstrate significant elevation. Occasionally, these "histo spots" may form peripheral depigmented linear streaks that suggest a choroidal vascular predilection (▶ Fig. 15.8).[32] The streaks are often equatorial in distribution and may be found in as many as 5% of patients with POHS. An absence of anterior chamber inflammation and vitreous cells is characteristic of POHS.

Patients with POHS are usually asymptomatic, but occasionally they present with sudden visual distortion or loss of vision. Visual symptoms are typically the result of macular CNV with secondary exudative changes (▶ Fig. 15.9 and ▶ Fig. 15.10).[33,34,35] The CNV is often visible ophthalmoscopically and appears

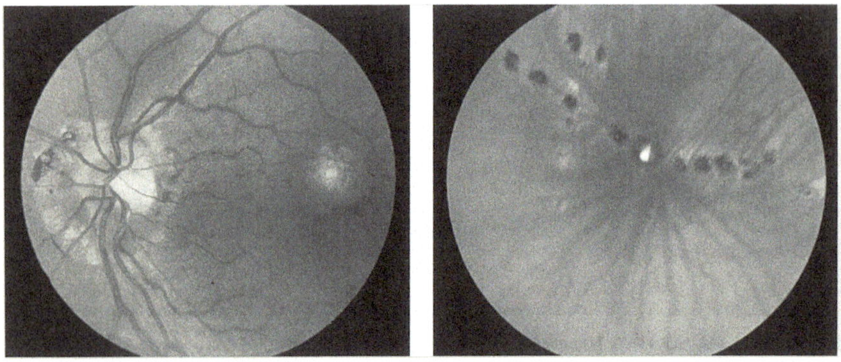

Fig. 15.7 Presumed ocular histoplasmosis syndrome: peripapillary chorioretinal scarring with patchy areas of hyperpigmentation and hypopigmentation. Just superior to the fovea is a flat, atrophic chorioretinal scar with associated intraretinal hemorrhage from underlying choroidal neovascularization.

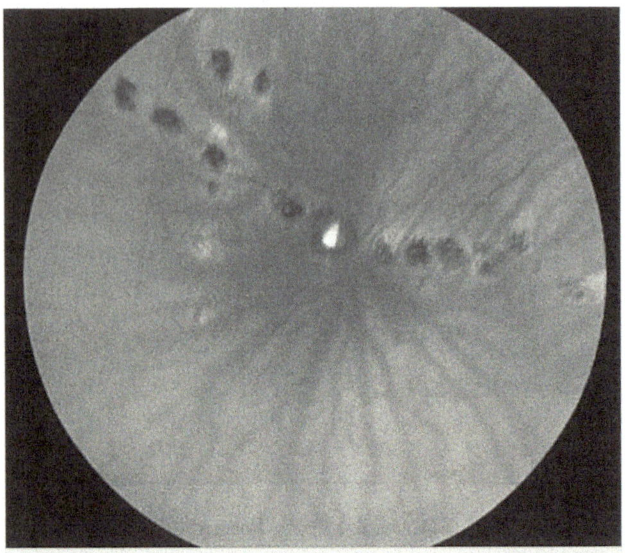

Fig. 15.8 Presumed ocular histoplasmosis syndrome: equatorial chorioretinal "histo spots" with typical atrophy and hyperpigmentation. The composite of spots comprises a peripheral linear streak. Peripheral linear streaks may also be observed in multifocal choroiditis and myopic degeneration.

under the neurosensory retina as a slightly elevated, gray-green lesion (▶ Fig. 15.9). FA usually shows the CNV to be well delineated, with classic early hyperfluorescence and late leakage. OCT findings may show subretinal or sub-RPE neovascular CNV with exudation as evident by subretinal and intraretinal fluid. The CNV lesions are most commonly classic on FA, and OCT shows type 2 lesions.

15.2.2 Diagnosis

The diagnosis of POHS is generally made in the setting of a suggestive exposure or geographic history and funduscopic features including at least two of the three components of the classic triad. Ophthalmoscopically, several other conditions may resemble POHS. In myopic degeneration, atrophic spots can be observed, but these are typically whiter and larger than POHS spots. Myopic degeneration also has peripapillary changes, but the myopic crescent often has a rim of pigment on the outer edge and not the inner edge, as observed in POHS. Furthermore, the optic disc in myopic degeneration is often tilted, but not in POHS. Lacquer cracks and Fuchs' spots would also not be expected in POHS.

Multifocal choroiditis is another condition that presents with multiple, atrophic "punched-out" lesions. The atrophic lesions in multifocal choroiditis, however, do not usually demonstrate marginal hyperpigmentation. Furthermore, there is often evidence of mild anterior uveitis or vitritis, not seen in POHS. Although both conditions can lead to CNV, multifocal choroiditis tends ultimately to be associated with more diffuse submacular fibrosis.

Pearls

- POHS may be confused with multifocal choroiditis. Patients with POHS, however, have no evidence of anterior chamber or vitreous inflammation.

Eyes with angioid streaks may have atrophic chorioretinal spots, but the spots tend to cluster in the equatorial region of the fundus, which does not occur in POHS. Although peripapillary changes and CNV are seen in both conditions, close inspection of the peripapillary retina should reveal the radially oriented subretinal streaks characteristic of angioid streaks.

Patients older than 50 years in whom CNV develops are more likely to have AMD than POHS. Drusen in the macula and the lack of punched-out peripheral lesions should lead to the correct diagnosis of AMD. Sometimes, however, CNV and exudative changes do develop in patients with POHS when they are older. In these cases, the CNV tends to behave in a more aggressive fashion than in those patients who present at an earlier age. Investigation of the natural history of POHS shows that visual acuity in eyes with POHS-associated CNV drops to less than 20/200 in the majority of patients within a few years.[36]

15.2.3 Pathogenesis and Histopathology

The syndrome is "presumed" secondary to infection with the fungus *H. capsulatum* because organisms are typically not found in the eyes of patients who manifest the classic clinical findings.[27] The exposure and acute infection are thought generally to be subclinical and take place years before the ophthalmoscopic presentation of disease.[31] The proposed pathogenesis is that a primary, subclinical pulmonary infection with *H. capsulatum* leads to the formation of multiple small granulomas throughout the body, including the choroid.[31,33,37] Lymphocytic infiltration of these granulomas is hypothesized to produce gradual enlargement of the scars to the point where they

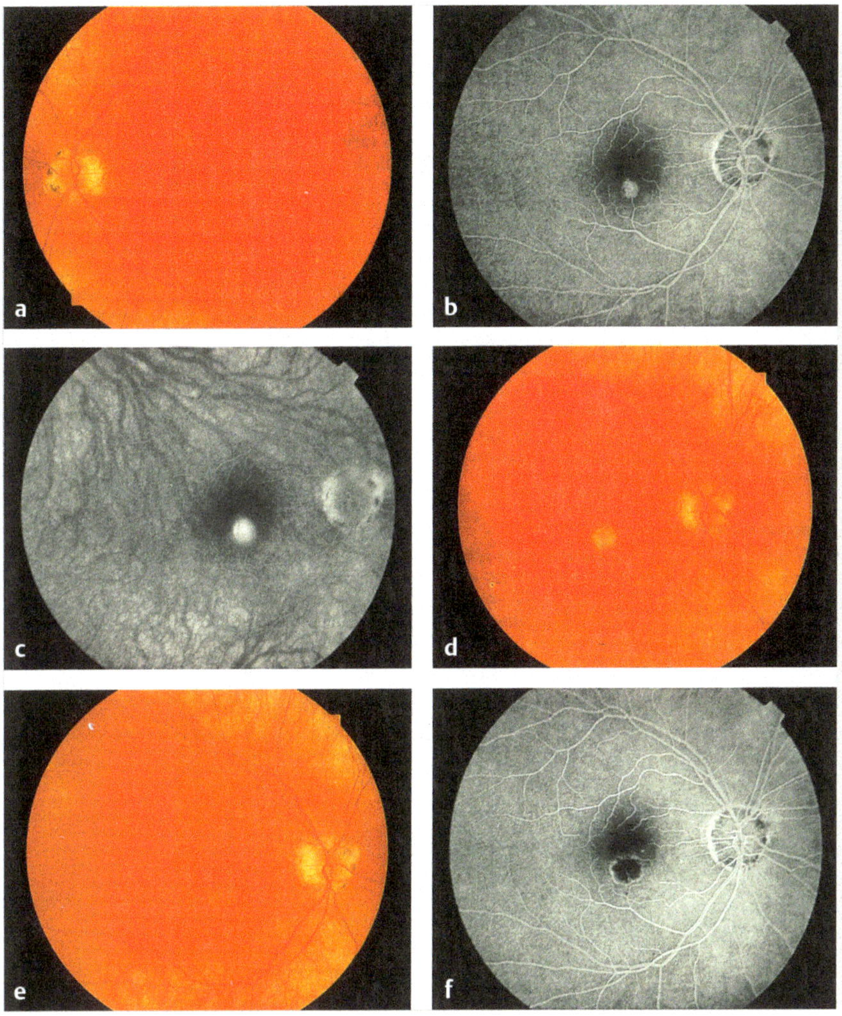

Fig. 15.9 Presumed ocular histoplasmosis syndrome. (a) A gray-green subretinal lesion with a small amount of surrounding fluid is present just inferior to the fovea. The corresponding fluorescein angiogram shows (b) early hyperfluorescence and (c) late leakage, consistent with choroidal neovascularization. It is well defined and juxtafoveal in location. (d) Fundus photograph taken immediately after laser photocoagulation treatment. Note the intense, gray-white, confluent laser mark covering the lesion. (e) Fundus photograph and (f) fluorescein angiogram approximately 1 month after treatment show a dry laser scar and no angiographic evidence of persistent neovascularization.

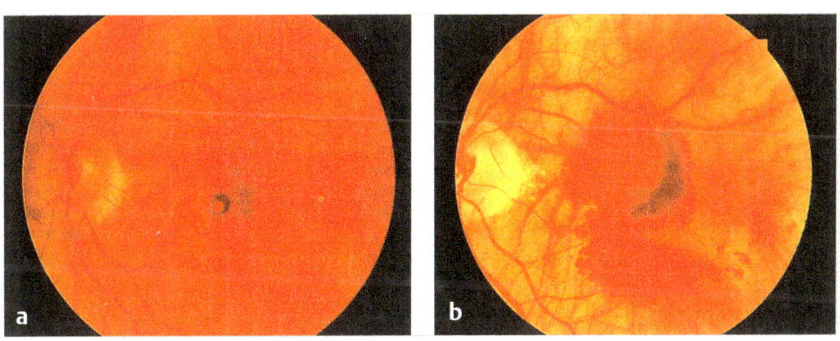

Fig. 15.10 Presumed ocular histoplasmosis syndrome. (a) A pigmented lesion suggestive of choroidal neovascularization with surrounding subretinal hemorrhage and fluid. The patient declined treatment and was observed. (b) During the course of 1 year, the lesion continued to grow and resulted in a large subretinal hemorrhage and a dramatic decline in visual acuity.

become typical “histo spots.”[38,39,40,41] Histopathologic studies have confirmed focal lymphocytic infiltrates beneath areas of submacular hemorrhage and CNV as well as in the areas of peripheral atrophic scars. The exact mechanism leading to CNV in POHS is not well understood, although it is assumed that the structural defects in Bruch’s membrane at the site of the “histo spots” likely contribute to neovascular ingrowth. CNV can occur many years following primary infection, often at the edges of “histo spots.” Studies have shown evidence of *H. capsulatum* DNA in these scars, indicating that there may be a role of chronic inflammation in the development of CNV.[42]

15.2.4 Management and Course

Asymptomatic patients with POHS must be educated about their disease. Patients with any “histo spots” in the macula, especially if one eye has any CNV-related maculopathy, are at highest risk for development of CNV and central vision loss. They should be instructed to monitor the integrity of their central vision with an Amsler grid on a daily basis and to report any new symptoms immediately. Regular funduscopic examinations should be performed, including SD-OCT of these macular lesions.

Clinical trials from the Macular Photocoagulation Study Group have demonstrated that laser photocoagulation of well-defined extrafoveal CNV in the setting of POHS is associated with a significantly reduced risk of severe visual acuity loss.[43,44] Laser photocoagulation of subfoveal CNV associated with POHS was *not* demonstrated to be beneficial.[45] Fortunately, fellow eyes can have a favorable prognosis (9% incidence within 5 years or about 2% per year) if there are no preexisting macular abnormalities. However, if there are any "histo spots" in the macula, typical or atypical, the risk for CNV in that eye is tripled.[46] PDT has also been investigated in the treatment of CNV secondary to POHS, especially in patients who did not benefit from laser photocoagulation (notably, patients with subfoveal CNV). There are only small case series investigating PDT for these lesions[47] that demonstrate possible efficacy. A prospective, uncontrolled study looked at 22 patients who completed 24-month follow-up. Patients were treated with initial PDT followed by retreatment at 3-month intervals if FA demonstrated evidence of leakage. At 24 months, median visual acuity improvement was + 6 letters. Additionally, 45% of patients gained at least 7 letters, while only 18% lost 8 or more letters.[48] PDT was a promising treatment for subfoveal lesions until the widespread adoption of anti-VEGF therapy. With the demonstration that anti-VEGF agents could not only preserve but also often improve vision in eyes with AMD-associated CNV, these agents have been used successfully in the treatment of other causes of CNV, including POHS. Case reports and case series have demonstrated the efficacy of intravitreal bevacizumab in the treatment of CNV secondary to POHS.[49,50,51,52] A retrospective, comparative case series investigated 150 eyes of 140 patients with subfoveal or juxtafoveal CNV secondary to POHS. The study compared intravitreal bevacizumab monotherapy versus combination therapy with intravitreal bevacizumab and PDT. Intravitreal bevacizumab monotherapy was used in 116 eyes and these patients showed a significant improvement in visual acuity from 20/83 at baseline to 20/54 at 2 years. Patients with subfoveal lesions showed a significant improvement from 20/132 at baseline to 20/63 at 2 years. Combination treatment (intravitreal bevacizumab and PDT) was performed in 34 eyes with subfoveal CNV and was associated with an improvement in visual acuity from 20/174 at baseline to 20/75 at 2 years. However, only 10 patients had 2-year follow-up, so the results were not statistically significant. In both groups, approximately 30% of patients gained three or more lines of vision with treatment. The monotherapy group received an average of 3.33 injections per year, while the combination group received an average of 2.42 injections per year. Although a key limitation of this study was the lack of standardized retreatment criteria, the study demonstrated that intravitreal bevacizumab as monotherapy or combined with PDT can stabilize and often improve visual acuity in patients with subfoveal CNV secondary to POHS.[53]

Pearls

- In POHS, the Macular Photocoagulation Study Group demonstrated a treatment benefit for patients with extrafoveal but not subfoveal CNV. However, recent studies favor anti-VEGF agents as the first-line treatment for subfoveal or juxtafoveal CNV associated with POHS.

Surgical extraction of subfoveal CNV was performed in the past, but with the advent of anti-VEGF agents, this technique has fallen out of favor. The Submacular Surgery Trial showed no significant benefit with surgery compared to observation, with 58% of patients in the surgery group having recurrence of CNV.[54]

Pearls

- In patients with POHS and a history of CNV in one eye, the risk for development of neovascularization in the fellow eye is much higher if any "histo spots" are present in the macula.

15.3 Angioid Streaks

Angioid streaks are irregular, tapering, linear breaks in Bruch's membrane that typically emanate from the optic disc. They were first described by Doyne in 1889[55] and termed *angioid* by Knapp[56] because of the vessel-like appearance of these lesions. Angioid streaks are of both ophthalmic and systemic interest because they are associated with an underlying, potentially serious systemic disease in approximately 50% of patients. Diagnostic work-up of 50 patients with angioid streaks demonstrated that one-half of the cases were idiopathic and the other half were associated in descending order with pseudoxanthoma elasticum, Paget's disease, sickle cell hemoglobinopathies, Ehlers–Danlos syndrome, and a variety of rare conditions.[57]

15.3.1 Clinical Features

Angioid streaks may appear light red-orange to dark red-brown, depending on the underlying color and pigmentation of the choroid (▶ Fig. 15.11). The radiating streaks are often joined

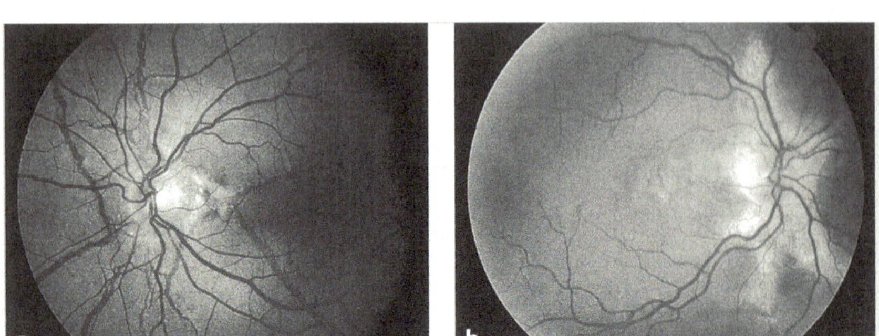

Fig. 15.11 Angioid streaks. **(a)** Typical angioid streaks radiating from the optic nerve head. **(b)** The streaks can vary in pigmentation and width, as seen in this fundus photograph.

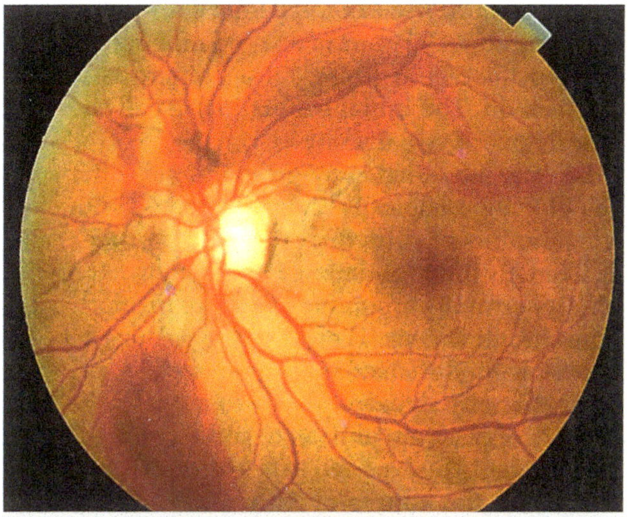

Fig. 15.12 Angioid streaks: minor blunt trauma to the left eye of a patient with angioid streaks. Multiple patches of subretinal hemorrhage are seen in the peripapillary area. (Image provided courtesy of Carl D. Regillo, MD.)

near the optic disc by a circumferential streak and may extend into the macula and occasionally the peripheral retina. The width of the streaks can vary from a thin line to four to five times the diameter of retinal vessels, and they typically taper as they extend away from the optic disc (▶ Fig. 15.11). They are usually bilateral.[58] In some instances, there is fibrovascular ingrowth or more diffuse overlying alterations of the RPE. Optic nerve head drusen or a mottled pigmentary appearance to the retina (*peau d'orange*) is also sometimes observed, particularly in association with pseudoxanthoma elasticum.[59] With time, some streaks may progressively enlarge and develop a more atrophic appearance, at which point the streaks become more difficult to discern.

CNV is the major cause of vision loss associated with angioid streaks.[59] The vision loss is usually abrupt and is caused by the presence of subretinal fluid or blood in the macula resulting from CNV that typically emanates from a streak. Occasionally, subretinal hemorrhage can occur without CNV. Relatively minor degrees of blunt ocular trauma can result in choroidal rupture, with an extension of the angioid streaks and subretinal hemorrhage in or around the macula (▶ Fig. 15.12).[58,59]

15.3.2 Diagnosis

Angioid streaks can be very subtle or very obvious, depending on the color contrast between the streak and the background fundus. The streaks are hyperfluorescent on FA, and this finding may be useful to help confirm their presence and make the diagnosis in some cases.[60] SD-OCT can show hyperreflectivity at the level of Bruch's membrane, suggestive of calcium deposits.[61] With the development of CNV, SD-OCT may show signs of exudation such as subretinal or intraretinal fluid. Choroidal thickness on SD-OCT has been correlated with risk of CNV development in eyes with angioid streaks. Choroidal thickness measurements were found to be less in patients who developed CNV compared to controls and those who did not develop CNV.[62] As noted previously, angioid streaks are associated with systemic findings of various diseases in about one-half of presentations.[57]

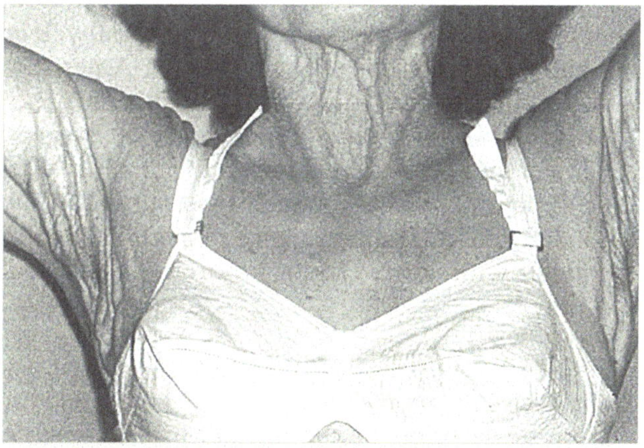

Fig. 15.13 Angioid streaks: the characteristic skin folds on the flexor aspects of the joints of a patient with pseudoxanthoma elasticum. (Image provided courtesy of the Wills Eye Hospital resident slide collection.)

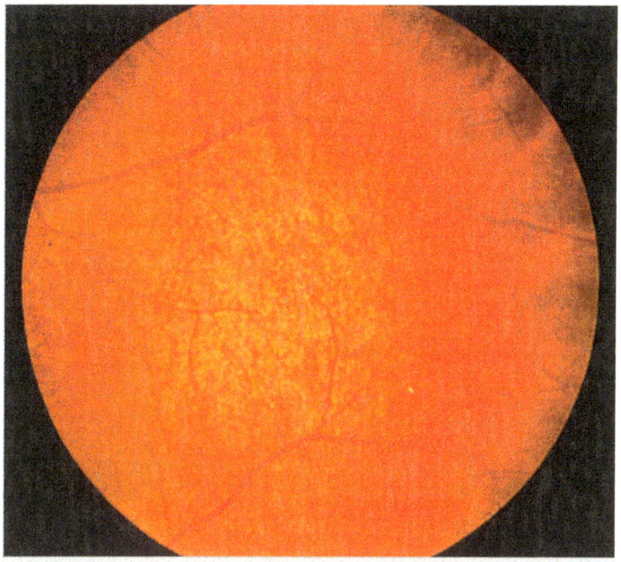

Fig. 15.14 Angioid streaks: The classic *peau d'orange* fundus of a patient with pseudoxanthoma elasticum. Note the multiple, yellow-orange lesions at the level of the retinal pigment epithelium.

Pseudoxanthoma Elasticum

Pseudoxanthoma elasticum is the most common disease associated with angioid streaks (▶ Fig. 15.13). Systemically, it is characterized by loose skin folds in the neck and on the flexor aspect of joints, potential cardiovascular disease, and an increased risk for gastrointestinal bleeding.[63] The appearance of the skin is likened to that of "chicken skin," with multiple yellow papules noted around the neck, flexor surfaces, and periumbilical areas. These skin manifestations are caused by abnormal dermal elastic tissue. This connective tissue abnormality also accounts for the increased risk of gastrointestinal and cardiovascular complications. Ophthalmoscopically, patients with pseudoxanthoma elasticum often demonstrate the *peau d'orange* fundus or orange skin appearance of the RPE (▶ Fig. 15.14). Such pigmentary changes are often seen in the temporal midperiphery. *Peau d'orange* is not characteristic for pseudoxanthoma elasticum, as it may also be observed with sickle cell hemoglobinopathy and Paget's disease.

Special Considerations

- In patients with angioid streaks, establishing the associated diagnosis of pseudoxanthoma elasticum is important, as these patients are at increased risk for potentially serious gastrointestinal and cardiovascular complications.

Paget's Disease

Paget's disease or osteitis deformans is a chronic, progressive disorder characterized by abnormal bone destruction and production. Common clinical characteristics include headaches, enlarged skull, enlarged digits, bone fractures, and cardiovascular complications. Serum alkaline phosphatase and urine calcium are elevated, but serum calcium is normal. Approximately 8 to 15% of patients with severe Paget's disease demonstrate evidence of angioid streaks late in the course of their disease.[59] Vision loss in Paget's disease is typically caused by CNV associated with angioid streaks; additionally, optic nerve compression caused by changes in bone surrounding the optic canal can result in optic atrophy and visual loss.

It is estimated that angioid streaks develop in approximately 1 to 2% of patients with *sickle cell hemoglobinopathy*.[64] The angioid streaks are unrelated to other findings observed in sickle cell retinopathy. It is unusual for CNV to develop in African American patients with sickle cell disease and angioid streaks.

Ehlers–Danlos Syndrome

Ehlers–Danlos syndrome is characterized by hyperelasticity of the skin and hyperflexibility of joints. The basic structural defect is related to abnormal collagen organization. The prevalence of angioid streaks in patients with Ehlers–Danlos syndrome is believed to be low.[65]

15.3.3 Pathogenesis and Histopathology

Angioid streaks represent dehiscences or breaks in what appears to be an abnormally brittle Bruch's membrane.[58] Regardless of the underlying associated systemic condition, Bruch's membrane has been found to be diffusely thickened and calcified. Disruption of the elastic lamina of Bruch's membrane is an early histopathologic finding. Degenerative changes in the choriocapillaris and RPE are likely to be secondary events that occur later in the course of the disease.

15.3.4 Management and Course

Patients with angioid streaks should be cautioned about the risk for Bruch's membrane ruptures and subretinal hemorrhage from incidental blunt trauma. Particularly as patients approach the fifth decade of life, they become at risk for CNV development and loss of vision from resultant exudative changes. Laser photocoagulation has been reported to obliterate extrafoveal CNV successfully.[66,67] PDT has been investigated for CNV secondary to angioid streaks and showed some promise for stabilization of vision.[68,69] Other studies showed a net loss in vision but suggested that PDT may slow down the vision loss, especially in eyes with subfoveal lesions. A prospective study of 23 eyes treated with PDT for CNV secondary to angioid streaks showed that vision in patients with subfoveal CNV went from a mean of 20/100 to 20/125 at 1 year, while the vision in patients with juxtafoveal CNV went from a mean of 20/50 to a mean of 20/100. Of those with juxtafoveal lesions, 57% progressed to subfoveal. With the advent of anti-VEGF treatment for CNV, many case series have demonstrated the efficacy of these agents, and they have now become the preferred treatment method. Following the first series published in 2006,[70] numerous small, retrospective case series have confirmed that intravitreal anti-VEGF agents can stabilize and often increase visual acuity in eyes with subfoveal CNV and in eyes with juxtafoveal or extrafoveal CNV.[71,72,73,74,75] Although there have been no randomized, controlled trials investigating the use of anti-VEGF agents in the treatment of CNV secondary to angioid streaks, several prospective trials have confirmed the impressive results from retrospective studies. A prospective study of 15 patients with CNV associated with angioid streaks reported that mean best-corrected visual acuity improved from 20/100 to 20/50 with a mean of 7.1 intravitreal ranibizumab injections over a year. In addition, 93% of patients had stabilization or improvement in visual acuity with a corresponding improvement in anatomy on OCT.[76] Another small, prospective study of seven patients with CNV associated with angioid streaks and pseudoxanthoma elasticum reported improvement in mean visual acuity from 20/63 at baseline to 20/32 at year 1.[77] For nonsubfoveal CNV lesions, PDT or laser photocoagulation may be beneficial in select cases, but a prospective study of 15 eyes showed the potential benefit of intravitreal bevacizumab. At 1-year follow-up, although mean best-corrected visual acuity did not change, only 2 of 15 eyes (13%) progressed to subfoveal lesions.[78]

Treatment protocols for intravitreal anti-VEGF treatment vary considerably in each series, including agent used, fixed versus PRN treatment, and retreatment criteria. None of the studies compared different approaches. Unlike CNV associated with AMD, which is often treated using a treat-and-extend protocol, CNV associated with angioid streaks is more commonly treated with one to three monthly injections followed by PRN retreatment based on clinical and SD-OCT evaluation (▶ Fig. 15.15). In a multicentered, randomized, prospective clinical trial of 30 patients with CNV not caused by AMD, patients were treated with intravitreal ranibizumab monthly or thrice monthly followed by PRN. In both groups, no patients lost more than 15 letters. At 12 months, 64 and 57% of patients gained 15 or more letters in the monthly and PRN groups, respectively.[79] This study suggests similar efficacy of monthly versus PRN treatment, but larger prospective studies would be needed to confirm these findings. It is important to counsel patients to use an Amsler grid on a regular basis and report any sudden changes in an attempt to detect CNV at its earliest stages. Furthermore, a general medical evaluation is warranted for patients who manifest angioid streaks to detect any of the associated systemic conditions that may be present.

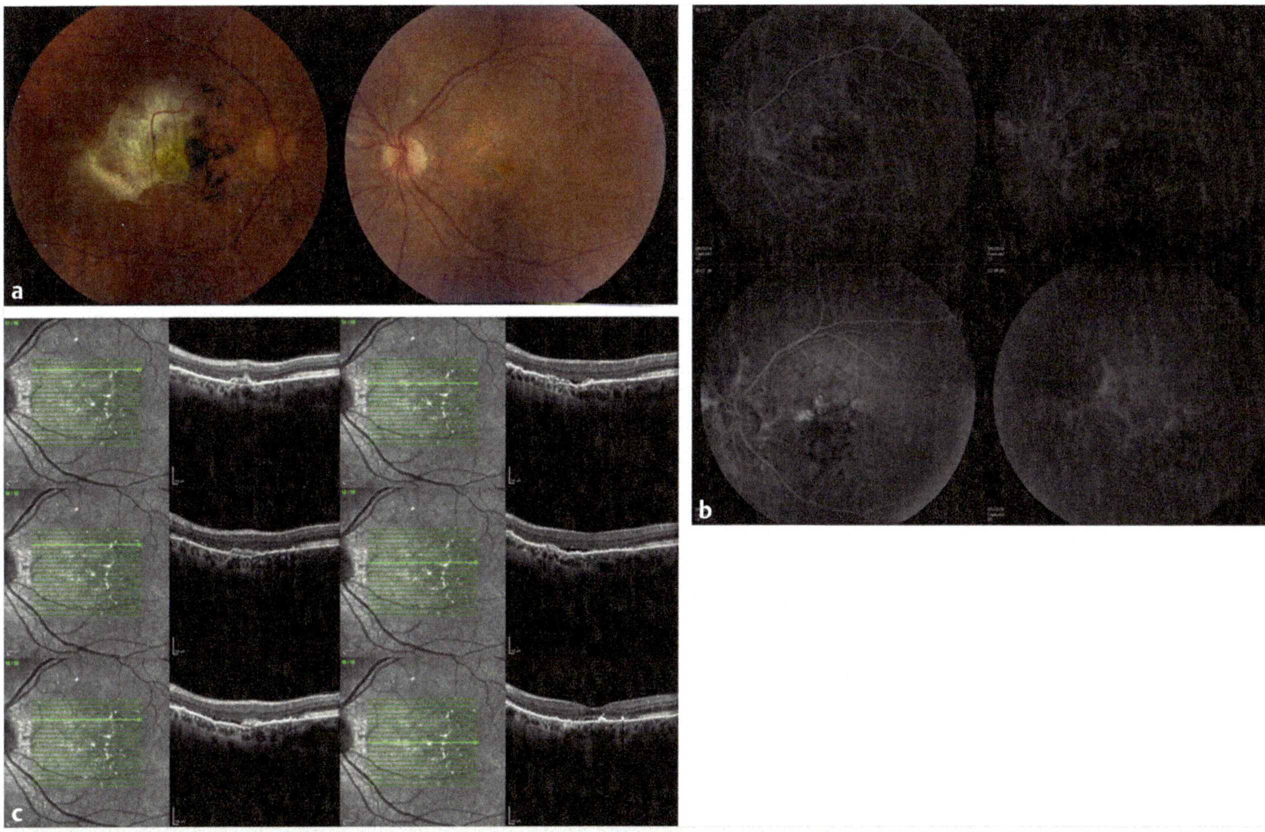

Fig. 15.15 (**a**) Pseudoxanthoma elasticum. Right eye shows chronic disciform scar. Left eye shows angioid streaks radiating from the optic nerve. There is a new retinal hemorrhage in a juxtafoveal location. (**b**) Fluorescein angiography of the left eye highlights the radially oriented angioid streaks. There is an area of hyperfluorescence that leaks in the later phases consistent with a choroidal neovascularization. (**c**) SD-OCT shows subretinal choroidal neovascularization with associated subretinal fluid.

15.4 Idiopathic Choroidal Neovascularization

Macular CNV in patients younger than 50 years is typically observed in association with a primary ophthalmic disease such as POHS, pathologic myopia, angioid streaks, traumatic choroidal rupture, or other causes of chorioretinal lesions in the macula. A distinct subset of patients exists, however, in whom CNV develops in the absence of any macular abnormalities. These patients manifest *idiopathic* CNV.[80,81,82,83]

15.4.1 Clinical Features

Patients with new-onset idiopathic CNV are young, averaging about 30 years of age and ranging from the teens to the 50 s at presentation. There is no gender predilection. The initial evaluation usually reveals some degree of visual acuity loss in the involved eye. A discrete, subretinal, gray-green lesion is often visible ophthalmoscopically and is associated with variable amounts of subretinal fluid, hemorrhage, and occasionally lipid exudation. It is common to observe RPE hypertrophy around the CNV, particularly with more chronic lesions. There is a conspicuous absence of myopic fundus changes, angioid streaks, peripapillary changes, drusen, or "histo spots." The vast majority of cases are unilateral and, therefore, the fellow eye would be expected to be completely normal.[83]

Early in the course of disease, FA will usually readily identify the CNV, showing it as a discrete area of early hyperfluorescence and late leakage. In this setting, as with the other diseases discussed in this chapter, ICG does not typically add much clinically useful information to what is already seen on FA. However, SD-OCT should be performed for all the diseases in this chapter and can show the extent of exudation and allow serial tracking of disease activity following treatment.

The extent of the exudative changes seen acutely and the area of RPE atrophy or subretinal fibrosis that results are typically smaller, on average, than those seen with AMD-related CNV. Patients may be able to fixate in the apparent area of atrophy and maintain good visual acuity throughout the evolution of the process. However, the natural history of idiopathic CNV can be highly unpredictable.[83]

15.4.2 Diagnosis

As noted earlier, the diagnosis of idiopathic CNV is made when a young patient manifests CNV without any other ophthalmic condition evident. By definition, patients are younger than 50 years and do not demonstrate stigmata of AMD, pathologic myopia, angioid streaks, intraocular inflammatory disease, or prior trauma.

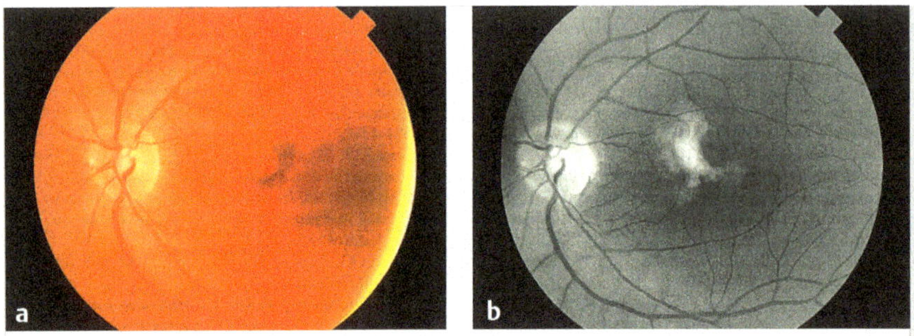

Fig. 15.16 Idiopathic choroidal neovascularization. **(a)** A fundus photograph of the left eye of a healthy 30-year-old woman who noted sudden blurred vision. The visual acuity was 20/60. A grayish green subretinal lesion beneath the fovea and associated neurosensory elevation were present. The lesion was observed. **(b)** Follow-up photograph (5 years later) shows evidence of subretinal fibrosis with discrete foci of hyperpigmentation and areas of retinal pigment epithelial atrophy at the inferior borders of the lesion. The vision improved spontaneously to 20/25.

15.4.3 Pathogenesis and Histopathologic

The pathogenesis of idiopathic CNV is not well understood. There is minimal histopathologic information on the subject, mainly because most patients are young when they manifest the condition. The disease is not hereditary and, being an overwhelmingly unilateral process, is unlikely to be caused by an occult, diffuse, degenerative process.

15.4.4 Management and Course

The Macular Photocoagulation Study trials have demonstrated that laser photocoagulation is effective in decreasing the risk for significant visual loss from idiopathic CNV that is either extrafoveal or juxtafoveal in location.[43,44,81,82] Interestingly, patients with subfoveal idiopathic CNV do not necessarily demonstrate a natural history that dooms them to profound loss of vision, such as that observed in AMD (▶ Fig. 15.16). A study of such patients with idiopathic CNV reported a best-corrected median visual acuity of 20/100 at presentation and 20/70 at final follow-up.[83] Visual acuity was stable or improved to some degree in 95% of patients, with only 5% experiencing a significant loss of vision. Based on such data, laser treatment of *subfoveal* idiopathic CNV is not advisable. PDT has been investigated for the treatment of idiopathic CNV,[84,85] showing efficacy for subfoveal lesions. A prospective study of 17 eyes treated with PDT for subfoveal idiopathic CNV resulted in 94% of patients having stabilized or improved vision at 12 months. However, like the other diseases causing CNV in this chapter, intravitreal anti-VEGF agents have created a paradigm shift in treatment. With the concerns of RPE atrophy with PDT, intravitreal anti-VEGF agents have largely replaced PDT for the treatment of CNV. Several small case series have demonstrated the efficacy of anti-VEGF agents in preserving visual acuity in eyes with idiopathic CNV.[86,87,88,89] A prospective trial with 40 patients with subfoveal idiopathic CNV demonstrated the efficacy of intravitreal bevacizumab.[90] Patients were treated with an initial intravitreal bevacizumab injection followed by PRN treatment based on clinical and OCT examinations. All patients exhibited stable or improved visual acuity with the mean best-corrected visual acuity improving from 20/68 at baseline to 20/39 at 12 months. In addition, 70% of eyes gained two or more lines of vision, and FA and OCT showed absence of disease activity in all eyes at 1 year. A small, retrospective study compared intravitreal anti-VEGF agents to PDT for subfoveal idiopathic CNV reported that all patients in the anti-VEGF group had stable or improved vision at 2 years, while 21% of patients in the PDT group had worsened visual acuity.[91] Anti-VEGF treatment is now the preferred treatment for idiopathic CNV.

Controversial Points

- Intravitreal anti-VEGF agents have been shown to stabilize or improve visual acuity in idiopathic CNV. PRN treatment is commonly utilized, although an optimal treatment protocol has not been determined.

References

[1] Sperduto RD, Seigel D, Roberts J, Rowland M. Prevalence of myopia in the United States. Arch Ophthalmol. 1983; 101(3):405–407

[2] Curtin BJ. Physiologic vs pathologic myopia: genetics vs environment. Ophthalmology. 1979; 86(5):681–691

[3] Soubrane G, Coscas G. Choroidal neovascularization membrane in degenerative myopia. In: Ryan SJ, ed. Retina. Vol. 2. St. Louis, MO: Mosby; 1989:201–215

[4] Ohno-Matsui K, Tokoro T. The progression of lacquer cracks in pathologic myopia. Retina. 1996; 16(1):29–37

[5] Hampton GR, Kohen D, Bird AC. Visual prognosis of disciform degeneration in myopia. Ophthalmology. 1983; 90(8):923–926

[6] Vander JF. Choroidal neovascularization associated with myopic macular degeneration. In: Tasman WS, ed. Clinical Decisions in Medical Retinal Disease. St. Louis, MO: Mosby; 1994:95–102

[7] Grossniklaus HE, Green WR. Pathologic findings in pathologic myopia. Retina. 1992; 12(2):127–133

[8] Borley WE, Snyder AA. Surgical treatment of high myopia; the combined lamellar scleral resection with scleral reinforcement using donor eye. Trans Am Acad Ophthalmol Otolaryngol. 1958; 62(6):791–801, discussion 801–802

[9] Vancea P. New concept in the treatment of progressive myopia. Ann Ophthalmol. 1971; 3(10):1105–1108

[10] Avila MP, Weiter JJ, Jalkh AE, Trempe CL, Pruett RC, Schepens CL. Natural history of choroidal neovascularization in degenerative myopia. Ophthalmology. 1984; 91(12):1573–1581

[11] Pece A, Brancato R, Avanza P, Camesasca F, Galli L. Laser photocoagulation of choroidal neovascularization in pathologic myopia: long-term results. Int Ophthalmol. 1995–1995; 18(6):339–344

[12] Soubrane G, Pison J, Bornert P, Perrenoud F, Coscas G. Subretinal neovessels in degenerative myopia: results of photocoagulation [in French]. Bull Soc Ophtalmol Fr. 1986; 86(3):269–272

[13] Jalkh AE, Weiter JJ, Trempe CL, Pruett RC, Schepens CL. Choroidal neovascularization in degenerative myopia: role of laser photocoagulation. Ophthalmic Surg. 1987; 18(10):721–725

[14] Verteporfin in Photodynamic Therapy Study Group. Photodynamic therapy of subfoveal choroidal neovascularization in pathologic myopia with verteporfin. 1-year results of a randomized clinical trial—VIP report no. 1. Ophthalmology. 2001; 108(5):841–852

[15] Blinder KJ, Blumenkranz MS, Bressler NM, et al. Verteporfin therapy of subfoveal choroidal neovascularization in pathologic myopia: 2-year results of a randomized clinical trial–VIP report no. 3. Ophthalmology. 2003; 110 (4):667–673

[16] Laud K, Spaide RF, Freund KB, Slakter J, Klancnik JM, Jr. Treatment of choroidal neovascularization in pathologic myopia with intravitreal bevacizumab. Retina. 2006; 26(8):960–963

[17] Tewari A, Dhalla MS, Apte RS. Intravitreal bevacizumab for treatment of choroidal neovascularization in pathologic myopia. Retina. 2006; 26(9):1093–1094

[18] Brown DM, Kaiser PK, Michels M, et al. ANCHOR Study Group. Ranibizumab versus verteporfin for neovascular age-related macular degeneration. N Engl J Med. 2006; 355(14):1432–1444

[19] Rosenfeld PJ, Brown DM, Heier JS, et al. MARINA Study Group. Ranibizumab for neovascular age-related macular degeneration. N Engl J Med. 2006; 355 (14):1419–1431

[20] Wang E, Chen Y. Intravitreal anti-vascular endothelial growth factor for choroidal neovascularization secondary to pathologic myopia: systematic review and meta-analysis. Retina. 2013; 33(7):1375–1392

[21] Wolf S, Balciuniene VJ, Laganovska G, et al. RADIANCE Study Group. RADIANCE: a randomized controlled study of ranibizumab in patients with choroidal neovascularization secondary to pathologic myopia. Ophthalmology. 2014; 121(3):682–92.e2

[22] Ruiz-Moreno JM, Arias L, Montero JA, Carneiro A, Silva R. Intravitreal anti-VEGF therapy for choroidal neovascularisation secondary to pathological myopia: 4-year outcome. Br J Ophthalmol. 2013; 97(11):1447–1450

[23] Martin DF, Maguire MG, Ying GS, Grunwald JE, Fine SL, Jaffe GJ, CATT Research Group. Ranibizumab and bevacizumab for neovascular age-related macular degeneration. N Engl J Med. 2011; 364(20):1897–1908

[24] Chakravarthy U, Harding SP, Rogers CA, et al. IVAN Study Investigators. Ranibizumab versus bevacizumab to treat neovascular age-related macular degeneration: one-year findings from the IVAN randomized trial. Ophthalmology. 2012; 119(7):1399–1411

[25] Yang HS, Kim JG, Kim JT, Joe SG. Prognostic factors of eyes with naïve subfoveal myopic choroidal neovascularization after intravitreal bevacizumab. Am J Ophthalmol. 2013; 156(6):1201–1210.e2

[26] Yoon JU, Kim YM, Lee SJ, Byun YJ, Koh HJ. Prognostic factors for visual outcome after intravitreal anti-VEGF injection for naive myopic choroidal neovascularization. Retina. 2012; 32(5):949–955

[27] Holland GN. Endogenous fungal infections of the retina and choroid. In: Ryan SJ, ed. Retina. Vol. 2. St. Louis, MO: Mosby; 1989:631

[28] Woods AC, Wahlen HE. The probable role of benign histoplasmosis in the etiology of granulomatous uveitis. Am J Ophthalmol. 1960; 49:205–220

[29] Macher A, Rodrigues MM, Kaplan W, et al. Disseminated bilateral chorioretinitis due to Histoplasma capsulatum in a patient with the acquired immunodeficiency syndrome. Ophthalmology. 1985; 92(8):1159–1164

[30] Ganley JP. Epidemiologic characteristics of presumed ocular histoplasmosis. Acta Ophthalmol Suppl. 1973; 119:1–63

[31] McDonald HR, Schatz H, Johnson RN, Madeira D. Acquired macular disease. In: Tasman WS, Jaeger EA, eds. Duane's Clinical Ophthalmology. Vol. 3. Philadelphia, PA: JB Lippincott; 1990

[32] Fountain JA, Schlaegel TF, Jr. Linear streaks of the equator in the presumed ocular histoplasmosis syndrome. Arch Ophthalmol. 1981; 99(2):246–248

[33] Lewis ML, Van Newkirk MR, Gass JDM. Follow-up study of presumed ocular histoplasmosis syndrome. Ophthalmology. 1980; 87(5):390–399

[34] Gutman FA. The natural course of active choroidal lesions in the presumed ocular histoplasmosis syndrome. Trans Am Ophthalmol Soc. 1979; 77:515–541

[35] Klein ML, Fine SL, Knox DL, Patz A. Follow-up study in eyes with choroidal neovascularization caused by presumed ocular histoplasmosis. Am J Ophthalmol. 1977; 83(6):830–835

[36] Macular Photocoagulation Study Group. Krypton laser photocoagulation for neovascular lesions of ocular histoplasmosis. Results of a randomized clinical trial. Arch Ophthalmol. 1987; 105(11):1499–1507

[37] Watzke RC, Claussen RW. The long-term course of multifocal choroiditis (presumed ocular histoplasmosis). Am J Ophthalmol. 1981; 91(6):750–760

[38] Makley TA, Jr, Craig EL, Long JW. Histopathology of presumed ocular histoplasmosis. Palestra Oftalmol Pan Am. 1977; 1:72–82

[39] Meredith TA, Green WR, Key SN, III, Dolin GS, Maumenee AE. Ocular histoplasmosis: clinicopathologic correlation of 3 cases. Surv Ophthalmol. 1977; 22(3):189–205

[40] Khalil MK. Histopathology of presumed ocular histoplasmosis. Am J Ophthalmol. 1982; 94(3):369–376

[41] Makley TA, Craig EL, Werling K. Histopathology of ocular histoplasmosis. In: Schlaegel TF, ed. Update on Ocular Histoplasmosis. International Ophthalmology Clinics, Vol 23. Boston, MA: Little Brown & Company; 1983:1–18

[42] Spencer WH, Chan CC, Shen DF, Rao NA. Detection of histoplasma capsulatum DNA in lesions of chronic ocular histoplasmosis syndrome. Arch Ophthalmol. 2003; 121(11):1551–1555

[43] Macular Photocoagulation Study Group. Argon laser photocoagulation for neovascular maculopathy. Five-year results from randomized clinical trials. Arch Ophthalmol. 1991; 109(8):1109–1114

[44] Macular Photocoagulation Study Group. Laser photocoagulation for juxtafoveal choroidal neovascularization. Five-year results from randomized clinical trials. Arch Ophthalmol. 1994; 112(4):500–509

[45] Fine SL, Wood WJ, Isernhagen RD, et al. Laser treatment for subfoveal neovascular membranes in ocular histoplasmosis syndrome: results of a pilot randomized clinical trial. Arch Ophthalmol. 1993; 111(1):19–20

[46] Macular Photocoagulation Study Group. Five-year follow-up of fellow eyes of individuals with ocular histoplasmosis and unilateral extrafoveal or juxtafoveal choroidal neovascularization. Arch Ophthalmol. 1996; 114(6):677–688

[47] Busquets MA, Shah GK, Wickens J, et al. Ocular photodynamic therapy with verteporfin for choroidal neovascularization secondary to ocular histoplasmosis syndrome. Retina. 2003; 23(3):299–306

[48] Rosenfeld PJ, Saperstein DA, Bressler NM, et al. Verteporfin in Ocular Histoplasmosis Study Group. Photodynamic therapy with verteporfin in ocular histoplasmosis: uncontrolled, open-label 2-year study. Ophthalmology. 2004; 111(9):1725–1733

[49] Nielsen JS, Fick TA, Saggau DD, Barnes CH. Intravitreal anti-vascular endothelial growth factor therapy for choroidal neovascularization secondary to ocular histoplasmosis syndrome. Retina. 2012; 32(3):468–472

[50] Schadlu R, Blinder KJ, Shah GK, et al. Intravitreal bevacizumab for choroidal neovascularization in ocular histoplasmosis. Am J Ophthalmol. 2008; 145 (5):875–878

[51] Mansour AM, Mackensen F, Arevalo JF, et al. Intravitreal bevacizumab in inflammatory ocular neovascularization. Am J Ophthalmol. 2008; 146 (3):410–416

[52] Ehrlich R, Ciulla TA, Maturi R, et al. Intravitreal bevacizumab for choroidal neovascularization secondary to presumed ocular histoplasmosis syndrome. Retina. 2009; 29(10):1418–1423

[53] Cionni DA, Lewis SA, Petersen MR, et al. Analysis of outcomes for intravitreal bevacizumab in the treatment of choroidal neovascularization secondary to ocular histoplasmosis. Ophthalmology. 2012; 119(2):327–332

[54] Hawkins BS, Bressler NM, Bressler SB, et al. Submacular Surgery Trials Research Group. Surgical removal vs observation for subfoveal choroidal neovascularization, either associated with the ocular histoplasmosis syndrome or idiopathic: I. Ophthalmic findings from a randomized clinical trial: Submacular Surgery Trials (SST) Group H Trial: SST Report No. 9. Arch Ophthalmol. 2004; 122(11):1597–1611

[55] Doyne RW. Choroidal and retinal changes. The result of blows on the eye. Trans Ophthalmol Soc U K. 1889; 9:128–40

[56] Knapp H. On the formation of dark angioid streaks as an unusual metamorphosis of retinal hemorrhages. Arch Ophthalmol. 1892; 21:289–292

[57] Clarkson JG, Altman RD. Angioid streaks. Surv Ophthalmol. 1982; 26(5):235–246

[58] Vander JF, Duker JS, Jaeger EA. Miscellaneous diseases of the fundus. In: Tasman WS, Jaeger EA, eds. Duane's Clinical Ophthalmology. Philadelphia, PA: JB Lippincott; 1990:1–14

[59] Gass JDM. Stereoscopic Atlas of Macular Diseases. 4th ed. St. Louis, MO: Mosby; 1997:118–123

[60] Smith JL, Gass JDM, Justice J, Jr. Fluorescein fundus photography of angioid streaks. Br J Ophthalmol. 1964; 48:517–521

[61] Arvas S, Akar S, Yolar M, Yetik H, Kizilkaya M, Ozkan S. Optical coherence tomography (OCT) and angiography in patients with angioid streaks. Eur J Ophthalmol. 2002; 12(6):473–481

[62] Ellabban AA, Tsujikawa A, Matsumoto A, et al. Macular choroidal thickness and volume in eyes with angioid streaks measured by swept source optical coherence tomography. Am J Ophthalmol. 2012; 153(6):1133–43.e1

[63] Connor PJ, Jr, Juergens JL, Perry HO, Hollenhorst RW, Edwards JE. Pseudoxanthoma elasticum and angioid streaks. A review of 106 cases. Am J Med. 1961; 30:537–543

[64] Nagpal KC, Asdourian G, Goldbaum M, Apple D, Goldberg MF. Angioid streaks and sickle haemoglobinopathies. Br J Ophthalmol. 1976; 60(1):31–34

[65] Green WR, Friedman-Kien A, Banfield WG. Angioid streaks in Ehlers-Danlos syndrome. Arch Ophthalmol. 1966; 76(2):197–204

[66] Lim JI, Bressler NM, Marsh MJ, Bressler SB. Laser treatment of choroidal neovascularization in patients with angioid streaks. Am J Ophthalmol. 1993; 116 (4):414–423

[67] Pece A, Avanza P, Galli L, Brancato R. Laser photocoagulation of choroidal neovascularization in angioid streaks. Retina. 1997; 17(1):12–16

[68] Shaikh S, Ruby AJ, Williams GA. Photodynamic therapy using verteporfin for choroidal neovascularization in angioid streaks. Am J Ophthalmol. 2003; 135 (1):1–6

[69] Karacorlu M, Karacorlu S, Ozdemir H, Mat C. Photodynamic therapy with verteporfin for choroidal neovascularization in patients with angioid streaks. Am J Ophthalmol. 2002; 134(3):360–366

[70] Teixeira A, Moraes N, Farah ME, Bonomo PP. Choroidal neovascularization treated with intravitreal injection of bevacizumab (Avastin) in angioid streaks. Acta Ophthalmol Scand. 2006; 84(6):835–836

[71] Bhatnagar P, Freund KB, Spaide RF, et al. Intravitreal bevacizumab for the management of choroidal neovascularization in pseudoxanthoma elasticum. Retina. 2007; 27(7):897–902

[72] Rinaldi M, Dell'Omo R, Romano MR, Chiosi F, Cipollone U, Costagliola C. Intravitreal bevacizumab for choroidal neovascularization secondary to angioid streaks. Arch Ophthalmol. 2007; 125(10):1422–1423

[73] Wiegand TW, Rogers AH, McCabe F, Reichel E, Duker JS. Intravitreal bevacizumab (Avastin) treatment of choroidal neovascularisation in patients with angioid streaks. Br J Ophthalmol. 2009; 93(1):47–51

[74] Neri P, Salvolini S, Mariotti C, Mercanti L, Celani S, Giovannini A. Long-term control of choroidal neovascularisation secondary to angioid streaks treated with intravitreal bevacizumab (Avastin). Br J Ophthalmol. 2009; 93(2):155–158

[75] Sawa M, Gomi F, Tsujikawa M, Sakaguchi H, Tano Y. Long-term results of intravitreal bevacizumab injection for choroidal neovascularization secondary to angioid streaks. Am J Ophthalmol. 2009; 148(4):584–590.e2

[76] Ladas ID, Kotsolis AI, Ladas DS, et al. Intravitreal ranibizumab treatment of macular choroidal neovascularization secondary to angioid streaks: one-year results of a prospective study. Retina. 2010; 30(8):1185–1189

[77] Finger RP, Charbel Issa P, Hendig D, Scholl HP, Holz FG. Monthly ranibizumab for choroidal neovascularizations secondary to angioid streaks in pseudoxanthoma elasticum: a one-year prospective study. Am J Ophthalmol. 2011; 152 (4):695–703

[78] Battaglia Parodi M, Iacono P, La Spina C, et al. Intravitreal bevacizumab for nonsubfoveal choroidal neovascularization associated with angioid streaks. Am J Ophthalmol. 2014; 157(2):374–377.e2

[79] Heier JS, Brown D, Ciulla T, et al. Ranibizumab for choroidal neovascularization secondary to causes other than age-related macular degeneration: a phase I clinical trial. Ophthalmology. 2011; 118(1):111–118

[80] Cleasby GW. Idiopathic focal subretinal neovascularization. Am J Ophthalmol. 1976; 81(5):590–599

[81] Macular Photocoagulation Study Group. Argon laser photocoagulation for idiopathic neovascularization. Results of a randomized clinical trial. Arch Ophthalmol. 1983; 101(9):1358–1361

[82] Macular Photocoagulation Study Group. Krypton laser photocoagulation for idiopathic neovascular lesions. Results of a randomized clinical trial. Arch Ophthalmol. 1990; 108(6):832–837

[83] Ho AC, Yannuzzi LA, Pisicano K, DeRosa J. The natural history of idiopathic subfoveal choroidal neovascularization. Ophthalmology. 1995; 102(5):782–789

[84] Chan WM, Lam DS, Wong TH, et al. Photodynamic therapy with verteporfin for subfoveal idiopathic choroidal neovascularization: one-year results from a prospective case series. Ophthalmology. 2003; 110(12):2395–2402

[85] Spaide RF, Martin ML, Slakter J, et al. Treatment of idiopathic subfoveal choroidal neovascular lesions using photodynamic therapy with verteporfin. Am J Ophthalmol. 2002; 134(1):62–68

[86] Chan WM, Lai TY, Liu DT, Lam DS. Intravitreal bevacizumab (avastin) for choroidal neovascularization secondary to central serous chorioretinopathy, secondary to punctate inner choroidopathy, or of idiopathic origin. Am J Ophthalmol. 2007; 143(6):977–983

[87] Gomi F, Nishida K, Oshima Y, et al. Intravitreal bevacizumab for idiopathic choroidal neovascularization after previous injection with posterior subtenon triamcinolone. Am J Ophthalmol. 2007; 143(3):507–510

[88] Mandal S, Garg S, Venkatesh P, Mithal C, Vohra R, Mehrotra A. Intravitreal bevacizumab for subfoveal idiopathic choroidal neovascularization. Arch Ophthalmol. 2007; 125(11):1487–1492

[89] Inoue M, Kadonosono K, Watanabe Y, et al. Results of 1-year follow-up examinations after intravitreal bevacizumab administration for idiopathic choroidal neovascularization. Retina. 2010; 30(5):733–738

[90] Zhang H, Liu ZL, Sun P, Gu F. Intravitreal bevacizumab for treatment of subfoveal idiopathic choroidal neovascularization: results of a 1-year prospective trial. Am J Ophthalmol. 2012; 153(2):300–306.e1

[91] Kang HM, Koh HJ. Intravitreal anti-vascular endothelial growth factor therapy versus photodynamic therapy for idiopathic choroidal neovascularization. Am J Ophthalmol. 2013; 155(4):713–719, 719.e1

16 Central Serous Chorioretinopathy

M. Ali Khan and Jason Hsu

16.1 Introduction

Central serous chorioretinopathy (CSC) is a complex chorioretinal disorder characterized by a circumscribed serous (exudative) retinal detachment that is usually confined to the posterior pole. The pathogenesis is incompletely understood but is generally thought to be due to alterations of the choroidal vasculature, resulting in a breakdown of the retinal pigment epithelium (RPE) barrier and subsequent leakage of fluid into the subretinal space.[1,2,3] While previously thought to be idiopathic, several systemic associations including elevated endogenous or exogenous corticosteroids,[4,5,6] pregnancy,[7] gastric *Helicobacter pylori* infection,[8,9] and Type A personality traits[10] have been described.

CSC most commonly affects otherwise healthy individuals between the ages of 30 and 50 years, with a male-to-female ratio of approximately 6:1.[11,12,13,14] The condition is most commonly reported in Asian and Caucasian populations.[12] While most cases are self-limited with recovery of visual function, others may be chronic or recurrent, leading to progressive visual decline from persistent serous macular detachment.

Insights from indocyanine green angiography (ICGA) and spectral-domain optical coherence tomography (OCT) have improved our understanding of this condition, but the precise pathophysiology remains elusive. Therapies for CSC are evolving, including modified photodynamic therapy (PDT) protocols, anti–vascular endothelial growth factor (anti-VEGF) therapy, and steroid hormone antagonists, but evidence from randomized, controlled trials remains limited.

16.2 Clinical Features

Common symptoms of CSC include a relative scotoma and distorted central vision. Visual acuity is usually reduced to between 20/30 and 20/60 and can be partially corrected with a low-plus lens, as the anteriorly displaced neurosensory retina results in a hyperopic shift. Some patients, particularly those with severe or recurrent disease, have visual acuities as low as 20/200. With the onset of macular subretinal fluid collection, patients describe symptoms of metamorphopsia, micropsia, persistent afterimages, altered color vision, and a central dimness in vision.

16.2.1 Typical Central Serous Chorioretinopathy

Typical CSC is the most common presentation, characterized by a solitary, round or oval-shaped neurosensory detachment of limited size located in the macula (▶ Fig. 16.1). The subretinal fluid is clear and well demarcated. The finding of turbid subretinal fluid or subretinal blood is unusual in CSC and suggests another diagnosis. In some cases, the neurosensory detachment can be very shallow and a hint to its presence will be the loss of the foveal reflex. Once suspected, the retinal elevation can be confirmed with OCT. Using a macular contact lens with a narrow slit beam directed at an angle, viewing the macula under red-free conditions, and using indirect ophthalmoscopy are helpful clinical examination techniques that may be employed when OCT is unavailable.

Small serous retinal pigment epithelial detachments (PEDs) are observed commonly in association with the neurosensory detachment. These serous PEDs are smooth, well-circumscribed, orange-colored elevations with a slightly darker, distinct rim. They may be under or adjacent to the neurosensory elevation.

16.2.2 Chronic Central Serous Chorioretinopathy

Chronic CSC is characterized by widespread RPE alterations in the posterior pole secondary to chronic subretinal fluid. This variant of CSC has been referred to as decompensated RPE.[12] Patients may have chronic disease resulting from one persistent episode of CSC or after multiple recurrences following initial resolution.

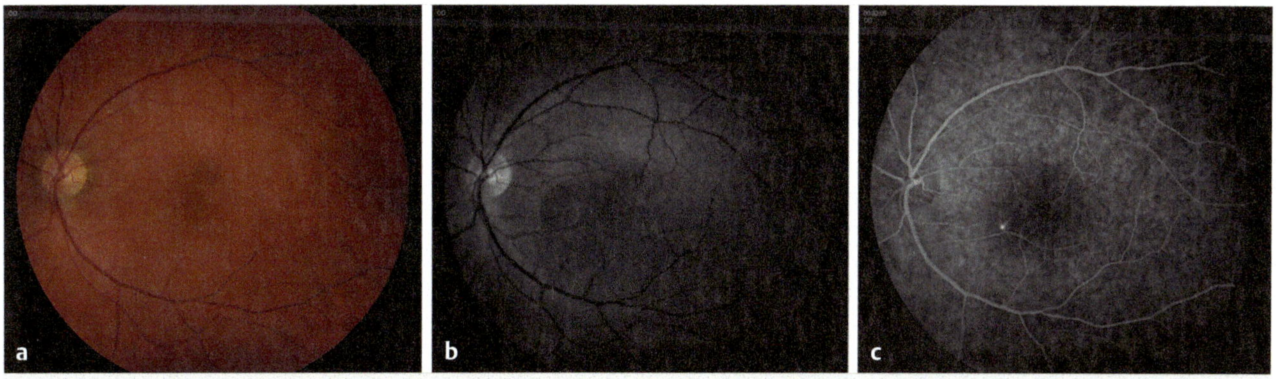

Fig. 16.1 Typical central serous chorioretinopathy. (**a**) Fundus photograph shows a well-circumscribed collection of clear subretinal fluid. (**b**) Red-free photograph demonstrates better delineation of the detachment borders. (**c**) Early-phase fluorescein angiogram reveals a pinpoint hyperfluorescent leakage site inferonasal to the foveal center.

Patients with chronic CSC generally have a more pronounced loss of visual acuity than those with typical CSC.[12] The following findings may, infrequently, be seen in patients with chronic CSC: retinal capillary telangiectasia or nonperfusion, cystoid macular edema, choriocapillaris atrophy, and secondary choroidal neovascularization (CNV).[15] Because of the extensive pigmentary alterations and chronically reduced visual acuity, these patients are sometimes misdiagnosed as having an inherited macular dystrophy or age-related macular degeneration.

16.2.3 Bullous Central Serous Chorioretinopathy

A third form of the disease is described by the presence of a large amount of subretinal fluid in the macula that extends into the inferior periphery.[16] The "bullous" appearance of the retinal detachment accounts for the name of this variant. Affected eyes may also have multiple, large PEDs. Bullous CSC is rare in the United States but appears to be more common in Japan.[17] It has also been reported in organ transplant patients and others treated with high doses of corticosteroids.[6]

16.2.4 Miscellaneous Fundus Findings

Eyes with CSC of any variant occasionally have fibrin or lipid deposited under the retina.[18] It appears as gray-white translucent dots or sheets on the undersurface of the detached retina. The fibrin is often located near the leakage site and occurs more commonly in eyes with PED and in patients who are pregnant or diabetic. Subretinal lipid has a yellow, hard-edged, waxy appearance. It is commonly found at the border of neurosensory detachments but also may be deposited in clumps in an apparently random distribution. Eyes with either type of subretinal deposits have been misdiagnosed as having retinitis, choroidal tumors, or CNV because of the presence of exudate.[12]

16.3 Imaging Modalities

16.3.1 Fluorescein Angiography

In acute cases of typical CSC, fluorescein angiography (FA) demonstrates at least one hyperfluorescent leak at the level of the RPE. Most commonly, the leakage of dye takes the form of an expanding dot (▸ Fig. 16.1). In a minority of cases (10–20%), the dye rises up under the neurosensory detachment as a "smokestack" leak (▸ Fig. 16.2). This pattern is thought to be related to the increased concentration of protein in the fluid accumulating in the detachment.[19] The new fluid entering into the detachment has less protein and, consequently, a lower specific gravity. The newly entering fluid rises up and then spreads out when it reaches the dome of the detachment.

Pearls

- Typical CSC will show an expanding dot or, less commonly, a "smokestack" leak on FA. The chronic variant will show widespread transmission defects and may often show multiple, subtle leakage sites.

16.3.2 Indocyanine Green Angiography

ICGA in eyes with CSC has demonstrated changes that appear to represent areas of possible decreased choroidal perfusion and overlapping or adjacent areas of choroidal vascular hyperpermeability.[20,21,22] Delayed choroidal filling has been reported in 63 to 100% of patients with CSC in certain series.[20,23] Dilated choroidal vasculature is observed in early phases, followed by multifocal, often bilateral choroidal vascular hyperpermeability in the mid to late phases of the angiographic evaluation. The later phases of ICGA show dispersion of leaked dye into hyperfluorescent patches.[22] Because the dye has cleared significantly from the circulation at this point, the large choroidal vessels in the region of the leak stand out as hypofluorescent channels. Interestingly, the areas of abnormal hyperfluorescence on ICGA are typically larger or more widespread than the abnormalities identified by FA (▸ Fig. 16.3).

16.3.3 Fundus Autofluorescence

Fundus autofluorescence (FAF) is an increasingly important imaging modality in the assessment of patients with CSC. In acute cases, the presence of subretinal fluid results in hyperautofluorescence in the area of neurosensory detachment. This hyperautofluorescence may persist even with resolution of subretinal fluid and, in this setting, is thought to be secondary to accumulation of damaged photoreceptor outer segments and/or unmasking of background RPE fluorescence in the presence of photoreceptor loss.[24,25] Ultimately, in chronic cases, progressive degeneration and atrophy of the RPE is later manifested as hypoautofluorescence (▸ Fig. 16.4).[24,25,26] Thus, the pattern of autofluorescence adds information regarding chronicity of disease, and in patients with chronic-recurrent CSC, a mixed autofluorescence pattern may exist.

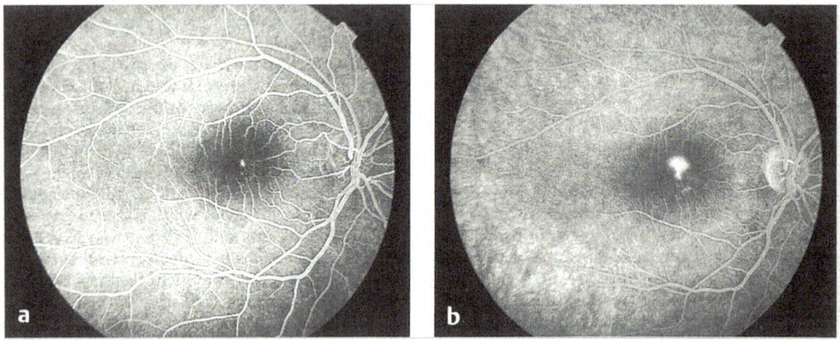

Fig. 16.2 (a) Early and (b) late phases of fluorescein angiogram show the classic "smokestack" leakage of dye under the neurosensory detachment of typical central serous chorioretinopathy.

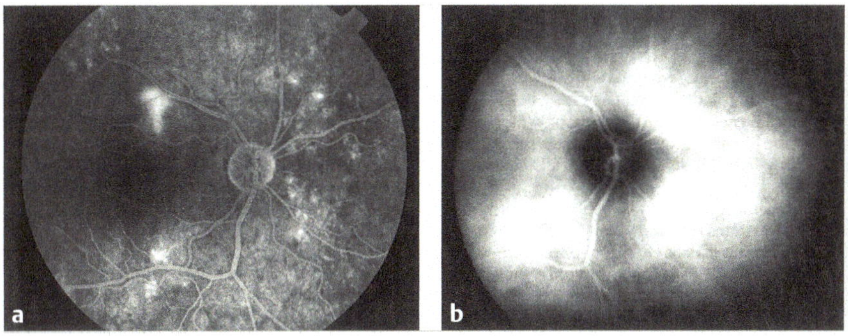

Fig. 16.3 (**a**) Midphase fluorescein angiogram shows a "smokestack" leak with several small window defects scattered around the optic disc. Clinically, subretinal fluid was confined to the central macular area. (**b**) Corresponding indocyanine green angiogram demonstrates multiple areas of ill-defined hyperfluorescence around the optic disc, consistent with widespread choroidal vascular hyperpermeability.

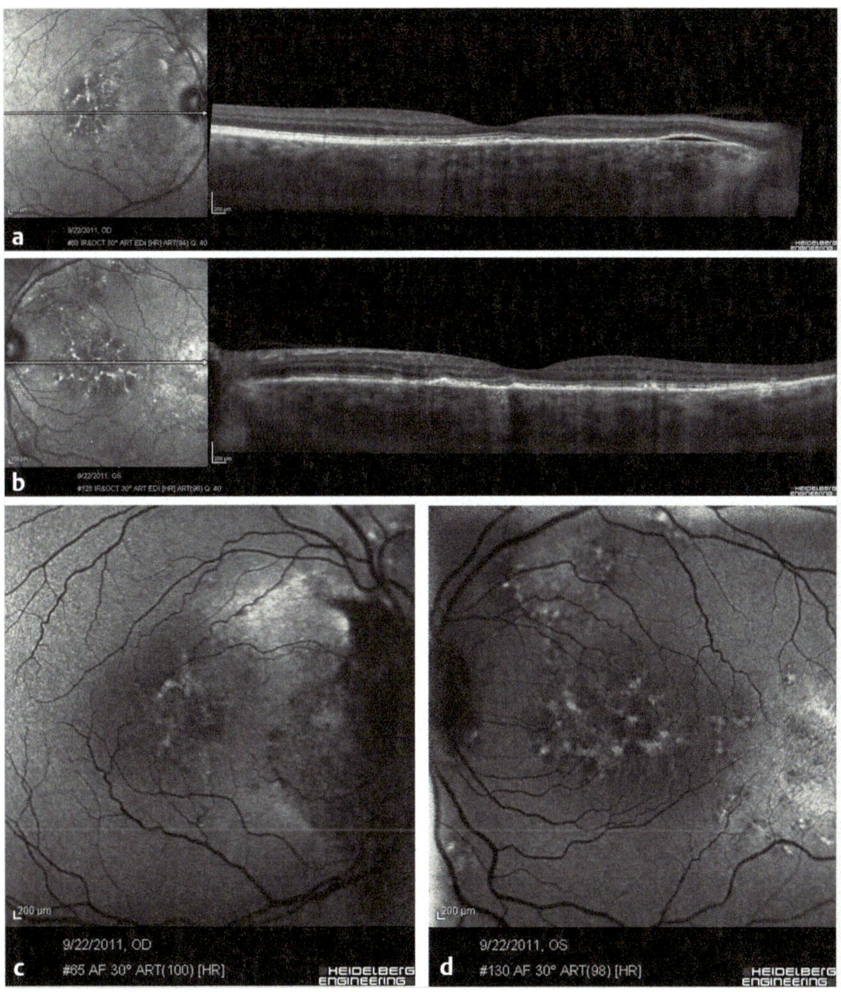

Fig. 16.4 Chronic central serous chorioretinopathy. Enhanced depth imaging optical coherence tomography of the (**a**) right eye and (**b**) left eye demonstrates increased choroidal thickness. A chronic pigment epithelial detachment is noted in the right eye, while ellipsoid layer abnormalities are pronounced in the left eye. Fundus autofluorescence of the (**c**) right eye and (**d**) left eye reveals central, granular hypoautofluorescence suggestive of chronic RPE damage. A "guttering" effect or descending tract is evident in the right eye inferior to the optic nerve.

Patterns of autofluorescence may also provide prognostic information. In one study, specific patterns of hypoautofluorescence, namely, granular or confluent patterns, were associated with poor visual outcomes on multiple regression analysis.[25] Furthermore, an additional study revealed FAF patterns correlated with best-corrected visual acuity and microperimetry results in patients with resolved CSC.[27]

Newer, ultra-widefield FAF allows for complete imaging of peripheral, gravitational tracts that may occur in patients with chronic CSC and, along with ultra-widefield ICGA, may help identify peripheral disease activity.[26]

16.3.4 Optical Coherence Tomography

OCT allows for fast, detailed, noninvasive assessment of patients with CSC (▶ Fig. 16.5). Neurosensory detachments and PEDs (▶ Fig. 16.6), and progression/resolution of fluid over time (▶ Fig. 16.7), are demonstrated readily on OCT. Cystoid macular edema and ellipsoid layer disruption, features described in patients with chronic CSC associated with poor visual outcome, are also detected readily with OCT.

Enhanced depth imaging (EDI) OCT reveals increased choroidal thickness in patients with CSC, consistent with choroidal

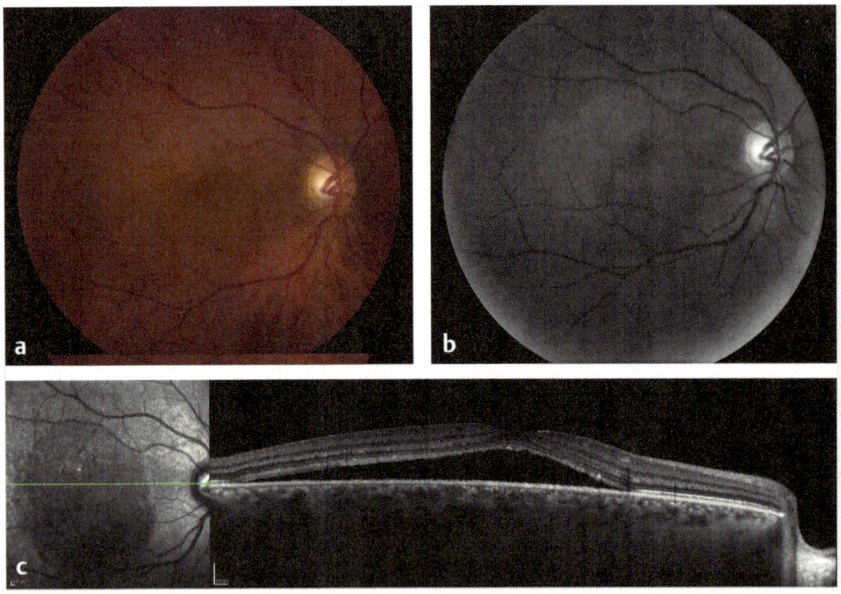

Fig. 16.5 Fundus photograph and (**b**) red-free photograph reveals a well-circumscribed serous retinal detachment consistent with typical central serous chorioretinopathy. (**c**) Enhanced depth imaging optical coherence tomography demonstrates the subretinal fluid.

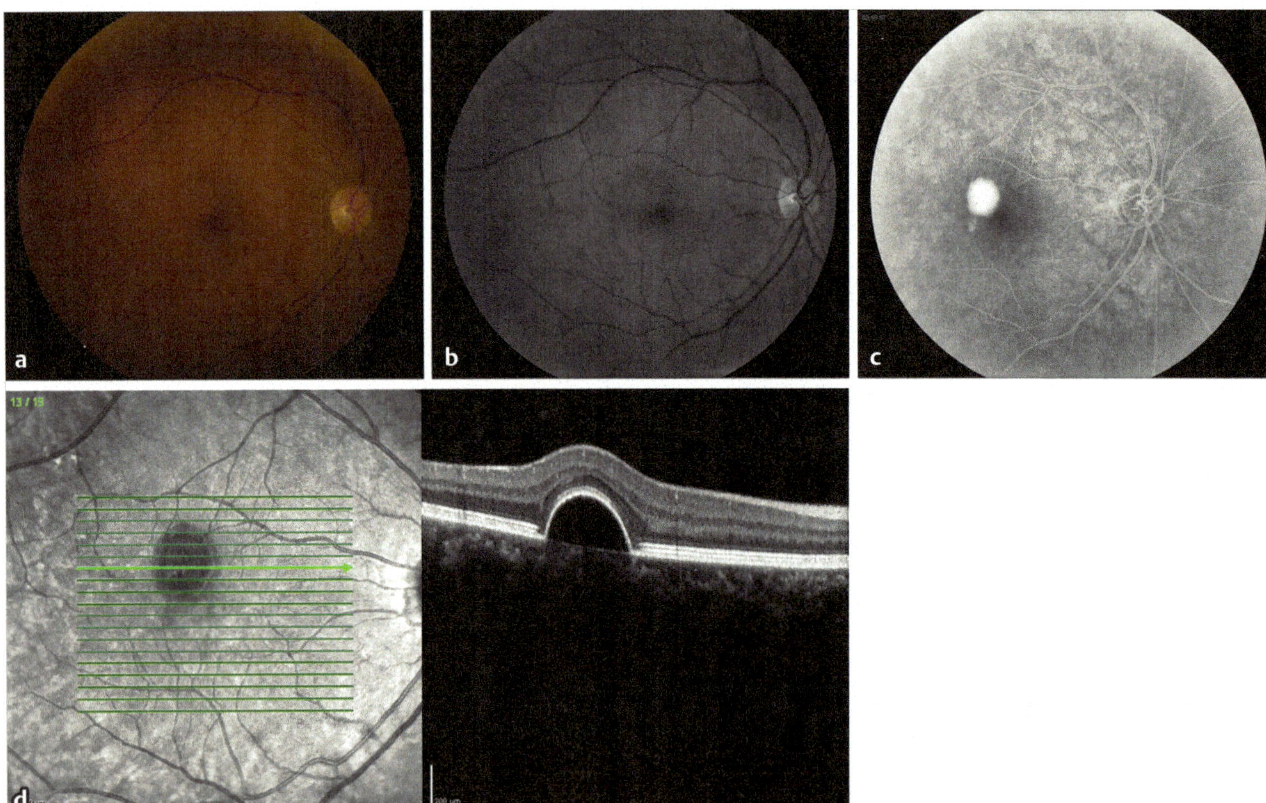

Fig. 16.6 (**a**) Fundus photograph and (**b**) red-free photograph demonstrate a pigment epithelial detachment (PED) superotemporal to the fovea in a patient with central serous chorioretinopathy. (**c**) Fluorescein angiography reveals pooling in the area of the PED in later frames. (**d**) Spectral-domain optical coherence tomography clearly demonstrates the PED.

changes noted on FA and ICGA.[28] Maruko et al demonstrated that, in patients with unilateral CSC, choroidal thickness as measured by EDI-OCT was significantly greater in the affected eye as compared to the unaffected fellow eye (414?± 109 vs. 350 ± 116 µm, respectively; $p < 0.001$).[29] Lending support to the idea that choroidal changes are present bilaterally in patients with CSC, Kim et al found choroidal thickness was increased in affected eyes (445.58 ± 100.25 µm) and unaffected fellow eyes (378.35 ± 117.44 µm) compared to healthy controls (266.80 ± 55.45 µm; $p < 0.001$ in both groups).[30] Choroidal thickness may be more pronounced in patients with chronic CSC. In a recent study, Hamzah et al reported mean EDI-OCT choroidal thickness to be 336.6 ± 91.6 µm in acute CSC and 388.0 ± 103.4 µm in chronic CSC.[31]

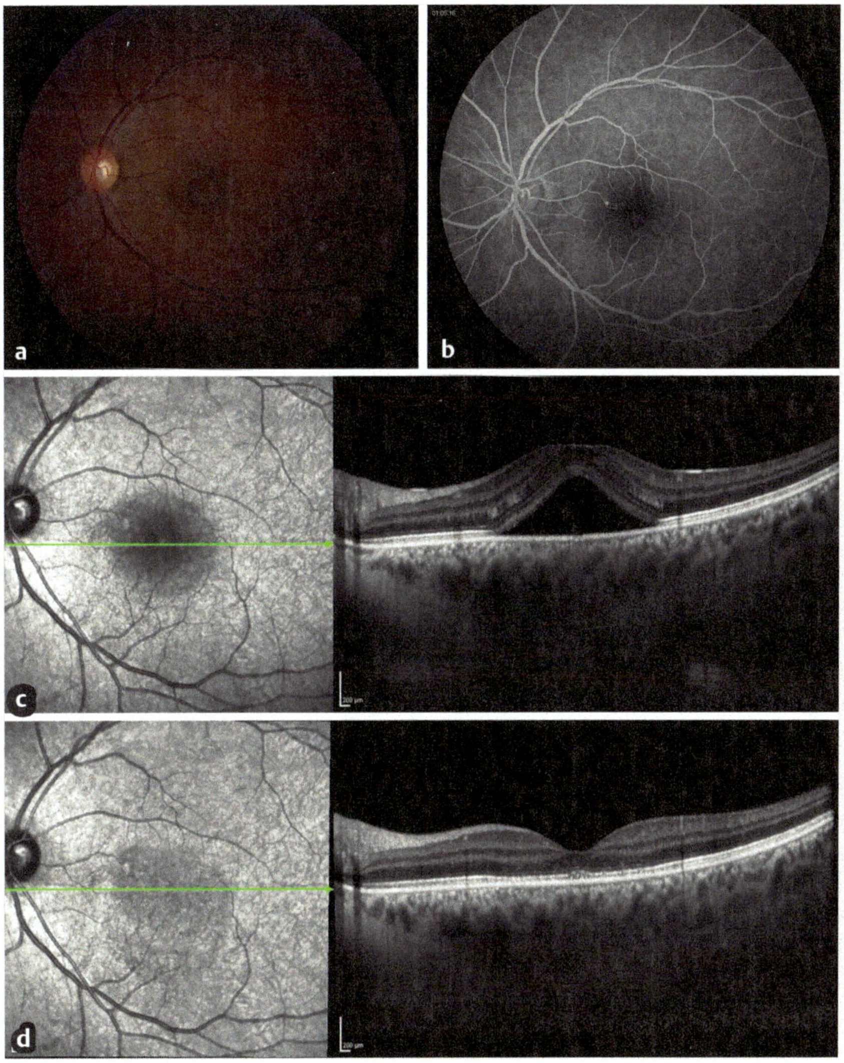

Fig. 16.7 (**a**) Fundus photograph reveals a well-circumscribed collection of clear subretinal fluid corresponding to (**b**) a pinpoint hyperfluorescent leakage site nasal to the foveal center consistent with central serous chorioretinopathy. (**c**) Enhanced depth imaging optical coherence tomography demonstrates subretinal fluid. (**d**) After 2 months of observational management, the fluid had resolved.

Similar to FA, OCT is helpful in differentiating CSC from other diagnoses, such as age-related macular degeneration. Newer OCT technology may provide information that was previously only available from FA or ICGA. In a recent study, en face swept-source OCT was able to identify RPE loss, enlarged choroidal vessels, and focal choroidal dilation in patients with chronic CSC.[32]

16.3.5 Multifocal Electroretinography and Microperimetry

Multifocal electroretinography (mERG) and microperimetry allow assessment of macular function and sensitivity in patients with CSC. Prior studies have shown reduced amplitudes of first- and second-order kernel mERG in patients with CSC,[33] with reduction of these amplitudes correlating with visual acuity. Microperimetry reveals reduction in macular sensitivity in acute CSC, with resolution of these changes with resolution of subretinal fluid.[34] However, in cases of chronic CSC with RPE atrophy and ellipsoid layer disruption on OCT, the reduction in macular sensitivity persists.[35]

16.4 Differential Diagnosis of Central Serous Chorioretinopathy

While clinical examination, FA, ICGA, FAF, and OCT make the diagnosis of CSC clear in most cases, a differential diagnosis must be considered in patients with serous retinal detachment and PEDs.

The principle condition that needs to be differentiated from CSC is CNV, which may arise from multiple disease entities. The ocular findings of CNV share many similarities with those of CSC; both diseases can manifest neurosensory detachment, PED, various RPE changes, and subretinal deposits of fibrin or lipid.[12] Eyes with CNV, however, often have thickening at the level of the RPE, turbid subretinal fluid, notched PED, RPE metaplasia, or subretinal blood, none of which is observed in eyes with CSC. In addition, eyes with CNV generally have associated macular lesions that predisposed them to the neovascular ingrowth. Such lesions include "punched-out" chorioretinal scars in presumed ocular histoplasmosis syndrome, lacquer cracks and areas of choroidal atrophy in degenerative myopia, breaks in Bruch's membrane resulting from traumatic choroidal ruptures, and drusen and RPE alterations in patients with age-related macular degeneration. In an older patient, it may not be possible to distinguish definitively the chronic CSC variant from age-related macular degeneration with occult CNV by ophthalmoscopy and FA alone.

Pearls

- Turbid subretinal fluid and subretinal blood are *not* features associated with CSC; their presence suggests underlying CNV.

The differential diagnosis of CSC also includes various infiltrative or inflammatory conditions of the choroid, congenital optic nerve abnormalities, and rhegmatogenous retinal detachment (see the following list).

- CNV
- Age-related macular degeneration
- Polypoidal choroidal vasculopathy
- Harada's (Vogt–Koyanagi–Harada) disease
- Optic nerve pit
- Posterior scleritis
- Choroidal tumors
- Rhegmatogenous retinal detachment

Infiltrative lesions of the choroid, such as leukemia, melanoma, and metastatic carcinoma, have a color different from that of the surrounding normal choroid, demonstrate thickening of the choroid by ultrasonography, and are not associated with serous PED. Eyes affected with inflammatory conditions, such as Harada's disease, show signs of intraocular inflammation with anterior chamber or vitreous cells and demonstrate numerous punctate leaking spots at the level of the RPE and staining of the optic nerve head on FA. Posterior scleritis can present with unilateral subretinal fluid in the macula similar to CSC, but B-scan ultrasonography reveals choroidal thickening associated with a characteristic zone of echolucency behind the globe. Eyes with congenital optic nerve pits commonly have serous detachments of the macula, but the optic nerve pit is generally readily visible and there are no leaks from the RPE on FA. In eyes with rhegmatogenous retinal detachment, there may be subretinal fluid in the macula that appears isolated from the peripheral detachment. Examination of just the posterior pole may lead to a misdiagnosis of CSC. However, standard peripheral retinal examination with indirect ophthalmoscopy will reveal the peripheral detachment and associated retinal break. In such eyes, FA would not show any leakage in the macula.

16.5 Pathophysiology

Integration of the clinical findings of CSC with recent research into the ICGA abnormalities of the choroidal circulation in patients with CSC has led to greater understanding of the pathophysiology of CSC. While FA may show a single leakage site, ICGA may show multiple, larger areas of increasing hyperfluorescence within the choroid. If these changes represent choroidal vascular hyperpermeability and subsequent increased hydrostatic pressure,[3,20,22,36,37] this excessive tissue hydrostatic pressure within the choroid could lead to PED, disruption of the RPE barrier, and abnormal egress of fluid under the retina. However, the pathophysiology underlying choroidal vascular hyperpermeability remains unknown.

16.6 Management and Course

The large majority of patients with CSC have complete, spontaneous resolution of subretinal fluid and good recovery of visual acuity,[38,39] both of which typically occur during a 2- to 4-month period. It is, however, not uncommon for visual recovery to lag behind the fluid resolution and for vision to continue to improve slightly for up to 6 months after the fluid is gone. Sometimes the macula appears normal after the neurosensory detachment resolves, but often some RPE stippling or clumping remains.

Pearls

- The majority of patients with CSC have complete, spontaneous resorption of the subretinal fluid and return of good central vision. Subjective or objective deficits in visual function, however, often persist.

When all CSC presentations are considered together, approximately 5% of eyes fail to achieve a final visual acuity of better than 20/40.[5] An important point in counseling patients with CSC is that affected eyes often will be left with a slight, permanent decrease in visual acuity, brightness, or color discrimination, even with a single episode of the typical variant. A lack of recovery of visual acuity to better than 20/40 is more often the result of the chronic, persistent presence of subretinal fluid or multiple recurrences that lead to extensive RPE disruption.

Recurrences are encountered in up to 50% of affected individuals.[40,41] Because the natural history of CSC is generally very good, most cases are never treated. Controversy still exists regarding optimal patient selection and timing of treatment for CSC. Treatment is usually reserved for patients with demands for high visual function, symptoms persisting beyond 3 months, or bilateral or recurrent disease.

16.6.1 Treatment Modalities

Observation

Given that the majority of patients experience resolution of subretinal fluid and achieve visual acuity of 20/40 or better, observation is the appropriate first-line therapy for most patients with CSC, particularly those with typical CSC and duration of symptoms less than 3 months. A thorough medical history should be taken and use of exogenous corticosteroids should be discontinued. Testing for endogenous corticosteroid levels may be considered in the appropriate clinical setting.

Thermal Laser Photocoagulation Therapy

Treatment of CSC with argon laser photocoagulation has been studied extensively. Laser photocoagulation directed to the site of leakage seen on FA shortens the duration of macular detachment in patients with typical CSC and leads to more rapid improvement of visual acuity[38,39] and a possible reduction in recurrence rate.[40,42] Although laser photocoagulation expedites visual recovery, most studies indicate that treatment of a focal leakage point does not improve the long-term visual outcome significantly,[14,43,44] which is understandable given the widespread choroidal vasculature changes noted on ICGA.

Complications of argon laser therapy include scar formation with resultant scotoma and possible secondary CNV development. Solitary, extrafoveal leakage sites are typically considered candidates for treatment. When considered, the area of leakage should be located more than 375 µm from the fovea and should be consistently in the same location on follow-up FA. Even if the neurosensory detachment has not changed during the months of observation before treatment, the original (baseline) fluorescein angiographic findings should not be used to guide the laser therapy.

In an attempt to avoid complications, treatment with subthreshold micropulse laser photocoagulation[45,46,47,48] has been explored, but data from controlled trials are lacking.

Photodynamic Therapy

Several prospective and retrospective studies have evaluated the efficacy of PDT for treatment of CSC, with promising results.

ICGA features have an important prognostic role when selecting candidates for PDT. PDT has been demonstrated to be more effective in eyes with intense hyperfluorescence on ICGA, with lack of hyperfluorescence associated with poor treatment response and a higher recurrence rate of subretinal fluid after treatment.[49] In appropriate patients, PDT therapy is associated with resolution of neurosensory detachment and improvement in visual acuity.[50,51]

Special Considerations

- Prior studies have revealed PDT is more effective in eyes with intense hyperfluorescence on ICGA, with lack of hyperfluorescence associated with poor treatment response and a higher recurrence rate of subretinal fluid after treatment.

In an effort to reduce complications associated with PDT, including choriocapillaris hypoperfusion, secondary CNV development, and RPE alterations,[52] modified PDT protocols have been evaluated in retrospective and prospective studies. Modifications include lower dose verteporfin and lower fluence PDT. Both lower dose verteporfin and lower fluence PDT were found to be effective in resolving subretinal fluid and improving visual acuity,[53,54] with one recent study suggesting that lower dose verteporfin may lead to faster resorption of subretinal fluid as compared with lower fluence PDT.[55] Moreover, studies[56,57,58,59] of lower dose verteporfin and lower fluence PDT have demonstrated fewer adverse effects compared to full-dose, standard-fluence PDT, including in regard to choriocapillaris hypoperfusion and development of CNV.

Comparative data, however, remain limited. In one study, half-dose PDT was associated with faster resolution of neurosensory detachment compared to laser photocoagulation, but no difference in anatomic and visual outcomes were observed at 3 months.[60] An additional study revealed lower fluence PDT was associated with a higher rate of fluid resorption without rescue treatment as compared to ranibizumab therapy in patients with chronic CSC.[61] Further prospective, randomized trials are needed to determine the optimal PDT protocol and compare effectiveness to other treatment modalities.

Intravitreal Anti–Vascular Endothelial Growth Factor Therapy

Use of intravitreal anti-VEGF therapy for acute and chronic CSC remains controversial. As an elevated VEGF level in the aqueous humor or plasma of patients with CSC has not been demonstrated,[62] the rationale for treatment with anti-VEGF therapy has been questioned.

Controversies

- Intravitreal anti-VEGF therapy has been used as a treatment modality for CSC. However, elevated VEGF levels have not been demonstrated in the aqueous humor or plasma of patients with CSC. Use of intravitreal anti-VEGF therapy for CSC remains controversial.

Case series of patients with CSC have suggested possible efficacy of intravitreal anti-VEGF therapy, including improvement of visual acuity, resolution of neurosensory detachment, and improvement of leakage on FA after treatment.[63,64] A recent meta-analysis of available studies regarding intravitreal bevacizumab as a treatment for CSC, however, did not reveal a clear benefit.[65] Data from randomized, controlled trials are necessary to assess the true utility of anti-VEGF treatment for CSC, while preclinical studies are warranted to investigate a mechanism for treatment response.

Other Therapies

Adrenergic receptor antagonists (metoprolol,[66] propranolol[67]), steroid hormone antagonists (ketoconazole,[68] mifepristone,[69] eplerenone,[70,71] finasteride[72]), carbonic anhydrase inhibitors (acetazolamide[73]), rifampin,[74] low-dose aspirin,[75] and *H. pylori* eradication antibiotic therapy[76] have been evaluated for the treatment of patients with CSC in case reports or case series. At this time, such therapies are considered exploratory.

16.7 Conclusion

CSC remains a complex, incompletely understood disease. While most patients have a good visual prognosis, significant vision loss may occur in patients with chronic disease. Insights from ICGA, FAF, and OCT are improving our understanding of CSC. Further study is required to determine the optimal treatment for patients with CSC, particularly regarding the optimal protocol for PDT and the role of anti-VEGF therapy.

References

[1] Spaide RF, Goldbaum M, Wong DWK, Tang KC, Iida T. Serous detachment of the retina. Retina. 2003; 23(6):820–846, quiz 895–896

[2] Pryds A, Sander B, Larsen M. Characterization of subretinal fluid leakage in central serous chorioretinopathy. Invest Ophthalmol Vis Sci. 2010; 51 (11):5853–5857

[3] Guyer DR, Yannuzzi LA, Slakter JS, Sorenson JA, Ho A, Orlock D. Digital indocyanine green videoangiography of central serous chorioretinopathy. Arch Ophthalmol. 1994; 112(8):1057–1062

[4] Zakir SM, Shukla M, Simi Z-U-R, Ahmad J, Sajid M. Serum cortisol and testosterone levels in idiopathic central serous chorioretinopathy. Indian J Ophthalmol. 2009; 57(6):419–422

[5] Gass J. Stereoscopic Atlas of Macular Diseases. St. Louis, MO: CV Mosby; 1987

[6] Friberg TR, Eller AW. Serous retinal detachment resembling central serous chorioretinopathy following organ transplantation. Graefes Arch Clin Exp Ophthalmol. 1990; 228(4):305–309

[7] Gass JD. Central serous chorioretinopathy and white subretinal exudation during pregnancy. Arch Ophthalmol. 1991; 109(5):677–681

[8] Cotticelli L, Borrelli M, D'Alessio AC, et al. Central serous chorioretinopathy and Helicobacter pylori. Eur J Ophthalmol. 2006; 16(2):274–278

[9] Misiuk-Hojlo M, Michalowska M, Turno-Krecicka A. Helicobacter pylori—a risk factor for the developement of the central serous chorioretinopathy. Klin Oczna. 2009; 111(1–3):30–32

[10] Yannuzzi LA. Type-A behavior and central serous chorioretinopathy. Retina. 1987; 7(2):111–131

[11] Kitzmann AS, Pulido JS, Diehl NN, Hodge DO, Burke JP. The incidence of central serous chorioretinopathy in Olmsted County, Minnesota, 1980–2002. Ophthalmology. 2008; 115(1):169–173

[12] Spaide RF, Campeas L, Haas A, et al. Central serous chorioretinopathy in younger and older adults. Ophthalmology. 1996; 103(12):2070–2079, discussion 2079–2080

[13] Castro-Correia J, Coutinho MF, Rosas V, Maia J. Long-term follow-up of central serous retinopathy in 150 patients. Doc Ophthalmol. 1992; 81(4):379–386

[14] Gilbert CM, Owens SL, Smith PD, Fine SL. Long-term follow-up of central serous chorioretinopathy. Br J Ophthalmol. 1984; 68(11):815–820

[15] Schatz H, Osterloh MD, McDonald HR, Johnson RN. Development of retinal vascular leakage and cystoid macular oedema secondary to central serous chorioretinopathy. Br J Ophthalmol. 1993; 77(11):744–746

[16] Gass JD. Bullous retinal detachment. An unusual manifestation of idiopathic central serous choroidopathy. Am J Ophthalmol. 1973; 75(5):810–821

[17] Tsukahara I, Uyama M. Central serous choroidopathy with bullous retinal detachment. Albrecht Von Graefes Arch Klin Exp Ophthalmol. 1978; 206 (3):169–178

[18] Ie D, Yannuzzi LA, Spaide RF, Rabb MF, Blair NP, Daily MJ. Subretinal exudative deposits in central serous chorioretinopathy. Br J Ophthalmol. 1993; 77 (6):349–353

[19] Shimizu K, Tobari I. Central serous retinopathy: dynamics of subretinal fluid. Mod Probl Ophthalmol. 1971; 9:152–157

[20] Prünte C, Flammer J. Choroidal capillary and venous congestion in central serous chorioretinopathy. Am J Ophthalmol. 1996; 121(1):26–34

[21] Okushiba U, Takeda M. Study of choroidal vascular lesions in central serous chorioretinopathy using indocyanine green angiography [in Japanese]. Nippon Ganka Gakkai Zasshi. 1997; 101(1):74–82

[22] Spaide RF, Hall L, Haas A, et al. Indocyanine green videoangiography of older patients with central serous chorioretinopathy. Retina. 1996; 16(3):203–213

[23] Kitaya N, Nagaoka T, Hikichi T, et al. Features of abnormal choroidal circulation in central serous chorioretinopathy. Br J Ophthalmol. 2003; 87(6):709–712

[24] Spaide RF, Klancnik JM, Jr. Fundus autofluorescence and central serous chorioretinopathy. Ophthalmology. 2005; 112(5):825–833

[25] Imamura Y, Fujiwara T, Spaide RF. Fundus autofluorescence and visual acuity in central serous chorioretinopathy. Ophthalmology. 2011; 118(4):700–705

[26] Pang CE, Shah VP, Sarraf D, Freund KB. Ultra-widefield imaging with autofluorescence and indocyanine green angiography in central serous chorioretinopathy. Am J Ophthalmol. 2014; 158(2):362–371.e2

[27] Oh J, Kim S-W, Kwon S-S, Oh IK, Huh K. Correlation of fundus autofluorescence gray values with vision and microperimetry in resolved central serous chorioretinopathy. Invest Ophthalmol Vis Sci. 2012; 53(1):179–184

[28] Yang L, Jonas JB, Wei W. Optical coherence tomography-assisted enhanced depth imaging of central serous chorioretinopathy. Invest Ophthalmol Vis Sci. 2013; 54(7):4659–4665

[29] Maruko I, Iida T, Sugano Y, Ojima A, Sekiryu T. Subfoveal choroidal thickness in fellow eyes of patients with central serous chorioretinopathy. Retina. 2011; 31(8):1603–1608

[30] Kim YT, Kang SW, Bai KH. Choroidal thickness in both eyes of patients with unilaterally active central serous chorioretinopathy. Eye (Lond). 2011; 25 (12):1635–1640

[31] Hamzah F, Shinojima A, Mori R, Yuzawa M. Choroidal thickness measurement by enhanced depth imaging and swept-source optical coherence tomography in central serous chorioretinopathy. BMC Ophthalmol. 2014; 14:145

[32] Ferrara D, Mohler KJ, Waheed N, et al. En face enhanced-depth swept-source optical coherence tomography features of chronic central serous chorioretinopathy. Ophthalmology. 2014; 121(3):719–726

[33] Lai TYY, Lai RYK, Ngai JWS, Chan W-M, Li H, Lam DSC. First and second-order kernel multifocal electroretinography abnormalities in acute central serous chorioretinopathy. Doc Ophthalmol. 2008; 116(1):29–40

[34] Reibaldi M, Boscia F, Avitabile T, et al. Functional retinal changes measured by microperimetry in standard-fluence vs low-fluence photodynamic therapy in chronic central serous chorioretinopathy. Am J Ophthalmol. 2011; 151 (6):953–960.e2

[35] Ojima Y, Tsujikawa A, Hangai M, et al. Retinal sensitivity measured with the micro perimeter 1 after resolution of central serous chorioretinopathy. Am J Ophthalmol. 2008; 146(1):77–84

[36] Piccolino FC, Borgia L, Zinicola E, Zingirian M. Indocyanine green angiographic findings in central serous chorioretinopathy. Eye (Lond). 1995; 9(Pt 3):324–332

[37] Piccolino FC, Borgia L. Central serous chorioretinopathy and indocyanine green angiography. Retina. 1994; 14(3):231–242

[38] Ross A, Ross AH, Mohamed Q. Review and update of central serous chorioretinopathy. Curr Opin Ophthalmol. 2011; 22(3):166–173

[39] Aggio FB, Roisman L, Melo GB, Lavinsky D, Cardillo JA, Farah ME. Clinical factors related to visual outcome in central serous chorioretinopathy. Retina. 2010; 30(7):1128–1134

[40] Yap EY, Robertson DM. The long-term outcome of central serous chorioretinopathy. Arch Ophthalmol. 1996; 114(6):689–692

[41] Fok ACT, Chan PPM, Lam DSC, Lai TYY. Risk factors for recurrence of serous macular detachment in untreated patients with central serous chorioretinopathy. Ophthalmic Res. 2011; 46(3):160–163

[42] Robertson DM, Ilstrup D. Direct, indirect, and sham laser photocoagulation in the management of central serous chorioretinopathy. Am J Ophthalmol. 1983; 95(4):457–466

[43] Brancato R, Scialdone A, Pece A, Coscas G, Binaghi M. Eight-year follow-up of central serous chorioretinopathy with and without laser treatment. Graefes Arch Clin Exp Ophthalmol. 1987; 225(3):166–168

[44] Ficker L, Vafidis G, While A, Leaver P. Long-term follow-up of a prospective trial of argon laser photocoagulation in the treatment of central serous retinopathy. Br J Ophthalmol. 1988; 72(11):829–834

[45] Ricci F, Missiroli F, Cerulli L. Indocyanine green dye-enhanced micropulsed diode laser: a novel approach to subthreshold RPE treatment in a case of central serous chorioretinopathy. Eur J Ophthalmol. 2004; 14(1):74–82

[46] Ricci F, Missiroli F, Regine F, Grossi M, Dorin G. Indocyanine green enhanced subthreshold diode-laser micropulse photocoagulation treatment of chronic central serous chorioretinopathy. Graefes Arch Clin Exp Ophthalmol. 2009; 247(5):597–607

[47] Lanzetta P, Furlan F, Morgante L, Veritti D, Bandello F. Nonvisible subthreshold micropulse diode laser (810 nm) treatment of central serous chorioretinopathy. A pilot study. Eur J Ophthalmol. 2008; 18(6):934–940

[48] Chen S-N, Hwang J-F, Tseng L-F, Lin C-J. Subthreshold diode micropulse photocoagulation for the treatment of chronic central serous chorioretinopathy with juxtafoveal leakage. Ophthalmology. 2008; 115(12):2229–2234

[49] Inoue R, Sawa M, Tsujikawa M, Gomi F. Association between the efficacy of photodynamic therapy and indocyanine green angiography findings for central serous chorioretinopathy. Am J Ophthalmol. 2010; 149(3):441–6.e1, 2

[50] Yannuzzi LA, Slakter JS, Gross NE, et al. Indocyanine green angiography-guided photodynamic therapy for treatment of chronic central serous chorioretinopathy: a pilot study. Retina. 2003; 23(3):288–298

[51] Silva RM, Ruiz-Moreno JM, Gomez-Ulla F, et al. Photodynamic therapy for chronic central serous chorioretinopathy: a 4-year follow-up study. Retina. 2013; 33(2):309–315

[52] Cardillo Piccolino F, Eandi CM, Ventre L, Rigault de la Longrais RC, Grignolo FM. Photodynamic therapy for chronic central serous chorioretinopathy. Retina. 2003; 23(6):752–763

[53] Ma J, Meng N, Xu X, Zhou F, Qu Y. System review and meta-analysis on photodynamic therapy in central serous chorioretinopathy. Acta Ophthalmol (Copenh). 2014; 92(8):e594–e601
[54] Alkin Z, Perente I, Ozkaya A, et al. Comparison of efficacy between low-fluence and half-dose verteporfin photodynamic therapy for chronic central serous chorioretinopathy. Clin Ophthalmol. 2014; 8:685–690
[55] Nicoló M, Eandi CM, Alovisi C, et al. Half-fluence versus half-dose photodynamic therapy in chronic central serous chorioretinopathy. Am J Ophthalmol. 2014; 157(5):1033–1037
[56] Chan W-M, Lai TYY, Lai RYK, Tang EWH, Liu DTL, Lam DSC. Safety enhanced photodynamic therapy for chronic central serous chorioretinopathy: one-year results of a prospective study. Retina. 2008; 28(1):85–93
[57] Lai TYY, Chan W-M, Li H, Lai RYK, Liu DTL, Lam DSC. Safety enhanced photodynamic therapy with half dose verteporfin for chronic central serous chorioretinopathy: a short term pilot study. Br J Ophthalmol. 2006; 90(7):869–874
[58] Reibaldi M, Cardascia N, Longo A, et al. Standard fluence versus low fluence photodynamic therapy in chronic central serous chorioretinopathy: a nonrandomized clinical trial. Am J Ophthalmol. 2010; 149(2):307–315.e2
[59] Shin JY, Woo SJ, Yu HG, Park KH. Comparison of efficacy and safety between half-fluence and full-fluence photodynamic therapy for chronic central serous chorioretinopathy. Retina. 2011; 31(1):119–126
[60] Lim JW, Kang SW, Kim Y-T, Chung SE, Lee SW. Comparative study of patients with central serous chorioretinopathy undergoing focal laser photocoagulation or photodynamic therapy. Br J Ophthalmol. 2011; 95(4):514–517
[61] Bae SH, Heo J, Kim C, et al. Low-fluence photodynamic therapy versus ranibizumab for chronic central serous chorioretinopathy: one-year results of a randomized trial. Ophthalmology. 2014; 121(2):558–565
[62] Lim JW, Kim MU, Shin M-C. Aqueous humor and plasma levels of vascular endothelial growth factor and interleukin-8 in patients with central serous chorioretinopathy. Retina. 2010; 30(9):1465–1471
[63] Lim SJ, Roh MI, Kwon OW. Intravitreal bevacizumab injection for central serous chorioretinopathy. Retina. 2010; 30(1):100–106
[64] Artunay O, Yuzbasioglu E, Rasier R, Sengul A, Bahcecioglu H. Intravitreal bevacizumab in treatment of idiopathic persistent central serous chorioretinopathy: a prospective, controlled clinical study. Curr Eye Res. 2010; 35(2):91–98
[65] Chung Y-R, Seo EJ, Lew HM, Lee KH. Lack of positive effect of intravitreal bevacizumab in central serous chorioretinopathy: meta-analysis and review. Eye (Lond). 2013; 27(12):1339–1346
[66] Avci R, Deutman AF. Treatment of central serous choroidopathy with the beta receptor blocker metoprolol (preliminary results) [in German]. Klin Monatsbl Augenheilkd. 1993; 202(3):199–205
[67] Tatham A, Macfarlane A. The use of propranolol to treat central serous chorioretinopathy: an evaluation by serial OCT. J Ocul Pharmacol Ther. 2006; 22 (2):145–149
[68] Golshahi A, Klingmüller D, Holz FG, Eter N. Ketoconazole in the treatment of central serous chorioretinopathy: a pilot study. Acta Ophthalmol (Copenh). 2010; 88(5):576–581
[69] Nielsen JS, Jampol LM. Oral mifepristone for chronic central serous chorioretinopathy. Retina. 2011; 31(9):1928–1936
[70] Bousquet E, Beydoun T, Zhao M, Hassan L, Offret O, Behar-Cohen F. Mineralocorticoid receptor antagonism in the treatment of chronic central serous chorioretinopathy: a pilot study. Retina. 2013; 33(10):2096–2102
[71] Breukink MB, den Hollander AI, Keunen JEE, Boon CJF, Hoyng CB. The use of eplerenone in therapy-resistant chronic central serous chorioretinopathy. Acta Ophthalmol (Copenh). 2014; 92(6):e488–e490
[72] Forooghian F, Meleth AD, Cukras C, Chew EY, Wong WT, Meyerle CB. Finasteride for chronic central serous chorioretinopathy. Retina. 2011; 31(4):766–771
[73] Pikkel J, Beiran I, Ophir A, Miller B. Acetazolamide for central serous retinopathy. Ophthalmology. 2002; 109(9):1723–1725
[74] Ravage ZB, Packo KH, Creticos CM, Merrill PT. Chronic central serous chorioretinopathy responsive to rifampin. Retin Cases Brief Rep. 2012; 6(1):129–132
[75] Caccavale A, Romanazzi F, Imparato M, Negri A, Morano A, Ferentini F. Low-dose aspirin as treatment for central serous chorioretinopathy. Clin Ophthalmol. 2010; 4:899–903
[76] Rahbani-Nobar MB, Javadzadeh A, Ghojazadeh L, Rafeey M, Ghorbanihaghjo A. The effect of Helicobacter pylori treatment on remission of idiopathic central serous chorioretinopathy. Mol Vis. 2011; 17:99–103

17 Macular Holes

John T. Thompson

17.1 Introduction

Gass stimulated interest in macular holes with his theory that tangential traction played a role in the development of macular holes.[1] The development of vitreoretinal surgical techniques for macular holes has allowed a majority of eyes to achieve successful closure of the hole with visual improvement. The landmark report by Kelly and Wendel[2] first demonstrated that vitrectomy with removal of the posterior cortical vitreous and injection of an intraocular gas bubble could be used to close macular holes (anatomic success) and improve visual acuity (functional success). Their report has stimulated much additional research and refinements in the techniques of macular hole surgery.

Visual improvement following successful treatment of macular holes led to a reevaluation of the etiology of visual loss in eyes with macular holes. It was realized that visual loss was not caused by irretrievable loss of photoreceptors but rather by dehiscence in the fovea with neurosensory detachment surrounding the macular hole.[3,4,5] This was confirmed using scanning laser microperimetry, which demonstrated that closure of the macular hole resulted in disappearance of the absolute scotoma and improved visual function of the photoreceptors within the area of the neurosensory retinal detachment.[3] The goal of macular hole surgery was to close the macular hole and cause the neurosensory retinal detachment to resolve. Successful closure of the macular hole and elimination of the intraretinal cystic changes near the edge of the macular hole and subretinal fluid around the edges of the macular hole led to visual improvement.

17.2 Clinical Features and Pathophysiology

In one study, the incidence of macular holes was reported to be 7.8 persons and 8.69 eyes per 100,000 population per year eyes in Olmsted County, Minnesota, which is predominantly Caucasian.[6] Macular holes have been reported to occur about 2 to 3 times more frequently in women compared to men in surgical series reports[7,8] and 3.3 times more frequently in women compared to men in a population-based study.[4] Idiopathic macular holes typically develop in the seventh or eighth decade of life. The mean age of patients with myopic macular holes is younger, and it is much younger in patients with traumatic macular hole due to increased incidence of ocular trauma in young individuals. The cause of the gender difference is unknown, although there may be anatomic variability between men and women with respect to the firmness of attachment of the collagen fibrils of the posterior hyaloid with the fovea. A macular hole develops in the fellow eye in about 7 to 12% of patients with macular holes.[6,9] Patients with macular holes usually report some degree of decreased vision or metamorphopsia. Patients note central scotomas much less frequently. Often, symptoms are first noticed when the patient incidentally covers the fellow eye. Approximately one-half of untreated eyes with macular holes have progressive loss of visual acuity by two or more lines in eyes followed up for < 3 years, 4 to 5 years, and > 6 years.[9]

The diagnosis of macular hole is usually straightforward. It may be identified on examination of the macula with a contact lens or hand-held indirect lens (e.g., 78-diopter lens) in conjunction with slit-lamp biomicroscopy. A fully developed macular hole appears as a dark, round defect in the fovea that is typically surrounded by a small cuff of neurosensory retinal detachment (▶ Fig. 17.1). Small, yellow dots are sometimes present in the center of the hole at the level of the retinal pigment epithelium (RPE). Prehole opacities (pseudo-opercula) may be present depending on the stage of the hole, as described later. The accuracy of diagnosing a macular hole is reasonably high with slit-lamp biomicroscopy but optical coherence tomography (OCT) has become an essential tool to confirm the diagnosis of a full-thickness macular hole.

The development of macular holes has been divided into four stages by Gass.[1,10] His classification helped to define the role of the vitreous in the pathophysiology of macular holes and appears to correlate well with clinical observations of macular holes, even though he did not have the benefit of OCT, which has helped to further refine our understanding of the pathophysiology of macular holes. Macular hole development is related primarily to tangential contraction of attached, prefoveolar cortical vitreous. This traction ultimately causes a break or dehiscence to occur at the umbo, the thinnest and weakest portion of the retina, and subsequent centrifugal movement of the foveolar tissue. Subsequent to Gass's publication, the importance of a perimacular posterior vitreous detachment was recognized by Spaide et al and Gaudric et al using early OCT imaging.[11,12] The localized vitreous separation around the fovea can lead to additional traction with ocular movements that helps to create the foveal dehiscence as the vitreous is inserted obliquely at the perimeter of the fovea where it can exert additional traction. The presumed sequence of events is illustrated

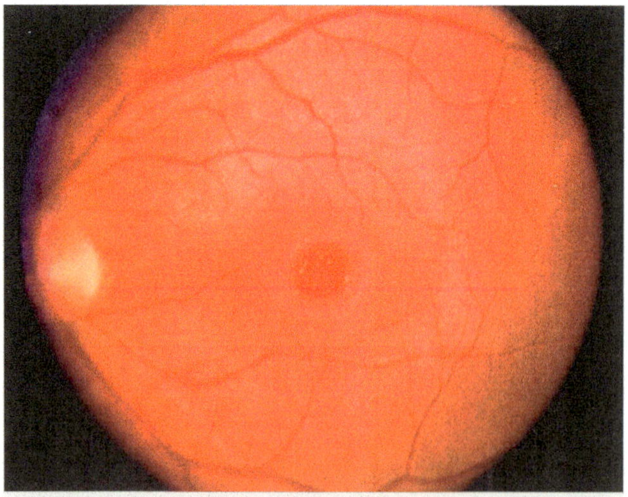

Fig. 17.1 A typical macular hole is characterized by a round defect in the foveal neurosensory retina surrounded by a cuff of neurosensory detachment. There are punctate drusen-like deposits within the macular hole.

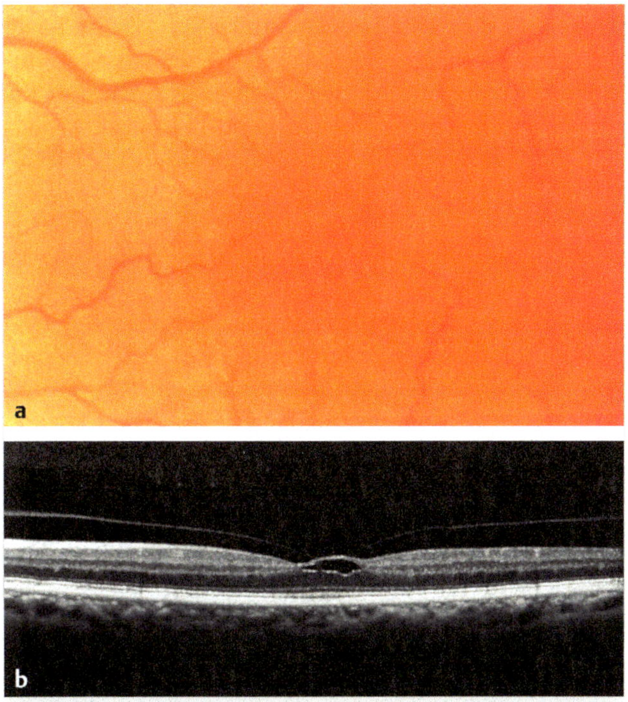

Fig. 17.2 (**a**) Stage 1 macular holes are rarely recognized clinically and are associated with only minimal metamorphopsia. Vitreous traction on the fovea produces a yellow ring of foveal elevation, and there is no defect in the central neurosensory retina by contact lens examination. (**b**) OCT of stage 1 macular hole shows vitreous traction on the fovea with cystic changes. This eye eventually developed a full-thickness macular hole.

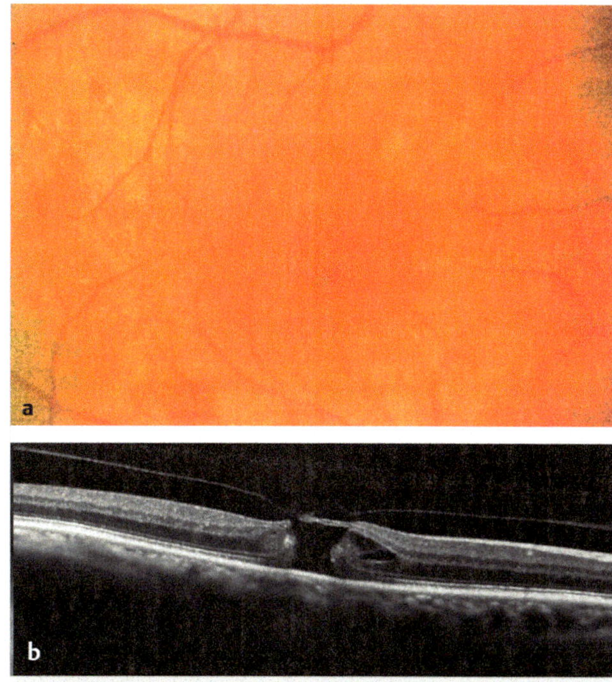

Fig. 17.3 (**a**) A stage 2 macular hole develops when there is a dehiscence in the fovea visible by contact lens biomicroscopy. This eye has an arcuate dehiscence in the fovea from the 5:30 to 8 o'clock position. (**b**) Spectral-domain OCT of a stage 2 macular hole shows a flap of retina with vitreomacular traction to the flap.

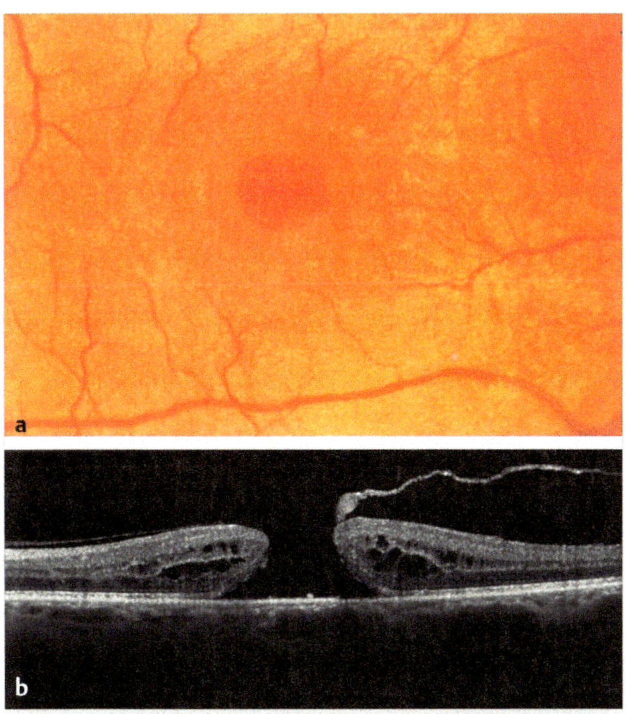

Fig. 17.4 (**a**) Stage 3 macular holes are typically 400 to 500 µm in size and usually have a readily identifiable surrounding neurosensory detachment. The posterior hyaloid (not visible in the photograph) is still attached at this stage. (**b**) OCT often shows intraretinal cystic changes near the edge of the macular hole.

in ► Fig. 17.2, ► Fig. 17.3, and ► Fig. 17.4, and the specific clinical features of each stage are as follows.

17.2.1 Stage 1 Macular Hole

Stage 1 macular hole is characterized by a yellow spot (stage 1A) or yellow ring (stage 1B), which is believed to represent a focal elevation of the fovea caused by tangential vitreous traction. Stage 1 macular holes do not represent true macular holes in that there is no dehiscence of the foveal photoreceptors. A few eyes with stage 1 macular hole have spontaneous separation of the posterior hyaloid from the macula and return to normal, although they most probably progress to stage 2 macular holes. Stage 1 macular holes are generally short-lived (lasting perhaps several weeks) and often minimally symptomatic, so they are only occasionally recognized clinically (► Fig. 17.2a) but can be recognized easily with OCT (► Fig. 17.2b).

17.2.2 Stage 2 Macular Holes

Stage 2 macular holes have a small central or arcuate perifoveal dehiscence (► Fig. 17.3a). Soon thereafter, a small cuff of surrounding neurosensory retinal detachment develops around the foveal dehiscence. Some eyes with stage 2 macular holes have a flap overlying the macular hole that can make the macular hole difficult to recognize with slit-lamp biomicroscopy alone; they are best seen with OCT (► Fig. 17.3b). The stage 2 macular hole enlarges gradually to form a stage 3 macular hole.

17.2.3 Stage 3 Macular Holes

Stage 3 macular holes are typically 400 µm or larger, and the posterior hyaloid/cortical vitreous is still attached around the fovea (▶ Fig. 17.4a, b). Some eyes may have persistence of a stage 3 macular hole for many months or even years. Some, but not all, eyes progress to stage 4 macular holes.

17.2.4 Stage 4 Macular Holes

Stage 4 macular holes differ from stage 3 holes only in that the posterior hyaloid has separated completely from the macula and optic nerve. Thus, a Weiss ring is present at this stage. Spectral-domain OCT has shown that most stage 3 macular holes have a perimacular posterior vitreous detachment; therefore, stage 4 macular holes are best described as eyes with a complete posterior vitreous detachment (▶ Fig. 17.5).

The "operculum" associated with some stage 3 and 4 macular holes appears to represent a pseudo-operculum, as it does not appear to contain photoreceptors.[13] There are reports of spontaneous closure of stage 2 and 3 macular holes, but this event is uncommon.[14,15] Most eyes with macular holes show progressive deterioration in visual acuity until the acuity stabilizes between 20/100 and 20/400. An updated classification system for vitreomacular traction and macular holes has been developed, and this is more useful in evaluating the surgical and visual acuity results than the Gass classification system. An updated classification scheme for macular holes has been proposed.[16] Macular holes are classified by size: small (=250 µm) (▶ Fig. 17.6a), medium (>250 to =400 µm) (▶ Fig. 17.6b), and large (>400 µm) (▶ Fig. 17.6c). Eyes are also classified by whether or not there is vitreous traction to the edges of the macular hole and whether the macular hole is primary or secondary.[16] Secondary macular holes include such causes as traumatic macular holes, myopic macular holes, macular holes secondary to choroidal neovascularization, macular schisis, and cystoid macular edema (CME).

Although OCT has become the standard method to confirm the diagnosis of a macular hole, several ancillary techniques also suggest the presence of a full-thickness macular hole (stage 2, 3, or 4). During biomicroscopic examination of the macula, a narrow slit beam of light can be directed at the hole. When asked to look at the beam, a patient with a full-thickness macular hole should typically report a break or focal constriction in the slit ("positive slit beam" or Watzke–Allen sign). Similarly, the hole can be demonstrated with a laser aiming beam of about 50 µm in size. When the beam is placed within the hole, the patient should not be able to see the beam ("positive laser beam" sign). Fluorescein angiography can also be useful diagnostically. With a macular hole, there is usually a central round window defect corresponding to the size of the hole. There may also be a rim of hypofluorescence around the hole representing the cuff of neurosensory detachment around the hole (▶ Fig. 17.7).

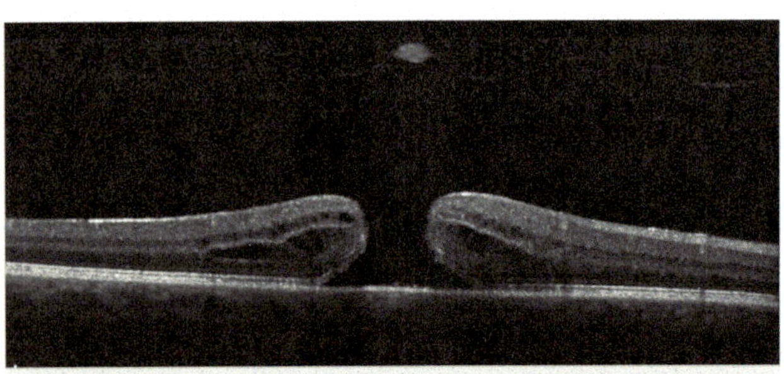

Fig. 17.5 Stage 4 macular hole is defined as a full-thickness macular hole in the setting of a complete posterior vitreous detachment. A pseudo-operculum may be visible anterior to the macular hole.

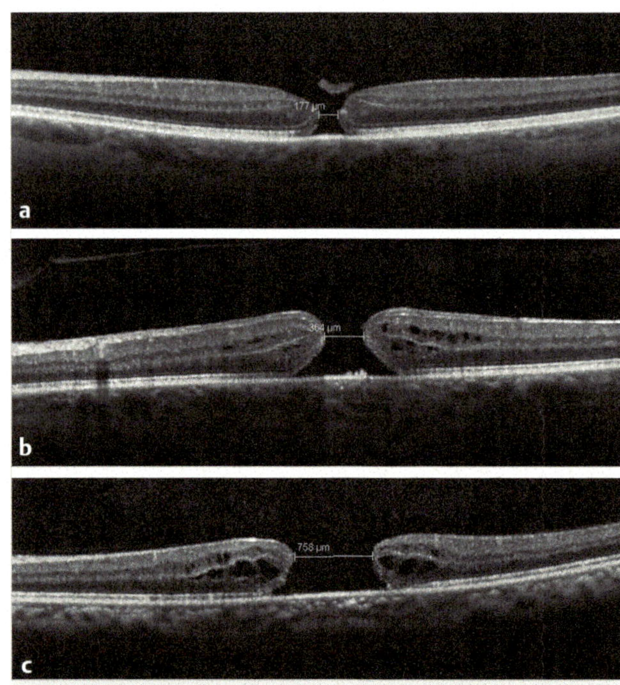

Fig. 17.6 Alternate classification of macular hole by size: **(a)** small (≤ 250 µm); **(b)** medium (250 to 400 µm); **(c)** large (≥ 400 µm).

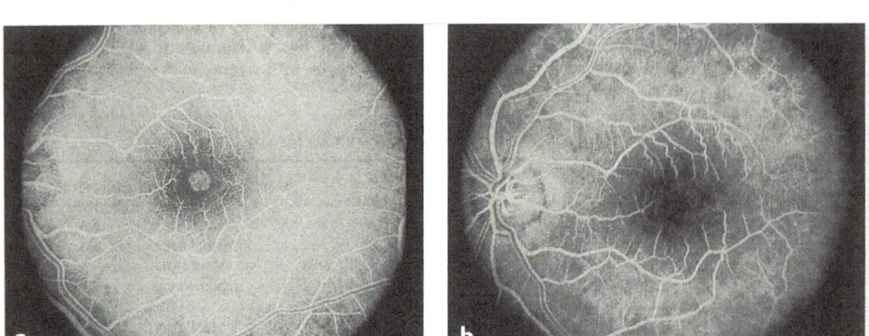

Fig. 17.7 **(a)** Fluorescein angiography of a macular hole shows a hyperfluorescent round window defect corresponding to the macular hole itself. There may be mild surrounding hypofluorescence corresponding to subretinal fluid surrounding the macular hole. **(b)** The central window defect disappears following successful closure of the macular hole. Some subtle abnormalities in the retinal pigment epithelium are noted in the fovea following closure of the macular hole.

17.3 Differential Diagnosis

The most common condition that mimics a macular hole is a macular pseudohole resulting from an epiretinal membrane or a lamellar macular hole.[17] The epiretinal membrane creates a white-yellow sheen surrounding the fovea, which makes the fovea appear dark like a macular hole (▶ Fig. 17.8a). OCT images of lamellar macular holes show thinning of the central fovea often with an epiretinal membrane causing thickening of the perifoveal retina (▶ Fig. 17.8b). Unless the macular distortion from the epiretinal membrane is severe, eyes with macular pseudoholes typically have a visual acuity in the range of 20/20 to 20/40, which is much better than would be expected for a true macular hole of the same size. In addition, a cuff of subretinal fluid is absent with a pseudohole. One would also not expect a positive slit beam or laser aiming beam sign, as there is no dehiscence of foveal neurosensory tissue with the pseudohole.

OCT has become the primary way to distinguish macular holes from lamellar macular holes and macular pseudoholes. Fluorescein angiography can also help to differentiate macular holes from macular pseudoholes/lamellar macular holes. Macular pseudoholes/lamellar macular holes usually lack the central, well-defined window defect corresponding to the defect in the neurosensory retina.

Several other macular pathologic entities can be confused with a macular hole. CME related to prior cataract surgery, retinal venous occlusive disease, or intraocular inflammation may mimic a macular hole when a prominent central cyst is present. OCT can easily distinguish a cyst from a hole, and fluorescein angiography will typically show diffuse leakage associated with macular edema. A small, round subfoveal hemorrhage related to choroidal neovascularization or Valsalva maneuver may resemble a macular hole. Subfoveal hemorrhages show up as localized areas of increased reflectivity on OCT and block fluorescence on fluorescein angiography, which readily differentiates them from a macular hole. The cherry-red spot associated with a central retinal artery occlusion may be confused with a macular hole. The visual acuity is much worse in eyes with a central retinal artery occlusion than would be expected in eyes with a macular hole. OCT will show increased reflectivity in the superficial retina from inner retinal ischemia and the absence of a central full-thickness defect.

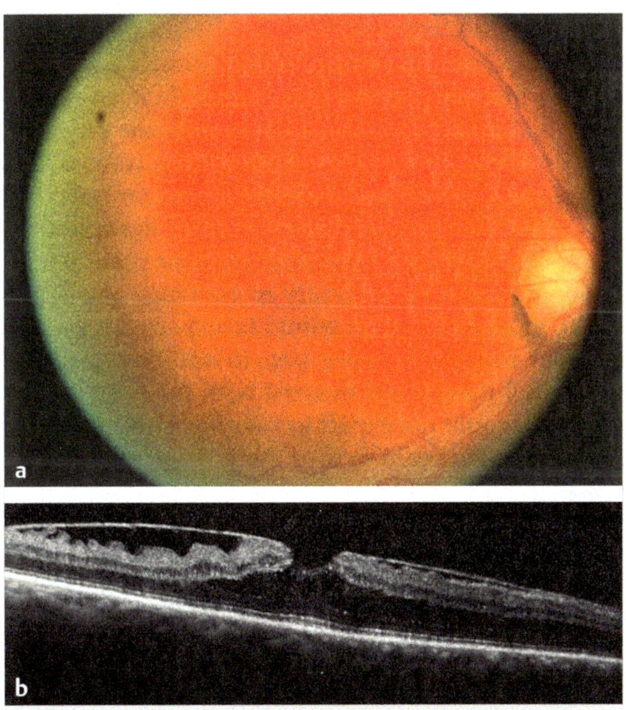

Fig. 17.8 (a) Macular pseudoholes resemble macular holes but are caused by an epiretinal membrane surrounding the fovea. The semiopaque membrane surrounds the fovea and is more transparent in the center of the fovea, giving the appearance of a central dark spot resembling a macular hole. (b) OCT of macular pseudohole with prominent epiretinal membrane and thickening of the perimacular retina.

Pearls

- OCT is essential in correctly diagnosing macular holes and distinguishing them from other macular diseases that may resemble macular holes.

17.4 Management and Course

17.4.1 Preoperative Considerations

In considering treatment, it is useful to subdivide macular holes into several categories based primarily on the age and etiology of the hole, as indicated in ▶ Table 17.1. The best anatomic and visual prognosis occurs in eyes with recent-onset macular holes of 250 μm or less (these are typically less than 6 months in duration), as these eyes presumably have less damage to the foveal photoreceptors than do eyes with older macular holes.

Table 17.1 Categories of macular holes

Types of holes	Macular hole surgery indicated?
Idiopathic	
Recent macular holes (< 250 μm and < 6-mo duration)	Almost all eyes
Intermediate macular holes (250–500 μm and 6–24 mo)	Most eyes
Chronic macular holes (> 500 μm and > 2-y duration)	Some eyes
Persistent macular holes	Most eyes
Recurrent macular holes	Most eyes
Secondary	
Traumatic macular holes	Most eyes
Macular holes secondary to cystoid macular edema	Few eyes
Vitreomacular traction syndrome	Almost all eyes (or try ocriplasmin)
Diabetic retinopathy (posterior hyaloid traction, traction retinal detachment)	Some eyes

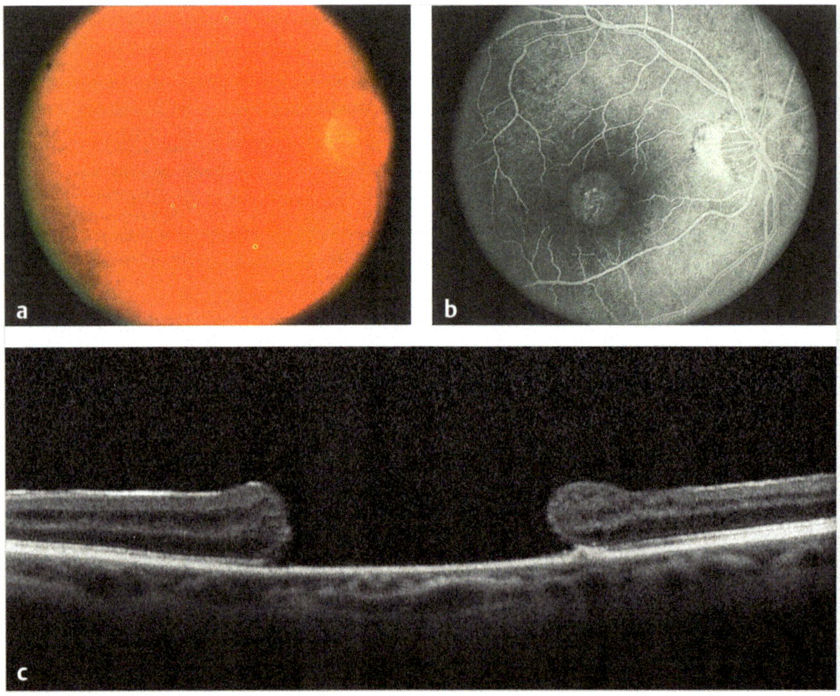

Fig. 17.9 (**a**) Chronic macular holes tend to be larger (500–1,000 µm) and may be surrounded by retinal pigment epithelial atrophy beneath the cuff of neurosensory detachment. Some chronic macular holes have a demarcation line (ring) at the border of the neurosensory detachment. (**b**) The fluorescein angiogram shows prominent retinal pigment epithelial atrophy around the central hyperfluorescent window defect in this eye with a 6-year-old macular hole. (**c**) An OCT of a very large, chronic macular hole of over 10 years' duration with a small cuff of subretinal fluid and more extensive disruption of the external limiting membrane and ellipsoid layers.

Some recent macular holes enlarge relatively rapidly to 300 to 500 µm, so the duration and size of the macular hole do not correlate precisely. This is why it is important for ophthalmologists and optometrists to recognize macular holes so they can be treated when they are of recent onset. Routine examination of the macula using slit-lamp biomicroscopy with a 78-diopter or contact lens is essential, as macular holes may be easily missed with indirect ophthalmoscopy only. Eyes with intermediate-duration macular holes (these are often 6–24 months in duration) still have a reasonably good prognosis and macular hole surgery is still indicated, but the visual results do not tend to be as good as in eyes with more recent macular holes. These macular holes are often in the range of 250 to 500 µm.

Chronic macular holes (more than 2 years' duration) are more difficult to close, and the visual results tend to be less favorable. Chronic macular holes are usually large (greater than 500 µm), and they may have a round demarcation line at the border of the neurosensory detachment (▶ Fig. 17.9a) or extensive RPE atrophy in the area of the cuff of subretinal fluid around the macular hole, which is best visualized with fluorescein angiography (▶ Fig. 17.9b) and OCT (▶ Fig. 17.9c). The decision whether or not to recommend vitreous surgery for an eye with a chronic macular hole is based on several factors, including the visual needs of the patient, status of the fellow eye, and estimated duration of the macular hole. The preoperative visual acuity of the patient and age of the macular hole, both of which are generally related to the size of the macular hole, are the most important prognostic factors for macular hole surgery. Macular holes older than 5 years can sometimes be closed successfully, but the visual acuity rarely improves substantially; therefore, in general, patients with such old macular holes should not receive surgery as most will not experience further decreases in visual acuity if nothing is done.

Persistent macular holes occur when the macular hole is noted to remain open soon after macular hole surgery has been performed. This usually represents primary failure of the macular hole to close and is noted when the intraocular gas bubble is small (less than 40%). Persistent macular holes may be missed unless the macula is examined by OCT 4 to 6 weeks following surgery. If the macular hole edges are visible after the gas bubble meniscus is above the macula, this is a strong suggestion that the macular hole has reopened, even if a neurosensory cuff has not yet formed. Recurrent macular holes are defined as cases in which the macular hole was definitely closed, as seen with OCT, after surgery, often with improvement in visual acuity. Recurrent macular holes may develop months to years following initially successful surgery. The causes of recurrent macular holes are variable and are associated most often with tangential traction from an epiretinal membrane in the macula but can occur after ocular trauma or cataract surgery complicated by postoperative CME. Repeat vitrectomy with removal of the epiretinal membrane/internal limiting membrane (ILM), if not removed previously, is generally the most effective treatment. There are reports of moderate success with fluid–gas exchange performed in the office, but this technique does not remove the source of tangential traction at the edge of the macular hole.

Macular holes may lead to an extensive retinal detachment in some eyes, especially those with high myopia. A peripheral retinal break must be ruled out, as many rhegmatogenous retinal detachments in eyes with macular holes actually result from a peripheral retinal break rather than the macular hole. Some of these macular holes are full-thickness macular holes and others are macular pseudoholes. When the macular hole is the cause of a large rhegmatogenous retinal detachment, then vitrectomy should be considered rather than a scleral buckle or pneumatic retinopexy to treat the retinal detachment. Traditional macular hole surgery is successful in treating these retinal detachments and macular holes in many eyes, but ancillary techniques such as macular buckle or long-term silicone oil tamponade can be considered to improve the success of closing the macular hole and treating the retinal detachment. Treatment of myopic macular holes with extensive retinal detachment will be discussed in more detail in the section "Myopic Macular Holes." The visual results of macular hole surgery are less favorable in eyes with associated rhegmatogenous retinal detachment because there is more extensive damage to the macular photoreceptors. Some eyes with high myopia have myopic macular degeneration which may also limit the visual recovery.

Secondary macular holes are associated with other abnormal conditions that lead to foveal traction or stretching and subsequent macular hole formation. Vitreomacular adhesions with vitreomacular traction syndrome may lead to macular holes and have an excellent prognosis if the traction is relieved. Intravitreal ocriplasmin may be considered as an alternative to surgery when there is vitreous traction to the edge of a small (< 400 µm) macular hole.[18] Trauma is a less common cause of macular hole but is important to recognize. Traumatic macular holes typically occur in boys and young male adults. The prognosis of vitreous surgery in eyes with traumatic macular holes is often determined by the extent of damage to macular RPE from the trauma. Traumatic macular holes have a higher rate of spontaneous closure compared to idiopathic macular holes, so it is best to wait 1 month after the trauma to see if the hole is closed on examination with OCT before considering vitreous surgery. Fluorescein angiography is a helpful tool to assess the extent of the traumatic macular damage, such as commotio retinae, choroidal rupture, and RPE atrophy. The results of vitreous surgery may be excellent in eyes with traumatic macular holes, so RPE atrophy and pigmentary changes in the macula should not be considered a contraindication to vitreous surgery (▶ Fig. 17.10). Macular holes may also form in eyes with chronic CME, although most of these "holes" are actually large cysts. OCT is essential to distinguish between a large cyst and a full-thickness macular hole. Eyes with diabetic retinopathy and posterior hyaloid traction syndrome, traction retinal detachment, or epiretinal membranes also have an increased risk of developing macular holes due to traction on the fovea. For eyes with chronic CME and macular holes associated with diabetic retinopathy, the continuity of the ellipsoid layer and external limiting membrane (ELM) on OCT should be evaluated carefully before recommending surgery. Chronic damage to the macula from CME and diabetic retinopathy often limits the visual acuity improvement even if the macular holes are closed successfully.

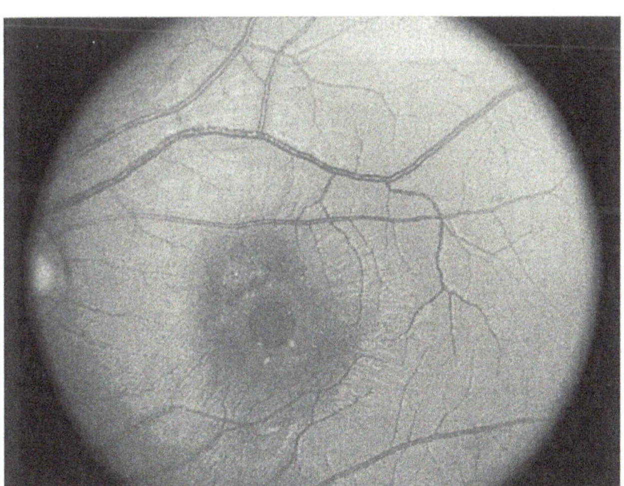

Fig. 17.10 This traumatic macular hole was caused by a baseball injury to the left eye. The visual acuity was reduced to 20/125 before surgery. There is some retinal pigment epithelial atrophy in the superior portion of the fovea resulting from the trauma. This macular hole was closed with vitreous surgery, and the visual acuity improved to 20/80.

17.4.2 Indications for Macular Hole Surgery

Functional criteria are very important in deciding whether or not to recommend macular hole surgery, as the patient measures the success of macular hole surgery by the improvement in vision rather than by the anatomic status of the macular hole (open or closed). Preoperative visual acuity is the most important prognostic factor for postoperative visual acuity in eyes with macular holes. Patients usually notice and complain of decreased vision by the time the visual acuity decreases to the level of 20/50 or worse. Some small stage 2 macular holes will close spontaneously, so it is reasonable to follow up a patient for a month with a small stage 2 macular hole, minimal symptoms, good visual acuity (20/30 or better), and vitreous traction to the flap at the edge of the macular hole. Spontaneous closure of the macular hole occurred spontaneously in 10.6% of eyes with injection of intravitreal saline in the ocriplasmin trial.[12] If the macular hole is monitored and increases in size with decreasing visual acuity, it is reasonable to consider vitrectomy. The visual needs of the patient and symptoms are important criteria that help to determine the recommended timing of macular hole surgery. The success rate for improving visual acuity following macular hole surgery is excellent, so almost all patients with symptomatic full-thickness macular holes should receive treatment. In about one-eighth of patients with unilateral macular holes, a macular hole eventually develops in the fellow eye.[6,7,19] Patients should be informed of this when they are presented with the treatment options for unilateral macular holes. ▶ Table 17.1 summarizes the general recommendations for surgery in eyes with different categories of macular holes.

Pearls

- Patients judge the success of macular hole surgery by the improvement in their vision, not by the anatomic status of the macular hole (open or closed).

Patients with bilateral macular holes of less than 2 years' duration should be considered for macular hole surgery in both eyes. The success of macular hole surgery cannot be predicted for each eye, so bilateral surgery gives the patient the best chance for maximal visual recovery. Patients who have bilateral macular holes and one eye with a chronic macular hole more than 2 years old generally benefit from treatment of the more recent macular hole. If the outcome is good, then the expectations for surgery in the fellow eye with a chronic macular hole can be discussed so that the patient can make an informed decision about the fellow eye.

Macular hole surgery is never an emergent procedure, and patients should be informed of the treatment options and allowed to decide whether or not to proceed with macular hole surgery electively. Most macular hole surgery can be scheduled within several weeks of initial presentation to the vitreoretinal surgeon. Some patients wish to wait longer periods of time, but prolonged waits (3 or more months) may reduce the chances of visual and anatomic success because the preoperative visual acuity and potential postoperative visual acuity typically decrease as the hole becomes older and enlarges. Macular hole surgery can typically be performed under local/monitored anesthesia using small-gauge vitrectomy instrumentation on an outpatient basis.

Some patients are less favorable candidates for macular hole surgery, but improvements in techniques allow many of these patients to have successful closure of the macular hole with improved visual acuity. If a patient is unwilling or unable to remain prone postoperatively, prior cataract surgery and a large, long-acting gas bubble will allow adequate tamponade to close most macular holes. Patients who are unreliable in returning for office visits, have very limited visual needs, or are noncompliant with following postoperative instructions may not be good candidates for surgery.

17.4.3 Surgical Technique

The basic steps of the technique for macular hole surgery are summarized in the following list.

Basic Steps for Macular Hole Surgery

1. Three-port pars plana vitrectomy
2. Creation of posterior vitreous detachment in eyes with incomplete vitreous detachment
3. Removal of detached posterior hyaloid and trimming of the vitreous to peripheral vitreous base
4. Removal of ILM around the macular hole (with or without staining of ILM)
5. Check periphery for retinal tears and treat tears with laser/cryopexy
6. Fluid–gas exchange
7. Prone positioning (if used)

A standard, three-port pars plana vitrectomy is performed with the goal of removing most of the vitreous (see Chapter 40). It is essential to identify and remove the attached posterior hyaloid in eyes with macular holes because the posterior hyaloid contributes to traction in stages 2 and 3 macular holes. Although it is already separated, removal of the posterior vitreous is also desirable in eyes with stage 4 macular holes to create room for a large intraocular gas bubble. It is not necessary to perform simultaneous scleral indentation during vitrectomy for aggressive shaving of the vitreous base, as this maneuver may increase the risk of creating peripheral retinal tears.

Several techniques can be used to identify adherent posterior cortical vitreous and separate it from the retina. A commonly employed technique involves the use of a cannula with a soft silicone tip. With active aspiration, the soft-tip cannula is used to "search" for the posterior cortical vitreous. If the flexible silicone tip is slowly brushed about 0.5 mm anterior to the retina near the fovea or over the optic nerve head, it will seem to jump to any residual cortical vitreous when plugged by the gel, the so-called fish strike sign (▶ Fig. 17.11). Once engaged, the gel is separated by gently pulling anteriorly. Because the cortical vitreous gel can be strongly adherent to the posterior pole, many surgeons opt to use larger, rigid cannulas or even the vitreous cutting/aspirating probe itself. The larger diameter openings of these instruments allow the vitreous gel to be grasped more firmly. If the vitreous is strongly adherent to the retina, which is especially common in traumatic macular holes in children/young adults, the infusion pressure can be increased and the aspiration suction increased to start the vitreous separation. Although fluidics has improved substantially with the newest generation of vitrectomy systems, care must be taken so that the eye does not collapse suddenly as aspiration suction is increased. The intravitreal instillation of triamcinolone in the course of the performing the vitrectomy is a popular way to help visual vitreous gel and insure complete removal from the posterior retina.

With all these separating techniques, the induced vitreous detachment is extended peripherally to about the equator by pulling the posterior hyaloid forward into the midvitreous cavity. The macular hole is observed as the posterior hyaloid is peeled from around the edges of the macular hole, to be certain that the hyaloid separates easily from the edges of the macular hole. The posterior hyaloid virtually always separates from the macular hole without visibly damaging the fovea. Occasionally, in an area of peripheral vitreoretinal adhesion such as lattice degeneration, a retinal tear will be created. The onset of mild vitreous bleeding as the posterior vitreous detachment is extended anteriorly strongly suggests a peripheral retinal break. The vitreous cutter is then used to remove the remaining posterior cortical vitreous and hyaloid to the posterior border of the vitreous base.

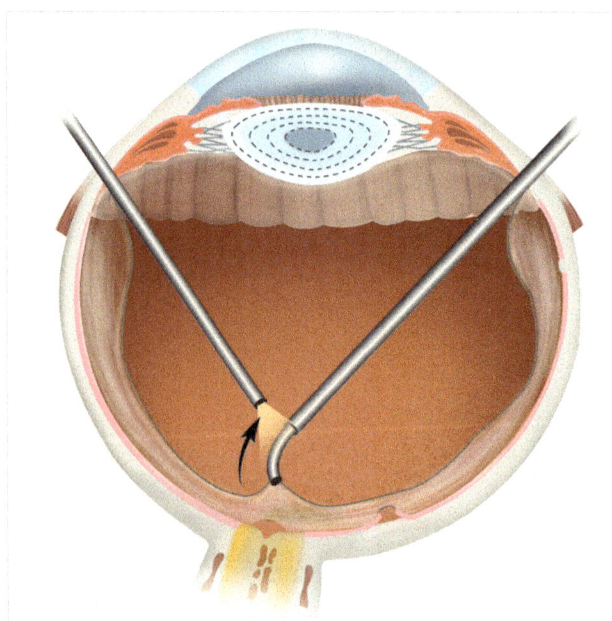

Fig. 17.11 A soft-tip silicone cannula attached to active aspiration being used to search for the attached, posterior cortical vitreous. Once the cortical vitreous is aspirated into the lumen of the cannula, the flexible portion of the cannula bends toward the vitreous as the cannula is moved (the so-called fish strike sign).

Almost all vitreoretinal surgeons routinely remove the ILM around the macular hole, as this has been shown in most studies to improve the success rate of closing the macular hole. A number of studies have confirmed that ILM peeling improves the chance of closing the macular hole with one surgery.[8,20,21,22,23,24,25] A meta-analysis of randomized clinical trials by the Cochrane Eyes and Vision Group found that ILM peeling was associated with improved anatomic success of closing macular holes and improved visual results at 3 months postoperatively.[26] There are three basic techniques to remove the ILM. The first is removal of the ILM with no staining. This can be difficult in some eyes, especially when the fundus is lightly pigmented. The ILM usually tends to fragment and it can be difficult to find the edge of the ILM. However, visual acuity results can be equivalent to eyes where indocyanine green (ICG) stain is used to peel the ILM.[27,28,29,30,31,32] Some studies have reported improved results with ICG staining compared to no staining of the ILM.[33,34,35,36] The second technique uses triamcinolone to delineate the surface of the retina (and ILM). The triamcinolone is dusted onto the surface of the macula. It does not stain the ILM but allows the surgeon to see where the ILM has been removed as removal of the ILM removes the triamcinolone particles on the surface of the retina.[37] The third technique is for surgeons to stain the ILM. The dye most commonly used to stain the ILM in the United States is ICG. This dye stains the ILM well but can cause retinal toxicity in some eyes, so the goal is to use a low concentration and only stain the ILM around the macular hole. A useful technique is to perform a fluid–air exchange just before instilling the ICG and place only one to three drops of ICG anterior to the macular hole. The ICG is then lavaged out of the eye when the air is removed. The second stain is brilliant blue G. This is not FDA approved in the United States but is commonly used in other parts of the world where it is approved by local authorities. It does not stain the ILM as well as ICG does but provides adequate staining in many eyes. The safety profile of brilliant blue G appears to be better than ICG. The third stain is trypan blue. Trypan blue does not stain the ILM very well, and it is often necessary to apply more trypan blue to restain the ILM if the staining is inadequate to see the ILM. Trypan blue appears to be relatively safe,[38,39,40] similar to brilliant blue G, but has largely fallen out of favor due to poor staining of the ILM. The literature is divided about whether ICG staining of the ILM is helpful or harmful. A number of studies have reported that visual acuity outcomes in eyes in which ICG was used are equivalent to visual acuity outcomes in eyes in which ICG was not used.[27,28,29,30,31,32,33,34,35,36,40] A few studies have found long-term ocular damage due to ICG, including RPE atrophy, visual field defects, and optic nerve atrophy.[41,42,43,44] The technique with which ICG is used to stain the ILM appears to be an important determining factor in whether or not ICG causes RPE toxicity.

Pearls

- Almost all vitreoretinal surgeons routinely remove the ILM around the macular hole, as this has been shown in most studies to improve the success rate of closing the macular hole.

A fluid–air exchange is then performed, draining fluid from anterior to the optic nerve. Care is taken to avoid touching the optic nerve or retina with the extrusion needle. If a larger gas fill is desired, then the surgeon can wait 5 to 10 minutes and aspirate anterior to the optic disc again to remove residual vitreous fluid that collects around the optic nerve, which can amount to as much as 0.4 mL of liquid.[45] If a longer acting gas bubble is used, the air can then be exchanged with a nonexpansile concentration of sulfur hexafluoride (SF_6) or perfluoropropane (C_3F_8). The sclerotomies are then checked for leakage after the instruments are removed and any leaking sclerotomies are closed to avoid early postoperative hypotony.

Adjunctive Agents for Macular Hole Surgery

Adjunctive agents used for macular hole surgery include transforming growth factor-beta 2,[46,47,48] autologous serum,[49] autologous blood, cryoprecipitate,[50] serum plus thrombin,[51] thrombin,[52] and autologous platelet concentrate.[53,54] Some surgeons have proposed that adjunctive agents enhance the formation of a stable chorioretinal adhesion between the edges of the macular hole and the RPE, although the use of adjunctive agents has fallen out of favor as current techniques with ILM removal allow excellent closure of the macular hole in over 90% of eyes. Histopathologic studies of successfully closed macular holes have demonstrated formation of a glial plug bridging the histopathologic defect in the neurosensory retina.[55,56] This glial plug appears to pull the edges of the macular hole in a centripetal direction, causing the defect in the neurosensory retina of the closed macular hole to be smaller histopathologically than in the clinical photographs of the preoperative macular hole. Removal of the ILM appears to help stimulate the glial plug to close the edges of the macular hole.

Controversial Points

- The use of ICG to stain the ILM remains controversial. Some surgeons obtain excellent visual success after use of ICG, yet other studies have shown better visual acuity results in eyes in which the ILM is stained with brilliant blue G.

Intraocular Gas Selection

Most surgeons still use SF_6 or C_3F_8 gas for prolonged internal tamponade of the macular hole, although some recent publications have advocated the use of air with only a few days of prone positioning. The premixed gas is lavaged into the vitreous cavity air from a syringe at the end of the procedure to achieve the desired gas concentration.

Postoperative Prone Positioning

Contact of the gas bubble with the macular hole for some period of time in the early postoperative period appears essential for successful closure of the macular hole. The controversy is primarily how long contact of the gas bubble is needed. Studies of serial OCT images in the first week following surgery have improved our understanding of the rate of macular hole closure.[55,57,58,59] Some surgeons have used OCT to determine how long patients must remain prone. Once the hole is closed on OCT through the gas bubble, prone positioning is discontinued.[58,59] If the patient is not going to remain prone, then a large gas bubble (at least 80% or larger) is needed for at least a few days so the bubble will be in apposition with the macular hole when the patient is sitting upright, looking straight ahead. A number of recent reports have shown good results with avoidance of prone positioning, with macular hole closure achieved in 60 to 100% of eyes.[60,61,62,63,64,65,66,67,68] Several studies including a Cochrane meta-analysis of multiple studies evaluating macular hole surgery with and without prone positioning found that results were similar when the macular holes were < 400 µm but that prone positioning was beneficial for larger macular holes.[69,70,71] Another approach is to use tamponade with silicone oil, which avoids prone positioning postoperatively, but this requires a second surgery to remove the oil, and visual outcomes are not as good as with the use of gas tamponade.[72,73,74,75] Macular holes that are difficult to close, such as myopic macular holes and chronic macular holes, have been reported to benefit from longer periods of prone positioning.[76] A large gas bubble is not as important if the patient is compliant with prone positioning, but a large gas bubble helps to ensure adequate contact of the bubble against the macular hole. A number of studies have demonstrated good results with short-duration tamponade using room air, SF_6, or C_2F_6.[77,78,79,80,81,82,83,84] Other authors have advocated use of longer acting gas bubbles such as 16% C_3F_8 or 25% SF_6 with short-duration prone positioning as the bubble will cover the macular hole if it is approximately 60% or greater.[85,86] Studies of compliance with prone positioning have shown that patients maintained prone positioning for only about half the time that the patients claimed they maintained but only 18% of the total time were patients positioned at greater than 45 degrees from upright.[87,88] A number of devices are being marketed that can assist patients with prone positioning in either a sitting or recumbent position.

Controversial Points

- The need for prone positioning and the optimal duration of prone positioning are unknown but greater duration of prone positioning does appear to increase the overall success of closing the macular hole with one surgery. A large percentage gas fill on the first postoperative day and a longer acting gas bubble help to compensate for suboptimal compliance with prone positioning.

17.4.4 Combined Macular Hole Surgery and Cataract Extraction

Some patients with macular holes have concomitant, visually significant cataracts, which must also be treated to allow good visualization during vitrectomy surgery. A pars plana vitrectomy and phacoemulsification through a corneal incision can be combined in one operation. Some have advocated combining macular hole surgery and cataract surgery even in eyes with minimal cataract formation, as significant nuclear sclerosis develops relatively soon after macular hole surgery alone in virtually all of patients older than 60 years.[48] This technique is used more commonly in regions where retinal surgeons perform cataract surgery routinely. This has the advantage of treating the macular hole and eventual cataract in phakic eyes with a single surgery. Simultaneous cataract and macular hole surgery has the disadvantage of an increased risk of postoperative CME that may prevent closure of the macular hole and iridocapsular adhesions causing impaired mobility of the pupil as a result of the gas bubble pushing the intraocular lens and capsule against the iris in the early postoperative period.

17.4.5 Nonsurgical Treatment of Macular Holes

An alternative treatment for relatively recent macular holes involves lysis of vitreous traction to the edge of the macular hole using the enzyme ocriplasmin. This technique is appropriate to consider in eyes with persisting vitreous attachment to the macular hole. The ocriplasmin is injected into the vitreous cavity and the eye is monitored for lysis of traction at the edge of the macular hole which will lead to macular hole closure in some eyes. In the phase 3 study of ocriplasmin, macular holes were successfully closed in 40.6% of eyes treated with ocriplasmin versus 10.6% of eyes treated with placebo (saline injection into the vitreous).[18] In eyes in which the macular hole did not close, the success of subsequent surgical treatment appeared to be equivalent to eyes without prior ocriplasmin use.

Special Considerations

- Ocriplasmin is a reasonable option for treating recent stage 2 macular holes associated with persistent vitreomacular traction on OCT, if the macular hole is less than 400 µm in size and there is no epiretinal membrane associated with the macular hole. Ocriplasmin has a lower success rate in eyes without vitreomacular traction, so vitreous surgery should be considered as the initial treatment in these eyes.

17.4.6 Persistent/Recurrent Macular Holes

The initial surgery to close a macular hole is not successful in all eyes, so some patients must face the decision about whether or not to undergo repeated surgery. As described previously, reopening of a macular hole typically occurs in two settings: early and late. The macular hole may remain open as soon as the gas bubble meniscus is above the macula. This is referred to as a persistent macular hole, even though early postoperative OCT through the intraocular gas bubble has shown that some of these holes close briefly but then reopen. This represents a primary failure of the retina to adhere to the RPE when the gas bubble no longer provides tamponade to the macular hole. A recurrent macular hole may occur many months or years later in eyes in which the macular hole was initially closed by OCT, usually with improved visual acuity. The hole then reopens and

Table 17.2 Selected studies of idiopathic macular hole surgery

Authors	Macular hole closed	Visual acuity measurement	Visual acuity change (lines)	Percentage of eyes improved by two or more lines
Kelly and Wendel[2]	30/52 (58%)	Snellen[a]	+ 3.5	22/52 (42%)
Wendel et al[94]	125/170 (73%)	Snellen[a]	NR	95/170 (56%)
Thompson et al[8]	85/90 (94%)	Refracted ETDRS	+ 2.6	NR
Freeman et al[89]	36/52 (69%)	Refracted ETDRS	+ 0.3	11/59 (19%)
Smiddy et al[9]	179/193 (93%)	Snellen[a]	NR	139/193 (72%)
Tognetto et al[21]	396/425 (93%)	Snellen[a]	+ 3.1	NR
Schaal and Barr[90]	205/240 (75%)	Snellen[a]	+ 3.0	NR
Tsipursky et al[91]	398/425 (93.6%)	Snellen[a]	~ + 3.5 overall	NR
Williamson and Lee[40]	275/351 (78.3%)	Snellen[a]	+ 3.1	NR

Abbreviations: ETDRS, Early Treatment Diabetic Retinopathy Study standardized visual acuity chart; NR, not reported.

[a]Nonrefracted Snellen chart visual acuity.

the visual acuity often decreases. OCT should be performed in patients with decreased acuity after previous successful macular hole surgery. Persistent macular holes occur in 5 to 10% of eyes (▶ Table 17.2).[8,9,21,40,89,90,91] Macular hole recurrences develop in as many as 4.8% of eyes,[92] although the rate of recurrence may be somewhat lower in recent years when ILM has been routinely peeled as part of the surgery.[93] Most late recurrences occur for unknown reasons but some occur in eyes with CME following cataract surgery or ocular trauma. This is why pseudophakic CME should be treated aggressively in eyes with prior macular hole surgery. Some surgeons advocate placing patients prophylactically on nonsteroidal anti-inflammatory drops prior to cataract surgery to try to minimize the risk of developing CME. Some recurrent macular holes also develop when the patient develops a macular epiretinal membrane which causes traction.

The decision about whether or not to treat a persistent or recurrent macular hole must be based on a number of factors. Persistent and recurrent macular holes are somewhat more difficult to close than a macular hole treated with surgery for the first time. Factors that are relevant when repeated surgery is considered for a macular hole include the following: (1) visual needs of the patient; (2) duration of the macular hole (recent macular holes respond more favorably to repeated surgery than chronic macular holes); (3) size of the macular hole (eyes with smaller macular holes and good visual acuity appear to have a better visual outcome than eyes with larger macular holes and poorer visual acuities); (4) macular holes in eyes with high myopia and posterior staphylomas are substantially more difficult to close if they fail the initial surgery; (5) status and stability of the fellow eye; and (6) patient compliance with prone positioning after the first surgery and willingness to remain in a prone position for 10 or more days.

Surgery for persistent and recurrent macular holes has a better success when performed in the operating room rather than injecting a gas bubble in the office followed by additional prone positioning. Vitrectomy in the operating room allows the surgeon to stain ILM to look for residual ILM around the macular hole. It is advisable to peel additional ILM around the macular hole,[95] as this may uncover fine epiretinal membranes that extend into the macula. A large, long-acting gas bubble such as 16% C_3F_8 can be placed in the operating room. Care should be taken to wait a few minutes after the fluid–air exchange to allow additional fluid to accumulate anterior to the disc and then aspirate the residual fluid to try to achieve a 90% or greater bubble on the first postoperative day. One of the reasons macular hole surgery fails is noncompliance with prone positioning, and the large, long-acting gas bubble will help improve the chances of closure if the bubble covers the macula completely even when the patient is not prone. Special techniques using autologous transplantation of ILM may be helpful in eyes with persistent macular holes.[96] The second approach consists of an in-office fluid–gas exchange. Some surgeons have advocated placing eight to nine 50-µm laser burns to the RPE just inside of the edge of the neurosensory retina, taking care to avoid the central fovea just before the fluid–gas exchange to try to encourage formation of a stable chorioretinal adhesion during the gas tamponade.[97]

17.4.7 Anatomic and Visual Results

Macular hole surgery is successful in closing the macular hole in most eyes. The round defect in the neurosensory retina within the fovea disappears following successful surgery (▶ Fig. 17.12a, b). There may be some subtle pigmentary changes in the RPE in the fovea where the macular hole was located. The round window defect visible on fluorescein angiography also disappears following successful closure of the macular hole. The most desirable type of closure is when the edges of the macular hole join together with a near-normal foveal contour (▶ Fig. 17.12c, d). Some eyes following macular hole surgery demonstrate reapposition of the edges of the macular hole against the RPE, but there remains a gap between the edges of the macular hole. This has been termed type 2 closure (▶ Fig. 17.13).[98] Many patients with macular holes complain of metamorphopsia (as well as decreased acuity), and metamorphopsia has also been shown to improve following successful closure of the macular hole.[99]

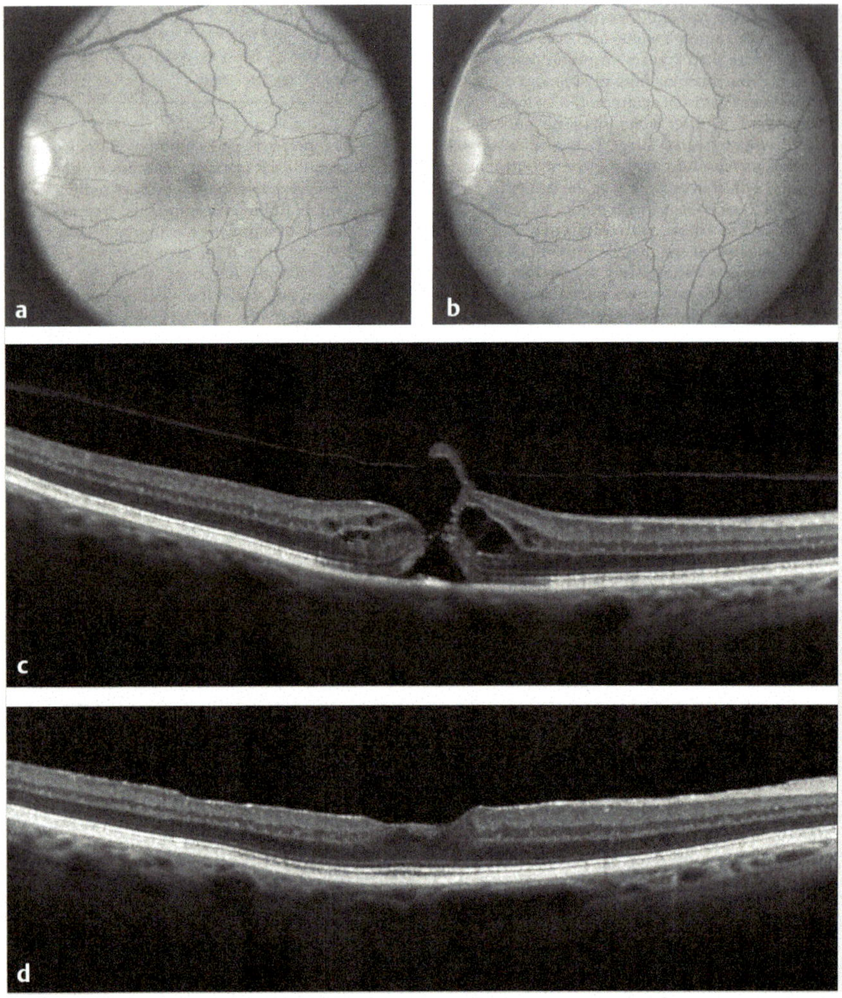

Fig. 17.12 (**a**) The preoperative appearance of a stage 3 macular hole in an eye with a visual acuity of 20/200. (**b**) This macular hole was closed successfully with vitreoretinal surgery, and the macular hole is no longer visible. Visual acuity improved to 20/63. (**c**) Preoperative OCT of another patient with a stage 2 macular hole and 20/40 acuity. (**d**) Postoperative appearance of successfully closed macular hole with virtually normal ellipsoid layer/external limiting membrane and a visual acuity of 20/20.

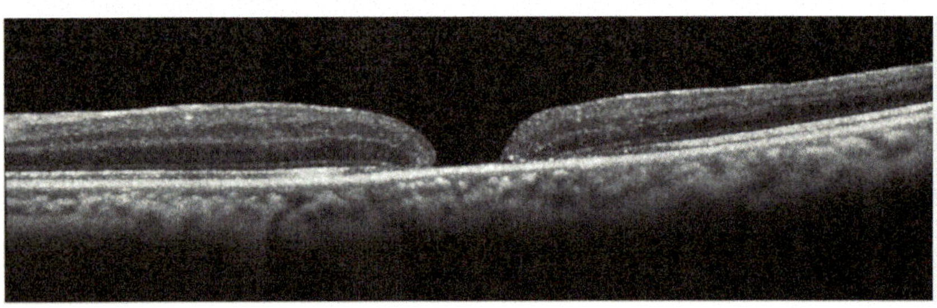

Fig. 17.13 Some macular holes close with reapposition of the neurosensory retina against the retinal pigment epithelium, but the two edges of the hole do not join. This has been termed type 2 macular hole closure to contrast this to the more typical macular hole closure shown in ▶ Fig. 17.12d.

The success of macular hole surgery has improved over the past 20 years, and most recent studies report macular hole closure in 90% of eyes or more, with visual acuity improvement of two lines or more in about two-thirds of eyes.[8,21] Findings on preoperative and postoperative OCT, particularly the integrity of the inner segment/outer segment (ELM/ellipsoid) layers, have reasonably good predictive value for visual acuity outcomes of macular hole surgery.[100] ▶ Table 17.2 summarizes the results of selected studies of surgery for idiopathic macular holes covering a range of studies from the earliest to most recent studies. These studies primarily reported on the results of vitreous surgery for recent and intermediate-duration macular holes (2 years or less). Patient age is not a limiting factor, as the results appear to be equivalent in patients younger and older than 80 years.[101] Vision-related quality of life also improves following macular hole surgery.[102,103] The visual acuity gains following macular hole surgery have been reported to be stable for 4 or more years.[74,104] Additional studies have examined the results of surgery for selected subgroups of macular holes, such as chronic, myopic, recurrent, and traumatic macular holes.

Chronic Macular Holes

Chronic macular holes have been assumed to be more difficult to close with vitreous surgery. An early study reported successful closure of three macular holes older than 3 years, with visual acuity improvement in two of three eyes.[105] A second report of macular hole surgery in 45 eyes with macular holes of more than 2 years' duration demonstrated closure of the macular hole in 71% and a two-line improvement in visual acuity in 47% of eyes.[106]

Controversial Points

- Macular hole surgery in eyes with recurrent or chronic macular holes is successful in closing the macular hole in a majority of eyes. The indications remain debatable because the visual results are generally not as favorable as in eyes with primary macular holes of recent onset.

Recurrent/Persistent Macular Holes

Recurrent/persistent macular holes may be treated successfully with repeated surgery. Although results are not as good as with primary closure, an early study reported closure in 12 of 12 eyes, with visual acuity improvement in 42% of eyes.[107] A larger study of 48 eyes with recurrent macular holes showed closure of the macular hole in 83% of eyes and a three-line visual acuity improvement in 52% of eyes.[108] Eyes with a visual acuity better than 20/80 preoperatively had a significantly better chance of achieving a good postoperative acuity (20/63 or better).[108] Overall, the results for repeated macular hole surgery are not as favorable as the results for primary surgery, but most eyes treated with a second surgery do have a successful outcome with improved visual acuity. There are occasional eyes that reopen after two macular hole surgeries. These are termed multiple recurrent macular holes. Surgery is most likely to be successful when the macular hole was closed temporarily by at least one of the prior surgeries.[109]

Myopic Macular Holes

Myopic macular holes are more difficult to close, and the success of macular hole surgery decreases with increasing axial length in highly myopic eyes, but reasonably good results may still be achieved.[110] Staining and removal of the ILM are especially helpful in closing these macular holes. Some myopic macular holes have a morphology similar to idiopathic macular holes and some eyes develop localized or extensive retinal detachments associated with their macular holes. Long-acting tamponade is very helpful and can include gas[110,111] or extended tamponade with silicone oil[111,112,113,114,115] to achieve closure of the macular hole. Michalewska and colleagues reported the inverted ILM flap technique which may further help with closure of the macular hole. The inverted ILM flap technique leaves a rim of ILM attached to the edge of the macular hole and this is folded onto the fovea so the ILM bridges the defect in the neurosensory retina. Using this technique, successful anatomic closure was achieved in 19/19 eyes with myopic macular holes.[116] Macular buckling can also be used in eyes with refractory retinal detachment associated with macular holes.[117]

Special Considerations

- Macular holes associated with high myopia and retinal detachment are more challenging to close. ILM removal using an ILM stain and long-acting tamponade, preferably with intraocular gas, is essential. The inverted ILM flap technique is helpful to improve the likelihood of closing the macular hole. The visual acuity improvement may be limited by macular atrophy, but most of these myopic eyes still benefit from surgery.

Trauma

Trauma represents an uncommon etiology of macular holes, but traumatic macular holes are an important cause of decreased vision in younger patients with ocular trauma. Spontaneous closure is more common in traumatic macular holes, and therefore surgery should be delayed for about a month to see if the hole closes. This also allows traumatic damage such as commotio retinae to resolve. If the traumatic macular hole remains open, then vitrectomy is generally indicated. Successful closure of traumatic macular holes has been reported in 92 to 96% of eyes with one or more surgeries.[118,119,120] Visual acuity improved two or more lines in 67% of eyes in one study.[113] Some larger traumatic macular holes may be difficult to close, but the visual acuity improvements can be substantial in these eyes, possibly because of the young age of a majority of these patients. Trauma-induced RPE changes in the fovea may limit visual recovery but are not a contraindication for this surgery. Cataract progression was substantially delayed following surgery in these patients because of their young age. Surgery should be considered in eyes with traumatic macular holes unless the damage to the macula is so extensive as to preclude the possibility of visual improvement.

17.4.8 Complications of Macular Hole Surgery

Macular hole surgery shares many of the same potential complications as vitrectomy surgery for other indications (see Chapter 40). Although rare, the most serious risk of surgery is *infectious endophthalmitis*, which develops in about 0.07% eyes undergoing vitrectomy for a variety of indications.[121] The risk for infectious endophthalmitis is probably increased when autologous blood products are used as adjunctive agents, and it is one of several reasons such agents are no longer used for macular hole surgery.[122] Eyes in which evidence of infectious endophthalmitis develops should be treated with intravitreal antibiotics. The protocols outlined in the Endophthalmitis Vitrectomy Study (EVS) should be used, even though the EVS studied eyes following cataract surgery as there are no randomized studies of endophthalmitis following vitrectomy for macular holes (see Chapter 35).[123] Furthermore, it may be advisable to remove the intraocular gas bubble to allow the antibiotics to diffuse freely within the vitreous cavity.

Elevated intraocular pressure (IOP) develops most commonly between the first day and several weeks following surgery. Elevated IOP often occurs in the first 48 hours following surgery and likely results from impaired aqueous outflow related to inflammation from the surgical procedure or expansion of the gas bubble when concentrations of C_3F_8 greater than 12 to 14% or SF_6 concentrations greater than 20% are used. In these eyes, the angle remains open. Treatment consists of aqueous suppressants such as dorzolamide, timolol, or brimonidine. A much smaller percentage of eyes with elevated IOP following macular hole surgery have angle closure with a shallow or flat anterior chamber. These eyes do not respond well to aqueous suppressants. These eyes can be treated with a YAG peripheral iridectomy that is best placed in the inferior peripheral iris at 6 o'clock position as this is where the fluid in the posterior chamber is located in a gas-filled eye. Reformation of the anterior chamber with saline may be required if the YAG peripheral iridectomy does not correct the flat anterior chamber. If the IOP is very high (> 40 mm Hg) and the vitreous cavity has a 100% gas bubble, the surgeon must consider the possibility that pure C_3F_8 or SF_6 was instilled into the vitreous by mistake. If this is suspected, the patient needs immediate decompression of the vitreous cavity and daily monitoring of the IOP as the remaining gas bubble may continue to expand as air enters the gas bubble over the first 48 to 72 hours following surgery.

Retinal Tears or Rhegmatogenous Retinal Detachments

Retinal tears or rhegmatogenous retinal detachments are an important cause of ocular morbidity in eyes undergoing macular hole surgery. The rate of retinal detachment is variable and ranges from 1.2% in one series[124] to 14% in another contemporaneous series using 20-gauge vitrectomy.[125] Meticulous examination of the peripheral retina is essential *before* fluid–gas exchange because the creation of a posterior vitreous detachment and 20-gauge vitrectomy is associated with retinal tears in 16% of eyes with macular holes.[124] A study comparing the creation of retinal breaks during 20-gauge versus 23-gauge vitrectomy found an incidence of 16.7% with 20-gauge vitrectomy compared to 7.8% for 23-gauge vitrectomy.[126] About two-thirds of these iatrogenic retinal breaks are located in the inferior retina and are created during creation or extension of a posterior vitreous detachment. These tears should be treated by cryopexy or laser photocoagulation. Occasionally, a retinal tear will be noted without retinal detachment within the first 2 weeks following surgery. Treatment with laser photocoagulation or cryopexy and appropriate prone positioning may prevent a retinal detachment in these eyes. It is very important to prevent a retinal detachment, as detachment of the macula may cause reopening of the macular hole.

Pearls

- In contrast to the retinal tears associated with most other vitrectomy operations, which are usually seen superiorly near the sclerotomies, nearly two-thirds of iatrogenic retinal breaks in macular hole surgery are located in the inferior retina.

RPE Alterations

RPE alterations in the macula following macular hole surgery were reported as a potential complication of macular hole surgery.[89,127,128] These RPE changes are a combination of RPE atrophy and pigment clumping. The pigment clumping is easily seen on fundus examination (▶ Fig. 17.14), and the RPE atrophy may be visualized best on fluorescein angiography. The three most common causes of the RPE atrophy are (1) mechanical damage to the macula with ILM peeling, (2) phototoxicity from the light pipe, and (3) ICG toxicity to the RPE. Mechanical damage to the RPE can occur with removal of the ILM. Care must be taken to not bump the retina when the ILM is grasped with forceps. This is why it is best to start the ILM peel at least 1,000 µm from the center of the fovea as an RPE "bruise" is most likely to occur where the ILM peel is started. On rare occasions, the ILM is very firmly adherent to the underlying neurosensory retina, and a perimacular full-thickness retinal tear can be created when removing the ILM. If the surgeon observes that the retina is starting to lift when the ILM is lifted, the ILM peel should be stopped and started in another area. Phototoxicity from the fiberoptic light pipe can also create RPE changes, but unlike a mechanical trauma during ILM peel, these RPE changes do not develop until a month or more following surgery. Keeping the light pipe away from the fovea (at least 5 mm) and limiting the amount of time the light pipe is held relatively close to the fovea may prevent this complication of macular surgery. A good rule of thumb is to not hold the light pipe close to the macula for longer than one can hold one's breath (about 60 seconds). The third cause of RPE changes in the macula is ICG toxicity. ICG is very helpful in staining the ILM but has the potential to cause toxicity and subsequent atrophy of the RPE. Care must be taken to use as little ICG as possible to stain the ILM. It is also important to not vigorously remove the viscous fluid within the macular hole (the subretinal fluid on OCT), as this fluid tends to prevent ICG from diffusing into the subretinal space during a short exposure of 30 to 60 seconds before the excess ICG is removed from the eye.

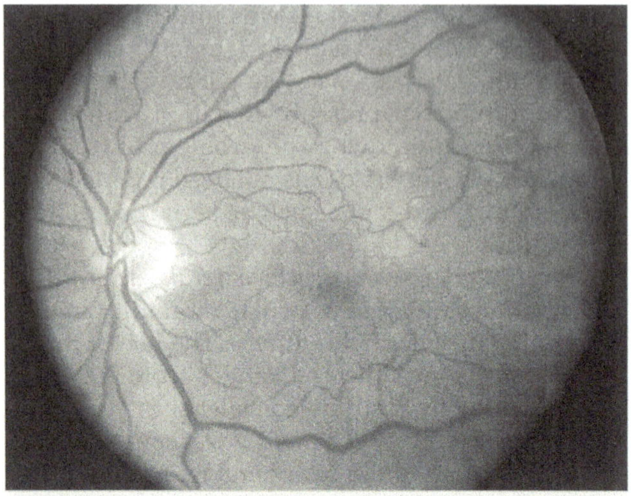

Fig. 17.14 Phototoxicity from the fiberoptic light pipe creates pigment clumping in the fovea and may develop following macular hole surgery when the light pipe is held too close to the fovea.

Visual Field Loss

Visual field loss is another complication of macular hole surgery.[129,130,131,132,133,134] Patients in whom visual field loss develops generally notice an inferotemporal visual field defect as the gas bubble is being absorbed. These visual field defects are usually due to dehydration injury to the macula and result from the jet stream of air from the infusion cannula against the nerve fiber layer.[135] It is desirable to have a large gas bubble in eyes with macular holes but care must be taken to not dry the surface of the retina excessively and repeatedly.

Persistent/Recurrent Macular Holes

Persistent/recurrent macular holes have been discussed previously and are among the most common complications of macular hole surgery. Sometimes the glial plug that normally closes the macular hole never develops, so the hole reopens once the macular hole is again exposed to a vitreous filled with fluid. Eyes in which there is traction on the macula, such as eyes which develop an epiretinal membrane or CME following cataract surgery, are especially prone to develop late recurrent macular holes.[136]

Nuclear Sclerotic Cataracts

The development of nuclear sclerotic cataracts is inevitable after macular hole surgery in phakic persons older than 50 years, and even younger patients will eventually develop increased nuclear sclerosis following vitrectomy. Increased oxidation of the lens from increased vitreous oxygen concentration following vitrectomy is the primary cause of these nuclear sclerotic cataracts.[137] One study showed that nuclear sclerosis progressed at least two grades in 55% of eyes followed up for at least 1 year and 71% of eyes followed up for 2 years or more following vitrectomy for macular hole.[48] Most patients older than 50 years with macular hole surgery require cataract extraction within 9 to 18 months of their macular hole surgery. Posterior subcapsular cataracts did not show substantial progression in a prior study,[48] although in a few eyes gas-induced posterior subcapsular cataracts do develop because of poor patient compliance with prone positioning.

17.5 Conclusion

The treatment of macular holes has improved dramatically in the past two decades. Current surgical techniques allow a majority of eyes with macular holes of less than 2 years' duration to be treated with vitreous surgery and gain two or more lines of visual acuity. Improved accuracy in the diagnosis of macular holes from use of OCT and recognition of macular holes by primary eye care providers with prompt referral of patients with macular holes to the retinal surgeon maximize the chances for improved visual acuity following surgery. The complication rate of macular hole surgery has decreased with improvement of surgical techniques. In the future, the main goals will center on finding safer dyes for ILM staining and decreasing the burden of prone positioning. Improved selection of the eyes most likely to benefit from surgery will help to improve the overall surgical results. Prevention of macular holes is an elusive goal, but improvements in our understanding of the pathophysiology of macular holes may help to recognize and preemptively treat the foveal traction associated with the perimacular posterior vitreous detachment that often precedes the macular hole. It is a testament to the research studies by many different investigators that substantial vision loss from macular holes is increasingly uncommon.

References

[1] Gass JDM. Idiopathic senile macular hole. Its early stages and pathogenesis. Arch Ophthalmol. 1988; 108(5):629–639

[2] Kelly NE, Wendel RT. Vitreous surgery for idiopathic macular holes. Results of a pilot study. Arch Ophthalmol. 1991; 109(5):654–659

[3] Sjaarda RN, Frank DA, Glaser BM, Thompson JT, Murphy RP. Resolution of an absolute scotoma and improvement of relative scotomata after successful macular hole surgery. Am J Ophthalmol. 1993; 116(2):129–139

[4] Johnson RN, Gass JDM. Idiopathic macular holes: observations, stages of formation, and implications for surgical intervention. Ophthalmology. 1988; 95 (7):917–924

[5] Guez JE, Le Gargasson JF, Massin P, Rigaudière F, Grall Y, Gaudric A. Functional assessment of macular hole surgery by scanning laser ophthalmoscopy. Ophthalmology. 1998; 105(4):694–699

[6] McCannel CA, Ensminger JL, Diehl NN, Hodge DN. Population-based incidence of macular holes. Ophthalmology. 2009; 116(7):1366–1369

[7] Chew EY, Sperduto RD, Hiller R, et al. Clinical course of macular holes: the Eye Disease Case-Control Study. Arch Ophthalmol. 1999; 117(2):242–246

[8] Thompson JT, Glaser BM, Sjaarda RN, Murphy RP, Hanham A. Effects of intraocular bubble duration in the treatment of macular holes by vitrectomy and transforming growth factor-beta 2. Ophthalmology. 1994; 101(7):1195–1200

[9] Smiddy WE, Feuer W, Cordahi G. Internal limiting membrane peeling in macular hole surgery. Ophthalmology. 2001; 108(8):1471–1476, discussion 1477–1478

[10] Gass JD. Reappraisal of biomicroscopic classification of stages of development of a macular hole. Am J Ophthalmol. 1995; 119(6):752–759

[11] Gaudric A, Haouchine B, Massin P, Paques M, Blain P, Erginay A. Macular hole formation: new data provided by optical coherence tomography. Arch Ophthalmol. 1999; 117(6):744–751

[12] Spaide RF, Wong D, Fisher Y, Goldbaum M. Correlation of vitreous attachment and foveal deformation in early macular hole states. Am J Ophthalmol. 2002; 133(2):226–229

[13] Madreperla SA, McCuen BW, II, Hickingbotham D, Green WR. Clinicopathologic correlation of surgically removed macular hole opercula. Am J Ophthalmol. 1995; 120(2):197–207

[14] Hikichi T, Trempe CL. Resolution of an absolute scotoma after spontaneous disappearance of idiopathic full-thickness macular hole. Am J Ophthalmol. 1994; 118(1):121–122

[15] Lewis H, Cowan GM, Straatsma BR. Apparent disappearance of a macular hole associated with development of an epiretinal membrane. Am J Ophthalmol. 1986; 102(2):172–175

[16] Duker JS, Kaiser PK, Binder S, et al. The International Vitreomacular Traction Study Group classification of vitreomacular adhesion, traction, and macular hole. Ophthalmology. 2013; 120(12):2611–2619

[17] Klein BR, Hiner CJ, Glaser BM, Murphy RP, Sjaarda RN, Thompson JT. Fundus photographic and fluorescein angiographic characteristics of pseudoholes of the macula in eyes with epiretinal membranes. Ophthalmology. 1995; 102 (5):768–774

[18] Stalmans P, Benz MS, Gandorfer A, et al. MIVI-TRUST Study Group. Enzymatic vitreolysis with ocriplasmin for vitreomacular traction and macular holes. N Engl J Med. 2012; 367(7):606–615

[19] Lewis ML, Cohen SM, Smiddy WE, Gass JD. Bilaterality of idiopathic macular holes. Graefes Arch Clin Exp Ophthalmol. 1996; 234(4):241–245

[20] Christensen UC, Krøyer K, Sander B, et al. Value of internal limiting membrane peeling in surgery for idiopathic macular hole stage 2 and 3: a randomised clinical trial. Br J Ophthalmol. 2009; 93(8):1005–1015

[21] Tognetto D, Grandin R, Sanguinetti G, et al. Macular Hole Surgery Study Group. Internal limiting membrane removal during macular hole surgery: results of a multicenter retrospective study. Ophthalmology. 2006; 113 (8):1401–1410

[22] Haritoglou C, Reiniger IW, Schaumberger M, Gass CA, Priglinger SG, Kampik A. Five-year follow-up of macular hole surgery with peeling of the internal limiting membrane: update of a prospective study. Retina. 2006; 26(6):618–622

[23] Sheidow TG, Blinder KJ, Holekamp N, et al. Outcome results in macular hole surgery: an evaluation of internal limiting membrane peeling with and without indocyanine green. Ophthalmology. 2003; 110(9):1697–1701

[24] Foulquier S, Glacet-Bernard A, Sterkers M, Soubrane G, Coscas G. Study of internal limiting membrane peeling in stage-3 and -4 idiopathic macular hole surgery [in French]. J Fr Ophtalmol. 2002; 25(10):1026–1031

[25] Brooks HL, Jr. Macular hole surgery with and without internal limiting membrane peeling. Ophthalmology. 2000; 107(10):1939–1948, discussion 1948–1949

[26] Spiteri Cornish K, Lois N, Scott NW, et al. Vitrectomy with internal limiting membrane peeling versus no peeling for idiopathic full-thickness macular hole. Ophthalmology. 2014; 121(3):649–655

[27] Nakamura Y, Kondo M, Asami T, Terasaki H. Comparison of macular hole surgery without internal limiting membrane peeling to eyes with internal limiting membrane peeling with and without indocyanine green staining: three-year follow-up. Ophthalmic Res. 2009; 41(3):136–141

[28] Nagai N, Ishida S, Shinoda K, Imamura Y, Noda K, Inoue M. Surgical effects and complications of indocyanine green-assisted internal limiting membrane peeling for idiopathic macular hole. Acta Ophthalmol Scand. 2007; 85 (8):883–889

[29] Lai MM, Williams GA. Anatomical and visual outcomes of idiopathic macular hole surgery with internal limiting membrane removal using low-concentration indocyanine green. Retina. 2007; 27(4):477–482

[30] Kumagai K, Furukawa M, Ogino N, Uemura A, Larson E. Long-term outcomes of internal limiting membrane peeling with and without indocyanine green in macular hole surgery. Retina. 2006; 26(6):613–617

[31] Slaughter K, Lee IL. Macular hole surgery with and without indocyanine green assistance. Eye (Lond). 2004; 18(4):376–378

[32] Kwok AK, Lai TY, Man-Chan W, Woo DC. Indocyanine green assisted retinal internal limiting membrane removal in stage 3 or 4 macular hole surgery. Br J Ophthalmol. 2003; 87(1):71–74

[33] Brasil OM, Brasil OF. Comparative analysis of macular hole surgery followed by internal limiting membrane removal with and without indocyanine green staining [in Portuguese]. Arq Bras Oftalmol. 2006; 69(2):157–160

[34] Ben Simon GJ, Desatnik H, Alhalel A, Treister G, Moisseiev J. Retrospective analysis of vitrectomy with and without internal limiting membrane peeling for stage 3 and 4 macular hole. Ophthalmic Surg Lasers Imaging. 2004; 35 (2):109–115

[35] Lochhead J, Jones E, Chui D, et al. Outcome of ICG-assisted ILM peel in macular hole surgery. Eye (Lond). 2004; 18(8):804–808

[36] Kwok AK, Lai TY, Yuen KS, Tam BS, Wong VW. Macular hole surgery with or without indocyanine green stained internal limiting membrane peeling. Clin Experiment Ophthalmol. 2003; 31(6):470–475

[37] Kumagai K, Furukawa M, Ogino N, Larson E, Uemura A. Long-term outcomes of macular hole surgery with triamcinolone acetonide-assisted internal limiting membrane peeling. Retina. 2007; 27(9):1249–1254

[38] Beutel J, Dahmen G, Ziegler A, Hoerauf H. Internal limiting membrane peeling with indocyanine green or trypan blue in macular hole surgery: a randomized trial. Arch Ophthalmol. 2007; 125(3):326–332

[39] Lee KL, Dean S, Guest S. A comparison of outcomes after indocyanine green and trypan blue assisted internal limiting membrane peeling during macular hole surgery. Br J Ophthalmol. 2005; 89(4):420–424

[40] Williamson TH, Lee E. Idiopathic macular hole: analysis of visual outcomes and the use of indocyanine green or brilliant blue for internal limiting membrane peel. Graefes Arch Clin Exp Ophthalmol. 2014; 252(3):395–400

[41] von Jagow B, Höing A, Gandorfer A, et al. Functional outcome of indocyanine green-assisted macular surgery: 7-year follow-up. Retina. 2009; 29 (9):1249–1256

[42] Yamashita T, Uemura A, Kita H, Nakao K, Sakamoto T. Long-term outcomes of visual field defects after indocyanine green-assisted macular hole surgery. Retina. 2008; 28(9):1228–1233

[43] Gass CA, Haritoglou C, Schaumberger M, Kampik A. Functional outcome of macular hole surgery with and without indocyanine green-assisted peeling of the internal limiting membrane. Graefes Arch Clin Exp Ophthalmol. 2003; 241(9):716–720

[44] Engelbrecht NE, Freeman J, Sternberg P, Jr, et al. Retinal pigment epithelial changes after macular hole surgery with indocyanine green-assisted internal limiting membrane peeling. Am J Ophthalmol. 2002; 133(1):89–94

[45] Rubin JS, Thompson JT, Sjaarda RN, Pappas SS, Jr, Glaser BM. Efficacy of fluid-air exchange during pars plana vitrectomy. Retina. 1995; 15(4):291–294

[46] Glaser BM, Michels RG, Kuppermann BD, Sjaarda RN, Pena RA. Transforming growth factor-beta 2 for the treatment of full-thickness macular holes. A prospective randomized study. Ophthalmology. 1992; 99(7):1162–1172, discussion 1173

[47] Lansing MB, Glaser BM, Liss H, et al. The effect of pars plana vitrectomy and transforming growth factor-beta 2 without epiretinal membrane peeling on full-thickness macular holes. Ophthalmology. 1993; 100(6):868–871, discussion 871–872

[48] Thompson JT, Glaser BM, Sjaarda RN, Murphy RP. Progression of nuclear sclerosis and long-term visual results of vitrectomy with transforming growth factor beta-2 for macular holes. Am J Ophthalmol. 1995; 119(1):48–54

[49] Liggett PE, Skolik DS, Horio B, Saito Y, Alfaro V, Mieler W. Human autologous serum for the treatment of full-thickness macular holes. A preliminary study. Ophthalmology. 1995; 102(7):1071–1076

[50] Pavan PR, Oteiza EE. Complications of autologous cryoprecipitates and thrombinar. Vitreous Society Abstracts, 1994

[51] Blumenkranz MS, Coll GE, Chang S, et al. Use of autologous plasma-thrombin mixture as adjuvant therapy for macular hole. Ophthalmology. 1994; 101 9A:7:69

[52] Johnson MW, Vine AK. Use of thrombin as mitogen therapy in macular hole surgery. Macula Society Abstracts, 1995

[53] Gaudric A, Massin P, Paques M, et al. Autologous platelet concentrate for the treatment of full-thickness macular holes. Graefes Arch Clin Exp Ophthalmol. 1995; 233(9):549–554

[54] Korobelnik JF, Hannouche D, Belayachi N, Branger M, Guez JE, Hoang-Xuan T. Autologous platelet concentrate as an adjunct in macular hole healing: a pilot study. Ophthalmology. 1996; 103(4):590–594

[55] Funata M, Wendel RT, de la Cruz Z, Green WR. Clinicopathologic study of bilateral macular holes treated with pars plana vitrectomy and gas tamponade. Retina. 1992; 12(4):289–298

[56] Madreperla SA, Geiger GL, Funata M, de la Cruz Z, Green WR. Clinicopathologic correlation of a macular hole treated by cortical vitreous peeling and gas tamponade. Ophthalmology. 1994; 101(4):682–686

[57] Yamashita T, Sakamoto T, Yamashita T, et al. Individualized, spectral domain-optical coherence tomography-guided facedown posturing after macular hole surgery: minimizing treatment burden and maximizing outcome. Retina. 2014; 34(7):1367–1375

[58] Masuyama K, Yamakiri K, Arimura N, Sonoda Y, Doi N, Sakamoto T. Posturing time after macular hole surgery modified by optical coherence tomography images: a pilot study. Am J Ophthalmol. 2009; 147(3):481–488.e2

[59] Eckardt C, Eckert T, Eckardt U, Porkert U, Gesser C. Macular hole surgery with air tamponade and optical coherence tomography-based duration of face-down positioning. Retina. 2008; 28(8):1087–1096

[60] Forsaa VA, Raeder S, Hashemi LT, Krohn J. Short-term postoperative non-supine positioning versus strict face-down positioning in macular hole surgery. Acta Ophthalmol (Copenh). 2013; 91(6):547–551

[61] Nadal J, Delas B, Piñero A. Vitrectomy without face-down posturing for idiopathic macular holes. Retina. 2012; 32(5):918–921

[62] Yorston D, Siddiqui MA, Awan MA, Walker S, Bunce C, Bainbridge JW. Pilot randomised controlled trial of face-down posturing following phacovitrectomy for macular hole. Eye (Lond). 2012; 26(2):267–271

[63] Lange CA, Membrey L, Ahmad N, et al. Pilot randomised controlled trial of face-down positioning following macular hole surgery. Eye (Lond). 2012; 26 (2):272–277

[64] Carvounis PE, Kopel AC, Kuhl DP, Heffez J, Pepple K, Holz ER. 25-gauge vitrectomy using sulfur hexafluoride and no prone positioning for repair of macular holes. Retina. 2008; 28(9):1188–1192

[65] Mittra RA, Kim JE, Han DP, Pollack JS. Sustained postoperative face-down positioning is unnecessary for successful macular hole surgery. Br J Ophthalmol. 2009; 93(5):664–666

[66] Rubinstein A, Ang A, Patel CK. Vitrectomy without postoperative posturing for idiopathic macular holes. Clin Experiment Ophthalmol. 2007; 35 (5):458–461

[67] Merkur AB, Tuli R. Macular hole repair with limited nonsupine positioning. Retina. 2007; 27(3):365–369

[68] Tranos PG, Peter NM, Nath R, et al. Macular hole surgery without prone positioning. Eye (Lond). 2007; 21(6):802–806

[69] Solebo AL, Lange CA, Bunce C, Bainbridge JW. Face-down positioning or posturing after macular hole surgery. Cochrane Database Syst Rev. 2011; 7(12): CD008228

[70] Guillaubey A, Malvitte L, Lafontaine PO, et al. Comparison of face-down and seated position after idiopathic macular hole surgery: a randomized clinical trial. Am J Ophthalmol. 2008; 146(1):128–134

[71] Tornambe PE, Poliner LS, Grote K. Macular hole surgery without face-down positioning. A pilot study. Retina. 1997; 17(3):179–185

[72] Couvillion SS, Smiddy WE, Flynn HW, Jr, Eifrig CW, Gregori G. Outcomes of surgery for idiopathic macular hole: a case-control study comparing silicone oil with gas tamponade. Ophthalmic Surg Lasers Imaging. 2005; 36(5):365–371

[73] Karia N, Laidlaw A, West J, Ezra E, Gregor MZ. Macular hole surgery using silicone oil tamponade. Br J Ophthalmol. 2001; 85(11):1320–1323

[74] Scott IU, Moraczewski AL, Smiddy WE, Flynn HW, Jr, Feuer WJ. Long-term anatomic and visual acuity outcomes after initial anatomic success with macular hole surgery. Am J Ophthalmol. 2003; 135(5):633–640

[75] Goldbaum MH, McCuen BW, Hanneken AM, Burgess SK, Chen HH. Silicone oil tamponade to seal macular holes without position restrictions. Ophthalmology. 1998; 105(11):2140–2147, discussion 2147–2148

[76] Conart JB, Selton J, Hubert I, et al. Outcomes of macular hole surgery with short-duration positioning in highly myopic eyes: a case-control study. Ophthalmology. 2014; 121(6):1263–1268
[77] Usui H, Yasukawa T, Hirano Y, Morita H, Yoshida M, Ogura Y. Comparative study of the effects of room air and sulfur hexafluoride gas tamponade on functional and morphological recovery after macular hole surgery: a retrospective study. Ophthalmic Res. 2013; 50(4):227–230
[78] Almeida DR, Wong J, Belliveau M, Rayat J, Gale J. Anatomical and visual outcomes of macular hole surgery with short-duration 3-day face-down positioning. Retina. 2012; 32(3):506–510
[79] Rayat J, Almeida DR, Belliveau M, Wong J, Gale J. Visual function and vision-related quality of life after macular hole surgery with short-duration, 3-day face-down positioning. Can J Ophthalmol. 2011; 46(5):399–402
[80] Malik A, Dooley I, Mahmood U. Single night postoperative prone posturing in idiopathic macular hole surgery. Eur J Ophthalmol. 2012; 22(3):456–460
[81] Hasegawa Y, Hata Y, Mochizuki Y, et al. Equivalent tamponade by room air as compared with SF(6) after macular hole surgery. Graefes Arch Clin Exp Ophthalmol. 2009; 247(11):1455–1459
[82] Krohn J. Duration of face-down positioning after macular hole surgery: a comparison between 1 week and 3 days. Acta Ophthalmol Scand. 2005; 83 (3):289–292
[83] Miura M, Elsner AE, Osako M, Iwasaki T, Okano T, Usui M. Dissociated optic nerve fiber layer appearance after internal limiting membrane peeling for idiopathic macular hole. Retina. 2003; 23(4):561–563
[84] Park DW, Sipperley JO, Sneed SR, Dugel PU, Jacobsen J. Macular hole surgery with internal-limiting membrane peeling and intravitreous air. Ophthalmology. 1999; 106(7):1392–1397, discussion 1397–1398
[85] Wickens JC, Shah GK. Outcomes of macular hole surgery and shortened face down positioning. Retina. 2006; 26(8):902–904
[86] Ellis JD, Malik TY, Taubert MA, Barr A, Baines PS. Surgery for full-thickness macular holes with short-duration prone posturing: results of a pilot study. Eye (Lond). 2000; 14 Pt 3A:307–312
[87] Verma D, Jalabi MW, Watts WG, Naylor G. Evaluation of posturing in macular hole surgery. Eye (Lond). 2002; 16(6):701–704
[88] Leitritz MA, Ziemssen F, Voykov B, Bartz-Schmidt KU. Usability of a gravity- and tilt-compensated sensor with data logging function to measure posturing compliance in patients after macular hole surgery: a pilot study. Graefes Arch Clin Exp Ophthalmol. 2014; 252(5):739–744
[89] Freeman WR, Azen SP, Kim JW, el-Haig W, Mishell DR, III, Bailey I, The Vitrectomy for Treatment of Macular Hole Study Group. Vitrectomy for the treatment of full-thickness stage 3 or 4 macular holes. Results of a multicentered randomized clinical trial. Arch Ophthalmol. 1997; 115(1):11–21
[90] Schaal S, Barr CC. Management of macular holes: a comparison of 1-year outcomes of 3 surgical techniques. Retina. 2009; 29(8):1091–1096
[91] Tsipursky MS, Heller MA, De Souza SA, et al. Comparative evaluation of no dye assistance, indocyanine green and triamcinolone acetonide for internal limiting membrane peeling during macular hole surgery. Retina. 2013; 33 (6):1123–1131
[92] Duker JS, Wendel R, Patel AC, Puliafito CA. Late re-opening of macular holes after initially successful treatment with vitreous surgery. Ophthalmology. 1994; 101(8):1373–1378
[93] Kumagai K, Furukawa M, Ogino N, Larson E. Incidence and factors related to macular hole reopening. Am J Ophthalmol. 2010; 149(1):127–132
[94] Wendel RT, Patel AC, Kelly NE, Salzano TC, Wells JW, Novack GD. Vitreous surgery for macular holes. Ophthalmology. 1993; 100(11):1671–1676
[95] Che X, He F, Lu L, et al. Evaluation of secondary surgery to enlarge the peeling of the internal limiting membrane following the failed surgery of idiopathic macular holes. Exp Ther Med. 2014; 7(3):742–746
[96] Morizane Y, Shiraga F, Kimura S, et al. Autologous transplantation of the internal limiting membrane for refractory macular holes. Am J Ophthalmol. 2014; 157(4):861–869.e1
[97] Del Priore LV, Kaplan HJ, Bonham RD. Laser photocoagulation and fluid-gas exchange for recurrent macular hole. Retina. 1994; 14(4):381–382
[98] Kang SW, Ahn K, Ham DI. Types of macular hole closure and their clinical implications. Br J Ophthalmol. 2003; 87(8):1015–1019
[99] Krøyer K, Christensen U, la Cour M, Larsen M. Metamorphopsia assessment before and after vitrectomy for macular hole. Invest Ophthalmol Vis Sci. 2009; 50(12):5511–5515
[100] Oh J, Smiddy WE, Flynn HW, Jr, Gregori G, Lujan B. Photoreceptor inner/outer segment defect imaging by spectral domain OCT and visual prognosis after macular hole surgery. Invest Ophthalmol Vis Sci. 2010; 51(3):1651–1658
[101] Thompson JT, Sjaarda RN. Results of macular hole surgery in patients over 80 years of age. Retina. 2000; 20(5):433–438
[102] Fukuda S, Okamoto F, Yuasa M, et al. Vision-related quality of life and visual function in patients undergoing vitrectomy, gas tamponade and cataract surgery for macular hole. Br J Ophthalmol. 2009; 93(12):1595–1599
[103] Hirneiss C, Neubauer AS, Gass CA, et al. Visual quality of life after macular hole surgery: outcome and predictive factors. Br J Ophthalmol. 2007; 91 (4):481–484
[104] Reiniger IW, Gass CA, Schaumberger M, Kampik A, Haritoglou C. Long-term functional results after macular hole surgery. Results of a prospective study [in German]. Ophthalmologe. 2006; 103(6):501–505
[105] Kokame GT. Macular hole surgery for chronic macular holes. Retina. 1996; 16(1):75 78
[106] Thompson JT, Sjaarda RN, Lansing MB. The results of vitreous surgery for chronic macular holes. Retina. 1997; 17(6):493–501
[107] Ie D, Glaser BM, Thompson JT, Sjaarda RN, Gordon LW. Retreatment of full-thickness macular holes persisting after prior vitrectomy. A pilot study. Ophthalmology. 1993; 100(12):1787–1793
[108] Smiddy WE, Sjaarda RN, Glaser BM, et al. Reoperation after failed macular hole surgery. Retina. 1996; 16(1):13–18
[109] Thompson JT, Sjaarda RN. Surgical treatment of macular holes with multiple recurrences. Ophthalmology. 2000; 107(6):1073–1077
[110] Sulkes DJ, Smiddy WE, Flynn HW, Feuer W. Outcomes of macular hole surgery in severely myopic eyes: a case-control study. Am J Ophthalmol. 2000; 130(3):335–339
[111] Mancino R, Ciuffoletti E, Martucci A, et al. Anatomical and functional results of macular hole retinal detachment surgery in patients with high myopia and posterior staphyloma treated with perfluoropropane gas or silicone oil. Retina. 2013; 33(3):586–592
[112] Scholda C, Wirtitsch M, Biowski R, Stur M. Primary silicone oil tamponade without retinopexy in highly myopic eyes with central macular hole detachments. Retina. 2005; 25(2):141–146
[113] Nishimura A, Kimura M, Saito Y, Sugiyama K. Efficacy of primary silicone oil tamponade for the treatment of retinal detachment caused by macular hole in high myopia. Am J Ophthalmol. 2011; 151(1):148–155
[114] Soheilian M, Ghaseminejad AK, Yazdani S, et al. Surgical management of retinal detachment in highly myopic eyes with macular hole. Ophthalmic Surg Lasers Imaging. 2007; 38(1):15–22
[115] Nadal J, Verdaguer P, Canut MI. Treatment of retinal detachment secondary to macular hole in high myopia: vitrectomy with dissection of the inner limiting membrane to the edge of the staphyloma and long-term tamponade. Retina. 2012; 32(8):1525–1530
[116] Michalewska Z, Michalewski J, Dulczewska-Cichecka K, Nawrocki J. Inverted internal limiting membrane flap technique for surgical repair of myopic macular holes. Retina. 2014; 34(4):664–669
[117] Alkabes M, Burés-Jelstrup A, Salinas C, et al. Macular buckling for previously untreated and recurrent retinal detachment due to high myopic macular hole: a 12-month comparative study. Graefes Arch Clin Exp Ophthalmol. 2014; 252(4):571–581
[118] Rubin JS, Glaser BM, Thompson JT, et al. Vitrectomy, fluid-gas exchange and transforming growth factor-beta-2 for the treatment of traumatic macular holes. Ophthalmology. 1995; 102:1840–1845
[119] Amari F, Ogino N, Matsumura M, Negi A, Yoshimura N. Vitreous surgery for traumatic macular holes. Retina. 1999; 19(5):410–413
[120] Chow DR, Williams GA, Trese MT, Margherio RR, Ruby AJ, Ferrone PJ. Successful closure of traumatic macular holes. Retina. 1999; 19(5):405–409
[121] Cohen SM, Flynn HW, Jr, Murray TG, Smiddy WE, The Postvitrectomy Endophthalmitis Study Group. Endophthalmitis after pars plana vitrectomy. Ophthalmology. 1995; 102(5):705–712
[122] Cohen SM, Hammer ME, Grizzard WS. Endophthalmitis after pars plana vitrectomy with or without autologous blood products for macular hole. Ophthalmology. 1996; 103 9A:161
[123] Haimann MH, Weiss H, Miller J, et al. Endophthalmitis Vitrectomy Study Group. Results of the Endophthalmitis Vitrectomy Study. A randomized trial of immediate vitrectomy and of intravenous antibiotics for the treatment of postoperative bacterial endophthalmitis. Arch Ophthalmol. 1995; 113 (12):1479–1496
[124] Sjaarda RN, Glaser BM, Thompson JT, Murphy RP, Hanham A. Distribution of iatrogenic retinal breaks in macular hole surgery. Ophthalmology. 1995; 102 9:1387–1392
[125] Park SS, Marcus DM, Duker JS, et al. Posterior segment complications after vitrectomy for macular hole. Ophthalmology. 1995; 102(5):775–781

[126] Jalil A, Ho WO, Charles S, Dhawahir-Scala F, Patton N. Iatrogenic retinal breaks in 20-G versus 23-G pars plana vitrectomy. Graefes Arch Clin Exp Ophthalmol. 2013; 251(6):1463–1467
[127] Poliner LS, Tornambe PE. Retinal pigment epitheliopathy after macular hole surgery. Ophthalmology. 1992; 99(11):1671–1677
[128] Charles S. Retinal pigment epithelial abnormalities after macular hole surgery. Retina. 1993; 13(2):176
[129] Hutton WL, Fuller DG, Snyder WB, Fellman RL, Swanson WH. Visual field defects after macular hole surgery. A new finding. Ophthalmology. 1996; 103(12):2152–2158, discussion 2158–2159
[130] Boldt HC, Munden PM, Folk JC, Mehaffey MG. Visual field defects after macular hole surgery. Am J Ophthalmol. 1996; 122(3):371–381
[131] Ezra E, Arden GB, Riordan-Eva P, Aylward GW, Gregor ZJ. Visual field loss following vitrectomy for stage 2 and 3 macular holes. Br J Ophthalmol. 1996; 80(6):519–525
[132] Pendergast SD, McCuen BW, II. Visual field loss after macular hole surgery. Ophthalmology. 1996; 103(7):1069–1077
[133] Kerrison JB, Haller JA, Elman M, Miller NR. Visual field loss following vitreous surgery. Arch Ophthalmol. 1996; 114(5):564–569
[134] Melberg NS, Thomas MA. Visual field loss after pars plana vitrectomy with air/fluid exchange. Am J Ophthalmol. 1995; 120(3):386–388
[135] Welch JC. Dehydration injury as a possible cause of visual field defect after pars plana vitrectomy for macular hole. Am J Ophthalmol. 1997; 124 (5):698–699
[136] Paques M, Massin P, Blain P, Duquesnoy AS, Gaudric A. Long-term incidence of reopening of macular holes. Ophthalmology. 2000; 107(4):760–765, discussion 766
[137] Holekamp NM, Shui YB, Beebe DC. Vitrectomy surgery increases oxygen exposure to the lens: a possible mechanism for nuclear cataract formation. Am J Ophthalmol. 2005; 139(2):302–310

18 Epiretinal Membrane and Vitreomacular Traction

Kevin R. Tozer and Mark W. Johnson

18.1 Epiretinal Membrane

18.1.1 Introduction

First described by Iwanoff[1] in 1865, the proliferation of fibrocellular membranes on the inner surface of the macula is a relatively common and well-studied phenomenon. The nomenclature used to describe these membranes has been extensive, including but not limited to *surface wrinkling retinopathy*,[2] *cellophane maculopathy*,[3] *preretinal macular gliosis*,[4] *premacular membrane*,[5] and *macular pucker*.[6] However, at present, the most commonly used terminology is *epiretinal membrane* (ERM). This chapter will review the epidemiology, clinical features and diagnosis, pathogenesis, mechanisms of visual impairment, and treatment options for this macular condition.

18.1.2 Epidemiology

With more than 30 million people affected in the United States alone, ERM is one of the most common vitreoretinal disorders. In the adult population, the overall prevalence has been reported to be between 6 and 11.8%.[7,8,9] The prevalence in the population older than 70 years has been reported to be as high as 15.1%.[9] Autopsy studies have shown similar rates, with a prevalence of approximately 6% that increases with age.[10] In healthy adults older than 50 years, the 5-year incidence of developing ERM is 5.3%.[11]

Several modifiable and nonmodifiable risk factors for ERM have been identified. Although ERMs have been described in young individuals,[12,13] the most significant risk factor is age and most cases are diagnosed after the age of 50 years.[14,15] While ERMs show no gender preference in adults,[7,9] boys are affected more frequently in the pediatric population.[16] Ethnicity plays only a minor role, with Asians (particularly Chinese) and Hispanics having a slightly higher prevalence of ERM than Caucasians or African Americans.[15,17] Presence of ERM in one eye is a major risk factor for its development in the fellow eye, with approximately 20 to 30% of cases being bilateral.[2,8,10,11,18] The 5-year incidence of developing ERM in one eye if the contralateral eye has ERM at baseline is 13.5%.[11] Other risk factors include high cholesterol, diabetes (with or without retinopathy), penetrating trauma, and smoking.[7,13,17] The incidence of symptomatic ERM following surgical repair of rhegmatogenous retinal detachment is between 4 and 8%.[19,20,21] Lower rates, around 1 to 2%, are seen following prophylactic repair of peripheral retinal breaks.[22]

18.1.3 Clinical Features and Diagnosis

The clinical manifestations of ERM are varied and depend largely on the thickness and contracture of the membrane. In its mildest form, the membrane is thin and virtually transparent with minimal contraction. This is commonly referred to as *cellophane maculopathy* due to the irregular cellophane-like reflection of light from the surface of the membrane.[3,18] Although this stage is frequently asymptomatic, symptoms such as metamorphopsia and decreased visual acuity commonly develop as the membrane progresses. Other symptoms less frequently reported include macropsia, photopsia, central binocular diplopia, and interference with vision in the fellow eye.[8,18] The majority of patients with ERMs have mild symptoms and remain stable or experience little progression over time.[23]

Pearls

- Patients with ERMs typically experience variable degrees of blur and metamorphopsia, often including macropsia.

At presentation, visual acuity is typically 20/30 to 20/70,[2,4] with only 15% of eyes having less than 20/70 vision.[24] Progression of ERM is uncommon but highly variable. One large prospective cohort showed a 28% rate of progression in terms of size of macular involvement over 5 years and a similar 25% rate of spontaneous improvement when classified as mild at presentation.[11] Cases that were more advanced at presentation were even less likely to progress. Other studies have shown similar rates for progression of vision loss, ranging from 13 to 29% over a 2- to 4-year follow-up period.[4,24] Less than 5% of all patients will progress to visual acuities of 20/200 or worse.[18] Cases associated with retinal tears are more likely to progress rapidly, although this is still rare.[25]

The diagnosis of ERM is clinical, but can be aided by ancillary testing. Biomicroscopic features begin with a glistening light reflex, which can be assessed more easily using red-free light. Later findings include wrinkling of the internal limiting membrane (ILM) and retinal striae (▶ Fig. 18.1a,b). Retinal vessels may show straightening toward the membrane and marked tortuosity under areas of membrane contracture (▶ Fig. 18.1c,d). The normal arcuate pattern of the major arcades may exhibit a reversal of its usual curvature, with vascular segments that point in a radiating fashion toward the contracted membrane. The retina underlying the ERM is typically thickened, sometimes folded, and occasionally demonstrates intraretinal hemorrhages or patches of retinal whitening similar to cotton-wool spots. Rarely, ectopia or even shallow traction detachment of the macula can result. There may be cystoid spaces and occasionally full-thickness holes in the fovea. Pseudoholes of the macula, caused by fenestrations in the ERM overlying or adjacent to the fovea, may also be present (▶ Fig. 18.2).

The most useful ancillary test for diagnosis and assessment of ERM is optical coherence tomography (OCT). OCT clearly highlights ERMs as a preretinal hyperreflective band of varying thickness (▶ Fig. 18.1b). A near-universal OCT finding in ERM is retinal thickening, which varies greatly in its severity.[26] Additional features that can be identified by OCT include multifocal retinal contraction centers,[27] intraretinal cystoid spaces, disruptions of the ellipsoid zone, and small accumulations of hyperreflective (vitelliform) material beneath the fovea (▶ Fig. 18.3). The ellipsoid zone has been of particular interest as disruptions in this layer appear to be predictive of poorer postoperative visual outcomes.[28,29,30,31]

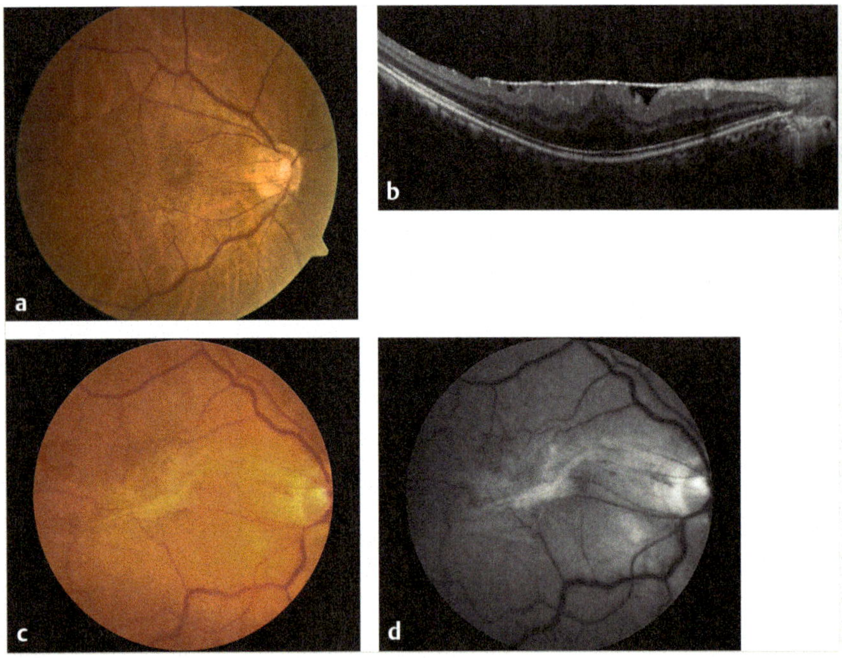

Fig. 18.1 (a) Color fundus photograph of a mild epiretinal membrane demonstrating wrinkling of the internal limiting membrane and retinal striae. (b) Optical coherence tomography of macula (the same retina as in (a)) demonstrating a hyper-reflective band characteristic of an epiretinal membrane with associated retinal thickening and distortion. (c) Color fundus photo of a severe epiretinal membrane (macular pucker) with more pronounced findings, including vascular distortion and retinal hemorrhages. (d) Red-free photo (the same retina as in (c)) highlighting the membrane and the associated retinal changes.

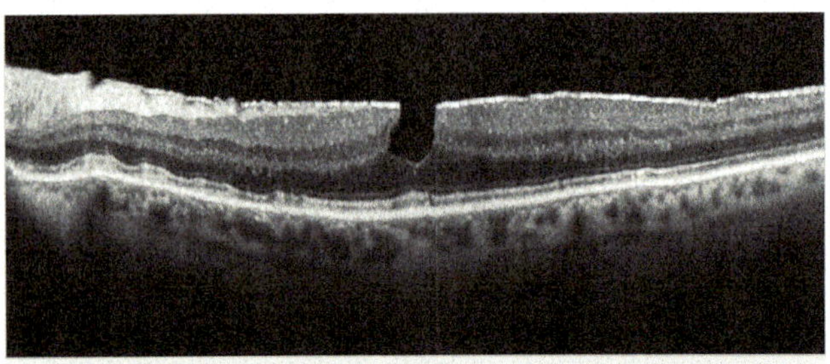

Fig. 18.2 Optical coherence tomography image demonstrating a macular pseudohole caused by contracture of a fenestrated epiretinal membrane.

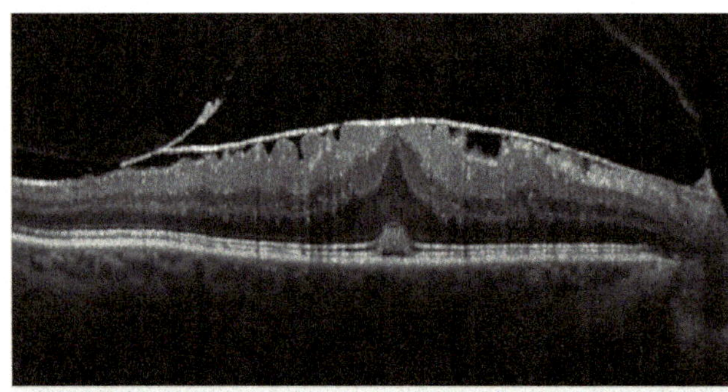

Fig. 18.3 Optical coherence tomography image demonstrating characteristic outer retinal changes caused by an epiretinal membrane, including ellipsoid layer disruptions and a subfoveal vitelliform deposit. Note also that the epiretinal membrane is growing onto the back surface of the partially detached posterior hyaloid.

Fluorescein angiography may also be a useful adjunct in evaluating ERMs. Fluorescein angiography typically shows alterations in the retinal vascular pattern, such as straightening of vessels and areas of increased vascular tortuosity (▶ Fig. 18.4). Late-phase angiograms may show varying amounts of fluorescein leakage resulting from traction-induced vascular permeability alterations. Additionally, fluorescein angiography may eliminate other possible retinal vascular anomalies that can be confused with ERM formation, such as pseudophakic cystoid macular edema and branch retinal vein occlusion. Finally, fluorescein angiography may rule out the presence of a choroidal neovascular membrane, which may lie occult beneath an ERM.[3]

Pearls

- Clinical evaluation includes slit-lamp biomicroscopy with monochromatic red-free illumination, OCT, and sometimes fluorescein angiography.

Gass classified ERMs according to the degree of distortion they create in the underlying retina.[3] In Gass's classification, cellophane maculopathy (grade 0) is defined as a thin transparent membrane without associated retinal distortion. Crinkled cellophane maculopathy (grade 1) denotes membranes that produce minimal distortion of the retina, causing radiating striae and some tortuosity of retinal vessels. Such membranes generally cause mild symptoms of visual blurring with or without metamorphopsia. Macular pucker (grade 2) refers to membranes that are more dense and contracted, often appearing as a grayish sheet and causing marked distortion of the underlying retina with significant metamorphopsia and reduction in central visual function. This grading system has been useful in clinical research but is not widely used in clinical practice.

An important clinical consideration is determining whether an ERM is primary or secondary to other pathology. Posterior vitreous detachment (PVD) is a near-universal precursor to primary or idiopathic ERM formation.[4,14,32,33,34] Features consistent with idiopathic ERM include older age and better visual acuity compared to secondary membranes.[35] Secondary ERMs can arise from a variety of underlying pathologies, including diabetic retinopathy, retinal vein occlusion, sickle cell disease,

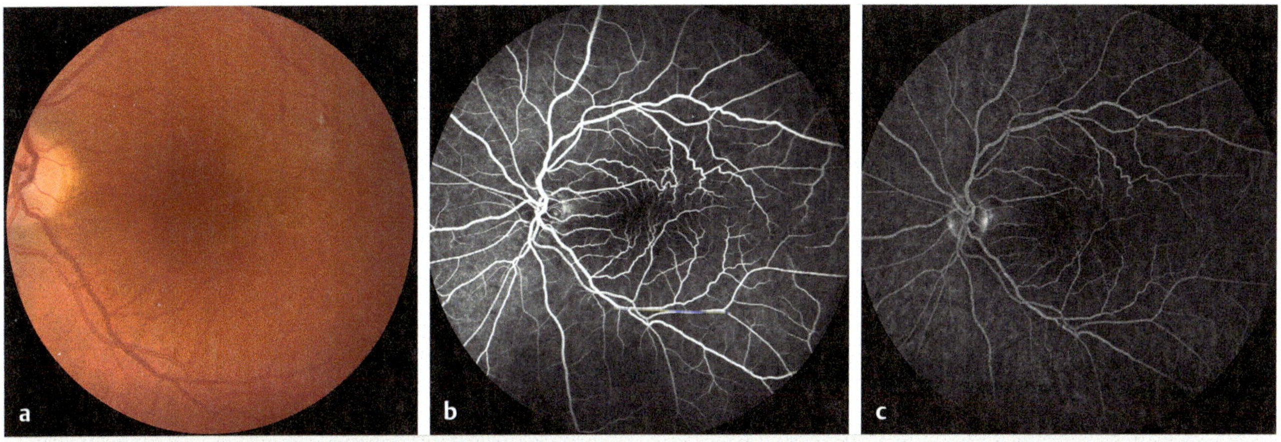

Fig. 18.4 (**a**) Color fundus photograph with (**b**) early- and (**c**) late-phase fluorescein angiogram images. Straightening/tortuosity of the retinal vessels and the sheen of an epiretinal membrane are visible in (**a**). The angiogram images demonstrate mild late leakage (**c**), which is present in variable amounts with epiretinal membranes.

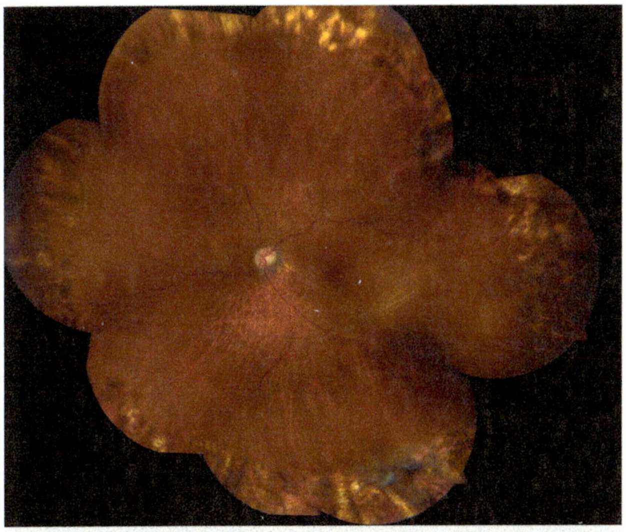

Fig. 18.5 Composite retinal photograph of a secondary epiretinal membrane that developed following retinal detachment repair with exuberant peripheral retinal laser photocoagulation.

retinal detachment, trauma, and ocular surgery (▶ Fig. 18.5).[21,35,36,37,38] Unlike primary ERMs, secondary membranes may be seen in younger patients[16] and portend a worse visual prognosis. An important structural difference between primary and secondary membranes is that primary membranes have a more fascial adherence to the retina, whereas secondary membranes are more focally adherent.[39] Additionally, secondary membranes are more frequently found to have associated cystoid macular edema,[35] which contributes to worse visual outcomes.

18.1.4 Pathogenesis and Pathology

The pathogenesis of ERMs is not clearly defined, and several theories exist. Additionally, idiopathic ERMs likely have a different pathogenesis than those secondary to other causes such as trauma or retinal detachment. The two prevailing modern theories for the formation of idiopathic ERMs are (1) glial cell migration through inner retinal microbreaks and (2) transdifferentiation of epiretinal vitreous remnants resulting from vitreoretinal separation with vitreoschisis. Both theories underscore the importance of PVD as the primary pathogenic event.

Idiopathic ERM has long been known to be strongly associated with age-related PVD.[34] Modern studies have documented PVD in 80 to 95% of all cases of ERM.[14,27,32,40] Even in cases where a complete separation of the vitreous from the retina is not seen, a partial PVD involving the perifoveal or entire macular area can almost always be identified on ultrasound or OCT imaging.[41,42] The perifoveal macula is typically the first site of vitreous detachment because the premacular vitreous liquefies early in life (resulting in a *premacular bursa* or *lacuna*) and because the perifoveal posterior hyaloid is weakly attached to the thin perifoveal ILM.[5,41,43,44]

An early theory concerning the formation of idiopathic ERMs involved migration of glial cells through microbreaks in the ILM. The microbreaks were presumed to be secondary to traction caused by a prior PVD.[10,45,46] Once the glial cells have access to the preretinal space, this theory proposes that they migrate along the retinal surface and proliferate to form patches or sheets of ERM. On histologic examination of ERMs, the cells resemble glial cells[47] and have similar immunofluorescence staining.[48] While it remains unclear whether the microbreak theory plays a role in most cases of idiopathic ERM, it is likely important in the setting of known retinal tears as retinal pigment epithelial cells are known to be present in higher numbers in membranes in these eyes.[48,49,50]

The second theory of pathogenesis of ERMs proposes that they arise from cells found within the vitreous cortex. This concept dates back to the 1960s,[51,52,53,54] but has been further elucidated more recently by Sebag.[55,56,57] Several pathology studies have demonstrated the presence of vitreous collagen interposed between the retina and ERM,[33,58,59,60] strongly suggesting a role for vitreous gel in ERM formation. The theory proposes that during the course of PVD, the posterior vitreous cortex splits and thin cortical remnants remain adherent to the ILM. This splitting has come to be known as "vitreoschisis" and occurs because of the well-documented lamellar structure of the posterior vitreous cortex (▶ Fig. 18.6).[40,56,61,62,63] The key

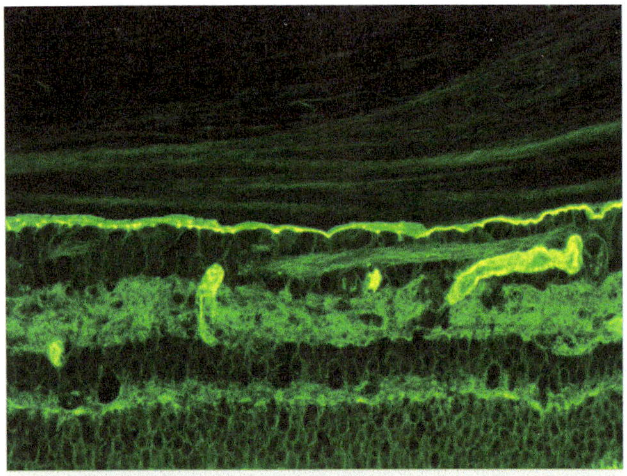

Fig. 18.6 Immunofluorescence imaging of the vitreoretinal interface in a monkey demonstrating the lamellar structure of the posterior vitreous cortex (magnification ~400×). (Reproduced with permission by BMJ Publishing Group Ltd. from Gupta P et al.[63])

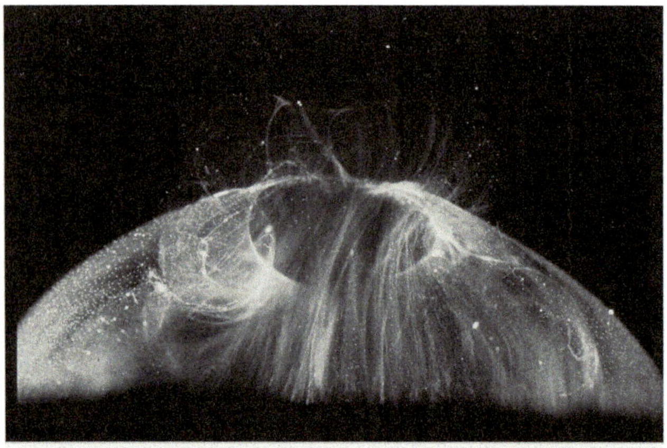

Fig. 18.7 Dark-field slit microscopy of the vitreous body from a 59-year-old human. Hyalocytes are visualized as small white dots embedded in the posterior vitreous cortex. Large dots represent debris. (Reproduced with permission by Springer from Sebag.[64])

cellular element responsible for ERM formation is thought to be the hyalocyte. Hyalocytes, which are embedded in the posterior vitreous cortex[64] (▶ Fig. 18.7), are capable not only of secreting collagen (the main structural component of ERMs) but also of transdifferentiation into myofibroblasts.[65,66,67] This would explain the ability of ERMs to contract and form the characteristic retinal wrinkling of macular pucker.

Although most authorities now believe that vitreoschisis is a critical step in the formation of ERMs, this theory is not accepted by all retinal specialists and investigators. Some studies have failed to show colocalization between areas of retained vitreous cortex following PVD and subsequent ERM formation.[68] Regardless of whether ERMs form due to retinal microbreaks or remnant hyalocyte proliferation, both theories emphasize the importance of PVD in the development of this disorder.

Pearls

- PVD (either complete or partial) is a crucial event in the pathogenesis of ERMs.

The histopathology of surgically removed and cadaveric ERM specimens unfortunately does not clarify the question of membrane origin. ERMs are composed of multiple cellular elements, including retinal pigment epithelial cells, astrocytes, inflammatory cells, and collagen. The collagen has been shown to be both newly synthesized and native vitreous collagen.[45,46,69] The precise determination of cell origin in specimens has been difficult, as many of the cells can undergo morphologic changes that make them appear similar in structure.[6] Furthermore, various authors have ascribed different names to what are likely the same cellular components. In his original studies, Foos suggested that astroglial cells were the predominant cell type in ERMs. Later, Snead and colleagues used the term *laminocytes* to describe these same cells.[48]

18.1.5 Mechanisms of Visual Impairment

It is important to understand that the tractional effects of ERMs are not limited to the inner retina. Multiple functional and structural analyses have documented deleterious effects of ERMs on all layers of the retina. This fact is critical to understanding the mechanisms by which ERMs impair visual function.

Retinal thickening is the most obvious structural change associated with ERM that has been explored as an indicator of disease severity and visual dysfunction. Even prior to the advent of OCT imaging, it was known that contracting membranes could induce retinal edema and thickening. Now, detailed studies have been performed with the high resolution of spectral-domain OCT to correlate central retinal thickness and visual acuity. While many studies do show a direct correlation, the bulk of the available data suggests that retinal thickening may only be a piece of the puzzle.[28,70]

More recently, attention has turned to outer retinal structures, such as the ellipsoid zone (previously referred to as the inner segment/outer segment junction), which is easily visible on OCT as a hyperreflective line just anterior to the retinal pigment epithelium (RPE). Disruption of the ellipsoid zone is felt to represent damage to the photoreceptors themselves. OCT-based studies have confirmed that ellipsoid line disruptions correlate with decreased visual acuity and increased metamorphopsia.[29,70] Similarly, Niwa and colleagues used focal macular electroretinography (ERG) in patients with ERMs to show decreased a-wave responses indicating outer retinal dysfunction.[28] The same study, however, showed that b-wave responses decreased before a-wave responses, suggesting that the inner retina is affected before the outer retina.

Aside from the photoreceptors, dysfunctions of Müller and bipolar cells have been proposed as important precursors to vision loss. One study used multifocal ERG to find predictive features of poor visual outcome following surgery for ERM. An abnormal positive peak (P1) value, which represents both Müller and bipolar cells, was found to be more accurate than ellipsoid zone disruptions in predicting poor postoperative visual outcomes.[31] Other studies, however, have shown ellipsoid zone disruption to correlate well with the postoperative visual acuity[71]

18.1.6 Management and Course

Most ERMs are mild or asymptomatic and require no treatment.[23] In cases where the ERM is secondary to an underlying retinal pathology, treatment of that condition may be indicated. Spontaneous separation of the membrane from the retina can occur, typically coincident with vitreomacular separation. This uncommon event is thought to be more likely when the membrane is associated with peripheral retinal vasculopathies such as retinal telangiectasis or hemangioblastoma, especially after treatment of the vascular abnormalities.[3] In idiopathic cases, spontaneous separation is rare, and when symptoms progress to a severity that interferes significantly with daily activities using the involved eye alone, surgery is the only current treatment option.

18.1.7 Preoperative Evaluation

Preoperative evaluation of surgical patients should include a comprehensive ophthalmic examination to be certain that there are no contraindications to intraocular surgery, such as acute external infection. It is also important to assess the degree of preexisting lens opacity and to examine the entirety of the retina, including its periphery. Preoperative evaluation should include careful slit-lamp biomicroscopy to determine the relationship of the membrane to the macula and to estimate areas where the membrane might be approached surgically. Biomicroscopy, OCT, and fluorescein angiography may be useful to detect associated retinal abnormalities, especially occult disorders such as choroidal neovascularization and retinal vascular occlusion with macular ischemia.

Surgical Procedure

The surgical procedure consists of pars plana vitrectomy followed by delamination of the ERM using various intraocular picks and forceps. In some patients, a discrete edge of the membrane is apparent, which can be lifted to begin the membrane peeling. In most patients with idiopathic ERM, there is no detectable margin and the membrane must be incised or pinched to begin the delamination. The application of a gentle tangential force combined with anterior traction generally achieves a safe delamination of the ERM. Multiple petechiae may occur during membrane peeling, but these are visually insignificant, dissipate rapidly, and require no treatment. It is not uncommon for membranes to extend further into the periphery than was expected clinically. It is important to recognize that whitish retinal patches, similar to cotton-wool spots, may be present before and after delamination of the ERM. The surgeon must be aware of these zones and avoid mistaking them for residual membrane, as attempts to achieve further dissection may result in retinal damage.[6] Rarely, focal areas of firm adhesion between the membrane and retina are found. If it is determined that further attempts to peel these areas carry an unacceptable risk of causing a retinal tear, cutting around the adhesion and leaving a patch of residual membrane may be preferable.

Special Considerations

- Gray-white zones similar in appearance to cotton-wool spots may be present before and immediately after delamination of ERMs. Surgeons should avoid mistaking these areas for residual membrane, as further dissection may result in retinal injury.

One of the major issues regarding surgical removal of an ERM involves determining the appropriate dissection plane. Many surgeons prefer to remove not only the ERM but also the underlying ILM. Removing the ILM enhances the surgeon's ability to remove the membrane completely, along with any vitreous cortex that may be interposed between the membrane and the retinal surface. Although there is no good evidence that ILM peeling improves postoperative visual outcomes, several studies have shown that removing this membrane reduces the incidence of recurrent ERM formation.[72,73] To enhance visualization of the ILM and ERM, some surgeons prefer to use vital dyes such as trypan blue,[74] indocyanine green (ICG),[75] or brilliant blue G.[76] Although the use of ICG in macular surgery has been shown to have a concentration-dependent retinal toxic effect, the dye has been used extensively in macular surgery without significant adverse effect, especially when the exposure of the dye during surgery is brief.[77]

Controversial Points

- Staining of the ILM with ICG remains a topic of debate. Potential advantages include improved membrane visualization and enhanced membrane removal, but there may be a risk of deleterious ICG-induced retinal toxicity. Valid evidence and many advocates support both sides of the argument in terms of both clinical utility and safety profile.

Surgical Procedure

After surgery, visual acuity improvement of two or more lines on a Snellen's chart occurs in approximately 75% of patients.[78] Some patients achieve visual acuity approaching 20/20. However, even those patients who experience dramatic improvement will routinely notice that postoperative vision in the treated eye is not equal to that in their fellow normal eye and will frequently continue to describe residual blur and metamorphopsia. While significant improvement of retinal structural abnormalities is expected after surgery, postoperative OCT imaging routinely shows persistent architectural abnormalities of the macula, such as irregular thickening (▶ Fig. 18.8). In general, patients with preoperative symptoms less than 1 year have better postoperative visual outcomes, but long-standing symptoms are not a contraindication to surgery.[78] Other predictors of better visual outcomes include preoperative visual acuity better than 20/100,[79] intact ellipsoid zone on OCT,[71] and short P1 times on multifocal ERG.[31] Poorer outcomes may be seen

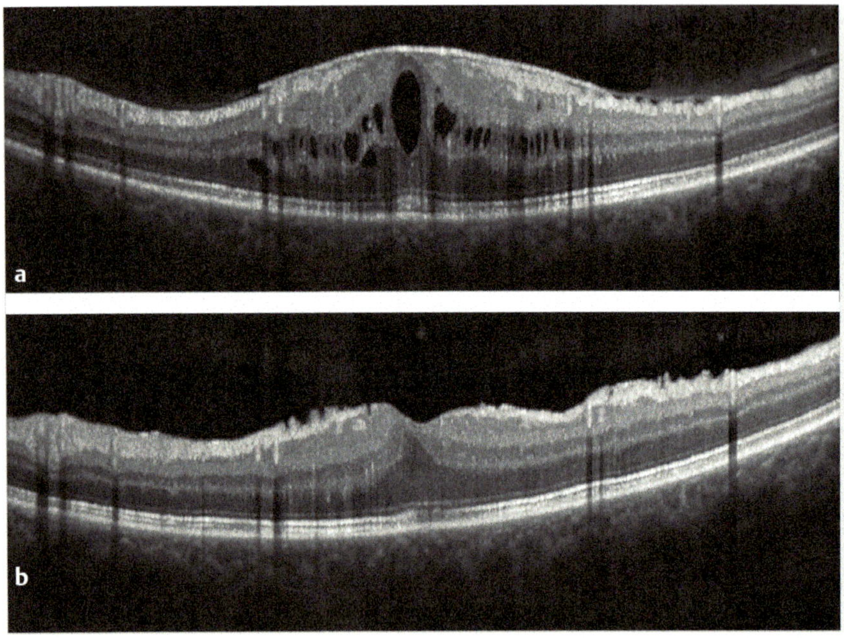

Fig. 18.8 Optical coherence tomography images of the same macula (**a**) before and (**b**) after surgical peeling of an epiretinal membrane. Despite removal of the membrane and resolution of much of the retinal distortion and cystic changes present in (**a**) there are persistent abnormalities in the architecture of the fovea in (**b**).

when there is preoperative cystoid macular edema.[80] In general, surgery is uncommonly offered to patients with visual acuity equal to or better than 20/40, except for individuals with exceedingly demanding visual requirements, severe metamorphopsia, or foveal ectopia with disabling central binocular diplopia. As a corollary, patients who have marked loss of vision—for instance, to the level of finger counting—are less likely to regain reading acuity following peeling of the ERM.

Pearls

- Following vitrectomy and successful peeling of ERM, patients generally experience visual improvement and a reduction in metamorphopsia. However, patients typically do not have complete resolution of symptoms and frequently report residual blur and distortion.

Complications of surgery include anesthetic sequelae, failure to accomplish complete removal of the ERM, retinal breaks, retinal detachment, progressive nuclear cataract, photic maculopathy, and, rarely, endophthalmitis or choroidal hemorrhage.[3] Posterior retinal breaks are uncommon and can generally be managed by means of gas tamponade with or without endolaser photocoagulation. Peripheral retinal breaks typically occur intraoperatively from vitreous traction associated with instrument passage through sclerotomies or surgical induction of PVD. The intraoperative onset of rivulets of vitreous hemorrhage that gravitate posteriorly from the periphery should be regarded as an indication that a peripheral retinal break may have occurred. Methodical examination of the fundus periphery with scleral depression is mandatory at the completion of vitrectomy to detect and allow treatment of such breaks. Additionally, at the time of postoperative evaluations, the far retinal periphery should again be examined carefully to facilitate early detection and treatment of retinal breaks or detachment.

Progressive nuclear cataract occurs postoperatively in nearly all patients older than 50 years and typically results in the need for cataract surgery within several years of vitrectomy.[3,81] Patients should be advised that the development of cataract is anticipated. Patients may initially be disappointed with the visual results of vitrectomy surgery because of the concomitant progression of cataract, and they often experience considerable improvement in visual acuity following cataract surgery. However, the cataract surgeon should be cautious when removing lenticular material, as an unusual degree of mobility of the posterior capsule may be encountered in a vitrectomized eye.

Recurrence of symptomatic ERM is uncommon and occurs at a rate of approximately 5%.[78] Recurrences are seen more frequently in younger patients[82] and less frequently if the ILM has been removed.[72,73] Recurrent membranes typically present with increased symptoms of metamorphopsia and blur. Visual improvement may often be achieved in such patients with repeated surgical delamination.

18.2 Vitreomacular Traction Syndrome

The vitreomacular traction syndrome (VMTS) is a condition characterized by partial separation of the posterior vitreous with persistent attachment to the macula and peripapillary retina. The area of vitreous detachment may be limited to the perifoveal posterior retina or extend throughout the fundus midperiphery to the posterior aspect of the vitreous base. In VMTS and the related vitreofoveal traction syndrome, the traction exerted on the macula is in an anteroposterior direction in contrast to the tangential traction seen in ERM.[56] VMTS is distinguished from simple vitreomacular adhesion by the fact that the latter has no morphological foveal disturbances, while VMTS features foveal anatomic deformations typically accompanied by visual symptoms. These traction-induced alterations may include foveal pseudocysts, cystoid or schisis-like foveal thickening, disruptions of the photoreceptor layer, and subretinal fluid or vitelliform accumulations (▶ Fig. 18.9a).

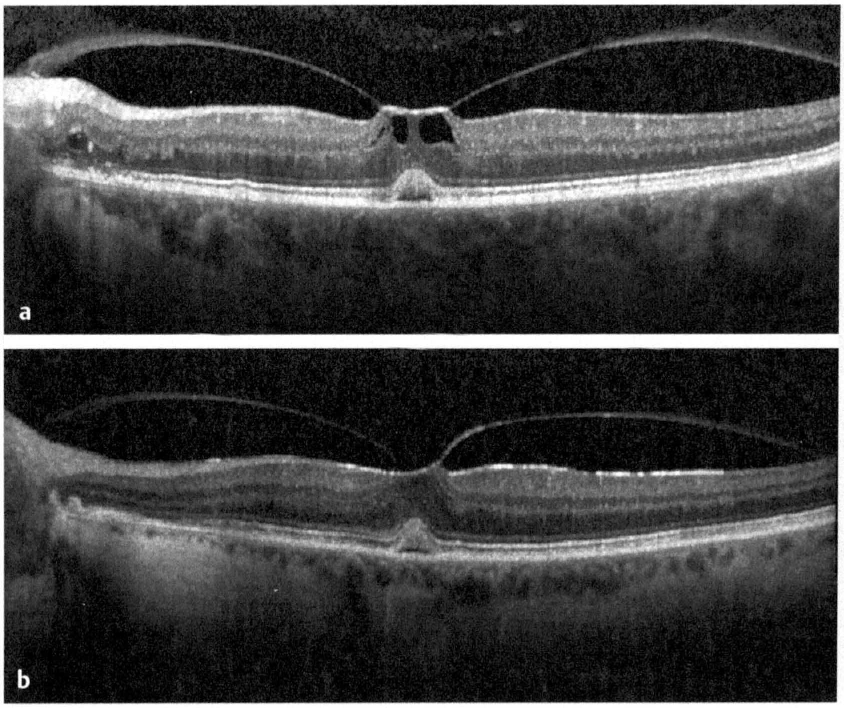

Fig. 18.9 (a,b) Optical coherence tomography images representative of vitreomacular traction syndrome (VMTS). In both (**a**) and (**b**), there is anteroposterior traction exerted by the partial hyaloidal separation with persistent vitreofoveal adhesion. This has caused focal detachment of the fovea with underlying accumulation of vitelliform material. Cystic changes of the fovea are also present in (**a**) and a mild epiretinal membrane, which is frequently but not universally seen in VMTS, is present in (**b**).

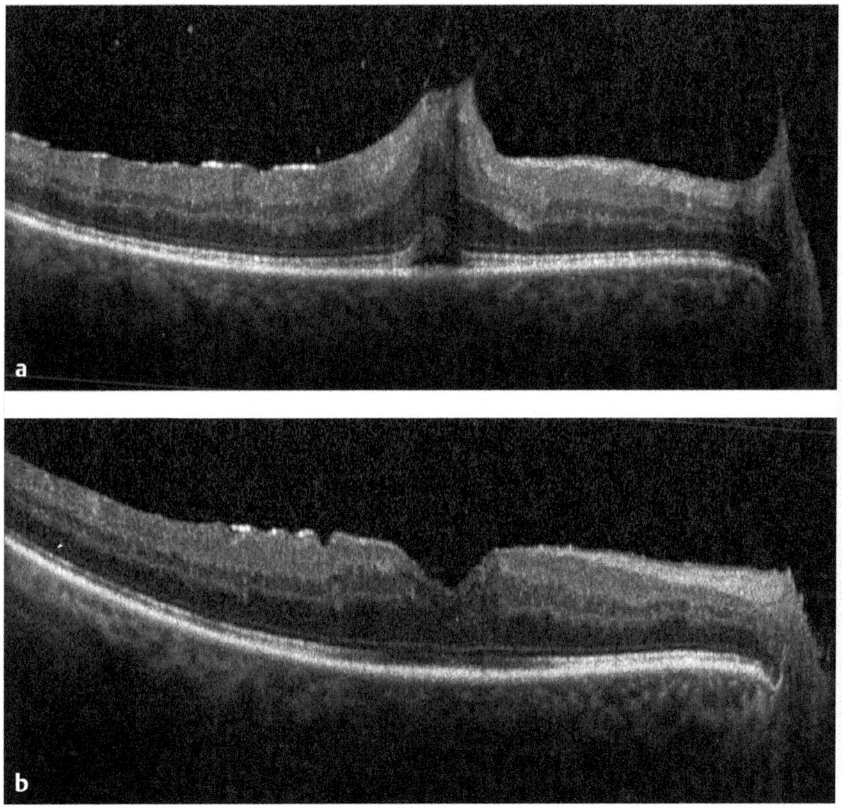

Fig. 18.10 Optical coherence tomography of the same retina (**a**) before and (**b**) after vitrectomy for treatment of vitreomacular traction syndrome.

VMTS can be classified by the diameter of the vitreous attachment to the macular surface. If the area of attachment is greater than 1,500 µm, it is classified as broad; if the area is less than 1,500 µm, it is classified as focal.[83] Although not present in all cases, ERM is a common component of VMTS (▶ Fig. 18.9b). As in cases of routine macular pucker, the ERM in this setting likely represents transdifferentiation of a vitreoschitic layer of vitreous remaining on the macular surface following perifoveal vitreous separation. Interestingly, the cellular make-up of the ERMs in these two settings differs somewhat, in that VMTS membranes have more myofibroblasts and fewer RPE cells than macular pucker membranes.[84] Importantly, in VMTS, the epiretinal fibrocellular membrane proliferates along the exposed retinal surface and continues onto the back surface of the detached posterior hyaloid. This configuration strengthens the vitreoretinal adhesion in VMTS, effectively anchoring the vitreous to the macula and reducing the chances for spontaneous or pharmacologic vitreous separation.[85,86,87]

Patients typically present with complaints of visual blur and distortion. Clinical findings on biomicroscopy may include separation of the perifoveal posterior hyaloid that may be visibly thickened, foveal or macular thickening and distortion, ERM, retinal striae, tractional macular detachment, and a peripapillary vitreoretinal traction ridge. Whereas some patients with vitreomacular traction may have spontaneous improvement associated with spontaneous vitreous separation and resolution of traction, many patients will have persistent symptoms that may or may not be progressive.[88] Although observation is appropriate for patients with mild visual symptoms, several treatment options are available for patients with significant associated visual loss. The gold standard treatment remains pars plana vitrectomy with surgical separation of the vitreomacular adhesion and peeling of any associated ERM.[86,89,90] Vitrectomy techniques generally relieve the traction and restore normal retinal architecture (▶ Fig. 18.10); however, published visual acuity results have been variable. Newer, evolving approaches include pneumatic and pharmacologic vitreolysis, in which vitreomacular separation is induced by injecting either an expansile gas bubble[91] or a vitreolytic drug such as ocriplasmin[87] into the vitreous cavity. These less invasive approaches appear to be most effective in eyes with small vitreomacular adhesion sizes and no significant ERM. However, efficacy and safety issues remain with both approaches, and more research is needed to better define their roles in the management of VMTS.

References

[1] Iwanoff A. Beiträge zur normalen und pathologischen Anatomie des Auges. Graefes Arch Clin Exp Ophthalmol. 1865; 11(1):135–170

[2] Scudder MJ, Eifrig DE. Spontaneous surface wrinkling retinopathy. Ann Ophthalmol. 1975; 7(3):333–336, 339–341

[3] Gass JDM. Stereoscopic atlas of macular diseases: diagnosis and treatment. St. Louis, MO: Mosby; 1987

[4] Sidd RJ, Fine SL, Owens SL, Patz A. Idiopathic preretinal gliosis. Am J Ophthalmol. 1982; 94(1):44–48

[5] Sebag J. Vitreous – from biochemistry to clinical relevance. In: Tasman W, Jaeger E, eds. Duane's Foundations of Clinical Ophthalmology. Philadelphia, PA: Lippincott Williams & Wilkins; 1998:1–34

[6] McDonald H, Shatz H, Johnson R. Introduction to epiretinal membranes. In: Ryan SJ, ed. Retina. 2nd ed. St. Louis, MO: Mosby; 1994:1819–1823

[7] Klein R, Klein BE, Wang Q, Moss SE. The epidemiology of epiretinal membranes. Trans Am Ophthalmol Soc. 1994; 92:403–425, discussion 425–430

[8] Mitchell P, Smith W, Chey T, Wang JJ, Chang A. Prevalence and associations of epiretinal membranes. The Blue Mountains Eye Study, Australia. Ophthalmology. 1997; 104(6):1033–1040

[9] McCarty DJ, Mukesh BN, Chikani V, et al. Prevalence and associations of epiretinal membranes in the visual impairment project. Am J Ophthalmol. 2005; 140(2):288–294

[10] Roth AM, Foos RY. Surface wrinkling retinopathy in eyes enucleated at autopsy. Trans-Am Acad Ophthalmol Otolaryngol. 1971; 75(5):1047–10–58

[11] Fraser-Bell S, Guzowski M, Rochtchina E, Wang JJ, Mitchell P. Five-year cumulative incidence and progression of epiretinal membranes: the Blue Mountains Eye Study. Ophthalmology. 2003; 110(1):34–40

[12] Banach MJ, Hassan TS, Cox MS, et al. Clinical course and surgical treatment of macular epiretinal membranes in young subjects. Ophthalmology. 2001; 108 (1):23–26

[13] Meyer CH, Rodrigues EB, Mennel S, Schmidt JC, Kroll P. Spontaneous separation of epiretinal membrane in young subjects: personal observations and review of the literature. Graefes Arch Clin Exp Ophthalmol. 2004; 242 (12):977–985

[14] Appiah AP, Hirose T, Kado M. A review of 324 cases of idiopathic premacular gliosis. Am J Ophthalmol. 1988; 106(5):533–535

[15] Fraser-Bell S, Ying-Lai M, Klein R, Varma R, Los Angeles Latino Eye Study. Prevalence and associations of epiretinal membranes in latinos: the Los Angeles Latino Eye Study. Invest Ophthalmol Vis Sci. 2004; 45(6):1732–1736

[16] Khaja HA, McCannel CA, Diehl NN, Mohney BG. Incidence and clinical characteristics of epiretinal membranes in children. Arch Ophthalmol. 2008; 126 (5):632–636

[17] Ng CH, Cheung N, Wang JJ, et al. Prevalence and risk factors for epiretinal membranes in a multi-ethnic United States population. Ophthalmology. 2011; 118(4):694–699

[18] Wise GN. Clinical features of idiopathic preretinal macular fibrosis. Schoenberg Lecture. Am J Ophthalmol. 1975; 79(3):349–7

[19] Hagler WS, Aturaliya U. Macular puckers after retinal detachment surgery. Br J Ophthalmol. 1971; 55(7):451–457

[20] Lobes LA, Jr, Burton TC. The incidence of macular pucker after retinal detachment surgery. Am J Ophthalmol. 1978; 85(1):72–77

[21] Uemura A, Ideta H, Nagasaki H, Morita H, Ito K. Macular pucker after retinal detachment surgery. Ophthalmic Surg. 1992; 23(2):116–119

[22] Michels RG, Wilkinson CP, Rice TA, Hengst TC. Retinal Detachment. St. Louis, MO: Mosby; 1990

[23] Margherio R, Margherio A. Epiretinal macular membranes. In: Albert DM, Jakobiec FA, eds. Principles and Practice of Ophthalmology. Philadelphia, PA: WB Saunders; 1994:919–926

[24] Wiznia RA. Natural history of idiopathic preretinal macular fibrosis. Ann Ophthalmol. 1982; 14(9):876–878

[25] Sheard RM, Sethi C, Gregor Z. Acute macular pucker. Ophthalmology. 2003; 110(6):1178–1184

[26] Michalewski J, Michalewska Z, Cisiecki S, Nawrocki J. Morphologically functional correlations of macular pathology connected with epiretinal membrane formation in spectral optical coherence tomography (SOCT). Graefes Arch Clin Exp Ophthalmol. 2007; 245(11):1623–1631

[27] Gupta P, Sadun AA, Sebag J. Multifocal retinal contraction in macular pucker analyzed by combined optical coherence tomography/scanning laser ophthalmoscopy. Retina. 2008; 28(3):447–452

[28] Niwa T, Terasaki H, Kondo M, Piao C-H, Suzuki T, Miyake Y. Function and morphology of macula before and after removal of idiopathic epiretinal membrane. Invest Ophthalmol Vis Sci. 2003; 44(4):1652–1656

[29] Oster SF, Mojana F, Brar M, Yuson RM, Cheng L, Freeman WR. Disruption of the photoreceptor inner segment/outer segment layer on spectral domain-optical coherence tomography is a predictor of poor visual acuity in patients with epiretinal membranes. Retina. 2010; 30(5):713–718

[30] Inoue M, Morita S, Watanabe Y, et al. Inner segment/outer segment junction assessed by spectral-domain optical coherence tomography in patients with idiopathic epiretinal membrane. Am J Ophthalmol. 2010; 150(6):834–839

[31] Kim JH, Kim YM, Chung EJ, Lee SY, Koh HJ. Structural and functional predictors of visual outcome of epiretinal membrane surgery. Am J Ophthalmol. 2012; 153(1):103–10.e1

[32] Johnson MW. Posterior vitreous detachment: evolution and complications of its early stages. Am J Ophthalmol. 2010; 149(3):371–82.e1

[33] Kishi S, Shimizu K. Oval defect in detached posterior hyaloid membrane in idiopathic preretinal macular fibrosis. Am J Ophthalmol. 1994; 118(4):451–456

[34] Wise GN. Relationship of idiopathic preretinal macular fibrosis to posterior vitreous detachment. Am J Ophthalmol. 1975; 79(3):358–362

[35] Yazici AT, Alagöz N, Çelik HU, et al. Idiopathic and secondary epiretinal membranes: do they differ in terms of morphology? An optical coherence tomography-based study. Retina. 2011; 31(4):779–784

[36] Appiah AP, Hirose T. Secondary causes of premacular fibrosis. Ophthalmology. 1989; 96(3):389–392

[37] Benichou C, Flament J. Epiretinal membrane and photocoagulation with argon laser. Discussion of 3 cases [in French]. Bull Soc Ophtalmol Fr. 1989; 89 (4):613–619

[38] Carney MD, Jampol LM. Epiretinal membranes in sickle cell retinopathy. Arch Ophthalmol. 1987; 105(2):214–217

[39] Mori K, Gehlbach PL, Sano A, Deguchi T, Yoneya S. Comparison of epiretinal membranes of differing pathogenesis using optical coherence tomography. Retina. 2004; 24(1):57–62

[40] Sebag J, Gupta P, Rosen RR, Garcia P, Sadun AA. Macular holes and macular pucker: the role of vitreoschisis as imaged by optical coherence tomography/

scanning laser ophthalmoscopy. Trans Am Ophthalmol Soc. 2007; 105:121–129, 129–131
[41] Johnson MW. Perifoveal vitreous detachment and its macular complications. Trans Am Ophthalmol Soc. 2005; 103:537–567
[42] Gallemore RP, Jumper JM, McCuen BW, II, Jaffe GJ, Postel EA, Toth CA. Diagnosis of vitreoretinal adhesions in macular disease with optical coherence tomography. Retina. 2000; 20(2):115–120
[43] Balazs EA, Denlinger J. Aging changes in the vitreous. In: Aging and Human Visual Function. Sekuler R, Kline D, Dismukes K, eds. New York, NY: Alan R Liss; 1982:45–47
[44] Sebag J. Ageing of the vitreous. Eye (Lond). 1987; 1(Pt 2):254–262
[45] Bellhorn MB, Friedman AH, Wise GN, Henkind P. Ultrastructure and clinicopathologic correlation of idiopathic preretinal macular fibrosis. Am J Ophthalmol. 1975; 79(3):366–373
[46] Foos RY. Vitreoretinal juncture; epiretinal membranes and vitreous. Invest Ophthalmol Vis Sci. 1977; 16(5):416–422
[47] Foos RY. Vitreoretinal juncture—simple epiretinal membranes. Albrecht Von Graefes Arch Klin Exp Ophthalmol. 1974; 189(4):231–250
[48] Snead DR, James S, Snead MP. Pathological changes in the vitreoretinal junction 1: epiretinal membrane formation. Eye (Lond). 2008; 22(10):1310–1317
[49] Snead DR, Cullen N, James S, et al. Hyperconvolution of the inner limiting membrane in vitreomaculopathies. Graefes Arch Clin Exp Ophthalmol. 2004; 242(10):853–862
[50] Cherfan GM, Smiddy WE, Michels RG, de la Cruz Z, Wilkinson CP, Green WR. Clinicopathologic correlation of pigmented epiretinal membranes. Am J Ophthalmol. 1988; 106(5):536–545
[51] Jaffe NS. Macular retinopathy after separation of vitreoretinal adherence. Arch Ophthalmol. 1967; 78(5):585–591
[52] Jaffe NS. Vitreous traction at the posterior pole of the fundus due to alterations in the vitreous posterior. Trans Am Acad Ophthalmol Otolaryngol. 1967; 71(4):642–652
[53] Jaffe NS. Complications of acute posterior vitreous detachment. Arch Ophthalmol. 1968; 79(5):568–571
[54] Tanenbaum HL, Schepens CL, Elzeneiny I, Freeman HM. Macular pucker following retinal detachment surgery. Arch Ophthalmol. 1970; 83(3):286–293
[55] Sebag J. Anomalous posterior vitreous detachment: a unifying concept in vitreo-retinal disease. Graefes Arch Clin Exp Ophthalmol. 2004; 242(8):690–698
[56] Sebag J. Vitreoschisis. Graefes Arch Clin Exp Ophthalmol. 2008; 246(3):329–332
[57] Sebag J. Vitreous anatomy, aging, and anomalous posterior vitreous detachment. In: Dartt D, Besharse J, Dana R, eds. Encyclopedia of the Eye. Vol. 4. Oxford: Elsevier; 2010:307–315
[58] Messmer EM, Heidenkummer HP, Kampik A. Ultrastructure of epiretinal membranes associated with macular holes. Graefes Arch Clin Exp Ophthalmol. 1998; 236(4):248–254
[59] Heilskov TW, Massicotte SJ, Folk JC. Epiretinal macular membranes in eyes with attached posterior cortical vitreous. Retina. 1996; 16(4):279–284
[60] Kishi S, Demaria C, Shimizu K. Vitreous cortex remnants at the fovea after spontaneous vitreous detachment. Int Ophthalmol. 1986; 9(4):253–260
[61] Balazs EA. Fine structure and function of ocular tissues. The vitreous. Int Ophthalmol Clin. 1973; 13(3):169–187
[62] Kakehashi A, Schepens CL, de Sousa-Neto A, Jalkh AE, Trempe CL. Biomicroscopic findings of posterior vitreoschisis. Ophthalmic Surg. 1993; 24 (12):846–850
[63] Gupta P, Yee KM, Garcia P, et al. Vitreoschisis in macular diseases. Br J Ophthalmol. 2011; 95(3):376–380
[64] Sebag J. Structure of the Vitreous. In Sebag J, ed. The Vitreous. New York, NY: Springer; 1989:35–58
[65] Sakamoto T, Ishibashi T. Hyalocytes: essential cells of the vitreous cavity in vitreoretinal pathophysiology? Retina. 2011; 31(2):222–228
[66] Kita T, Hata Y, Kano K, et al. Transforming growth factor-ß2 and connective tissue growth factor in proliferative vitreoretinal diseases: possible involvement of hyalocytes and therapeutic potential of Rho kinase inhibitor. Diabetes. 2007; 56(1):231–238
[67] Kohno RI, Hata Y, Kawahara S, et al. Possible contribution of hyalocytes to idiopathic epiretinal membrane formation and its contraction. Br J Ophthalmol. 2009; 93(8):1020–1026
[68] Chen TY, Yang CM, Liu KR. Intravitreal triamcinolone staining observation of residual undetached cortical vitreous after posterior vitreous detachment. Eye (Lond). 2006; 20(4):423–427
[69] Clarkson JG, Green WR, Massof D. A histopathologic review of 168 cases of preretinal membrane. Am J Ophthalmol. 1977; 84(1):1–17
[70] Okamoto F, Sugiura Y, Okamoto Y, Hiraoka T, Oshika T. Associations between metamorphopsia and foveal microstructure in patients with epiretinal membrane. Invest Ophthalmol Vis Sci. 2012; 53(11):6770–6775
[71] Suh MH, Seo JM, Park KH, Yu HG. Associations between macular findings by optical coherence tomography and visual outcomes after epiretinal membrane removal. Am J Ophthalmol. 2009; 147(3):473–480.e3
[72] Bovey EH, Uffer S, Achache F. Surgery for epimacular membrane: impact of retinal internal limiting membrane removal on functional outcome. Retina. 2004; 24(5):728–735
[73] Park DW, Dugel PU, Garda J, et al. Macular pucker removal with and without internal limiting membrane peeling: pilot study. Ophthalmology. 2003; 110 (1):62–64
[74] Haritoglou C, Eibl K, Schaumberger M, et al. Functional outcome after trypan blue-assisted vitrectomy for macular pucker: a prospective, randomized, comparative trial. Am J Ophthalmol. 2004; 138(1):1–5
[75] Hillenkamp J, Saikia P, Gora F, et al. Macular function and morphology after peeling of idiopathic epiretinal membrane with and without the assistance of indocyanine green. Br J Ophthalmol. 2005; 89(4):437–443
[76] Enaida H, Hisatomi T, Hata Y, et al. Brilliant blue G selectively stains the internal limiting membrane/brilliant blue G-assisted membrane peeling. Retina. 2006; 26(6):631–636
[77] Narayanan R, Kenney MC, Kamjoo S, et al. Toxicity of indocyanine green (ICG) in combination with light on retinal pigment epithelial cells and neurosensory retinal cells. Curr Eye Res. 2005; 30(6):471–478
[78] Margherio RR, Cox MS, Jr, Trese MT, Murphy PL, Johnson J, Minor LA. Removal of epimacular membranes. Ophthalmology. 1985; 92(8):1075–1083
[79] de Bustros S, Thompson JT, Michels RG, Rice TA, Glaser BM. Vitrectomy for idiopathic epiretinal membranes causing macular pucker. Br J Ophthalmol. 1988; 72(9):692–695
[80] Rice TA, De Bustros S, Michels RG, Thompson JT, Debanne SM, Rowland DY. Prognostic factors in vitrectomy for epiretinal membranes of the macula. Ophthalmology. 1986; 93(5):602–610
[81] Cherfan GM, Michels RG, de Bustros S, Enger C, Glaser BM. Nuclear sclerotic cataract after vitrectomy for idiopathic epiretinal membranes causing macular pucker. Am J Ophthalmol. 1991; 111(4):434–438
[82] Benhamou N, Massin P, Spolaore R, Paques M, Gaudric A. Surgical management of epiretinal membrane in young patients. Am J Ophthalmol. 2002; 133 (3):358–364
[83] Duker JS, Kaiser PK, Binder S, et al. The International Vitreomacular Traction Study Group classification of vitreomacular adhesion, traction, and macular hole. Ophthalmology. 2013; 120(12):2611–2619
[84] Gandorfer A, Rohleder M, Kampik A. Epiretinal pathology of vitreomacular traction syndrome. Br J Ophthalmol. 2002; 86(8):902–909
[85] Chang LK, Fine HF, Spaide RF, Koizumi H, Grossniklaus HE. Ultrastructural correlation of spectral-domain optical coherence tomographic findings in vitreomacular traction syndrome. Am J Ophthalmol. 2008; 146(1):121–127
[86] Johnson MW. Tractional cystoid macular edema: a subtle variant of the vitreomacular traction syndrome. Am J Ophthalmol. 2005; 140(2):184–192
[87] Stalmans P, Benz MS, Gandorfer A, et al. MIVI-TRUST Study Group. Enzymatic vitreolysis with ocriplasmin for vitreomacular traction and macular holes. N Engl J Med. 2012; 367(7):606–615
[88] John VJ, Flynn HW, Jr, Smiddy WE, et al. Clinical course of vitreomacular adhesion managed by initial observation. Retina. 2014; 34(3):442–446
[89] Melberg NS, Williams DF, Balles MW, et al. Vitrectomy for vitreomacular traction syndrome with macular detachment. Retina. 1995; 15(3):192–197
[90] Smiddy WE, Michels RG, Glaser BM, deBustros S. Vitrectomy for macular traction caused by incomplete vitreous separation. Arch Ophthalmol. 1988; 106 (5):624–628
[91] Rodrigues IA, Stangos AN, McHugh DA, Jackson TL. Intravitreal injection of expansile perfluoropropane (c(3)f(8)) for the treatment of vitreomacular traction. Am J Ophthalmol. 2013; 155(2):270–276.e2

19 Macular Dystrophies

Anita Agarwal

19.1 Macular Dystrophies

A collection of various inherited macular disorders is grouped under the term *macular dystrophies*. Most are isolated conditions that involve the macular region and are not genetically related to each other.

19.1.1 Vitelliform Dystrophies (VMD2 Gene Dystrophy)

Bestrophin 1 (*BEST1*) gene has been implicated in autosomal dominant Best's disease, autosomal dominant vitreoretinochoroidopathy (ADVIRC), autosomal dominant microcornea rod–cone degeneration syndrome (ADMRCS), and autosomal recessive bestrophinopathy (ARB).

Best's Vitelliform Macular Dystrophy

Best's disease (vitelliform macular dystrophy) is an autosomal dominantly inherited disorder with variable penetrance and expressivity.[1,2,3,4,5,6,7,8,9,10,11,12,13,14,15,16,17,18,19,20,21,22,23,24,25,26,27] The gene responsible for Best's vitelliform macular dystrophy (BVMD) was cloned by Petrukhin and colleagues in 1998 and named the *Bestrophin 1* (*BEST1*) gene.[28] It consists of 11 exons and 585 amino acids, and spans 15 kilobases of genomic DNA. The gene is expressed predominantly in the retinal pigment epithelial (RPE) cells and the bestrophin protein is located mainly on the basolateral plasma membrane of the RPE and to a small extent within the RPE cells. The protein is believed to function as an intracellular Ca^{2+}-dependent Cl^- channel and a HCO_3^- channel.[29,30,31,32] Disruption of the ion conductance across the RPE by abnormal *Bestrophin 1* is likely responsible for the absence of light peak response in the electro-oculogram (EOG) in both patients and unaffected carriers of Best's disease.[14,19,26,33,34] The disease appears to affect primarily the RPE. The clinical appearance of the condition can be divided into five stages.

Previtelliform or Carrier Stage

Although vitelliform lesions have been observed as early as the first week of life, the fundi of most patients probably are normal during the first few months or years of life. Many carriers never manifest a change in the fundus and they are incidentally found when other family members with the typical vitelliform lesions are seen. They exhibit low Arden ratios on EOG testing.

Vitelliform Stage

In infancy or in early childhood, patients may develop a sharply circumscribed subretinal lesion that has been likened to the yolk of a sunny-side-up fried egg (▶ Fig. 19.1). Visual acuity at this stage of the disease is usually normal. Early in the disease, little or no elevation of the retina occurs. Subsequently, the lesion appears elevated as the yellow material increases in amount and is found in the outer photoreceptor zone, subretinal space, and within the RPE layer.[29,35] The color and pattern of the RPE surrounding the lesion are usually normal. Variations in size and stage of development of the lesion may be present in the eyes of the same patient. The lesion initially may be evident only in one eye. In some patients, the fellow eye may remain near-normal with 20/20 acuity throughout life.[36] The vitelliform lesion may occasionally disappear spontaneously. The lesions may be eccentrically located and may be multiple.[37] In a few patients, they may be unusually large and geographic in shape. Some patients may show a finely mottled pattern of yellowish change in the RPE throughout the fundus.

Pseudohypopyon Stage

Usually by the time the patient reaches puberty, the yellowish lesion shows evidence of disruption (▶ Fig. 19.2). It appears that the yellow material is partly taken up by the RPE cells and the heavier material gravitates inferiorly in the subretinal space. There is thinning of the RPE and occasionally some clumping of pigment in the superior portion of these lesions.

With further disruption of the vitelliform lesion, multiple irregular yellowish subretinal deposits produce a picture likened to a scrambled egg (▶ Fig. 19.3). Multifocal yellow deposits may occasionally be arranged in a more orderly ring distribution near the periphery of these lesions. The visual acuity is often decreased to the level of 20/30 to 20/40 in the presence of extensive scrambling of the vitelliform lesion.

Atrophic Stage

Eventually all of the yellow pigment may disappear and leave an oval area of atrophic RPE.

Cicatricial and Choroidal Neovascular Stage

Many patients develop evidence of one or more plaques of white subretinal fibrous tissue, and in some cases there is

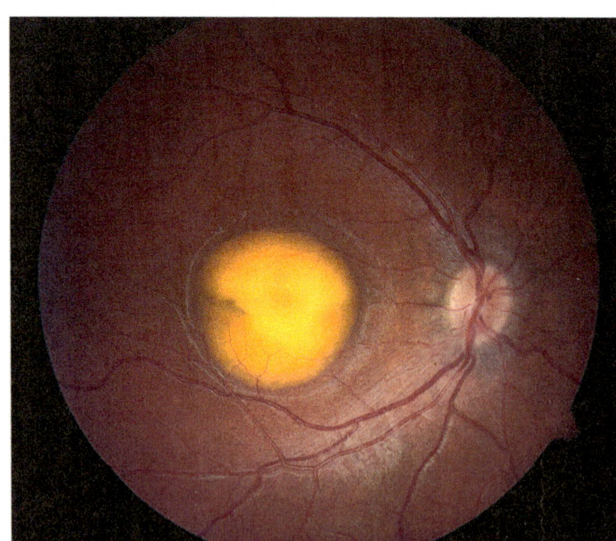

Fig. 19.1 Egg yolk–like lesion in an 8-year-old girl with Best's vitelliform macular dystrophy

evidence of choroidal neovascularization and hemorrhagic detachment of the macula.[6,12] These latter patients eventually develop a white or partly pigmented disciform scar. The central vision is generally 20/100 or less at this stage of the disease. Serous detachment of the retina may occur at any stage of the development of vitelliform lesions (▶ Fig. 19.4). This "Best's space" may never collapse even after the vitelliform material has been absorbed or broken down.

In the vitelliform stage, the early phases of angiography demonstrate complete obstruction of the choroidal fluorescence by the lesion.[12,18] There is no generalized obscuration of the choroidal fluorescence such as occurs in Stargardt's disease. During the later stages of angiography, the vitelliform lesion may appear nonfluorescent or may appear to fluoresce slightly. As the yellow pigment gravitates inferiorly, angiography in the area vacated by the yellow material reveals evidence of early fluorescence secondary to depigmentation and late staining of the altered RPE (▶ Fig. 19.5). Angiography permits detection of choroidal neovascularization and shows evidence of staining of fibrous tissue if present in the subretinal space. It is probable that occult choroidal neovascularization is present within some of the subretinal plaques of fibrous tissue. The vitelliform lesions are brightly hyperautofluorescent (▶ Fig. 19.6).

Peripheral visual fields, electroretinographic findings, and dark adaptation in these patients are normal. Color vision in the late stages of the disease may be mildly disturbed. The EOG is markedly abnormal, with the light-to-dark ratio (Arden ratio) usually being below 1.50.[8,14,19] EOGs of carriers of the disease usually yield a subnormal result. Patients who are both homozygous and heterozygous for the *BEST1* gene show low Arden ratio, thus making this feature most characteristic of the condition. The disease is inherited as an autosomal dominant trait. Best's disease usually occurs in Caucasian patients but may occur occasionally in Africans and Asians.[38]

Visual prognosis is moderate to good for at least the first six decades of life.[5] Most patients retain reading vision in at least one eye throughout life. The progression of visual loss is slow and occurs for the most part beyond the age of 40 years.[16] Acute and permanent loss of central vision may occur in association with bleeding from subretinal new vessels. A macular hole may occasionally occur in patients with Best's disease.

Histopathologic findings in Best's disease included a periodic acid–Schiff (PAS)-positive, acid mucopolysaccharide–negative, electron-dense, finely granular material in the inner segments of the degenerating photoreceptors and Müller cells recently identified predominantly as A2E[39]; an abnormal fibrillar

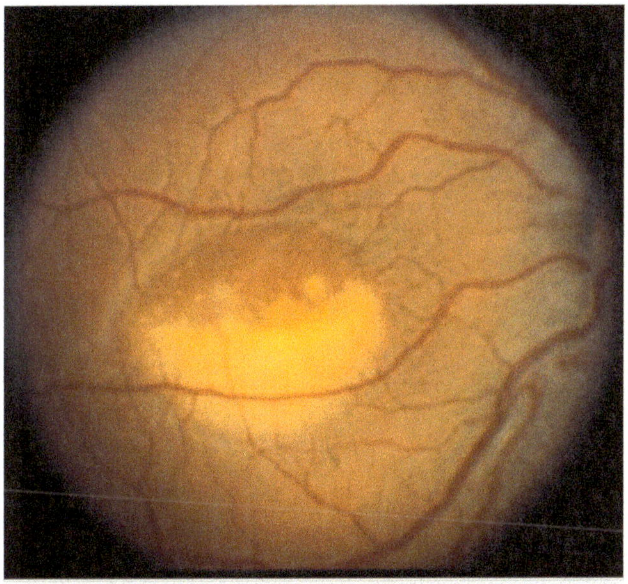

Fig. 19.2 Pseudohypopyon stage of Best's vitelliform macular dystrophy

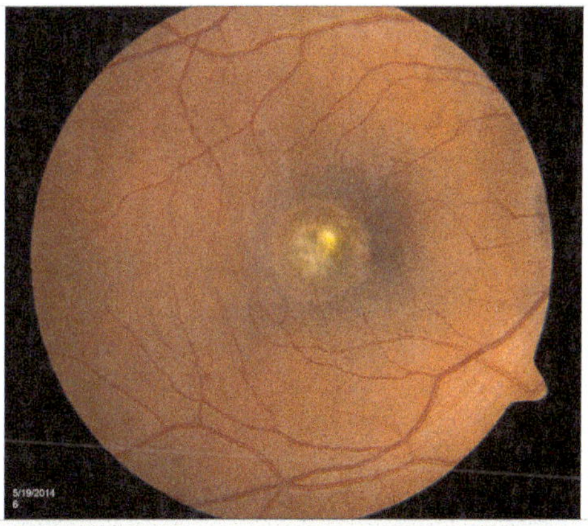

Fig. 19.3 Scrambled egg stage of Best's vitelliform macular dystrophy

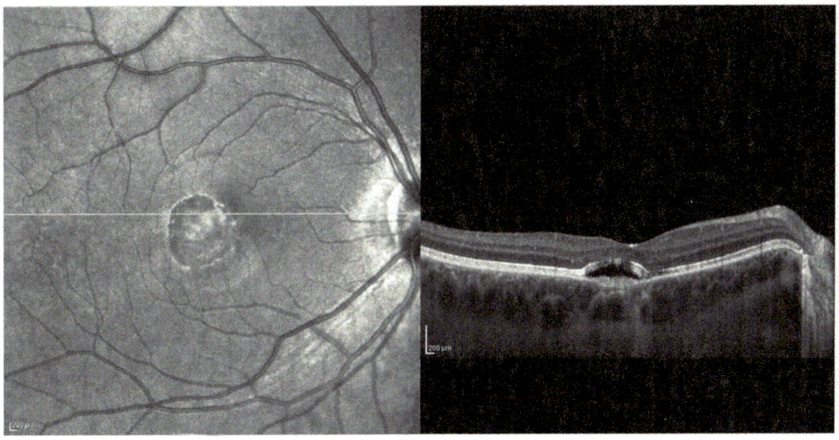

Fig. 19.4 Persistence of "Best's space" even after resolution of vitelliform material.

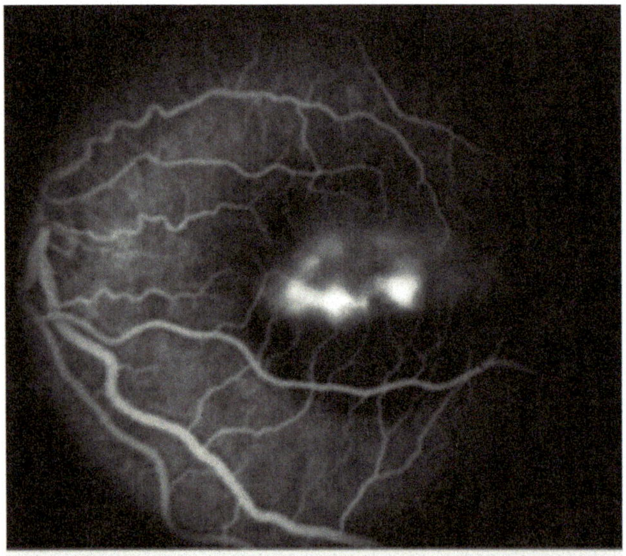

Fig. 19.5 Staining of the RPE in the area above the pseudohypopyon.

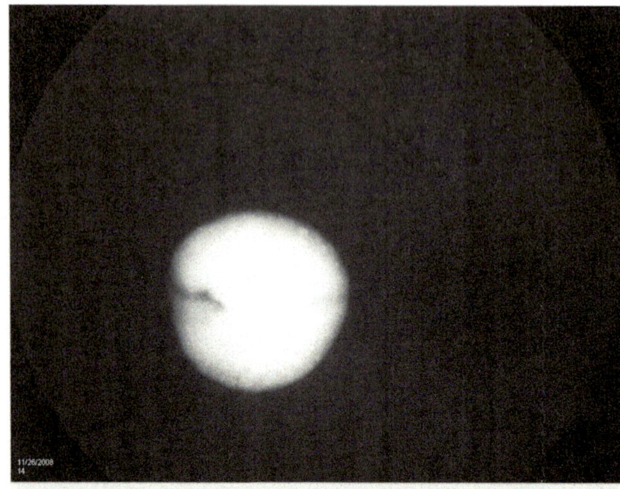

Fig. 19.6 The vitelliform material is brilliantly autofluorescent.

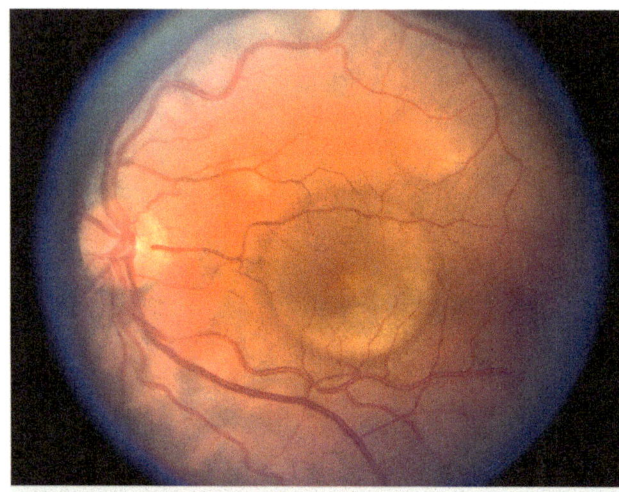

Fig. 19.7 Multifocal Best's disease.

material beneath the RPE cells in the region of photoreceptor cell loss; and normal choriocapillaris.[13] Breaks in Bruch's membrane and choroidal neovascularization have been demonstrated.[1,13] These studies, together with the in vivo demonstration of autofluorescence of vitelliform lesions in Best's disease by Miller,[7,29,35,40] suggest that the yellow pigment may at least in part be caused by lipofuscin. Histopathologic examination of an 86-year-old homozygous for *BEST1* gene showed accumulation of lipofuscin, a large component of it made up of A2E, within the RPE cells. Other RPE granules were melanoliposomes. Extraction of the granules in this eye and another 81-year-old's eye heterozygous for the gene showed the lipofuscin to be mostly made up of A2E similar to that found in diseases caused by the *ABCR* transport gene abnormality.[39]

The vitelliform stage of Best's disease should be differentiated from other diseases that cause solitary yellowish macular lesions—for example, dominantly inherited adult-onset vitelliform foveomacular dystrophy (pattern dystrophy), basal laminar drusen with vitelliform detachment, acute polymorphous exudative vitelliform maculopathy, paraneoplastic vitelliform maculopathy in metastatic melanoma, and fundus flavimaculatus (Stargardt's disease) with large central flecks. The early age of development of the yellow lesion and the progressive vitelliruptiform changes are essential findings to differentiate patients with Best's disease from those with adult-onset vitelliform foveomacular dystrophy (pattern dystrophy), because the latter disease may be associated with subnormal EOGs in one-third of cases and because both are dominantly inherited. Four other yellow lesions that simulate Best's disease include vitelliform detachment in some patients with basal laminar drusen, focal serous RPE detachments containing dehemoglobinized blood pigment, some cases of central serous retinopathy with subretinal fibrin, and resolving subretinal hematomas. Gene testing for the *BEST1* gene with the presence of these features confirms the diagnosis. Future identification of specific gene defects and the nature of the vitelliform material will help elucidate the pathogenic relationship of the various disorders that demonstrate similar yellow lesions in the macula.[41,42]

Multifocal vitelliform lesions may occur in patients with Best's disease (▶ Fig. 19.7). The lesions may vary in size and may be several disc diameters or larger in size and often have some irregularity to their contour. These larger lesions frequently demonstrate partial resolution or disruption of the yellow material.

Pearls

- Atypical presentations of Best's disease include multifocal vitelliform lesions, normal fundus and reduced EOG in family members manifesting incomplete penetrance, and unilateral vitelliform lesion with bilateral reduced EOG.

BEST1 gene has also been implicated in ADVIRC, ADMRCS, and ARB, all with extraretinal features implicating that the gene may be involved in ocular development.[29]

19.1.2 Autosomal Dominant Vitreoretinochoroidopathy

Autosomal dominant vitreoretinochoroidopathy (ADVIRC) is an autosomal dominantly inherited pigmentary retinopathy described by Kaufman et al in 1982.[43] It is characterized by an annular peripheral pigmentary retinopathy for 360 degrees with a distinct posterior boundary near the equator (▶ Fig. 19.8) associated with punctate whitish opacities in the superficial retina along with vitreous cells and fibrillary condensation. Peripheral retinal arteriolar narrowing and occlusion, evidence of retinal neovascularization, choroidal atrophy, and presenile cataracts can be present. Evidence of blood–retinal barrier breakdown is seen by cystoid macular edema.

These patients usually do not have symptoms of night blindness. The electroretinogram (ERG) is normal or only slightly reduced. The EOG is variably affected, with Arden ratio ranging from normal to subnormal. There have been a few cases with late cone dystrophy.[44] The gene defect has been localized to the *BEST1* gene with missense mutations and exon skipping on the long arm of chromosome 11.[29,45,46]

19.1.3 Autosomal Dominant Microcornea Rod–Cone Dystrophy, Cataract with Staphyloma

A subgroup of patients who have all or some features of ADVIRC may also have microcornea and shallow anterior chamber with evidence of subacute or acute angle-closure glaucoma. Some of these patients show posterior staphyloma and some are myopic.[47] The inheritance pattern is autosomal dominant, with a mutation in the *BEST1* gene.[29,45] The EOG is abnormal in all patients with ADMRCS syndrome. A full-field ERG may show subnormal photopic and scotopic responses. With time, these patients show progressive ERG changes with severe rod and cone photoreceptor dysfunction, unlike ADVIRC that is relatively stable. The ADMRCS syndrome is generally more severe than ADVIRC. However, there are family members who have overlapping findings of the two conditions.[29]

19.1.4 Autosomal Recessive Bestrophinopathy

Autosomal Recessive Bestrophinopathy (ARB), first described by Burgess et al in 2008,[48] usually starts with central visual loss, with an age of onset ranging from 4 to 40 years (mean, 25 years). The visual acuity often deteriorates to less than 20/60 in both eyes within a few years. Patients are generally hyperopic with shallow anterior chambers and may present with subacute or acute angle-closure glaucoma. Fundus examination shows irregular RPE alterations with yellow-white subretinal deposits that are seen throughout the retina, preferentially in the macula and midperiphery (▶ Fig. 19.9). They resemble multifocal Best's disease. Intraretinal and subretinal fluid may be observed in the macula that can be confirmed by optical coherence tomography (OCT). The macular lesions may evolve into atrophic scars, causing a further decline in vision.[48] The EOG is severely reduced or absent to light rise. The macular focal pattern ERG and multifocal ERG are markedly abnormal, indicating severe macular dysfunction. The full-field ERG shows reduced and delayed rod and cone responses indicating panretinal photoreceptor dysfunction. On angiography, there is widespread patchy hyperfluorescence due to RPE atrophy and retinal edema. These areas correspond to areas of increased fundus autofluorescence (▶ Fig. 19.10), suggesting lipofuscin accumulation in the pigment epithelium. The areas of RPE loss show decreased fundus autofluorescence. High-resolution OCT of the macula shows photoreceptor detachment from the pigment epithelium, disruption of the photoreceptor layer, and intraretinal cysts but persevered inner retinal layers (▶ Fig. 19.11).[29,48] Those patients who are heterozygous to the mutation are entirely normal clinically and electrophysiologically.

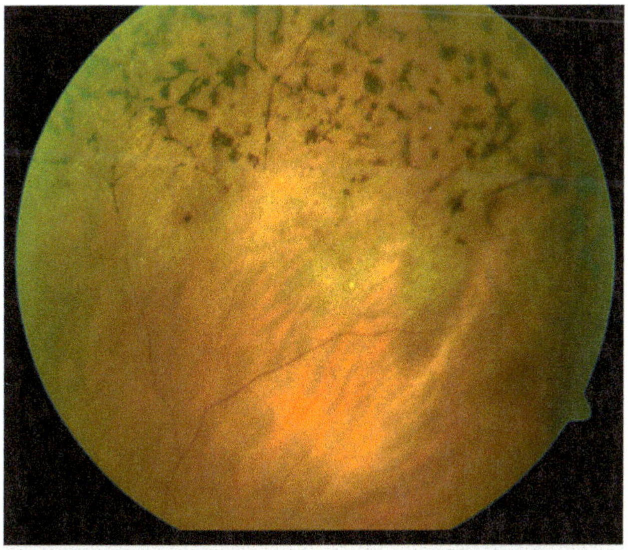

Fig. 19.8 Sharp demarcation between the pigmentary retinopathy zone and posterior fundus in the vicinity of the equator. (Image courtesy of Dr. Ranjit Dhaliwal.)

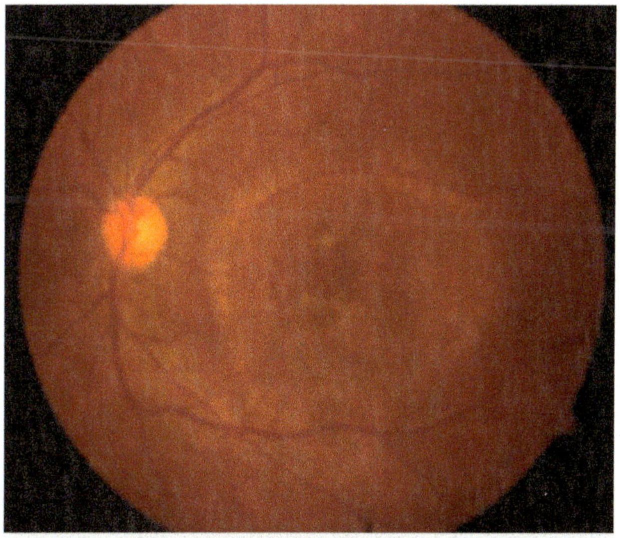

Fig. 19.9 Fundus appearance of a 38-year-old woman with gradual decline in vision over 8 years showing multifocal subretinal yellow lesions arranged in a ring in both macula. (Image is provided courtesy of Dr. Deeksha Katoch.)

All three conditions described earlier are caused by mutations in the *BEST1* gene, the same gene that causes BVMD. Whereas Best's, ADVIRC, and ADMRCS syndromes are autosomal dominant, ARB occurs in the presence of homozygous or compound heterozygous *BEST1* mutation.

Nearly all mutations identified in BVMD and adult-onset foveal macular vitelliform dystrophy, a type of pattern dystrophy, are missense mutations. Those mutations causing ADVIRC and the MRCS syndrome are splice mutations,[29,46,48] leading to in-frame deletions or duplications. The null phenotype of ARB is caused by homozygous or compound heterozygous nonsense or missense *BEST1* mutation.[29,49] The variable expressivity and penetrance probably account for the wide variation in the phenotype of these conditions. It is likely they are also dependent on other genetic or environmental modifiers to manifest all features of the condition.

19.2 Pattern Dystrophy

Pattern dystrophies constitute a group of disorders that was initially believed to have autosomal dominant inheritance. However, several sporadic cases and their association sometimes with certain genetically inherited systemic diseases indicate a variable genetic association and a lot more yet to be learned about this group of dystrophies.

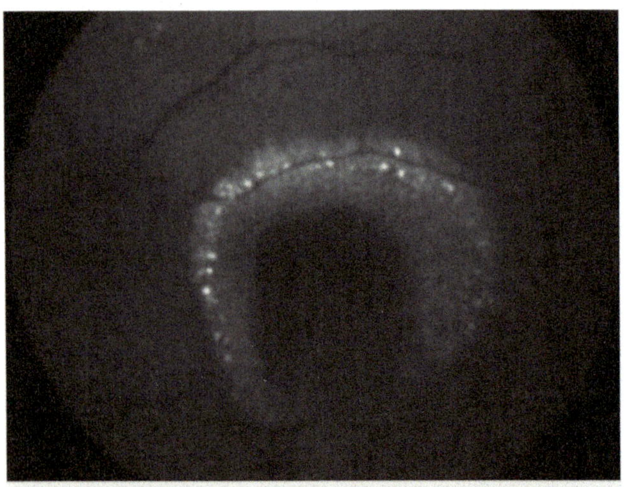

Fig. 19.10 The macular lesions in a patient with autosomal recessive bestrophinopathy are hyperautofluorescent and stain on fluorescein angiography (Image is provided courtesy of Dr. Deeksha Katoch).

Patients present usually in midlife with mild disturbances of central vision associated with a variety of patterns of yellow, orange, or gray pigment deposits in the macular area.[12,21,50,51,52,53,54,55,56,57,58,59,60,61,62,63,64,65,66,67,68,69,70,71,72,73,74,75,76,77,78,79,80,81,82,83,84,85,86,87,88] The prognosis for retention of good central vision in at least one eye until late adulthood is good. The ERG is typically normal, but the EOG may be slightly or moderately subnormal. These dystrophies are usually inherited as an autosomal dominant trait. Mutations of the peripherin/*RDS* and slow gene (Pro 210 ARG) and codon 167 of the *RDS* gene were first demonstrated in family members of patients with dominantly inherited pattern dystrophy.[88,89,90,91,92] Since then, several other mutations of the peripherin/*RDS* gene have been found in families and sporadic cases of pattern dystrophy.[86,87,88] Of importance are the varying phenotypes, often within families seen with the same genetic mutation.[31,93,94,95,96,97] In addition to the association with different phenotypes of pattern dystrophy, peripherin/*RDS* gene mutations are associated with central areolar choroidal dystrophy, autosomal dominant retinitis pigmentosa, autosomal dominant cone and cone–rod dystrophy, retinitis punctata albescens, and digenic retinitis pigmentosa.[96,98,99,100,101] The peripherin/*RDS* gene localizes to chromosome 6p21.2, spans 26 kilobases of genomic DNA, and contains three exons. The gene product of peripherin/*RDS* is an integral membrane protein peripherin/*RDS* within rods and cones, and plays an important role in the photoreceptor outer-segment morphogenesis by managing disc formation, alignment, and shedding. Other gene that has been associated with pattern dystrophy includes VMD2.

Based on the pattern of pigment distribution, pattern dystrophies have been subdivided clinically into five principal groups. A few patients may show different patterns in the two eyes. Some may show progression from one pattern to another over time. For these reasons, it is probable that these are closely related, if not expressions of the same disorder.

19.2.1 Group 1: Adult-Onset Foveomacular Vitelliform Dystrophy

Patients with adult-onset foveomacular vitelliform dystrophy are visually asymptomatic or suffer mild visual blurring and metamorphopsia in one or both eyes, usually with the onset between ages 30 and 50 years. Symmetric, solitary, usually 1/3 to 1 disc diameter size, round or oval, slightly elevated, yellow subretinal lesions, often with a central pigmented area in each eye are characteristic of the condition (▶ Fig. 19.12).

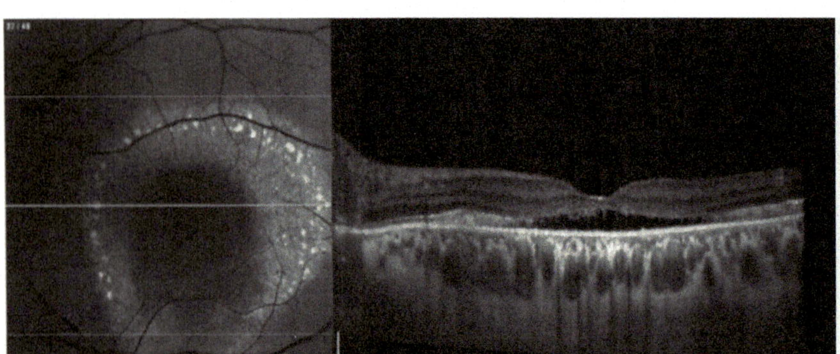

Fig. 19.11 OCT shows loss of photoreceptor nuclei and outer segments and accumulation of material in the subretinal space around the fovea. (Image courtesy of Dr. Deeksha Katoch.)

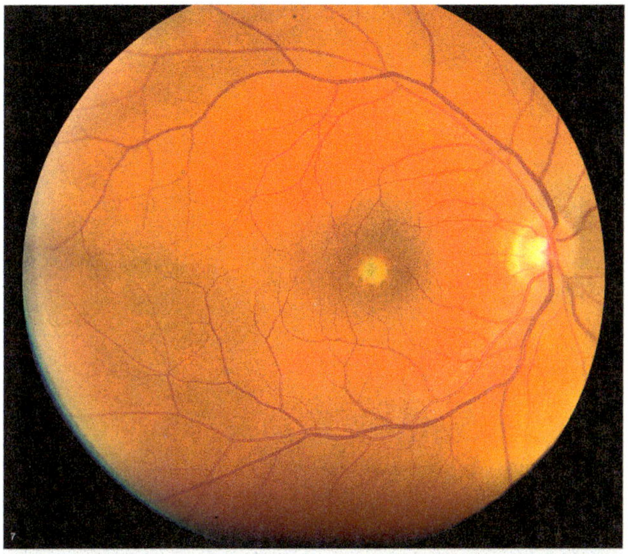

Fig. 19.12 Solitary vitelliform lesion in the right fovea with central pigmentation.

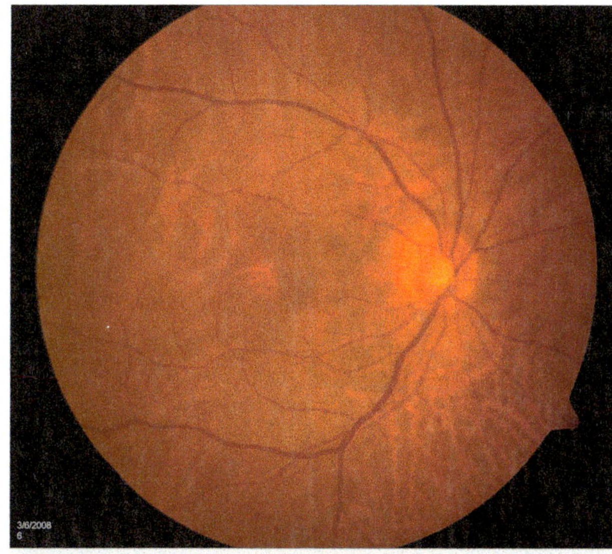

Fig. 19.13 Loss of vitelliform material revealing depigmented RPE in the fovea.

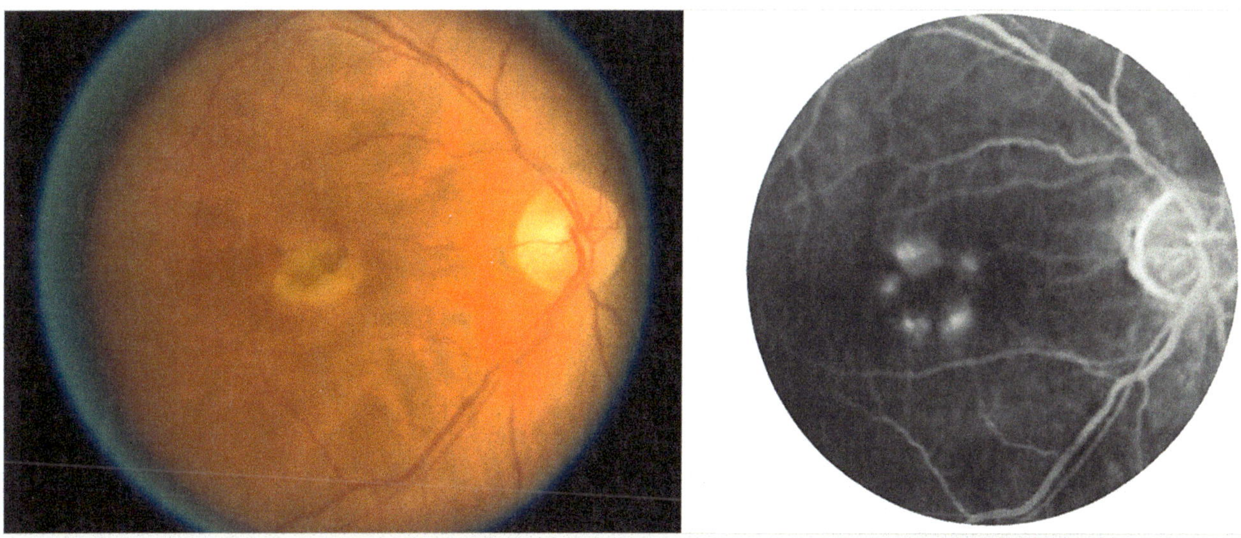

Fig. 19.14 Solitary vitelliform lesion with (a) central pigmentation that blocks fluorescence centrally and (b) has a halo of hyperfluorescence surrounding it.

Additional small yellow flecks may sometimes be present in the paracentral region.[12,51,52,53,55,57,59,60,61,67,69,70,72,73,74,79,84] Initially, the yellow lesion may be present in only one eye. Although most of the foveal lesions are approximately 1/3 disc diameter in size, occasionally they may be larger and misdiagnosed as the "sunny-side-up" stage of BVMD or as bilateral serous detachment of the RPE. Later, the foveal lesions may fade and leave an irregular oval or round area of depigmentation of the RPE (▶ Fig. 19.13). Some patients eventually develop additional paracentral yellow deposits, often in a triradiate pattern. Fluorescein angiography during the early stages of the disease shows either a nonfluorescent lesion or, more typically, a small irregular ring (halo) of hyperfluorescence surrounding a central nonfluorescent spot (▶ Fig. 19.14). Some of the extrafoveal small yellow lesions show discrete staining, similar to drusen, and others are either nonfluorescent or have a halo of fluorescence surrounding them. The yellow and gray components of the lesions are brightly autofluorescent and the depigmented RPE in late lesions are hypoautofluorescent.

This form of pattern dystrophy was first observed in female patients in three successive generations in one family at the Bascom Palmer Eye Institute and reported by Gass.[72] Recently, a mutation of the peripherin RDS gene has been demonstrated in two of these patients.[91]

Unlike those in BVMD, the vitelliform lesions in patients with pattern dystrophy usually first appear in the fourth decade or beyond, are generally smaller, and do not show disruption and layering of the yellow pigment in the dependent portion of the lesions. In some families, there is an overlap in the features of Best's disease and pattern dystrophy.[102]

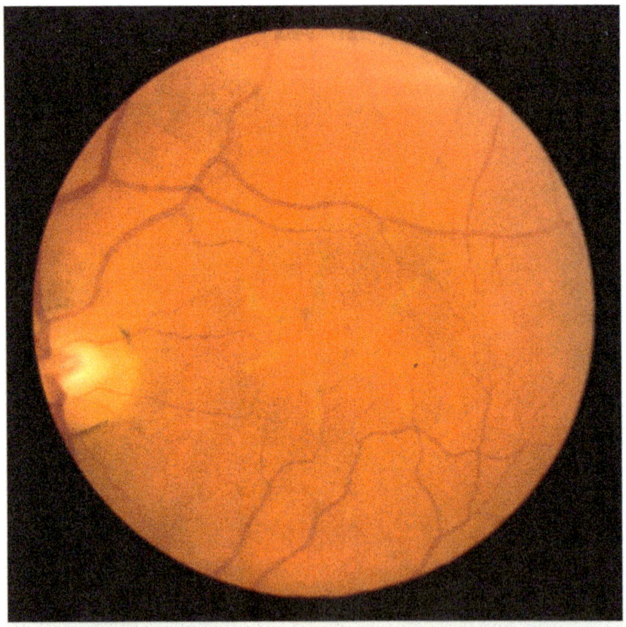

Fig. 19.15 Butterfly type of pattern dystrophy with yellow material radiating from the center.

19.2.2 Group 2: Butterfly-Shaped Pigment Dystrophy

Gray-brown or yellow pigment is arranged in a well-organized triradiate pattern confined to the center of the macula in a symmetric fashion, likened to the shape of a butterfly (▶ Fig. 19.15).[62,71,78] A zone of depigmentation occurs around this pigment figure. The optic disc and vessels are normal. Some patients have a reticular pigmentary pattern of drusen in the periphery. The early phases of angiography show hypofluorescence of the central pigment lines with hyperfluorescent borders. The shapes of the central yellow lesions in pattern dystrophies vary considerably and may simulate a variety of inanimate or animate objects.

19.2.3 Group 3: Reticular Dystrophy of the RPE

In patients with reticular dystrophy, the pattern of yellow pigment extends into the periphery of the macula and resembles coarse, knotted fishnet or chicken wire.[56,63,66,76,77,82] It begins in the foveal area and gradually extends 4 or 5 disc diameters from the macula in all directions. The midperiphery and the periphery of the fundus are unaffected early in the disease. The network may be more apparent angiographically than ophthalmoscopically. It usually fades with age and may be replaced by extensive atrophic changes in the RPE in later life. Patients with reticular dystrophy may show an autosomal recessive as well as autosomal dominant inheritance.

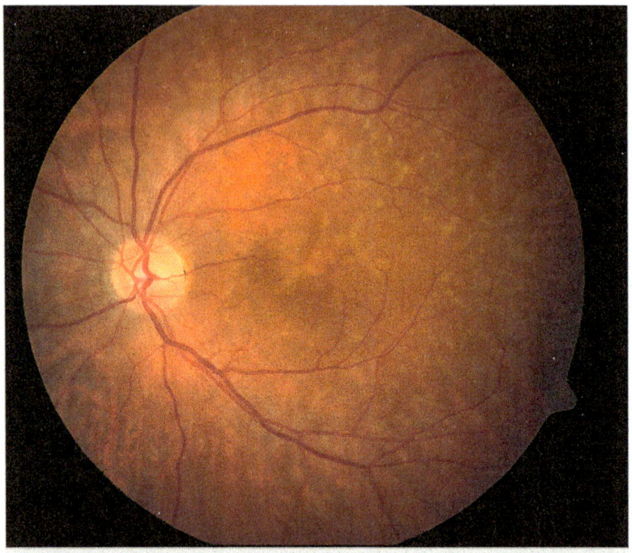

Fig. 19.16 Multiple flecks of "fundus flavimaculatus" type of pattern dystrophy with 20/20 vision in a 55-year-old woman.

19.2.4 Group 4: Multifocal Pattern Dystrophy Simulating Fundus Flavimaculatus

Some patients develop multiple irregular or triradiate yellow lesions centrally or eccentrically, and in some cases these are widely scattered and partly interconnected in a triradiate fashion that may simulate those in fundus flavimaculatus (Stargardt's disease) (▶ Fig. 19.16).[103,104,105] These patients, who do not show fluorescein angiographic evidence of a dark choroid suggesting lipofuscin storage, have been recently reported as examples of dominantly inherited fundus flavimaculatus. Unlike most patients with fundus flavimaculatus, these patients have good visual acuity and a more favorable visual prognosis. However, some of these patients with an exaggerated phenotype can show progressive loss of the yellow material and RPE/photoreceptor thinning and atrophy resulting in islands of, or confluent, geographic atrophy (▶ Fig. 19.17). Choroidal neovascular membranes can rarely occur. Histopathologic and electron microscopic studies of the eye of a patient with this type of pattern dystrophy have demonstrated that the flecks are not caused by abnormal lipofuscin storage.[105]

19.2.5 Group 5: Coarse Pigment Mottling in the Macula (Fundus Pulverulentus)

Patients with fundus pulverulentus typically display mild visual loss associated with a prominent, coarse, punctate mottling of the pigment epithelium in the central macular area (▶ Fig. 19.18a,b).[54,61,65] This pattern is most often seen in patients with pseudoxanthoma elasticum.[106] They simulate pigment mottling seen in patients with resolved central serous chorioretinopathy.

Although it is convenient to subdivide patients with pattern dystrophy into these five groups, it is important to realize that the fundus findings in some patients do not fall precisely into one group. Some may show one pattern in one eye and another pattern in the fellow eye. Others may show one or more eccentric triradiate yellow or darkly pigmented lesions. Some may have one or more lesions in only one eye early in their course. The fundus findings in patients with pattern dystrophy and an asymmetric distribution of triradiate pigment figures must be differentiated from similar findings that may develop in some patients with recurrent idiopathic central serous chorioretinopathy/organ transplant retinopathy and in patients with Elschnig's spots caused by hypertensive choroidopathy, for example, in a patient with toxemia of pregnancy.

The visual prognosis is good in all subgroups of pattern dystrophy.[73,107] Late geographic atrophy (▶ Fig. 19.17) and choroidal neovascularization may occur in any of the subgroups and are responsible for visual loss. Choroidal neovascularization occurs only infrequently.[90] Absence of a dark choroid angiographically and good visual function suggest pattern dystrophy rather than fundus flavimaculatus.[103,105] An occasional cause of loss of vision in these patients is the development of a macular hole.[108]

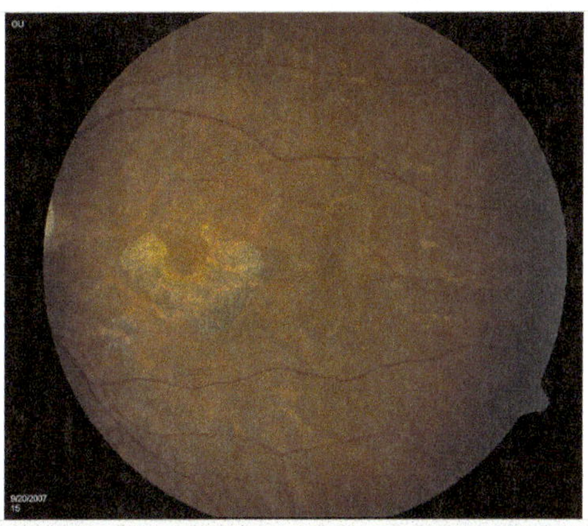

Fig. 19.17 Central geographic atrophy in a 52 year old woman with fundus flavimaculatus type of pattern dystrophy.

Histopathologic examination of the eyes of two patients with almost identical lesions revealed similar findings.[60,109] In one case, however, the eye showed evidence of a high concentration of lipofuscin, which may be responsible for the central yellow lesion.[60] A report of the histopathologic and ultrastructural findings in two eyes of a 51-year-old man with a pattern of flecks suggesting fundus flavimaculatus and normal macula and visual acuity found no evidence of lipofuscin storage or acid mucopolysaccharide accumulation in the RPE—these are characteristic findings in fundus flavimaculatus.[105] Elevated aggregates of enlarged RPE cells with apices distended by accumulated lipid membranes with a tubulovesicular appearance were responsible for the flecks. The findings in this patient suggest that the yellow flecks in the pattern dystrophies, although they clinically appear similar to those in Stargardt's disease and fundus flavimaculatus, are not caused by focal lipofuscin storage in the RPE. The same may prove true in the case of vitelliform lesions in Best's disease. Unlike patients with Stargardt's disease, patients with Best's disease and adult-onset vitelliform foveomacular dystrophy do not show the angiographic feature of obstruction of the normal background choroidal fluorescence (silent choroid) that is caused by diffuse heavy deposition of lipofuscin material in the RPE.

19.2.6 Systemic Diseases Associated with Pattern Dystrophy

Macular changes typical of pattern dystrophy occur in 70%[106] of patients with pseudoxanthoma elasticum. The fundus

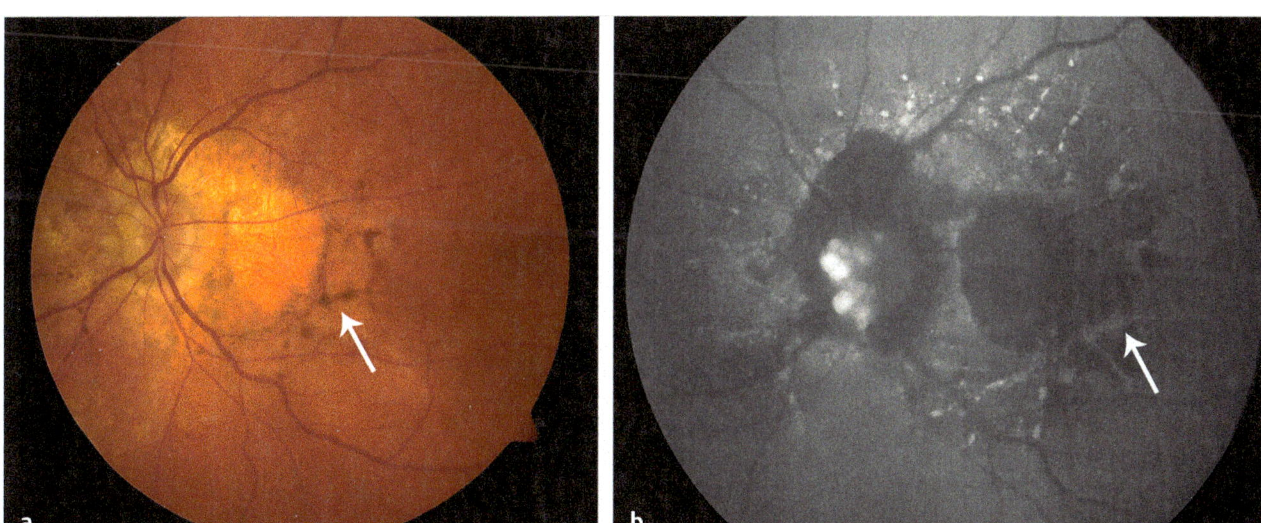

Fig. 19.18 **(a)** Disc drusen, angioid streaks, geographic atrophy, and punctate pigment dots of "fundus pulverulentus" type of pattern dystrophy in a patient with pseudoxanthoma elasticum. **(b)** The pigment dots of fundus pulverulentus pattern dystrophy are hyperautofluorescent (arrows).

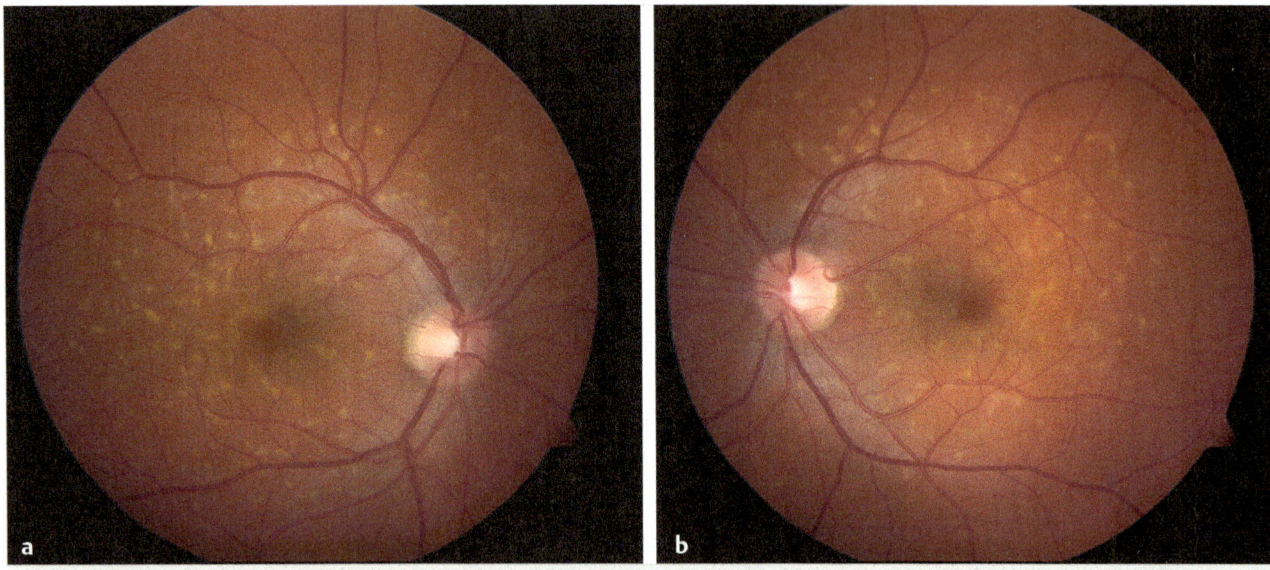

Fig. 19.19 (**a**) Right and (**b**) left fundus of a 39-year-old asymptomatic man with triradiate or pisciform flecks at the RPE level. He was ABCA4 positive.

pulverulentus pattern is most frequently observed, although all five types of pattern are seen.[106,110,111,112] Pattern dystrophy has also been observed in patients with myotonic dystrophy, hereditary spastic paraplegia (Kjellin's syndrome), and maternally inherited mitochondrial myopathies (Maternally inherited diabetes and deafness [MIDD], Myopathy, encephalopathy, lactic acidosis, and stroke like syndrome [MELAS], Myopathy, encephalopathy, ragged red fibers [MERRF]) and in one patient with McArdle's disease, a glycogen storage disease in which a deficiency of muscle phosphorylase inhibits the ability of striated muscle to use its stored glycogen.[113]

Pearls

- Pattern dystrophy is relatively common, can be sporadic or dominant in inheritance, can be bilateral or unilateral, and can mimic several disorders. Ruling out other causes of the clinical appearance may be necessary to establish the diagnosis. Occasionally, patients diagnosed with exudative age-related macular degeneration may have underlying pattern dystrophy by itself or associated with pseudoxanthoma elasticum. Careful evaluation of the fluorescein angiogram and autofluorescence imaging and absence of drusen help make the diagnosis.

Stargardt's Disease (Fundus Flavimaculatus)

In 1909, Stargardt described seven patients from two families, with visual loss beginning in the first two decades of life and with a normal fundus, who later developed macular atrophy and yellowish deep retinal flecks.[114] In 1965, Franceschetti described similar patients who also had flecks that extended into the peripheral fundus.[115,116] This was termed *fundus flavimaculatus*. Stargardt's disease and fundus flavimaculatus are names now used interchangeably in the literature.

Patients with Stargardt's disease develop visual loss that may be unassociated with any evidence of flecks or RPE atrophy during childhood or early adulthood (but soon afterward develop atrophic macular changes and the appearance of "pisciform" yellowish RPE flecks; ▶ Fig. 19.19a,b). They appear somewhat similar to, but should be differentiated from, drusen. These flecks are variable in size, shape, and distribution. When located in the midperiphery, they are often arranged in a triradiate or reticular pattern that has been likened to a forked fishtail. As they begin to fade, their color changes from yellow to gray, partly due to loss of RPE substance, and they may appear larger and less discrete. Fluorescein angiography is important in differentiating the flecks in Stargardt's disease (fundus flavimaculatus) from drusen. Whereas drusen show a pattern of hyperfluorescence corresponding precisely with their size, the yellow flecks in fundus flavimaculatus either appear nonfluorescent when the lipofuscin is intracellular or show an irregular pattern of fluorescence with disruption or atrophy of RPE cells.[117]

Most patients with this disease experience loss of central vision first in childhood or young adulthood. Some, however, become symptomatic in midlife or beyond. Loss of central vision may be accompanied by symptomatic as well as electrophysiologic evidence of significant cone dysfunction.[118,119] Some patients, particularly those who develop widespread flecks extending into the periphery, may develop evidence of rod as well as cone dysfunction.[120] Patients with Stargardt's disease can be subdivided into the four groups based on the fundus and fluorescein angiographic findings at the time of presentation.

Group 1: Vermillion Fundi and Hidden Choroidal Fluorescence

Some patients with subnormal visual acuity have relatively normal-appearing fundi except for the easy-to-overlook heavily pigmented RPE that in most lightly pigmented patients imparts a vermillion color and obscures most of the details of the choroid from view. Angiographically, the retinal vessels are displayed prominently on a dark background of minimal choroidal fluorescence.

Group 2: Atrophic Maculopathy with or without Flecks

In some patients, the loss of pigment in the macula may be so minimal that only with angiography can this be demonstrated with certainty. These patients and those in group 1 may be misdiagnosed either as having functional complaints or as having a lesion involving the optic pathways. Particularly in young children, the flecks may not be present or may be quite small and limited in number. Likewise, the vermillion fundus and dark choroid angiographically may not be present in early life as the accumulation of abnormal lipofuscin occurs with age. On subsequent follow-up, flecks as well as evidence of diffuse lipofuscin storage in the RPE occur. The flecks may be confined to the macula or may extend into the midperiphery of the fundi. Fluorescein angiography demonstrates a dark choroid due to blockage of choroidal hyperfluorescence by the thickened RPE cells with abnormal lipofuscin (▶ Fig. 19.20). The degree and pattern of atrophy of the RPE in the central macular area vary and do not always correlate with the degree of visual loss. The RPE may show only mild loss of its normal color, a beaten-metal appearance, or marked geographic atrophy. A diffuse oval or bull's-eye pattern of atrophy occurs commonly. The lipofuscin within the flecks accounts for the increased autofluorescence, which may be surrounded by regions of decreased autofluorescence from the adjacent atrophic RPE. The autofluorescence pattern can resemble chronic idiopathic central serous chorioretinopathy, mitochondrial myopathies, and flecks of pattern dystrophy (▶ Fig. 19.21). Patients with the bull's-eye change may be mistaken for cone dystrophy. Varying degrees of atrophy of the RPE surround and extend between the flecks. This is always more evident angiographically than biomicroscopically. The optic disc and retinal vessels in patients in groups 1 and 2 are normal.

Patients with widespread flecks may develop in one or occasionally both eyes well-defined zone of reactive RPE changes that includes hypertrophy, hyperplasia, fibrous metaplasia, and atrophy. This is due to disruption of the swollen RPE cells filled with abnormal lipofuscin from mild trauma. Patients may occasionally develop subretinal neovascularization and disciform detachment of the macula.[121,122,123]

Color vision testing usually shows a mild red–green dyschromatopsia. Many patients show prolongation in rod dark adaptation and selective prolongation of the later segment of rod recovery.[124,125,126] Electroretinographic findings are usually normal or slightly disturbed. The EOG is subnormal in some cases. Some patients may develop photophobia, loss of color vision, and electroretinographic evidence of a cone dystrophy.

Group 3: Atrophic Maculopathy with Late Signs and Symptoms of Retinitis Pigmentosa

Patients in group 3 are similar to those in group 2 but in addition show signs and symptoms of retinitis pigmentosa,

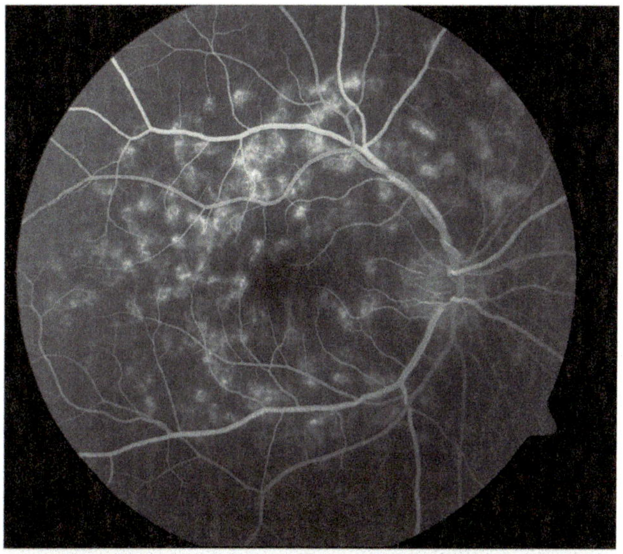

Fig. 19.20 Fluorescein angiogram showing dark background choroid and hyperfluorescence of the flecks in a patient without macular atrophy.

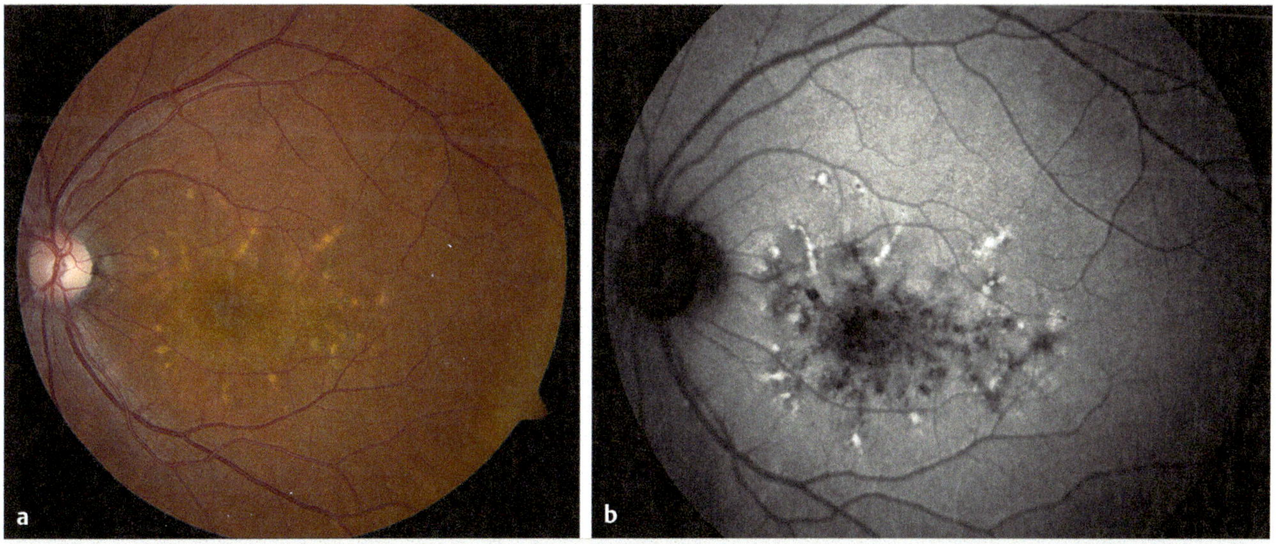

Fig. 19.21 (**a**) Fundus photograph and (**b**) autofluorescence imaging of the left eye of patient with fundus flavimaculatus reveal some of the flecks to be hyperautofluorescent and others atrophic.

including nyctalopia, diffuse loss of pigment from the RPE, narrowing of the retinal vessels, and abnormalities of both the scotopic and photopic ERG.[118]

Group 4: Flecks Not Associated with Macular Atrophy

Patients may have paracentral and central flecks associated with minimal biomicroscopic and angiographic evidence of atrophy of the RPE between the flecks. Visual acuity may be normal if flecks do not involve the center of the fovea. Most patients with a large fleck in the foveola have subnormal acuity. Fluorescein angiography shows a dark choroid, obstruction of the background fluorescence by the flecks with minimal hyperfluorescence in a small area immediately surrounding the flecks. In the absence of information concerning other family members, and in eyes showing borderline evidence of a dark choroid, it may be difficult or impossible to differentiate some patients in group 4 from patients with fundus flavimaculatus type of pattern dystrophy.[127,128]

Whereas the fundus findings and the degree and rate of visual loss are usually symmetric, the atrophic changes and visual loss in some patients may be more advanced in one eye.

There is considerable evidence that Stargardt's disease and fundus flavimaculatus are the same disease and that the latter probably represents a more advanced and widespread stage of lipofuscin storage and RPE damage. The age of onset of visual loss and the severity of visual loss are generally greater in patients with widespread flecks (fundus flavimaculatus).[129] The electro-oculographic and electroretinographic findings are more likely to be subnormal in patients who either have or are destined to develop widespread flecks in the fundi and other signs and symptoms of a more widespread tapetoretinal dystrophy.[120,129,130] The electrophysiologic studies therefore are probably of some prognostic value, particularly in younger patients who have only minimal flecks.

Histopathologic examination reveals that the RPE cells posterior to the equator are enlarged and densely packed with an intensely PAS-positive substance with ultrastructural, autofluorescent, and histochemical properties consistent with an abnormal form of lipofuscin.[124,131,132,133,134,135,136] The greatest concentration of this lipopigment is located in the posterior fundus. Scanning electron microscopy has shown evidence that focal areas of marked hypertrophy of RPE cells, as well as aggregates of cells containing lipofuscin, are responsible for the nonfluorescent yellow flecks.[133,134]

In most patients who show clinical evidence of lipofuscin storage, fundus flavimaculatus is inherited as an autosomal recessive trait. A similar phenotype, however, occurs in some families showing evidence of dominant inheritance.[133,137] In families with dominantly inherited fundus flavimaculatus, gene mutations have been mapped to the short arm of chromosome 1 and to chromosome 13q34.[128,138] Linkage to chromosome 6q has also been established.[127] The patients in this latter family did not show angiographic evidence of lipofuscin storage. The author believes that patients with a fundus flavimaculatus–like distribution of flecks, absence of a dark choroid, autosomal dominant inheritance, and generally a more favorable visual prognosis are more appropriately classified as having pattern dystrophy rather than Stargardt's disease.

Pattern dystrophy is not the only disorder that may simulate fundus flavimaculatus. A similar pattern of flecks may develop within weeks or several months in one or both eyes of patients with idiopathic uveal effusion, bilateral diffuse uveal melanocytic proliferation, renal or other organ transplantation and chronic central serous chorioretinopathy, collagen vascular disease, and vitreoretinal (large cell) lymphoma.

19.3 Malattia Leventinese (Doyne's Honeycomb Macular Dystrophy)

A family with dominantly inherited radial pattern of innumerable, small to large basal laminar drusen was initially reported from the Leventine valley in Switzerland.[139,140,141,142,143] Doyne described the same condition as dominantly inherited honeycomb retinal dystrophy in 1899.[144] The drusen are nodular, varying in size from small to large in the macular region, and are typically arranged in a radial pattern in the temporal macula (▶ Fig. 19.22). With time, the overlying RPE may show atrophy and/or fibrous metaplasia. The visual acuity is often excellent in spite of the fibrous metaplastic changes. The radial drusen demonstrate early discrete fluorescence similar to that of basal laminar drusen (▶ Fig. 19.23). The nodular drusen are hyperautofluorescent (▶ Fig. 19.24). On indocyanine green angiography, the lesions mask the fluorescence early and the central drusen stain late with hypofluorescence of its edge.[145] High-resolution OCT shows conical or globular deposits between the RPE and the Bruch's membrane (▶ Fig. 19.25) and in late stages secondary disruption of the outer nuclear layer.[146,147] Choroidal neovascularization is known to occur and responds to anti–vascular endothelial growth factor antibodies

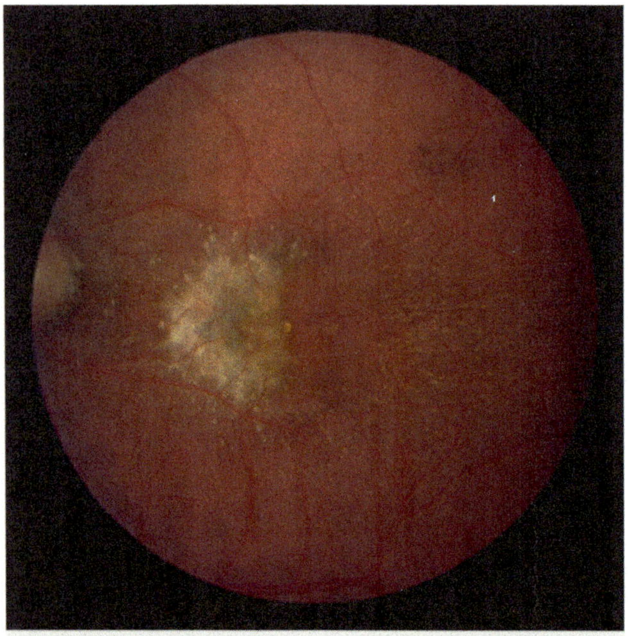

Fig. 19.22 Nodular drusen with central fibrosis in a 31-year-old man. The temporal drusen are radial in arrangement. From Agarwal, A. Gass' Atlas of Macular Diseases, 5th edition. Elsevier, Saunders; 2012.

and photodynamic therapy.[148,149] Even though the typical appearance is of nodular drusen that fill the macula and often the area nasal to the disc (▶ Fig. 19.26), phenotypic heterogeneity is seen in some families, showing less extensive drusen or predominant fibrous change rather than drusen (▶ Fig. 19.27).[144,150] Mutation in the *EFEMP1* gene (Arg345Trp) is responsible for the condition.[151,152,153] There has been a family diagnosed clinically as malattia leventinese, without the Arg345Trp mutation, suggesting other gene defects may also cause this phenotype.[150] Light and electron microscopic findings in one patient demonstrated evidence that these drusen are caused by thickening of the basement membrane of the RPE.[154]

Pearls

- Malattia leventinese and Doyne's honeycomb macular dystrophy constitute the same disorder. Although more common with Swiss ancestry, the disorder has been found worldwide. Even though large nodular drusen found extensively throughout the macula and nasal to the disc are the typical appearance, some patients may have a mild, smaller phenotype.

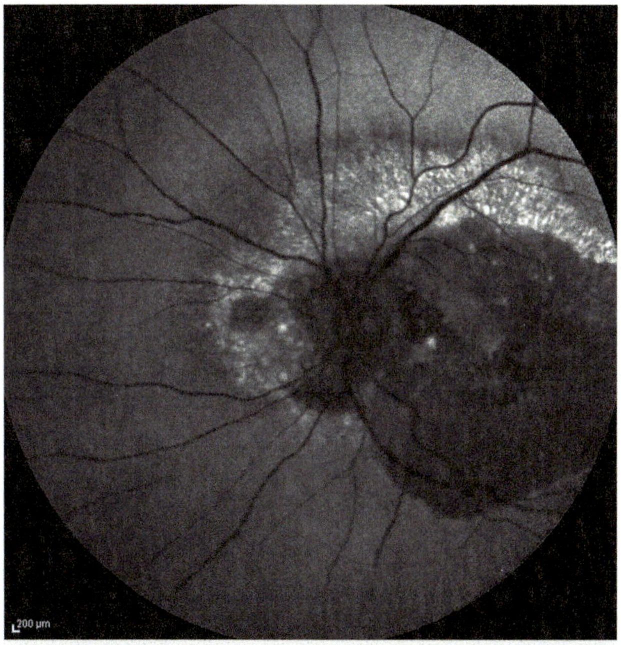

Fig. 19.24 The nodular drusen are hyperautofluorescent.

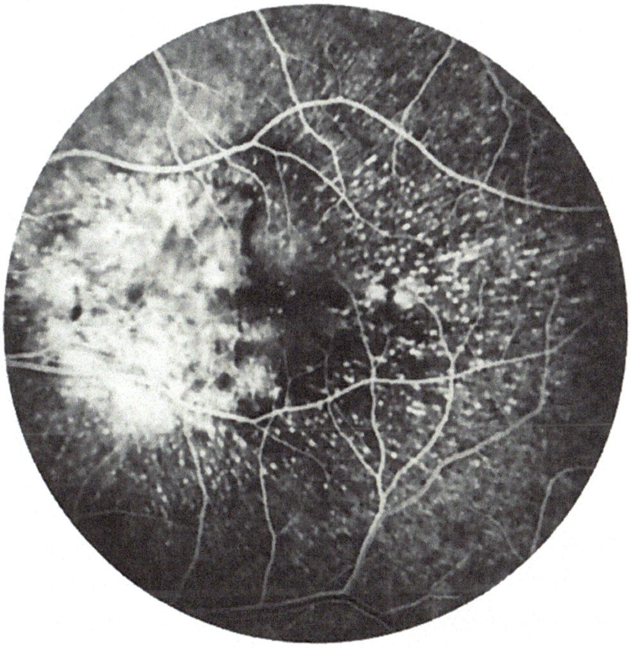

Fig. 19.23 Fluorescein angiogram reveals the radial arrangement of the drusen more distinctly. From Agarwal, A. Gass' Atlas of Macular Diseases, 5th edition. Elsevier, Saunders; 2012.

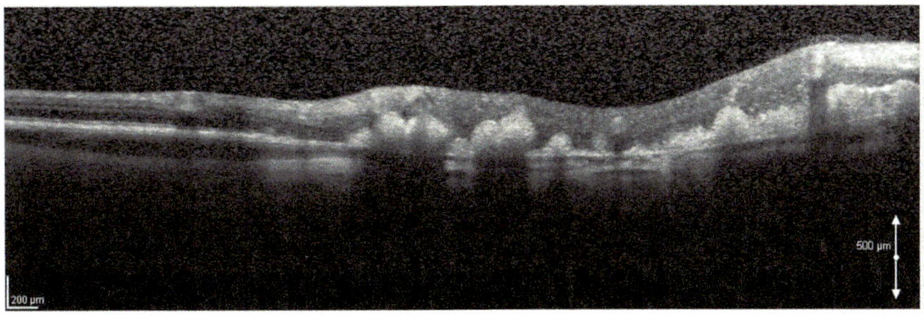

Fig. 19.25 The drusen show nodular thickening at the level of the RPE on OCT. From Agarwal, A. Gass' Atlas of Macular Diseases, 5th edition. Elsevier, Saunders; 2012.

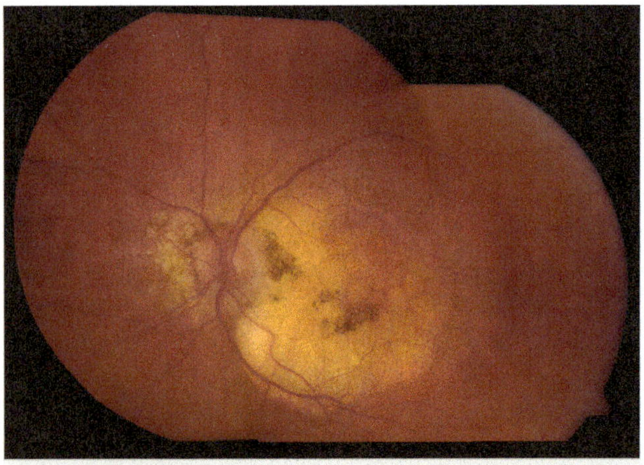

Fig. 19.26 Nodular drusen also seen nasal to disc in both eyes of a 64-year-old woman. From Agarwal, A. Gass' Atlas of Macular Diseases, 5th edition. Elsevier, Saunders; 2012.

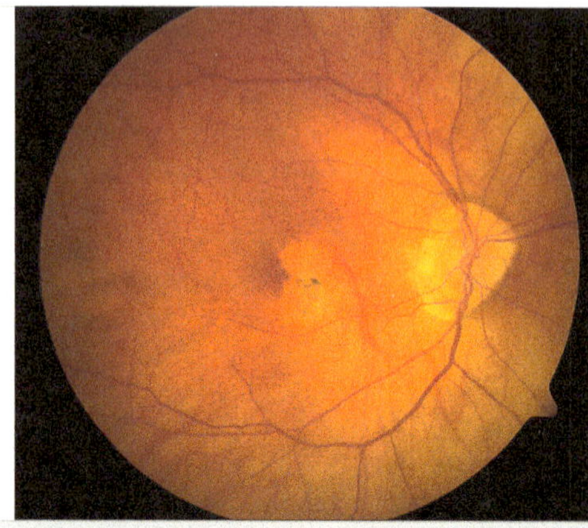

Fig. 19.27 The older sister of the patient in ▶ Fig. 19.26 had a much milder phenotype even though both had the same genetic mutation in the *EFEMP1* gene.

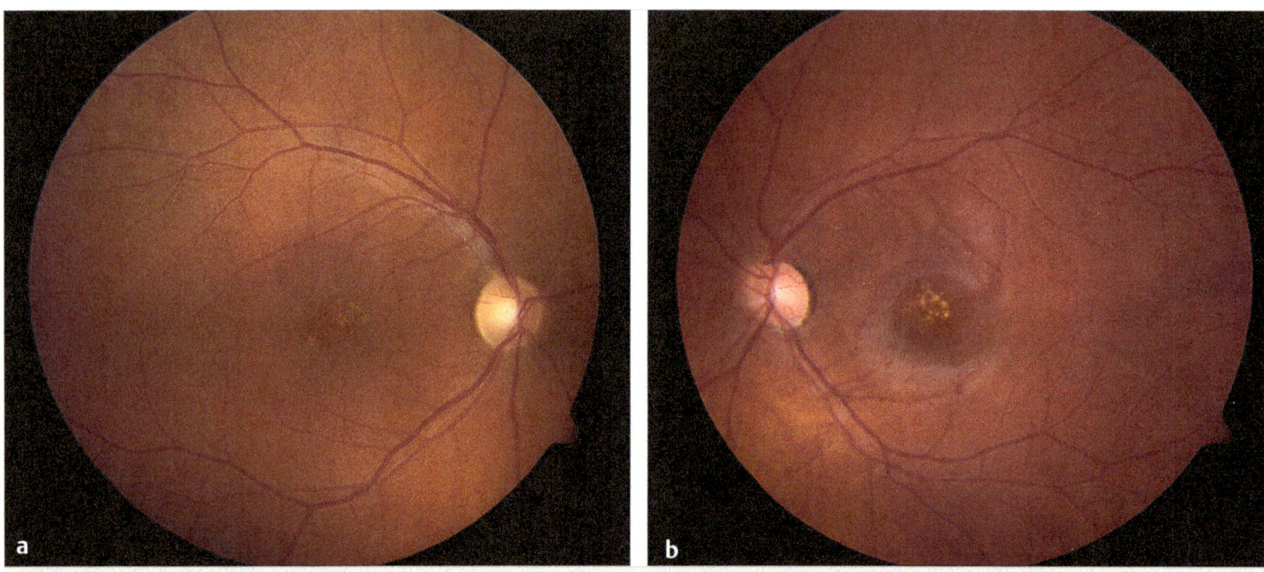

Fig. 19.28 (a) Asymptomatic 39 year old mother and (b) 15 year old daughter with drusen limited to the central fovea.

19.4 North Carolina Macular Dystrophy

North Carolina macular dystrophy (NCMD) is an autosomal dominantly inherited disorder that has its onset in infancy. Two main phenotypes make up the disorder: one characterized by small drusen-like changes arranged compactly in the central macula (▶ Fig. 19.28a,b; mother and daughter) and the second an excavated "staphyloma-like" lesion in the macula (▶ Fig. 19.29). Patients with the drusen-like phenotype are mostly asymptomatic, and the lesion tends to remain unchanged throughout life unless secondary choroidal neovascularization develops. The lesions are hyperfluorescent early on fluorescein angiography and fade late. They are not visible on OCT, and the overlying photoreceptors and inner retina are normal. The staphyloma-like lesion appears as a yellow-white excavation in the central macula with thinning and outward bowing of the retina, RPE, choroid, and sclera. Again, these lesions seem to remain stable and show little progressive thinning or reduction in visual acuity. They are hypofluorescent on fluorescein angiography and on autofluorescence imaging (▶ Fig. 19.30) due to absence of choriocapillaris. On OCT, the retina, RPE, and choroid are thinned out. Some eyes show intrachoroidal cavitations (ICCs) similar to those seen in high myopia (▶ Fig. 19.31).[155,156] It is likely the phenotypes are developmental in origin for several reasons. First, the macular lesions are seen as early as 2 months of age. Second, the remarkably good vision despite the macular appearance suggests eccentric fixation that likely develops early in life. A review of one large family revealed that all patients followed up for 30 years maintained stable visual acuity (excluding those that developed choroidal neovascularization). Furthermore, the staphyloma-like appearance is similar to congenital lesions such as

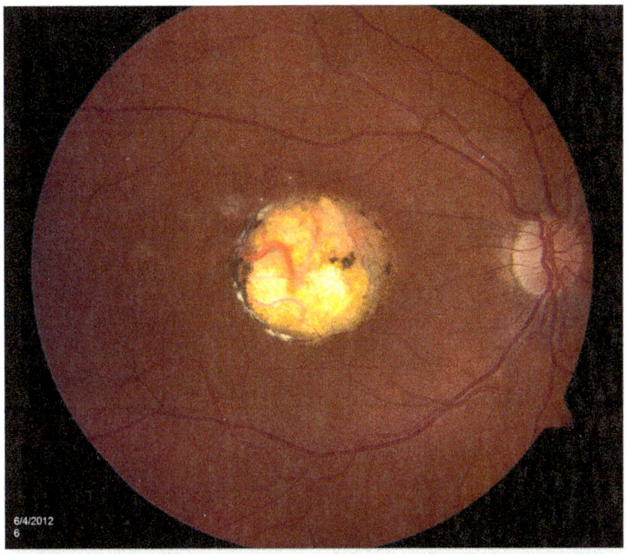

Fig. 19.29 Right fundus of a 19-year-old girl with "staphyloma-like" appearance showing yellow excavated lesion.

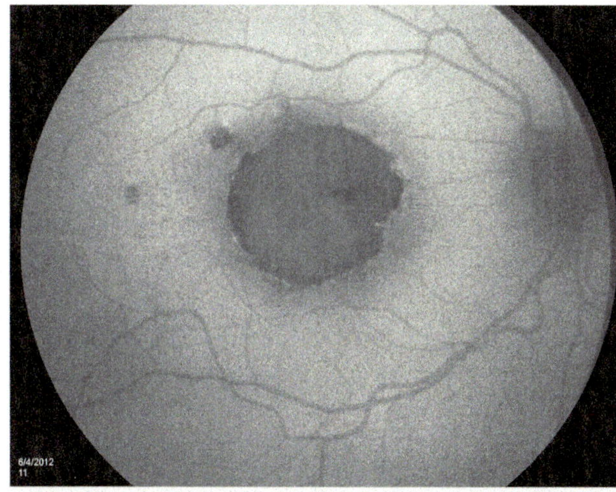

Fig. 19.30 The lesion is hypoautofluorescent due to thinning and loss of RPE.

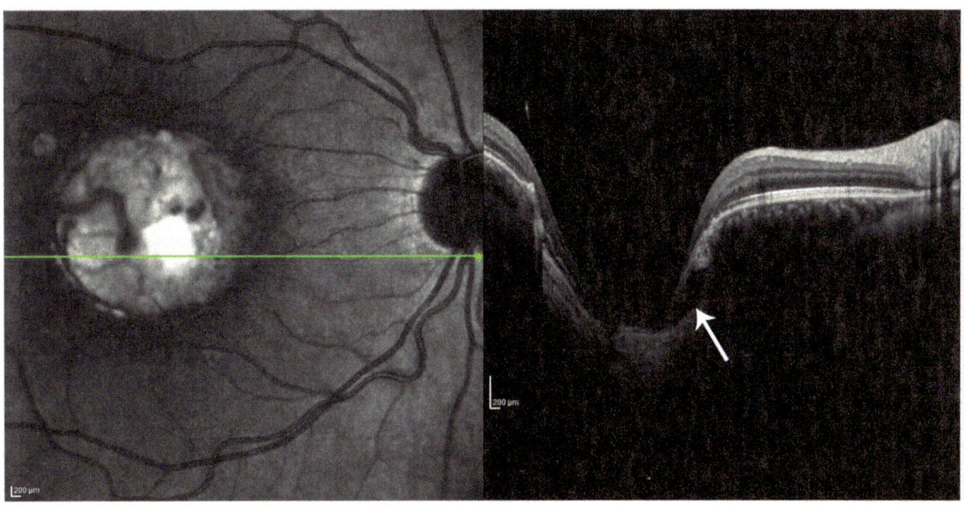

Fig. 19.31 OCT shows posterior bowing of the retina, choroid, and sclera with thinning and intra-choroidal cavitation (arrow). The left eye had a similar appearance and so did her mother.

toxoplasmosis. In the developing human eye, the RPE begins to differentiate at day 30. At 6 weeks, the choroid and Bruch's membrane start to form, and at 12 weeks, the sclera forms in the posterior pole. The development and maintenance of the RPE, choroid, and sclera are highly interdependent.[157,158] In animal models, the absence of normal RPE leads to a failure of induction of the choroid and sclera. Macular RPE is likely the primary developmental abnormality in all grades of NCMD. The staphyloma-like lesion is a more severe phenotype likely owing to an earlier in utero developmental abnormality of the posterior pole, affecting the nearby retina, choroid, and sclera. The ICCs likely also result during this process. The secondary vitreous is derived from the inner retina beginning at gestational week 9, near the ocular wall. This occurs around the same time as the RPE, choroid, and sclera develop. The inner retina is abnormal, and secondary vitreous may develop erroneously and ICCs may represent sequestered vitreous.[156]

The NCMD gene (*MCDR1*) is mapped to the 6q14-q16.2 region and the disease-causing gene was very recently identified as the PRDM13 gene. Dysregulation of the PRDM13 protein which is involved in macular development seems to explain the developmental phenotype of NCMD.[59] Although initially described in inhabitants of North Carolina with their descendancy traced to three Irish brothers, the phenotype has been found in Caucasian patients outside North Carolina and the United States,[160,161,162] in African American,[163] Belize,[164] and Korean patients.[165]

19.5 North Carolina–like Dominant Macular Dystrophy

Three families with an autosomal dominant inheritance and lesions resembling those of NCMD have been recently described; however, each of their gene defect localizes to chromosome 5, region p13.1-p15.33 (MCDR3), chromosome 14q with additional sensorineural deafness, or 6q14 between loci for cone-rod dystrophy 7 (CORD7) and NCMD (MCDR1).[166,167]

19.6 Sorsby's Fundus Dystrophy

Sorsby and associates described five families with autosomal dominant inheritance of drusen, choroidal neovascularization, and subretinal hemorrhages beginning in the fifth decade of life, with multiple recurrences and eventual disciform scarring resembling age-related macular degeneration. Progressive loss of peripheral and night vision associated with choroidal and RPE changes that resemble reticular pseudodrusen occurs over time. A thick deposit of lipid-laden material within the Bruch's membrane and under the RPE causes the yellow drusen/pseudodrusen-like change. Overlying RPE and photoreceptors and the underlying choriocapillaris degenerate over time, leaving areas of geographic atrophy. The condition has high penetrance and is characterized by recurrent choroidal neovascularization resulting in significant loss of vision. Those with extensive peripheral changes will have reduced electroretinographic function. Some patients are known to have reduced Arden ratio on EOG testing. Overall, the fundus appearance and manifestations resemble an earlier onset, widespread and progressive phenotype of severe age-related exudative macular degeneration (▶ Fig. 19.32).

The genetic defect is in the *TIMP 3* gene on chromosome 22q12.3 gene that normally inhibits matrix metalloproteases and other proteins that are enzymes which degrade and catalyze shedding of ectodomains of cell surface proteins. *TIMP 3* is secreted by the RPE and deposited into the Bruch's membrane and regulates extracellular matrix. *TIMP3* also has antiangiogenic and proapoptotic activity and regulates inflammation. Most mutations occur at the exon 5 site of the C-terminal domain of the protein. Most recently, a novel mutation Ser38Cys substitution was found in two unrelated patients in exon 1 of the N-terminal domain.[168]

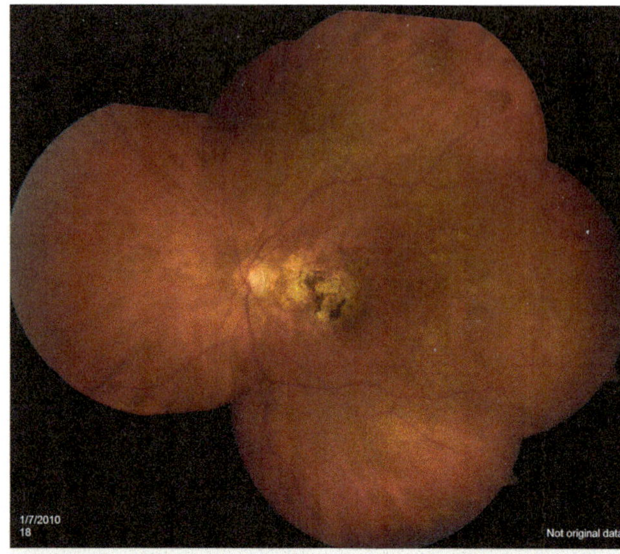

Fig. 19.32 Posterior pole and wide-field photograph of the left eye of a 54-year-old woman with extensive macular scarring from recurrent choroidal neovascularization. Yellow lesions at the level of the RPE/Bruch's membrane gradually increased and extended anterior to the equator. She was positive for a Ser38Cys mutation at exon 1 of the N-terminal end of the *TIMP3* gene.

Pearls

- Early recognition of the condition in patients who present with signs of exudative age-related macular degeneration in their 40 s and have a strong family history helps in regular monitoring and prompt institution of antiangiogenic therapy at the onset of choroidal neovascularization.

19.7 Autosomal Dominant Central Areolar Chorioretinal Dystrophy

This dystrophy is characterized by the development of fine, mottled depigmentation in the macular region, usually in late childhood or early adulthood in the absence of any symptoms. Visual acuity, visual fields, ERG, and dark adaptation are normal early in the course. Multifocal ERG shows abnormal central function and late stages may sometimes show more widespread cone and rod dysfunction.[169,170] The EOG may be subnormal. Fluorescein angiography is helpful in detecting the earliest pigmentary changes of the macular region that may eventually have a bull's-eye configuration. Associated is the gradual development of symmetric, sharply outlined, bull's-eye oval or round areas of geographic atrophy of the RPE in the macula in the absence of any flecks or drusen. There is slow, mild deterioration of visual acuity during the fourth and fifth decades of life. Families with earlier age of onset of visual acuity changes are known.[171] The area of geographic depigmentation of the RPE enlarges concentrically but usually does not exceed 3 to 4 disc diameters. In some patients, geographic atrophy of the RPE in the peripapillary region accompanies the macular changes. As the patient lives beyond the fifth decade, the reddish orange color of the large choroidal vessels within the area of RPE atrophy is replaced by a yellow-white color. Serous and hemorrhagic disciform detachment occurs rarely, if at all. Visual acuity in the range of 20/100 to 20/200 may be retained even during the seventh and eighth decades of life. The optic disc, retinal vessels, and RPE outside the macular area are usually normal in appearance.

Initially, a relative (but later an absolute) central scotoma corresponding to the area of RPE atrophy can be demonstrated. Peripheral fields are normal. Fluorescein angiography demonstrates varying degrees of loss of the choriocapillaris within the area of RPE atrophy that correlates well with the degree of loss of visual function.[12] There usually is minimal evidence of atrophy of the large choroidal vessels throughout the course of the disease.

Dominantly inherited central areolar chorioretinal dystrophy occurs infrequently and has been confused in the literature with a variety of other more prevalent diseases associated with geographic atrophy of the RPE or other disorders that cause a bull's-eye pattern of pigment epithelial atrophy such as benign concentric annular macular dystrophy, and chloroquine and hydroxychloroquine toxicity. Examination of two or more generations of patients is necessary to make the diagnosis.

Mutation in the peripherin/*RDS* gene on chromosome 6 is the most common cause of autosomal dominant central areolar choroidal dystrophy, although the disease is genetically heterogeneous.[100,172,173,174] Five different mutations have so far been found, the commonest being arginine 195 leucine mutation.[173,175]

19.8 Sveinsson's Helicoid Peripapillary Chorioretinal Dystrophy ("Choroiditis Areata")

This is a rare, distinct bilateral autosomal dominant fundus disorder characterized by sharply demarcated, wing- or propeller-like atrophic chorioretinal lesions radiating away from the optic disc, in the absence of evidence of inflammation (serpiginous choroiditis), angioid streaks, myopic degeneration, and paravenous retinochoroidal atrophy.[176,177,178,179,180,181] Mild astigmatism is common.[177,181] It was first described in Iceland in 1939 by Sveinsson,[180] who named it "choroiditis areata"; Franceschetti in 1962[178] renamed it helicoid peripapillary chorioretinal degeneration due to the lack of inflammation, and Sveinsson redescribed four affected successive generations in 1979 demonstrating dominant inheritance and progression with age.[177,181] The lesions can be seen at birth and progress slowly with late macular involvement. The topography of the lesions suggests that they may result from tearing of Bruch's membrane and RPE.[177] All cases so far have been described from Iceland, and the ones seen in Canada, Denmark, France, Germany, Norway, Sweden, Switzerland, the United Kingdom, and the United States all have ancestors in Iceland who are members of the extended Icelandic pedigree. In order to prevent ambiguity associated with the term helicoid peripapillary chorioretinal dystrophy, the name Sveinsson's chorioretinal atrophy has been proposed.[182] The defect has been mapped to the 11p15 region by linkage analysis.[182,183]

19.9 Occult Macular Dystrophy

The condition originally described by Miyake et al[184] with autosomal dominant inheritance presents with progressive central visual loss, normal fundus and fluorescein angiographic appearance (▶ Fig. 19.33), progressive color vision defect, and normal full-field ERG but an abnormal pattern and multifocal ERG.[185,186,187] Since the original reports, several sporadic cases have been reported, suggesting the disorder may have multiple etiologies or variable penetrance.[188] The age of presentation varies from 11 to 45 years, although most present after age 25 years. Patients note gradual difficulty with central vision and ability to discern colors. Often they are unable to distinguish traffic light colors and are known to run through red lights. Fundus examination and fluorescein angiography are normal. However, OCT shows granularity/fragmentation of the cone outer segment line and variable decreased signal intensity of the outer nuclear layer, ellipsoid, and cone outer segment tips (COST) lines (▶ Fig. 19.34).[189,190,191,192] Full-field ERG is normal but the central hexagons of multifocal ERG show reduced amplitudes. A defect in the *RP1L1* gene has been found in some families of autosomal dominant occult macular dystrophy.[193,194] This gene is also known to be associated with some types of retinitis pigmentosa. Even though the condition is most often reported in Japan, families and sporadic cases have been found in Italy, rest of Europe, the United States, Korea, and other Southeast Asian countries.

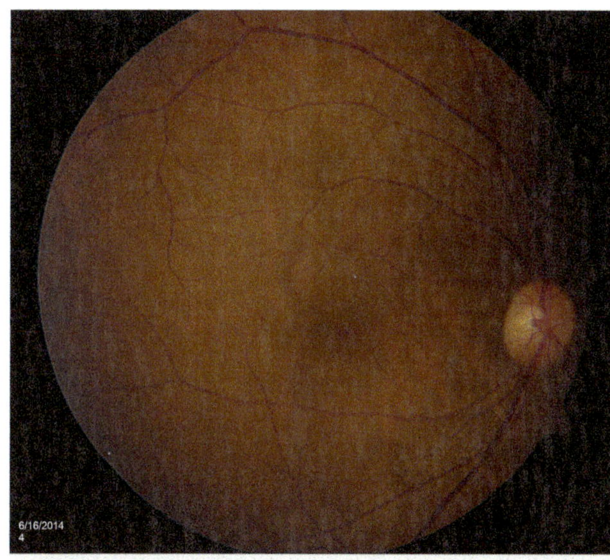

Fig. 19.33 Normal fundus appearance of a 42-year-old Korean woman with difficulty in discerning traffic lights and reduction of vision to 20/70.

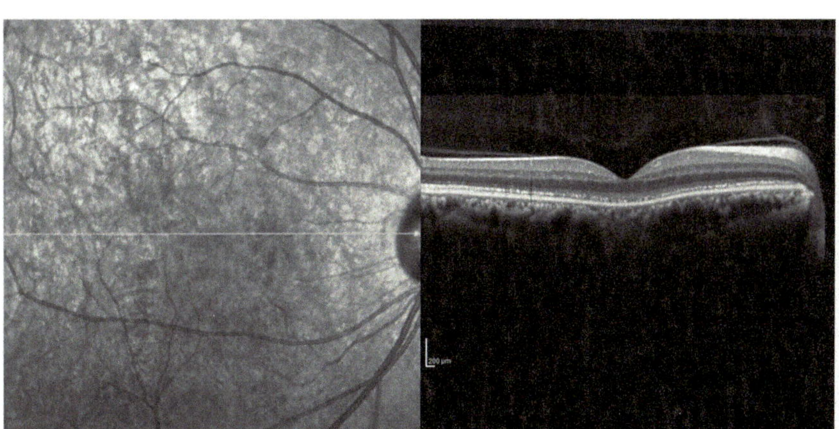

Fig. 19.34 Central cone photoreceptors were reduced in number and the ellipsoid and COST line show fragmentation.

19.10 Dominant Cystoid Macular Edema

Deutman et al in 1976 first described in three pedigrees signs of typical cystoid macular edema due to leaking perimacular capillaries. Other features were diffuse retinal capillary leakage all over the posterior pole, whitish punctate deposits in the vitreous, a normal ERG, a subnormal EOG, and moderate to high hyperopia. In more advanced stages, the macula developed a central zone of "beaten bronze" atrophy and strabismus occurred frequently.[195] Subsequently, Fishman et al confirmed similar findings in four patients of Greek ancestry.[196]

The condition begins in early childhood with accumulation of fluid-filled cystic spaces in the macula usually in patients younger than 20 years (stage 1). In stage 2, mild to moderate chorioretinal atrophy begins and the cystic spaces reduce in size and number. By stage 3, most patients are in their 50 s and show marked macular atrophy and hyperpigmented deposits.[197] The genetic locus has been mapped to 7p15.3 but the gene is yet to be found.

Diagnosis is based on examining members of multiple generations within a family. The condition can easily be mistaken for central areolar choroidal dystrophy, which is also autosomal dominant in inheritance pattern, Stargardt's disease without flecks, cone dystrophy, and advanced toxic maculopathy for hydroxychloroquine and chloroquine. A family history suggestive of dominant inheritance and finding cystoid spaces in the younger members of the family are necessary in making the diagnosis.[198]

References

[1] Weingeist TA, Kobrin JL, Watzke RC. Histopathology of Best's macular dystrophy. Arch Ophthalmol. 1982; 100(7):1108–1114

[2] Pece A, Gaspari G, Avanza P, Magni R, Brancato R. Best's multiple vitelliform degeneration. Int Ophthalmol. 1992; 16(6):459–464

[3] Noble KG, Scher BM, Carr RE. Polymorphous presentations in vitelliform macular dystrophy: subretinal neovascularisation and central choroidal atrophy. Br J Ophthalmol. 1978; 62(8):561–570

[4] Morse PH, MacLean AL. Fluorescein fundus studies in hereditary vitelliruptive macular degeneration. Am J Ophthalmol. 1968; 66(3):485–494

[5] Mohler CW, Fine SL. Long-term evaluation of patients with Best's vitelliform dystrophy. Ophthalmology. 1981; 88(7):688–692

[6] Miller SA, Bresnick GH, Chandra SR. Choroidal neovascular membrane in Best's vitelliform macular dystrophy. Am J Ophthalmol. 1976; 82(2):252–255

[7] Miller SA. Fluorescence in Best's vitelliform dystrophy, lipofuscin, and fundus flavimaculatus. Br J Ophthalmol. 1978; 62(4):256–260

[8] Massof RW, Fleischman JA, Fine SL, Yoder F. Flicker fusion thresholds in Best macular dystrophy. Arch Ophthalmol. 1977; 95(6):991–994

[9] Maloney WF, Robertson DM, Duboff SM. Hereditary vitelliform macular degeneration: variable fundus findings within a single pedigree. Arch Ophthalmol. 1977; 95(6):979–983

[10] Krill AE, Morse PA, Potts AM, Klien BA. Hereditary vitelliruptive macular degeneration. Am J Ophthalmol. 1966; 61(6):1405–1415

[11] Kraushar MF, Margolis S, Morse PH, Nugent ME. Pseudohypopyon in Best's vitelliform macular dystrophy. Am J Ophthalmol. 1982; 94(1):30–37

[12] Gass JDM. Stereoscopic Atlas of Macular Diseases—Diagnosis and Treatment. 2nd ed. St. Louis, MO: CV Mosby; 1977

[13] Frangieh GT, Green WR, Fine SL. A histopathologic study of Best's macular dystrophy. Arch Ophthalmol. 1982; 100(7):1115–1121

[14] François J, De Rouck A, Fernandez-Sasso D. Electro-oculography in macular degeneration [in French]. Bull Soc Belge Ophtalmol. 1966; 143:547–552

[15] Fishman GA, Ward LM, Rusin MM. Vitreous fluorophotometry in patients with Best's macular dystrophy. Retina. 1990; 10(2):102–104

[16] Fishman GA, Baca W, Alexander KR, Derlacki DJ, Glenn AM, Viana M. Visual acuity in patients with best vitelliform macular dystrophy. Ophthalmology. 1993; 100(11):1665–1670

[17] Deutman AF. The Hereditary Dystrophies of the Posterior Pole of the Eye. Assen: Van Gorcum; 1971:198

[18] Curry HF, Jr, Moorman LT. Fluorescein photography of vitelliform macular degeneration. Arch Ophthalmol. 1968; 79(6):705–709

[19] Cross HE, Bard L. Electro-oculography in Best's macular dystrophy. Am J Ophthalmol. 1974; 77(1):46–50

[20] Cavender JC. Best's macular dystrophy. Arch Ophthalmol. 1982; 100(7):1067

[21] Birndorf LA, Dawson WW. A normal electrooculogram in a patient with a typical vitelliform macular lesion. Invest Ophthalmol. 1973; 12(11):830–833

[22] Best F. Über eine hereditäre Maculaaffektion; Beitrag zur Vererbungslehre. Z Augenheilkd. 1905; 13:199–212

[23] Berkley WL, Bussey FR. Heredodegeneration of the macula. Am J Ophthalmol. 1949; 32(3):361–365

[24] Benson WE, Kolker AE, Enoch JM, Van Loo JA, Jr, Honda Y. Best's vitelliform macular dystrophy. Am J Ophthalmol. 1975; 79(1):59–66

[25] Barricks ME. Vitelliform lesions developing in normal fundi. Am J Ophthalmol. 1977; 83(3):324–327

[26] Bard LA, Cross HE. Genetic counseling of families with Best macular dystrophy. Trans Sect Ophthalmol Am Acad Ophthalmol Otolaryngol. 1975; 79(6): OP865–OP873

[27] Anderson SR, ed. Ocular pathology in hereditary (vitelliform) macular degeneration. In: European Ophthalmic Pathology Society meeting; May 28, 1970; Ghent, Belgium

[28] Petrukhin K, Koisti MJ, Bakall B, et al. Identification of the gene responsible for Best macular dystrophy. Nat Genet. 1998; 19(3):241–247

[29] Boon CJ, Klevering BJ, Leroy BP, Hoyng CB, Keunen JE, den Hollander AI. The spectrum of ocular phenotypes caused by mutations in the BEST1 gene. Prog Retin Eye Res. 2009; 28(3):187–205

[30] Yu K, Qu Z, Cui Y, Hartzell HC. Chloride channel activity of bestrophin mutants associated with mild or late-onset macular degeneration. Invest Ophthalmol Vis Sci. 2007; 48(10):4694–4705

[31] Boon CJ, Klevering BJ, den Hollander AI, et al. Clinical and genetic heterogeneity in multifocal vitelliform dystrophy. Arch Ophthalmol. 2007; 125 (8):1100–1106

[32] Bakall B, Marknell T, Ingvast S, et al. The mutation spectrum of the bestrophin protein—functional implications. Hum Genet. 1999; 104(5):383–389

[33] Hartzell HC, Qu Z, Yu K, Xiao Q, Chien LT. Molecular physiology of bestrophins: multifunctional membrane proteins linked to best disease and other retinopathies. Physiol Rev. 2008; 88(2):639–672

[34] Hartzell C, Qu Z, Putzier I, Artinian L, Chien LT, Cui Y. Looking chloride channels straight in the eye: bestrophins, lipofuscinosis, and retinal degeneration. Physiology (Bethesda). 2005; 20:292–302

[35] Spaide RF, Noble K, Morgan A, Freund KB. Vitelliform macular dystrophy. Ophthalmology. 2006; 113(8):1392–1400

[36] Schachat AP, de la Cruz Z, Green WR, Patz A. Macular hole and retinal detachment in Best's disease. Retina. 1985; 5(1):22–25

[37] Miller SA. Multifocal Best's vitelliform dystrophy. Arch Ophthalmol. 1977; 95(6):984–990

[38] Thu T, Chan WM, Dung D, Huan P, Lam DS. A large macular hole in a young patient with Best's disease. Clin Experiment Ophthalmol. 2003; 31(6):539–540

[39] Bakall B, Radu RA, Stanton JB, et al. Enhanced accumulation of A2E in individuals homozygous or heterozygous for mutations in BEST1 (VMD2). Exp Eye Res. 2007; 85(1):34–43

[40] Spaide R. Autofluorescence from the outer retina and subretinal space: hypothesis and review. Retina. 2008; 28(1):5–35

[41] Forsman K, Graff C, Nordström S, et al. The gene for Best's macular dystrophy is located at 11q13 in a Swedish family. Clin Genet. 1992; 42(3):156–159

[42] Yoder FE, Cross HE, Chase GA, et al. Linkage studies of Best's macular dystrophy. Clin Genet. 1988; 34(1):26–30

[43] Kaufman SJ, Goldberg MF, Orth DH, Fishman GA, Tessler H, Mizuno K. Autosomal dominant vitreoretinochoroidopathy. Arch Ophthalmol. 1982; 100 (2):272–278

[44] Chen CJ, Goldberg MF. Progressive cone dysfunction and geographic atrophy of the macula in late stage autosomal dominant vitreoretinochoroidopathy (ADVIRC). Ophthalmic Genet. 2016; 37(1):81–85

[45] Yardley J, Leroy BP, Hart-Holden N, et al. Mutations of VMD2 splicing regulators cause nanophthalmos and autosomal dominant vitreoretinochoroidopathy (ADVIRC). Invest Ophthalmol Vis Sci. 2004; 45(10):3683–3689

[46] Burgess R, MacLaren RE, Davidson AE, et al. ADVIRC is caused by distinct mutations in BEST1 that alter pre-mRNA splicing. J Med Genet. 2009; 46 (9):620–625

[47] Reddy MA, Francis PJ, Berry V, et al. A clinical and molecular genetic study of a rare dominantly inherited syndrome (MRCS) comprising of microcornea, rod-cone dystrophy, cataract, and posterior staphyloma. Br J Ophthalmol. 2003; 87(2):197–202

[48] Burgess R, Millar ID, Leroy BP, et al. Biallelic mutation of BEST1 causes a distinct retinopathy in humans. Am J Hum Genet. 2008; 82(1):19–31

[49] Gerth C, Zawadzki RJ, Werner JS, Héon E. Detailed analysis of retinal function and morphology in a patient with autosomal recessive bestrophinopathy (ARB). Doc Ophthalmol. 2009; 118(3):239–246

[50] Fletcher RC, Jampol LM, Rimm W. An unusual presentation of Best's disease. Br J Ophthalmol. 1977, 61(11).719–721

[51] Wiznia RA, Perina B, Noble KG. Vitelliform macular dystrophy of late onset. Br J Ophthalmol. 1981; 65(12):866–868

[52] Watzke RC, Folk JC, Lang RM. Pattern dystrophy of the retinal pigment epithelium. Ophthalmology. 1982; 89(12):1400–1406

[53] Vine AK, Schatz H. Adult-onset foveomacular pigment epithelial dystrophy. Am J Ophthalmol. 1980; 89(5):680–691

[54] Slezak H, Hommer K. Fundus pulverulentus [in German]. Albrecht Von Graefes Arch Klin Exp Ophthalmol. 1969; 178(2):176–182

[55] Skalka HW. Vitelliform macular lesions. Br J Ophthalmol. 1981; 65(3):180–183

[56] Sjögren H. Dystrophia reticularis laminae pigmentosae retinae, an earlier not described hereditary eye disease. Acta Ophthalmol (Copenh). 1950; 28 (3):279–295

[57] Singerman LJ, Berkow JW, Patz A. Dominant slowly progressive macular dystrophy. Am J Ophthalmol. 1977; 83(5):680–693

[58] Shiono T, Ishikawa A, Hara S, Tamai M. Pattern dystrophy of the retinal pigment epithelium. Retina. 1990; 10(4):251–254

[59] Sabates R, Pruett RC, Hirose T. Pseudovitelliform macular degeneration. Retina. 1982; 2(4):197–205

[60] Patrinely JR, Lewis RA, Font RL. Foveomacular vitelliform dystrophy, adult type. A clinicopathologic study including electron microscopic observations. Ophthalmology. 1985; 92(12):1712–1718

[61] O'Donnell FE, Schatz H, Reid P, Green WR. Autosomal dominant dystrophy of the retinal pigment epithelium. Arch Ophthalmol. 1979; 97(4):680–683

[62] Mejia JR, Gieser RG. Sporadic butterfly macular dystrophy. Ann Ophthalmol. 1981; 13(11):1253–1254

[63] Mesker RP, Oosterhuis JA, Delleman JW. A retinal lesion resembling Sjögren's dystrophia reticularis laminae pigmentosae retinae. In: Winkelman JE, Crone RA, eds. Perspectives in Ophthalmology. Vol. II. Amsterdam: Excerpta Medica; 1970: 40–5

[64] Marmor MF. "Vitelliform" lesions in adults. Ann Ophthalmol. 1979; 11 (11):1705–1712

[65] Marmor MF, Byers B. Pattern dystrophy of the pigment epithelium. Am J Ophthalmol. 1977; 84(1):32–44

[66] Kingham JD, Fenzl RE, Willerson D, Aaberg TM. Reticular dystrophy of the retinal pigment epithelium. A clinical and electrophysiologic study of three generations. Arch Ophthalmol. 1978; 96(7):1177–1184

[67] Kingham JD, Lochen GP. Vitelliform macular degeneration. Am J Ophthalmol.. 1977; 84:526–5–31

[68] Hsieh RC, Fine BS, Lyons JS. Patterned dystrophies of the retinal pigment epithelium. Arch Ophthalmol. 1977; 95(3):429–435

[69] Hodes BL, Feiner LA, Sherman SH, Cunningham D. Progression of pseudovitelliform macular dystrophy. Arch Ophthalmol. 1984; 102(3):381–383

[70] Hittner HM, Ferrell RE, Borda RP, Justice J, Jr. Atypical vitelliform macular dystrophy in a 5-generation family. Br J Ophthalmol. 1984; 68(3):199–207

[71] Gutman I, Walsh JB, Henkind P. Vitelliform macular dystrophy and butterfly-shaped epithelial dystrophy: a continuum? Br J Ophthalmol. 1982; 66 (3):170–173

[72] Gass JD. A clinicopathologic study of a peculiar foveomacular dystrophy. Trans Am Ophthalmol Soc. 1974; 72:139–156

[73] Gass JDM. Dominantly inherited adult form of vitelliform foveomacular dystrophy. In: Fine SL, Owens SL, eds. Management of Retinal Vascular and Macular Disorders. Baltimore, MD: Williams & Wilkins; 1983:182–186

[74] Girard P, Setbon G, Forest A, Coscas G. Macroreticular and butterfly shaped dystrophies of the retinal pigment epithelium [author's transl.; in French]. J Fr Ophtalmol. 1980; 3(2):101–108

[75] Fishman GA, Trimble S, Rabb MF, Fishman M. Pseudovitelliform macular degeneration. Arch Ophthalmol. 1977; 95(1):73–76

[76] Fishman GA, Woolf MB, Goldberg MF, Busse B. Reticular tapeto-retinal dystrophy. As a possible late stage of Sjögren's reticular dystrophy. Br J Ophthalmol. 1976; 60(1):35–40

[77] Deutman AF, Rümke AML. Reticular dystrophy of the retinal pigment epithelium. Dystrophia reticularis laminae pigmentosa retinae of H. Sjogren. Arch Ophthalmol. 1969; 82(1):4–9

[78] Deutman AF, van Blommestein JDA, Henkes HE, Waardenburg PJ, Solleveld-van Driest E. Butterfly-shaped pigment dystrophy of the fovea. Arch Ophthalmol. 1970; 83(5):558–569

[79] Epstein GA, Rabb MF. Adult vitelliform macular degeneration: diagnosis and natural history. Br J Ophthalmol. 1980; 64(10):733–740

[80] de Jong PTVM, Delleman JW. Pigment epithelial pattern dystrophy. Four different manifestations in a family. Arch Ophthalmol. 1982; 100(9):1416–1421

[81] Cortin P, Archer D, Maumenee IH, Feiock K, Speros P. A patterned macular dystrophy with yellow plaques and atrophic changes. Br J Ophthalmol. 1980; 64(2):127–134

[82] Chopdar A. Reticular dystrophy of retina. Br J Ophthalmol. 1976; 60(5):342–344

[83] Burgess D. Subretinal neovascularization in a pattern dystrophy of the retinal pigment epithelium. Retina. 1981; 1(3):151–155

[84] Bloom LH, Swanson DE, Bird AC. Adult vitelliform macular degeneration. Br J Ophthalmol. 1981; 65(11):800–801

[85] Ayazi S, Fagan R. Pattern dystrophy of the pigment epithelium. Retina. 1981; 1(4):287–289

[86] Renner AB, Fiebig BS, Weber BH, et al. Phenotypic variability and long-term follow-up of patients with known and novel PRPH2/RDS gene mutations. Am J Ophthalmol. 2009; 147(3):518–530.e1

[87] Zhuk SA, Edwards AO. Peripherin/RDS and VMD2 mutations in macular dystrophies with adult-onset vitelliform lesion. Mol Vis. 2006; 12:811–815

[88] Wells J, Wroblewski J, Keen J, et al. Mutations in the human retinal degeneration slow (RDS) gene can cause either retinitis pigmentosa or macular dystrophy. Nat Genet. 1993; 3(3):213–218

[89] Nichols BE, Sheffield VC, Vandenburgh K, Drack AV, Kimura AE, Stone EM, et al. Butterfly-shaped pigment dystrophy of the fovea caused by a point mutation in codon 167 of the RDS gene. Nat Genet. 1993; 3(3):202–207

[90] Feist RM, White MF, Jr, Skalka H, Stone EM. Choroidal neovascularization in a patient with adult foveomacular dystrophy and a mutation in the retinal degeneration slow gene (Pro 210 Arg). Am J Ophthalmol. 1994; 118(2):259–260

[91] Gorin MB, Jackson KE, Ferrell RE, et al. A peripherin/retinal degeneration slow mutation (Pro-210-Arg) associated with macular and peripheral retinal degeneration. Ophthalmology. 1995; 102(2):246–255

[92] Weleber RG, Carr RE, Murphey WH, Sheffield VC, Stone EM. Phenotypic variation including retinitis pigmentosa, pattern dystrophy, and fundus flavimaculatus in a single family with a deletion of codon 153 or 154 of the peripherin/RDS gene. Arch Ophthalmol. 1993; 111(11):1531–1542

[93] Gamundi MJ, Hernan I, Muntanyola M, et al. High prevalence of mutations in peripherin/RDS in autosomal dominant macular dystrophies in a Spanish population. Mol Vis. 2007; 13:1031–1037

[94] Testa F, Marini V, Rossi S, et al. A novel mutation in the RDS gene in an Italian family with pattern dystrophy. Br J Ophthalmol. 2005; 89(8):1066–1068

[95] Francis PJ, Schultz DW, Gregory AM, et al. Genetic and phenotypic heterogeneity in pattern dystrophy. Br J Ophthalmol. 2005; 89(9):1115–1119

[96] Yang Z, Li Y, Jiang L, et al. A novel RDS/peripherin gene mutation associated with diverse macular phenotypes. Ophthalmic Genet. 2004; 25(2):133–145

[97] van Lith-Verhoeven JJ, van den Helm B, Deutman AF, et al. A peculiar autosomal dominant macular dystrophy caused by an asparagine deletion at codon 169 in the peripherin/RDS gene. Arch Ophthalmol. 2003; 121(10):1452–1457

[98] Boon CJ, den Hollander AI, Hoyng CB, Cremers FP, Klevering BJ, Keunen JE. The spectrum of retinal dystrophies caused by mutations in the peripherin/RDS gene. Prog Retin Eye Res. 2008; 27(2):213–235

[99] Conley S, Nour M, Fliesler SJ, Naash MI. Late-onset cone photoreceptor degeneration induced by R172W mutation in Rds and partial rescue by gene supplementation. Invest Ophthalmol Vis Sci. 2007; 48(12):5397–5407

[100] Keilhauer CN, Meigen T, Stöhr H, Weber BH. Late-onset central areolar choroidal dystrophy caused by a heterozygous frame-shift mutation affecting codon 307 of the peripherin/RDS gene. Ophthalmic Genet. 2006; 27(4):139–144

[101] Yang Z, Lin W, Moshfeghi DM, et al. A novel mutation in the RDS/Peripherin gene causes adult-onset foveomacular dystrophy. Am J Ophthalmol. 2003; 135(2):213–218

[102] Giuffrè G. Autosomal dominant pattern dystrophy of the retinal pigment epithelium. Intrafamilial variability. Retina. 1988; 8(3):169–173
[103] Aaberg TM, Han DP. Evaluation of phenotypic similarities between Stargardt flavimaculatus and retinal pigment epithelial pattern dystrophies. Trans Am Ophthalmol Soc. 1987; 85:101–119
[104] Lopez PF, Aaberg TM. Phenotypic similarities between Stargardt's flavimaculatus and pattern dystrophies. Aust N Z J Ophthalmol. 1992; 20(3):163–171
[105] McDonnell PJ, Kivlin JD, Maumenee IH, Green WR. Fundus flavimaculatus without maculopathy. A clinicopathologic study. Ophthalmology. 1986; 93 (1):116–119
[106] Agarwal A, Patel P, Adkins T, Gass JD. Spectrum of pattern dystrophy in pseudoxanthoma elasticum. Arch Ophthalmol. 2005; 123(7):923–928
[107] Lim JI, Enger C, Fine SL. Foveomacular dystrophy. Am J Ophthalmol. 1994; 117(1):1–6
[108] Noble KG, Chang S. Adult vitelliform macular degeneration progressing to full-thickness macular hole. Arch Ophthalmol. 1991; 109(3):325
[109] Jaffe GJ, Schatz H. Histopathologic features of adult-onset foveomacular pigment epithelial dystrophy. Arch Ophthalmol. 1988; 106(7):958–960
[110] Finger RP, Charbel Issa P, Ladewig MS, et al. Pseudoxanthoma elasticum: genetics, clinical manifestations and therapeutic approaches. Surv Ophthalmol. 2009; 54(2):272–285
[111] Li Volti S, Avitabile T, Li Volti G, et al. Optic disc drusen, angioid streaks, and mottled fundus in various combinations in a Sicilian family. Graefes Arch Clin Exp Ophthalmol. 2002; 240(9):771–776
[112] McDonald HR, Schatz H, Aaberg TM. Reticular-like pigmentary patterns in pseudoxanthoma elasticum. Ophthalmology. 1988; 95(3):306–311
[113] Leonardy NJ, Harbin RL, Sternberg P, Jr. Pattern dystrophy of the retinal pigment epithelium in a patient with McArdle's disease. Am J Ophthalmol. 1988; 106(6):741–742
[114] Stargardt K. Über familiäre, progressive Degeneration in der Maculagegend des Auges. Albrecht Von Graefes Archiv für Ophthalmologie. 1909; 71 (3):534–550
[115] Franceschetti A. Über tapeto-retinale Degenerationen im Kindesalter Dritter Fortbildungskurs der Deutschen Ophthalmologischen Gesellschaft, Hamburg, 1962. In: Sautter H, ed. Entwicklung und Fortschritt in der Augenheilkunde. Stuttgart: Enke; 1963:107
[116] Franceschetti A. A special form of tapetoretinal degeneration: fundus flavimaculatus. Trans Am Acad Ophthalmol Otolaryngol. 1965; 69(6):1048–1053
[117] Anmarkrud N. Fundus fluorescein angiography in fundus flavimaculatus and Stargardts disease. Acta Ophthalmol (Copenh). 1979; 57(2):172–182
[118] Leys A, Van De Sompel W. Dark choroid in cone-rod dystrophy. Eur J Ophthalmol. 1992; 2(1):39–40
[119] Iijima H, Gohdo T, Hosaka O. Fundus flavimaculatus with severely reduced cone electroretinogram. Jpn J Ophthalmol. 1992; 36(3):249–256
[120] Hadden OB, Gass JDM. Fundus flavimaculatus and Stargardt's disease. Am J Ophthalmol. 1976; 82(4):527–539
[121] Bottoni F, Fatigati G, Carlevaro G, De Molfetta V. Fundus flavimaculatus and subretinal neovascularization. Graefes Arch Clin Exp Ophthalmol. 1992; 230 (5):498–500
[122] Leveille AS, Morse PH, Burch JV. Fundus flavimaculatus and subretinal neovascularization. Ann Ophthalmol. 1982; 14(4):331–334
[123] Klein R, Lewis RA, Meyers SM, Myers FL. Subretinal neovascularization associated with fundus flavimaculatus. Arch Ophthalmol. 1978; 96(11):2054–2057
[124] Klien BA, Krill AE. Fundus flavimaculatus. Clinical, functional and histopathologic observations. Am J Ophthalmol. 1967; 64(1):3–23
[125] Krill AE, Klien BA. Flecked retina syndrome. Arch Ophthalmol. 1965; 74 (4):496–508
[126] Fishman GA, Farbman JS, Alexander KR. Delayed rod dark adaptation in patients with Stargardt's disease. Ophthalmology. 1991; 98(6):957–962
[127] Stone EM, Nichols BE, Kimura AE, Weingeist TA, Drack A, Sheffield VC. Clinical features of a Stargardt-like dominant progressive macular dystrophy with genetic linkage to chromosome 6q. Arch Ophthalmol. 1994; 112 (6):765–772
[128] Zhang K, Bither PP, Park R, Donoso LA, Seidman JG, Seidman CE. A dominant Stargardt's macular dystrophy locus maps to chromosome 13q34. Arch Ophthalmol. 1994; 112(6):759–764
[129] Moloney JBM, Mooney DJ, O'Connor MA. Retinal function in Stargardt's disease and fundus flavimaculatus. Am J Ophthalmol. 1983; 96(1):57–65
[130] Itabashi R, Katsumi O, Mehta MC, Wajima R, Tamai M, Hirose T. Stargardt's disease/fundus flavimaculatus: psychophysical and electrophysiologic results. Graefes Arch Clin Exp Ophthalmol. 1993; 231(10):555–562
[131] Steinmetz RL, Garner A, Maguire JI, Bird AC. Histopathology of incipient fundus flavimaculatus. Ophthalmology. 1991; 98(6):953–956
[132] Newell FW, Krill AE, Farkas TG. Drusen and fundus flavimaculatus: clinical, functional, and histologic characteristics. Trans Am Acad Ophthalmol Otolaryngol. 1972; 76(1):88–100
[133] Lopez PF, Maumenee IH, de la Cruz Z, Green WR. Autosomal-dominant fundus flavimaculatus. Clinicopathologic correlation. Ophthalmology. 1990; 97 (6):798–809
[134] Eagle RC, Jr, Lucier AC, Bernardino VB, Jr, Yanoff M. Retinal pigment epithelial abnormalities in fundus flavimaculatus: a light and electron microscopic study. Ophthalmology. 1980; 87(12):1189–1200
[135] Birnbach CD, Järveläinen M, Possin DE, Milam AH. Histopathology and immunocytochemistry of the neurosensory retina in fundus flavimaculatus. Ophthalmology. 1994; 101(7):1211–1219
[136] Maumenee IH, Maumenee AE, eds. Fundus flavimaculatus; clinical, genetic, and pathologic observations. Blutzirkulation in der Uvea, in der Netzhaut und im Sehnerven (Physiologie und Pathologie). In: 5th Congress of the European Society of Ophthalmology; April 5–9, 1976; Hamburg. Stuttgart: Enke; 1978:80–82
[137] Cibis GW, Morey M, Harris DJ. Dominantly inherited macular dystrophy with flecks (Stargardt). Arch Ophthalmol. 1980; 98(10):1785–1789
[138] Kaplan J, Gerber S, Larget-Piet D, et al. A gene for Stargardt's disease (fundus flavimaculatus) maps to the short arm of chromosome 1. Nat Genet. 1993; 5 (3):308–311
[139] Forni S, Babel J. Clinical and histological study of the disease of Leventina. Disease belonging to the group of hyaline degenerescences of the posterior pole [in French]. Ophthalmologica. 1962; 143:313–322
[140] Gass JDM. Stereoscopic Atlas of Macular Diseases—Diagnosis and Treatment. 3rd ed. St. Louis, MO: CV Mosby; 1987
[141] Haimovici R, Wroblewski J, Piguet B, et al. Symptomatic abnormalities of dark adaptation in patients with EFEMP1 retinal dystrophy (Malattia Leventinese/Doyne honeycomb retinal dystrophy). Eye (Lond). 2002; 16(1):7–15
[142] Miyanaga Y, Mizutani T, Yamanishi R. A pedigree of Doyne's honeycomb macular degeneration. Jpn J Clin Ophthalmol. 1977; 31:431–435
[143] Piguet B, Haimovici R, Bird AC. Dominantly inherited drusen represent more than one disorder: a historical review. Eye (Lond). 1995; 9(Pt 1):34–41
[144] Evans K, Gregory CY, Wijesuriya SD, et al. Assessment of the phenotypic range seen in Doyne honeycomb retinal dystrophy. Arch Ophthalmol. 1997; 115(7):904–910
[145] Souied EH, Leveziel N, Querques G, Darmon J, Coscas G, Soubrane G. Indocyanine green angiography features of Malattia leventinese. Br J Ophthalmol. 2006; 90(3):296–300
[146] Gerth C, Zawadzki RJ, Werner JS, Héon E. Retinal microstructure in patients with EFEMP1 retinal dystrophy evaluated by Fourier domain OCT. Eye (Lond). 2009; 23(2):480–483
[147] Souied EH, Leveziel N, Letien V, Darmon J, Coscas G, Soubrane G. Optical coherent tomography features of malattia leventinese. Am J Ophthalmol. 2006; 141(2):404–407
[148] Pager CK, Sarin LK, Federman JL, et al. Malattia leventinese presenting with subretinal neovascular membrane and hemorrhage. Am J Ophthalmol. 2001; 131(4):517–518
[149] Dantas MA, Slakter JS, Negrao S, Fonseca RA, Kaga T, Yannuzzi LA. Photodynamic therapy with verteporfin in mallatia leventinese. Ophthalmology. 2002; 109(2):296–301
[150] Toto L, Parodi MB, Baralle F, Casari G, Ravalico G, Romano M. Genetic heterogeneity in Malattia Leventinese. Clin Genet. 2002; 62(5):399–403
[151] Stone EM, Lotery AJ, Munier FL, et al. A single EFEMP1 mutation associated with both Malattia Leventinese and Doyne honeycomb retinal dystrophy. Nat Genet. 1999; 22(2):199–202
[152] Fu L, Garland D, Yang Z, et al. The R345 W mutation in EFEMP1 is pathogenic and causes AMD-like deposits in mice. Hum Mol Genet. 2007; 16(20):2411–2422
[153] Matsumoto M, Traboulsi EI. Dominant radial drusen and Arg345Trp EFEMP1 mutation. Am J Ophthalmol. 2001; 131(6):810–812
[154] Dusek J, Streicher T, Schmidt K. Hereditary drusen of Bruch's membrane. II: Studies of semi-thin sections and electron microscopy results [in German]. Klin Monatsbl Augenheilkd. 1982; 181(2):79–83
[155] Agarwal A, Schoenberger SD. Macular caldera in North Carolina macular dystrophy—reply. JAMA Ophthalmol. 2014; 132(6):787
[156] Schoenberger SD, Agarwal A. Intrachoroidal cavitation in North Carolina macular dystrophy. JAMA Ophthalmol. 2013; 131(8):1073–1076

[157] Zhao S, Overbeek PA. Regulation of choroid development by the retinal pigment epithelium. Mol Vis. 2001; 7:277–282
[158] Seko Y, Tanaka Y, Tokoro T. Scleral cell growth is influenced by retinal pigment epithelium in vitro. Graefes Arch Clin Exp Ophthalmol. 1994; 232 (9):545–552
[159] Small KW, DeLuca AP, Whitmore SS, et al. North Carolina Macular Dystrophy Is Caused by Dysregulation of the Retinal Transcription Factor PRDM13. Ophthalmology. 2016; 123:9–18
[160] Rohrschneider K, Blankenagel A, Kruse FE, Fendrich T, Völcker HE. Macular function testing in a German pedigree with North Carolina macular dystrophy. Retina. 1998; 18(5):453–459
[161] Reichel MB, Kelsell RE, Fan J, et al. Phenotype of a British North Carolina macular dystrophy family linked to chromosome 6q. Br J Ophthalmol. 1998; 82(10):1162–1168
[162] Small KW, Puech B, Mullen L, Yelchits S. North Carolina macular dystrophy phenotype in France maps to the MCDR1 locus. Mol Vis. 1997; 3:1
[163] Kiernan DF, Shah RJ, Hariprasad SM, et al. Thirty-Year follow-up of an African American family with macular dystrophy of the retina, locus 1 (North Carolina macular dystrophy). Ophthalmology. 2011; 118(7):1435–1443
[164] Rabb MF, Mullen L, Yelchits S, Udar N, Small KW. A North Carolina macular dystrophy phenotype in a Belizean family maps to the MCDR1 locus. Am J Ophthalmol. 1998; 125(4):502–508
[165] Kim SJ, Woo SJ, Yu HG. A Korean family with an early-onset autosomal dominant macular dystrophy resembling North Carolina macular dystrophy. Korean J Ophthalmol. 2006; 20(4):220–224
[166] Michaelides M, Johnson S, Tekriwal AK, et al. An early-onset autosomal dominant macular dystrophy (MCDR3) resembling North Carolina macular dystrophy maps to chromosome 5. Invest Ophthalmol Vis Sci. 2003; 44 (5):2178–2183
[167] Francis PJ, Johnson S, Edmunds B, et al. Genetic linkage analysis of a novel syndrome comprising North Carolina-like macular dystrophy and progressive sensorineural hearing loss. Br J Ophthalmol. 2003; 87(7):893–898
[168] Schoenberger SD, Agarwal A. A novel mutation at the N-terminal domain of the TIMP3 gene in Sorsby fundus dystrophy. Retina. 2013; 33(2):429–435
[169] Lotery AJ, Silvestri G, Collins AD. Electrophysiology findings in a large family with central areolar choroidal dystrophy. Doc Ophthalmol. 1998–1999; 97 (2):103–119
[170] Hartley KL, Blodi BA, VerHoeve JN. Use of the multifocal electroretinogram in the evaluation of a patient with central areolar choroidal dystrophy. Am J Ophthalmol. 2002; 133(6):852–854
[171] Mansour AM. Central areolar choroidal dystrophy in a family with pseudoachondroplastic spondyloepiphyseal dysplasia. Ophthalmic Paediatr Genet. 1988; 9(1):57–65
[172] Ouechtati F, Belhadj Tahar O, Mhenni A, et al. Central areolar choroidal dystrophy associated with inherited drusen in a multigeneration Tunisian family: exclusion of the PRPH2 gene and the 17p13 locus. J Hum Genet. 2009; 54(10):589–594
[173] Boon CJ, Klevering BJ, Cremers FP, et al. Central areolar choroidal dystrophy. Ophthalmology. 2009; 116(4):771–782, 782.e1
[174] Klevering BJ, Deutman AF, Maugeri A, Cremers FP, Hoyng CB. The spectrum of retinal phenotypes caused by mutations in the ABCA4 gene. Graefes Arch Clin Exp Ophthalmol. 2005; 243(2):90–100
[175] Keilhauer CN, Meigen T, Weber BH. Clinical findings in a multigeneration family with autosomal dominant central areolar choroidal dystrophy associated with an Arg195Leu mutation in the peripherin/RDS gene. Arch Ophthalmol. 2006; 124(7):1020–1027
[176] Babel J. Geographic and helicoid choroidopathies. Clinical and angiographic study; attempted classification [in French]. J Fr Ophtalmol. 1983; 6(12):981–993
[177] Brazitikos PD, Safran AB. Helicoid peripapillary chorioretinal degeneration. Am J Ophthalmol. 1990; 109(3):290–294
[178] Franceschetti A. A curious affection of the fundus oculi: helicoid peripapillar chorioretinal degeneration. Its relation to pigmentary paravenous chorioretinal degeneration. Doc Ophthalmol. 1962; 16:81–110
[179] Rubino A. Su una particolare anomalia bilaterale e simmetrica dello strato pigmentato retinico. Boll Oculist. 1940; 19:318–322
[180] Sveinsson K. Choroiditis areata. Acta Ophthalmol. 1939; 17:73–80
[181] Sveinsson K. Helicoidal peripapillary chorioretinal degeneration. Acta Ophthalmol (Copenh). 1979; 57(1):69–75
[182] Fossdal R, Jonasson F, Kristjansdottir GT, et al. A novel TEAD1 mutation is the causative allele in Sveinsson's chorioretinal atrophy (helicoid peripapillary chorioretinal degeneration). Hum Mol Genet. 2004; 13(9):975–981
[183] Fossdal R, Magnússon L, Weber JL, Jensson O. Mapping the locus of atrophia areata, a helicoid peripapillary chorioretinal degeneration with autosomal dominant inheritance, to chromosome 11p15. Hum Mol Genet. 1995; 4 (3):479–483
[184] Miyake Y, Horiguchi M, Tomita N, et al. Occult macular dystrophy. Am J Ophthalmol. 1996; 122(5):644–653
[185] Wildberger H, Niemeyer G, Junghardt A. Multifocal electroretinogram (mfERG) in a family with occult macular dystrophy (OMD). Klin Monatsbl Augenheilkd. 2003; 220(3):111–115
[186] Piao CH, Kondo M, Tanikawa A, Terasaki H, Miyake Y. Multifocal electroretinogram in occult macular dystrophy. Invest Ophthalmol Vis Sci. 2000; 41 (2):513–517
[187] Fujii S, Escaño MF, Ishibashi K, Matsuo H, Yamamoto M. Multifocal electroretinography in patients with occult macular dystrophy. Br J Ophthalmol. 1999; 83(7):879–880
[188] Lyons JS. Non-familial occult macular dystrophy. Doc Ophthalmol. 2005; 111 (1):49–56
[189] Kitaguchi Y, Kusaka S, Yamaguchi T, Mihashi T, Fujikado T. Detection of photoreceptor disruption by adaptive optics fundus imaging and Fourier-domain optical coherence tomography in eyes with occult macular dystrophy. Clin Ophthalmol. 2011; 5:345–351
[190] Sisk RA, Berrocal AM, Lam BL. Loss of foveal cone photoreceptor outer segments in occult macular dystrophy. Ophthalmic Surg Lasers Imaging. 2010:1–3
[191] Kiernan DF, Mieler WF, Hariprasad SM. Spectral-domain optical coherence tomography: a comparison of modern high-resolution retinal imaging systems. Am J Ophthalmol. 2010; 149(1):18–31
[192] Koizumi H, Maguire JI, Spaide RF. Spectral domain optical coherence tomographic findings of occult macular dystrophy. Ophthalmic Surg Lasers Imaging. 2009; 40(2):174–176
[193] Hayashi T, Gekka T, Kozaki K, et al. Autosomal dominant occult macular dystrophy with an RP1L1 mutation (R45W). Optom Vis Sci. 2012; 89(5):684–691
[194] Akahori M, Tsunoda K, Miyake Y, et al. Dominant mutations in RP1L1 are responsible for occult macular dystrophy. Am J Hum Genet. 2010; 87 (3):424–429
[195] Deutman AF, Pinckers AJ, Aan de Kerk AL. Dominantly inherited cystoid macular edema. Am J Ophthalmol. 1976; 82(4):540–548
[196] Fishman GA, Goldberg MF, Trautmann JC. Dominantly inherited cystoid macular edema. Ann Ophthalmol. 1979; 11(1):21–27
[197] Saksens NT, van Huet RA, van Lith-Verhoeven JJ, den Hollander AI, Hoyng CB, Boon CJ. Dominant cystoid macular dystrophy. Ophthalmology. 2015; 122(1):180–191
[198] Schadlu R, Shah GK, Prasad AG. Optical coherence tomography findings in autosomal dominant macular dystrophy. Ophthalmic Surg Lasers Imaging. 2008; 39(1):69–72

20 Hereditary Retinal Degenerations

Angela M. Herro and Byron L. Lam

20.1 Introduction

The hereditary retinal degenerations are a group of disorders that both phenotypically and genotypically span a wide spectrum of ophthalmic presentations. In this chapter, the clinical presentation, diagnostic evaluation, treatment, and prognostic factors for each of the more common hereditary retinal degenerations will be discussed. The clinical manifestations of Stargardt's disease will be touched on; however, more detailed description of disease and management is found in Chapter 19, Macular Dystrophies.

20.2 Rod-Cone Retinal Degenerations

20.2.1 Retinitis Pigmentosa

Retinitis pigmentosa (RP) is a group of genetically heterogeneous inherited retinal degenerative disorders characterized by early rod photoreceptor dysfunction followed by progressive rod and cone photoreceptor dysfunction and death. It affects approximately 1 in 4,000 individuals worldwide and may be inherited as an autosomal dominant, autosomal recessive (most common), or X-linked pattern. Nearly 50% of patients with RP have no family history of RP, with the vast majority of these sporadic cases being autosomal recessive. Over 85 genes have been identified in association with RP, which has a wide range of clinical features and severity. Mutations in more than 20 genes are associated with the autosomal dominant form of RP; 20 to 30% are related to mutations in the *RHO* (rhodopsin) gene.[1] The most common gene involved in the autosomal recessive form is *USH2A*, which makes up 10 to 15% of autosomal recessive cases. Lastly, the X-linked form is associated with at least six genes, but mutations in *RPGR* and *RP2* genes account for the majority.

Clinical Features

The most common form of RP begins with night blindness, or nyctalopia, which may be described as either an inability to visually adapt or a very slow rate of visual adaptation at night. Difficulty seeing in dark conditions can be a problem from early childhood, but in some patients it may not be noticed until the third or fourth decade. RP may also manifest as difficulty with peripheral vision, sometimes expressed by the patient or family members as clumsiness. Visual field loss usually occurs early in the midperiphery ("ring" scotoma) because the midperipheral regions of the retina have the highest concentration of rods. A small central area of vision typically results eventually with disease progression.

Central vision may be good for very long periods of time in many forms of RP. However, there is a general trend of better central vision in the autosomal dominant form and an earlier loss of central vision in the X-linked recessive and autosomal recessive forms. In addition, cystoid macular edema (CME) and posterior subcapsular cataracts are frequent late complications in all genetic varieties of RP, and are important reasons for counseling patients regarding the importance of regular follow-up.[2] Refractive error can contribute to the evaluation of inheritance pattern, as those with X-linked disease are more likely to have 2 diopters or more of myopia, whereas those with a dominant form are usually hyperopic. Color vision can also be helpful with diagnosis, as most patients with isolated RP will have either normal red/green color vision or an acquired deficiency in blue cone function or tritanopia.[1]

Pearls

- Although central vision is usually preserved until late in the course of RP, the development of cataracts and CME can lead to earlier and potentially treatable visual acuity loss.

The classic fundus appearance of RP includes what is often referred to as waxy pallor of the disc, caused by either gliosis over the disc or attenuated vessels on the disc; a generalized mottling or "moth-eaten" pattern to the retinal pigment epithelium (RPE); a refractile (tapetum-like) appearance to the retina; narrowed arterioles; and pigment within the retina, as a generalized granularity, more discrete pigment clumps, or pigment deposits appearing as bone spicules (▶ Fig. 20.1). Histologic studies suggest that the source of the pigment is the RPE and that the pigment deposition is secondary to the degenerative process and not a contributing factor to the progress of the disease itself. With the passage of time, there may be progressive atrophy of the RPE and choriocapillaris in both the peripheral retina and the macula, a greater degree of disc pallor, further narrowing of the retinal arterioles until they may resemble white threads, and an increase in pigmentary retinal deposits. Although the majority of patients with typical RP show many

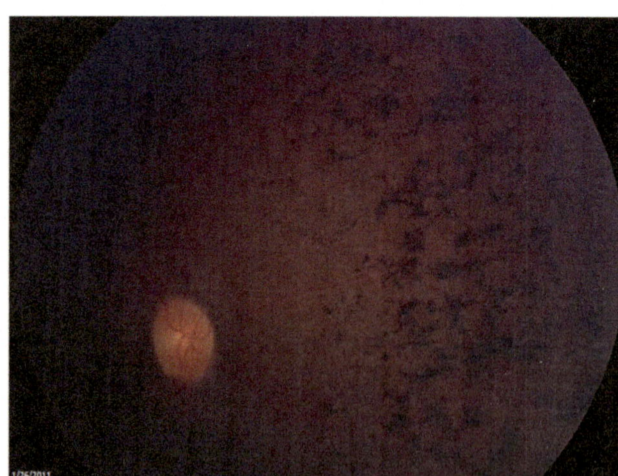

Fig. 20.1 Typical fundus appearance of retinitis pigmentosa with narrowed arterioles, peripheral bone spicule pigment clumping, and a "moth-eaten" appearance to the retina.

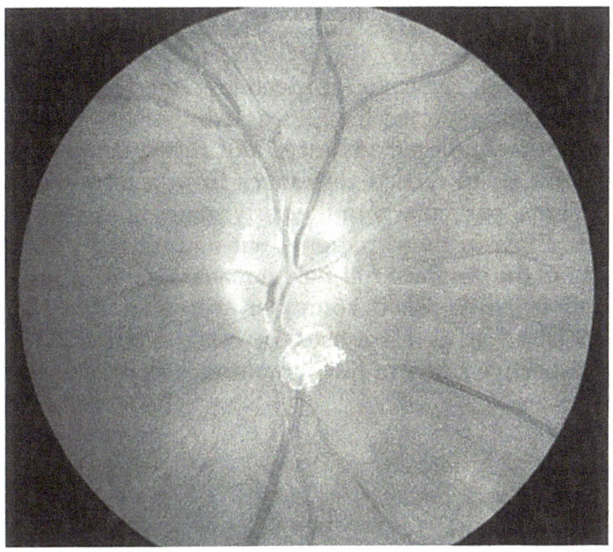

Fig. 20.2 Optic disc photograph of a 17-year-old boy with retinitis pigmentosa demonstrating optic nerve head drusen.

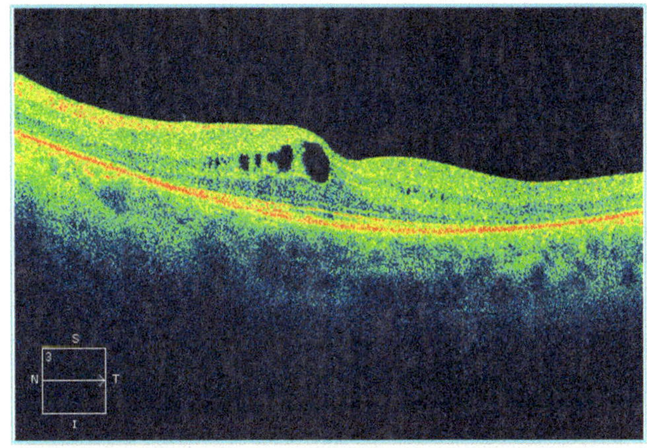

Fig. 20.3 Ocular coherence tomography (OCT) of a patient with retinitis pigmentosa showing cystoid macular edema.

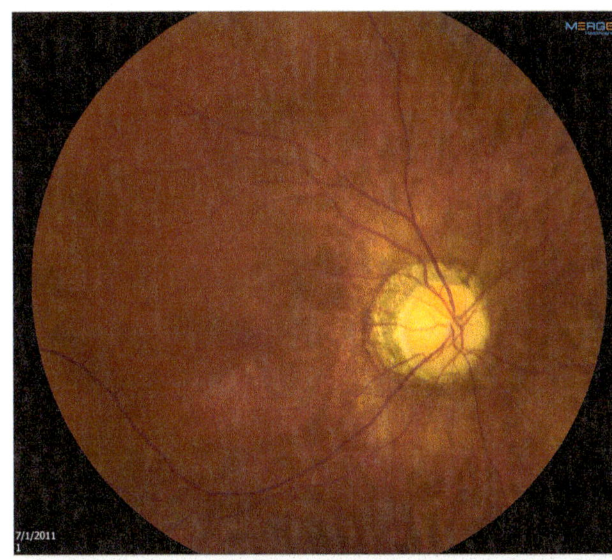

Fig. 20.4 Fundus photograph of a known X-linked retinitis pigmentosa carrier showing narrowed arterioles and waxy pallor of the optic nerve.

or all of the above-mentioned funduscopic changes, there are morphologic variations that may make the diagnosis more difficult on funduscopic evaluation alone. Some patients with RP do not have classic pigmentary clumping in the fundus, and this was formerly referred to as *retinitis sine pigmento*, which is likely on the spectrum of disease presentation, just observed at an earlier phase of RP.[2]

Optic nerve head drusen have been reported to be present more often in patients with RP than in the general population[3] (▶ Fig. 20.2). Histology in one case showed that these were true disc drusen and not astrocytic hamartomas.[4]

Diagnostic Testing

Visual field testing provides information regarding the rate of visual decline. Commonly used automated visual field strategies are mesopic, confined to the central 55 degrees, and may not provide an accurate assessment of patients' visual field function.

CME and macular atrophy are easily detectable by optical coherence tomography (OCT) when central vision is affected (▶ Fig. 20.3). The structure–function relationship between the appearances of the photoreceptors in the outer retina on OCT can also help to predict the degree of visual disability including visual field and visual acuity.[5]

The full-field electroretinography (ERG) responses are decreased markedly in early stages of RP, making full-field ERG an important diagnostic tool in the diagnosis of RP. Adherence to ERG international standards is essential. Given its dynamic range in RP, the full-field ERG may be near barely detectable levels even at the time of diagnosis in some patients, indicating its limitations in following up patients with RP. While most full-field ERG responses in RP show rod-cone dysfunction where rod responses are affected more severely than cone responses, cone-rod dysfunction also occurs. Of interest, a nondetectable full-field ERG in RP patients does not necessarily imply a total loss of retinal function. For instance, advanced RP patients with a small island of 20/20 vision often have nondetectable full-field ERG responses.[2]

Although the above-mentioned findings can be seen in typical cases of RP, there are general differences among the genetic varieties with respect to the rate of progression of the disease and the effect on central vision.[6] The autosomal dominant form of the disease generally progresses more slowly, with a greater retention of visual field as well as preservation of central vision. The X-linked recessive variety seems the most rapidly progressive, with marked peripheral loss by the second decade and severe central vision loss by the mid-30 s.[2]

In the X-linked recessive form of RP, the female carriers may show a wide spectrum of changes on the basis of lyonization. The majority of patients have no ocular complaints, but there may be a variety of retinal changes. The retina ranges from a normal appearance, to a diffuse pigment mottling, to isolated patches of RPE loss with pigment migration (▶ Fig. 20.4). Some carriers show a tapetum-like change in the parafoveal area.

There may be progression of these retinal changes with age, with visual function affected in some patients.

Berson et al[7] have demonstrated the importance of ERG testing to determine the X-linked female carrier. In 95% of such cases, one or both of the following ERG abnormalities will be found: (1) an increased cone b-wave implicit time; (2) a reduction in the amplitude of the dark-adapted response. These studies are important in terms of genetic counseling for those patients who have no retinal abnormalities but may be carriers of the X-linked form of RP.

Genetic testing of known RP genotypes is commercially available from several sources. Because not all RP genotypes are known and because of differences in genotypes tested among laboratories, negative results may be encountered. A comprehensive family tree and determination of hereditary pattern allow a higher yield of positive results.

Management and Course

Patients with RP often feel that complete blindness will be the eventual outcome; however, the majority of such patients never become completely blind, and a small percentage may retain very useful daytime vision all their lives. At present, it is not possible to separate or predict these categories in the early stages of disease. It is equally important to treat patients' misconceptions and fears as much as to treat the disease itself.

As with all patients with hereditary retinal degenerations, a comprehensive family tree to include affected, unaffected, and potential carrier family members is drawn out to determine potential hereditary pattern. Patient concerns of the disease affecting other family members or future offspring are addressed. Genetic testing is considered depending on the needs of the patient.

Patients with RP are followed up at least every 1 to 2 years if stable. In addition to performing a standard ocular evaluation, a spectral-domain OCT is obtained, particularly in the face of any precipitous loss in vision, as this may signal the possibility of either CME or cataract.

Acetazolamide (Diamox) at a dosage of 125 mg twice a day has been found to be effective in a number of RP patients with CME. A trial for a period of a few months is reasonable to ascertain its effect, which may take up to 6 months to reach maximum effectivity.[8] This dose varies widely from 125 mg every other day to 500 mg daily across many studies. Alternative systemic and local medications for RP-associated CME have been used, such as methazolamide, oral steroid therapy using a derivative of prednisolone, intravitreal corticosteroids, and intravitreal anti–vascular endothelial growth factor agents.[9] In a comprehensive review article by Salvatore et al, the outcomes of each therapy are nicely summarized, ranging from no effect, to morphologic effect only, to a significant improvement in visual acuity.[9] These studies are not limited to patients with RP but include those with juvenile X-linked retinoschisis, Usher's syndrome, and choroideremia, among others.[10,11] Most have a shared multifactorial mechanism including anatomic abnormalities, impairment of the blood–retinal barrier, tangential vitreous traction, and mutations in retinoschin.[9,10,11] The patient may have rebound edema while on the medication, in which case a trial of holiday from the treatment and reinstatement may be associated with a resumption of its effect.[12]

Posterior subcapsular cataracts are seen in approximately 50% of patients with RP and may lead to severe glare and reduction of vision. Although glare itself is often not a sufficient reason to perform cataract surgery, as this can be a common symptom in patients with RP even in the absence of cataracts, the combination of increased glare and decreased vision may make cataract surgery a reasonable option. Such patients should have their potential acuity measured before a decision is made to proceed with cataract surgery because degenerative macular changes may preclude visual improvement. Patients with RP have a higher incidence of zonular instability, so it is important to evaluate for this before surgery and be prepared to insert a capsular tension ring. Finally, there is a higher incidence of posterior capsular opacification in patients with RP, with a rate of 80% reported in one study with approximately 50% of eyes requiring capsulotomy.[13]

The most consistent way of following up patients with RP is with visual field evaluation, with the Goldmann's perimeter being more useful than a more restrictive computerized field. Although certain laboratories have the capability of following up such patients by performing serial ERGs using summated computer 30-Hz cone flicker responses, this is not available in many places.

There has been considerable discussion regarding the pros and cons of therapy with vitamins A, and Berson et al[14] reported that patients with RP who were treated with 15,000 IU of vitamin A per day, in the form retinyl palmitate, had a slower mean rate of decline of retinal function than those who were not treated with vitamin A. The investigators suggested a negative effect of taking 400 IU of vitamin E daily on the course of RP. This report prompted a number of letters,[15] many of which doubted the conclusions of the authors, as much of the conclusion was drawn from ERG testing and not visual fields or visual acuity. At present, it seems that this mode of therapy is still open to question. Another nutritional treatment option for these patients is docosahexaenoic acid (DHA), an omega-3 fatty acid important for photoreceptor function. In a 4-year study of patients with X-linked recessive RP, a dose of 400 mg/day of DHA was not associated with any identifiable safety risks.[16] Another larger study did not show a clear benefit of taking DHA supplements for RP; however, there was a trend toward slower progression of the visual field defect with higher blood concentrations of DHA.[1] A recent Cochrane database review from 2013 concluded that there is no clear evidence for the benefit of treatment with vitamin A and/or DHA for people with RP; however, the Cochrane review did not report on a potential adverse effect of vitamin E.[17] Many patients are well aware of this study, and the conclusions and controversy should be explained to patients before they begin vitamin A treatment or are advised against the use of vitamin E. It is safe to advise a patient that they can avoid supplementation with vitamin E but should not attempt to remove it from their diet. Similarly, patients should be counseled that if they would like to try vitamin A therapy, they should take the retinyl palmitate form and not exceed 15,000 IU daily.

There are ongoing trials to evaluate the efficacy and safety of gene therapy and stem cell therapy in patients with retinal degenerations. The first FDA-humanitarian-approved treatment for RP is the use of an implanted retinal prosthesis known as the Argus II system. This device uses a video camera and implanted retinal chip to relay images via electrical impulses that are transmitted through the optic nerve and down the visual pathway. It is currently approved on a humanitarian basis for those patients with profound RP with bare or no light perception.[18] The device allows patients to perceive high-contrast images and movement, affording them a better circadian rhythm as well as identifying the location or movement of objects or people. Some of the activities tested included locating and touching a square on a white field, recognizing large letters or words, detecting street curbs, and matching black, grey, and white socks.[18]

Further treatment includes occupational therapy in low-vision clinics, magnifiers, closed-circuit television, and increased lighting as well as preventative measures such as the use of UVA and UVB blocking sunglasses and the use of CPF 550 lenses to reduce glare and increase adaptation when moving from light to dark.

20.2.2 Syndromic Retinitis Pigmentosa

Although often occurring in isolation, RP can be associated with a systemic disease in approximately 20 to 30% of cases.[1] A list of many of the syndromes associated with RP or a retinal degeneration similar to RP is provided in the following.

Systemic Diseases Associated with Retinitis Pigmentosa

Metabolic disorders:

- Lipid abnormalities
  1. Bassen–Kornzweig syndrome
  2. Refsum's disease (infantile and adult)
  3. Neuronal ceroid lipofuscinosis (Batten's disease)
     a) Hagberg–Santavuori (early infancy)
     b) Jansky–Bielschowsky (late infancy)
     c) Spielmeyer–Vogt (juvenile)
  4. Miscellaneous rare associations
     a) Hooft's disease
     b) Letterer–Siwe disease
     c) Pelizaeus–Merzbacher disease
     d) Mucolipidosis IV
- Mucopolysaccharide storage disorders (MPSs)
  1. MPS I-H (Hurler)
  2. MPS I-S (Scheie)
  3. MPS I-H/S (Hurler–Scheie)
  4. MPS II (Hunter)
  5. MPS III (Sanfilippo)
- Miscellaneous rare associations
  1. Oxalosis
  2. Albinism
  3. Cystinuria

Neurologic disorders:

- Laurence–Moon syndrome
- Bardet–Biedl syndrome
- Hereditary ataxias
  1. Friedreich
  2. Pierre Marie
  3. Spastic paraplegia
  4. Pallidal degeneration
  5. Cerebellar (autosomal dominant)
- Mitochondrial myopathy (Kearns–Sayre syndrome)
- Usher's syndrome
- Alström's disease
- Miscellaneous rare associations
  1. Cockayne's syndrome
  2. Charcot–Marie–Tooth syndrome
  3. Flynn–Aird syndrome
  4. Marinesco–Sjögren syndrome

Renal or hepatic disorders:

- Medullary cystic disease (juvenile nephronophthisis; Senior–Løken syndrome; Fanconi's syndrome)
- Alagille's syndrome
- Zellweger's syndrome (cerebrohepatorenal syndrome)
- Adrenoleukodystrophy

In some instances, these are known metabolic disorders, and as such they may provide insight into the basic pathogenetic mechanisms of the retinal disease. Likewise, knowledge of the associations may lead the ophthalmologist to the appropriate systemic disorder. A few of the more common disorders as well as certain disorders for which some therapeutic assistance may be available are discussed. A more complete description of all of them is found in the review article of Bateman et al[19] and in Chapter 22.

20.2.3 Usher's Syndrome

Usher's syndrome is defined as the association of congenital deafness with RP and is the most common syndromic form of RP. It is the most common form of inherited deaf-blindness with an autosomal recessive pattern and is caused by mutations in at least nine genes.

Although Usher's syndrome is most commonly divided into three subtypes based primarily on the audiologic clinical presentation,[20] types I and II account for the majority of cases. Type I is defined as profound deafness, usually congenital, vestibular symptoms, and early-onset RP. Patients with type I Usher's syndrome often do not walk until the age of 18 months. Type II is associated with partial deafness, intact vestibular function, and a milder form of RP.[20] These first two types are heterogeneous and can be caused by eight different genes, while type III has only been associated with one gene to date.[21] Type III is characterized by progressive hearing loss, vestibular function, and retinal changes.[22] Other syndromes of RP with associated deafness are listed as follows.

The exact incidence of Usher's syndrome is difficult to determine, but surveys among individuals with RP suggest that up to 17% of patients with RP have profound deafness,[21] that 4% of children in schools for the deaf have RP,[23] and that 50% of blind-deaf persons have Usher's syndrome.[24] The prevalence of Usher's syndrome in the general population has been estimated to be between 1.8 and 4.4 cases per 100,000.[24] It is important to remember that these patients may also experience vision loss related to CME that is amenable to treatment with topical dorzolamide therapy.[11]

Syndromes with Deafness and Retinal Degeneration

- Usher
- Alport
- Alström
- Cockayne
- Enamel dysplasia (Albers-Schönberg)
- Refsum (adult and infantile)
- Waardenburg
- Bardet–Biedl
- Flynn–Aird
- Friedreich's ataxia
- Kearns–Sayre
- Hurler (MPS I)
- Marshall

20.2.4 Bardet–Biedl Syndrome

In 1920, Bardet[25] described a patient with RP, obesity, and polydactyly; in 1922, Biedl[26] added two other features—namely, mental retardation and hypogenitalism. This now seems a distinct entity from that described by Laurence and Moon[27] 60 years earlier—four patients with RP with paraplegia but without polydactyly or obesity, although these were once classified together as Laurence-Moon-Bardet-Biedl syndrome.[28]

Most patients do not demonstrate all five features, but for the diagnosis to be established, four of the five, including RP, should be present. It is often inherited in an autosomal recessive form, and more than 10 genes have been identified in causality.

The retinal degeneration usually presents atypically, with central degenerative changes and associated early loss of central vision. Although the peripheral retina may appear relatively normal, often showing the more typical RP changes only later in life, the ERG provides evidence of a generalized retinal degeneration at all stages. Renal abnormalities are also quite common, in one report being present in 90% of autopsy subjects.[29]

20.2.5 Neuronal Ceroid Lipofuscinosis (Batten's Disease)

At present, Batten's disease includes five distinct entities, all inherited in an autosomal recessive fashion and separated on the basis of clinical and electromicrographic (EM) features.[30] Although the biochemical abnormalities are unknown, there appears to be a difference in the stored lipopigments.[31]

The EM features serve to identify the disorders, and gene mapping has placed these disorders at separate chromosomal regions. Of the five types, the two most likely to present to the ophthalmologist are the late infantile form (Jansky–Bielschowsky) and the juvenile form (Spielmeyer–Vogt). All the disorders are characterized by an accumulation of autofluorescent lipopigments in neurons as well as in nonneural tissues. Investigators initially believed that the storage material was the aging pigment lipofuscin and that the yellow pathologic storage lipopigment was ceroid, thus leading to the term *neuronal ceroid lipofuscinosis*. However, it is now recognized that the storage material is neither ceroid nor lipofuscin but instead contains autofluorescent lipopigments.[32] Histologically, the diagnosis can be made through biopsy of skin or bulbar conjunctiva.[33]

There are clinical differences among the varieties. The infantile type typically shows mental and motor abnormalities between the ages of 1 and 1.5 years. Very early visual loss resulting from a generalized retinal degeneration in a child who had been visually normal should suggest this disorder. In addition to a brownish discoloration of the macula and findings of a generalized retinal degeneration, optic atrophy is also observed. The late infantile type has its onset between the ages of 2 and 4 years with seizures and psychomotor deterioration. In this variant, there is both optic atrophy and a generalized degeneration of the retina.[31] The juvenile form is the most common of the variants, and the initial manifestation of the disorder may be decreased vision. The ophthalmoscopic findings of macular degeneration or a bull's eye maculopathy may lead to the erroneous diagnosis of Stargardt's disease. However, an ERG will give evidence of widespread photoreceptor degeneration, and eventually an RP-like picture will develop. Somatically, there is progressive mental deterioration and occasionally seizures, with the average age of death being 17 years.

20.2.6 Bassen–Kornzweig Syndrome (Abetalipoproteinemia)

Manifestations of this syndrome, initially described in two siblings in 1950,[34] include malformed erythrocytes (acanthocytosis), neuromuscular disturbances with ataxia, fat intolerance, and RP. The funduscopic changes described in some of the reported cases vary from the typical fundus picture of RP to one with associated scattered deep white deposits. Strabismus and associated nystagmus have also been observed in several patients and may well be related to the central nervous system defect. All psychophysical and electrophysiologic findings are similar to those in any of the generalized retinal degenerations.

Although this autosomal recessive disorder was initially believed to be caused by an absence of beta-lipoprotein,[35] later evidence revealed the metabolic disorder to be more widespread and caused by a mutation in the gene encoding a microsomal triglyceride transfer protein resulting in deficiencies in apolipoprotein (apo) B.[36,37] In addition to low serum levels of fats and cholesterol, there is a concomitant lowering of the fat-soluble vitamins, including vitamins A and E, due to malabsorption. Studies have shown that vitamin A and E supplements, in sufficient amounts to raise the serum vitamin A and E to normal levels, lead to normal dark-adapted thresholds and a return of the previously reduced ERG, and help slow the progression of the retinopathy.[38,39] It is not known, however, if the retinal degeneration is solely related to vitamin A deficiency or if there is additional causality of the mutation itself. However, the reversal of these changes concurrent with administration of large doses of vitamin A indicates that this may be a treatable form of retinal degeneration. It is important for the ophthalmologist to recognize the possibility of this disease and refer patients for appropriate testing such as a stool sample, blood smear, and lipid workup.

Controversial Points

- Normalizing serum vitamin A levels with oral vitamin A supplementation can reverse the psychophysical and electrophysiologic abnormalities of Bassen–Kornzweig syndrome. Although the effects on the clinical course of disease are not known, such reversal suggests that this may be a treatable form of RP.

In several respects, the clinical course of the retinal changes in this condition resembles that expected in a retinal deficiency of vitamin A. In both conditions, rod vision deteriorates at an earlier stage than cone vision. This is thought to be a consequence of the fact that the cone visual pigments are synthesized more rapidly than rod pigments, so that when vitamin A is in short supply the needs of the cones are satisfied more effectively than those of the rods.

To establish whether vitamin A deficiency alone is responsible for the retinal degeneration in abetalipoproteinemia, it is important to maintain normal serum vitamin A levels in patients with this disease from the earliest possible age and to use a sensitive index of retinal function, such as the ERG, to check for evidence of retinal dysfunction. Frequent measurements of serum vitamin A levels are also necessary, as these may fluctuate.

20.2.7 Refsum's Disease

Refsum's disease (heredopathia atactica polyneuritiformis) is an autosomal recessive disorder predominantly affecting the nervous system. First described in 1945,[40] the characteristic findings in this syndrome are atypical RP with night blindness and constriction of the visual fields, chronic polyneuritis with progressive paresis of the distal parts of the extremities, dry skin, elevated cerebrospinal fluid protein levels, and ataxia with other cerebellar signs. Less frequently observed findings include anosmia, pupillary abnormalities, cataracts, deafness, alteration of the electrocardiogram, and skeletal abnormalities.

Nyctalopia is present in nearly all patients studied and is the most common initial ocular symptom, usually occurring before the third decade of life. The retinal pigmentation is usually a mottled, nondescript type, although a typical bone spicule configuration has sometimes been observed.

In 1963, an abnormal long-chain fatty acid was detected in the serum, urine, kidney, and liver of a patient with Refsum's disease.[41] This fatty acid—3, 7, 11,15-tetramethylhexadecenoic (phytanic) acid—was subsequently found in other patients with this syndrome. An interesting relationship has been suggested between the abnormal fatty acid and the associated atypical RP. Baum et al[42] hypothesized that palmitic acid, found in its esterified form in high concentration in normal retina, is structurally similar to phytanic acid. There may be an interference, possibly enzymatic, with fatty acid metabolism concomitant with or preceding the incorporation of palmitic acid into the vitamin A ester of the rhodopsin cycle.

Most patients with Refsum's disease have a deficiency of phytanoyl-coenzyme A (CoA) hydroxylase enzyme activity, leading to an accumulation of phytanic acid, and diagnosis can be made with plasma levels of phytanic acid greater than 200 umol/L. A study of patients with severe neurologic handicaps associated with Refsum's syndrome showed a remarkable recovery of neurologic function following use of a low-phytanic-acid diet and normalization of their phytanic acid levels.[1,43] Although this report makes no mention of patients' ocular status, more recent studies in such patients have shown some return of retinal function and apparent cessation of the disease process.[44] The infantile form has been described with early RP[45]; however, dietary restriction in this group of patients was not associated with improvement in retinal function. Despite the lack of long-term follow-up, this disorder may also prove to be one of the treatable forms of RP.

Controversial Points

- Normalization of the elevated phytanic acid levels in Refsum's disease by a low-phytanic-acid diet may improve retinal function and halt or slow the progression of disease.

20.2.8 Kearns–Sayre Syndrome (Mitochondrial Myopathy)

Kearns–Sayre syndrome is one of the mitochondrial myopathies in which the mitochondria are increased in number and distorted, accumulating in skeletal muscle (including the extraocular muscles), RPE, and heart.

Chronic progressive external ophthalmoplegia is most often the presenting clinical manifestation, and symptoms usually present before the age of 20 years. Histologically, the affected muscles will show "ragged-red fibers," a finding caused by the accumulation of mitochondria beneath the plasma membrane and between myofibrils. In the majority of cases of mitochondrial myopathy, there are no other ocular findings. In about one-third of patients,[46] however, there will be evidence of pigmentary retinopathy, but with extremely variable findings. These can range from a salt-and-pepper appearance, either throughout the retina or just in the periphery, to macular degeneration or an RP-like appearance, with all the attendant psychophysical and electrophysiologic changes.

In 1958, Kearns and Sayre[47] reported several patients with RP, external ophthalmoplegia, and complete heart block, and a later, more expansive article by Kearns[48] noted the frequent association of this disorder with cardiomyopathy. There is currently no disease-modifying therapy available; however, patients suspected of having this disease should be referred for EKG testing.[49]

Pearls

- The finding of an RP picture with chronic progressive external ophthalmoplegia should alert the clinician to investigate associated cardiac abnormalities. The constellation of these signs is known as the *Kearns–Sayre syndrome*.

Case Report

A 26-year-old Caucasian woman had a 6-year history of noting blank areas in her peripheral visual field. Visual fields were difficult to obtain and results were considered unreliable when she was first tested. Because of the absence of any demonstrable ocular abnormalities and the continuation of complaints in this very anxious woman, she was referred to a psychiatrist. One year later, a visual field examination was again performed, and a temporal scotomatous region was noted. The patient then had an extreme anxiety reaction, manifested by continual complaints with regard to her vision, and she was once again referred for psychotherapy. When she was seen 1 year later, narrowed arterioles were visible in the retinal periphery of her fundus. There was no evidence of any bone corpuscular pigmentary changes. A fluorescein angiogram was normal. Visual fields again were impossible to evaluate because of poor cooperation. The suspected diagnosis of RP was borne out by the ERG, which showed an absent response under all test conditions. There is little doubt than an ERG performed early in the clinical course would have immediately provided the correct diagnosis of RP.

20.2.9 Leber's Congenital Amaurosis

Leber's congenital amaurosis (LCA) is characterized by a congenital generalized retinal dysfunction and is usually inherited in an autosomal recessive pattern. Leber's original description[50] included a group of children, younger than 1 year, who presented with nystagmus, decreased vision, and either normal fundi or a wide variety of fundus changes indicative of a generalized retinal degeneration (▶ Fig. 20.5). LCA can result from mutations in at least 14 genes associated with retinal development and include *CEP290, CRB1, GUCY2D,* and *RPE65*, among others. The visual changes are usually stable or very slowly progressive, unlike many other retinal degenerations discussed in this chapter. The visual acuity varies widely from 20/30 to 20/200 to light perception and, as such, may have associated sensory nystagmus.[51] Pupillary examination may show sluggish reactions and light-near dissociation. A profoundly abnormal or extinguished ERG is the electrophysiologic hallmark of the disorder. However, certain associated disorders, such as keratoconus (often contributed to by the Franceschetti's oculodigital poking behavior), high hyperopia, mental retardation, skeletal abnormalities, renal disease, and neurologic abnormalities, have been described with LCA. Some of these somatic problems may also be seen in specific systemic disorders associated with RP, such as infantile Refsum's disease,[45] neuronal ceroid lipofuscinosis,[52] and the renal-retinal syndromes.[53] Thus, the use of the term *Leber's congenital amaurosis* in these complicated cases tends to obscure the true meaning of the disorder.

Targets for therapy at this time are centered on gene therapy in forms with a reduction or absence of a protein with an essential function such as the *RPE65* form of disease. Studies are ongoing for gene therapy using viral vectors with the human *RPE65* gene. Thus far, these studies have found improvement in visual acuity despite continued degeneration of the retina including progressive outer retinal thinning, and more studies are necessary to better understand the multifactorial pathology of this disease.[51,54]

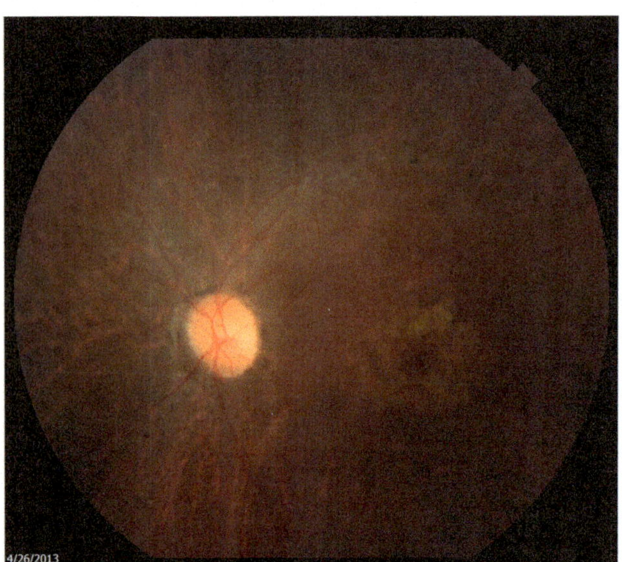

Fig. 20.5 Fundus photograph of a patient with Leber's congenital amaurosis showing mottled appearance of the macula with patchy "moth-eaten" appearance of the peripheral retina with some pigment clumping and relative sparing of the periarteriolar area.

20.2.10 Childhood-Onset Retinitis Pigmentosa

This should be differentiated from the congenital form, described earlier, by normal vision, the absence of nystagmus, and good visual function in infancy. It is most important when seeing a child with early-onset RP (i.e., ages 3–10 years) to exclude the systemic diagnosis of neuronal ceroid lipofuscinosis or Batten's disease since the associated symptoms, morbidity, and potential for treatment are very different.

Case Report

A 7-year-old boy was initially seen by an ophthalmologist at age 5 years because of difficulty seeing the blackboard at school. The parents had noted no prior problems. At the initial examination, a vision of 20/50 in each eye was found, and the ophthalmologist noted "yellow, circular lesions involving the macula" in both eyes. The child was referred for electrodiagnostic testing 1 month later, and the vision had fallen to 20/80 in each eye. The examining physician noted pale discs, an atrophic retina, and an "unusual reddish disclike disturbance" of the macula. The ERG was essentially extinguished and a diagnosis of LCA was made.

Because of a progressive loss in vision, the child was referred to our center 4 months after his initial examination. The history confirmed that the child had seen well in infancy and had no nystagmus. The vision had fallen to 10/400 in the right eye and 20/400 in the left eye. The retina showed a generalized granularity, narrowed arterioles, temporal disc pallor, and mild parafoveal depigmentation. No pigment clumps were noted.

The patient was referred to the neurology department, and studies confirmed the suspected diagnosis of neuronal ceroid lipofuscinosis.

Comment

In a young child with previously good vision and no nystagmus, a diagnosis of LCA should not be entertained. With the

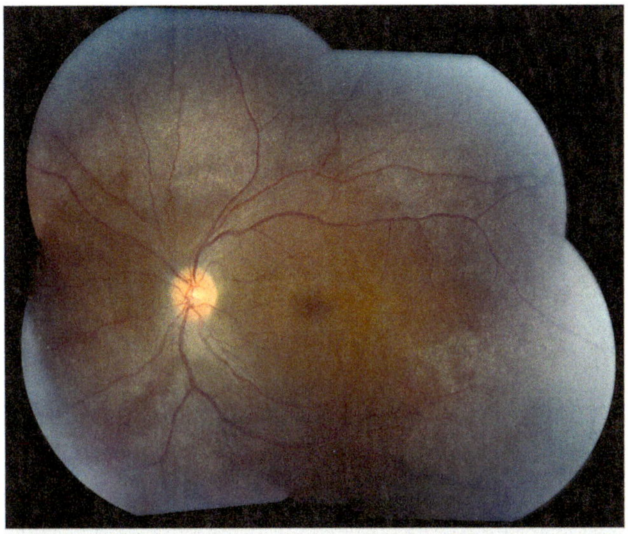

Fig. 20.6 Fundus photograph of a patient with a nonspecific rod-cone dystrophy demonstrating the clinical sign of preserved para-arteriolar retinal pigment epithelium.

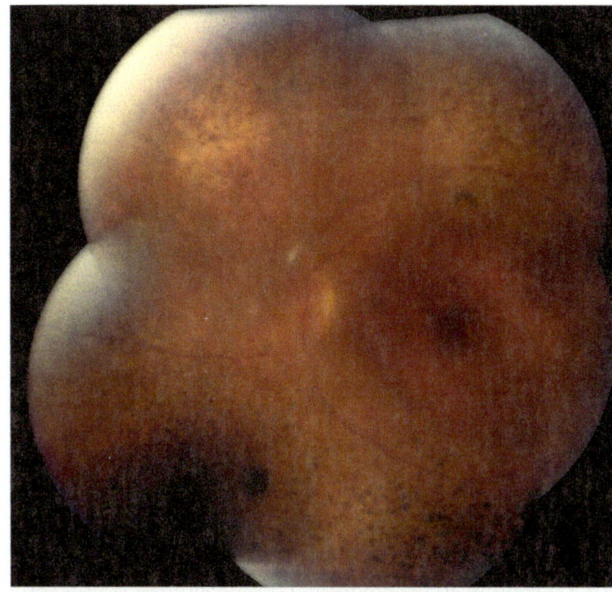

Fig. 20.7 Montage color fundus photograph of a patient with enhanced S-cone syndrome demonstrating retinal pigmentary change, particularly around the vascular arcades, and macular mottling due to active or resolved cystoid macular edema.

additional findings of a very rapid visual loss and an ERG indicative of a generalized retinal degeneration, one must rule out neuronal ceroid lipofuscinosis. The suspicion of this disorder is further heightened by the unusual macular changes in this patient, as this is a key feature of Batten's disease.

20.2.11 Preserved Para-Arteriolar Retinal Pigment Epithelium

This is more of a descriptive sign of disease rather than a distinct entity. Preserved para-arteriolar RPE[55] is most closely described as an autosomal recessive form of LCA, mapped to chromosome 1, gene *CRB1*, that has an aggressive course with early-onset blindness from associated macular changes.[56] The hallmark of the disorder is the relative preservation of the RPE adjacent to and underlying the retinal arterioles (▶ Fig. 20.6). With time, such preserved areas disappear and are included in the disease process.

20.2.12 Enhanced S-Cone Syndrome

This syndrome, so-named because of a unique hypersensitivity of the S (blue)-cone system,[57] is a retinal disorder characterized by increased sensitivity to blue light, poor night vision, and an unusual type of ERG. It is inherited in an autosomal recessive pattern from gene *NR2E3* on chromosome 15q23. The eponym Goldmann–Favre syndrome has been given to this disorder when retinal degeneration is more severe and accompanied by a liquefied vitreous body. Although some of the ERG responses in this syndrome are similar to what is seen in most forms of RP (an absent dark-adapted rod response to blue light and a markedly reduced cone flicker response), the following ERG responses distinguish this form of RP: the ERG responses to single flashes of white light are similar under both light- and dark-adapted conditions, and relatively larger responses are seen to stimuli from the blue end of the spectrum than from the longer wavelengths. Night blindness occurs early in life, and the fundus abnormalities include cystoid macular changes and pigment disturbances near the vascular arcades (▶ Fig. 20.7). This can also be seen using OCT imaging of the schisis or cystoid cavities as well as using fundus autofluorescence which can demonstrate hyperautofluorescence along the arcades.[58] There is currently no treatment to prevent the retinal degeneration; however, as in many hereditary retinal dystrophies, treatment with topical and/or oral carbonic anhydrase inhibitors can be used for CME in these patients as well.[9]

20.2.13 Cone Dystrophy

Cone dystrophy will be discussed briefly here; however, because of the increased density of cones in the macula, this will also be covered in Chapter 19, Macular Dystrophies. Cone dystrophy is a progressive dystrophy caused by the gene *GUCA1A* on chromosome 6. This mutation has also been linked to cone–rod dystrophy, which is clinically very similar to the former. Patients usually present in childhood or early adult life with photophobia, loss of color and central vision, and distinctive ERG findings. Clinically, one can see pigment stippling and a classic bull's eye pattern of atrophy later in the course of disease. On ERG testing, there is a low or unrecordable single-flash photopic wave and 30-Hz flicker. In most cases, the scotopic ERG and electro-oculogram (EOG) are normal. There is currently no treatment for this disease; however, gene therapy trials are ongoing for similar degenerative conditions and may show promise for cone dystrophy as well.

20.2.14 Stargardt's Disease

Although not classically a hereditary degenerative retinopathy, Stargardt's disease shares some features of RP and, in certain stages, can be confused clinically with RP. Stargardt's disease is usually inherited in an autosomal recessive pattern caused by the *ABCA4* gene on chromosome 1. It often presents in the first or second decade of life with symptoms of gradually decreasing central visual acuity. It is characterized by discrete pisciform flecks at the level of the RPE, which may or may not involve the macula and can sometimes manifest as a ring scotoma on visual field testing, making it similar to RP. It is the degeneration of the RPE that often leads to the photoreceptor loss in this disease, as well as other acquired macular degenerations. OCT imaging can help detect early macular pathology when the diagnosis is unclear, and pattern ERG can help isolate the layers that have reduced function.[59] On electrophysiologic testing, the full-field ERG is usually normal depending on the severity of the flecks and atrophy, and the EOG is often mildly affected. Dark adaptation may be delayed as the *ABCA4* gene affects rods preferentially to cones. There are ongoing clinical trials for gene therapy and human embryonic stem cell (hESC) therapy that show promise for the treatment of this disease. Preliminary results of subretinal treatment with hESC-derived RPE in these patients demonstrated safety over approximately 3-year follow-up, improvement or stabilized visual acuity in most eyes, and lack of abnormal proliferation of cells.[60] The study included two groups of patients—those with Stargardt's disease and those with age-related macular degeneration—and three dose cohorts in each group. Research is ongoing to use the subretinal space as a site of treatment using complex biological treatments including gene therapy.[60] More details of diagnosis and management of this disease can be found in Chapter 19, Macular Dystrophies.

20.2.15 Disorders Associated with Early Abnormalities of the Choriocapillaris

This group of diseases demonstrates an early associated abnormality of the choriocapillaris. However, it is still not understood whether the primary abnormality is in the choriocapillaris or the RPE–photoreceptor complex. The absence of the choriocapillaris on fluorescein angiography distinguishes this from RP and other disorders in the previous section.

Choroideremia

This generalized, progressive, retinal degeneration was first distinguished from typical RP in 1871,[61] and the X-linked recessive mode of inheritance was firmly grounded by McCulloch and McCulloch[62]; thus, the condition occurs most commonly in males. The syndrome has been mapped to gene *CHM*, and genetic testing is available. The onset of symptoms usually occurs in the first or second decade of life, with the major complaint being poor night vision.

The initial fundus appearance (▶ Fig. 20.8) is a "salt-and-pepper" pigment mottling in the equator and posterior pole; it has been reported as early as age 22 months.[63] Even at this stage, the ERG is abnormal, showing reduced or absent scotopic components. Below the pigment mottling, the underlying choroid may appear ophthalmoscopically normal, although fluorescein angiography may show a patchy loss of the choriocapillaris and choroidal vessels (▶ Fig. 20.9). Later, small areas of RPE atrophy in the midperiphery eventually coalesce and progress centrally until the prototypical prominence of the orange-red

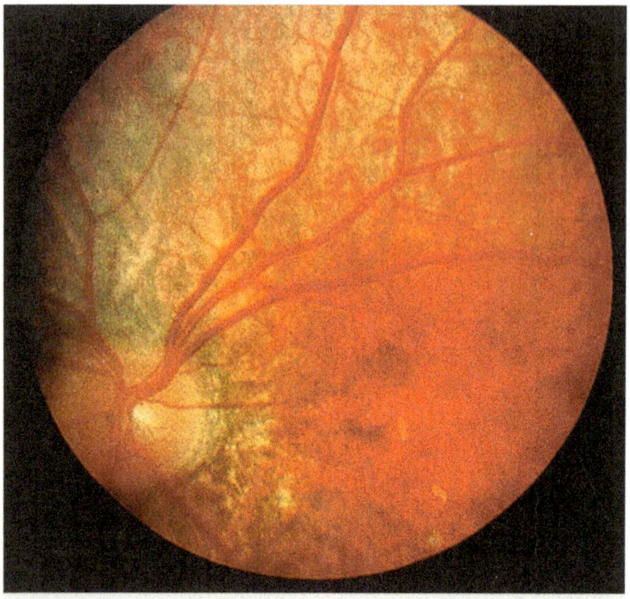

Fig. 20.8 Choroideremia: Early changes in a 14-year-old boy. There is prominence of the choroidal vasculature and patchy loss of retinal pigment epithelium of the posterior pole.

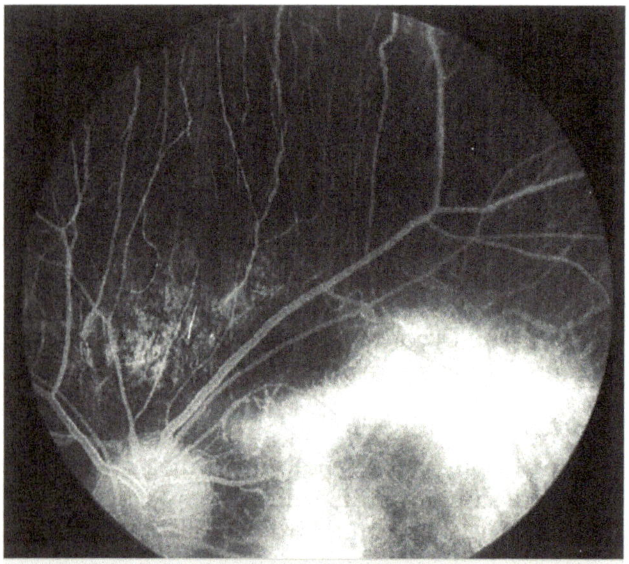

Fig. 20.9 Choroideremia: Fluorescein angiogram shows loss of choriocapillaris with isolated patches of retained retinal pigment epithelium and choriocapillaris.

choriocapillaris is seen clinically; the macula is affected last, and relatively good vision is preserved until late in the disease. In the final stage, the entire fundus, with perhaps the exception of the macula, shows the diffuse yellow-white reflex of the underlying sclera (▶ Fig. 20.10). At this stage, the fundus may resemble that of gyrate atrophy, making ophthalmoscopic distinction between the two diseases difficult. Furthermore, these patients can also experience cystic macular edema in up to 60% of eyes; the CME is often seen only with OCT imaging (▶ Fig. 20.11).[64] It is unclear whether the edema responds to traditional treatment for RP, for example, with oral or topical

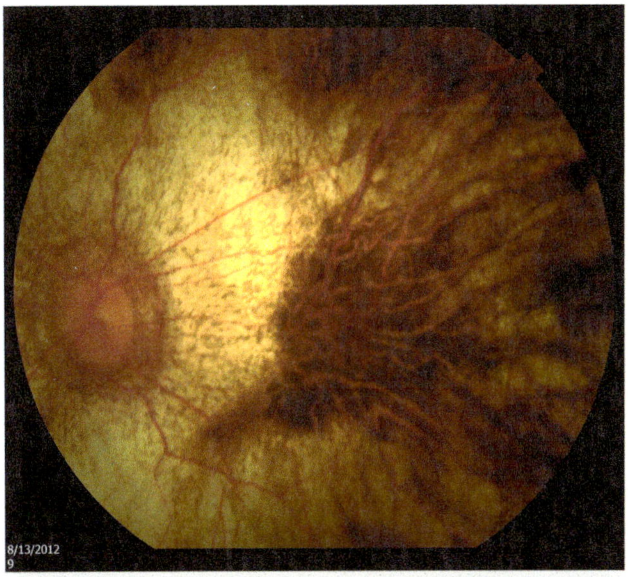

Fig. 20.10 Fundus photograph of a patient with late stages of choroideremia showing diffuse visualization of the yellow-white reflex of the underlying sclera and relative preservation of the macula.

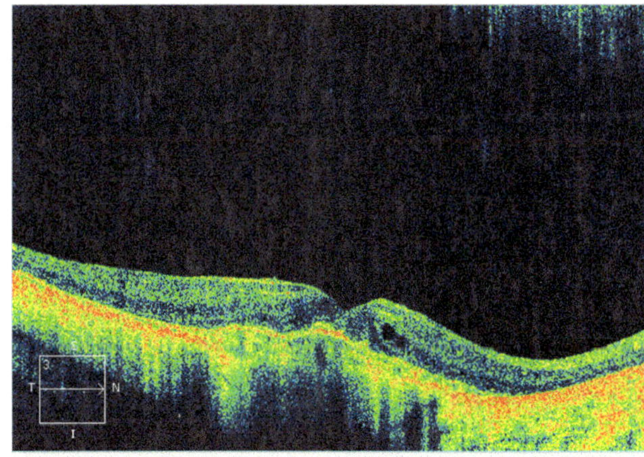

Fig. 20.11 Optical coherence tomography of a patient with choroideremia demonstrating macular edema and overall retinal thinning.

carbonic anhydrase inhibitors. Although the rate of progression may vary within a pedigree, most patients with this disorder lose virtually all vision by 35 years of age.[62]

A characteristic of most X-linked diseases is that the female carrier shows specific signs; in choroideremia, the fundus changes of the carrier are unique and pathognomonic of the disease. Typically, these changes resemble those seen in the early stages of male disease—that is, a generalized pigment mottling, particularly noticeable in the midperiphery and macular area (▶ Fig. 20.12). Despite the fundus appearance similar to that of the affected male, visual function is usually normal in the female carrier and remains so throughout life.[65] The fundus signs are usually stationary, and fluorescein angiography shows no loss of the choriocapillaris.[66] However, there are some reports in which the female carrier may show a severe functional deficit and marked abnormalities on the fluorescein angiogram (▶ Fig. 20.13). The Lyon hypothesis of female mosaicism accounts for these rare occurrences.[62,65] There are ongoing trials for gene therapy but, to date, there is no established treatment for this disease.[67]

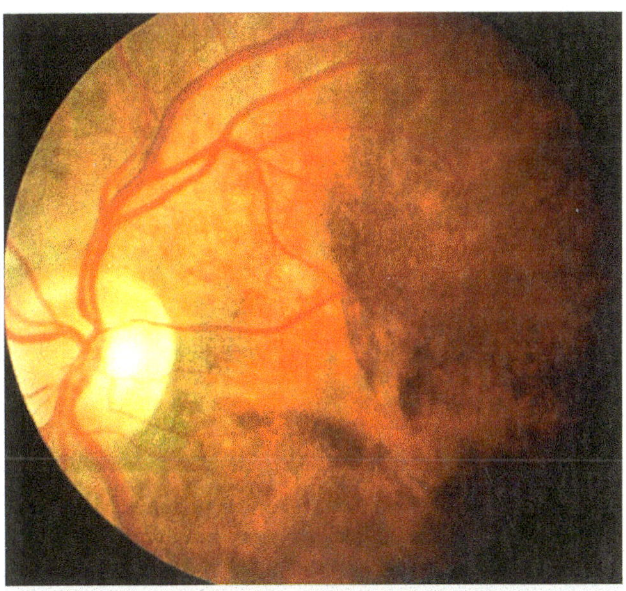

Fig. 20.12 Fundus photograph of a female carrier of choroideremia showing irregular pigment in the retina; however, vision remained 20/20 with a normal electroretinogram.

Gyrate Atrophy

Gyrate atrophy is a rare choroidal disease, usually inherited as an autosomal recessive disorder, mapped to the ornithine aminotransferase gene on chromosome 10. Symptoms usually appear in the second and third decades of life and consist of poor night vision and constricted visual fields. Myopia is present invariably, and cataracts are seen in a high proportion of patients.[68]

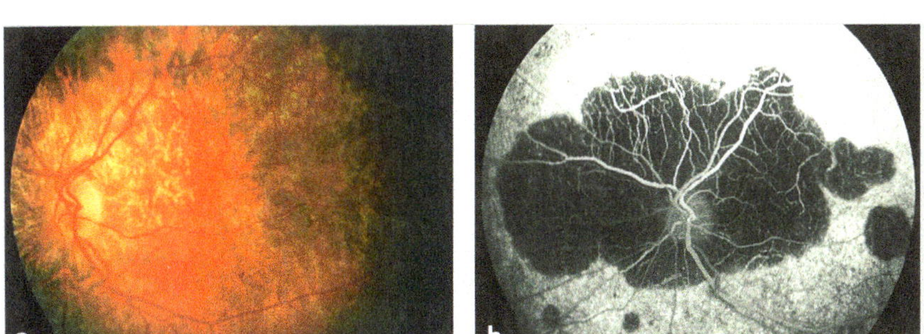

Fig. 20.13 Choroideremia: 61-year-old female carrier of choroideremia who has had a progressive decrease in vision over 10 years. Acuity is now 20/70 in the right eye and 20/100 in the left eye. (**a**) Fundus photograph shows peripapillary loss of retinal pigment epithelium. (**b**) Fluorescein angiogram shows marked loss of the peripapillary choriocapillaris with small patches of loss seen elsewhere, indicative of retinal mosaicism.

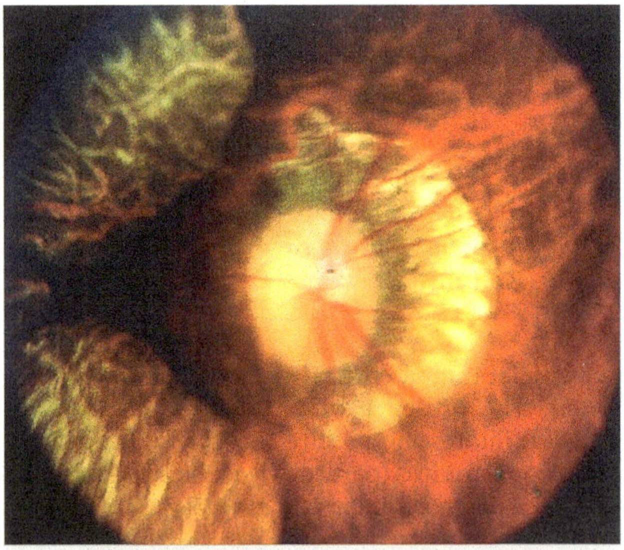

Fig. 20.14 Gyrate atrophy in a 27-year-old man: Vision is 20/50 in the right eye and 20/30 in the left eye. There is a sharp demarcation between normal and abnormal retina.

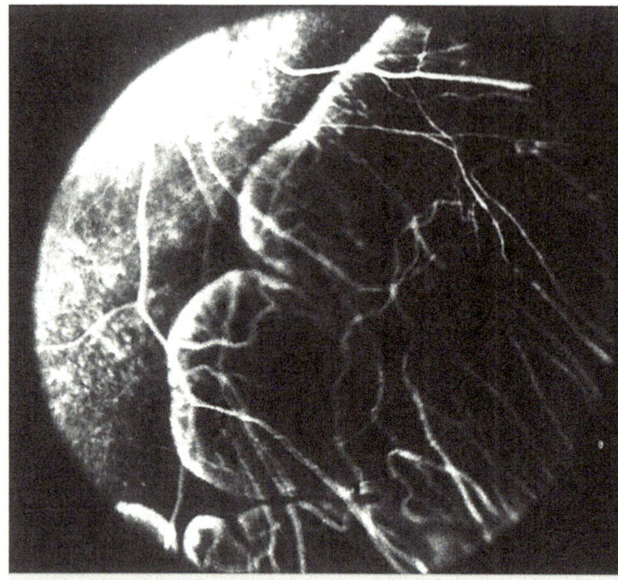

Fig. 20.15 Gyrate atrophy: Fluorescein angiogram of the affected area shows a loss of the choriocapillaris and a sharp border next to the more normal-appearing retina.

The fundus abnormality begins in the midperiphery with a thinning and transparency of the RPE; the underlying choroid may appear either normal or sclerotic. Affected areas are separated from normal-appearing retina by scalloped borders, which begin as isolated islands and then merge to assume the form of a garland. Because of pigment accumulation, the scalloped borders have a darker appearance, thus increasing the contrast between the adjacent normal and abnormal retinal tissues (▶ Fig. 20.14). Fluorescein angiography shows a loss of the choriocapillaris in the affected areas (▶ Fig. 20.15).

As the disease progresses, pigment clumping and choriocapillaris atrophy are noted; eventually, there is disappearance of the entire choroid, exposing the white sclera. The optic discs and retinal vessels may be normal in the initial stages, but with time the vessels show gradual narrowing. In the very late stages, choroidal atrophy may be seen from the periphery to the posterior pole, but usually the macula is spared.

Electricophysiologic and psychophysical studies indicate the presence of a generalized retinal degeneration, even in the early stages of the disorder. The late stages of gyrate atrophy can be remarkably similar to the late stages of choroideremia, but the different mode of genetic transmission for the two diseases is an important distinguishing feature. Also, as noted previously, the female carrier in choroideremia shows distinctive funduscopic changes that help differentiate these two disorders.

In 1973, Simell and Takki[69] discovered that all patients with gyrate atrophy had elevated levels of ornithine, an amino acid derived from intake of arginine, in urine and plasma. This was discovered to be caused by an absence or near absence of the pyridoxine-dependent mitochondrial matrix enzyme ornithine aminotransferase, which is necessary for the breakdown of excess ornithine in humans.[70,71] Although it was felt initially that only the eye was affected, later studies noted abnormalities in skeletal muscle and the liver.[72] Some patients treated only with pyridoxine (vitamin B_6) showed a lowering of their plasma ornithine levels,[73] whereas other patients responded to a low-protein diet, with improvement in visual acuity and visual fields without a change in the clinical appearance of the retina.[74] Other studies have suggested that proline supplements[75] or a low-arginine diet may be effective in halting the disorder's progression. There are indications that the reduction of plasma ornithine leads to improvement in dark-adapted retinal sensitivity, a slight increase in the size of the visual field, improved color discrimination, and an enhancement of the ERG response.[76] However, other investigators could not find any improvement. The possibility that abnormalities in the ornithine cycle may lead to retinal degeneration is further borne out by the finding of two siblings with presumed LCA who had elevated ornithine and serum threonine levels.[77]

Pearls

- The late stages of gyrate atrophy can be remarkably similar to advanced choroideremia, but the different mode of genetic transmission for the two diseases is an important distinguishing feature.

Bietti's Crystalline Retinopathy

In this relatively rare disorder, initially described in 1937,[78] crystalline deposits are observed in all layers of the retina and are associated with varying degrees of choriocapillaris and RPE loss (▶ Fig. 20.16). It is included here, as there can be a degenerative response to the crystals, leading to flattening of the ERG and poor night vision. In some cases, superficial limbal corneal crystals have also been observed. The presence of retinal crystals and the unusual fluorescein picture showing areas of focal choriocapillaris loss (particularly in the posterior pole) make the diagnosis relatively easy (▶ Fig. 20.17). The fundus changes can be those of a generalized degenerative disorder, or only

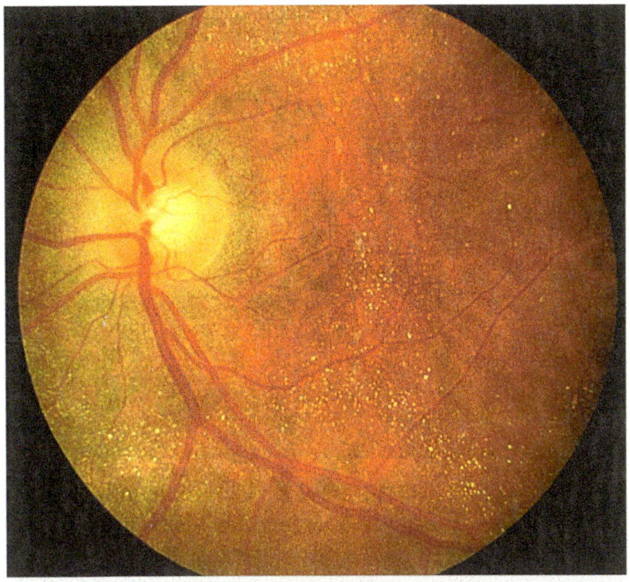

Fig. 20.16 Bietti's crystalline retinopathy: Crystalline deposits are scattered irregularly in the posterior pole.

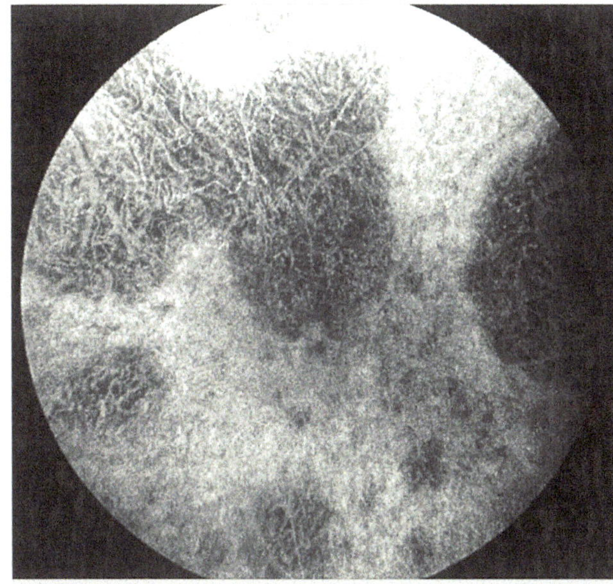

Fig. 20.17 Bietti's crystalline retinopathy: Fluorescein angiogram shows islands of choriocapillaris loss.

focal areas of the retina may be involved. The size and location of the affected regions determine the degree to which visual acuity, night vision, and the ERG recordings are disturbed.[79] The inheritance is presumed to be autosomal recessive, with some pedigrees showing two siblings affected.

Controversial Points

- Lowering plasma ornithine levels, as with pyridoxine supplements and low-protein or low-arginine diets, may be effective in halting the progression of gyrate atrophy in some individuals.

20.3 Disorders Associated with Vitreous Abnormalities

Although most patients with RP show vitreous cells or "dust particles" consisting of pigment or macrophages and, in some instances, large amorphous globules in the vitreous, the disorders discussed in the following have in common very profound alterations of the vitreous associated with varying degrees of chorioretinal atrophy, retinal detachments, retinal vascular abnormalities, cataracts, and vitreoretinal bands.

20.3.1 Heredoretinal Degenerations Associated with Vitreous Abnormalities

- Goldmann–Favre disease (autosomal recessive)
- Wagner's disease (autosomal dominant)
- Stickler's syndrome (autosomal dominant)
- Jansen's disease (autosomal dominant)
- Autosomal dominant vitreoretinochoroidopathy (ADVIRC) (autosomal dominant)
- Erosive vitreoretinopathy (autosomal dominant)
- Autosomal dominant neovascular inflammatory vitreoretinopathy (autosomal dominant)

The hallmark vitreous change is that of early liquefaction or syneresis, the so-called optically empty vitreous. In only a few instances are these disorders associated with ERG and psychophysical findings, but a brief summary of each disorder in this group is noted here. (The major disorders of this group are discussed in detail in Chapter 23.)

20.3.2 Wagner's Disease

In 1938, Wagner[80] described an autosomal dominant vitreoretinal disorder characterized by an empty vitreous with avascular membranes, strands and veils, lattice degeneration of the retina, chorioretinal atrophy, and secondary cataracts. This has since been mapped to the gene *VCAN* on chromosome 5q14. The disorder appears in childhood and is progressive in nature, with the chorioretinal atrophy causing significant visual loss and visual field defects in the fourth and fifth decades of life. The ERG amplitudes reflect the degree of chorioretinal degeneration. In several vitreoretinal disorders, a high proportion of patients have rhegmatogenous retinal detachment; however, this is not a prominent feature of this group. Peripheral traction retinal detachment appears to be a common problem, however, occurring in more than 50% of patients older than 45 years.

20.3.3 Stickler's Syndrome

In 1965, Stickler et al[81] described a family with vitreous syneresis, high myopia, frequent retinal detachments, and the associated somatic finding of a progressive, severe arthropathy. Later reports noted facial flattening and various abnormalities of the soft palate and association with the Pierre Robin's syndrome.[82]

There is no evidence of a generalized retinal degeneration, but patients may show perivascular pigmentary changes. Presenile cataracts, usually described as wedge or fleck, can be seen in approximately 50% of patients with this disease, along with progressive myopia in 90% and retinal detachment in 60%, based on a questionnaire in 2001 sent to UK and U.S. support groups. Some have reported association with congenital or open-angle glaucoma; however, the exact incidence is not known.[83] Although reports in the past argued the point of whether or not Wagner's disease and Stickler's syndrome are part of a continuum, the finding of a gene mutation in the procollagen II locus *(COL2A1)* on chromosome 12[84] separates patients with Stickler's syndrome.

20.3.4 Jansen's Disease

In 1961, Jansen[85] described an autosomal dominant disorder in the Netherlands and assumed that it was similar to the Wagner pedigree. Indeed, it is similar in all respects, with the exception of a very high incidence of retinal detachment. Its exact relationship to Wagner's disease is unknown but gene studies linked the original family to chromosome 5q14 where genes for Wagner's syndrome also reside.[86]

20.3.5 Autosomal Dominant Vitreoretinopathies

Autosomal Dominant Vitreoretinochoroidopathy

This disorder, as the name implies, is inherited in an autosomal dominant pattern and is associated with preretinal white opacities, retinal arteriolar narrowing and occlusion, diffuse vascular incompetence, CME, and cataracts.[87] It shares a gene with many other retinal dystrophies, the bestrophin gene on chromosome 11. In later stages, peripheral chorioretinal atrophy may be observed. The vitreous is fibrillar with some cells. The ERG is normal initially and shows a reduction in tandem with the degree of chorioretinal atrophy.

Autosomal Dominant Neovascular Inflammatory Vitreoretinopathy (ADNIV)

This disease, similar to ADVIRC, is mapped to chromosome 11 and is an adult-onset progressive disorder in which affected individuals exhibit noninfectious uveitis, early loss of the ERG b-wave, and pigmentary retinal degeneration with increasing severity with time.[88] Initially, the changes are seen in the retinal periphery, with closure of retinal vessels, some retinal pigmentation, and vitreous cells. With increasing age, the pigmentation becomes more prominent and spreads posteriorly, with associated RPE atrophy. Neovascularization of the disc and peripheral retina may occur and lead to vitreous hemorrhage and traction retinal detachment and may progress toward the appearance of phthisis bulbi. Patients can experience profound visual loss and further complications such as peripheral retinal scarring and neovascular glaucoma because of this.[88] The disease is thought to be an autoimmune, T-cell-mediated condition and does not seem to be related to antiretina antibody B-cell response.[89]

20.4 Congenital Stationary Night Blindness Disorders

The group of disorders known collectively as *congenital stationary night blindness* (CSNB) can often be confused with generalized forms of retinal degeneration. Making a differential diagnosis may prove difficult because the ERG is in some way abnormal in all types of CSNB. However, the nature of the ERG change and some characteristic clinical features will help distinguish each of the CSNB disorders from the hereditary retinal degenerations. In particular, the forms of CSNB with a normal fundus are simple to distinguish from other degenerations with classic retinal changes. Furthermore, the forms that demonstrate fundus findings are distinct because of their characteristic appearance. The visual impairment is much less severe than many forms of RP and patients only lose rod function, which affects their vision in low light conditions; their cone function remains relatively preserved.[90]

There are many forms of this disease with inheritance patterns spanning autosomal recessive, autosomal dominant, and X-linked recessive. These disorders can be divided into two groups: (1) those with a normal fundus appearance and (2) those with an abnormal fundus appearance (Oguchi's disease, fundus albipunctatus).

20.4.1 Congenital Stationary Night Blindness with Normal Fundi

The most common forms of congenital stationary night blindness (CSNB) and most true to the name are those with a normal fundus. The fundus is completely normal, as are the visual fields, two important findings that allow differentiation between CSNB and various types of RP. The dark-adaptation curves show an absent rod segment as there is partial or total absence of rods which is demonstrated clinically by the invariable presence of nyctalopia.

The X-linked form of the disease is most often caused by a mutation in the *NYX* gene on chromosome Xp11 and can be divided into two categories based on electroretinographic and clinical signs and symptoms. The first form, *Schubert–Bornschein*, has decreased b-wave to a greater degree than the a-wave, and clinically these patients have decreased vision and nystagmus (▶ Fig. 20.18). This is distinguished from *Riggs* where the vision is normal and there is an absence of nystagmus, and on ERG testing, the reduction of a- and b-waves is symmetric (▶ Fig. 20.19).[91] The autosomal dominant form has been mapped to the *GNAT* gene on chromosome 3, and is most famously described by the Nougaret family and is often referred to as the Nougaret subtype. The clinical features are similar to that of the *Riggs* form with normal acuity, visual fields, and fundus with poor night vision. Because of the confusion with various forms of disease, many classify the X-linked forms into complete (CSNB1) and incomplete (CSNB2). In CSNB1, there is complete absence of the rod response as compared to CSNB2 with slight preservation of rod function, usually demonstrated by a detectable a-wave. It can be separated clinically from rod monochromatism and LCA because of the normal fundus, including normal-sized retinal arterioles, and the classic negative waveform on ERG.

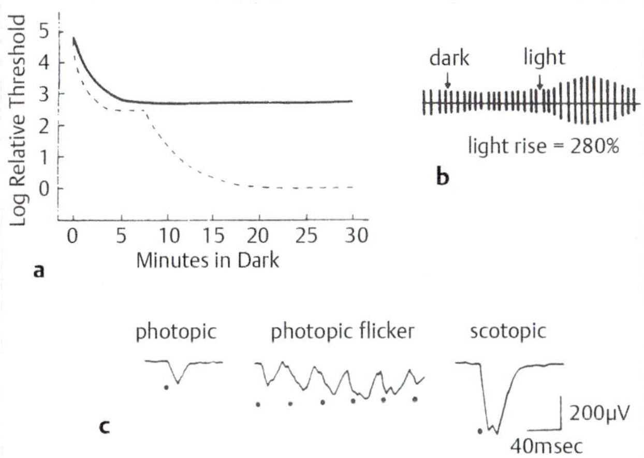

Fig. 20.18 Congenital stationary night blindness with normal fundus (type I): a 19-year-old man with poor night vision all his life. Visual acuity was 20/20 in each eye. (**a**) Dark-adaptation curve comparing the patient (solid line) with a normal subject (dashed line). The patient shows no evidence of a rod branch of the adaptation curve. The cone thresholds are slightly elevated. (**b**) Normal electro-oculogram light rise. (**c**) Electroretinogram shows only a negative (a-wave) response of normal amplitude, with no positive component.

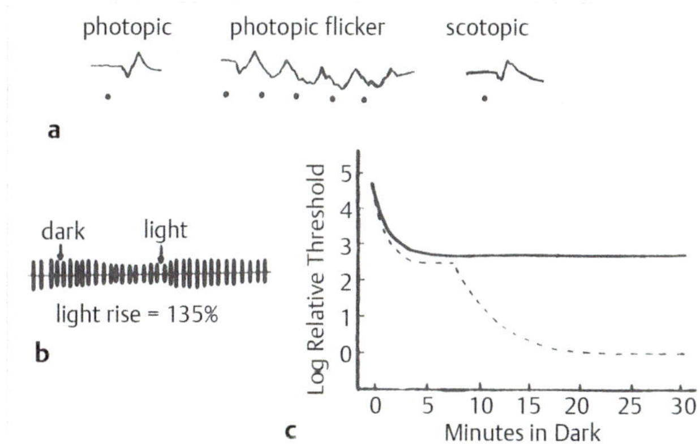

Fig. 20.19 Congenital stationary night blindness with normal fundus (type II). A 32-year-old woman reported poor night vision all her life. There is a family history of night blindness; her father and one sister, as well as one of her (affected) sister's sons, were similarly affected. (**a**) Electroretinogram shows a small, brisk response under photopic conditions that remains unchanged in the dark. (**b**) Electro-oculogram shows an abnormal light rise. (**c**) Patient's dark-adaptation data (solid line) show no evidence of rod adaptation compared with those of the normal subject (dashed line). The cone thresholds are slightly elevated.

In vivo measurements of rhodopsin in both CSNB1 and CSNB2 have shown that the amount of rhodopsin and the speed at which it regenerates after being bleached away are normal.[91] Thus, the concept that the defect in this condition either is postreceptoral (type I) or involves some membrane property of the receptor (type II) is strongly reinforced.

20.4.2 Congenital Stationary Night Blindness with Abnormal Fundi

There are two forms of CSNB with abnormal fundi: *Oguchi's disease* and *fundus albipunctatus*. Associated with each condition are unique fundus alterations that are almost unequivocal diagnostic indicators.[91]

The first type of CSNB with distinctive retinal changes is fundus albipunctatus (▶ Fig. 20.20). This can be inherited in an autosomal dominant or recessive pattern and has a fundus appearance similar to that of Bietti's crystalline dystrophy. This form of CSNB is often confused with the progressive, generalized degeneration with scattered white deposits in RP, formerly known as retinitis punctata albescens. However, the visual fields and retinal arterioles are normal in fundus albipunctatus but not in retinitis punctata albescens. Nonetheless, one should be aware that unless the patient with fundus albipunctatus is given sufficient time to dark-adapt, ERG recordings may appear very diminished. In fact, the major diagnostic finding in fundus albipunctatus is the very slow adaptation properties of the rods and cones. ▶ Fig. 20.21 shows that it may take longer than 1 hour for the cone system to reach normal thresholds, and the rod thresholds may stay elevated for as long as 2 to 3 hours before eventually attaining normal levels.[92] Fundus albipunctatus is unlike any other form of CSNB in that the slow recovery of sensitivity, as well as the prolonged period of darkness required to obtain normal ERGs and EOGs, goes hand in hand with retarded rod and cone photopigment regeneration.[2]

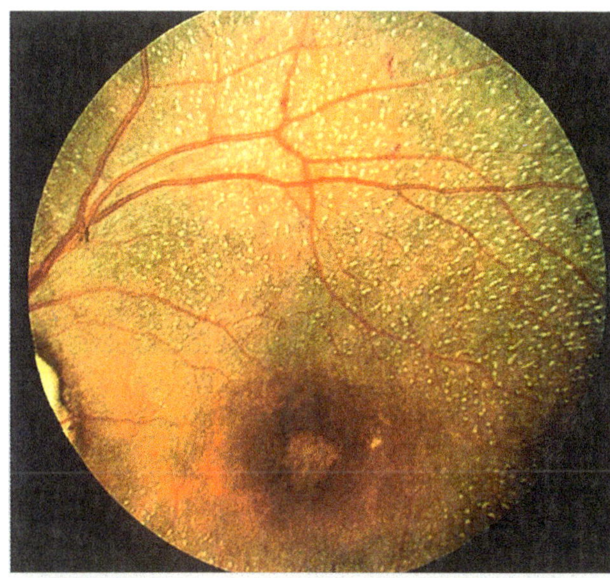

Fig. 20.20 Fundus albipunctatus in a 23-year-old woman: Multiple small, yellow-white spots are present throughout retina. Vision is 20/20 in each eye.

In the second type, *Oguchi's disease* (▶ Fig. 20.22), the retina has a peculiar silvery metallic sheen, with the retinal vessels standing out in marked contrast against this reflective background. This is a rare disease, inherited in an autosomal recessive pattern, which has been localized to the rhodopsin kinase gene on chromosome 13. This unusual picture can be seen throughout the retina or may be found only in the posterior pole or the periphery. Such striking retinal changes should of themselves provide a sufficient clue to the diagnosis, but several other findings should also be noted. For example, the retinal sheen in Oguchi's disease may disappear if the eye is kept in total darkness for about 3 hours (*Mizuo–Nakamura*

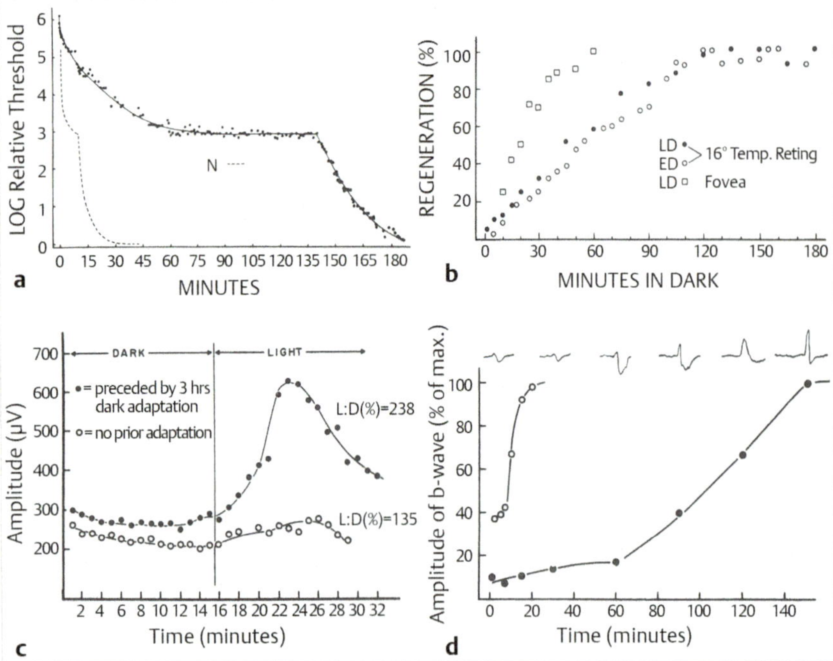

Fig. 20.21 Fundus albipunctatus in a 34-year-old man whose brother is similarly affected. Vision is 20/20 in each eye. **(a)** Dark adaptation. Normal (N) is dashed line. Note the slow fall to normal levels of both cones and rods. **(b)** Fundus reflectometry at the fovea and in the periphery. There is a marked delay in regeneration of the cones (normal half-time is about 55 seconds) and rods (normal half-time is about 4 minutes). In this patient, the half-time for the cones was 25 minutes and for the rods 60 minutes. **(c)** Electro-oculogram findings. When the dark testing cycle is only 15 minutes, there is no true light rise, only baseline fluctuations. When the dark cycle is increased to 3 hours, the light rise is normal. **(d)** Electroretinogram shows dark-adapted, low-intensity white flash. Open circles show that the rise to near-maximum amplitude in a normal person occurs within 30 minutes. The patient shows almost no change for 60 minutes and then a slow rise to a normal amplitude. Electroretinogram records during the course of adaptation are noted on top.

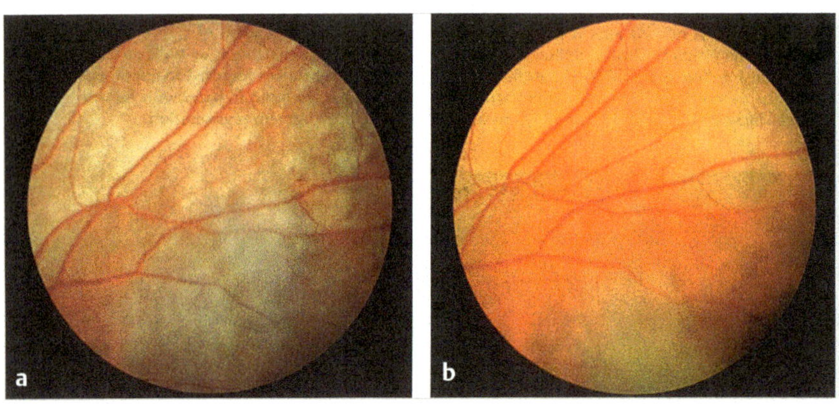

Fig. 20.22 Oguchi's disease. A 29-year-old man has had problems with dark adaptation all his life. He did, however, note that after prolonged periods in the dark, his sensitivity seemed as good as that of other people. A brother is similarly affected. **(a)** Appearance of the retina following light adaptation. There is a metallic sheen to the entirety of the retina; the retinal vessels stand out in dark relief against this unusual background. **(b)** Same area of the retina following 3 hours in the dark; the metallic reflex is gone and this same area now appears normal.

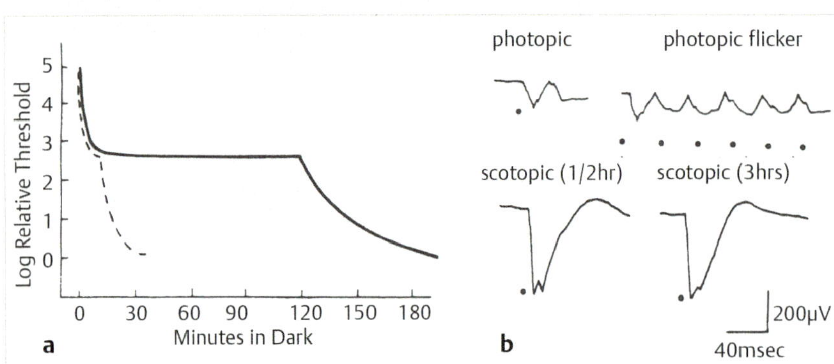

Fig. 20.23 Oguchi's disease. **(a)** Recovery of dark adaptation was followed for 180 minutes (note the compressed time scale on the abscissa). The cone system of the patient quickly attains normal sensitivity levels (normal curve shown by dashed lines) but remains at that level for up to 2 hours. The rod system finally intrudes at the 2-hour mark, and after another hour, normal thresholds are recorded. **(b)** Electroretinogram showing a normal-amplitude a-wave and a reduced b-wave under scotopic conditions. There is little change in the waveform, even after 3 hours of adaptation.

phenomenon). Even more important is the fact that the dark-adapted thresholds, which rapidly reach normal cone levels, remain on the cone plateau for about 2 hours and then require 3 or more hours of darkness to return to normal dark-adapted levels.[2] There is no known association between the slow rate of rod adaptation and the fundus coloration changes wrought by darkness. However, in a study looking at OCT imaging of patients with Oguchi's disease, there is an absence of the inner segment/outer segment line in the light-adapted or partially dark-adapted macula that emerges after prolonged dark adaptation, suggesting that the microarchitecture of the rod photoreceptors changes with improvement in function.[93] As shown in ▶ Fig. 20.23, both photopic and scotopic ERGs have an abnormal appearance, similar to that of the negative-type ERG obtained in patients with type I CSNB with normal fundus. Interestingly, even after the dark-adapted thresholds have returned to normal levels, the ERG b-wave may still be absent. Oguchi's disease, like all the forms of CSNB discussed thus far, shows rhodopsin in normal amounts and with normal photopigment kinetics, an indication that some form of malfunction within the phototransduction cascade is responsible for this prolonged return of rod sensitivity.

Pearls

- In fundus albipunctatus, standard psychophysical and electrophysiologic tests show abnormalities, but results become normal after prolonged dark adaptation. In contrast, these tests do not ever normalize in progressive retinal degenerations.

References

[1] Hartong DT, Berson EL, Dryja TP. Retinitis pigmentosa. Lancet. 2006; 368 (9549):1795–1809

[2] Lam BL. Electrophysiology of Vision. Boca Raton, FL: Taylor & Francis; 2005

[3] Drusen GS. Arch Ophthalmol. 1985; 103(9):1283

[4] Novack RL, Foos RY. Drusen of the optic disk in retinitis pigmentosa. Am J Ophthalmol. 1987; 103(1):44–47

[5] Yoon CK, Yu HG. The structure-function relationship between macular morphology and visual function analyzed by optical coherence tomography in retinitis pigmentosa. J Ophthalmol. 2013; 2013:821460

[6] Szlyk JP, Fishman GA, Alexander KR, Peachey NS, Derlacki DJ. Clinical subtypes of cone-rod dystrophy. Arch Ophthalmol. 1993; 111(6):781–788

[7] Berson EL, Rosen JB, Simonoff EA. Electroretinographic testing as an aid in detection of carriers of X-chromosome-linked retinitis pigmentosa. Am J Ophthalmol. 1979; 87(4):460–468

[8] Ikeda Y, Yoshida N, Notomi S, et al. Therapeutic effect of prolonged treatment with topical dorzolamide for cystoid macular oedema in patients with retinitis pigmentosa. Br J Ophthalmol. 2013; 97(9):1187–1191

[9] Salvatore S, Fishman GA, Genead MA. Treatment of cystic macular lesions in hereditary retinal dystrophies. Surv Ophthalmol. 2013; 58(6):560–584

[10] Pacella E, Arrico L, Santamaria V, et al. Dorzolamide chlorhydrate versus acetazolamide in the management of chronic macular edema in patients with retinitis pigmentosa: description of three case reports. Ophthalmol Eye Dis. 2014; 6:21–26

[11] Genead MA, Fishman GA. Efficacy of sustained topical dorzolamide therapy for cystic macular lesions in patients with retinitis pigmentosa and usher syndrome. Arch Ophthalmol. 2010; 128(9):1146–1150

[12] Thobani A, Fishman GA. The use of carbonic anhydrase inhibitors in the retreatment of cystic macular lesions in retinitis pigmentosa and X-linked retinoschisis. Retina. 2011; 31(2):312–315

[13] Dikopf MS, Chow CC, Mieler WF, Tu EY. Cataract extraction outcomes and the prevalence of zonular insufficiency in retinitis pigmentosa. Am J Ophthalmol. 2013; 156(1):82–88.e2

[14] Berson EL, Rosner B, Sandberg MA, et al. A randomized trial of vitamin A and vitamin E supplementation for retinitis pigmentosa. Arch Ophthalmol. 1993; 111(6):761–772

[15] Fielder AR. A randomized trial of vitamin A and vitamin E supplementation for retinitis pigmentosa. Arch Ophthalmol. 1993; 111(11):1463–, author reply 1463–1466

[16] Wheaton DH, Hoffman DR, Locke KG, Watkins RB, Birch DG. Biological safety assessment of docosahexaenoic acid supplementation in a randomized clinical trial for X-linked retinitis pigmentosa. Arch Ophthalmol. 2003; 121 (9):1269–1278

[17] Rayapudi S, Schwartz SG, Wang X, Chavis P. Vitamin A and fish oils for retinitis pigmentosa. Cochrane Database Syst Rev. 2013; 12:CD008428

[18] FDA. FDA approves first retinal implant for adults with rare genetic eye disease. FDA News Release 2013. Available online at: http://www.fda.gov/NewsEvents/Newsroom/PressAnnouncements/ucm339824.htm (Accessed September 1, 2014)

[19] Bateman JB, Lang GE, Maumenee IH. Multisystem genetic disorders associated with retinal dystrophies. In: Ryan SJ, ed. Retina. 2nd ed. Vol. 1. St. Louis, MO: Mosby; 1994:467–491

[20] Merin S, Abraham FA, Auerbach E. Usher's and Hallgren's syndromes. Acta Genet Med Gemellol (Roma). 1974; 23:49–55

[21] Williams DS. Usher syndrome: animal models, retinal function of Usher proteins, and prospects for gene therapy. Vision Res. 2008; 48(3):433–441

[22] Pakarinen L, Karjalainen S, Simola KO, Laippala P, Kaitalo H. Usher's syndrome type 3 in Finland. Laryngoscope. 1995; 105(6):613–617

[23] Fraser GR. Profound childhood deafness. J Med Genet. 1964; 1(2):118–151

[24] Boughman JA, Vernon M, Shaver KA. Usher syndrome: definition and estimate of prevalence from two high-risk populations. J Chronic Dis. 1983; 36 (8):595–603

[25] Bardet G. On congenital obesity syndrome with polydactyly and retinitis pigmentosa (a contribution to the study of clinical forms of hypophyseal obesity). 1920. Obes Res. 1995; 3(4):387–399

[26] Biedl A. A pair of siblings with adiposo-genital dystrophy. 1922. Obes Res. 1995; 3(4):404

[27] Laurence JZ, Moon RC. Four cases of "retinitis pigmentosa" occurring in the same family, and accompanied by general imperfections of development. Ophthal Rev. 1866; 2:32–41

[28] Bocchini CA. Laurence-Moon Syndrome.NMS. Online Mendelian Inheritance in Man. Johns Hopkins University. Mar 2015. Web. 5 May 2015

[29] Bauman ML, Hogan GR. Laurence-Moon-Biedl syndrome. Report of two unrelated children less than 3 years of age. Am J Dis Child. 1973; 126(1):119–126

[30] Zeman W. The certoid lipofuscinoses. In: Zimmerman HM, ed. Progress in Neuropathology. Vol. 3. New York, NY: Grune & Stratton; 1976:203–223

[31] Zeman W. Batten disease: ocular features, differential diagnosis and diagnosis by enzyme analysis. In: Bergsma D, Bron AJ, Cotlier E, eds. The Eye and Inborn Errors of Metabolism. New York, NY: Alan R Liss; 1976:441–453

[32] Garg HS, Awasthi YC, Srivastava SK. Studies in neuronal ceroid-lipofuscinosis: heterogeneous nature of neuronal autofluorescent lipopigments. J Neurosci Res. 1981; 6(6):771–783

[33] Arsenio-Nunes ML, Goutières F, Aicardi J. An ultramicroscopic study of skin and conjunctival biopsies in chronic neurological disorders of childhood. Ann Neurol. 1981; 9(2):163–173

[34] Bassen FA, Kornzweig AL. Malformation of the erythrocytes in a case of atypical retinitis pigmentosa. Blood. 1950; 5(4):381–387

[35] Salt HB, Wolff OH, Lloyd JK, Fosbrooke AS, Cameron AH, Hubble DV. On having no beta-lipoprotein. A syndrome comprising a-beta-lipoproteinaemia, acanthocytosis, and steatorrhoea. Lancet. 1960; 2(7146):325–329

[36] Gotto AM, Levy RI, John K, Fredrickson DS. On the protein defect in abetalipoproteinemia. N Engl J Med. 1971; 284(15):813–818

[37] Zamel R, Khan R, Pollex RL, Hegele RA. Abetalipoproteinemia: two case reports and literature review. Orphanet J Rare Dis. 2008; 3:19

[38] Gouras P, Carr RE, Gunkel RD. Retinitis pigmentosa in abetalipoproteinemia: effects of vitamin A. Invest Ophthalmol. 1971; 10(10):784–793

[39] Runge P, Muller DP, McAllister J, Calver D, Lloyd JK, Taylor D. Oral vitamin E supplements can prevent the retinopathy of abetalipoproteinaemia. Br J Ophthalmol. 1986; 70(3):166–173

[40] Refsum S. Heredopathia atactica polyneuritiformis phytanic-acid storage disease, Refsum's disease:" a biochemically well-defined disease with a specific dietary treatment. Arch Neurol. 1981; 38(10):605–606

[41] Richterich R, Kahlke W, Rossi E, van Mechelen P. Refsum's syndrome (heredopathia atactica polyneuritiformis): congenital disorder of lipid metabolism with storage of 3,7,11,15-tetramethyl-hexadecanoic acid [in German]. Klin Wochenschr. 1963; 41:800–801

[42] Baum JL, Tannenbaum M, Kolodny EH. Refsum's syndrome with corneal involvement. Am J Ophthalmol. 1965; 60(4):699–708

[43] Eldjarn L, Try K, Stokke O, et al. Dietary effects on serum-phytanic-acid levels and on clinical manifestations in heredopathia atactica polyneuritiformis. Lancet. 1966; 1(7439):691–693

[44] Grant CA, Berson EL. Treatable forms of retinitis pigmentosa associated with systemic neurological disorders. Int Ophthalmol Clin. 2001; 41(1):103–110

[45] Weleber RG, Tongue AC, Kennaway NG, Budden SS, Buist NR. Ophthalmic manifestations of infantile phytanic acid storage disease. Arch Ophthalmol. 1984; 102(9):1317–1321

[46] Mullie MA, Harding AE, Petty RK, Ikeda H, Morgan-Hughes JA, Sanders MD. The retinal manifestations of mitochondrial myopathy. A study of 22 cases. Arch Ophthalmol. 1985; 103(12):1825–1830

[47] Kearns TP, Sayre GP. Retinitis pigmentosa, external ophthalmophegia, and complete heart block: unusual syndrome with histologic study in one of two cases. AMA Arch Opthalmol. 1958; 60(2):280–289

[48] Kearns TP. External ophthalmoplegia, pigmentary degeneration of the retina, and cardiomyopathy: a newly recognized syndrome. Trans Am Ophthalmol Soc. 1965; 63:559–625

[49] Phadke M, Lokeshwar MR, Bhutada S, et al. Kearns Sayre Syndrome—case report with review of literature. Indian J Pediatr. 2012; 79(5):650–654

[50] Leber T. Uber retinitis pigmentosa und angeboren Amaurose. Albrecht Von Graefes Arch Klin Exp Ophthalmol.. 1869; 15:1–25

[51] Cideciyan AV. Leber congenital amaurosis due to RPE65 mutations and its treatment with gene therapy. Prog Retin Eye Res. 2010; 29(5):398–427

[52] Zeman W. The neuronal ceroid lipofuscinoses. In: Zimmerman HM, ed. Progress in Neuropathology. Vol. 3. New York, NY: Grune & Stratton; 1976:203–223

[53] Carr RE. Familial juvenile nephronophthisis. In: Gold DH, Weingeist TA, eds. The Eye in Systemic Disease. Philadelphia, PA: JB Lippincott; 1990:502–504

[54] Cideciyan AV, Jacobson SG, Beltran WA, et al. Human retinal gene therapy for Leber congenital amaurosis shows advancing retinal degeneration despite enduring visual improvement. Proc Natl Acad Sci U S A. 2013; 110(6):E517–E525

[55] Heckenlively JR. Preserved para-arteriole retinal pigment epithelium (PPRPE) in retinitis pigmentosa. Br J Ophthalmol. 1982; 66(1):26–30

[56] van den Born LI, van Soest S, van Schooneveld MJ, Riemslag FC, de Jong PT, Bleeker-Wagemakers EM. Autosomal recessive retinitis pigmentosa with preserved para-arteriolar retinal pigment epithelium. Am J Ophthalmol. 1994; 118(4):430–439

[57] Jacobson SG, Marmor MF, Kemp CM, Knighton RW. SWS (blue) cone hypersensitivity in a newly identified retinal degeneration. Invest Ophthalmol Vis Sci. 1990; 31(5):827–838

[58] Hull S, Arno G, Sergouniotis PI, et al. Clinical and molecular characterization of enhanced S-cone syndrome in children. JAMA Ophthalmol. 2014; 132 (11):1341–1349

[59] Lenassi E, Jarc-Vidmar M, Glavac D, Hawlina M. Pattern electroretinography of larger stimulus field size and spectral-domain optical coherence tomography in patients with Stargardt disease. Br J Ophthalmol. 2009; 93(12):1600–1605

[60] Schwartz SD, Regillo CD, Lam BL, et al. Human embryonic stem cell-derived retinal pigment epithelium in patients with age-related macular degeneration and Stargardt's macular dystrophy: follow-up of two open-label phase 1/2 studies. Lancet. 2015; 385(9967):509–516

[61] Mauthner L. Ein Fall von Choroideremia. Berd Naturw Med Ver Innsbruch. 1871; 2:191

[62] McCulloch C, McCulloch RJ. A hereditary and clinical study of choroideremia. Trans Am Acad Ophthalmol Otolaryngol. 1948; 52:160–190

[63] Kurstjens IH. Choroideremia and gyrate atrophy of the choroid and retina. Doc Ophthalmol. 1965; 19:1–122

[64] Kaur S, Sachdev N. Ocular coherence tomography findings in a case of choroideremia. Int Ophthalmol. 2014; 34(2):297–299

[65] Goodman G, Ripps H, Siegel IM. Sex-linked ocular disorders: trait expressivity in males and carrier females. Arch Ophthalmol. 1965; 73:387–398

[66] Noble KG, Carr RE, Siegel IM. Fluorescein angiography of the hereditary choroidal dystrophies. Br J Ophthalmol. 1977; 61(1):43–53

[67] Black A, Vasireddy V, Chung DC, et al. Adeno-associated virus 8-mediated gene therapy for choroideremia: preclinical studies in in vitro and in vivo models. J Gene Med. 2014; 16(5–6):122–130

[68] Kaiser-Kupfer MI, Ludwig IH, de Monasterio FM, Valle D, Krieger I. Gyrate atrophy of the choroid and retina. Early findings. Ophthalmology. 1985; 92 (3):394–401

[69] Simell O, Takki K. Raised plasma-ornithine and gyrate atrophy of the choroid and retina. Lancet. 1973; 1(7811):1031–1033

[70] Valle D, Kaiser-Kupfer MI, Del Valle LA. Gyrate atrophy of the choroid and retina: deficiency of ornithine aminotransferase in transformed lymphocytes. Proc Natl Acad Sci U S A. 1977; 74(11):5159–5161

[71] Akaki Y, Hotta Y, Mashima Y, et al. A deletion in the ornithine aminotransferase gene in gyrate atrophy. J Biol Chem. 1992; 267(18):12950–12954

[72] McCulloch C, Marliss EB. Gyrate atrophy of the choroid and retina: clinical, ophthalmologic, and biochemical considerations. Trans Am Ophthalmol Soc. 1975; 73:153–171

[73] Weleber RG, Kennaway NG, Buist NR. Vitamin B6 in management of gyrate atrophy of choroid and retina. Lancet. 1978; 2(8101):1213

[74] Kaiser-Kupfer MI, de Monasterio FM, Valle D, Walser M, Brusilow S. Gyrate atrophy of the choroid and retina: improved visual function following reduction of plasma ornithine by diet. Science. 1980; 210(4474):1128–1131

[75] Hayasaka S, Saito T, Nakajima H, Takahashi O, Mizuno K, Tada K. Clinical trials of vitamin B6 and proline supplementation for gyrate atrophy of the choroid and retina. Br J Ophthalmol. 1985; 69(4):283–290

[76] Kaiser-Kupfer MI, de Monasterio F, Valle D, Walser M, Brusilow S. Visual results of a long-term trial of a low-arginine diet in gyrate atrophy of choroid and retina. Ophthalmology. 1981; 88(4):307–310

[77] Berson EL, Shih VE, Sullivan PL. Ocular findings in patients with gyrate atrophy on pyridoxine and low-protein, low-arginine diets. Ophthalmology. 1981; 88(4):311–315

[78] Bietti GB. Uber familiares Vorkommen von "retinitis punctata albescens" (verbunden mit "Dystrophia marginalis cristalinea carnes."), Glitzern des Glasköpers und anderen degenerativen Augenveranderungen. Klin Monatsbl Augenheilkd. 1937; 99:737–756

[79] Traboulsi EI, Faris BM. Crystalline retinopathy. Ann Ophthalmol. 1987; 19 (4):156–158

[80] Wagner H. Ein bisher unbekanntes Erbleiden des Auges (Degeneration hyaloideoretinalis hereditaria), beobachtet in Kanton Zurich. Klin Monatsbl Augenheilkd. 1938; 100:840–857

[81] Stickler GB, Belau PG, Farrell FJ, et al. Hereditary progressive arthro-ophthalmopathy. Mayo Clin Proc. 1965; 40:433–455

[82] Weingeist TA, Hermsen V, Hanson JW, Bumsted RM, Weinstein SL, Olin WH. Ocular and systemic manifestations of Stickler's syndrome: a preliminary report. Birth Defects Orig Artic Ser. 1982; 18(6):539–560

[83] Stickler GB, Hughes W, Houchin P. Clinical features of hereditary progressive arthro-ophthalmopathy (Stickler syndrome): a survey. Genet Med. 2001; 3 (3):192–196

[84] Brown DM, Nichols BE, Weingeist TA, Sheffield VC, Kimura AE, Stone EM. Procollagen II gene mutation in Stickler syndrome. Arch Ophthalmol. 1992; 110 (11):1589–1593

[85] Jansen LM. Degeneratio hyaloideo-retinalis herditaria. Ophthalmologica. 1962; 144:458–464

[86] Ryan SJ, Schachat AP, Wilkinson CP, Hinton DR, Sadda SR, Wiedermann P. Chromosome 5q retinopathies. Retina. 5th ed. Philidelphia: Elsevier; 2013:840–842.

[87] Kaufman SJ, Goldberg MF, Orth DH, Fishman GA, Tessler H, Mizuno K. Autosomal dominant vitreoretinochoroidopathy. Arch Ophthalmol. 1982; 100 (2):272–278

[88] Bennett SR, Folk JC, Kimura AE, Russell SR, Stone EM, Raphtis EM. Autosomal dominant neovascular inflammatory vitreoretinopathy. Ophthalmology. 1990; 97(9):1125–1135, discussion 1135–1136

[89] Mahajan VB, Vallone JG, Lin JH, et al. T-cell infiltration in autosomal dominant neovascular inflammatory vitreoretinopathy. Mol Vis. 2010; 16:1034–1040

[90] McAlear SD, Kraft TW, Gross AK. 1 rhodopsin mutations in congenital night blindness. Adv Exp Med Biol. 2010; 664:263–272

[91] Carr RE. Congenital stationary nightblindness. Trans Am Ophthalmol Soc. 1974; 72:448–487

[92] Carr RE, Ripps H, Siegel IM, Weale RA. Rhodopsin and the electrical activity of the retina in congenital night blindness. Invest Ophthalmol. 1966; 5(5):497–507

[93] Yamada K, Motomura Y, Matsumoto CS, Shinoda K, Nakatsuka K. Optical coherence tomographic evaluation of the outer retinal architecture in Oguchi disease. Jpn J Ophthalmol. 2009; 53(5):449–451

21 Sickle Retinopathy

Royce W. S. Chen, Harry W. Flynn Jr., Sharon Fekrat, and Morton F. Goldberg

21.1 Sickle Cell Hemoglobinopathies

Sickle cell hemoglobinopathies originated in Central and West Africa. They have since become the most common hemoglobinopathy affecting humans and are now found throughout the world, including North America (▶ Table 21.1) and Mediterranean countries, such as Italy, Greece, Saudi Arabia, and Israel.

Of those individuals with sickle hemoglobinopathies, proliferative retinopathy occurs in about 45% with sickle cell hemoglobin C disease (SC), 17% with sickle thalassemia hemoglobinopathy (SThal), and 14% with sickle cell disease (SS) (▶ Table 21.1).[1] In individuals with sickle cell trait (AS) and hemoglobin C trait (AC), proliferative retinopathy may also develop; however, the incidence is likely to be very low.[2,3] The incidence of proliferative disease associated with homozygous hemoglobin C (CC) is not known. The development of proliferative disease is not only genotype dependent but also age dependent. In some eyes, proliferative sickle cell retinopathy may be clinically detectable in the first 10 years of life, but it is most likely to become manifest between 15 and 30 years of age.[4] The greatest risk of proliferative sickle cell retinopathy in individuals with SC is between 20 and 34 years of age, and in individuals with SS is between 40 and 50 years of age.

21.2 Pathogenesis and Genetics

In the erythrocytes of healthy individuals, hemoglobin A possesses two alpha and two beta polypeptide chains, each with a ferroprotoporphyrin heme ring. The two alpha genes, located on chromosome 16, and the one beta gene, located on chromosome 11, encode these chains.

The word *hemoglobinopathy* refers to those diseases associated with structurally abnormal hemoglobin. In persons with sickle cell hemoglobinopathies, hemoglobin A is abnormal; the glutamic acid residue, in at least one of the beta polypeptide chains, is replaced by either valine to form hemoglobin S or lysine to form hemoglobin C. When this abnormal hemoglobin occurs in combination with normal hemoglobin A or abnormal hemoglobin S or C, a variety of sickle cell hemoglobinopathies may develop (▶ Table 21.1). A thalassemia may result when there is an inadequate rate of synthesis of either the alpha or beta chain; an SThal hemoglobinopathy is diagnosed when sickle hemoglobin is also present.

Table 21.1 Prevalence of sickle hemoglobinopathies in North America

Hemoglobinopathy	Prevalence (%)	Proliferative retinopathy (%)
Any sickle hemoglobin	10	N/A
Sickle cell trait (AS)	8	Uncommon
Hemoglobin C trait (AC)	2	Uncommon
Sickle cell homozygote (SS)	0.4	14[a]
Sickle cell hemoglobin C (SC)	0.2	45[a]
Sickle cell thalassemia (SThal)	0.03	17[a]
Homozygous C (CC)	0.016	Unknown

[a]Approximate.

When an erythrocyte with abnormal hemoglobin is exposed to hypoxic, acidotic, or hyperosmolar conditions, it may assume a sickle shape. The sickled red blood cell is less pliable than a normal erythrocyte. Consequently, blood viscosity increases, and vasoocclusive events may occur. Vasoocclusion in the peripheral retinal vasculature initiates the cascade of events in proliferative sickle cell retinopathy that may culminate in vitreous hemorrhage or retinal detachment.

Pearls

- Vasoocclusion in the peripheral retinal vasculature initiates the cascade of events in proliferative sickle cell retinopathy that may culminate in vitreous hemorrhage or retinal detachment.

Individuals with larger quantities of abnormal hemoglobin in their red blood cells and a greater likelihood for the abnormal hemoglobin to sickle under less than ideal conditions may be more likely to have systemic manifestations of the disease.[5] Systemic morbidity is greater in SS homozygotes than in persons with other hemoglobinopathies; this may be partly attributed to the high concentration (more than 90%) of hemoglobin S within the red blood cells of these patients. Intravascular sickling may develop in the microvascular circulations of subjects with SS disease, leading to erythrocyte sludging, hemolysis, shorter survival, and anemia despite increased red blood cell synthesis. Repeated infarcts of the bone marrow may lead to bony sclerosis and trabeculation, demonstrated on skull, vertebral, and long-bone X-ray films, as well as aseptic necrosis of the femoral head. Sickling in precapillary arterioles may lead to abdominal discomfort, pulmonary infarcts, joint aches, and strokes.

Systemic findings are less common in individuals with SC, SThal, and AS hemoglobinopathies. SC and SThal heterozygotes usually have a mild or unremarkable systemic course with very few crises annually and a slightly depressed hematocrit level. Despite minimal systemic manifestations, however, patients with SC and SThal are more likely than patients with SS to have retinal manifestations of their disease (▶ Table 21.1). The discrepancy between the severity of systemic and retinal findings in the various hemoglobinopathies is not well understood. The AS heterozygote rarely suffers either systemic or retinal morbidity, except under severe hypoxic stress, because only about half of the hemoglobin is abnormal. Nevertheless, in the AS heterozygote, a hyphema may result in ocular morbidity that may be just as severe as in the eyes of patients with other hemoglobinopathies.[6]

Special Considerations

- Even though an AS heterozygote may rarely suffer systemic or retinal morbidity, a hyphema may result in serious ocular complications that may be just as severe as in the eyes of patients with other hemoglobinopathies.

Proliferative sickle cell retinopathy is more likely to develop in individuals with SC and SThal hemoglobinopathies than in those with other hemoglobinopathies, and an explanation for this has not been well documented. The sickling rate, blood viscosity, and hematocrit are interrelated variables that are believed to be important in the pathogenesis of sickle retinopathy.[5,7] Erythrocyte sickling tends to occur when red blood cells with sickle hemoglobin encounter relatively acidotic, deoxygenated, or hyperosmolar environments. The decreased pliability of sickled cells hinders effective circulation through the microvascular network, leading to increased blood viscosity. In the retinal microvasculature, blood viscosity is determined largely by the red blood cell concentration. Therefore, an even higher viscosity results when individuals with higher hematocrits have a sickling episode; this contributes to additional vasoocclusions. For example, the hematocrit in SC and SThal heterozygotes is significantly higher than in SS patients. Consequently, SC or SThal heterozygotes have a higher blood viscosity than SS patients and, therefore, may be subject to a greater number of vasoocclusive events in the retinal microvasculature, where erythrocyte characteristics play a pivotal role. Even though SS individuals have an increased number of sickled erythrocytes, the lower hematocrit, and presumably lower viscosity, may offer relative protection against the occurrence of vasoocclusive events in the retinal vasculature.

21.3 Clinical Features and Histopathology

Sickling of red blood cells may occur in any microvascular system of the eye. The various signs and symptoms along with any effect on the visual outcome depend on the anatomic location of the vasoocclusive event.

Anteriorly, microvascular occlusions in the bulbar conjunctiva produce various clinically evident small-vessel irregularities. Among them is the classic *comma sign*. The presence of these comma-shaped vascular segments, although not pathognomonic for sickle cell disease, can be a useful diagnostic finding.[8] In general, conjunctival vascular changes are seen in about 70% of SS, 34% of SC, and 17% of SThal patients.[8] They are completely asymptomatic.

Occlusions of iris vessels can also occur. Clinically, these typically present as asymptomatic, white, atrophic patches on the iris surface. If extensive, there can be pupillary irregularity.

Pearls

- Vasoocclusive events in the bulbar conjunctival vasculature produce the characteristic *comma sign*, a subtle but potentially useful diagnostic finding.

The presence of a hyphema, surgical or traumatic in nature, has special significance in a patient with any type of sickle hemoglobinopathy.[6] In general, there is greater potential for ocular damage with a hyphema in these eyes than in eyes of individuals without sickle cell disease. This is mainly because the relatively low oxygenation and high ascorbate levels of the anterior chamber promote sickling. Compared with normal red blood cells, sickled cells are more prone to block aqueous outflow through the trabecular meshwork and lead to higher increases in intraocular pressure. Furthermore, blood flow through the central retinal artery and to the optic nerve may be more likely to be compromised for a given level of increased intraocular pressure in patients with sickle cell disease. Therefore, the intraocular pressure must be monitored closely and not allowed to remain higher than about 24 mm Hg for longer than 24 hours.[6] If intraocular pressure control is not adequate with medical management, surgical intervention to evacuate the hyphema and quickly lower the eye pressure is needed. Of note is that it is best to avoid repetitive use of carbonic anhydrase inhibitors, particularly acetazolamide, and osmotic agents in this setting, as they may promote sickling by causing acidosis and hemoconcentration.

Posteriorly, the retinal findings are most important and may be subdivided into nonproliferative and proliferative manifestations. Related nonproliferative changes include abnormalities of the optic nerve head, macula, choroid, and vitreoretinal interface, all of which are detailed in the following paragraphs.

21.3.1 Nonproliferative Manifestations

Salmon patch hemorrhages, iridescent spots, and black sunburst lesions characterize nonproliferative or background sickle cell retinopathy. These three manifestations may be pathogenetically related.

Salmon Patch Hemorrhage

A salmon patch hemorrhage is an oval-shaped aggregation of superficial intraretinal or preretinal blood. Such patches are usually found next to medium-sized retinal arterioles in the equatorial retina and may be up to one disc diameter in size.[9] They have well-demarcated boundaries and a dome-shaped or flattened appearance. They initially appear red in color, but after several days often take on a more pink or orange (salmon-colored) tint (▶ Fig. 21.1). The hemorrhages usually remain localized on or within the retina, but they can extend into either the subretinal space or vitreous cavity. Unless blood breaks through into the vitreous cavity, the hemorrhages are usually asymptomatic. Sudden arteriolar occlusion by sickled red blood cells with later rupture of the arteriole is thought to be the mechanism of salmon patch formation.

Iridescent Spots

As the salmon patch hemorrhage resolves, the retina may return to normal. In some cases, however, a faint dip or depression develops in the area of the hemorrhage after it resorbs. In others, particularly those with a significant intraretinal component, a small retinoschisis cavity containing yellowish spots may form M. These glistening specks have been referred to as

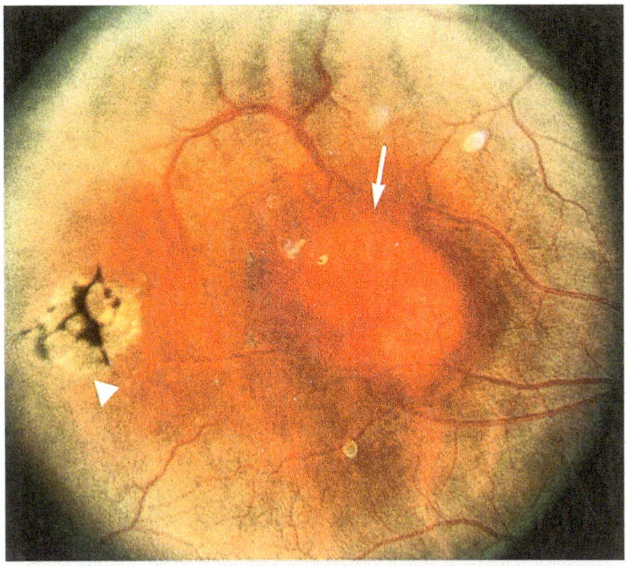

Fig. 21.1 A salmon patch hemorrhage with the distinct pink-orange coloration (arrow), and a black sunburst lesion (arrowhead) with characteristic spiculated or stellate borders from perivascular pigment accumulation.

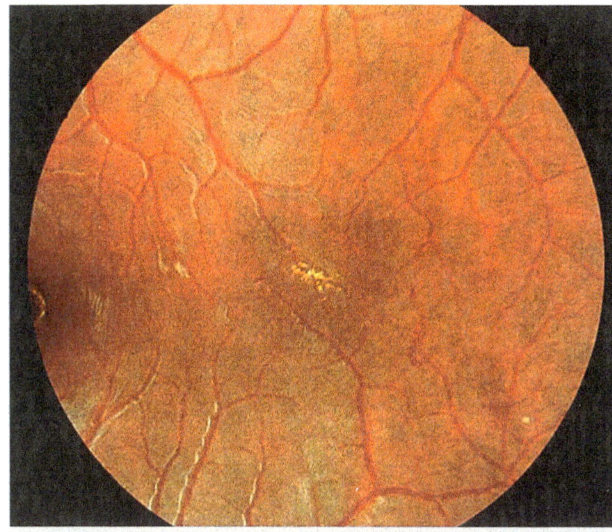

Fig. 21.2 Iridescent spots in a localized small retinoschisis cavity, both of which presumably formed after resorption of an intraretinal salmon patch hemorrhage.

iridescent spots and represent multiple hemosiderin-laden macrophages (▶ Fig. 21.2).[10] The reported incidence varies within the literature, but such schisis cavities have been found in up to 33% of SC, 18% of SThal, and 13% of SS individuals.[2,7,11,12] Histopathologically, the schisis space is lined posteriorly by the neurosensory retina and anteriorly by the internal limiting membrane.

Black Sunburst Lesion

The black sunburst lesion is an oval or round collection of retinal pigment epithelium (RPE) that has migrated into the neurosensory retina.[7] These focal pigmented spots classically have spiculated or stellate borders resulting from accumulation of the pigment around small, branching blood vessels (▶ Fig. 21.1). Refractile granules, similar to iridescent spots, may also be seen within the lesions. The location and size of black sunbursts are similar to those of salmon patch hemorrhages. The reported incidence of black sunburst lesions is up to 41% in SC heterozygotes, 35% in SS patients, and 20% in SThal individuals.[11,12]

Histopathologically, black sunbursts show focal RPE hyperplasia, hypertrophy, and intraretinal migration. The overlying retina may also be degenerated and thinned. Diffuse deposits of iron, melanin pigment and hemosiderin-laden macrophages may coexist.[10]

Controversial Points

- The black sunburst lesion may evolve directly from a salmon patch hemorrhage, from underlying CNV, or from a focal choroidal occlusion. The most common pathogenesis is not known.

Black sunbursts may come about in several ways. They may evolve from a salmon patch hemorrhage that has dissected into the subretinal space and promoted a localized RPE reaction.[13] They may also represent secondary RPE changes from choroidal neovascularization (CNV).[14] Lastly, they may form as a result of a focal choroidal occlusion.[14]

Special Considerations

- Salmon patch hemorrhages are nonproliferative lesions that may occasionally extend into the vitreous, resulting in floaters and decreased visual acuity. In rare instances, these lesions can result in significant visual compromise, necessitating surgical evacuation of the hemorrhage.

21.3.2 Optic Disc

The *sickle disc sign* is the presence of small reddish dots on the surface of the optic disc and represents epipapillary arterioles and capillaries clogged with sickled red blood cells. These dots may be Y-shaped or linear and generally are visually asymptomatic. In one study,[15] the finding was present in 9 of 80 (11%) individuals with sickle cell hemoglobinopathies, 7 of who had SS disease. Frank neovascularization of the disc, unlike with other vasoocclusive retinopathies, is very rare in sickle hemoglobinopathies.[3,11,16] This is probably because the postequatorial retina is not significantly ischemic.

21.3.3 Macula

Microvascular changes in the macula and along the temporal raphe have been observed in 36% of SC, 32% of SS, and 20% of SThal patients.[17] These abnormalities include foveal avascular zone (FAZ) irregularities, enlarged precapillary arterioles and capillaries, microaneurysm-like dots, cotton-wool spots, and hairpin-shaped venular loops with adjacent capillary nonperfusion. Changes in the parafoveal vascular network may represent the initial vasoocclusive process that can progress to FAZ enlargement and, rarely, macular infarction (▶ Fig. 21.3).[18] Central retinal thinning (or atrophy) can result, and this may manifest ophthalmoscopically as a dark oval or circular concavity with a bright central reflex, the so-called macular depression sign. Unless the parafoveal vascular disruption is extensive, visual acuity is often not significantly affected.

The temporal vascular raphe begins at the fovea and extends temporally toward the periphery. The end-arteriolar branches that meet at the raphe may also become plugged with sickled red blood cells. Spectral-domain optical coherence tomography (SD-OCT) of the retina of sickle cell patients often demonstrates focal thinning of the macula in this area, revealing structural changes due to subclinical vascular occlusions (▶ Fig. 21.4).[19] No definite relationship between the extent of nonperfusion along the raphe and that in the periphery exists, despite the vascular similarities in these regions.[17]

21.3.4 Retinal Vessels

In the posterior pole, the major retinal vessels are usually normal, particularly in AS and SThal patients. However, large-vessel tortuosity may be present in up to 32% of SC and 47% of SS patients.[7] Vasoocclusion or arteriovenous shunting in the retinal periphery (discussed later) may play a role in the development of posterior vascular tortuosity.

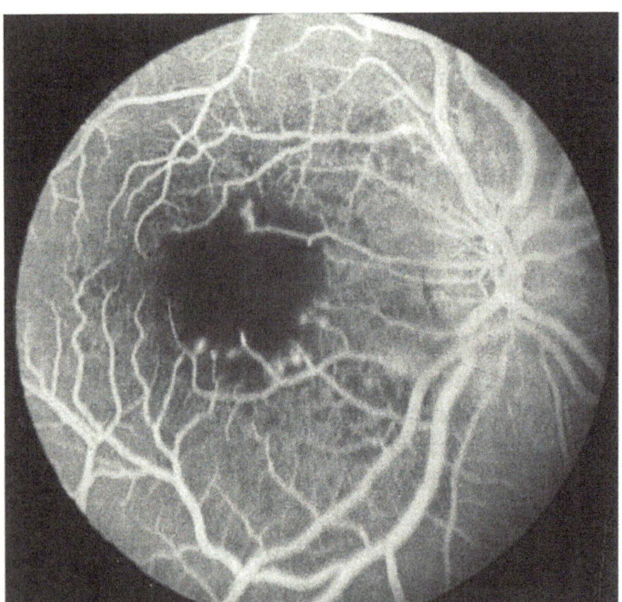

Fig. 21.3 Arteriolar occlusion and capillary nonperfusion in the central macula of a patient with sickle cell disease. The abrupt termination of the parafoveal capillaries has produced an enlarged foveal avascular zone.

Major arterial occlusive events, such as branch and central retinal artery obstructions, are well-described associations of sickle cell disease.[11,20] They may result in transient or permanent loss of vision and can occur in both eyes simultaneously.[20] Retinal venous occlusive disease, on the other hand, is rare in patients with sickle hemoglobinopathies. Because of this, an additional underlying ocular or systemic disease should be sought in a patient with sickle hemoglobinopathy and a retinal vein occlusion.

21.3.5 Angioid Streaks

Angioid streaks are irregular, gray lines deep to the retina that extend radially from the optic nerve head. In general, they may occur in up to 6% or more of patients with various sickle hemoglobinopathies.[21] However, they appear to be more common in patients with SS disease, particularly those of older age. In a series of Jamaican individuals with SS disease, angioid streaks were documented in 2% of those younger than 40 years and almost 22% of those older than 40 years.[21]

The pathogenesis of angioid streaks in sickle cell disease is not well understood. Chronic hemolysis with secondary iron deposition, causing a brittle Bruch's membrane, was a suggested mechanism; however, histopathologic examination in an SS homozygote demonstrated heavy calcification of Bruch's membrane without iron or hemosiderin. The natural history is generally unremarkable[21]; secondary CNV is a relatively uncommon complication.

21.3.6 Choroidal Occlusions

Focal choroidal vascular nonperfusion can occur and lead to overlying RPE hypertrophy and outer retinal atrophy. Histopathologically, choroidal vessels clogged with red blood cells and platelet-fibrin thrombi have been documented.[22] As discussed previously, such occlusions may also be pathogenetically related to the development of peripheral CNV and the black sunburst lesions of patients with sickle cell hemoglobinopathies.[14,22,23]

21.3.7 Vitreoretinal Interface

Peripheral retinal whitening, similar to white-without-pressure lesions, may be observed in eyes of patients with sickle hemoglobinopathy and may represent zones of abnormal or stronger vitreoretinal adhesion.[22] The peripheral whitening may be present in up to 82% of SThal, 83% of SC, and 93% of SS individuals. This abnormality may be similar to white-without-pressure lesions observed in the general population instead of being a distinct entity characteristic of individuals with sickle cell disease.[24]

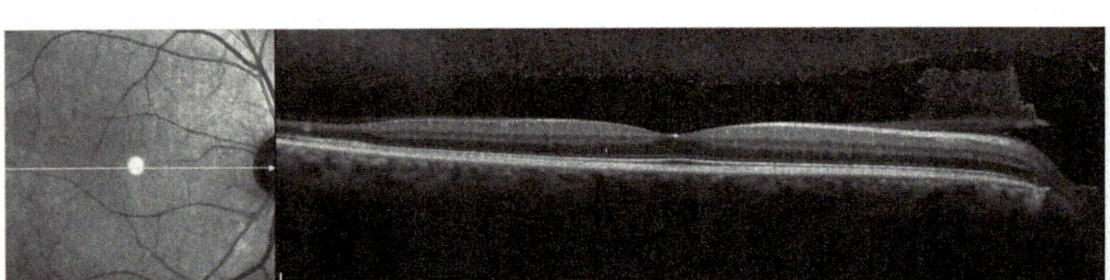

Fig. 21.4 Spectral-domain optical coherence tomography showing an area of focal retinal thinning in the temporal raphe.

Dark-without-pressure lesions, brown patches within the fundus, have been described in SC and SS patients.[25] These homogeneous, brown lesions appear flat and geographic and may be transiently observed in the equatorial retina and posterior pole, without leaving a remnant of their existence after spontaneously disappearing. The pathogenesis of these lesions is unknown. Ophthalmoscopically and angiographically, the underlying choroid appears unaffected. Consequently, these lesions are not thought to be associated with hemorrhage, as previously suggested.[11,25]

21.4 Proliferative Retinal Manifestations

Peripheral retinal arteriolar occlusion is the initiating pathogenetic event of proliferative sickle cell retinopathy, often resulting in "sea fan" retinal neovascularization (▸ Fig. 21.5). Flat sea fans are less likely than elevated ones to result in vitreous hemorrhage and the tractional vitreous membrane formation that may predispose to tractional and/or rhegmatogenous retinal detachment.[26]

A five-stage clinical classification of proliferative sickle cell retinopathy was originally described by Goldberg[27] and has since been widely accepted. Fluorescein angiography nicely demonstrates the peripheral retinal manifestations of both the preproliferative and proliferative stages.

21.4.1 Stage I

Stage I is characterized by peripheral arteriolar occlusion (▸ Fig. 21.6), the precursor of proliferative sickle retinopathy. Slower arteriovenous transit times and decreased blood flow in the peripheral retinal vasculature may predispose to sickling and vasoocclusion. Vasoocclusive events usually occur in the precapillary arterioles, as observed on fluorescein angiography and in more recent dual-perspective histologic analyses.[22] The sickled red blood cells are functionally similar to microemboli and interfere with blood flow, contributing to the formation of intravascular thromboses. Blood flow within the retinal arteriolar system ceases, and the capillaries and venules that supply the affected region are no longer perfused. Consequently, zones of peripheral capillary nonperfusion result.

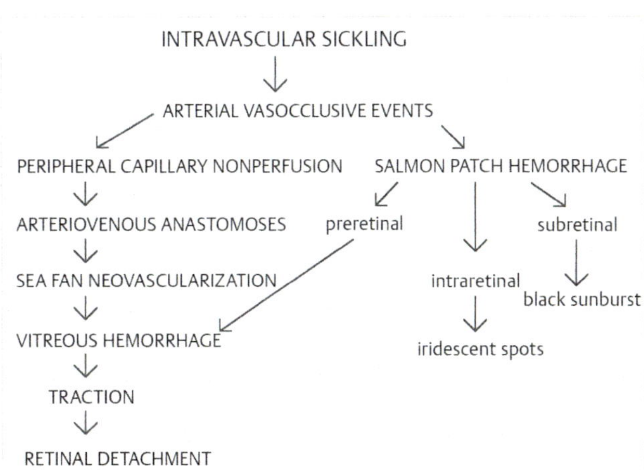

Fig. 21.5 The cascade of events in eyes with proliferative sickle retinopathy.

21.4.2 Stage II

Stage II is characterized by the formation of arteriovenous anastomoses at the junction of perfused and nonperfused peripheral retina (▸ Fig. 21.7, temporal periphery). The abnormal vascular connections shunt blood, often at slow velocities, from occluded arterioles to adjacent medium-sized veins. Fluorescein angiography differentiates these anastomotic channels, which do not leak fluorescein, from true neovascularization, which almost always leaks fluorescein dye. The vascular connections may have formed from the preexisting retinal vasculature by the enlargement and dilation of retinal capillaries.[16] The sluggish blood flow through this network contributes to red blood cell deoxygenation during one passage and may contribute to further sickling and vasoocclusive events. The development of these abnormal arteriovenous anastomoses may be a hydrostatic response to the distal occlusion and appears to contribute to the evolution of sea fan neovascularization.[16]

21.4.3 Stage III

Stage III is characterized by peripheral retinal neovascularization, or sea fans (▸ Fig. 21.8). (The term *sea fan* is used to describe the neovascular frond in sickle cell disease because it

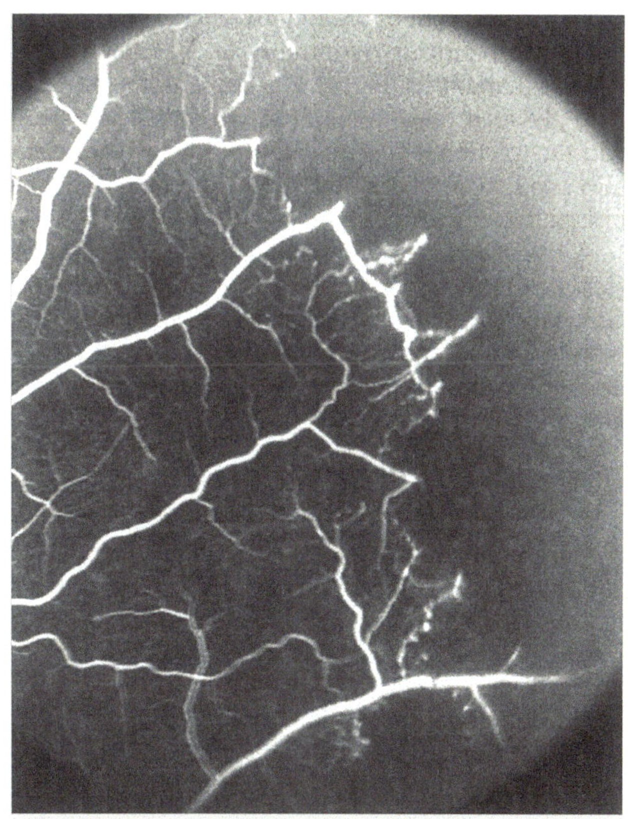

Fig. 21.6 Stage I proliferative sickle cell retinopathy: Peripheral arteriolar occlusions. In affected areas, retinal arteriolar flow ends abruptly and creates a zone of peripheral capillary nonperfusion as demonstrated by fluorescein angiography.

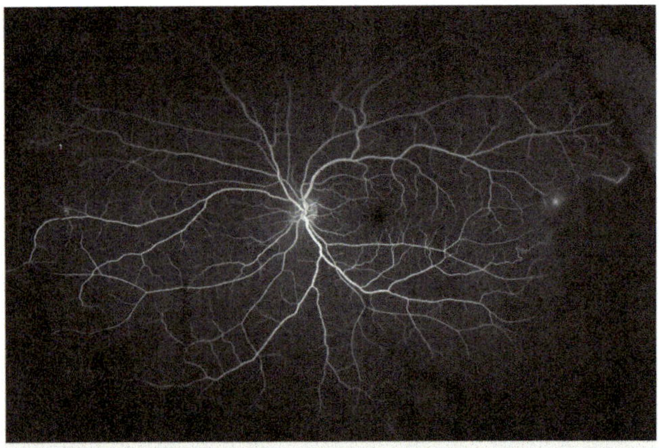

Fig. 21.7 Ultrawide-field fluorescein angiography of proliferative sickle retinopathy. Peripheral nonperfusion, arteriovenous anastomoses, and peripheral neovascular lesions are present in a single image.

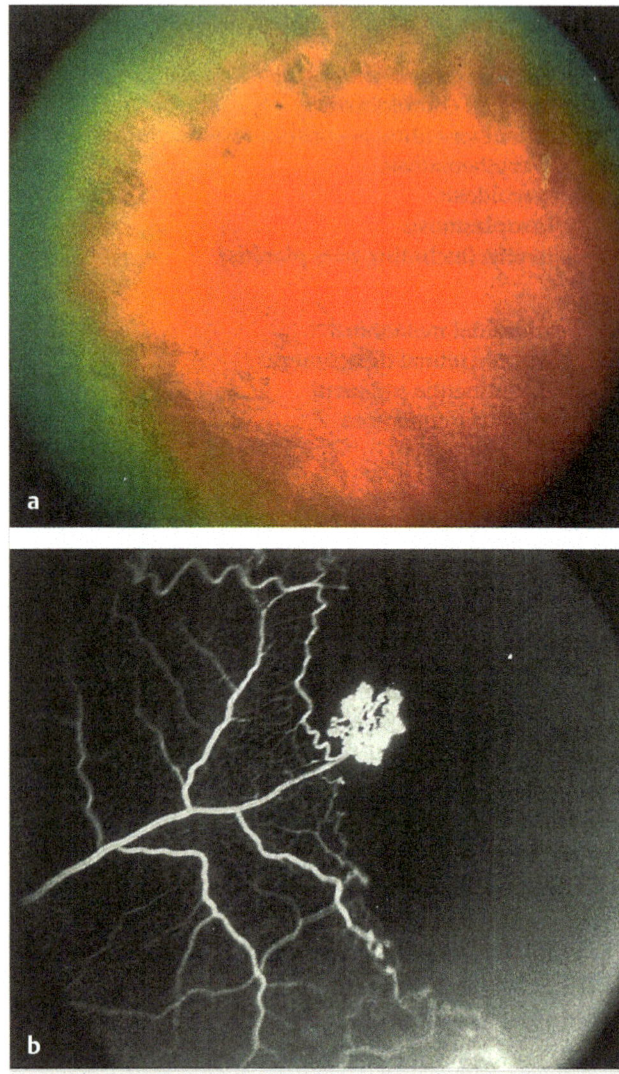

Fig. 21.8 Stage III proliferative sickle cell retinopathy: Peripheral retinal neovascularization ("sea fan"). (**a**) Clinical and (**b**) angiographic appearance of another active neovascular frond. Note the growth of neovascularization toward the peripheral, nonperfused retina.

bears a resemblance to the marine invertebrate *Gorgonia flabellum.*) Following the development of arteriovenous anastomoses, neovascularization occurs about 18 months later, with an approximate incidence of 14% per year in SC heterozygotes.[16] The neovascular tissue often sprouts from the venous side of the anastomosis, proliferating toward peripheral nonperfused retina (▶ Fig. 21.8). The nonperfused peripheral retina is ischemic and is thought to produce angiogenic substances that stimulate and foster the development of the neovascular tissue. Increased levels of basic fibroblast growth factor have been documented in peripheral nonperfused regions.[28] Elevated levels of both pigment epithelium-derived factor (PEDF), an inhibitor of angiogenesis, and vascular endothelial growth factor (VEGF) have been demonstrated in active neovascular lesions.[29] In regressed sea fans, only PEDF is elevated, suggesting that the activity and progression of angiogenesis may be dependent on the relative levels of PEDF and VEGF.[29]

Vasoocclusive events in precapillary arterioles may lead to altered blood flow patterns that result in further sickling and vasoocclusions elsewhere in the retinal vascular system, including the venous system.[22] Vasoocclusion within a venous segment may produce increased intravascular pressure within a proximal vessel and, consequently, focal vascular extrusion.[22] The intraluminal diameter of the distended vessel may continue to increase as the intravascular pressure remains high. Deformation of the vascular anatomy may induce endothelial cell proliferation and contribute to neovascularization.[30]

Sea fans form most commonly in the peripheral superotemporal quadrant, and less commonly in the inferotemporal, superonasal, and inferonasal quadrants. Sea fans begin to develop as new capillaries proliferate, forming fine red channels that may be difficult to identify with indirect ophthalmoscopy. The sea fan is initially flat and proliferates on the retinal surface between the internal limiting membrane and posterior hyaloid. One feeding arteriole and one draining venule may supply the neovascular frond, and these may possess large luminal diameters in some retinas. A large, arborizing sea fan may develop and acquire more than one feeding and draining vessel (▶ Fig. 21.8). Growth of sea fans usually occurs circumferentially, rather than radially toward the ora serrata or posterior pole, and they may extend around the entire peripheral retina. Fibroglial tissue, accompanying the circumferential growth, may contribute to the formation of a peripheral traction band. Chronic transudation into the vitreous from the incompetent blood–retinal barrier of the neovascular tissue may induce premature syneresis and collapse of the vitreous, creating tractional forces on the retina that can lead to vitreous hemorrhage, retinal breaks, and retinal detachment of stages IV and V.

21.4.4 Stage IV

Stage IV is characterized by vitreous hemorrhage. Vitreous hemorrhage occurs in about 20% of SC individuals and about 3% of SS homozygotes.[7,11] In those with other sickle cell hemoglobinopathies, vitreous hemorrhage may be less common.[7] Risk factors for the development of a vitreous hemorrhage in an untreated eye with sickle retinopathy include any vitreous hemorrhage on initial examination, greater than 60 total degrees of active sea fans, and the presence of SC disease.[31]

Sea fans may be pulled into the central vitreous cavity by adherent vitreous that can induce sufficient traction on the neovascular frond to cause bleeding. Hemorrhage may occur sporadically through the years because of vitreous movement, vitreous syneresis, contraction of preexisting vitreous bands, or minimal ocular trauma. The hemorrhage may be unnoticed by the patient and localized to the region around the sea fan or may become dispersed in the vitreous cavity, causing symptoms of floaters or decreased vision. Blood and plasma may repeatedly ooze from the sea fans and stimulate the formation of vitreous bands and membranes, culminating in retinal detachment (stage V) in some cases.

Pearls

- Risk factors for the development of a future vitreous hemorrhage in an untreated eye with sickle retinopathy include any vitreous hemorrhage on initial examination, greater than 60 total degrees of active sea fans, and the presence of SC disease.

21.4.5 Stage V

Rhegmatogenous and/or traction retinal detachment characterizes stage V. Because proliferative disease is most common in SC individuals, retinal detachment occurs most commonly in this hemoglobinopathy population.[7] Retinal detachment occurs less frequently in association with SS disease.[11]

Retinal traction caused by fibroglial membranes and vitreous bands may produce a retinal break and detachment. The membranes and bands result from chronic transudation into the vitreous and recurrent vitreous hemorrhage from neovascular proliferation. A retinal break, usually located adjacent to the fibrovascular lesion, may be masked by these lesions and can be challenging to identify in some eyes. Retinal ischemia may lead to retinal atrophy and retinal break formation with detachment of the retina, even in the absence of significant vitreoretinal traction.

21.5 Differential Diagnosis

Peripheral retinal neovascularization has been associated with numerous diseases (see the following list).[32]

Differential Diagnosis of Peripheral Retinal Neovascularization

- Retinal vascular diseases with retinal ischemia
  - Ocular ischemic syndromes
  - Carotid–cavernous sinus fistulas
  - Eales' disease
  - Familial exudative vitreoretinopathy
  - Hyperviscosity states, including chronic myelogenous leukemia
  - Idiopathic occlusive arteriolitis
  - Multiple sclerosis
  - Proliferative diabetic retinopathy
  - Retinal vein occlusion
  - Retinal artery occlusion
  - Retinal embolization (including talc retinopathy)
  - Retinopathy of prematurity
  - Sickling hemoglobinopathies
- Inflammatory diseases with possible ischemia
  - Birdshot choroidopathy
  - Retinal vasculitis (including systemic lupus erythematosus)
  - Sarcoidosis
  - Toxoplasmosis
  - Uveitis (including pars planitis)
- Other
  - Choroidal melanoma
  - Chronic retinal detachment
  - Incontinentia pigmenti
  - Retinitis pigmentosa

Source: Adapted from Jampol et al.[32]

A complete patient evaluation, including a family history and clinical examination, may be needed to make the correct diagnosis.

Sickle cell screening tests, such as the sickle prep (metabisulfite slide test) and the more commonly used solubility test (Sickledex; Orthodiagnostics), will identify the presence of sickle hemoglobin. A positive result from one of these tests should be supplemented with quantitative hemoglobin electrophoresis to differentiate homozygous and heterozygous states.

21.6 Management and Course

Spontaneous nonperfusion or autoinfarction of sea fans may occur during the proliferative phase of sickle cell retinopathy in up to 60% of lesions and peaks about 24 months after the development of proliferative disease.[3,33,34,35,36] Although autoinfarction may lead to regression of the sea fan and a decreased risk for significant vitreous hemorrhage, vitreoretinal traction may still develop at any time and lead to retinal detachment. Furthermore, in a single eye, various sea fans may behave differently; one sea fan may autoinfarct, while a sea fan elsewhere in the same retina increases progressively in size and causes complications.

The mechanism of sea fan autoinfarction is not well understood. Spontaneous regression of the neovascular lesion may result from vitreous traction with kinking or avulsion of the sea fan vascular supply, decreased concentration of angiogenic factors, or recurrent sickling and thrombosis within the sea fan lesion.[34,35] Some combination of mechanisms is probably at play.

21.6.1 Indications for Treatment

Treatment is typically not indicated for any of the nonproliferative retinal manifestations of sickle hemoglobinopathies. Regular, careful retinal examinations should be performed to detect progression to proliferative disease. Ultrawide-field fluorescein angiography can identify peripheral neovascularization at its earliest stages (▶ Fig. 21.7).[37]

The primary goal in managing sickle eye disease is to detect and treat the neovascularization (stage III disease) early on, before it leads to the more advanced complications that characterize stages IV and V. Once significant vitreous hemorrhage or retinal detachment occurs, more aggressive and invasive management, such as vitrectomy, may be needed. As discussed later, surgery performed in a patient with sickle cell hemoglobinopathy carries a higher risk for both ocular and systemic complications than if performed in a patient without sickle cell disease.[38,39,40]

General treatment guidelines are outlined in the following text box.

Proliferative sickle cell retinopathy: guidelines for therapeutic intervention:

- Large, elevated sea fan(s).
- Rapid enlargement of sea fan(s).
- Bilateral proliferative sickle cell disease.
- Evidence of vitreous hemorrhage or retinal detachment.
- Advanced proliferative retinopathy and complications in fellow eye.

Note that treatment is not necessarily performed in all eyes with stage III retinopathy because, as discussed earlier, progressive sea fan growth is not the rule and autoinfarction of sea fans occurs relatively frequently. Close observation, for example, is reasonable if the patient can reliably return for follow-up examinations and manifests only a few, small, flat neovascular fronds in one eye.[31] In such cases, treatment would be performed in the case of sea fan growth or any secondary hemorrhage.

The primary treatment modality used to promote regression of neovascularization is laser photocoagulation. The most common laser treatment strategies are local scatter laser photocoagulation and peripheral circumferential scatter photocoagulation.[34,41,42] Historically, cryotherapy and direct feeder vessel photocoagulation were also used to control proliferative disease; however, due to a higher incidence of retinal tears and detachments, the latter two methods have largely been replaced by scatter and circumferential photocoagulation.[43,44]

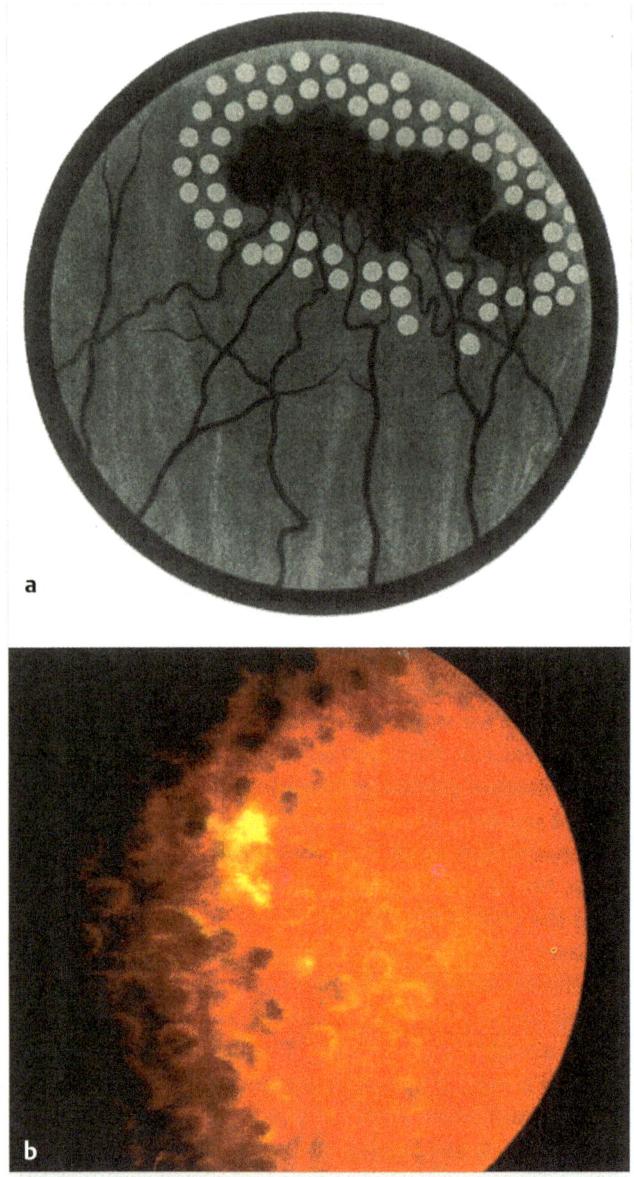

Fig. 21.9 The application of local scatter laser photocoagulation around active sea fan neovascularization. (a) Schematic drawing of the laser technique and (b) good posttreatment regression of the sea fan. (Adapted with permission from Goldberg and Jampol.[38])

21.6.2 Laser Photocoagulation

Local Scatter Laser Photocoagulation

In eyes with proliferative retinopathy, scatter photocoagulation to the retina surrounding each sea fan is effective in decreasing the risk for vitreous hemorrhage and visual loss.[34] A randomized, clinical trial evaluating this technique demonstrated partial or complete regression in about 80% of sea fans after one treatment, compared with a regression rate of 46% in control eyes.[34] Furthermore, the study showed a low rate of complications from the treatment.

Laser is applied using either a slit-lamp or indirect ophthalmoscope delivery system. The spots are placed about one burn width apart around each sea fan in a scatter pattern (▶ Fig. 21.9) with the following settings: 0.1- to 0.2-second duration, 500-µm spot size, and 200 milliwatts (mW) of power; the parameters are titrated to create a mild-to-moderate intensity burn. The area encompassed by the scatter laser photocoagulation typically extends about one to two disc diameters both anterior and posterior to the lesion and about 1 clock hour to either side. Through ablation of some of the surrounding ischemic retina, the treatment is thought to work by decreasing the amount of vasoproliferative factor(s) produced around the sea fan, thereby promoting its involution. The chorioretinal adhesions created by the laser spots may also help minimize or prevent subsequent retinal detachment.

Peripheral Circumferential Scatter Laser Photocoagulation

This technique involves applying laser spots in a scatter fashion to the entire 360-degree zone of peripheral retinal capillary nonperfusion. The laser delivery systems and parameters are similar to those used with the local scatter treatment. Although the efficacy of this approach has not been evaluated in a randomized clinical trial, the reported neovascular regression rates appear favorable.[45] Furthermore, the rate of new neovascular frond development during follow-up of eyes treated in this fashion is very low, at around 1.5%, implying an additional prophylactic benefit of laser applied to the entire avascular area.[42,45]

A 360-degree treatment, however, is probably not necessary in many cases. Current evidence does not confirm that circumferential treatment is superior to the other techniques.[33,38,41] Furthermore, applying more laser spots would theoretically increase the risk for the various complications seen with laser treatments in general, such as bleeding and formation of retinal holes and epiretinal membranes. However, in practice, complications from this approach are still very low, and if the patient is not likely to return for follow-up examinations, it may be the treatment of choice.

21.6.3 Anti-VEGF Intravitreal Injection

Intravitreal injections have not been widely adopted for proliferative sickle retinopathy, despite the now common use of anti-VEGF agents in other conditions, such as age-related macular degeneration, retinal vein occlusion, and diabetic retinopathy. In experimental case reports, one patient experienced a rapid resolution of vitreous hemorrhage with regression of neovascularization following off-label intravitreal bevacizumab,[46] while another patient developed a secondary hyphema following bevacizumab.[47] Anti-VEGF agents may be used less frequently in proliferative sickle retinopathy both because of the high rate of spontaneous autoinfarction of neovascular complexes and because the angiogenic process itself remains incompletely understood. Because of the limited evidence, the efficacy of anti-VEGF agents in proliferative sickle retinopathy remains unknown.

21.6.4 Surgical Management

Pars plana vitrectomy is indicated for eyes with dense, nonclearing vitreous hemorrhage; visually significant macular pathology, including epiretinal membranes and macular holes; and retinal detachments. Initially, dense hemorrhage should be observed to allow for spontaneous clearing.[38] Serial B-scan ultrasonography is utilized to exclude any coexisting retinal detachment, a finding that would prompt more urgent surgical intervention. At each follow-up visit, a search is made to identify the source of the hemorrhage using ophthalmoscopy and, sometimes, fluorescein angiography. Photocoagulation may be attempted if a source of bleeding is visualized. If the vitreous hemorrhage remains relatively dense after an initial trial of observation, and if laser photocoagulation has not been possible, vitrectomy with endolaser or indirect laser photocoagulation is indicated.[38] The visual prognosis is generally favorable in these eyes.[48]

Surgical intervention is usually needed for rhegmatogenous detachments, as these can progress quickly. However, for pure traction retinal detachments, surgery may be delayed or deferred indefinitely if the detachment remains peripheral and stationary. In early surgical reports on proliferative sickle retinopathy, anterior segment ischemia was a common complication, prompting recommendations of preoperative exchange transfusions and avoidance of an encircling scleral buckle.[49] Because of the potential to contract the human immunodeficiency virus and hepatitis B or C, exchange transfusions are no longer utilized routinely.[40] Recent surgical series with and without scleral buckling have also reported a much lower incidence of anterior segment ischemia following vitreoretinal surgery, suggesting that current scleral buckling techniques may be safely combined with pars plana vitrectomy if significant anterior vitreoretinal traction necessitates greater peripheral support.[40,48,50] Eyes with significant anterior traction retinal detachments carry a guarded prognosis.[48]

Pearls

- Vitreoretinal surgery in eyes with vitreous hemorrhage alone generally results in favorable surgical outcomes, while eyes with traction retinal detachments, especially those with anterior pathology, often require more than one procedure and carry a more guarded prognosis.

Despite improvements in both surgical techniques and outcomes, surgical intervention in this population continues to introduce an increased risk for intraoperative and postoperative complications in comparison with patients without sickle cell hemoglobinopathies undergoing similar surgery.[38] Potential complications include intraoperative systemic sickle cell crises during the administration of general anesthesia, anterior segment ischemia, and macular and optic nerve infarction from sustained intraocular pressure elevation.

Preventive measures should be incorporated into patient care to decrease the chance of such systemic and ocular morbidity from surgery. From a systemic standpoint, a preoperative hematologic consultation should be considered. Keeping the patient well hydrated and oxygenated in the perioperative period should help minimize generalized sickling complications. As with hyphema management, repetitive use of carbonic anhydrase inhibitors should be avoided. Intraoperative hyperbaric oxygen has been recommended as an alternative to exchange transfusions, but this is not widely available.

Special Considerations

- Anterior segment ischemia as a consequence of vitreoretinal surgery is rarely encountered with current surgical techniques. Scleral buckling may be employed to complement vitrectomy when necessary.

To minimize ischemic injury to the globe in the perioperative period, perfusion must be optimized. This is accomplished most readily by taking measures to prevent significant rises in intraocular pressure. With scleral buckling repair of a retinal detachment, it is preferable to drain the subretinal fluid to prevent the intraocular pressure from rising significantly when the buckle is secured in place. During vitrectomy, the intraocular pressure should be kept at lower-than-usual levels, a task made easier with the valved cannulas and current vitrectomy systems. Maximizing preoperative neovascularization regression is also important, as this reduces the chances of intraocular bleeding during vitrectomy and obviates the need to raise the ocular pressure purposefully to gain control of hemorrhaging. The use of large volumes or expansile concentrations of intraocular gases should be limited. Heavy applications of laser should also be avoided, as anterior segment ischemia following panretinal photocoagulation has been reported.[51] Hyperoxygenation in the perioperative period is a valuable adjunct.

21.7 Acknowledgments

This chapter was supported in part by an unrestricted grant from Research to Prevent Blindness, Inc., and Core Grant No. P30-EY014801 from the National Eye Institute.

References

[1] Clarkson JG. The ocular manifestations of sickle-cell disease: a prevalence and natural history study. Trans Am Ophthalmol Soc. 1992; 90:481–504

[2] Abrams LS, Goldberg MF. Retinopathy associated with hemoglobin AC. Arch Ophthalmol. 1994; 112(11):1410–1411

[3] Nagpal KC, Asdourian GK, Patrianakos D, et al. Proliferative retinopathy in sickle cell trait. Report of seven cases. Arch Intern Med. 1977; 137(3):325–328

[4] Condon PI, Serjeant GR. Behaviour of untreated proliferative sickle retinopathy. Br J Ophthalmol. 1980; 64(6):404–411

[5] Goldberg MF. Sickle cell retinopathy. In: Duane TD, Jaeger EA, eds. Clinical Ophthalmology. Vol. 3. Philadelphia, PA: Harper & Row; 1985:1–45

[6] Goldberg MF. Sickled erythrocytes, hyphema, and secondary glaucoma: I. The diagnosis and treatment of sickled erythrocytes in human hyphemas. Ophthalmic Surg. 1979; 10(4):17–31

[7] Welch RB, Goldberg MF. Sickle-cell hemoglobin and its relation to fundus abnormality. Arch Ophthalmol. 1966; 75(3):353–362

[8] Paton D. The conjunctival sign in sickle cell disease. Arch Ophthalmol. 1962; 68:627–632

[9] Gagliano DA, Goldberg MF. The evolution of salmon-patch hemorrhages in sickle cell retinopathy. Arch Ophthalmol. 1989; 107(12):1814–1815

[10] Romayanada N, Goldberg MF, Green WR. Histopathology of sickle cell retinopathy. Trans Am Acad Ophthalmol Otolaryngol. 1973; 77(5):OP642–OP676

[11] Condon PI, Serjeant GR. Ocular findings in homozygous sickle cell anemia in Jamaica. Am J Ophthalmol. 1972; 73(4):533–543

[12] Condon PI, Serjeant GR. Ocular findings in hemoglobin SC disease in Jamaica. Am J Ophthalmol. 1972; 74(5):921–931

[13] van Meurs JC. Evolution of a retinal hemorrhage in a patient with sickle cell-hemoglobin C disease. Arch Ophthalmol. 1995; 113(8):1074–1075

[14] Lutty GA, McLeod DS, Pachnis A, Costantini F, Fabry ME, Nagel RL. Retinal and choroidal neovascularization in a transgenic mouse model of sickle cell disease. Am J Pathol. 1994; 145(2):490–497

[15] Goldbaum MH. Retinal depression sign indicating a small retinal infarct. Am J Ophthalmol. 1978; 86(1):45–55

[16] Raichand M, Goldberg MF, Nagpal KC, Goldbaum MH, Asdourian GK. Evolution of neovascularization in sickle cell retinopathy. A prospective fluorescein angiographic study. Arch Ophthalmol. 1977; 95(9):1543–1552

[17] Asdourian GK, Nagpal KC, Busse B, et al. Macular and perimacular vascular remodelling sickling haemoglobinopathies. Br J Ophthalmol. 1976; 60 (6):431–453

[18] Cusick M, Toma HS, Hwang TS, Brown JC, Miller NR, Adams NA. Binasal visual field defects from simultaneous bilateral retinal infarctions in sickle cell disease. Am J Ophthalmol. 2007; 143(5):893–896

[19] Hoang QV, Chau FY, Shahidi M, Lim JI. Central macular splaying and outer retinal thinning in asymptomatic sickle cell patients by spectral-domain optical coherence tomography. Am J Ophthalmol. 2011; 151(6):990–994.e1

[20] Acacio I, Goldberg MF. Peripapillary and macular vessel occlusions in sickle cell anemia. Am J Ophthalmol. 1973; 75(5):861–866

[21] Nagpal KC, Asdourian G, Goldbaum M, et al. Angioid streaks and sickle hemoglobinopathies. Br J Ophthalmol. 1976; 60:31–34

[22] McLeod DS, Goldberg MF, Lutty GA. Dual-perspective analysis of vascular formations in sickle cell retinopathy. Arch Ophthalmol. 1993; 111(9):1234–1245

[23] Dizon RV, Jampol LM, Goldberg MF, Juarez C. Choroidal occlusive disease in sickle cell hemoglobinopathies. Surv Ophthalmol. 1979; 23(5):297–306

[24] Nagpal KC, Huamonte F, Constantaras A, Asdourian G, Goldberg MF, Busse B. Migratory white-without-pressure retinal lesions. Arch Ophthalmol. 1976; 94(4):576–579

[25] Nagpal KC, Goldberg MF, Asdourian G, Goldbaum M, Huamonte F. Dark-without-pressure fundus lesions. Br J Ophthalmol. 1975; 59(9):476–479

[26] Jampol LM, Green JL, Jr, Goldberg MF, Peyman GA. An update on vitrectomy surgery and retinal detachment repair in sickle cell disease. Arch Ophthalmol. 1982; 100(4):591–593

[27] Goldberg MF. Classification and pathogenesis of proliferative sickle retinopathy. Am J Ophthalmol. 1971; 71(3):649–665

[28] Lutty GA, Merges C, Crone S, McLeod DS. Immunohistochemical insights into sickle cell retinopathy. Curr Eye Res. 1994; 13(2):125–138

[29] Kim SY, Mocanu C, Mcleod DS, et al. Expression of pigment epithelium-derived factor (PEDF) and vascular endothelial growth factor (VEGF) in sickle cell retina and choroid. Exp Eye Res. 2003; 77(4):433–445

[30] van Meurs JC. Ocular findings in sickle cell disease on Curacao [Thesis]. Nijmegen, the Netherlands: Catholic University of Nijmegen; 1990

[31] Condon P, Jampol LM, Farber MD, Rabb M, Serjeant G. A randomized clinical trial of feeder vessel photocoagulation of proliferative sickle cell retinopathy. II. Update and analysis of risk factors. Ophthalmology. 1984; 91(12):1496–1498

[32] Jampol LM, Ebroon DA, Goldbaum MH. Peripheral proliferative retinopathies: an update on angiogenesis, etiologies and management. Surv Ophthalmol. 1994; 38(6):519–540

[33] Jacobson MS, Gagliano DA, Cohen SB, et al. A randomized clinical trial of feeder vessel photocoagulation of sickle cell retinopathy. A long-term follow-up. Ophthalmology. 1991; 98(5):581–585

[34] Farber MD, Jampol LM, Fox P, et al. A randomized clinical trial of scatter photocoagulation of proliferative sickle cell retinopathy. Arch Ophthalmol. 1991; 109(3):363–367

[35] Nagpal KC, Patrianakos D, Asdourian GK, Goldberg MF, Rabb M, Jampol L. Spontaneous regression (autoinfarction) of proliferative sickle retinopathy. Am J Ophthalmol. 1975; 80(5):885–892

[36] Downes SM, Hambleton IR, Chuang EL, Lois N, Serjeant GR, Bird AC. Incidence and natural history of proliferative sickle cell retinopathy: observations from a cohort study. Ophthalmology. 2005; 112(11):1869–1875

[37] Cho M, Kiss S. Detection and monitoring of sickle cell retinopathy using ultra wide-field color photography and fluorescein angiography. Retina. 2011; 31 (4):738–747

[38] Goldberg MF, Jampol LM. Treatment of neovascularization, vitreous hemorrhage, and retinal detachment in sickle cell retinopathy. In: Symposium on Medical and Surgical Diseases of the Retina and Vitreous: Transactions of the New Orleans Academy of Ophthalmology. CV Mosby, St. Louis: 1983:53–81

[39] Cohen SB, Fletcher ME, Goldberg MF, Jednock NJ. Diagnosis and management of ocular complications of sickle hemoglobinopathies: Part V. Ophthalmic Surg. 1986; 17(6):369–374

[40] Pulido JS, Flynn HW, Jr, Clarkson JG, Blankenship GW. Pars plana vitrectomy in the management of complications of proliferative sickle retinopathy. Arch Ophthalmol. 1988; 106(11):1553–1557

[41] Rednam KRV, Jampol LM, Goldberg MF. Scatter retinal photocoagulation for proliferative sickle cell retinopathy. Am J Ophthalmol. 1982; 93(5):594–599

[42] Kimmel AS, Magargal LE, Stephens RF, Cruess AF. Peripheral circumferential retinal scatter photocoagulation for the treatment of proliferative sickle retinopathy. An update. Ophthalmology. 1986; 93(11):1429–1434

[43] Goldbaum MH, Fletcher RC, Jampol LM, Goldberg MF. Cryotherapy of proliferative sickle retinopathy, II: triple freeze-thaw cycle. Br J Ophthalmol. 1979; 63(2):97–101

[44] Jampol LM, Goldberg MF. Retinal breaks after photocoagulation of proliferative sickle cell retinopathy. Arch Ophthalmol. 1980; 98(4):676–679

[45] Dizon-Moore RV, Jampol LM, Goldberg MF. Chorioretinal and choriovitreal neovascularization. Their presence after photocoagulation of proliferative sickle cell retinopathy. Arch Ophthalmol. 1981; 99(5):842–849

[46] Siqueira RC, Costa RA, Scott IU, Cintra LP, Jorge R. Intravitreal bevacizumab (Avastin) injection associated with regression of retinal neovascularization caused by sickle cell retinopathy. Acta Ophthalmol Scand. 2006; 84(6):834–835

[47] Babalola OE. Intravitreal bevacizumab (Avastin) associated with secondary hyphaema in a case of proliferative sickle cell retinopathy. BMJ Case Rep. 2010; 2010. DOI: 10.1136/bcr.11.2009.2441

[48] Chen RW, Flynn HW, Jr, Lee WH, et al. Vitreoretinal management and surgical outcomes in proliferative sickle retinopathy: a case series. Am J Ophthalmol. 2014; 157(4):870–875.e1

[49] Ryan SJ, Goldberg MF. Anterior segment ischemia following scleral buckling in sickle cell hemoglobinopathy. Am J Ophthalmol. 1971; 72(1):35–50

[50] Williamson TH, Rajput R, Laidlaw DA, Mokete B. Vitreoretinal management of the complications of sickle cell retinopathy by observation or pars plana vitrectomy. Eye (Lond). 2009; 23(6):1314–1320

[51] Leen JS, Ratnakaram R, Del Priore LV, Bhagat N, Zarbin MA. Anterior segment ischemia after vitrectomy in sickle cell disease. Retina. 2002; 22(2):216–219

22 Retinal Manifestations of Metabolic Disease

Katherine E. Talcott, James D. Palmer, and Shizuo Mukai

22.1 Introduction

While the genetic basis and systemic manifestations of many metabolic diseases are quite diverse, their range of retinal expression can be divided into two main categories. Those causing cherry-red spot (▶ Fig. 22.1) are listed in List 1; those resulting in pigmentary retinopathy (▶ Fig. 22.2) are given in List 2. Pigmentary changes in the temporal macula at the insertion of the long ciliary nerve can be seen in infants and young children and are sometimes confused for an "eccentric cherry-red spot" (▶ Fig. 22.3). This is a normal finding and typically is not seen as the fundus pigmentation increases with age. A cherry-red spot is always at the fovea. A summary of the genetic etiologies of these metabolic diseases can be found in ▶ Table 22.1.

Diseases Causing Cherry-Red Spots

- Storage diseases
  - GM_1 gangliosidosis
  - GM_2 gangliosidosis (Tay–Sachs and Sandhoff)
  - Niemann–Pick types A and B
  - Sialidoses
  - Farber's lipogranulomatosis
- Other etiologies
  - Central retinal artery occlusion
  - Traumatic retinal edema
  - Macular hole with surrounding cuff of subretinal fluid

Metabolic Diseases Causing Pigmentary Retinopathy

- Lysosomal storage diseases
  - Mucopolysaccharidoses
  - Hurler–Scheie syndrome
  - Hunter's syndrome
  - Sanfilippo's disease
- Peroxisomal diseases
  - Zellweger's spectrum disorders (Zellweger, neonatal adrenoleukodystrophy, infantile Refsum)
  - Refsum's disease
  - Primary hyperoxaluria
- Disorders of amino acid and lipoprotein metabolism
  - Cystinosis
  - Gyrate atrophy
  - Abetalipoproteinemia
  - Hypobetalipoproteinemia
- Others
  - Mucolipidosis IV
  - Ceroid lipofuscinoses

22.2 Lipidoses

The sphingolipidoses are a type of lysosomal storage disease in which glycolipids with a sphingosine base are not degraded properly, leading to an accumulation in cytoplasmic vesicles.

22.2.1 GM_2 Gangliosidoses (Tay–Sachs disease and Sandhoff's disease)

Tay–Sachs and Sandhoff's diseases are characterized by storage of GM_2 ganglioside in the lysosomes of neuronal tissue, which results in progressive loss of neurologic function. Tay–Sachs disease is most prevalent in Ashkenazi Jews, with a carrier rate

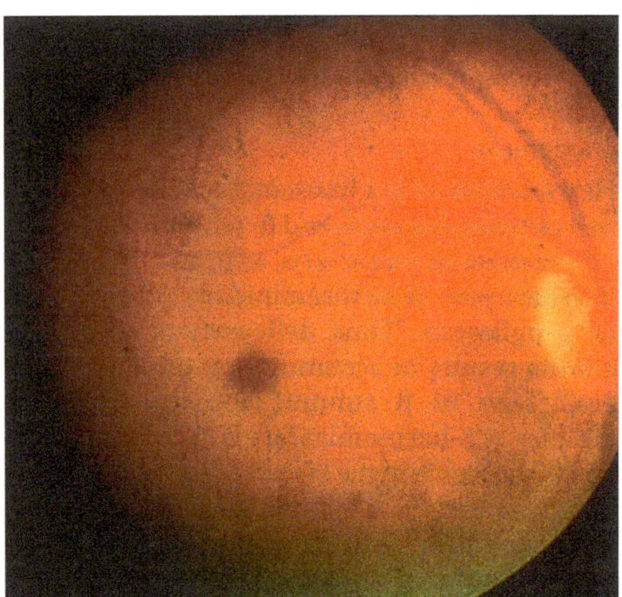

Fig. 22.1 Cherry-red spot in the macula of a patient with lipidosis. (Image courtesy of Craig A. Mckeown, MD.)

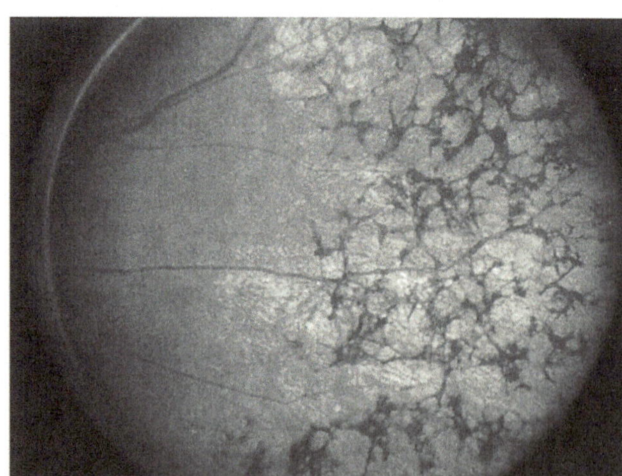

Fig. 22.2 Pigmentary retinopathy indistinguishable from retinitis pigmentosa can be seen in some metabolic disorders. (Image courtesy of Robert Petersen, MD.)

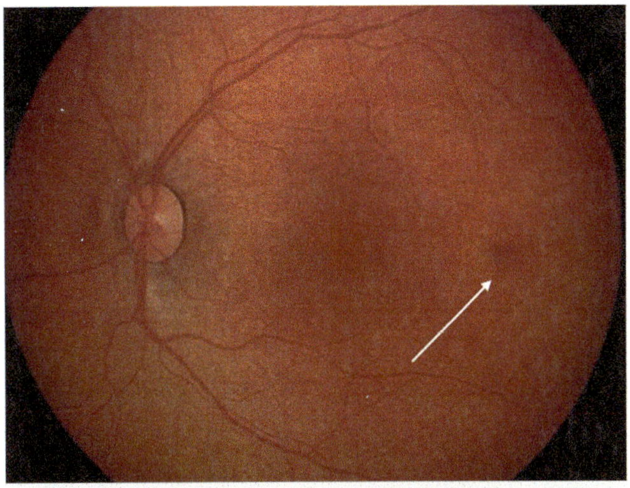

Fig. 22.3 Normal pigmentary changes at the insertion of the long ciliary nerve in an infant appear as an "eccentric cherry-red spot." (arrow).

estimated to be 1 in 30 to 1 in 40 among European Jews living in the United States, compared with 1 in 300 among non-Jews.[1] It is also more common in individuals of Pennsylvania Dutch, Southern Louisiana Cajun, or Eastern Quebec French Canadian descent.[1] No single ethnic group has an increased rate of Sandhoff's disease. Instead, several geographically or demographically isolated populations have higher incidences, such as in the town of Cordoba in Argentina, where 36 cases in 15 families have been detected in 3 years.[2]

Clinical Features

Infantile Tay–Sachs is the archetype of the gangliosidoses. It is characterized by early onset, at age 3 to 5 months; hyperirritability; and advancing weakness. These infants rapidly lose motor and intellectual skills after the age of 1 year and may crawl but never walk. The natural course leads to a decerebrate, vegetative state by the second to fourth year of life. Visual inattentiveness is frequently the presenting complaint, and the ocular stigma, a macular cherry-red spot, is found early in all patients. Additionally, infants are commonly macrocephalic from accumulation of storage material in the brain. A juvenile form of Tay–Sachs exists; this has a later onset and slower course but a similar constellation of signs and symptoms. The mildest form of the disease, the adult subtype, has its onset in the 20 s or 30 s. Presenting manifestations include ataxia, dysarthria, muscle weakness, and psychosis. One final variant, dubbed *chronic*, presents between ages 2 and 5 years and has a more gradual course, with patients surviving well into adulthood. The vast majority of patients have the infantile form.[3,4]

Pearls

- In Tay–Sachs disease, the genetic deficiency of ß -hexosaminidase A results in abnormal accumulation of GM_2 gangliosides in the lysosomes of neuronal cells. The macular cherry-red spot, a consistent and early finding, is caused by swelling and opacification of the ganglion cells around the fovea.

Although biochemically distinct, Sandhoff's disease has a similar range of presentations and clinical features. However, patients with Sandhoff's disease may also have organomegaly and occasional bony abnormalities.[2]

Diagnosis

Diagnosis of the GM_2 gangliosidoses is accomplished by assaying for the activity of individual ß-hexosaminidase isoenzymes in serum or cultured cells from affected individuals. Deficiency in the ß-hexosaminidase A isoenzyme is found in Tay–Sachs disease, whereas deficiency in ß -hexosaminidase A and B isoenzymes is detected in Sandhoff's disease. Heterozygous carriers can be detected by a reduced level of activity for ß-hexosaminidase.[1] In addition to biochemical testing, carrier state testing can be performed by DNA analysis. This is especially true in the Ashkenazi Jewish population, in which three mutations appear to be responsible for the vast majority of cases. Testing identifies 99.9% of carriers in the Ashkenazi Jewish population, with a false-negative rate of less than 2%.[5]

Pathogenesis

ß-Hexosaminidase is a lysosomal acid hydrolase composed of two subunits, a and ß, which can pair to create three isomeric forms: a/a, a/ß, and ß/ß. Only the a/ß isoenzyme, ß-hexosaminidase A, can degrade GM_2 gangliosides. Thus, deficiency of either a or ß subunits results in accumulation of GM_2 gangliosides.[3] Loss of ß subunit activity also causes deficiency of ß-hexosaminidase B (ß/ß) and accumulation of globoside in the viscera.[6] Tay–Sachs disease is caused by mutations in the a subunit gene on chromosome 15, and Sandhoff's disease results from mutations in the ß subunit gene on chromosome 5. The onset and severity of the disease process correlate directly with the amount of residual enzymatic activity in the mutant subunit. Any mutations that cause complete loss of enzymatic activity in the homozygous state, such as a frameshift, splicing, or premature stop codon mutation, lead to the severe, rapidly progressing, infantile phenotype. Individuals with point mutations resulting in single amino acid substitutions often retain some enzymatic activity and, therefore, have a later onset and more gradual course of the juvenile or adult phenotype. Intermediate expressions may also occur in patients who are heterozygous for two mutant alleles, one severe and one mild.[3]

Gangliosides are most plentiful in the gray matter; it is not surprising, then, that most of the clinical manifestations and pathology center on the nervous system. Meganeurites, neurons distended with storage material, are the pathologic hallmark of the GM_2 gangliosidoses and are found throughout the nervous system. In the retina, ganglion cells and amacrine cells are swollen with storage material. The concentration of enlarged, opacified ganglion cells encircling the fovea results in the cherry-red spot. The storage material in Tay–Sachs disease is composed ultrastructurally of membranous cytoplasmic bodies with concentrically arranged layers.[2] In contrast, the storage material in Sandhoff's disease is more pleomorphic, containing fibrogranular vacuoles, membranous cytoplasmic bodies, and zebra bodies with stacked lamellae.[6]

Table 22.1 Genetic etiologies of metabolic diseases

Metabolic disease	Genetic etiology	Retinal findings
Lipidoses		
Tay–Sachs disease	Hexosaminidase A (*HEXA*)	Macular cherry-red spot
Sandhoff's disease	Hexosaminidase B (*HEXB*)	Macular cherry-red spot
GM_1 gangliosidosis	ß-Galactosidase 1 (*GLB1*)	Macular cherry-red spot, tortuous retinal vessels, retinal hemorrhages
Gaucher's disease	Glucocerebrosidase (*GBA*)	Posterior retinal white spots
Sphingomyelin lipidoses		
Niemann–Pick disease	Acid sphingomyelinase gene (*SMPD1*)	Macular cherry-red spots, macular halos
Mucopolysaccharidoses		
Mucopolysaccharidoses type I (Hurler's and Scheie's syndromes)	a-L-iduronidase (*IDUA*)	Retinal dystrophy with bone spicules
Mucopolysaccharidosis type II (Hunter's syndrome)	Iduronate 2-sulfatase (IDS)	Retinal degeneration
Mucopolysaccharidosis type III (Sanfilippo's syndrome)	N-sulfoglucoasmine sulfohydrolase (*SGSH*); N-acetyl-alpha-D-glucosaminidase (*NAGLU*); acetyl-CoA:alpha-glucosaminide N-acetyltransferase (*HGSNAT*); N-acetylglucosamine-6-sulfate sulfatase (*GNS*)	Retinal degeneration with bone spicules and vascular attenuation
Amino acid disorders		
Cystinosis	Cystinosin (*CTNS*)	RPE mottling and clumping, deep retinal crystals
Gyrate atrophy	Ornithine aminotransferase (*OAT*)	Demarcated areas of chorioretinal atrophy
Mucolipidosis		
Mucolipidosis IV	Mucolipin 1 (*MCOLN1*)	Retinal dystrophy
Ceroid lipofuscinoses		
Infantile, late infantile, juvenile, and adult types	Multiple genes implicated, including *CLN1*, *2*, and *3*	Granular perifovea, peripheral hypopigmentation, bone spicules, vascular attenuation
Peroxisomal disorders		
Zellweger spectrum disorders	Peroxins (majority in *PEX1* or *PEX6* genes)	Pigmentary retinopathy, vascular attenuation
Refsum disease	Phytanoyl-CoA hydroxylase (*PHYH*)	Pigmentary retinopathy, vascular attenuation
Adrenoleukodystrophy	ATP-binding cassette, subfamily D, member (*ABCD1*)	Macular pigmentary mottling
Primary hyperoxaluria type I	Alanine:glyoxylate aminotransferase (*AGXT*)	Crystalline retinopathy
Abetalipoproteinemia	Microsomal triglyceride transfer protein (*MTP*)	Pigmentary retinopathy

Management and Course

Management is mostly supportive. It is unknown whether bone marrow transplantation would alter the neurologic consequences of these diseases significantly.

22.2.2 GM_1 Gangliosidosis

GM_1 gangliosidosis is a rare, autosomal recessive disorder with an unknown incidence.[7]

Clinical Features

GM_1 gangliosidosis has a broad range of clinical expressions, which are divided by age of onset into infantile, juvenile, and adult forms. The infantile form is the most common and severe phenotype. Afflicted infants appear normal at birth but suffer developmental arrest and then regression by 3 to 6 months of age. Failure to thrive, hypotonia, hyperirritability, and seizures are prevalent manifestations. Hepatosplenomegaly, dysmorphic facies, and dysostosis multiplex are found less consistently.

Death ensues by the age of 2 years. The juvenile form has a later onset and more gradual course but similar clinical features. The chronic adult form is dominated by spastic ataxia; the dysmorphic and visceral expressions are less severe. In terms of ocular findings, a macular cherry-red spot is found in about 50% of affected infants and has been reported in some juvenile cases.[4,7] Additional ocular findings include visual inattentiveness, corneal clouding, tortuous retinal vessels, retinal hemorrhages, and optic atrophy.[8]

Morquio type B disease shares the same biochemical error but is clinically distinct from GM_1 gangliosidosis. Patients are normal at birth, but growth retardation and progressive, generalized skeletal dysplasia develop in the first decade of life. The nervous system is not involved, and patients are of normal intelligence. Corneal clouding is the only ocular expression of the disease.[7]

Diagnosis

Diagnosis is based primarily on markedly decreased or absent ß-galactosidase activity in cultured leukocytes or fibroblasts. Tears may also be used for enzyme assays. Prenatal diagnosis can be made by assaying enzyme activity in cultured amniocytes or chorionic villus cells. Morquio type B is differentiated from GM_1 gangliosidosis by the predominance of skeletal abnormalities in the absence of neurologic involvement and the high concentrations of keratan sulfate in the urine.[7]

Pathophysiology and Histopathology

Mutations in the ß-galactosidase 1 (*GLB1*) gene on chromosome 3 result in accumulation of ganglioside GM_1. The gangliosides are the major storage compounds in GM_1 gangliosidosis, whereas keratan sulfate is the dominant storage substance in Morquio B disease. Thus, the phenotypic differences between GM_1 gangliosidosis and Morquio B may be the result of altered enzymatic substrate specificity. Higher levels of residual enzyme activity correlate roughly with the later onset and milder phenotype.

By light microscopy, meganeurites similar to those seen in Tay–Sachs disease are found throughout the central nervous system. The ultrastructural characteristics of the storage material are also similar.[7] In the retina, there is extensive ganglion cell loss, and the remaining cells are greatly distended with storage vesicles. Electron microscopy demonstrates numerous clear vacuoles in the cell bodies of rods and cones and membranous cytoplasmic bodies in the bipolar and ganglion cells.[9]

Management and Course

No therapy has proved effective in GM_1 gangliosidosis. Bone marrow transplants in a canine model failed to alter the course of the disease.[7]

22.2.3 Gaucher's Disease

Gaucher's disease is the most common of the lysosomal storage diseases, with an incidence of 1 in 10,000 to 20,000 Americans. Type 1 is the most prevalent (90% of cases) and occurs with greater frequency in the Ashkenazi Jewish population, while types 2 and 3 are less common and occur across all ethnic groups.[10,11]

Clinical Features

Affected patients are divided into three categories: type I, nonneuropathic (adult); type II, acute neuropathic (infantile); and type III, subacute neuropathic (juvenile). As in GM_2 gangliosidoses, an earlier onset coincides with more severe disease and rapid course. These categories are actually arbitrary divisions in a continuous clinical spectrum; thus, there is considerable variation within each group. Type I patients may be completely asymptomatic or may display some or all of the following: anemia, thrombocytopenia, hepatosplenomegaly, and bone lesions. The adult-onset type is most common among the Ashkenazi Jewish population. The infantile, neuropathic form, type II, is much rarer and occurs panethnically. Infants with type II disease present in the early months of life with hepatosplenomegaly and neurologic deterioration. Death usually occurs before the age of 2 years. Patients with the juvenile type of disease demonstrate neuronal and visceral involvement; the neurologic complaints develop later in life and progress more slowly than in the infantile form.[3,9,12] The most consistent ocular finding reported is that of scattered, superficial, retinal white spots concentrated in the posterior pole, especially along the inferior vascular arcade (▶ Fig. 22.4). In older patients, a peculiar, pigmented, brown, triangular pingueculum may develop that contains Gaucher's cells, which are characteristic macrophages with foamy, lipid-laden cytoplasm.[13]

Pearls

- Gaucher's disease is the most common lysosomal storage disorder. The most common fundus finding is that of multiple, superficial white dots in the posterior retina, particularly around the inferior vascular arcade.

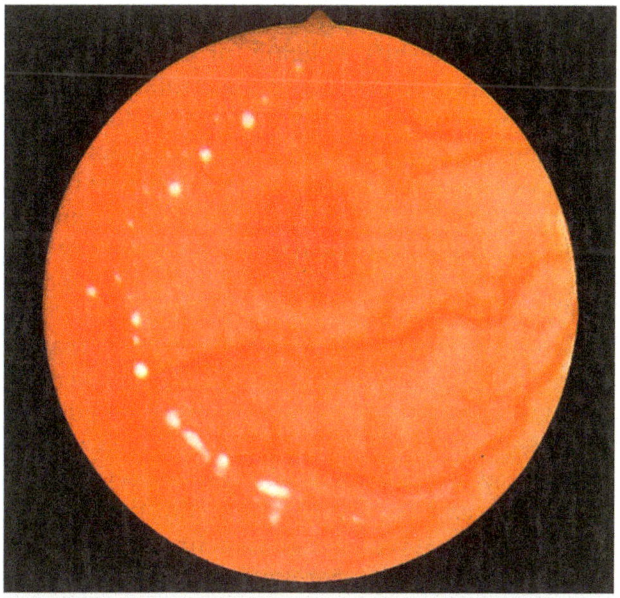

Fig. 22.4 Scattered white spots in the retina of a patient with Gaucher's disease. (Image courtesy of Robert Petersen, MD.)

Diagnosis

Diagnosis is made by analyzing leukocyte acid ß-glucosidase glucocerebrosidase activity. Although heterozygotes have, on average, 50% of the activity of normal subjects, the range of normal is so wide that the usefulness of enzyme assays to detect heterozygotes is limited. The finding of large numbers of Gaucher's cells on bone marrow aspirate is characteristic.[12] Mutation analysis can also confirm the diagnosis, predict clinical manifestations, and identify undiagnosed family members and carriers.[14]

Pathogenesis and Histopathology

Gaucher's disease is caused by mutations in the glucocerebrosidase (also called acid ß-glucosidase, *GBA*) gene on chromosome 1q21. More than 200 different mutations have been identified, with greater than 80% of them single-nucleotide substitutions.[15] Mutations in this lysosomal enzyme glucocerebrosidase lead to an accumulation of glucocerebroside within macrophage lysosomes.[16] Clinical manifestations result in the accumulation of lipid-laden macrophages in the spleen, liver, bone marrow, and bone, among other tissues/organs.[17] Gaucher's disease is a spectrum of disease manifestations, related to specific mutations rather than a disorder with separate subtypes. Recombination and insertion or deletion mutations cause neuropathic disease, whereas point mutations may cause either neuropathic or nonneuropathic disease.[12] This makes sense conceptually, because point mutations are more likely to result in enzymes with residual activity. In fact, considerable phenotypic variability can be found in siblings with identical genotypes, implying that environmental or other associated genetic factors can modify phenotypic expression.[9] Afflicted individuals may also be heterozygous, possessing two different mutant alleles for Gaucher's disease. These patients usually have an intermediate age of onset and rate of progression compared with what is predicted for homozygotes of each allele.[3]

Although the glucocerebrosidase deficiency exists in all cells, the phenotype is expressed only in the macrophage/monocyte system in the nonneuropathic forms, and also in the neurons in the neuropathic form.[12] By light microscopy, abnormal macrophages, called *Gaucher's cells*, which are filled with foamy, lipid-laden cytoplasm, are found in bone marrow, spleen, and liver. Histologically and ultrastructurally, the white spots in the fundus represent Gaucher's cells.[10,18]

Management and Course

Nonneuropathic Gaucher's disease is an ideal candidate for a variety of treatment approaches because it affects mainly macrophages, which are derived from bone marrow stem cells and are in constant contact with the bloodstream. Enzyme-replacement therapy (ERT) with recombinant glucocerebrosidase (imiglucerase, velaglucerase alfa, and taliglucerase alfa) is recommended for symptomatic children and those with severe manifestations of nonneuropathic (type 1) Gaucher's disease. It is also recommended for those with neuropathic type 3 disease with severe visceral symptoms and those at risk for type 3 disease (genotype or family history). It is not recommended for type 2 disease because it unfortunately does not alter the fatal neurologic outcomes.[19,20,21,22,23,24,25,26] Overall, ERT is individualized to each patient. Its high cost (> $400,000 per year) also makes it necessary to determine lowest effective initial and maintenance dose.[9] Hematopoietic stem cell transplantation was a treatment option previously but, given the associated morbidity and mortality, has been largely replaced by ERT.[27,28]

22.3 Sphingomyelin Lipidoses

22.3.1 Niemann-Pick Disease

All the sphingomyelin lipidoses, types A through F, are characterized biochemically by accumulation of sphingomyelin, particularly in the reticuloendothelial system. Only types A and B consistently have macular findings. The disease is panethnic but has the highest frequency among the Ashkenazi Jewish population, in which the incidences of types A and B disease are 1 in 40,000 and 1 in 80,000, respectively.[29,30,31]

Clinical Features

Type A, the acute neuropathic form, has its onset in early infancy. Affected infants exhibit progressive psychomotor retardation with massive hepatosplenomegaly and usually die by 3 years of age. The nonneuropathic type B has a slightly later onset in infancy than type A, and affected individuals manifest only visceral symptoms. Pancytopenia may occur secondary to hypersplenism, and pulmonary compromise can result from alveolar involvement.[30,31]

The ocular stigmata of the acute neuropathic form include corneal stromal opacities, cataracts, and cherry-red spots.[32] Macular cherry-red spots are eventually present in all affected individuals with type A, although they may not be observed initially. Macular halos, the mildest expression of a macular cherry-red spot, may be present in children with type B disease[33] (▶ Fig. 22.5).

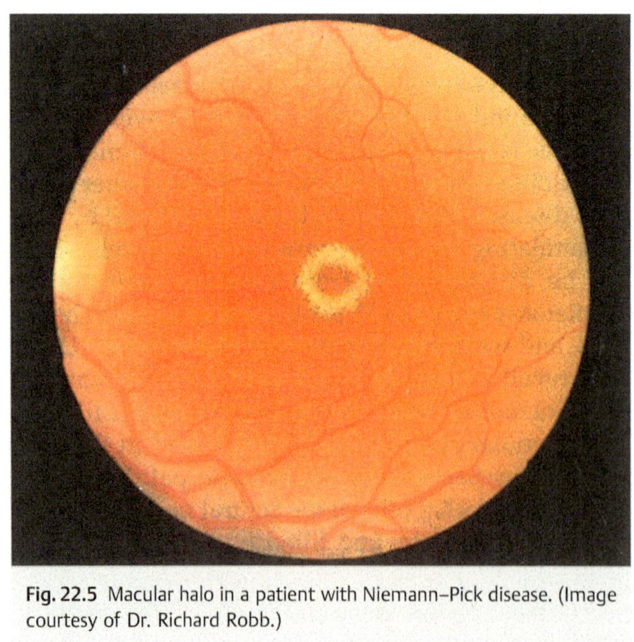

Fig. 22.5 Macular halo in a patient with Niemann–Pick disease. (Image courtesy of Dr. Richard Robb.)

Pearls

- In Niemann–Pick disease, only types A and B have clinically evident retinal changes. Cherry-red spots and macular halos are found in the neuropathic and nonneuropathic types, respectively.

Diagnosis

The diagnosis is based on the clinical findings, course of the disease, and testing for deficiency of sphingomyelinase activity in leukocytes.[3] The presence of Niemann-Pick cells (described later) in bone marrow aspirates supports the diagnosis of Niemann–Pick disease, but the diagnosis should be confirmed by enzyme assays. Definitive diagnosis of types A and B requires residual acid sphingomyelinase activity that is less than 10% of controls.[34] Prenatal diagnosis can be made by enzymatic or molecular analysis of cultured amniocytes or cells from chorionic villi.[35]

Pathogenesis and Histopathology

Niemann–Pick types A and B are caused by mutations in the acid sphingomyelinase gene (*SMPD1*) on chromosome 11p15. Mutations associated with type A disease result in complete absence of acid sphingomyelinase activity, leading to lysosomal accumulation of sphingomyelin.[36,37,38] Mutations associated with type B disease result in acid sphingomyelinase deficiency with some residual activity of the enzyme.[37,38,39] Comparison of enzymatic activity found that type B had 4% of normal acid sphingomyelinase activity while type A had undetectable activity.[37,39]

Distinctive foam cells, labeled *Niemann–Pick cells*, can be found in all affected tissues. However, their presence is not pathognomonic because similar cells can be observed in Tay–Sachs and several other metabolic diseases. Niemann–Pick cells are formed by lipid accumulating in bone marrow progenitor cells. They can be distinguished from Gaucher's cells by the smaller size, positive test for cholesterol, and weak staining for acid phosphatase. Ultrastructurally, Niemann–Pick cells contain granular lipid inclusions that may appear lamellar, like the membranous cytoplasmic bodies found in the neurons of patients with Tay–Sachs disease. In neuropathic disease, ganglion and glial cells of the central nervous system are distended, pale, and filled with large vacuoles. The glial cells may resemble foam cells.[35] In type A disease, membranous cytoplasmic bodies have been found in numerous ocular tissues, including keratocytes; endothelial cells; lens; retinal pigment epithelium (RPE); and fibroblasts of choroid, sclera, and extraocular muscles.[40]

Special Considerations

- The foam cells of Niemann–Pick disease are not pathognomonic for the condition, as similar cells can be observed histopathologically in Tay–Sachs and other metabolic diseases.

Management and Course

Unfortunately, the management of all forms of Niemann–Pick disease is supportive.

22.4 Mucopolysaccharidoses

The mucopolysaccharide (MPS) storage disorders are lysosomal storage disorders caused by a deficiency of enzymes required for the breakdown of glycosaminoglycans (GAGs) leading to the accumulation of partially degraded GAGs intracellularly and extracellularly in many tissues and in the urine.[41,42,43] All are progressive disorders and are inherited as an autosomal recessive trait except for Hunter's syndrome, which is an X-linked recessive trait. Of the six types, MPS I, II, and III exhibit retinal degeneration, whereas MPS I, IV, VI, and VII display corneal clouding.

22.4.1 Mucopolysaccharidosis Type I-H (MPS I-H, Hurler's Syndrome) and Type I-S (MPS I-S, Scheie's Syndrome)

Mucopolysaccharidosis type I (MPS I) is caused by a deficiency of the lysosomal hydrolase, alpha-L-iduronidase (*IDUA* gene), which is needed for the degradation of heparin sulfate and dermatan sulfate.[44] MPS I includes Hurler (MPS I-H), Hurler–Scheie (MPS I-H/S), and Scheie (MPS I-S) that represent a spectrum of severity.[45] The incidence of Hurler's syndromes in British Columbia is estimated to be 1 in 10,000 births.[46] Scheie's syndrome is very rare, with an incidence of 1 in 600,000 in British Columbia.[41]

Clinical Features

The Hurler's and Scheie's syndromes are now recognized to share the same biochemical defect and represent the extremes of a continuous spectrum of disease. In early infancy, patients with Hurler's syndromes often appear normal, but within the first year of life they manifest abnormalities such as coarse facies, large head, thick lips, enlarged tongue, airway problems, cardiac disease, hydrocephalus, hepatosplenomegaly, stiff joints, dysostosis multiplex, umbilical hernias, deafness, and mental retardation. Short stature becomes apparent by 2 to 3 years of age. Premature death usually ensues by the age of 10 years from cardiorespiratory failure.[41,47]

Corneal clouding associated with photophobia is often the first ocular manifestation of the MPS I-H and may progress to a point at which the fundus is obscured from view. It is caused by structural changes in the corneal stroma, including abnormalities of size, spacing, and arrangement of collagen fibrils.[48] Glaucoma has also been reported.[49,50] A retinal dystrophy with bone spicules develops, and the electroretinogram (ERG) is reduced or extinct.[50,51] Optic nerve head edema and subsequent optic atrophy are frequently observed. Enlargement of the optic nerve is caused by accumulation of acid mucopolysaccharides and leads to compression of the optic nerve at the lamina cribrosa or optic canal.[52]

The systemic manifestations of Scheie's syndrome are similar to those of Hurler's syndrome but less severe. Patients with Scheie's disease have a later onset of symptoms, which appear by 5 to 7 years of age. In one series of 10 patients, the most common presenting features were joint stiffness and corneal clouding.[45] Patients with Scheie's syndrome have normal stature, intelligence, and life expectancy. The diagnosis is made most commonly in the second decade of life. In a milder form, they share with Hurler's patients coarse facies, stiff joints, dysostosis multiplex, hernia, and deafness. Because of their longer life span, they also frequently are affected by carpal tunnel syndrome and aortic valvular disease, which result from accumulation of acid mucopolysaccharides at these sites. Orthopedic complications often dominate the long-term clinical picture. Crippling loss of hand function occurs secondary to carpal tunnel syndrome and progressive joint stiffness. Spondylolisthesis can lead to chronic back pain and occasionally results in spinal cord compression.[47]

The ocular features in Scheie's syndrome, like the systemic features, have a delayed but similar presentation to those of Hurler's syndrome. Corneal clouding becomes apparent in the second decade of life. It is most prominent peripherally and tends to be slowly progressive. Glaucoma frequently develops in the fourth and fifth decades of life. The retinal degeneration manifests as nyctalopia by age 20 to 30 years, and the fundus changes mimic those of retinitis pigmentosa.[50]

Diagnosis

Measurement of urinary GAG concentration, fractionation of GAG by electrophoresis or chromatography, and analysis of oligosaccharides can identify the type of MPS, oligosaccharidosis, or other storage disorders. Definitive diagnosis requires assay of alpha-L-iduronidase enzyme activity, usually in peripheral blood leukocytes. Differentiation between MPS type I Hurler and Scheie is based on the differences in clinical features and course (i.e., later onset, and lack of neurologic impairment in Scheie's disease). Carriers can also be detected by this method, as they have 50% or less of the a-L-iduronidase activity of normal controls. Prenatal diagnosis can be made by assaying cultured amniotic fluid cells by similar methods.[41,53] Conjunctival biopsy with ultrastructural study can assist in the diagnosis of storage diseases, but the changes are not specific to any one entity.[54] Mutation analysis is limited by the high frequency of "private" mutations, although analysis can be performed when the suspected mutation is known.[55,56,57,58]

Pathogenesis and Histopathology

The loss of a-L-iduronidase activity results in the buildup of intracellular heparin sulfate and dermatan sulfate, which are acid mucopolysaccharides that cannot be degraded and are deposited in swollen lysosomes.[49] Although the correlation between a-L-iduronidase activity and clinical severity is not absolute, most patients with severe disease have no detectable enzyme activity. The a-L-iduronidase gene (*IDUA*) has been cloned, and several mutant alleles have been analyzed. As expected, the more serious mutations resulting in frameshifts or premature stop codons are associated with little or no active enzyme and result in the more severe Hurler's phenotype. Point mutations frequently are associated with enzyme production and residual activity and result in the milder Scheie's phenotype.[3]

Chan and colleagues found abnormalities by electron microscopy in all ocular tissues of two patients without clinically detectable retinal degeneration.[54] They observed multimembranous inclusions in retinal ganglion cells and optic nerve astrocytes as well as fine fibrogranular inclusions in the RPE.

Management and Course

Currently, the only available therapy for MPS I is an allogenic bone marrow transplant. Patients with Hurler's disease receiving such transplants have improved visceral symptoms but show no improvement in skeletal abnormalities. The neurologic and intelligence outcomes have been variable, but a small number of patients who received early bone marrow transplants, before the age of 2 years, have developed normally, even though their genotypes would predict a severe Hurler's phenotype.[41] HLA-matched bone marrow transplants from siblings have the best chance of success, but when engraftment is achieved, unrelated donor transplants have been equally efficacious for visceral and neurologic symptoms.[59] Short of bone marrow transplant, treatment is limited to management of the disabling systemic and ocular manifestations, such as orthopedic problems, glaucoma, and corneal clouding.

22.4.2 Mucopolysaccharidosis Type II (MPS II, Hunter's Syndrome)

The incidence of Hunter's syndrome is estimated to be 1 in 150,000 in British Columbia and 1 in 67,500 in Israel.[46,60] Hunter's syndrome and adrenoleukodystrophy are the only two X-linked traits discussed in this chapter.

Clinical Features

Hunter's syndrome shares many features with the MPS type I syndromes. It presents in two forms: a severe, infantile form in which symptoms develop by 1 year of age and a less severe, childhood form with an older age of onset, at about 4 years. The infantile form is predominant. Affected individuals are generally mentally retarded and die before 15 years of age. Those with the childhood form have near-normal intelligence and life span. In both forms, coarse facies, immobile joints, short stature, airway problems, and hoarse voice gradually develop. The skeletal involvement tends to be milder in Hunter's syndrome than in Hurler's syndrome. One distinctive but rare feature of Hunter's syndrome is ivory-colored, nodular skin lesions affecting the neck, back, pectoral regions, upper arms, and thighs. The mildly afflicted patients often have cervical myelopathy in later life resulting from dural hyperplasia and thickening of the ligamenta flava.[41,47]

A progressive retinal degeneration with reduced ERG responses is the major ocular manifestation of Hunter's syndrome. The corneal clouding characteristic of the MPS type I syndromes is absent.[50] Chronic optic nerve head edema has been observed in the childhood form of Hunter.[41]

Diagnosis

Diagnosis is made by assaying for activity of iduronate sulfatase in cultured leukocytes.[41]

Pathogenesis and Histopathology

Hunter's syndrome is caused by a deficiency of iduronate 2-sulfatase, the gene of which (*IDS* gene) is located on chromosome Xq28, and results in lysosomal accumulation of heparin and dermatan sulfate.[61] Deletion of contiguous genes has been reported in patients with severe Hunter's syndrome.[62] Histologically, the retinal findings are indistinguishable from those of retinitis pigmentosa, with loss of photoreceptors and thinning of inner nuclear, outer nuclear, and ganglion cell layers. The RPE demonstrates pigmentary loss and migration. Fibrillogranular and multimembranous vacuoles are found in all ocular tissues examined by electron microscopy.[54]

Management and Course

No specific treatment has been proven effective in Hunter's syndrome.

22.4.3 Mucopolysaccharidosis Type III (MPS III, Sanfilippo's Syndrome)

MPS III is the most common mucopolysaccharidosis and is estimated to have a frequency of 1 in 24,000 in the Netherlands. Although it has less phenotypic variation than other mucopolysaccharidoses, it is biochemically heterogeneous. Defects in any one of four different enzymes may cause clinically similar disease.[41]

Clinical Features

The onset occurs between the ages of 2 and 6 years; affected children present with behavioral disorders and mental regression. The neurologic deterioration is profound and associated with progressive loss of developmental milestones, gait disturbances, deafness, and occasionally seizures. By contrast, the somatic stigmata of coarse facies, moderately short stature, hepatosplenomegaly, stiff joints, and hirsutism are less severe. Some mildly affected patients may even have normal features as adults. Death commonly occurs before the age of 20 years.

Corneal clouding is absent, but retinal degeneration closely resembling that of retinitis pigmentosa, with nyctalopia, bone spicules, vascular attenuation, and optic atrophy, is characteristic.[50] The ERG typically becomes extinct.[51]

Diagnosis

The diagnosis and subtyping of MPS III is made by assaying for the activity of the specific enzymes (see later) capable of causing the syndrome in cultured leukocytes or fibroblasts.[41]

Pathogenesis and Histopathology

MPS III can occur in four forms caused by different enzymatic deficiencies involved in the degradation of heparin sulfate and leading to its accumulation. Clinically, they are indistinguishable, except that type A disease tends to be more severe and associated with a shorter life span. Excessive heparan sulfate but not dermatan sulfate is excreted in the urine for all types of MPS III. MPS III A results from mutations in the gene encoding heparan sulfate sulfatase (also known as N-sulfoglucoasmine sulfohydrolase; *SGSH* gene) on 17q25.3.[63] MPS III B results from mutations in the gene encoding N-acetyl-alpha-D-glucosaminidase (*NAGLU* gene) at 17q21.[64] MPS III C results from deficiency of acetyl-CoA:alpha-glucosaminide N-acetyltransferase (*HGSNAT* gene), at 8p11.1.[65,66] Finally, MPS III D is caused by mutations in the gene encoding N-acetylglucosamine-6-sulfate sulfatase (*GNS* gene) at 12q14.[67] Del Monte and colleagues examined the eyes of a patient with MPS III and found the multimembranous cytoplasmic vacuoles typical of all mucopolysaccharidoses in the cornea, trabecular meshwork, iris, lens, RPE, retinal ganglion cells, and optic nerve. They also reported pathologic changes identical to those found in retinitis pigmentosa.[60,68]

Management and Course

No specific treatment has been proven effective in Sanfilippo's syndrome.

22.5 Amino Acid Disorders

22.5.1 Cystinosis

Cystinosis, characterized by an accumulation of cysteine in different organs and tissues, is an autosomal recessive disorder with infantile, juvenile, and adult forms. In France, the infantile form has been estimated to have a frequency of 1 in 326,000.[69]

Clinical Features

Affected individuals with the infantile (nephropathic) form appear normal for the first several months of life, then manifest failure to thrive, growth retardation, fever, aminoaciduria, and recurrent episodes of dehydration resulting from glomerular and renal tubular dysfunction. Renal transplant is often necessary before the teenage years. The juvenile (intermediate) type has a slightly later onset with milder course and symptoms. In the adult (benign) form, renal function is not impaired and onset occurs after the second decade of life. Affected individuals have a normal life expectancy.[70,71]

Photophobia is a common complaint of all patients with cystinosis because of the formation of cysteine crystals in the cornea, conjunctiva, and iris. The crystalline corneal accumulations can lead to recurrent erosions and incapacitating blepharospasm.[71] Late complications include posterior synechiae, corneal ulcerations, and visual impairment resulting from the corneal or retinal involvement.

Only individuals with the nephropathic form exhibit retinal findings, and these may precede the appearance of the corneal changes. Peripheral retinal pigment epithelial mottling and clumping are usually evident by 7 years of age. They eventually expand to involve the macula. Occasionally, yellow macular discoloration and deep retinal crystals also may be observed.[72,73] The visual fields, dark-adaptation curves, and electrophysiologic studies may be normal or reduced in patients with funduscopic changes.[74] Hemorrhagic retinopathy and visual impairment may occur.[71,73,75]

Diagnosis

Cystinosis can be confirmed by determining the cysteine content of peripheral blood leukocyte or fibroblasts.[76] Amniocytes may be used for prenatal diagnosis. Heterozygotes also have elevated levels of free cysteine in their leukocytes. Conjunctival biopsy specimens studied by electron microscopy show diagnostic membrane-bound inclusions in fibroblasts and histocytes.[77]

Pathogenesis and Histopathology

Derived from protein degradation within the lysosomes of cells, cystine is normally transported through the lysosomal membrane to the cytosol. In cystinosis, however, cystine accumulates within lysosomes because of a defect in the transport system and crystallizes.[77,78,79,80,81] The gene for nephropathic (or infantile) cystinosis, *CTNS*, encodes cystinosin, a lysosomal membrane protein that appears to be a hydrogen ion–driven transporter that exports cystine from lysosomes.[82,83,84,85] Various phenotypes of cystinosis are correlated with various mutations.[86] Histopathologic studies of autopsy eyes in the nephropathic form have revealed intracellular crystalline deposits in conjunctiva, cornea, sclera, iris, ciliary body, choroid, and RPE. Retinal pigment epithelial loss in the periphery accounts for the pigmentary changes observed on funduscopy.[71]

Management and Course

Cysteamine is the recommended treatment for all patients as soon as the diagnosis of cystinosis is confirmed. In a cohort of 86 adult patients with nephropathic cystinosis, initiating therapy before 5 years of age significantly decreased the incidence and delayed the onset of end-stage renal disease; delayed the onset of hypothyroidism, diabetes, and neuromuscular disorders; and improved life expectancy.[87] Cysteamine enters cells and concentrates within lysosomes, where it reacts with cystine to form both cysteine and a cysteine–cysteamine complex that is able to leave the lysosome.[88,89] The oral treatment does not improve corneal symptoms, but topical cysteamine drops have proved effective in clearing corneal crystals and reducing photophobia and blepharospasm.[90] Gel formulations of topical cysteamine have been shown to be superior to cysteamine drops.[91]

22.5.2 Gyrate Atrophy

Gyrate atrophy was first described by Jacobsohn in 1888 as an atypical retinitis pigmentosa and characterized by Fuchs in 1896. The biochemical basis for the disease was elucidated by Simell and Takki in 1973.[92] It is an autosomal recessive disorder with the highest incidence in Finland, about 1 in 50,000.[93]

Clinical Features

Most affected individuals appear clinically normal except for characteristically thin, straight, sparse hair. Less consistent findings include abnormal electroencephalogram (EEG), muscle weakness, abnormal electrocardiogram (ECG), and seizures.[50,94,95]

Nyctalopia is often the presenting feature, beginning in the first decade of life. During the second decade of life, sharply demarcated circular areas of chorioretinal atrophy develop, beginning in the midperiphery (▶ Fig. 22.6). The atrophic areas become confluent with time and extend anteriorly and posteriorly. The macular region is spared until late in the disease process; hence, central vision is usually maintained into the fourth or fifth decade of life. Loss of peripheral vision corresponds to the expanding zones of chorioretinal atrophy. Crystalline structures have been observed in the narrow pigmented septa separating the atrophic zones. The retinal vessels may become attenuated or remain of normal caliber. High myopia and astigmatism occur in 90% of affected individuals. Posterior subcapsular cataracts develop in the second or third decade of life. The amplitude of the ERG is diminished or abolished, and the electrooculogram (EOG) is abnormal.[95] There are reports of cystoid macular edema in patients with gyrate atrophy as well, with a short-term therapeutic effect seen with 4-mg intravitreal triamcinolone acetonide injection.[96,97,98]

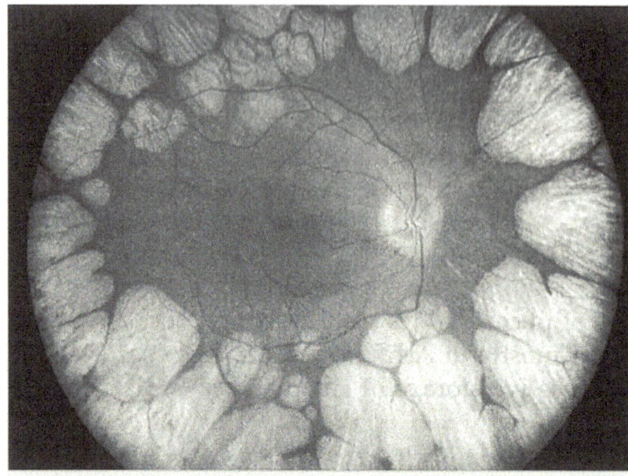

Fig. 22.6 Sharply demarcated circular areas of chorioretinal atrophy in gyrate atrophy.

Diagnosis

Diagnosis is made by observation of the characteristic fundus findings, demonstration of elevated plasma ornithine levels, and markedly decreased ornithine aminotransferase (OAT) activity in cultured fibroblasts or leukocytes. Heterozygotes have a reduced OAT activity, to about 50% of that of normal controls.[93]

Pathogenesis and Histopathology

The biochemical defect is decreased OAT activity, and several different mutations of the *OAT* gene, located on chromosome 10, have been documented.[93] OAT is a mitochondrial-encoded enzyme with pyridoxal phosphate (vitamin B6) enzyme as a cofactor that catalyzes the interconversion of ornithine, glutamate, and proline. Deficiencies increase plasma ornithine concentration.[99,100,101] The connection between hyperornithemia and gyrate atrophy is unclear, as other metabolic diseases causing hyperornithemia do not create gyrate-like fundus changes.[50] Histopathologic examination of affected eyes reveals atrophic regions of choriocapillaris, RPE, and photoreceptors immediately adjacent to normal-appearing tissue. Electron micrographic studies reveal swollen mitochondria in photoreceptors, corneal epithelium, nonpigmented ciliary epithelium, and iris. Earliest changes appear in the RPE cells with sporadic degeneration of scattered cells followed by more diffuse abnormalities of the RPE with accumulation of large phagosomes and crystalloid inclusions.[102] Similar changes are seen in liver mitochondria, and tubular aggregates are found ultrastructurally in type II muscle fibers.[93]

Controversial Points

- The biochemical defect in gyrate atrophy is decreased OAT activity. The relationship between the resulting hyperornithemia and gyrate atrophy, however, is unclear, as other diseases that cause hyperornithemia do not cause gyrate-like fundus changes.

Management and Course

Several treatment approaches have been successful in reducing plasma ornithine levels and preserving visual function in patients with gyrate atrophy. Supplemental pyridoxine can increase the activity of residual OAT in a small percentage of patients and results in a corresponding improvement in ERG, dark adaptation, and EOG. A strict, low-arginine diet has also been successful in stabilizing or slowing down progression of visual loss.[103,104]

Pearls

- Oral pyridoxine supplements and a diet low in arginine may help preserve or improve visual function in some patients with gyrate atrophy.

22.6 Mucolipidosis

22.6.1 Mucolipidosis V

Mucolipidosis IV is an autosomal recessive disorder found mostly in Ashkenazi Jews. It is characterized by excessive storage of gangliosides and mucopolysaccharides.

Clinical Features

In early infancy, affected individuals present with hypotonia, developmental delay, and progressive psychomotor retardation. Growth retardation becomes apparent by the age of 4 years, and facial features start to become coarse in the second decade. Patients with mucolipidosis type IV do not advance developmentally beyond the level of a typical 12- to 15-month-old infant. Visceral stigmata common to the other storage diseases are absent, and no mucopolysacchariduria is detected.[105]

Corneal epithelial clouding may be present at birth.[106] A retinal dystrophy that closely resembles that of retinitis pigmentosa can be observed.[107] Occasionally, it may be necessary to scrape the corneal epithelium to obtain a view of the fundus. Less common features include nystagmus, strabismus, and puffy eyelids.[105]

Diagnosis

Extracts of cultured fibroblasts demonstrate high levels of GM_3 and GD_3 gangliosides.[108] Prenatal diagnosis can be made by confirming the presence of characteristic inclusions on transmission electron microscopy of amniocytes.[109]

Pathogenesis and Histopathology

Mucolipidosis type IV involves a mutation of the mucolipin 1 gene (*MCOLN1*) on the short arm of chromosome 19.[110] MCOLN1 is thought to be part of the family of transient receptor channels, with mutations possibly leading to calcium efflux.[111] Histology of autopsy eyes revealed markedly disorganized and atrophic retina with loss of photoreceptor and ganglion cells.[107] Intraretinal pigment migration and severe optic atrophy were also seen. The remaining ganglion cells contained numerous cytoplasmic vacuoles. Ultrastructural studies of these vacuoles demonstrated membrane-limited cytoplasmic vacuoles containing a fine granular substance and concentric, lamellar, membranous structures. The granular vacuoles are consistent with MPS, and the lamellar vacuoles are consistent with phospholipid storage.

Management and Course

No specific therapy is available at present.

22.7 Ceroid Lipofuscinoses

22.7.1 Lipopigment Storage Disorders

Lipopigment storage disorders, characterized by accumulation of complex storage material within lysosomes, were first described early this century, but it was not until the 1960s that they were clearly identified as separate entities from Tay-Sachs disease, and the distinct electron microscopic features of the different forms were described.[112] The four types, infantile (Hagberg-Santavuori's syndrome), late infantile (Jansky–Bielschowsky syndrome), juvenile (Spielmeyer–Vogt or Batten's disease), and adult (Kufs's disease), are distinguished by age of onset and electron microscopic features. All are inherited as autosomal recessive traits, save for Kufs, which can be also be autosomal dominant. They share the characteristic of progressive neurologic degeneration. Visual loss is a prominent feature in the infantile, late infantile, and juvenile types. As a group, they have a global incidence of 1 in 12,500 per year.[113]

Clinical Features

Patients with the infantile onset form (INCL), also called Hagberg-Santavuori, initially appear normal but begin to lose developmental landmarks, manifesting ataxia and muscular hypotonia between 8 and 24 months of age. Eventually they progress to a vegetative state. Visual inattentiveness is apparent in the early stages. Examination of the fundus demonstrates a brownish coloration of the macula, hypopigmentation of the peripheral fundus, and optic atrophy. Late in the course, narrowing of the vessels is evident.[114,115] On ERG, rod responses are severely subnormal, but scotopic ERG shows a normal a-wave with a subnormal b-wave, suggesting an effect from proximal photoreceptors to optic nerve bipolar cells.[116,117]

In the late infantile-onset form (LINCL, also called Jansky–Bielschowsky) occurs in early childhood at 2 to 4 years, with rapid mental and motor deterioration. The presenting symptom is often a change in behavior. Visual inattentiveness usually becomes apparent after commencement of mental deterioration. Severe, intractable seizures are characteristic and often lead to death from aspiration pneumonia in early childhood. Funduscopic stigmata of granular perifoveal appearance, loss of foveal reflex, peripheral depigmentation, retinal vascular attenuation, and optic atrophy have been described.[118] ERG responses may be reduced.[119,120,121]

The most common presenting complaint of the juvenile-onset form (JNCL), Spielmeyer–Vogt or Batten's disease, is loss of central acuity between 6 and 8 years of age. Mental deterioration becomes evident shortly after the visual loss and is frequently associated with behavioral problems. Patients gradually progress to a vegetative state, and vision diminishes to no light perception. Patients usually survive to 15 to 25 years of age. The ophthalmic changes begin most often with granular macular pigmentary changes or bull's-eye macular pigmentary changes, which may be confused with Stargardt's disease.[122] Bone spicule formation and arteriolar narrowing may develop late in the course, mimicking retinitis pigmentosa.[123] ERG is abnormal early and advances to extinction.[121,124]

Patients with the adult-onset disorder (ANCL), or Kufs's disease, acquire advancing psychomotor deterioration in their third to fourth decades of life. No clinical ocular abnormalities have been described, but histologic abnormalities have been observed on autopsy.[125]

Diagnosis

Diagnosis is made on the basis of the clinical presentation and characteristic deposits visualized by electron microscopy. Historically, brain biopsies were performed but examination of conjunctiva, white blood cells, skin, rectal tissues, and muscle can be used. The deposits have a granular matrix in the infantile form, a curvilinear pattern in the late infantile type, a fingerprint design in the juvenile form, and a heterogeneous pattern in the adult type.[126,127,128]

Pathogenesis and Histopathology

A large number of genes causing ceroid lipofuscinoses have been identified, including *CLN1*, *2*, and *3*, but there does not appear to be a common mechanism and it is still unclear how mutations in these genes lead to the defining pathology. More than a dozen genes containing nearly 400 mutations have been identified. Although the end result is lysosomal storage body accumulation (including the subunit c of mitochondrial ATP synthase or sphingolipid activator proteins in lysosome-derive organelles), it does not appear to be the cause of the neurodegeneration.[129,130] In all ceroid lipofuscinoses, the pathologic hallmark is the presence of autofluorescent lipopigments within most tissues—the storage material resembles ceroid and lipofuscin, but it is actually lipoproteins and hydrophobic peptides.[131,132] Neuronal tissues are particularly heavily involved. The ultrastructural characteristics distinguishing the different types are discussed earlier.[50]

The pathologic characteristics of the infantile type were studied in ten autopsy eyes of five patients by Tarkkanen and colleagues.[124] They found severe degeneration of the retina with loss of cells in all retinal layers, glial proliferation, retinal pigment epithelial loss, pigmentary migration, and optic atrophy. The late infantile form also demonstrates extensive loss of photoreceptors and pigmentary migration.[133] Similar changes were described in the juvenile type.[128] In the adult form, severe ganglion cell loss was seen in a patient with a normal ophthalmologic examination.[125]

Management and Course

No specific therapy is available.

22.8 Peroxisomal Disorders

Peroxisomes are ubiquitous, single-membrane, cellular organelles present in all cells except for erythrocytes. They have a wide array of catabolic and anabolic functions. Disorders traced to peroxisomal dysfunction can be classified as single-enzyme defects or errors in peroxisomal assembly causing multiple enzymatic deficiencies and markedly reduced or absent peroxisomes.[134,135] They are a heterogenous group that typically result in neurologic dysfunction. Six peroxisomal disorders are consistently associated with retinal degenerations. With the exception of X-linked adrenoleukodystrophy, all peroxisomal disorders are inherited in an autosomal recessive pattern.[136]

22.8.1 Zellweger Spectrum Disorders (Zellweger's Syndrome, Neonatal Adrenoleukodystrophy, and Infantile Kefsum's Disease)

Clinical Features

These three disorders of peroxisomal assembly are now thought to represent a continuum, with Zellweger's syndrome the most severe, neonatal adrenoleukodystrophy intermediate in severity, and infantile Refsum's disease the least severe. Infants with classic Zellweger's syndrome, or cerebrohepatorenal syndrome, have a characteristic craniofacial dysmorphism consisting of high forehead, epicanthal folds, and hypoplastic supraorbital ridge and nose bridge. Other common features include deafness, seizures, hypotonia, psychomotor retardation, hepatomegaly, and cortical renal cysts. Magnetic resonance imaging (MRI) shows diffuse cortical and white matter abnormalities. Infants rarely survive beyond 6 months.[137] Patients with neonatal adrenoleukodystrophy typically have mild facial dysmorphism and no renal cortical cysts but otherwise manifest the same systemic findings as those with Zellweger's syndrome. MRI shows severe white matter deficiency.[137] The course is milder, with patients living an average of 4 years. Adrenocortical atrophy is typically present but rarely causes adrenal insufficiency.[135,136,138] Patients with infantile Refsum's disease also have either mild or no facial dysmorphism and lack renal cortical cysts. They typically present with severe developmental delay and can have systemic findings of Zellweger's syndrome, including hepatomegaly with cirrhosis, but are less likely to have seizures or hypotonia. Many affected individuals survive into adolescence.[135,136,137,139]

The ocular expressions of each disorder are similar, with pigmentary retinopathy, retinal vascular attenuation, and waxy optic nerve head pallor developing in most cases. The pigmentary retinopathy of Zellweger's syndrome mimics the pattern of classic retinitis pigmentosa, whereas the changes in neonatal adrenoleukodystrophy and infantile Refsum's disease are less classic, consisting of depigmentation of the perifoveal area and pigment clumping rather than bone spicules in the periphery.[136,140] All three syndromes demonstrate a reduced or extinguished ERG.[136,141,142] Additional ocular changes in Zellweger's syndrome are corneal clouding, cataract, and glaucoma.[142] Cataracts may also be found in neonatal adrenoleukodystrophy and rarely in infantile Refsum's disease.[135,140,141]

Diagnosis

The diagnosis of a peroxisomal assembly disorder should be considered for any neonate with hypotonia, seizures, failure to thrive, and/or dysmorphic features. In early childhood, patients with psychomotor retardation, progressive neurologic deficits, deafness, liver dysfunction, and retinal pigmentary degeneration should also be screened for peroxisomal assembly defects. Elevated plasma levels of very long-chain fatty acids (VLCFA) are found in all disorders of peroxisomal biogenesis, so measurement of plasma VLCFA levels can serve as an initial screening study. Other diagnostic findings include cytosolic localization of catalase activity and absent or reduced numbers of peroxisomes in liver biopsy specimens. Prenatal diagnosis can be made on cultured amniocytes or chorionic villus samples.[143] A "Pex Gene Screen" is also available and provides an algorithm permitting the identification of the molecular defect in these disorders.[144]

Pathogenesis and Histopathology

Zellweger's spectrum disorders are caused by mutations in genes cording for peroxins (PEX), proteins required for peroxisome formation, and lead to a generalized loss of peroxisomal functions. They have been linked to mutations in at least 12 different genes, with the majority in *PEX1* or *PEX6* genes that encode ATPases needed to import protein from the cytosol into peroxisomes. Severe defects in one of these PEX genes result in an absence of functional peroxisomes and typically the Zellweger's syndrome, while the neonatal adrenoleukodystrophy and infantile Refsum's disease phenotypes are often associated with partially functional peroxisomes.[133,145,146,147,148]

In Zellweger's syndrome, the most striking pathologic change is marked loss of photoreceptors. Retinal neurons, ganglion cells, and retinal pigment epithelial cells are reduced in number as well. There are numerous pigment-containing macrophages in the retina and subretinal space. When examined ultrastructurally, these macrophages contain bileaflet cytoplasmic inclusions consisting of cholesterol esters of VLCFA. Identical inclusions are found in the brain and RPE. The pathologic changes in adrenoleukodystrophy are indistinguishable from those seen in Zellweger's syndrome.[149,150] In infantile Refsum's disease, neuronal loss in all retinal layers was found on pathologic examination of an autopsy eye.[136]

Management and Course

The severe malformations and defects that evolve during fetal development are unlikely to be amenable to postnatal treatment. For some patients with mild phenotypes, dietary treatment with supplementation of ether lipid and restriction of phytanic acid and VLCFA could potentially stabilize disease progression.[143] Another approach is normalizing the concentration of docosahexaenoic acid (DHA), which is low in the brain and retina in these disorders and may contribute to neurologic abnormalities. One review of 20 individuals with Zellweger's spectrum disorders treated with DHA ethyl ester reported improved vision in half of those treated as well as increased muscle tone, and improved myelination on MRI. Benefits of this treatment, however, are still debated.[151,152]

22.8.2 Refsum Disease

Clinical Features

Patients affected with Refsum's disease commonly present with complaints of nyctalopia, gait disturbance, or extremity weakness before the age of 20 years. Systemic manifestations are frequent and include cerebellar ataxia, peripheral polyneuropathy, anosmia, nerve deafness, epiphyseal dysplasia, ichthyosis, cardiac conduction defects, and elevated cerebrospinal fluid protein without pleocytosis. Retinal degeneration with bone spicule pigmentary changes, retinal vascular attenuation, and optic atrophy is characteristic. ERG is diminished or extinguished, and visual field testing demonstrates progressive narrowing or a ring scotoma. Dark adaptation is delayed.[144,153,154]

Diagnosis

Diagnosis can be made by finding the classic tetrad of retinitis pigmentosa, peripheral polyneuropathy, cerebellar ataxia, and elevated cerebrospinal fluid protein in the absence of pleocytosis. The diagnosis is confirmed by elevated plasma concentration of phytanic acid and mutation analysis.[155] Fibroblasts can also be cultured and examined for documentation of reduced phytanic acid oxidase activity. Heterozygotes demonstrate a 50% reduction in phytanic acid oxidase activity compared with normal controls. Elevated levels of phytanic acid in the plasma are found in untreated Refsum patients and in patients with disorders of peroxisomal biogenesis and, therefore, are not specific on their own.[156]

Pearls

- Refsum's disease is characterized by the classic clinical tetrad of retinitis pigmentosa, peripheral polyneuropathy, cerebellar ataxia, and elevated cerebrospinal fluid protein. The biochemical defect is a reduced activity of phytanic acid oxidase, and dietary restriction of phytanate precursors may slow down or stabilize the retinal degeneration.

Pathogenesis and Histopathology

Refsum's disease is typically caused by mutations in the gene (*PAHX* or *PHYH*) encoding the enzyme phytanoyl-CoA hydroxylase, located on chromosome 10pter-p11.2.[155,157,158] Phytanoyl-CoA hydroxylase is a peroxisomal enzyme that catalyzes the first step of phytanic acid alpha-oxidation. Mutations in the

PEX7 gene, which encodes the peroxisomal type 2 targeting signal receptor, have also been shown to cause Refsum's disease.[159] Phytanic acid originates from exogenous sources and is absorbed from the diet. It is typically metabolized by activation to its CoA ester, phytanoyl-CoA, and then alpha-oxidation to pristanic acid, but patients with Refsum's disease are unable to degrade phytanic acid. The connection between the accumulation of phytanic acid and clinical manifestations is not clear. Possibly, incorporation of excess phytanic acid into cellular membrane and myelin disturbs normal function.[156]

Loss of photoreceptors, pigmentary migration, and accumulation of fatty acids in the outer layers of the retina and some retinal vessels have been reported in histopathologic studies of eyes from patients with Refsum's disease.[160]

Management and Course

Dietary restriction of phytanate precursors in meat, fish oils, and dairy products has been used to treat both forms of phytanic acid storage disease. In Refsum's disease, dietary restrictions have resulted in improvement of peripheral neuropathy and have slowed down or stabilized retinal degeneration.[144,156,161]

22.8.3 Adrenoleukodystrophy (Addison-Schilder's Disease)

Clinical Features

Adrenoleukodystrophy is the most common peroxisomal disorder and is inherited in an X-linked recessive fashion. There are two main phenotypes: a childhood form and an adult form, which is also called *adrenomyeloneuropathy*. The onset of the childhood form occurs between 5 and 10 years of age and manifests as behavioral changes, scholastic failure, or increased skin pigmentation, frequently precipitated by a viral syndrome. Adrenal insufficiency may precede neurologic symptoms by several years. Clinical features include progressive dementia, gait disturbance, blindness, and adrenocortical failure leading to skin pigmentation and hypoadrenalism. Death commonly takes place in adolescence.[162] Neuroimaging of affected children shows demyelinating lesions in the parietooccipital regions resembling those found in multiple sclerosis.[163] The adult form usually presents in the third decade of life with slowly progressive stiffness and weakness of the legs and sphincter disturbances.[164]

Visual loss in childhood adrenoleukodystrophy occurs years after the onset of systemic symptoms and is rapidly progressive, with both visual field and acuity loss. Optic atrophy and ocular motility disturbances are also frequently found. Macular pigmentary mottling is seen less frequently. The visually evoked potentials are typically abnormal, but ERG may be normal or reduced.[162] The adult variant (adrenomyeloneuropathy) is rarely associated with symptomatic visual loss, but pattern-reversal, visually evoked potentials and neuroimaging studies demonstrate involvement of the visual system in 63% of patients.[164]

Diagnosis

Children with behavioral changes and visual loss should be screened for elevated plasma levels of VLCFA including levels of hexacosanoic acid (C 26:0).[165] The demyelinating lesions found on neuroimaging studies are also useful diagnostically.[163] The diagnosis should also be confirmed by mutation analysis of the *ABCD1* gene. Given the concomitant adrenal insufficiency that can occur, all individuals with suspected or known adrenoleukodystrophy should be evaluated periodically for adrenal insufficiency.[166]

Pathogenesis and Histopathology

Adrenoleukodystrophy is caused by mutations in the ATP-binding cassette, subfamily D, member 1 gene (*ABCD1* gene), which is located at Xq28 and encodes an ABC transporter. This ABC transporter helps form the channel through which VLCFA can move into the peroxisome, probably as CoA-esters.[167,168] Prevention of VLCFA normal transport prevents beta-oxidation and leads to accumulation of abnormal VLCFA in affected organs including central nervous system, Leydig's cells of the testes, and adrenal cortex, underlying the pathology of adrenoleukodystrophy. Patients with adrenoleukodystrophy amass long-chain fatty acids and cholesterol esters, which results in adrenal dysfunction and demyelination. In terms of central nervous system effect, adrenoleukodystrophy is characterized by inflammatory demyelination, which results in symmetric loss of myelin in the cerebral and cerebellar white matter. The parietooccipital regions of the brain are usually affected first, with progression of the lesions toward the frontal or temporal lobes.[169,170] Visual loss is thought to be primarily a consequence of demyelinating lesions along the central visual tracts, but the findings of ganglion cell loss and gliosis of the inner retinal layers on histopathology suggest that primary retinal ganglion cell degeneration may be a contributing factor.[149]

Management and Course

Hematopoietic cell transplantation is recommended for patients with cerebral adrenoleukodystrophy as well as those with few to no neurologic symptoms, suggesting that they are early in their disease course. A case series of 12 boys with childhood cerebral adrenoleukodystrophy treated with hematopoietic cell transplantation were found to have plasma VLCFA concentration decreased by 55% with three demonstrating improvement or reversal in MRI changes.[171] Individuals with adrenoleukodystrophy but without clinical or MRI evidence of cerebral involvement are recommended to have dietary treatment with restriction of VLCFA intake and supplementation with Lorenzo's oil, a 4:1 mixture of glyceryl trioleate and glyceryl trierucate that inhibits endogenous synthesis of VLCFA.[172,173] However, this treatment has not demonstrated a clinically significant effect on the rate of neurologic progression in symptomatic patients of the childhood or adult phenotypes.

22.8.4 Primary Hyperoxaluria Type I Clinical Manifestations

Primary hyperoxaluria type I is an autosomal recessive disorder that becomes evident in early childhood or adulthood through renal failure or nephrolithiasis. Onset in childhood indicates a more rapid and severe course.[136] Oxalate crystals are deposited in many tissues, including the heart, testes, central nervous system, thyroid, adipose tissue, lymph nodes, muscles, skin, arterial walls, and bones.

Controversial Points

- Although dietary measures can normalize the levels of VLCFA in the plasma of patients with adrenoleukodystrophy, it does not appear to alter the natural course of disease. Bone marrow transplantation may be a more promising treatment modality.

A crystalline retinopathy is present in about 30% of patients. The crystalline flecks are often in a periarterial distribution, and hyperplastic clumps or rings of RPE with bright white or yellow centers are frequently observed in the central macular area. The visual acuity is usually unaffected by the pigmentary changes, but it can be reduced if optic atrophy or choroidal neovascularization develops.[164,174,175]

Diagnosis

Diagnosis is established by increased urinary oxalate excretion, liver biopsy demonstrating absence or significant reduction in alanine:glyoxylate aminotransferase activity, and confirmation by molecular genetic testing demonstrating a mutation in the responsible gene.[176]

Pathogenesis and Histopathology

Primary hyperoxaluria type 1 is due to defects in the *AGXT* gene that encodes the hepatic peroxisomal enzyme alanine:glyoxylate aminotransferase, which is involved in the conversion of glyoxylate to glycine.[177,178] This leads to an increase in the glyoxylate pool and overproduction of oxalate. In the eye, the pathologic findings consist of calcium oxalate crystals in the RPE, choroid, ciliary body, retina, episclera, conjunctiva, iris, and ocular muscles. The black macular pigmentary changes are believed to represent retinal pigment epithelial hypertrophy or hyperplasia in response to the irritative effects of the oxalate crystals.[136] Spectral domain OCT shows hyperreflective lesions within the RPE, correlating with the calcium oxalate crystals seen on pathology.[179]

Management and Course

Current treatment is limited to renal and/or liver transplantation for calcium oxalate-induced nephropathy.

22.8.5 Abetalipoproteinemia (Bassen-Kornzweig's Syndrome)

Abetalipoproteinemia has an autosomal recessive pattern of inheritance. Hypobetalipoproteinemia, which is clinically indistinguishable, has an autosomal dominant pattern of inheritance.[180]

Clinical Features

The onset of symptoms, with failure to thrive and steatorrhea, occurs most often in the first few years of life. The characteristic systemic features are spinal cerebellar ataxia; intestinal malabsorption with steatorrhea; cardiac abnormalities; erythrocyte acanthocytosis; and low levels of all serum lipids, lipoproteins, and fat-soluble vitamins.[180,181]

Nyctalopia is frequently the first ocular symptom. A ring scotoma may subsequently develop. On funduscopy, one observes atypical pigmentary retinal degeneration with waxy disc pallor, atrophic RPE changes, and pigment migration. Ptosis, strabismus, nystagmus, and ophthalmoplegia have also been associated with abetalipoproteinemia. Bilateral optic disc swelling has also be described.[182] The ERG becomes abnormal early in the course of disease and often progresses to extinction.[180,181]

Hypobetalipoproteinemia in the heterozygous state manifests only minimal symptoms, such as mild fat malabsorption, diminished deep tendon reflexes, and, rarely, ataxia or proprioceptive deficits. Homozygotes are clinically indistinguishable from persons with abetalipoproteinemia.[180]

Diagnosis

The diagnosis of abetalipoproteinemia is based on clinical features and the laboratory findings of uniformly depressed levels of all serum lipoproteins, absence of apolipoprotein B, and acanthocytosis. Hypobetalipoproteinemia can be distinguished from abetalipoproteinemia biochemically and genetically by the detection of low serum levels of lipoproteins in heterozygotes (usually the parent of the affected individual).[180]

Pathogenesis and Histopathology

The biochemical abnormality in abetalipoproteinemia is failure of assembly and/or secretion of chylomicrons and very low-density lipoproteins (VLDL). Each class of lipoprotein contains a characteristic B apoprotein, which forms the identification tag of the lipoprotein. Apo B-100 is the apoprotein for VLDL and low-density lipoprotein (LDL). A shorter version of the same apoprotein, apo B-48, is the apoprotein for chylomicrons. In patients with abetalipoproteinemia, the apoproteins are formed normally but accumulate intracellularly and are not secreted. Abetalipoproteinemia is caused by mutations encoding the microsomal triglyceride transfer protein (*MTP* gene), which is essential for the formation and secretion of apo B lipoproteins, both from the intestine (chylomicrons) and liver (LDL and VLDL).[181,183,184,185] Clinical manifestations result from the inability to absorb and transport vitamins A and E. Molecular genetic testing for *MTP* gene mutations is not currently commercially available.[186] In hypobetalipoproteinemia, the defect is in the apo B gene itself. The steatorrhea is caused by the inability of the enterocytes to secrete chylomicrons. The resulting accumulation of lipid within the intestinal mucosa causes a yellow discoloration, with lipid droplets visible ultrastructurally within the enterocyte cytoplasm. The fatty malabsorption prevents uptake of fat-soluble vitamins, particularly vitamin E, which depends largely on chylomicrons and VLDL for transport.[180]

On histopathologic examination, the ocular changes in abetalipoproteinemia resemble those of retinitis pigmentosa. There is extensive loss of photoreceptors, pigment migration, and abnormal granules in the RPE that stain with periodic acid–Schiff. Ultrastructurally, lamellar inclusions and abnormal amounts of lipofuscin are observed in the RPE.[187] The *MTP* gene has been shown to be expressed in the RPE and retinal ganglion cells, and its absence likely has negative consequences for Bruch's membrane.[188]

Management and Course

Chronic diarrhea responds well to a low-fat diet. The neurologic manifestations can be prevented by high-dose oral supplementation with vitamin E. Retinal degeneration was previously thought to be halted or prevented by this supplementation, and high doses of vitamin A were shown to reverse ERG and dark adaptation in early stages.[180,181,189] However, a longitudinal study of patients with abetalipoproteinemia and hypobetalipoproteinemia showed that retinal pigmentary and ERG changes may still occur despite early vitamins A and E treatment.[190]

Pearls

- In abetalipoproteinemia, neurologic manifestations can be prevented by high-dose oral vitamin E supplements. Retinal degeneration may be stabilized or minimized.

References

[1] Kaback M, Lim-Steele J, Dabholkar D, Brown D, Levy N, Zeiger K, The International TSD Data Collection, Network. Tay-Sachs disease—carrier screening, prenatal diagnosis, and the molecular era. An international perspective, 1970 to 1993. JAMA. 1993; 270(19):2307–2315

[2] Sandhoff KCE, Conzelmann E, Neufeld EF, et al. The GM2 gangliosidoses. In: Scriver CR, Beaudet AL, Sly WS, Valle D, eds. The Metabolic Basis of Inherited Disease, 6th ed., Vol. II. New York: McGraw-Hill; 1989:1807–1839

[3] Gieselmann V. Lysosomal storage diseases. Biochim Biophys Acta. 1995; 1270(2–3):103–136

[4] Pennock CA. Lysosomal storage disease. In: Holton JB, ed. The Inherited Metabolic Diseases, 2nd ed. Longdon: Churchill Livingstone; 1994:223–224

[5] Bach G, Tomczak J, Risch N, Ekstein J. Tay-Sachs screening in the Jewish Ashkenazi population: DNA testing is the preferred procedure. Am J Med Genet. 2001; 99(1):70–75

[6] Brownstein S, Carpenter S, Polomeno RC, Little JM. Sandhoff's disease (GM2 gangliosidosis type 2). Histopathology and ultrastructure of the eye. Arch Ophthalmol. 1980; 98(6):1089–1097

[7] Suzuki YSH, Oshima A. Beta-galactosidase deficiency (b-galactosidase): GM1 gangliosidosis and Morquio B disease. In: Scriver CR, Beaudet AL, Sly WS, Valle D, eds. The Metabolic Basis of Inherited Disease, 6th ed. New York: McGraw-Hill; 1989:2785–2827

[8] Chen H, Chan AY, Stone DU, Mandal NA. Beyond the cherry-red spot: Ocular manifestations of sphingolipid-mediated neurodegenerative and inflammatory disorders. Surv Ophthalmol. 2014; 59(1):64–76

[9] NIH Technology Assessment Panel on Gaucher Disease. Gaucher disease. Current issues in diagnosis and treatment. JAMA. 1996; 275(7):548–553

[10] Grabowski GA. Gaucher disease: gene frequencies and genotype/phenotype correlations. Genet Test. 1997; 1(1):5–12

[11] Koprivica V, Stone DL, Park JK, et al. Analysis and classification of 304 mutant alleles in patients with type 1 and type 3 Gaucher disease. Am J Hum Genet. 2000; 66(6):1777–1786

[12] Cogan DG, Chu FC, Gittinger J, Tychsen L. Fundal abnormalities of Gaucher's disease. Arch Ophthalmol. 1980; 98(12):2202–2203

[13] Ueno H, Ueno S, Kajitani T, et al. Clinical and histopathological studies of a case with juvenile form of Gaucher's disease. Jpn J Ophthalmol. 1977; 21:98–108

[14] Baldellou A, Andria G, Campbell PE, et al. Paediatric non-neuronopathic Gaucher disease: recommendations for treatment and monitoring. Eur J Pediatr. 2004; 163(2):67–75

[15] Cormand B, Montfort M, Chabás A, Vilageliu L, Grinberg D. Genetic fine localization of the beta-glucocerebrosidase (GBA) and prosaposin (PSAP) genes: implications for Gaucher disease. Hum Genet. 1997; 100(1):75–79

[16] Messner MC, Cabot MC. Glucosylceramide in humans. Adv Exp Med Biol. 2010; 688:156–164

[17] Cox TM. Gaucher disease: understanding the molecular pathogenesis of sphingolipidoses. J Inherit Metab Dis. 2001; 24 Suppl 2:106–121, discussion 87–88

[18] Zimran A, Elstein D, Levy-Lahad E, et al. Replacement therapy with imiglucerase for type 1 Gaucher's disease. Lancet. 1995; 345(8963):1479–1480

[19] Pastores GM, Weinreb NJ, Aerts H, et al. Therapeutic goals in the treatment of Gaucher disease. Semin Hematol. 2004; 41(4) Suppl 5:4–14

[20] Cox TM, Aerts JM, Belmatoug N, et al. Management of non-neuronopathic Gaucher disease with special reference to pregnancy, splenectomy, bisphosphonate therapy, use of biomarkers and bone disease monitoring. J Inherit Metab Dis. 2008; 31(3):319–336

[21] Martins AM, Valadares ER, Porta G, et al. Brazilian Study Group on Gaucher Disease and other Lysosomal Storage Diseases. Recommendations on diagnosis, treatment, and monitoring for Gaucher disease. J Pediatr. 2009; 155(4) Suppl:S10–S18

[22] Ben Turkia H, Gonzalez DE, Barton NW, et al. Velaglucerase alfa enzyme replacement therapy compared with imiglucerase in patients with Gaucher disease. Am J Hematol. 2013; 88(3):179–184

[23] Gonzalez DE, Turkia HB, Lukina EA, et al. Enzyme replacement therapy with velaglucerase alfa in Gaucher disease: results from a randomized, double-blind, multinational, Phase 3 study. Am J Hematol. 2013; 88(3):166–171

[24] Zimran A, Brill-Almon E, Chertkoff R, et al. Pivotal trial with plant cell-expressed recombinant glucocerebrosidase, taliglucerase alfa, a novel enzyme replacement therapy for Gaucher disease. Blood. 2011; 118 (22):5767–5773

[25] Zimran A, Pastores GM, Tylki-Szymanska A, et al. Safety and efficacy of velaglucerase alfa in Gaucher disease type 1 patients previously treated with imiglucerase. Am J Hematol. 2013; 88(3):172–178

[26] Pastores GM, Rosenbloom B, Weinreb N, et al. A multicenter open-label treatment protocol (HGT-GCB-058) of velaglucerase alfa enzyme replacement therapy in patients with Gaucher disease type 1: safety and tolerability. Genet Med. 2014; 16(5):359–366

[27] Steward CG, Jarisch A. Haemopoietic stem cell transplantation for genetic disorders. Arch Dis Child. 2005; 90(12):1259–1263

[28] Somaraju UR, Tadepalli K. Hematopoietic stem cell transplantation for Gaucher disease. Cochrane Database Syst Rev. 2012; 7:CD006974

[29] Levran O, Desnick RJ, Schuchman EH. Niemann-Pick disease: a frequent missense mutation in the acid sphingomyelinase gene of Ashkenazi Jewish type A and B patients. Proc Natl Acad Sci U S A. 1991; 88(9):3748–3752

[30] Levran O, Desnick RJ, Schuchman EH. Niemann-Pick type B disease. Identification of a single codon deletion in the acid sphingomyelinase gene and genotype/phenotype correlations in type A and B patients. J Clin Invest. 1991; 88(3):806–810

[31] Walton DS, Robb RM, Crocker AC. Ocular manifestations of group A Niemann-Pick disease. Am J Ophthalmol. 1978; 85(2):174–180

[32] Matthews JD, Weiter JJ, Kolodny EH. Macular halos associated with Niemann-Pick type B disease. Ophthalmology. 1986; 93(7):933–937

[33] Schuchman EHDR. Niemann-Pick disease type A and B: sphingomyelinase deficiencies. In: Scriver CR, Beaudet AL, Sly WS, Valle D, eds. The Metabolic and Molecular Basis of Inherited Disease, 7th ed. New York: McGraw-Hill; 1995:2601–2624

[34] van Diggelen OP, Voznyi YV, Keulemans JL, et al. A new fluorimetric enzyme assay for the diagnosis of Niemann-Pick A/B, with specificity of natural sphingomyelinase substrate. J Inherit Metab Dis. 2005; 28(5):733–741

[35] Robb RM, Kuwabara T. The ocular pathology of type A Niemann-Pick disease. A light and electron microscopic study. Invest Ophthalmol. 1973; 12 (5):366–377

[36] da Veiga Pereira L, Desnick RJ, Adler DA, Disteche CM, Schuchman EH. Regional assignment of the human acid sphingomyelinase gene (SMPD1) by PCR analysis of somatic cell hybrids and in situ hybridization to 11p15.1-—p15.4. Genomics. 1991; 9(2):229–234

[37] Graber D, Salvayre R, Levade T. Accurate differentiation of neuronopathic and nonneuronopathic forms of Niemann-Pick disease by evaluation of the effective residual lysosomal sphingomyelinase activity in intact cells. J Neurochem. 1994; 63(3):1060–1068

[38] Takahashi T, Suchi M, Desnick RJ, Takada G, Schuchman EH. Identification and expression of five mutations in the human acid sphingomyelinase gene causing types A and B Niemann-Pick disease. Molecular evidence for genetic heterogeneity in the neuronopathic and non-neuronopathic forms. J Biol Chem. 1992; 267(18):12552–12558

[39] Vanier MT, Rousson R, Garcia I, et al. Biochemical studies in Niemann-Pick disease. III. In vitro and in vivo assays of sphingomyelin degradation in cultured skin fibroblasts and amniotic fluid cells for the diagnosis of the various forms of the disease. Clin Genet. 1985; 27(1):20–32

[40] Vellodi A, Hobbs JR, O'Donnell NM, Coulter BS, Hugh-Jones K. Treatment of Niemann-Pick disease type B by allogeneic bone marrow transplantation. Br Med J (Clin Res Ed). 1987; 295(6610):1375–1376

[41] Wraith JE. The mucopolysaccharidoses: a clinical review and guide to management. Arch Dis Child. 1995; 72(3):263–267

[42] Muenzer J. Mucopolysaccharidoses. Adv Pediatr. 1986; 33:269–302

[43] Wenger DA, Coppola S, Liu SL. Insights into the diagnosis and treatment of lysosomal storage diseases. Arch Neurol. 2003; 60(3):322–328

[44] Scott HS, Bunge S, Gal A, Clarke LA, Morris CP, Hopwood JJ. Molecular genetics of mucopolysaccharidosis type I: diagnostic, clinical, and biological implications. Hum Mutat. 1995; 6(4):288–302

[45] Vijay S, Wraith JE. Clinical presentation and follow-up of patients with the attenuated phenotype of mucopolysaccharidosis type I. Acta Paediatr. 2005; 94(7):872–877

[46] Neufeld EFMJ. The mucopolysaccharidoses. In: Scriver CR, Beaudet AL, Sly WS, Valle D, eds. The Metabolic and Molecular Basis of Inherited Disease, 7th ed. New York: McGraw-Hill; 1995:2465–2494

[47] Klintworth G. Disorders of glycosaminoglycans (mucopolysaccharides) and proteoglycan. In: Garner A, Klintworth GK, eds. Pathobiology of Ocular Disease: A Dynamic Approach, Part B. New York: Marcel Dekker; 1982:863

[48] Alroy J, Haskins M, Birk DE. Altered corneal stromal matrix organization is associated with mucopolysaccharidosis I, III and VI. Exp Eye Res. 1999; 68 (5):523–530

[49] François J. Metabolic tapetoretinal degenerations. Surv Ophthalmol. 1982; 26(6):293–333

[50] Caruso RC, Kaiser-Kupfer MI, Muenzer J, Ludwig IH, Zasloff MA, Mercer PA. Electroretinographic findings in the mucopolysaccharidoses. Ophthalmology. 1986; 93(12):1612–1616

[51] Mailer C. Gargoylism associated with optic atrophy. Can J Ophthalmol. 1969; 4(3):266–271

[52] Hall CW, Liebaers I, Di Natale P, Neufeld EF. Enzymic diagnosis of the genetic mucopolysaccharide storage disorders. Methods Enzymol. 1978; 50:439–456

[53] McDonnell JM, Green WR, Maumenee IH. Ocular histopathology of systemic mucopolysaccharidosis, type II-A (Hunter syndrome, severe). Ophthalmology. 1985; 92(12):1772–1779

[54] Chan CC, Green WR, Maumenee IH, et al. Ocular ultrastructural studies of two cases of the Hurler syndrome (systemic mucopolysaccharidosis I-H). Ophthalmic Paediatr Genet. 1983; 2(1):3–19

[55] Fensom AH, Benson PF. Recent advances in the prenatal diagnosis of the mucopolysaccharidoses. Prenat Diagn. 1994; 14(1):1–12

[56] Cleary MA, Wraith JE. Antenatal diagnosis of inborn errors of metabolism. Arch Dis Child. 1991; 66(7 Spec No):816–822

[57] Bunge S, Steglich C, Lorenz P, et al. Prenatal diagnosis and carrier detection in mucopolysaccharidosis type II by mutation analysis. A 47,XXY male heterozygous for a missense point mutation. Prenat Diagn. 1994; 14(9):777–780

[58] Peters C, Balthazor M, Shapiro EG, et al. Outcome of unrelated donor bone marrow transplantation in 40 children with Hurler syndrome. Blood. 1996; 87(11):4894–4902

[59] Schaap T, Bach G. Incidence of mucopolysaccharidoses in Israel: is Hunter disease a "Jewish disease"? Hum Genet. 1980; 56(2):221–223

[60] Del Monte MA, Maumenee IH, Green WR, Kenyon KR. Histopathology of Sanfilippo's syndrome. Arch Ophthalmol. 1983; 101(8):1255–1262

[61] Hopwood JJ, Bunge S, Morris CP, et al. Molecular basis of mucopolysaccharidosis type II: mutations in the iduronate-2-sulphatase gene. Hum Mutat. 1993; 2(6):435–442

[62] Brusius-Facchin AC, De Souza CF, Schwartz IV, et al. Severe phenotype in MPS II patients associated with a large deletion including contiguous genes. Am J Med Genet A. 2012; 158A(5):1055–1059

[63] Scott HS, Blanch L, Guo XH, et al. Cloning of the sulphamidase gene and identification of mutations in Sanfilippo A syndrome. Nat Genet. 1995; 11 (4):465–467

[64] Zhao HG, Li HH, Bach G, Schmidtchen A, Neufeld EF. The molecular basis of Sanfilippo syndrome type B. Proc Natl Acad Sci U S A. 1996; 93(12):6101–6105

[65] Fan X, Zhang H, Zhang S, et al. Identification of the gene encoding the enzyme deficient in mucopolysaccharidosis IIIC (Sanfilippo disease type C). Am J Hum Genet. 2006; 79(4):738–744

[66] Hrebícek M, Mrázová L, Seyrantepe V, et al. Mutations in TMEM76* cause mucopolysaccharidosis IIIC (Sanfilippo C syndrome). Am J Hum Genet. 2006; 79(5):807–819

[67] Robertson DA, Callen DF, Baker EG, Morris CP, Hopwood JJ. Chromosomal localization of the gene for human glucosamine-6-sulphatase to 12q14. Hum Genet. 1988; 79(2):175–178

[68] Bois E, Feingold J, Frenay P, Briard ML. Infantile cystinosis in France: genetics, incidence, geographic distribution. J Med Genet. 1976; 13(6):434–438

[69] Read J, Goldberg MF, Fishman G, Rosenthal I. Nephropathic cystinosis. Am J Ophthalmol. 1973; 76(5):791–796

[70] Sanderson PO, Kuwabara T, Stark WJ, Wong VG, Collins EM. Cystinosis. A clinical, histopathologic, and ultrastructural study. Arch Ophthalmol. 1974; 91(4):270–274

[71] Dufier JL, Dhermy P, Gubler MC, Gagnadoux MF, Broyer M. Ocular changes in long-term evolution of infantile cystinosis. Ophthalmic Paediatr Genet. 1987; 8(2):131–137

[72] Wong VG, Lietman PS, Seegmiller JE. Alterations of pigment epithelium in cystinosis. Arch Ophthalmol. 1967; 77(3):361–369

[73] Kaiser-Kupfer MI, Caruso RC, Minkler DS, Gahl WA. Long-term ocular manifestations in nephropathic cystinosis. Arch Ophthalmol. 1986; 104(5):706–711

[74] Gahl WASJ, Aula PP. Lysosomal transport disorders: cystinosis and sialic acid storage disorders. In: Scriver CR, Beaudet AL, Sly WS, Valle D, eds. The Metabolic and Molecular Basis of Inherited Disease, 7th ed. New York: McGraw-Hill; 1995:3763–3797

[75] Schneider JA, Katz B, Melles RB. Update on nephropathic cystinosis. Pediatr Nephrol. 1990; 4(6):645–653

[76] Oshima RG, Willis RC, Furlong CE, Schneider JA. Binding assays for amino acids. The utilization of a cystine binding protein from Escherichia coli for the determination of acid-soluble cystine in small physiological samples. J Biol Chem. 1974; 249(19):6033–6039

[77] Gahl WA, Bashan N, Tietze F, Bernardini I, Schulman JD. Cystine transport is defective in isolated leukocyte lysosomes from patients with cystinosis. Science. 1982; 217(4566):1263–1265

[78] Gahl WA, Tietze F, Bashan N, Steinherz R, Schulman JD. Defective cystine exodus from isolated lysosome-rich fractions of cystinotic leucocytes. J Biol Chem. 1982; 257(16):9570–9575

[79] Jonas AJ, Smith ML, Allison WS, Laikind PK, Greene AA, Schneider JA. Proton-translocating ATPase and lysosomal cystine transport. J Biol Chem. 1983; 258(19):11727–11730

[80] Jonas AJ, Smith ML, Schneider JA. ATP-dependent lysosomal cystine efflux is defective in cystinosis. J Biol Chem. 1982; 257(22):13185–13188

[81] Thoene JG, Oshima RG, Ritchie DG, Schneider JA. Cystinotic fibroblasts accumulate cystine from intracellular protein degradation. Proc Natl Acad Sci U S A. 1977; 74(10):4505–4507

[82] Town M, Jean G, Cherqui S, et al. A novel gene encoding an integral membrane protein is mutated in nephropathic cystinosis. Nat Genet. 1998; 18 (4):319–324

[83] Haq MR, Kalatzis V, Gubler MC, et al. Immunolocalization of cystinosin, the protein defective in cystinosis. J Am Soc Nephrol. 2002; 13(8):2046–2051

[84] Cherqui S, Kalatzis V, Trugnan G, Antignac C. The targeting of cystinosin to the lysosomal membrane requires a tyrosine-based signal and a novel sorting motif. J Biol Chem. 2001; 276(16):13314–13321

[85] Kalatzis V, Cherqui S, Antignac C, Gasnier B. Cystinosin, the protein defective in cystinosis, is a H(+)-driven lysosomal cystine transporter. EMBO J. 2001; 20(21):5940–5949

[86] Gahl WA, Thoene JG, Schneider JA. Cystinosis. N Engl J Med. 2002; 347 (2):111–121

[87] Brodin-Sartorius A, Tête MJ, Niaudet P, et al. Cysteamine therapy delays the progression of nephropathic cystinosis in late adolescents and adults. Kidney Int. 2012; 81(2):179–189

[88] Markello TC, Bernardini IM, Gahl WA. Improved renal function in children with cystinosis treated with cysteamine. N Engl J Med. 1993; 328(16):1157–1162

[89] Kimonis VE, Troendle J, Rose SR, Yang ML, Markello TC, Gahl WA. Effects of early cysteamine therapy on thyroid function and growth in nephropathic cystinosis. J Clin Endocrinol Metab. 1995; 80(11):3257–3261

[90] Kaiser-Kupfer MI, Fujikawa L, Kuwabara T, Jain S, Gahl WA. Removal of corneal crystals by topical cysteamine in nephropathic cystinosis. N Engl J Med. 1987; 316(13):775–779

[91] Labbé A, Baudouin C, Deschênes G, et al. A new gel formulation of topical cysteamine for the treatment of corneal cystine crystals in cystinosis: the Cystadrops OCT-1 study. Mol Genet Metab. 2014; 111(3):314–320

[92] Simell O, Takki K. Raised plasma-ornithine and gyrate atrophy of the choroid and retina. Lancet. 1973; 12(1):1031–3

[93] Kaiser-Kupfer MI, Kuwabara T, Askanas V, et al. Systemic manifestations of gyrate atrophy of the choroid and retina. Ophthalmology. 1981; 88(4):302–306

[94] Takki K. Gyrate atrophy of the choroid and retina associated with hyperornithinaemia. Br J Ophthalmol. 1974; 58(1):3–23

[95] Kaiser-Kupfer MI, Caruso RC, Valle D. Gyrate atrophy of the choroid and retina. Long-term reduction of ornithine slows retinal degeneration. Arch Ophthalmol. 1991; 109(11):1539–1548

[96] Feldman RB, Mayo SS, Robertson DM, Jones JD, Rostvold JA. Epiretinal membranes and cystoid macular edema in gyrate atrophy of the choroid and retina. Retina. 1989; 9(2):139–142

[97] Oliveira TL, Andrade RE, Muccioli C, Sallum J, Belfort R, Jr. Cystoid macular edema in gyrate atrophy of the choroid and retina: a fluorescein angiography and optical coherence tomography evaluation. Am J Ophthalmol. 2005; 140(1):147–149

[98] Vasconcelos-Santos DV, Magalhães EP, Nehemy MB. Macular edema associated with gyrate atrophy managed with intravitreal triamcinolone: a case report. Arq Bras Oftalmol. 2007; 70(5):858–861

[99] Kaiser-Kupfer MI, de Monasterio FM, Valle D, Walser M, Brusilow S. Gyrate atrophy of the choroid and retina: improved visual function following reduction of plasma ornithine by diet. Science. 1980; 210(4474):1128–1131

[100] Valle D, Walser M, Brusilow S, Kaiser-Kupfer MI, Takki K. Gyrate atrophy of the choroid and retina. Biochemical considerations and experience with an arginine-restricted diet. Ophthalmology. 1981; 88(4):325–330

[101] Valle D, Walser M, Brusilow SW, Kaiser-Kupfer M. Gyrate atrophy of the choroid and retina: amino acid metabolism and correction of hyperornithinemia with an arginine-deficient diet. J Clin Invest. 1980; 65(2):371–378

[102] Wang T, Milam AH, Steel G, Valle D. A mouse model of gyrate atrophy of the choroid and retina. Early retinal pigment epithelium damage and progressive retinal degeneration. J Clin Invest. 1996; 97(12):2753–2762

[103] Weleber RG, Kennaway NG. Clinical trial of vitamin B6 for gyrate atrophy of the choroid and retina. Ophthalmology. 1981; 88(4):316–324

[104] Chitayat D, Meunier CM, Hodgkinson KA, et al. Mucolipidosis type IV: clinical manifestations and natural history. Am J Med Genet. 1991; 41(3):313–318

[105] Merin S, Nemet P, Livni N, Lazar M. The cornea in mucolipidosis IV. J Pediatr Ophthalmol. 1976; 13(5):289–295

[106] Riedel KG, Zwaan J, Kenyon KR, Kolodny EH, Hanninen L, Albert DM. Ocular abnormalities in mucolipidosis IV. Am J Ophthalmol. 1985; 99(2):125–136

[107] Bach G, Cohen MM, Kohn G. Abnormal ganglioside accumulation in cultured fibroblasts from patients with mucolipidosis IV. Biochem Biophys Res Commun. 1975; 66(4):1483–1490

[108] Kohn G, Livni N, Ornoy A, et al. Prenatal diagnosis of mucolipidosis IV by electron microscopy. J Pediatr. 1977; 90(1):62–66

[109] Zeman W, Donahue S. Fine structure of the lipid bodies in juvenile amaurotic idiocy. Acta Neuropathol. 1963; 3:144–149

[110] Bach G, Webb MB, Bargal R, Zeigler M, Ekstein J. The frequency of mucolipidosis type IV in the Ashkenazi Jewish population and the identification of 3 novel MCOLN1 mutations. Hum Mutat. 2005; 26(6):591

[111] Bach G. Mucolipin 1: endocytosis and cation channel—a review. Pflugers Arch. 2005; 451(1):313–317

[112] Rider JA, Rider DL. Batten disease: past, present, and future. Am J Med Genet Suppl. 1988; 5:21–26

[113] Raitta C, Santavuori P. Ophthalmological findings in infantile type of so-called neuronal ceroid lipofuscinosis. Acta Ophthalmol (Copenh). 1973; 51 (6):755–763

[114] Santavuori P, Vanhanen SL, Sainio K, et al. Infantile neuronal ceroid-lipofuscinosis (INCL): diagnostic criteria. J Inherit Metab Dis. 1993; 16(2):227–229

[115] Pampiglione G, Harden A. So-called neuronal ceroid lipofuscinosis. Neurophysiological studies in 60 children. J Neurol Neurosurg Psychiatry. 1977; 40 (4):323–330

[116] Weleber RG. The dystrophic retina in multisystem disorders: the electroretinogram in neuronal ceroid lipofuscinoses. Eye (Lond). 1998; 12 Pt 3b:580–590

[117] Weleber RG, Gupta N, Trzupek KM, Wepner MS, Kurz DE, Milam AH. Electroretinographic and clinicopathologic correlations of retinal dysfunction in infantile neuronal ceroid lipofuscinosis (infantile Batten disease). Mol Genet Metab. 2004; 83(1–2):128–137

[118] Goebel HH, Gerhard L, Kominami E, Haltia M. Neuronal ceroid-lipofuscinosis—late-infantile or Jansky-Bielschowsky type—revisited. Brain Pathol. 1996; 6 (3):225–228

[119] Hittner HM, Ziller RS. Ceroid-lipofuscinosis (Batten disease). Fluorescein angiography, electrophysiology, histopathology, ultrastructure, and a review of amaurotic familial idiocy. Arch Ophthalmol. 1975; 93(3):178–183

[120] Boustany RM. Neurology of the neuronal ceroid-lipofuscinoses: late infantile and juvenile types. Am J Med Genet. 1992; 42(4):533–535

[121] Spalton DJ, Taylor DS, Sanders MD. Juvenile Batten's disease: an ophthalmological assessment of 26 patients. Br J Ophthalmol. 1980; 64(10):726–732

[122] Dom R, Brucher JM, Ceuterick C, Carton H, Martin JJ. Adult ceroid-lipofuscinosis (Kufs' disease) in two brothers. Retinal and visceral storage in one; diagnostic muscle biopsy in the other. Acta Neuropathol. 1979; 45(1):67–72

[123] Goebel HH. The neuronal ceroid-lipofuscinoses. Semin Pediatr Neurol. 1996; 3(4):270–278

[124] Tarkkanen A, Haltaj M, Merenmies L. Ocular pathology in infantile type of neuronal ceroid-lipofuscinosis. J Pediatr Ophthalmol. 1977; 12(4):235–41

[125] Goebel HH, Klein H, Santavuori P, Sainio K. Ultrastructural studies of the retina in infantile neuronal ceroid-lipofuscinosis. Retina. 1988; 8(1):59–66

[126] Baumann RJ, Markesbery WR. Santavuori disease: diagnosis by leukocyte ultrastructure. Neurology. 1982; 32(11):1277–1281

[127] Traboulsi EI, Green WR, Luckenbach MW, de la Cruz ZC. Neuronal ceroid lipofuscinosis. Ocular histopathologic and electron microscopic studies in the late infantile, juvenile, and adult forms. Graefes Arch Clin Exp Ophthalmol. 1987; 225(6):391–402

[128] Vesa J, Hellsten E, Verkruyse LA, et al. Mutations in the palmitoyl protein thioesterase gene causing infantile neuronal ceroid lipofuscinosis. Nature. 1995; 376(6541):584–587

[129] Palmer DN, Barry LA, Tyynelä J, Cooper JD. NCL disease mechanisms. Biochim Biophys Acta. 2013; 1832(11):1882–1893

[130] Warrier V, Vieira M, Mole SE. Genetic basis and phenotypic correlations of the neuronal ceroid lipofusinoses. Biochim Biophys Acta. 2013; 1832 (11):1827–1830

[131] Libert J. Diagnosis of lysosomal storage diseases by the ultrastructural study of conjunctival biopsies. Pathol Annu. 1980; 15(Pt 1):37–66

[132] Arsenio-Nunes ML, Goutières F, Aicardi J. An ultramicroscopic study of skin and conjunctival biopsies in chronic neurological disorders of childhood. Ann Neurol. 1981; 9(2):163–173

[133] Wanders RJ, Waterham HR. Biochemistry of mammalian peroxisomes revisited. Annu Rev Biochem. 2006; 75:295–332

[134] Moser AB, Rasmussen M, Naidu S, et al. Phenotype of patients with peroxisomal disorders subdivided into sixteen complementation groups. J Pediatr. 1995; 127(1):13–22

[135] Folz SJ, Trobe JD. The peroxisome and the eye. Surv Ophthalmol. 1991; 35 (5):353–368

[136] Brown FR, III, McAdams AJ, Cummins JW, et al. Cerebro-hepato-renal (Zellweger) syndrome and neonatal adrenoleukodystrophy: similarities in phenotype and accumulation of very long chain fatty acids. Johns Hopkins Med J. 1982; 151(6):344–351

[137] Percy AK, Rutledge SL. Adrenoleukodystrophy and related disorders. Ment Retard Dev Disabil Res Rev. 2001; 7(3):179–189

[138] Scotto JM, Hadchouel M, Odievre M, et al. Infantile phytanic acid storage disease, a possible variant of Refsum's disease: three cases, including ultrastructural studies of the liver. J Inherit Metab Dis. 1982; 5(2):83–90

[139] Weleber RG, Tongue AC, Kennaway NG, Budden SS, Buist NR. Ophthalmic manifestations of infantile phytanic acid storage disease. Arch Ophthalmol. 1984; 102(9):1317–1321

[140] Budden SS, Kennaway NG, Buist NR, Poulos A, Weleber RG. Dysmorphic syndrome with phytanic acid oxidase deficiency, abnormal very long chain fatty acids, and pipecolic acidemia: studies in four children. J Pediatr. 1986; 108 (1):33–39

[141] Hittner HM, Kretzer FL, Mehta RS. Zellweger syndrome. Lenticular opacities indicating carrier status and lens abnormalities characteristic of homozygotes. Arch Ophthalmol. 1981; 99(11):1977–1982

[142] Lazarow PB, Moser HW. Disorders of peroxisome biogenesis. In: The Metabolic and Molecular Basis of Inherited Disease, 7th ed. New York: McGraw-Hill;1995:2287–2315

[143] Shimozawa N, Tsukamoto T, Suzuki Y, et al. A human gene responsible for Zellweger syndrome that affects peroxisome assembly. Science. 1992; 255 (5048):1132–1134

[144] Steinberg S, Chen L, Wei L, et al. The PEX Gene Screen: molecular diagnosis of peroxisome biogenesis disorders in the Zellweger syndrome spectrum. Mol Genet Metab. 2004; 83(3):252–263

[145] Ebberink MS, Mooijer PA, Gootjes J, Koster J, Wanders RJ, Waterham HR. Genetic classification and mutational spectrum of more than 600 patients with a Zellweger syndrome spectrum disorder. Hum Mutat. 2011; 32(1):59–69

[146] Weller S, Gould SJ, Valle D. Peroxisome biogenesis disorders. Annu Rev Genomics Hum Genet. 2003; 4:165–211

[147] Furuki S, Tamura S, Matsumoto N, et al. Mutations in the peroxin Pex26p responsible for peroxisome biogenesis disorders of complementation group 8 impair its stability, peroxisomal localization, and interaction with the Pex1p x Pex6p complex. J Biol Chem. 2006; 281(3):1317–1323

[148] Geisbrecht BV, Collins CS, Reuber BE, Gould SJ. Disruption of a PEX1-PEX6 interaction is the most common cause of the neurologic disorders Zellweger syndrome, neonatal adrenoleukodystrophy, and infantile Refsum disease. Proc Natl Acad Sci U S A. 1998; 95(15):8630–8635

[149] Garner A, Fielder AR, Primavesi R, Stevens A. Tapetoretinal degeneration in the cerebro-hepato-renal (Zellweger's) syndrome. Br J Ophthalmol. 1982; 66 (7):422–431

[150] Claridge KG, Gibberd FB, Sidey MC. Refsum disease: the presentation and ophthalmic aspects of Refsum disease in a series of 23 patients. Eye (Lond). 1992; 6(Pt 4):371–375

[151] Martinez M. Restoring the DHA levels in the brains of Zellweger patients. J Mol Neurosci. 2001; 16(2–3):309–316, discussion 317–321

[152] Paker AM, Sunness JS, Brereton NH, et al. Docosahexaenoic acid therapy in peroxisomal diseases: results of a double-blind, randomized trial. Neurology. 2010; 75(9):826–830

[153] Wierzbicki AS, Lloyd MD, Schofield CJ, Feher MD, Gibberd FB. Refsum's disease: a peroxisomal disorder affecting phytanic acid alpha-oxidation. J Neurochem. 2002; 80(5):727–735

[154] Wierzbicki AS, Mitchell J, Lambert-Hammill M, et al. Identification of genetic heterogeneity in Refsum's disease. Eur J Hum Genet. 2000; 8(8):649–651

[155] Jansen GA, Ofman R, Ferdinandusse S, et al. Refsum disease is caused by mutations in the phytanoyl-CoA hydroxylase gene. Nat Genet. 1997; 17 (2):190–193

[156] Singh I, Pahan K, Singh AK, Barbosa E. Refsum disease: a defect in the alpha-oxidation of phytanic acid in peroxisomes. J Lipid Res. 1993; 34(10):1755–1764

[157] Jansen GA, Hogenhout EM, Ferdinandusse S, et al. Human phytanoyl-CoA hydroxylase: resolution of the gene structure and the molecular basis of Refsum's disease. Hum Mol Genet. 2000; 9(8):1195–1200

[158] Mihalik SJ, Morrell JC, Kim D, Sacksteder KA, Watkins PA, Gould SJ. Identification of PAHX, a Refsum disease gene. Nat Genet. 1997; 17(2):185–189

[159] van den Brink DM, Brites P, Haasjes J, et al. Identification of PEX7 as the second gene involved in Refsum disease. Am J Hum Genet. 2003; 72(2):471–477

[160] Refsum S. Heredopathia atactica polyneuritiformis phytanic-acid storage disease, Refsum's disease:" a biochemically well-defined disease with a specific dietary treatment. Arch Neurol. 1981; 38(10):605–606

[161] Traboulsi EI, Maumenee IH. Ophthalmologic manifestations of X-linked childhood adrenoleukodystrophy. Ophthalmology. 1987; 94(1):47–52

[162] Moser HW. Clinical and therapeutic aspects of adrenoleukodystrophy and adrenomyeloneuropathy. J Neuropathol Exp Neurol. 1995; 54(5):740–745

[163] Kaplan PWKB, Kruse B, Tusa RJ, Shankroff J, Rignani J, Moser HW. Visual system abnormalities in adrenomyeloneuropathy. Ann Neurol. 1995; 37 (4):550–552

[164] Small KW, Pollock S, Scheinman J. Optic atrophy in primary oxalosis. Am J Ophthalmol. 1988; 106(1):96–97

[165] Moser AB, Kreiter N, Bezman L, et al. Plasma very long chain fatty acids in 3,000 peroxisome disease patients and 29,000 controls. Ann Neurol. 1999; 45(1):100–110

[166] Dubey P, Raymond GV, Moser AB, Kharkar S, Bezman L, Moser HW. Adrenal insufficiency in asymptomatic adrenoleukodystrophy patients identified by very long-chain fatty acid screening. J Pediatr. 2005; 146(4):528–532

[167] Moser HW, Raymond GV, Dubey P. Adrenoleukodystrophy: new approaches to a neurodegenerative disease. JAMA. 2005; 294(24):3131–3134

[168] Berger J, Gärtner J. X-linked adrenoleukodystrophy: clinical, biochemical and pathogenetic aspects. Biochim Biophys Acta. 2006; 1763(12):1721–1732

[169] Powers JM. Adreno-leukodystrophy (adreno-testiculo-leukomyelo-neuropathic-complex). Clin Neuropathol. 1985; 4(5):181–199

[170] Ferrer I, Aubourg P, Pujol A. General aspects and neuropathology of X-linked adrenoleukodystrophy. Brain Pathol. 2010; 20(4):817–830

[171] Dubey P, Fatemi A, Huang H, et al. Diffusion tensor-based imaging reveals occult abnormalities in adrenomyeloneuropathy. Ann Neurol. 2005; 58 (5):758–766

[172] Bezman L, Moser HW. Incidence of X-linked adrenoleukodystrophy and the relative frequency of its phenotypes. Am J Med Genet. 1998; 76(5):415–419

[173] Moser HW, Moser AB, Hollandsworth K, Brereton NH, Raymond GV. "Lorenzo's oil" therapy for X-linked adrenoleukodystrophy: rationale and current assessment of efficacy. J Mol Neurosci. 2007; 33(1):105–113

[174] Small KW, Letson R, Scheinman J. Ocular findings in primary hyperoxaluria. Arch Ophthalmol. 1990; 108(1):89–93

[175] Meredith TA, Wright JD, Gammon JA, Fellner SK, Warshaw BL, Maio M. Ocular involvement in primary hyperoxaluria. Arch Ophthalmol. 1984; 102 (4):584–587

[176] Milliner DS. The primary hyperoxalurias: an algorithm for diagnosis. Am J Nephrol. 2005; 25(2):154–160

[177] Danpure CJ. Advances in the enzymology and molecular genetics of primary hyperoxaluria type 1. Prospects for gene therapy. Nephrol Dial Transplant. 1995; 10 Suppl 8:24–29

[178] Monico CG, Rossetti S, Schwanz HA, et al. Comprehensive mutation screening in 55 probands with type 1 primary hyperoxaluria shows feasibility of a gene-based diagnosis. J Am Soc Nephrol. 2007; 18(6):1905–1914

[179] Querques G, Bouzitou-Mfoumou R, Soubrane G, Souied EH. Spectral-domain optical coherence tomography visualisation of retinal oxalosis in primary hyperoxaluria. Eye (Lond). 2010; 24(5):941–943

[180] Runge P, Muller DP, McAllister J, Calver D, Lloyd JK, Taylor D. Oral vitamin E supplements can prevent the retinopathy of abetalipoproteinaemia. Br J Ophthalmol. 1986; 70(3):166–173

[181] Wetterau JR, Aggerbeck LP, Bouma ME, et al. Absence of microsomal triglyceride transfer protein in individuals with abetalipoproteinemia. Science. 1992; 258(5084):999–1001

[182] Nasr MB, Symeonidis C, Mikropoulos DG, et al. Disc swelling in abetalipoproteinemia: a novel feature of Bassen-Kornzweig syndrome. Eur J Ophthalmol. 2011; 21(5):674–676

[183] Sharp D, Blinderman L, Combs KA, et al. Cloning and gene defects in microsomal triglyceride transfer protein associated with abetalipoproteinaemia. Nature. 1993; 365(6441):65–69

[184] Shoulders CC, Brett DJ, Bayliss JD, et al. Abetalipoproteinemia is caused by defects of the gene encoding the 97 kDa subunit of a microsomal triglyceride transfer protein. Hum Mol Genet. 1993; 2(12):2109–2116

[185] Rampoldi L, Danek A, Monaco AP. Clinical features and molecular bases of neuroacanthocytosis. J Mol Med (Berl). 2002; 80(8):475–491

[186] Kayden HJ, Traber MG. Absorption, lipoprotein transport, and regulation of plasma concentrations of vitamin E in humans. J Lipid Res. 1993; 34(3):343–358

[187] Bishara S, Merin S, Cooper M, Azizi E, Delpre G, Deckelbaum RJ. Combined vitamin A and E therapy prevents retinal electrophysiological deterioration in abetalipoproteinaemia. Br J Ophthalmol. 1982; 66(12):767–770

[188] Li CM, Presley JB, Zhang X, et al. Retina expresses microsomal triglyceride transfer protein: implications for age-related maculopathy. J Lipid Res. 2005; 46(4):628–640

[189] Gouras P, Carr RE, Gunkel RD. Retinitis pigmentosa in abetalipoproteinemia: Effects of vitamin A. Invest Ophthalmol. 1971; 10(10):784–793

[190] Chowers I, Banin E, Merin S, Cooper M, Granot E. Long-term assessment of combined vitamin A and E treatment for the prevention of retinal degeneration in abetalipoproteinaemia and hypobetalipoproteinaemia patients. Eye (Lond). 2001; 15(Pt 4):525–530

23 Hyaloideoretinopathies

William Tasman

23.1 X-Linked Juvenile Retinoschisis

X-linked juvenile retinoschisis (XLJR) is a bilateral ocular disorder that occurs in males and classically demonstrates a stellate maculopathy and peripheral retinal dehiscences in the nerve fiber layer.[1,2,3] The clinical features were first described by Haas in 1898.[4] It has since become well recognized and has been seen in all races throughout the world. Although in general it is a relatively rare eye condition, it is thought to be one of the most common forms of juvenile macular degenerations[5] with a prevalence of 1:15,000 to 1:30,000.[1,3] It is caused by the RS1 mutation. To date, more than 196 different mutations of the *RS1* gene have been associated with XLJS.[5,6] Thus, the gene mutations for XLJS are multiple and different phenotypes may be expressed.[6]

23.1.1 Clinical Features

Affected males usually present in early childhood when reading difficulties at school are first detected.[6,7,8,9,10] Occasionally, the diagnosis is made earlier when there is a family history of disease and formal screening examinations are performed. Rarely, it is diagnosed in infancy when a secondary complication leads to poor fixation, white pupillary reflex, or strabismus.

The macular changes in XLJR are characteristic and account for the mild-to-moderate decrease in visual acuity that is apparent in affected children.[1,2,6,7,8,9,10] Most commonly, the macula has the so-called stellate or spoke-wheel appearance, with superficial, radiating striae of the fovea (▶ Fig. 23.1a, b). The condition is often best appreciated under red-free viewing conditions, and although it may look like cystoid macular edema, it does not exhibit leakage of dye on fluorescein angiography.

In adult life, it is not unusual for this hallmark foveal change to disappear, leaving only a blunted foveal reflex and underlying retinal pigmentary epithelial changes that can be mistaken for age-related macular degeneration.[10] Furthermore, even in some young patients, this classic stellate appearance may not be apparent because it is obscured by a superimposed complication, such as macular dragging (▶ Fig. 23.2a, b) or extension of the peripheral schisis cavity into the posterior pole. Once again, alterations in the pigment epithelium of the fovea may be all that is appreciated. Regardless of the appearance, some form or degree of maculopathy should be expected in nearly all affected individuals.[1,10]

Peripheral retinoschisis is present in about 50 to 70% of eyes.[1,2,10] It is most common in the inferior quadrants, particularly inferotemporally, and is characterized by a gross splitting of the retina at the level of the nerve fiber layer, although occasionally inner retinal layers are included.[11] The peripheral schisis is usually not present at birth but typically develops during a period of 2 to 3 years in early childhood before stabilizing. In general, it is the peripheral schisis that is the source for the major, sight-threatening complications seen in XLJR.[12,13,14,15]

Pearls

- The stellate maculopathy of juvenile retinoschisis is the hallmark ophthalmoscopic feature of the disease. However, with increasing patient age, this classic foveal change may fade and leave only a blunted light reflex and underlying pigmentary alterations in the central macular area.

Occasionally, bullous elevation of the inner retinal layers can simulate a retinal detachment. Multiple breaks often develop in the thin inner layer, many of which become quite large. Indeed, in some instances, only small remnants of the inner layer remain, a finding referred to in the older literature as *vitreous veils*. With large inner wall holes, retinal blood vessels may be found coursing through this unsupported diaphanous layer.[13,15] The nerve fiber layer may then develop breaks (▶ Fig. 23.3). Breaks can also occur in the outer retinal layer or elsewhere in full-thickness retina and lead to rhegmatogenous retinal detachments.[12,15] Rarely, traction or exudative retinal detachment, macular ectopia with either temporal or nasal dragging, and schisis that progresses into the macula can also be seen and

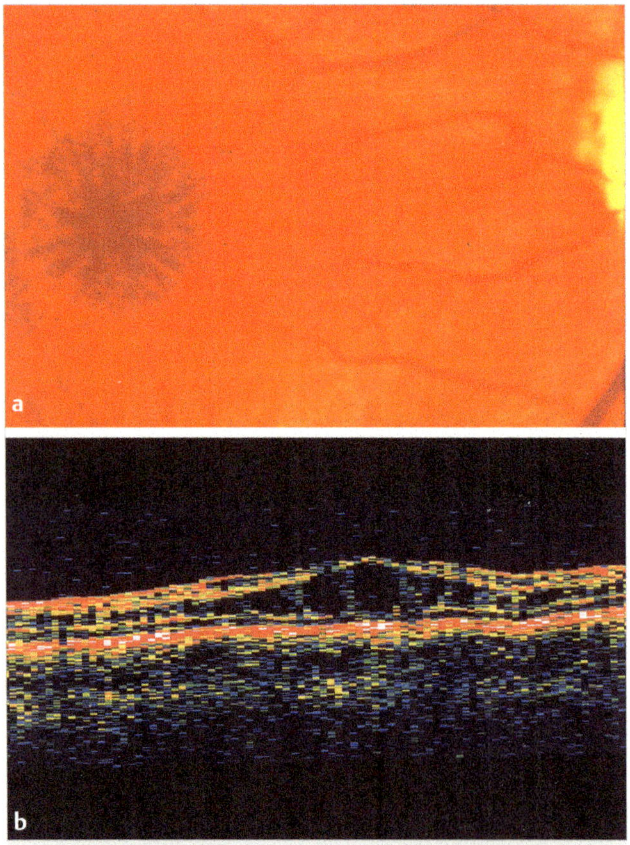

Fig. 23.1 (**a**) Stellate macular appearance in a 6-year-old boy with X-linked juvenile retinoschisis. (**b**) OCT showing macular cystic changes.

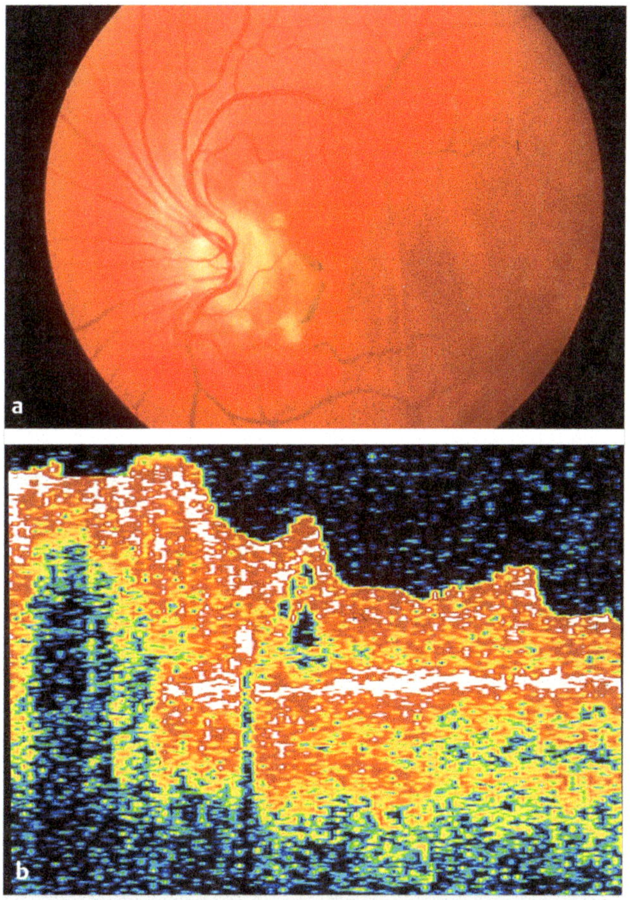

Fig. 23.2 (a) Nasal displacement of the retinal vessels and distortion of the macula in a 10-year-old boy with X-linked juvenile retinoschisis. (b) Vestige of macular cystic change is still visible.

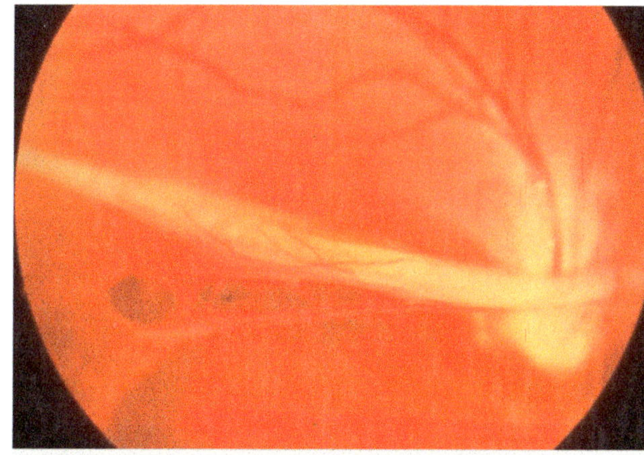

Fig. 23.3 Scrolled up nerve fiber layer with dehiscence in a 3-year-old boy with X-linked juvenile retinoschisis.

lead to further loss of vision.[5,14,15] Most of these complications are likely to manifest within the first decade of life.[6,10,12,14,15]

Vitreous hemorrhage is the most common secondary complication and has been reported to occur, to some degree, in up to 40% of affected individuals.[2,3,8,10,11,12,13,14,15] In many cases, it is mild and clears spontaneously or is confined to the schisis cavity and is not of visual significance. However, in some, it can be dense and nonclearing. The source is usually an unsupported retinal blood vessel that tears, but rarely, it can come about from disc or retinal neovascularization.[5]

Rhegmatogenous retinal detachment is the next most common problem leading to severe vision loss in XLJR, being observed in up to 22% of patients.[1,2,3,10,12] In some cases, the retinal detachment can be difficult to recognize, as the fluid beneath the outer layer is often shallow. As mentioned earlier, the detachment occurs either because outer wall breaks form in the presence of inner wall breaks or because full-thickness flap tears develop in the peripheral retina outside the schisis cavity.[15] Rhegmatogenous retinal detachments and their repair may be associated with a relatively high rate of proliferative vitreoretinopathy.[15]

Other associated clinical findings of XLJR include hypermetropia, strabismus, tapetoretina-like sheen, and cataract formation.[5] In some cases, the development of cataracts may be related to recurrent vitreous hemorrhage, but cataract has also been observed in children with XLJR who have not bled or undergone any surgical procedures.

23.1.2 Diagnosis

The constellation of macular and peripheral retinal findings usually allows the examiner to arrive readily at the diagnosis of XLJR. Family members should be examined, as finding other affected males will help confirm the diagnosis by demonstrating the X-linked mode of inheritance. Electroretinography (ERG) can also help establish the diagnosis by showing the characteristic decreased b-wave under both scotopic and photopic conditions.[16] This ERG finding is present in most affected individuals whether or not any peripheral schisis formation is present. Occasional cases have been reported in females, and I had the opportunity to examine two young women with clinically typical XLJS during a visit to Bogota, Colombia.

Pearls

- The characteristic ERG abnormality in juvenile retinoschisis is a decreased b-wave. It is a consistent finding, being present whether or not there is any peripheral retinoschisis.

23.1.3 Differential Diagnosis

The differential diagnostic considerations in XLJR include retinopathy of prematurity (ROP), Goldmann-Favré's disease, retinitis pigmentosa (RP), and familial exudative vitreoretinopathy (FEVR).

Patients with ROP usually have a gestational age of less than 29 weeks and a birth weight of less than 1,000 g. The disorder affects both male and female infants. Peripheral and posterior pole retinal pigmentation is common, and dragging of the retina is frequent. Peripheral retinoschisis resembling acquired or degenerative retinoschisis may occur, but dehiscences at the level of the nerve fiber layer do not develop in ROP.

Goldmann-Favré's disease is inherited as an autosomal recessive trait. Foveal schisis is often present and, as in XLJR, fluorescein angiography does not show cystoid leakage. The vitreous

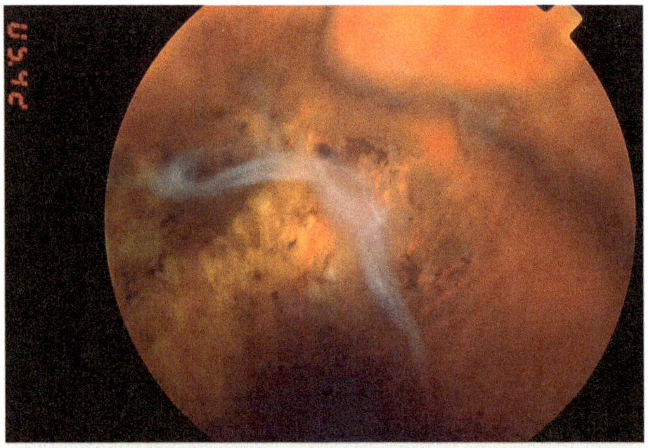

Fig. 23.4 Peripheral retinal pigmentary changes and associated preretinal membrane formation in a female patient with Goldmann-Favré's disease.

is liquefied, and pigmentary changes resembling those of RP are typically apparent (▶ Fig. 23.4). Rhegmatogenous retinal detachments are seen in both conditions. Unlike the ERG in XLJR, the ERG in Goldmann-Favré's disease shows both a-wave and b-wave involvement and is often flat.

RP is characterized by peripheral retinal pigmentary alterations, disc pallor, attenuated retinal vessels, and an abnormal ERG. X-linked retinoschisis may have associated scattered pigmentation in the retina, but it does not show the classic bone spicule pigmentary changes of RP. The ERG findings also differ between the two conditions. In patients with RP, true cystoid macular edema may develop, and this presentation may cause some diagnostic confusion between the two conditions if the mode of RP inheritance is X-linked. The fluorescein angiogram, however, would show leakage of dye in the fovea with RP if cystoid changes are present. FEVR is discussed later.

23.1.4 Pathogenesis and Genetics

Although the pathogenesis of XLJR is unknown, histopathologic and electrophysiologic data suggest that the clinical manifestations of XLJR result from a diffuse Müller's cell abnormality. Müller's cells, for example, are thought to play an important role in the initiation of the b-wave, and so the early and consistent ERG finding of a reduced b-wave lends support to the theory of a primary Mueller's cell dysfunction.[16]

Special Considerations

The differential diagnosis of XLJR includes mainly the following:

- ROP
- Goldmann-Favré's disease
- RP
- FEVR

Recently, linkage studies have localized the retinoschisis gene to the distal short arm of the X chromosome (Xp22.1–p22.3).[17,18] In contrast to the female carriers of most other X-linked hereditary eye diseases, the female carriers do not usually have any signs or symptoms of the condition. With current genetic technology, it is now possible to help confirm carriers and affected members of families suspected of having or being at risk for the disease through analysis of peripheral blood samples with DNA probes.[19,20]

23.1.5 Management and Course

Observation of XLJR is the primary course of management. Most patients have mild-to-moderate visual loss that remains stable or exhibits only minimal progression until late adulthood. Beyond the sixth decade of life, some further deterioration of central vision may occur.[10]

When the disease is first diagnosed, family screening and genetic counseling are in order. Any refractive error, amblyopia, or strabismus needs to be addressed to maximize visual function. Close follow-up, particularly during the first decade of life, is needed for early detection and prompt management of secondary complications. There are no effective prophylactic techniques; attempts to flatten peripheral retinoschisis with photocoagulation resulted in a high incidence of complications.[21]

Surgery is indicated for rhegmatogenous retinal detachment or visually significant vitreous hemorrhage.[12,15,22,23] In some retinal detachment cases, scleral buckling alone may suffice, but because the detachments may be associated with hemorrhage or proliferative vitreoretinopathy, relatively advanced vitrectomy techniques may be necessary.[15,23,24] Intraoperatively, unsupported retinal vessels should be cauterized and divided to prevent postoperative bleeding. Furthermore, with the cortical vitreous typically firmly adherent to nerve fiber layer remnants, a so-called inner layer retinectomy may need to be performed to relieve vitreoretinal traction adequately and achieve retinal reattachment; excising the separated nerve fiber layer of the peripheral schisis cavity has not been found to have significant adverse consequences.[13,23,24]

23.2 Familial Exudative Vitreoretinopathy

In 1969, Criswick and Schepens[25] first described what is now known as *familial exudative vitreoretinopathy (FEVR)*. They reported six cases from two families that exhibited bilateral vitreoretinal abnormalities that closely resembled various stages of ROP but lacked a history of premature birth. The major ocular findings from these original cases included peripheral retinal neovascularization with traction retinal detachments, lipid exudation, falciform folds, and macular dragging.

Subsequently, in 1971, Gow and Oliver[26] reported 22 patients from three generations who exhibited similar abnormalities and, with this large pedigree, confirmed an autosomal dominant mode of inheritance. By the mid-1970s, peripheral retinal nonperfusion was well demonstrated as both an early and consistent clinical feature of the condition.[27,28,29] This lent support to the current concept of the disease as a primary, peripheral retinal vascular defect that, with progression, causes secondary vitreoretinal traction phenomena, similar to ROP. Recently, cases of FEVR with an X-linked mode of inheritance have been identified.[30]

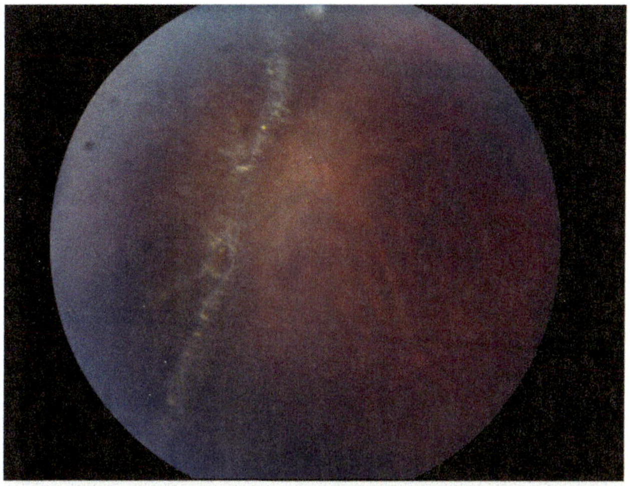

Fig. 23.5 Retinal vessels mark the edge of the vascularized retina in the periphery of an asymptomatic young woman with familial exudative vitreoretinopathy.

23.2.1 Clinical Features

The clinical features of FEVR vary considerably among affected individuals, even those of the same pedigree.[26,28,29,31,32] Furthermore, although the condition is bilateral, it can be very asymmetric and so symptoms that do manifest can be unilateral at presentation. A majority of affected individuals are asymptomatic through most or all of their lives and, therefore, maintain good visual acuity (▶ Fig. 23.5).[32] In these patients, the condition is diagnosed incidentally on routine examinations or through screening examinations after a family member presents with the disease. Symptoms of decreased vision, indicative of significant disease progression or secondary complications, can occur at any age, and when they come about early in life, the presenting features may be poor fixation, strabismus, or a white pupillary reflex.

The hallmark of the disease is the avascular peripheral retina (▶ Fig. 23.6).[27,32] This is an early and consistent finding. The zone of avascularity is variable in size but usually most prominent temporally and often present for 360 degrees. This finding, along with some subtle, associated nonproliferative vascular changes such as peripheral vascular sheathing, dilation, and shunt formation, represents the mildest form of disease which is typically asymptomatic.[32] It can be very subtle, and its detection is often facilitated by viewing with red-free light, or it may manifest as nonperfusion on fluorescein angiography or angioscopy. Of note is that in FEVR, but not in ROP, the peripheral zone of avascular retina is permanent; it never vascularizes with time.[29]

Progression is characterized by the development of varying degrees of peripheral fibrovascular proliferation or neovascularization and related complications.[26,28,29,31,32] The neovascularization occurs at the border of perfused and nonperfused retina. It, in turn, can lead to retinal detachment, macular dragging, and vitreous hemorrhage. The sometimes prominent intraretinal and subretinal lipid exudative response that was recognized in the earliest reports is the reason for the name used for the condition. Exudation may become so extensive as to detach the entire retina, a presentation that resembles advanced Coats' disease. Traction retinal detachments are relatively common and vary from localized, peripheral detachments that may be asymptomatic to large detachments that involve the macula.[32,33,34] The vitreoretinal traction forces can also cause full-thickness retinal breaks and lead to combined traction-rhegmatogenous detachments. In general, nonrhegmatogenous detachments (traction or exudative) tend to be more common in younger patients, whereas rhegmatogenous detachments are seen more frequently in older patients.[34] Tangentially directed traction can either drag the macula or cause a falciform fold that involves the macula.(▶ Fig. 23.7)[29,32] Vitreous hemorrhage is a surprisingly rare finding in FEVR, but does occur.

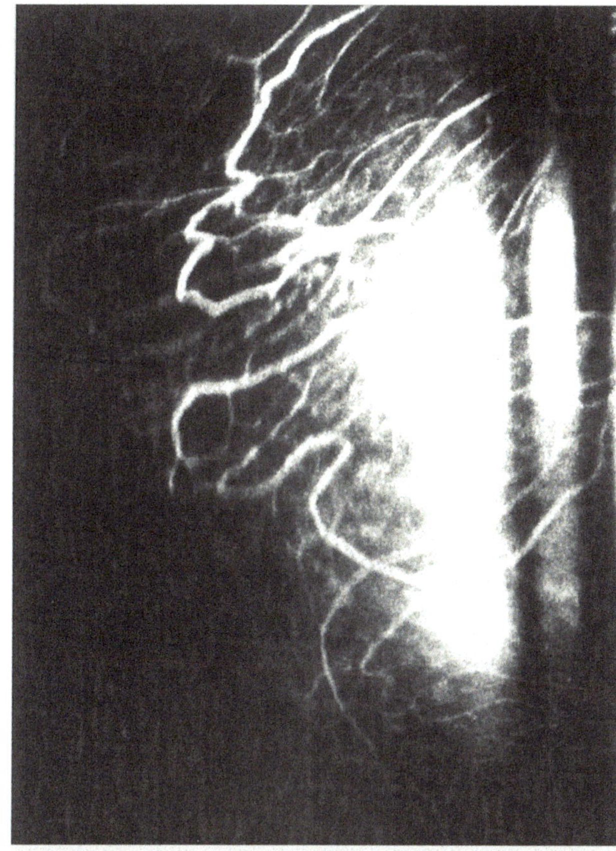

Fig. 23.6 Fluorescein angiogram showing the fibrillar termination of the retinal vessels at the border of perfused and nonperfused retina.

Neovascular glaucoma, cataract formation, and band keratopathy may also occur in FEVR. They are seen mainly in very severely affected eyes and probably represent the end-stage sequelae of long-standing, total retinal detachment.[29] There is otherwise nothing intrinsically abnormal with the anterior segment in FEVR.

23.2.2 Differential Diagnosis

The conditions that can resemble FEVR most closely include ROP, XLJR, incontinentia pigmenti (IP), and Norrie's disease (▶ Table 23.1). As a group, these disorders are lifetime diseases in which sight-threatening complications such as retinal detachment can arise at any age. Other than Norrie's disease, these conditions are described in detail in Chapter 12.

Pearls

- The peripheral avascular zone in FEVR is permanent and represents a rare, but ongoing risk for neovascularization and associated complications.

Norrie's disease is a rare, X-linked disease that can closely resemble the advanced stages of FEVR, with bilateral retinal detachments or falciform folds in infancy. Unlike FEVR, Norrie's disease may be associated with corneal opacification and microphthalmia in addition to the systemic findings of deafness and mental retardation.[35,36] Histopathologically, retinal dysplasia is present with Norrie's disease and not with FEVR.[29]

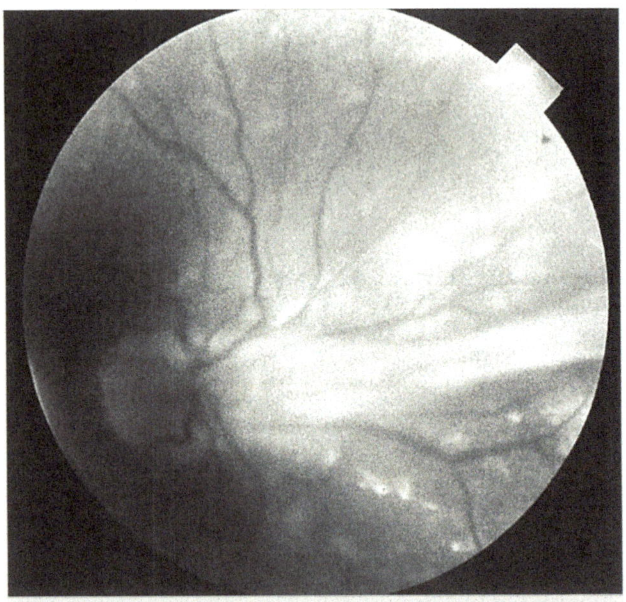

Fig. 23.7 Temporal retinal fold involving the macula in the granddaughter (and daughter) of the patients shown in (▶ Fig. 23.6).

Of note, there is recent evidence that the X-linked variants of FEVR and Norrie's disease result from defects of the same gene on the X chromosome.[37,38] It has been postulated that the two conditions may be different only in the timing of genetic insult, which occurs early in gestation with Norrie's disease and late in gestation with FEVR.[37] This would possibly explain the more widespread ocular and systemic abnormalities associated with Norrie's disease.

Rarely, there may be diagnostic confusion with FEVR and Coats' disease or persistent hyperplastic primary vitreous (PHPV), as all these conditions can present in infancy with leukocoria and total retinal detachment. The unilateral nature of Coats' disease and PHPV usually allows for the conditions to be differentiated readily from FEVR. Furthermore, neither Coats' disease nor PHPV is inherited, and so family history and ocular examinations of family members should be negative for these conditions.

23.2.3 Pathogenesis and Genetics

The cessation of peripheral retinal vascularization appears to be the primary, clinically evident abnormality of FEVR. The specific mechanism for this maldevelopment, however, is not known. Pathophysiologically, peripheral retinal ischemia and the liberation of neovascular growth factors are likely to be at play after birth because the larger the area of avascularity, the more frequently and earlier do neovascularization and its complications tend to develop.[32]

As determined originally, FEVR is most often inherited in an autosomal dominant pattern.[26] Linkage analysis suggests that the gene for the dominant form of the disease lies on the long arm of chromosome 11.[39] As mentioned earlier, there have also been recent reports of an X-linked mode of inheritance, and this too has been confirmed with linkage analysis.[30,38] This has caused some confusion clinically in differentiating certain cases of FEVR from XLJR and Norrie's disease, as described earlier. Further advances in the realm of molecular biology are likely to bring about techniques that will allow for the rapid and specific diagnosis of these entities in the near future. It is also likely that

Table 23.1 Differential diagnosis of familial exudative vitreoretinopathy

Feature	Familial exudative retinopathy	Retinopathy of prematurity	Incontinentia pigmenti	Norrie's disease	X-linked juvenile retinoschisis
Sex	Males–females	Males–females	Females only	Males only	Males only
Inheritance	Dominant or X-linked recessive	None	X-linked dominant	X-linked recessive	X-linked recessive
Prematurity	No	Yes	No	No	No
Laterality	Bilateral	Bilateral	Bilateral	Bilateral	Bilateral
Microphthalmia	No	No	No	+/–	No
Avascular periphery	Yes	Yes	Yes	+/–	No
Retinal detachment	Yes	Yes	Yes	Yes	Yes
Retinal folds or macular dragging	Yes	Yes	Yes	Yes	Yes
Systemic associations	No	+/–	Yes	Yes	No

Source: Adapted from Regillo.[30]

genetic-based diseases, in general, will be reclassified more by genotype than by phenotype.

23.2.4 Management and Course

Although initially FEVR was thought to be universally progressive resulting in a poor visual prognosis, more recent data suggest that the course of FEVR shows great intrapatient and interpatient variation.[32] In general, however, the rate and extent of progression are typically greatest when patients are young, and the younger the age at onset of symptoms, the worse the visual outcome.[32]

All family members of an affected individual must be examined. Asymptomatic patients should be followed up at regular intervals, approximately every 6 to 12 months. Patients must be followed up for life and never be considered free of risk for potentially serious complications.

Small tufts of neovascular tissue without any associated signs of leakage, bleeding, or detachment should be observed, as spontaneous regression can occur.[32] However, treatment with cryotherapy or laser photocoagulation is indicated with any progression (▸ Fig. 23.8)[28,29,32] of fibrovascular tissue or development of associated complications. With thick lipid exudation, laser uptake is poor and cryotherapy is preferred.

Surgical intervention is reserved for cases progressing to retinal detachment or vitreous hemorrhage affecting or threatening the macula. Both scleral buckling and vitrectomy techniques have been utilized with varying degrees of success.[25,30,31,32,40] The exact approach depends on the nature and configuration of the detachment and the presence or absence of associated features such as hemorrhage or proliferative vitreoretinopathy. The goal is to relieve vitreoretinal traction around abnormal vessels and any retinal breaks. Furthermore, to maximize the chances of long-term resolution of any associated exudative manifestations, all abnormal vessels under traction must be well treated with either laser or cryotherapy.[40] Anti-vascular endothelial growth factor (anti-VEGF) agents also may play a role in management.

23.3 Incontinentia Pigmenti

Incontinentia pigmenti (IP) is a rare, hereditary condition characterized by ocular, skin, central nervous system, skeletal, and other systemic abnormalities.[41,42,43] Although named after the histopathologic findings observed with the skin changes that manifest in infancy, the most serious aspects of IP are the retinal and intracranial changes that may occur.[43] IP is an X-linked dominant disease that is lethal in males and, therefore, it is almost exclusively a clinical disease of females.

23.3.1 Clinical Features

Overall, about one-third of individuals with IP have eye findings, most of which involve the posterior segment.[41,42,43] A variety of fundus abnormalities can be observed and include peripheral retinal avascularity with arteriovenous anastomoses and neovascularization, foveal hypoplasia, abnormal blood vessels traversing the macula, branch arterial occlusions, neovascularization of the disc retinal dragging and detachments (traction and rhegmatogenous), falciform folds, vitreous hemorrhage, and optic pallor.[43] Widespread retinal pigmentary alterations can also be observed, and in some cases these may result from spontaneous retinal reattachment. Cataracts, conjunctival pigmentation, and strabismus are other possible findings on ocular examination.

Fundus changes can manifest in infancy or later in life and can be relatively rapid in progression, especially when presenting within the first year of life.[44] The ocular abnormalities, however, are often extremely asymmetric. Bilateral retinal detachments may occur, but in many cases with advanced disease in one eye, the other eye shows only nonperfused peripheral retina similar to that seen in FEVR (▸ Fig. 23.9). The

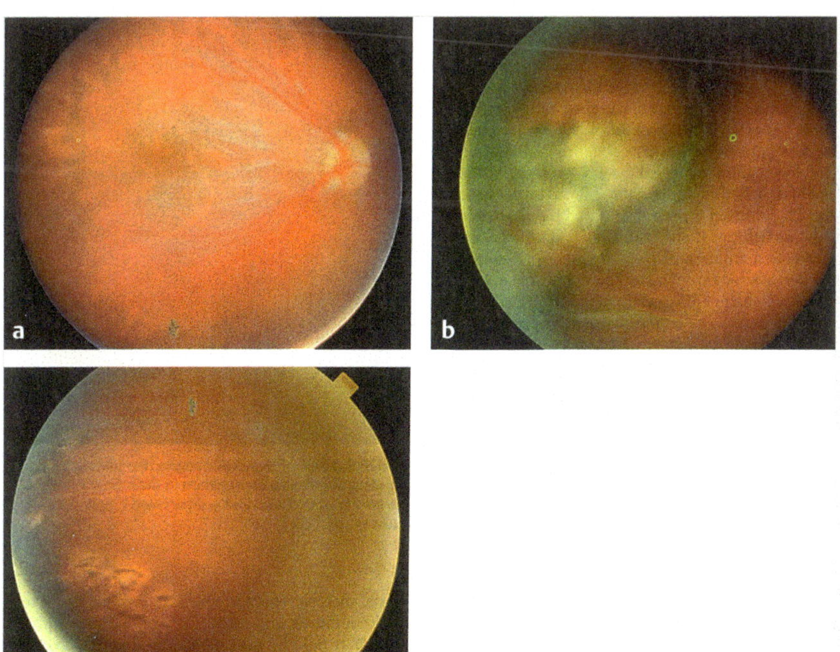

Fig. 23.8 A 5-year-old boy with familial exudative vitreoretinopathy: There is **(a)** macular ectopia and **(b)** exudation in the temporal periphery. **(c)** The lipid exudate completely resorbed within several months after laser photocoagulation to the peripheral avascular zone.

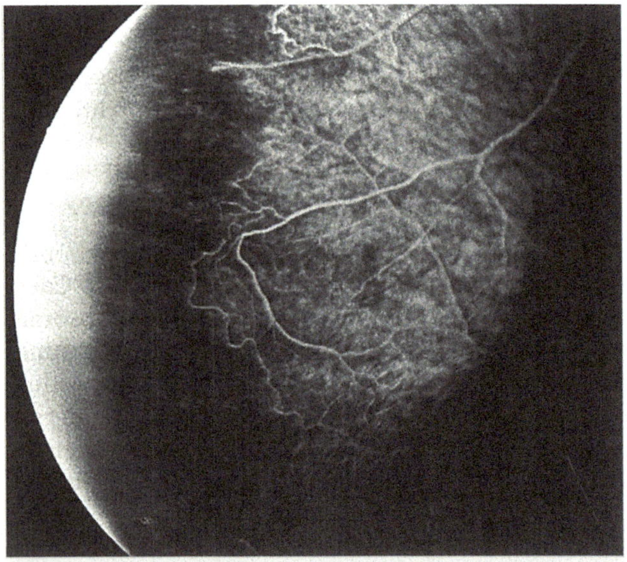

Fig. 23.9 Fluorescein angiogram showing the peripheral retinal avascular zone in an asymptomatic female patient with incontinentia pigmenti.

changes in the contralateral eye may be so subtle as to be easily overlooked without close scrutiny of the peripheral vasculature.

The characteristic skin changes start within days after birth. They initially consist of a widespread erythematous and blistering process that evolves into a verrucous stage at around 2 months of age (▶ Fig. 23.10). Within a few more months, a whorled or marbled pigmentation to the skin develops. Over years, the hyperpigmented areas typically fade to some degree, and by middle or late childhood, it is not unusual for the skin changes to be fairly inapparent; sometimes even subtle hypopigmentation develops. Some stage of the skin involvement is expected in nearly all affected individuals, but the history may be difficult to elicit if the episode was mild or mistaken for another type of neonatal rash. There is incomplete dentition and some teeth are peg shaped (▶ Fig. 23.11).

Pearls

- The acute, blistering skin rash of IP occurs shortly after birth. The pigmentary changes that follow typically fade with age and may be difficult to detect when the ocular and neurologic problems manifest sometimes years later. Therefore, the characteristic dermatologic feature of the syndrome may be apparent only by history.

Other systemic associated findings include various neurologic abnormalities, incomplete dentition, and focal alopecia on the crown of the skull. Varying degrees of cerebral ischemia, edema, hemorrhage, and atrophy have been described.[43] As a result, there can be mental retardation, seizures, and motor disturbances. Occipital damage may be a source of blindness in the absence of significant ocular abnormalities. Neuroimaging allows for documentation of central nervous system involvement, which occurs in about one-third of cases and aids in the diagnosis of the syndrome. Dental abnormalities are common, being observed in about 65% of cases, and consist most often of missing or cone-shaped teeth (▶ Fig. 23.11).[41,43,45] The presence of such changes helps confirm the diagnosis of IP.

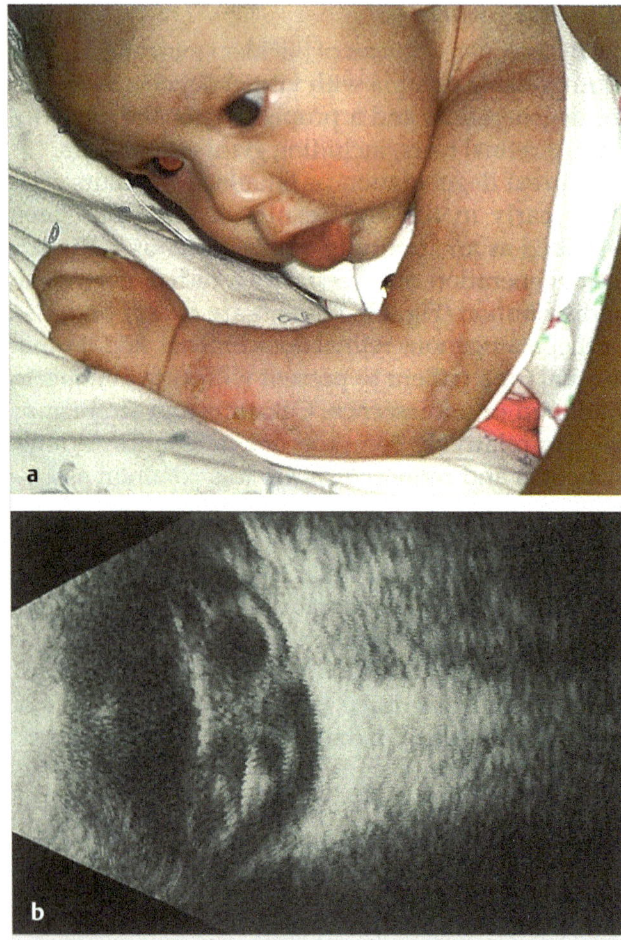

Fig. 23.10 Incontinentia pigmenti: (**a**) Typical, resolving blistering skin lesions on the arm of an affected infant. Note also the white pupillary reflex in the left eye. (**b**) B-scan ultrasonography of the left eye showed a total retinal detachment with retinal macrocysts.

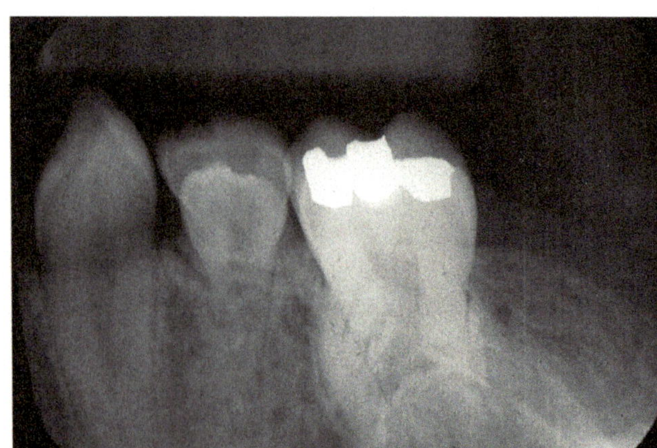

Fig. 23.11 Patient with Stickler's syndrome has incomplete dentition and one cone or pegged tooth.

23.3.2 Differential Diagnosis

IP should be included in the differential diagnosis of female patients with peripheral retinal nonperfusion, preretinal neovascularization, infantile retinal detachment, foveal hypoplasia, and dragging of the retina. A history of a blistering skin rash and any associated dental and central nervous system abnormalities are highly suggestive of IP.

23.3.3 Pathogenesis and Genetics

The pathogenesis of IP, like that of the other conditions described in this chapter, is unknown. Catalano[45] proposed that the underlying chromosomal defect somehow results in an autologous inflammatory disorder directed against an altered gene product that is normally responsible for differentiation of retinal and other structural elements. The specific genetic defect of the X chromosome has yet to be determined.

23.3.4 Management and Course

Most patients with IP can be observed. The most aggressive ocular courses usually manifest in infancy.[41,43,44] Therefore, very young patients (if the condition is diagnosed at such an early age) should be followed up particularly closely, as progressive neovascular proliferation may respond to cryotherapy or laser photocoagulation.[44] Traction retinal detachments are best handled with closed vitrectomy techniques.[46]

Unfortunately, in many cases a diagnosis is made only after one eye presents with end-stage, irreparable disease manifested as total retinal detachment and extensive retrolental fibrovascular tissue. However, significant ocular asymmetry is common, and although progression in the other eye can be seen later in life, progression to a severe degree that affects vision is unusual. Therefore, even if one eye is lost, the chances of retaining normal vision in the fellow eye are usually good.

23.4 Stickler's Syndrome (Hereditary Arthro-Ophthalmopathy)

Stickler's syndrome, or hereditary arthro-ophthalmopathy, is an autosomal dominant connective tissue disorder that has potentially severe and debilitating ocular, skeletal, and other systemic abnormalities.[3,47] The incidence of the disease is about 1 in 10,000. As with other dominantly inherited conditions, the clinical manifestations of Stickler's syndrome vary considerably, which is an area of potential concern regarding accurate diagnosis, appropriate genetic counseling, and effective intervention for those affected. A precise diagnosis before counseling is ideal, but accurate ophthalmic diagnosis is not sufficient to clarify the inheritance owing to the intrafamilial variability of the phenotype.

23.4.1 Clinical Features

The main ocular features of Stickler's syndrome consist of progressive myopia with vitreal degeneration, lattice degeneration, and a propensity for the development of retinal tears, including giant retinal tears.[17,48,49,50,51] The vitreal degeneration or liquefaction occurs relatively early in life and results in what has been described as an "optically empty vitreous." The lattice degeneration often assumes a radial, perivascular distribution (▶ Fig. 23.12). Patients are at very high risk for rhegmatogenous retinal detachments, and it is not unusual for a patient to present with detachments in childhood or adolescence. Cataracts and strabismus are also relatively common ocular manifestations. Glaucoma and retinoschisis are less common associated abnormalities.

Systemic findings include progressive hearing loss, cleft palate, and mandibular hypoplasia.[47,50] A characteristic flat facial appearance is often present. The syndrome also is associated with joint changes that typically consist of hypermobility, epiphyseal dysplasia, and degenerative changes similar to those of osteoarthritis. Many of the facial and skeletal features manifest before the ocular signs come to diagnosis. The arthritis and hearing loss are progressive and, as noted earlier, can become disabling problems. Other, less common systemic abnormalities include thoracic kyphoscoliosis, genu valgum, and marfanoid habitus.

23.4.2 Differential Diagnosis

The main differential diagnoses of Stickler's syndrome are Wagner's disease and Goldmann-Favré's disease (see "X-Linked Juvenile Retinoschisis" section). In the past, Wagner's disease and Stickler's syndrome were often grouped together because they are both autosomal dominant conditions that share the ocular findings of myopia, optically empty vitreous, and perivascular pigmentary changes.[3] However, Wagner's disease does not have any systemic associations, and there is no apparent increased risk for retinal detachment.[52,53] Furthermore, myopia is less pronounced and cataract formation appears to be more common in Wagner's disease. Finally, it is now known that Wagner's disease is genetically distinct from Stickler's syndrome.[53,54,55,56]

In 1972, Irene Maumenee reexamined and photographed the surviving patients with Wagner's disease in Switzerland.[54,55] Overall, Maumenee felt that Wagner's disease had more similarities to RP than Stickler's syndrome with which it had often

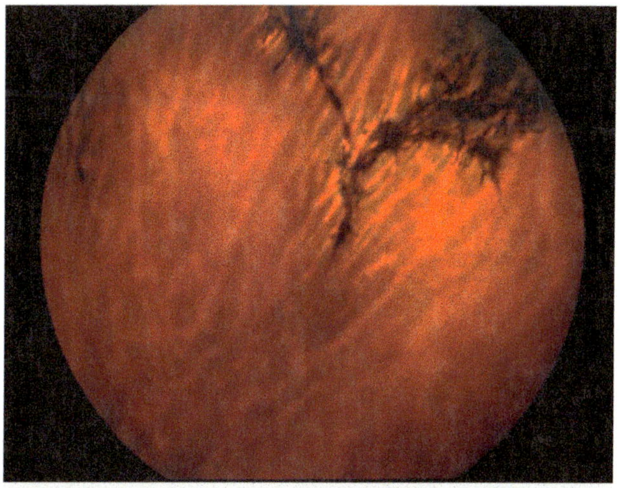

Fig. 23.12 Fundus photograph showing typical radial, perivascular lattice in an adult male with Stickler's syndrome.

been linked previously. Furthermore, the two conditions had separate mutations.

Pearls

- Wagner's disease and Goldmann-Favré's disease can have ocular findings that most closely resemble those of RP.

23.4.3 Pathogenesis and Genetics

Type II collagen is the main structural protein of secondary vitreous and hyaline cartilage. Stickler's syndrome has been recently shown to be caused by mutations in the type II procollagen gene (COL2A1) located on chromosome 12.[56] Exactly how this defective gene product leads to premature vitreous syneresis and other findings in Stickler's syndrome is not yet known. Interestingly, there have been reports of other disorders sharing clinical features of Stickler's syndrome that either had none of the ocular findings and were linked to the COL2A1 gene locus or had a subset of only the ocular findings with no other systemic findings, such as Wagner's disease with linkage to other genes (e.g., 5q13–14).[56]

Diagnostic tests for such a predisposition to Stickler's syndrome based on identification of the mutation in the *COL2A1* gene make possible genetic counseling and prophylactic treatment or early intervention for retinal detachment in affected people.

23.4.4 Management and Course

In an autosomal condition with variable expressivity but almost complete penetrance, it is important that every family member be examined. The youngest patient with Stickler's syndrome and a retinal detachment whom I have personally managed was 9 months old.

All retinal breaks and predisposing vitreoretinal pathology, such as lattice degeneration, should be treated with laser photocoagulation and/or cryotherapy. Freeman[52] has even advocated a prophylactic scleral buckle for the fellow eye of patients with Stickler's disease who have had a giant tear in the first eye.

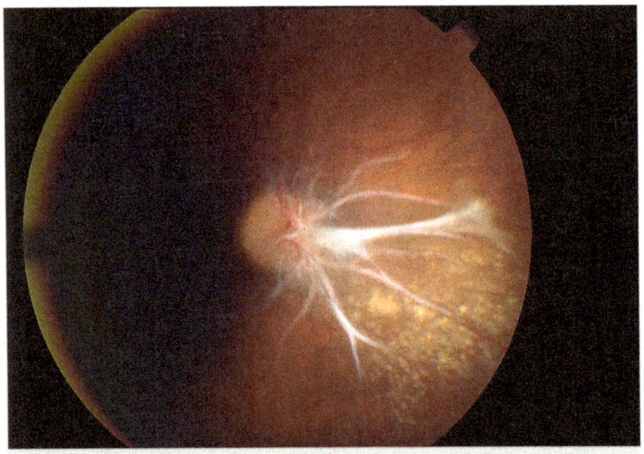

Fig. 23.13 Right eye of a female patient who underwent pars plana vitrectomy for toxocariasis at the age of 4 as it appears 22 years later.

More recently, a study from Cambridge, England, has advocated prophylactic cryotherapy to lattice in the fellow eye of patients with a retinal detachment.[53]

Retinal detachments in this disease often represent a challenging management issue, as it is not unusual to encounter multiple or posterior retinal breaks. A scleral buckle, vitrectomy, or both may be required to reattach the retina.

23.5 Toxocariasis

Toxocara Cani and Toxocara Cati seem less prevalent than it was 40 years ago (▸ Fig. 23.13). Still, it is important to differentiate toxocariasis from retinoblastoma which can now be done more precisely than in the past when far advanced cases presented with leukocoria. The enzyme-linked immunosorbent assay, when negative, can be helpful in ruling out toxocariasis, while eosinophilia and/or recovery of eosinophils supports the diagnosis of toxocariasis.

References

[1] Deutman AF. The Hereditary Dystrophies in the Posterior Pole of the Eye. Assen, The Netherlands: Van Gorcum; 1971:48–99

[2] Kim JE, Ruttum MS, Koeberl MJ, Hassemer EL, Sidjanin DJ. Genetic and clinical evaluation of juvenile retinoschisis. J AAPOS. 2009; 13(2):215–217

[3] Tasman WS. The vitreous. In: Duane TD, ed. Duane's Clinical Ophthalmology, Vol. 3 (38). Philadelphia, PA: JB Lippincott; 1984:7–10

[4] Haas J. Ueber das Zusammenvorkommen von Veränderungen der Retina und Choroidea. Arch Augenheilkd. 1898; 37:343–348

[5] George ND, Yates JR, Moore AT. X linked retinoschisis. Br J Ophthalmol. 1995; 79(7):697–702

[6] Kim DY, Mukai S. X-linked juvenile retinoschisis (XLRS): a review of genotype-phenotype relationships. Semin Ophthalmol. 2013; 28(5–6):392–396

[7] Ewing CC, Ives EJ. Juvenile hereditary retinoschisis. Trans Ophthalmol Soc U K. 1970; 89:29–39

[8] Harris GS, Yeung J. Maculopathy of sex-linked juvenile retinoschisis. Can J Ophthalmol. 1976; 11(1):1–10

[9] Forsius H, Krause U, Helve J, et al. Visual acuity in 183 cases of X-chromosomal retinoschisis. Can J Ophthalmol. 1973; 8(3):385–393

[10] Lisch W. Hereditary vitreoretinal degenerations: sex-linked juvenile retinoschisis. Dev Ophthalmol. 1983; 8:19–32

[11] George NDL, Yates JRW, Moore AT. Clinical features in affected males with X-linked retinoschisis. Arch Ophthalmol. 1996; 114(3):274–280

[12] Yanoff M, Kertesz Rahn E, Zimmerman LE. Histopathology of juvenile retinoschisis. Arch Ophthalmol. 1968; 79(1):49–53

[13] Verdaguer J, Pan American Association of Ophthalmology and American Journal of Ophthalmology Lecture. Juvenile retinal detachment. Am J Ophthalmol. 1982; 93(2):145–156

[14] Conway BP, Welch RB. X-chromosone-linked juvenile retinoschisis with hemorrhagic retinal cyst. Am J Ophthalmol. 1977; 83(6):853–855

[15] Greven CM, Moreno RJ, Tasman W. Unusual manifestations of X-linked retinoschisis. Trans Am Ophthalmol Soc. 1990; 88:211–225, discussion 226–228

[16] Regillo CD, Tasman WS, Brown GC. Surgical management of complications associated with X-linked retinoschisis. Arch Ophthalmol. 1993; 111(8):1080–1086

[17] Peachey NS, Fishman GA, Derlacki DJ, Brigell MG. Psychophysical and electroretinographic findings in X-linked juvenile retinoschisis. Arch Ophthalmol. 1987; 105(4):513–516

[18] Alitalo T, Kruse TA, de la Chapelle A. Refined localization of the gene causing X-linked juvenile retinoschisis. Genomics. 1991; 9(3):505–510

[19] Sieving PA, Bingham EL, Roth MS, et al. Linkage relationship of X-linked juvenile retinoschisis with Xp22.1-p22.3 probes. Am J Hum Genet. 1990; 47 (4):616–621

[20] Dahl N, Pettersson U. Use of linked DNA probes for carrier detection and diagnosis of X-linked juvenile retinoschisis. Arch Ophthalmol. 1988; 106 (10):1414–1416

[21] Kaplan J, Pelet A, Hentati H, et al. Contribution to carrier detection and genetic counselling in X linked retinoschisis. J Med Genet. 1991; 28(6):383–388

[22] Turut P, François P, Castier P, Milazzo S. Analysis of results in the treatment of peripheral retinoschisis in sex-linked congenital retinoschisis. Graefes Arch Clin Exp Ophthalmol. 1989; 227(4):328–331

[23] Schulman J, Peyman GA, Jednock N, Larson B. Indications for vitrectomy in congenital retinoschisis. Br J Ophthalmol. 1985; 69(7):482–486

[24] Trese MT, Ferrone PJ. The role of inner wall retinectomy in the management of juvenile retinoschisis. Graefes Arch Clin Exp Ophthalmol. 1995; 233 (11):706–708

[25] Regillo CD, Custis PH. Surgical management of retinoschisis. Curr Opin Ophthalmol. 1997; 8(3):80–86

[26] Criswick VG, Schepens CL. Familial exudative vitreoretinopathy. Am J Ophthalmol. 1969; 68(4):578–594

[27] Gow J, Oliver GL. Familial exudative vitreoretinopathy. An expanded view. Arch Ophthalmol. 1971; 86(2):150–155

[28] Canny CL, Oliver GL. Fluorescein angiographic findings in familial exudative vitreoretinopathy. Arch Ophthalmol. 1976; 94(7):1114–1120

[29] Tasman W, Augsburger JJ, Shields JA, Caputo A, Annesley WH, Jr. Familial exudative vitreoretinopathy. Trans Am Ophthalmol Soc. 1981; 79:211–226

[30] Regillo CD. Familial exudative vitreoretinopathy. In: Yannuzzi LA, Guyer DR, Chang S, Shields J, Green WR, eds. Retina, Vitreous, Macula: A Comprehensive Text. Philadelphia, PA: WB Saunders; 1997

[31] Plager DA, Orgel IK, Ellis FD, Hartzer M, Trese MT, Shastry BS. X-linked recessive familial exudative vitreoretinopathy. Am J Ophthalmol. 1992; 114 (2):145–148

[32] Laqua H. Familial exudative vitreoretinopathy. Albrecht Von Graefes Arch Klin Exp Ophthalmol. 1980; 213(2):121–133

[33] Benson WE. Familial exudative vitreoretinopathy. Trans Am Ophthalmol Soc. 1995; 93:473–521

[34] van Nouhuys CE. Juvenile retinal detachment as a complication of familial exudative vitreoretinopathy. Fortschr Ophthalmol. 1989; 86(3):221–223

[35] Hashimoto K, Miyakubo H, Inohara N, Tada H. Juvenile retinal detachment and familial exudative vitreoretinopathy. Jpn J Clin Ophthalmol. 1983; 37:797–803

[36] Townes PL, Roca PD. Norrie's disease (hereditary oculo-acoustic-cerebral degeneration). Report of a United States family. Am J Ophthalmol. 1973; 76 (5):797–803

[37] Jacklin HN. Falciform fold, retinal detachment, and Norrie's disease. Am J Ophthalmol. 1980; 90(1):76–80

[38] Chen Z-Y, Battinelli EM, Fielder A, et al. A mutation in the Norrie disease gene (NDP) associated with X-linked familial exudative vitreoretinopathy. Nat Genet. 1993; 5(2):180–183

[39] Fullwood P, Jones J, Bundey S, Dudgeon J, Fielder AR, Kilpatrick MW. X linked exudative vitreoretinopathy: clinical features and genetic linkage analysis. Br J Ophthalmol. 1993; 77(3):168–170

[40] Li Y, Fuhrmann C, Schwinger E, Gal A, Laqua H. The gene for autosomal dominant familial exudative vitreoretinopathy (Criswick-Schepens) on the long arm of chromosome 11. Am J Ophthalmol. 1992; 113(6):712–713

[41] Machemer R, Williams JM, Sr. Pathogenesis and therapy of traction detachment in various retinal vascular diseases. Am J Ophthalmol. 1988; 105 (2):170–181

[42] Carney RG. Incontinentia pigmenti. A world statistical analysis. Arch Dermatol. 1976; 112(4):535–542

[43] Watzke RC, Stevens TS, Carney RG, Jr. Retinal vascular changes of incontinentia pigmenti. Arch Ophthalmol. 1976; 94(5):743–746

[44] Goldberg MF, Custis PH. Retinal and other manifestations of incontinentia pigmenti (Bloch-Sulzberger syndrome). Ophthalmology 1993;100:1645–1654.

[45] Rahi J, Hungerford J. Early diagnosis of the retinopathy of incontinentia pigmenti: successful treatment by cryotherapy. Br J Ophthalmol. 1990; 74 (6):377–379

[46] Catalano RA. Incontinentia pigmenti. Am J Ophthalmol. 1990; 110(6):696–700

[47] Wald KJ, Mehta MC, Katsumi O, Sabates NR, Hirose T. Retinal detachments in incontinentia pigmenti. Arch Ophthalmol. 1993; 111(5):614–617

[48] Stickler GB, Belau PG, Farrell FJ, et al. Hereditary progressive arthro-ophthalmopathy. Mayo Clin Proc. 1965; 40:433–455

[49] Opitz JM, France T, Herrmann J, Spranger JW. The Stickler syndrome. N Engl J Med. 1972; 286(10):546–547

[50] Blair NP, Albert DM, Liberfarb RM, Hirose T. Hereditary progressive arthro-ophthalmopathy of Stickler. Am J Ophthalmol. 1979; 88(5):876–888

[51] Nielsen CE. Stickler's syndrome. Acta Ophthalmol (Copenh). 1981; 59 (2):286–295

[52] Freeman HM. Fellow eyes of giant retinal breaks. Trans Am Ophthalmol Soc. 1978; 76:343–382

[53] Fincham GS, Pasea L, Carroll C, et al. Prevention of retinal detachment in Stickler syndrome: the Cambridge Prophylactic Cryotherapy Protocol. Ophthalmology 2014;121(8):1588–1597

[54] Wagner H. Einbisher unbekanntes Erbleiden des Anges (Degeneratio hyaloideoretinalis hereditaria), beobachtet im Kanton Zurich. Klin Monatsbl Augenheilkd. 1938; 100:840–856

[55] Maumenee IH, Stoll HU, Mets MB. The Wagner syndrome versus hereditary arthroophthalmopathy. Trans Am Ophthalmol Soc. 1982; 80:349–365

[56] Ahmad NN, Ala-Kokko L, Knowlton RG, et al. Stop codon in the procollagen II gene (COL2A1) in a family with the Stickler syndrome (arthro-ophthalmopathy). Proc Natl Acad Sci U S A. 1991; 88(15):6624–6627

24 Infectious Chorioretinal Inflammatory Conditions

Janet L. Davis

24.1 Introduction

Bacterial, viral, protozoan, and helminthic infections of the posterior segment have characteristic ophthalmoscopic features that help clinicians deduce the type of infection and apply appropriate treatment. Some organisms possess such distinctive patterns of growth that a diagnosis can be made by fundus examination alone. The best example of this is cytomegalovirus (CMV) retinitis. Pattern recognition is relatively easy in the posterior segment of the eye because of the flat architecture, transparency of the retina, and multiplicity of tissues that may be affected differentially before full-thickness infection of all ocular coats occurs.[1]

Visual diagnosis of posterior segment infections (▶ Table 24.1) is assisted by an understanding of the fundamental characteristics of each infection: route of infection and preferential tissue of infection, host factors in susceptibility, characteristics of specific infections, and response to medication. In ocular inflammatory disease of infectious causes, compared with most other types of uveitis, diagnosis is the critical step leading to specific therapies that may be curative. Sampling of serum or intraocular fluids to determine the presence of host antibodies and non-host DNA, culture of intraocular fluids or tissue, histopathologic analysis, identification of infection in another body site, and response to therapy may all be used to confirm the suspected diagnosis.

24.2 Pathogenesis and Natural History

24.2.1 Route of Infection

Nonsurgical, nontraumatic infections of the posterior segment of the eye are typically blood borne. In acutely ill, septic patients, an endogenous endophthalmitis is considered with presentation of a red, painful, opacified eye. Bacterial culture of blood, urine, sputum, cerebrospinal fluid, or other suspected infected sites may help confirm the diagnosis when cultures of the ocular fluids are not obtainable or negative. The older publications on bacterial endogenous endophthalmitis mainly concern acutely ill patients, many of whom were likely treated only with intravenous antibiotics, which can be successful therapy due to the breakdown of the blood–retinal barrier.[11,12] Okada et

Table 24.1 Posterior segment infections with focal fundus lesions

Infection	Color	Level	Size and location	Other
Focal bacterial endogenous endophthalmitis	Yellow-white	Flat or slightly elevated, full-thickness retina with variable RPE involvement	Small; larger lesions produce diffuse infection	Uncommon presentation of endogenous endophthalmitis
Syphilis	Yellow to orange	Outer retina and choroid[2]	Outer temporal macula or diffuse retinal involvement	Minimal RPE involvement and scarring
Tuberculosis	White	Choroidal nodules; periphlebitis; Serpiginous-like lesions[3,4]	Miliary to large nodules; geographic	May be solitary; panophthalmitis also occurs
Bartonella henselae infection (cat-scratch disease)	Yellow-white	Irregular retinal infiltrates, thicker than cotton-wool spot	Miliary to small patches; may be solitary or sparse[5]	May be associated with branch retinal artery and vein occlusions[6] or neuroretinitis[7]
CMV retinitis	Yellow to white, usually with hemorrhage	Superficial, granular, with central pigmentary scarring	Variable; often 15% of retina or more at diagnosis	May be multifocal or solitary expanding patch
Necrotizing herpetic retinitis[8]	White to yellow	Thick layer of necrosis with vascular occlusions and pigment disruption	Peripheral, confluent, with rapid centripetal spread	Variable arteritis and optic neuritis
Toxoplasmosis	Variable gray to white or pale yellow	Thick layer of inflammatory swelling	Usually small recurrence at edge of pigmented scar; may take diffuse spreading form[9]	Acquired disease without preexisting scar is possible. Characteristic OCT appearance of full-thickness retinal opacification
Candidiasis	White	Subretinal base with penetration through retina and vitreous extension[10]	Small to moderate retinal lesions and focal vitreous opacities	May be solitary or multiple. Panophthalmitis may occur
Aspergillus infection	Yellow-white	Chorioretinal plaque with vasculitis	Predilection to involve macula	Intense inflammation and intravascular spread

Abbreviations: CMV, cytomegalovirus; OCT, optical coherence tomography; RPE, retinal pigment epithelium;

al summarized the sites cultured and the bacterial organisms isolated in a case series from 1994.[13]

Gram-positive organisms continue to account for the majority of bacterial endogenous endophthalmitis,[14] but the underlying source of infection has shifted, with fewer cases attributable to meningitis and more cases attributable to the expanded use of indwelling medical devices. *Klebsiella* is an emerging source of endogenous endophthalmitis in Asia and in the Western Hemisphere, often associated with liver abscess.[15] Fungal infection remains the most important cause of endogenous endophthalmitis. Earlier use of antifungal agents is decreasing the incidence of fungal endophthalmitis in medical settings.[16] Nine percent of patients in a multicenter study had signs of fungal choroiditis when examined within 72 hours of positive candidal blood cultures in 1994[17] compared to less than 1% in 2011.[15]

There appear to be two mechanisms by which blood-borne infection of the eye occurs. The first is through direct infection of the retina via the retinal blood vessels. CMV infection of the endothelium of a large retinal vessel with subsequent spread to surrounding tissues is the classic example of this type of entry (▶ Fig. 24.1). Retinal hemorrhages and cotton-wool spots are also common in septicemia and may be a *forme fruste* of endophthalmitis.[18] In general, endogenous bacterial endophthalmitis infects surrounding retina and vitreous so rapidly that the exact site of intravascular infection and penetration into the retina is usually not identified except at the time of vitrectomy. However, low-pathogenicity organisms can cause discrete, focal lesions of bacterial retinitis before producing a diffuse and destructive infection. *Listeria monocytogenes* and *Staphylococcus aureus* are the classic examples of this type of infection (▶ Fig. 24.2). One characteristic of retinal vascular entry is that the retinal pigment epithelium (RPE) is relatively spared. Unusual organisms such as *Corynebacterium* species or *Rhodococcus equi* may also produce this type of focal infection.[19,20]

The second type of entry into the eye is via the choroidal circulation. Enhanced depth ocular coherence tomography can detect choroidal masses in fungal endophthalmitis.[10] Yeasts are the predominant species producing endogenous endophthalmitis, affecting 39 patients compared to 14 patients infected with molds in a 22-year retrospective study.[21] Risk factors for mold infection were iatrogenic immunosuppression and organ transplantation. Mold-infected eyes were more likely to have hypopyon, shorter duration before presentation, and worse visual acuity.

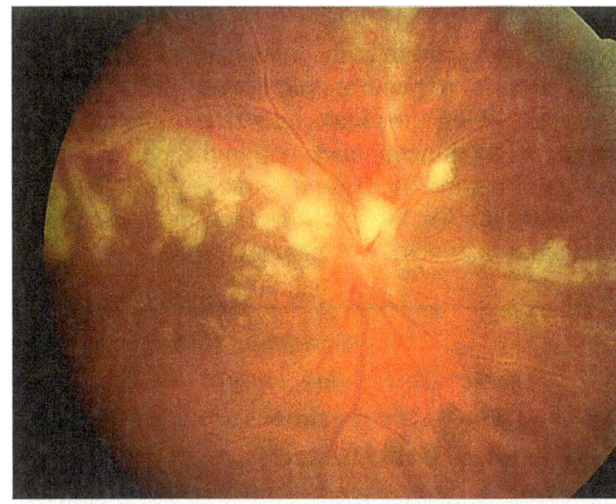

Fig. 24.1 Untreated cytomegalovirus retinitis: The retina superior to the superotemporal vein is atrophic from prior disease, which has now cicatrized. Some atrophy is also seen below the arcade. The white border at the 12:30 o'clock position corresponds to the nasal extent of the confluent retinitis. Multiple vessels are thickly cuffed with inflammatory cells; in some areas, retina adjacent to the inflamed vessels is also infected with cytomegalovirus.

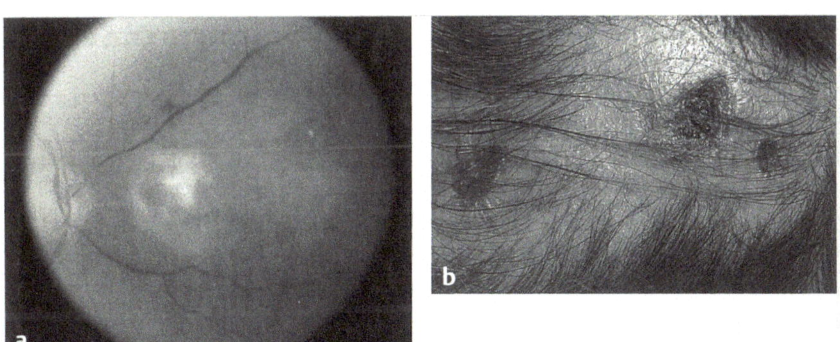

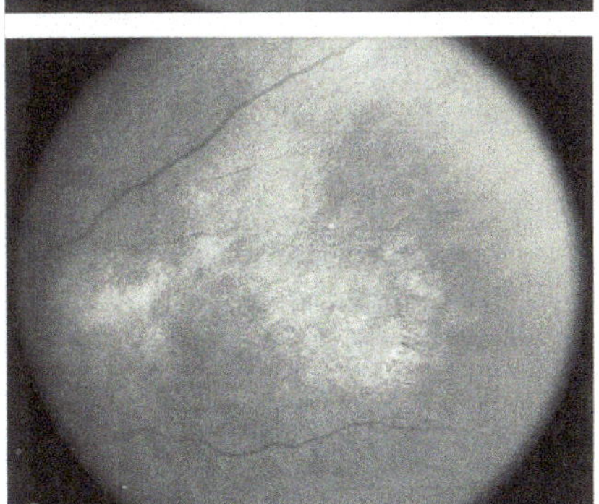

Fig. 24.2 (**a**) Focal inflammatory lesion in a patient with vitritis and 20/60 vision: The left eye had a similar but smaller lesion. The patient was receiving renal dialysis because of diabetic complications. A stitch abscess in the lower abdominal wall was drained and the patient was started on ceftriaxone and vancomycin. (**b**) Chronic scalp ulcers grew *Staphylococcus aureus*, a gram-negative rod, and an atypical mycobacterium. (**c**) Healing of the retinal lesions was achieved with ceftriaxone and vancomycin before amikacin was started for the atypical mycobacterium. *Staphylococcus aureus* is the presumed cause of this focal bacterial endophthalmitis.

Special Considerations

- Endogenous endophthalmitis presents with a spectrum of severity. Culture of extraocular sites and intravenous treatment, vitreous tap and injection, or therapeutic vitrectomy with intravitreal antibiotics may all be appropriate in certain settings. The Endophthalmitis Vitrectomy Study (EVS) findings cannot be extrapolated directly to endogenous endophthalmitis.

Routes of entry other than the blood are less common. Acute necrotizing herpetic retinitis (acute retinal necrosis [ARN]) appears to begin as a neural infection. This assumption is based on the latency of varicella-zoster and herpes simplex virus (HSV) within nerve ganglia and on animal models that document transmission of herpetic infection from one eye to the other via the anterior visual and pupillary pathways.[22] The confluent, peripheral, circumferential infection with centripetal spread represents death of the neurons in the retina at their termini and a dying back of neurons to the center. The fact that a strict neural pattern is not preserved is presumed to relate to lysis of infected cells with infection of adjacent elements (▶ Fig. 24.3).

The course of infection varies widely among infectious agents, from the potentially years-long course of diffuse unilateral subacute neuroretinitis (DUSN) to the acute endophthalmitis. Presentation depends on factors such as the replication speed of the organisms: never for the nematodal agents of DUSN, hours for viruses and fungi, and minutes for bacteria. Toxins, such as the lytic enzymes produced by streptococci and bacillus species, also modify the course of disease.

Understanding the pattern of disease assists clinicians in forming a provisional diagnosis and initiating treatment. It may be difficult to culture for all classes of organisms with small amounts of intraocular fluid. Spirochetes and toxoplasmosis[23] can be cultured only in living cells, and organisms sequestered in the retina may require chorioretinal biopsy rather than vitreous fluid sampling to be identified. Pattern recognition is powerful, but when characteristic patterns have been obliterated by dissemination within the eye and opacification of the media, ancillary diagnostic studies are essential. Analysis of aqueous humor is now routine for the diagnosis of viral retinitis and extensive toxoplasmosis.[24,25] Syphilis can be diagnosed by either aqueous humor polymerase chain reaction (PCR)[26] or by antibody determinations. The following text box displays an algorithm for the diagnosis and initial treatment of posterior segment disease.

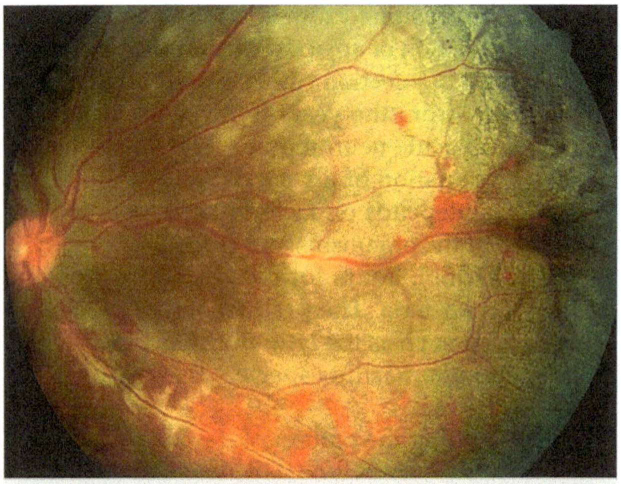

Fig. 24.3 Necrotizing herpetic retinitis in a patient with HIV infection: The lack of inflammation makes the typical features of the infection easier to see. Vessels are occluded in the area of retinal necrosis. In the far periphery, full-thickness necrosis has led to retinal hole formation and detachment. Large satellite lesions extend a great distance beyond the thick, confluent border of retinitis.

Pearls for the Initial Management of Infectious Posterior Uveitis

Chorioretinitis

- Treat classic recurrent toxoplasma chorioretinitis according to current guidelines with optional serology for toxoplasma
- Treat neuroretinitis according to current guidelines for *Bartonella* infection and obtain serology
- For other chorioretinitis, obtain specimens for diagnostic testing
  - Blood for quantitative RPR, FTA-ABS, human immunodeficiency virus (HIV), CMV, toxoplasmosis
  - Aqueous humor for PCR studies as indicated
    1. CMV, HSV 1, HSV 2, varicella, toxoplasma
- • Day 1: Start empiric therapy for viral infection
  - Intravitreal antiviral injection in affected eye(s)
  - Oral acyclovir or valacyclovir
- Day 3 to 4: Check RPR and FTA results
  - If RPR positive, HIV negative
    1. Aqueous procaine pen G IM 2.4 million u/d for 10 days with probenecid 500 mg four times a day or intravenous therapy
    2. Suspend antiviral treatment
    3. Lumbar puncture
  - If RPR or FTA-ABS positive and HIV positive
    1. Admit for intravenous aqueous penicillin
    2. Suspend antiviral treatment
    3. Lumbar puncture
  - If RPR and FTA-ABS negative
    1. Continue antiviral treatment and reinject
    2. Consider sending aqueous humor for syphilis antibody
- Day 5 to 10: Assess response to empiric therapy
  - Adjust therapy according to PCR results
  - Consider diagnostic vitrectomy if diagnosis is uncertain—this may include aspiration or biopsy of retinal and subretinal lesions

Panuveitis with Suspected Infection: For diffuse inflammation without prominent focal lesions or no view

- Day 1
  - RPR, FTA-ABS
  - Detailed review of systems and medical history
  - Culture of other infected sites, blood, and urine
  - Consider chest X-ray and echocardiography
  - Consider diagnostic vitrectomy for cytology and culture
  - Delay therapy until after diagnostic specimens obtained if possible

Pearls

- Plan carefully for the specimens to be taken during a diagnostic vitrectomy. Undiluted specimens are used for cytology and immunohistochemistry, culture, PCR, and antibody studies. Diluted specimens are ideal for flow cytometry and can be concentrated for bacterial and fungal culture or injected into aerobic and anaerobic blood culture bottles.

24.2.2 Host Factors

Intraocular infection may occur because a large number of organisms are circulating in the blood, or they may be circulating for a long time or intermittently, as in intravenous drug abusers, thereby increasing the chances of inoculation of the eye. Individuals most likely to experience overwhelming infection are, in general, those least able to mount defenses. If endogenous infection is suspected, a complete medical history of the past several months must be taken into consideration to see if instrumentation of intravascular structures has occurred, if intravascular medical devices have been implanted, or if intravenous drugs have been abused. Risk factors for HIV infection should be queried. In the case of fungal endophthalmitis, the active systemic infection may be remote and the eye may be the only site of residual infection.

The asymptomatic, uninstrumented patient is a diagnostic challenge. Dental work or colonic polyps may lead to brief seeding of the bloodstream and endogenous infection (▶ Fig. 24.4). Bronchiectasis or sinusitis may create prolonged reservoirs of infection. Usually, the number of organisms that enter the bloodstream from these sources is so small that the immune system rapidly clears the offenders. Subacute bacterial endocarditis with intermittent seeding of the bloodstream may also be difficult to diagnose. Transesophageal echography is useful to detect small vegetations on heart valves.

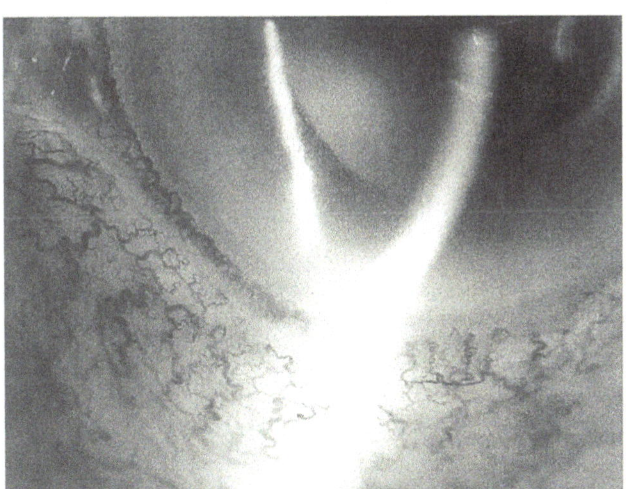

Fig. 24.4 This otherwise asymptomatic man was treated for several days with topical corticosteroids before endogenous endophthalmitis was diagnosed. Vitreous cultures grew a microaerophilic streptococcus that is a commensal organism of the mouth and gastrointestinal tract. Fibrin and hypopyon are present with no view of the fundus. He had no predisposing instrumentation other than a dental cleaning and no heart valve abnormality or chronic disease. Cultures from other sites were negative. Months after treatment, gastrointestinal bleeding from colonic polyps led to partial colectomy; erosion of a polyp was proposed as another possible inciting event for the endophthalmitis.

HIV infection has produced several interesting exceptions to the standard rules regarding infectious disorders. Syphilis in patients with acquired immunodeficiency syndrome (AIDS) may be difficult to treat even with high-dose penicillin.[27] Recurrences are common and not always accompanied by a positive quantitative RPR.[28] Prolonged impairment of the cellular immune system with depletion of CD4- and CD8-bearing lymphocytes appears to lead to susceptibility to viruses of the herpes class, especially CMV,[29] which can grow in a multitude of cell types and organs. Some individuals may have an unusual predisposition to a specific opportunistic infection that is based not on any global index of immunosuppression but on quite specific defects in the immunologic repertoire that, at present, cannot be measured. Functional assays of CMV-specific CD4- and CD8-positive T lymphocytes do not predict which HIV patients are likely to develop CMV retinitis during follow-up.[30] Improvement in CMV-specific T-cell responses is associated with treatment with highly active antiretroviral therapy (HAART) and immune recovery as well as resistance to recurrence of CMV retinitis.[31] Empirically, sustained elevation of CD4 + T lymphocytes greater than 100 cells per microliter for 6 months supports discontinuation of CMV-specific antiviral therapy.[32]

24.3 Specific Infections

24.3.1 Viral Retinitis

Cytomegalovirus Retinitis

Cytomegalovirus (CMV) retinitis is generally a slow-growing infection that produces an expanding lesion with a granular border and a central, atrophic zone (▶ Fig. 24.5). The virus propagates every 18 hours and spreads from cell to cell within the

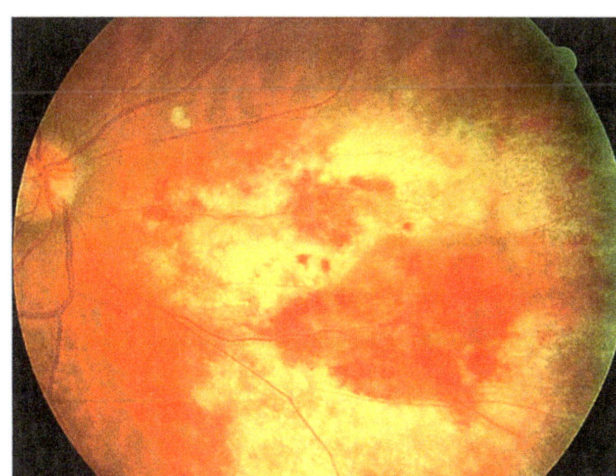

Fig. 24.5 Central clearing with scarring is typical of large cytomegalovirus lesions, which progress slowly enough to heal in their wake. Lack of central clearing in untreated cases can be seen in small, fresh cytomegalovirus lesions, rapidly progressing infections such as herpetic necrotizing retinitis, and infections that heal slowly (toxoplasmosis) or not at all (fungus).

retina and probably within the RPE. Infection originates in endothelial cells.[33] In the HAART era, progression of the active border by greater than or equal to 0.5 disc diameter occurred at a rate of 1.4/100 person-years of follow-up in patients with treated disease and immune recovery versus 28/100 person-years in newly diagnosed and untreated patients.

First described as a complication of organ transplantation, CMV retinitis occurred in only 1% of solid organ recipients from 1995 to 2005, presumably due to improved immunosuppression regimens and CMV surveillance programs with prophylactic treatment of recipients of organs from CMV-positive donors.[34] The incidence of CMV retinitis has also fallen in HIV-positive individuals in the HAART era and, in 2012, was reported to be 0.36/100 person-years in the Longitudinal Study of the Ocular Complications of AIDS.[35]

Any part of the retina can be infected, although most patients have relatively posterior disease at the time their disease is diagnosed.[36] Posterior disease may have the so-called fulminant appearance with secondary exudative retinal detachments (▶ Fig. 24.6). The degree of hemorrhage within lesions is variable; hemorrhage is more common with untreated posterior lesions, whereas a granular, nonhemorrhagic retinitis is more common in peripheral disease. In the HAART era, overall mortality of patients with CMV retinitis remains high at 9.8 deaths/100 person-years on a U.S. prospective multicenter study of 503 patients.[37] The rate of retinitis progression in that study was 7/100 person-years and rate of retinal detachment was 2.3/100 person-years.[37] Poor long-term visual outcomes after retinal detachment repair with silicone oil are of increasing importance in the HAART era[38] because patients will likely live longer after surgery. Silicone oil removal should be attempted in patients with stable repairs.

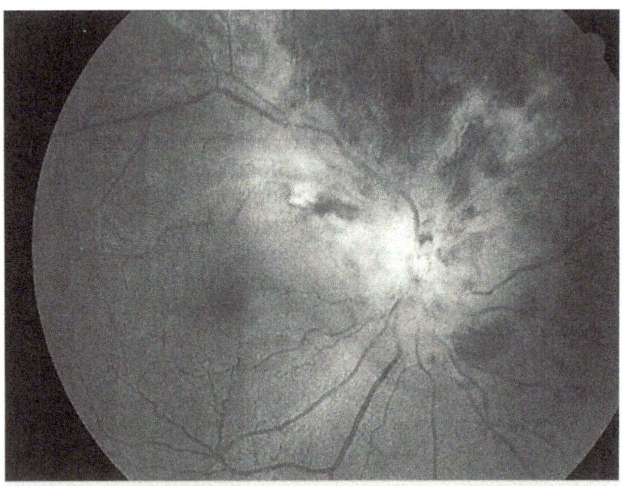

Fig. 24.6 The fulminant, edematous appearance characteristic of untreated cytomegalovirus retinitis involving the posterior pole: Vision was relatively good because the serous detachment did not reach the fovea. The optic nerve was not seriously impaired despite papillitis.

Treatment of CMV retinitis is generally with oral valganciclovir rather than intravenous ganciclovir or foscarnet. Intravenous ganciclovir and foscarnet are equivalent in time to remission[39] and intravenous ganciclovir and valganciclovir are also equivalent. The ganciclovir implant is superior to either,[40] but was taken off the market in 2013. Weekly intravitreal therapy with ganciclovir (2 mg per dose) provides excellent intraocular drug levels.[41] Intravitreal therapy is acceptable for induction, maintenance, or salvage therapy. ▶ Table 24.2 summarizes common dosing regimens for these agents. All three drugs require dosage adjustment for renal function; foscarnet is nephrotoxic. Shorter treatment courses of specific anti-CMV therapy are typical in the era of HAART.[32]

With improvement in the immune status of most HIV-positive patients, CMV retinitis is no longer a common retinal infection, although CMV is a common virus with increasing prevalence with aging.[42] Although better prophylaxis after organ transplantation has reduced the frequency of retinitis, CMV retinitis remains a clinical problem for patients with other types of iatrogenic immunosuppression and the elderly, who may have lost their specific immunity to CMV. Because CMV is a virus that propagates initially in the vascular endothelium, it may increase the risk of occlusions of the retinal circulation, especially if there is concomitant cardiovascular disease.[43,44] Such infections can be difficult to diagnose, in part because suspicion for CMV retinitis is low in the non–HIV-infected population and in part because the retinitis itself can be indolent and difficult to recognize. Diagnosis by PCR followed by oral valganciclovir for 3 months may be adequate treatment[45]; intravitreal injections of antivirals are also helpful in treatment. Interestingly, there are case reports of CMV retinitis occurring de novo after intravitreal injection of triamcinolone.[46]

Necrotizing Herpetic Retinitis

This disorder was named *acute retinal necrosis* before infections with varicella-zoster[47] or HSV types 1 and 2[48,49] were proven to be the cause. There is recognition that vertical transmission of HSV type 2 may play a role in many cases of HSV type 2 ARN in young persons.[50] The original description is that of a young,

Table 24.2 Standard doses of commonly used anticytomegalovirus drugs

Drug	Phase	Route	Dose	Systemic monitoring during treatment
Ganciclovir	Induction	Intravenous	5 mg/kg twice daily	Blood count, neutrophil count, creatinine
	Maintenance	Intravenous	5 mg/kg daily	
Valganciclovir	Induction	Oral	900 mg twice daily	Same as intravenous ganciclovir
	Maintenance	Oral	900 mg daily	
Foscarnet	Induction Maintenance	Intravenous Intravenous	90 mg/kg twice daily 90–120 mg/kg daily	Blood counts, creatinine, calcium, magnesium, phosphate

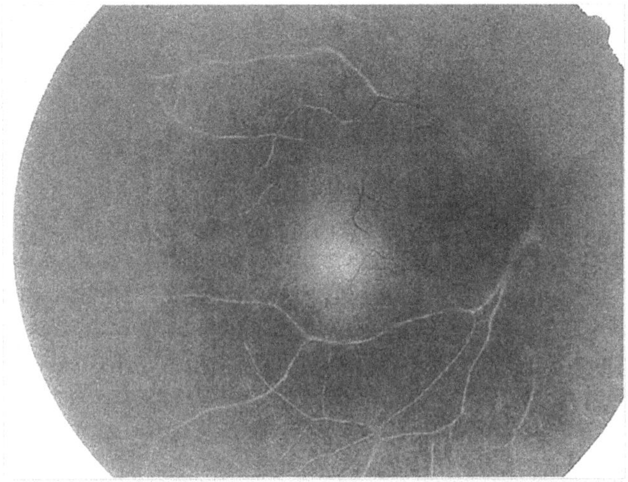

Fig. 24.7 Fluorescein angiogram, 26.1 seconds, demonstrating extensive closure of retinal arterioles in an immunocompetent, elderly patient with a small, 2-clock-hour sector of necrotizing herpetic retinitis: Vision is 20/400. The vascular closure is presumed to be a result of herpetic arteritis and occurred while the patient was on treatment with intravenous acyclovir. Oral prednisone was added and oral acyclovir was continued; vascular closure was reversed and the vision improved to 20/40 after several weeks.

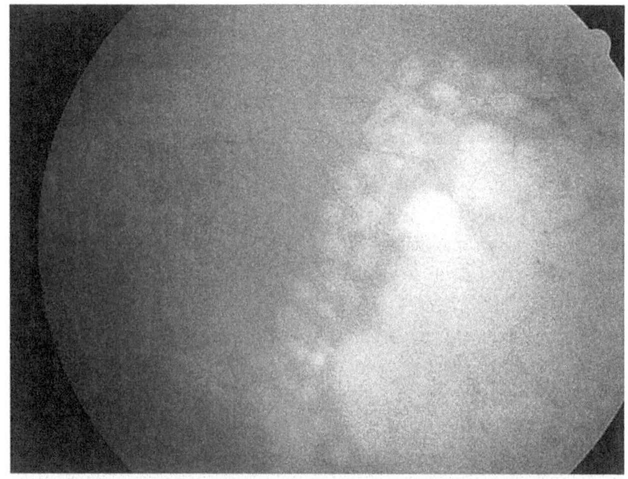

Fig. 24.8 Prophylactic treatment of the borders of necrotizing herpetic retinitis with laser photocoagulation may reduce the risk for later retinal detachment. No retinal detachment occurred in this eye. Vision was 20/25 after subsequent treatment of cataract and macular edema secondary to the viral infection.

healthy person with a bilateral, confluent, rapidly progressive, necrotizing retinitis starting in the periphery and spreading centripetally. Intense vitritis, granulomatous iritis, and episcleritis are common associated features. Generally, the patient has consulted an ophthalmologist and received treatment for iritis or episcleritis for 7 to 10 days before the posterior segment lesions are recognized and treated. The retinal whitening in the far periphery may be difficult to see in the early stages or may not exist in the early stages. After the retinitis is established, optic neuritis and retinal arteriolitis with vascular occlusion may occur (▶ Fig. 24.7). Decreases in velocity in the central retinal artery suggest a reduction in retinal blood flow.[51] Retinal ischemia contributes to vision loss. It is not clear whether aspirin or pentoxifylline treatment can alter the visual outcome by reducing vascular occlusions or improving retinal blood flow.

Combination therapy with both systemic and intravitreal foscarnet has been reported to be more effective than systemic therapy alone in decreasing the risk of retinal detachment and severe vision loss.[52]

Infection may be bilateral in up to two-thirds of affected individuals. If infection of the second eye occurs, it is usually within 6 weeks, although markedly delayed cases have been described.[53] One of the principal benefits of systemic antiviral treatment may be to reduce the final rate of infection of the second eye from roughly 65% to about 17%, based on one retrospective series.[53] Infections of the second eye are generally less severe than those of the first, perhaps because of prompt recognition and treatment. A 3-month course of 400 to 800 mg of oral acyclovir three to five times daily or valacyclovir 500 to 1,000 mg one to three times daily may provide important prophylaxis during the period of greatest risk for fellow eye involvement.[54]

There is a high risk for retinal detachment 8 to 12 weeks after onset of ARN. Whether retinal detachment occurs or not seems to be a principal determinant of visual outcome.[55] Inflammation, preretinal membrane formation, and hypotony can compromise surgical results. Prophylactic treatment with laser photocoagulation to demarcate the borders of the retinitis may reduce the rate of retinal detachment (▶ Fig. 24.8).[56]

In patients with AIDS, necrotizing herpetic retinitis is commonly associated with prior herpes zoster dermatitis, including ipsilateral herpes zoster ophthalmicus,[57] and a high incidence of bilaterality with rapid progression to retinal detachment and blindness.[58] The infection is often not controlled by intravenous acyclovir in the usual doses of 10 mg/kg three times daily for 7 to 10 days. Improved results with ganciclovir or ganciclovir and foscarnet as intravenous combined therapy have been reported.[57] Intravitreal injection of antiviral agents, either ganciclovir 2 mg three times per week for 2 to 3 weeks and then weekly as needed or foscarnet 2.4 mg on the same schedule is likely more effective than systemic treatment alone. The known involvement of the central nervous system during active necrotizing herpetic retinitis[49] and a report of progressive, extensive involvement of visual pathways in the brain[59] in an AIDS patient underscore the need for concomitant systemic treatment. The ideal duration of treatment is uncertain; once the virus resumes a latent state, it may be easier to maintain in remission than CMV or require less intensive medication to treat. However, recurrences have been reported as medication is reduced.[60] Intravenous or oral ganciclovir may provide adequate maintenance therapy and also provide prophylaxis against CMV disease.

In cases in which the diagnosis is unclear, amplification of DNA by the PCR[24] or comparative serology in aqueous humor and serum for varicella immunoglobulin G (IgG) antibody and HSV IgG antibody may be useful.[61] A disproportionately high titer of intraocular antibody supports a specific etiologic diagnosis. In patients with AIDS who have no inflammatory reaction, antibody titers are less likely to be positive; PCR is less likely to be positive more than 1 week after onset.[24]

Other Viral Infections

Epstein–Barr virus may produce a uveitis with retinal vasculitis.[62] Measles (rubeola) virus produces retinal infiltrates and loss of vision during the course of subacute sclerosing panencephalitis. Cases in immunosuppressed individuals have been reported.[63] Congenital rubella produces a classic "salt-and-pepper" pigmentation of the fundus[64]; although some progression of the pigmentary mottling may occur in early childhood, active retinal disease has only rarely been described. Human herpes virus 6 has been isolated from retinal tissues; appreciation of its role in uveitis is expanding.[65]

24.3.2 Protozoal Infections

Toxoplasma Chorioretinitis

Worldwide, toxoplasmic chorioretinitis is probably the most common posterior segment infection because of the prevalence of the causative organism in the food chain and its ability to encyst in body tissues, especially immunologically protected sites such as the brain and eye.

Toxoplasmic chorioretinitis is classically described as a unifocal lesion of full-thickness retinal and choroidal inflammation that leaves a scar with variable pigmentation. Because many clinically important cases represent reactivation from a preexistent scar, an acute inflammatory lesion at the border of a healed chorioretinal scar is virtually pathognomonic for toxoplasmic chorioretinitis. There is usually a focal vitreous inflammatory reaction directly over the lesion, which is useful in diagnosis. Compaction of vitreous strands (cylinders) coated with inflammatory cells is another characteristic feature. Prominent iritis with large keratic precipitates and ocular hypertension occurs with chronicity.

Formerly, all toxoplasmosis was assumed to be congenital. A survey in France reports that the incidence of congenital toxoplasmosis in 2007 was 2.9 (95% confidence interval [CI]: 2.5–3.2) per 10,000 live births; the incidence of symptomatic cases was estimated to be 0.34 (95% CI: 0.2–0.5) cases per 10,000 live births.[66] Seventy percent of congenitally infected but untreated children in Chicago had new chorioretinal lesions develop, often after the age of 10 years.[67] In contrast, the same group reported new lesions in only 31% (95% CI: 23–41%) of patients with congenital infection who were treated in the first year of life; the new lesions also often occurred after the first decade.[68] Newly acquired disease in children may be difficult to detect because symptoms are not reported. In adults, acquired disease without a prior pigmented scar may be misdiagnosed. Very small encystations that have never reactivated may also lack pigmentation and confound the clinician (▶ Fig. 24.9). Many of these small lesions are in the posterior pole and will become visually symptomatic from tissue swelling before vitreous reaction occurs, confusing the picture even more.

Episodes recur unpredictably and take 3 or 4 months to resolve without treatment. During periods of activation, the tachyzoites replicate by endodyogeny, or vertical splitting. Treatment of the inflammatory component with corticosteroids without treating the infectious component may be worse for the patient than no treatment, because natural immune defenses can stop the replication of new organisms and promote reencystation in most individuals. In immunocompromised patients and the elderly, delay of antibiotic treatment can lead to a spreading form of the disease that resembles an ARN (▶ Fig. 24.10).[9,69]

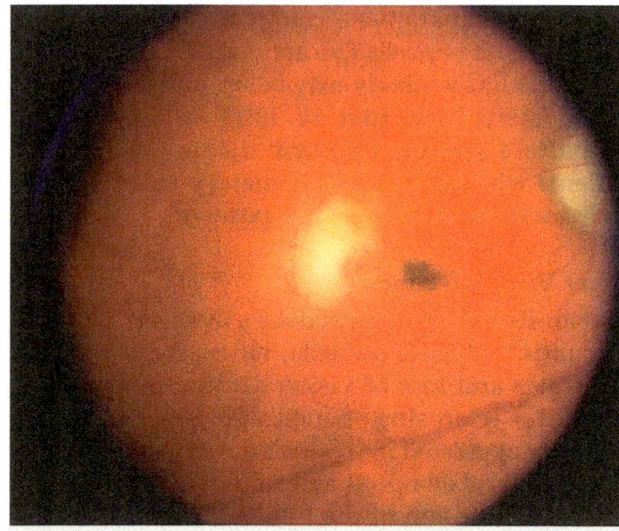

Fig. 24.9 This active lesion of toxoplasmic chorioretinitis may have developed from a small or nonpigmented focus and was, therefore, hidden by the subsequent inflammatory reaction. The pigmented chorioretinal lesion adjacent to the active focus is evidence that this is recurrent disease. Toxoplasmosis was initially rejected as a diagnosis because of lack of contiguous pigment; however, good resolution was obtained with antitoxoplasmic medications.

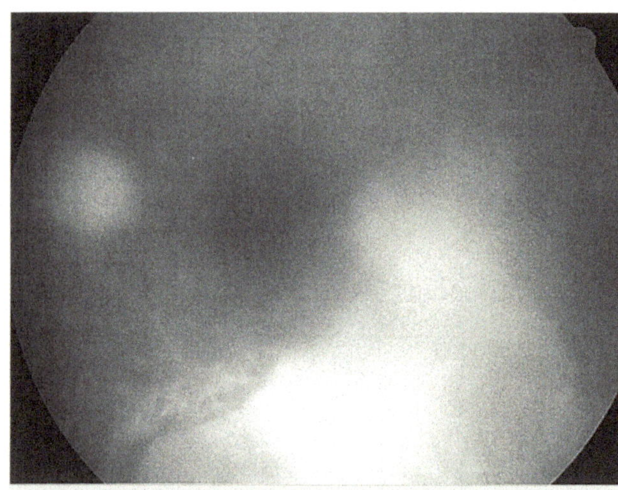

Fig. 24.10 The spreading form of toxoplasmosis can produce severe visual loss. Multiple courses of doxycycline were used to induce and maintain a remission of the toxoplasmic chorioretinitis in this elderly woman, but optic atrophy limited the vision to hand motions.

The diagnosis of toxoplasmic chorioretinitis is usually made clinically and is based on appearance of the fundus lesion. First episodes should be documented with determination of serum IgM antibody titers to *Toxoplasma* to detect recently acquired infection. IgG antibody should be present in all cases to indicate prior exposure; there are isolated reports in which it is not. The presence of *Toxoplasma* antibody in a patient with uveitis without characteristic features of retinochoroiditis does not confirm a diagnosis of toxoplasmosis. More precise diagnosis can be

Table 24.3 Regimens for treating ocular toxoplasmosis

Indication	Drug	Dose and route[a]	Comments
Monotherapy	Trimethoprim-sulfamethoxazole	Double-strength tablet twice daily	Inexpensive; risk for allergic reactions
	Clindamycin Atovaquone Azithromycin Doxycycline[d]	150–300 mg four times daily 750 mg three times daily 500 mg daily 100 mg two times daily	Increases risk of *Clostridium difficile*–associated colitis expensive; well tolerated; concern for time to healing; appropriate for some intolerant patients
Combined therapy	Pyrimethamine -plus-	25–75 mg orally daily	Folinic acid 5 mg three to seven times per week reduces risk for bone marrow toxicity
	Sulfadiazine - or -	1 g orally four times daily	Risk for allergic reactions; poorly tolerated; expensive
	Clindamycin -or- azithromycin	See above See above	See above See above
	Trimethoprim-sulfamethoxazole -plus-	See above	See above
	Clindamycin	See above	See above
	Atovaquone -plus- Clarithromycin or azithromycin	See above 1 g twice daily	See above
Pregnancy[b]	Clindamycin - or -	300–600 mg orally four times a day	Consult with obstetrician
First trimester	Spiramycin[c]	3 g orally in three to four doses	Consult with obstetrician
Second and third trimesters	Pyrimethamine - plus -	25–50 mg daily for 3 wk	Use with folinic acid 5 mg daily
	Sulfadiazine - alternating with	2–3 g/d in four divided doses for 3 wk	Consult with obstetrician
	Spiramycin[c]	3 g orally in three to four divided doses for 3 wk	

[a]Check drug reference manual for pediatric doses.

[b]Strong maternal indication needed unless there is risk for maternal-fetal transmission, in which case drug therapy may benefit the infant as well. Azithromycin is another possible agent, although not proved to be safe. Tetracyclines are contraindicated in pregnancy.

[c]Available from the Division of Anti-infective Drug Products, FDA; (301) 443–4310.

[d]Do not use tetracyclines for children younger than 8 years.

made by analysis of intraocular fluids.[9,24,25] Toxoplasmosis in HIV-infected and other immunocompromised patients is more likely to be multifocal, bilateral, associated with intracranial lesions, and relentlessly progressive and may require long-term antibiotics.[9,70]

Pearls

- Rising serum titers are not necessary for the diagnosis of posterior infectious uveitis and will not generally be present as the majority of infections are recurrences from latent infection. Similarly, a high level of serum antibody is not diagnostic as the ocular inflammation will not necessarily stimulate a marked serum antibody response. The presence of serum antibodies against a suspected infectious agent is useful confirmation of prior exposure.

Treatment of toxoplasmic chorioretinitis can be accomplished by a variety of antibiotic regimens during an approximately 6-week course (▶ Table 24.3). Classic "triple therapy" is pyrimethamine, sulfadiazine, folinic acid, and prednisone.[71] Trimethoprim–sulfamethoxazole with or without clindamycin and prednisone was popularized by Opremcak et al and is better tolerated and cheaper than triple therapy.[72] Evidence for superiority of one treatment over another is lacking.[73] Multiple alternative regimens are available. Atovaquone or azithromycin is generally better tolerated than sulfa-containing antibiotics or clindamycin. Prolonged time to lesion healing has been reported for azithromycin[74]; in contrast, atovaquone may prolong the time to recurrence.[75] Tetracyclines are also used. Newer treatments combine intravitreal dexamethasone with concomitant intravitreal clindamycin and are comparable in effectiveness to oral therapy.[76,77,78] Maintenance therapy with trimethoprim–sulfamethoxazole prevented recurrences for 1

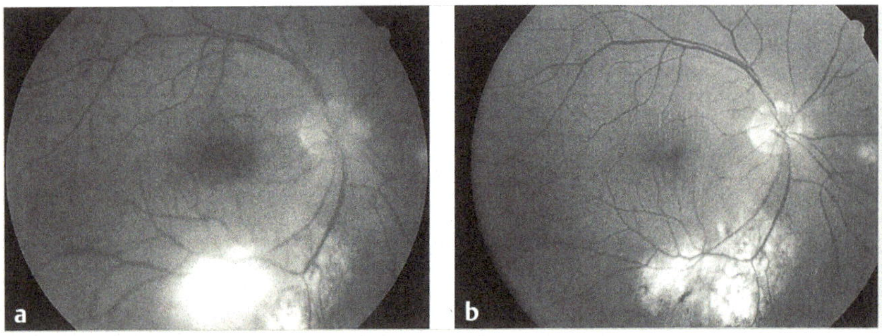

Fig. 24.11 (**a**) Toxoplasmic chorioretinitis in an HIV-infected man: Recurrence from a pigmented chorioretinal scar has a typical appearance. The other eye contained a central macular scar from toxoplasmosis. (**b**) Excellent healing was obtained after treatment with clarithromycin and atovaquone. Multiple drug allergies precluded the use of more conventional antibiotics.

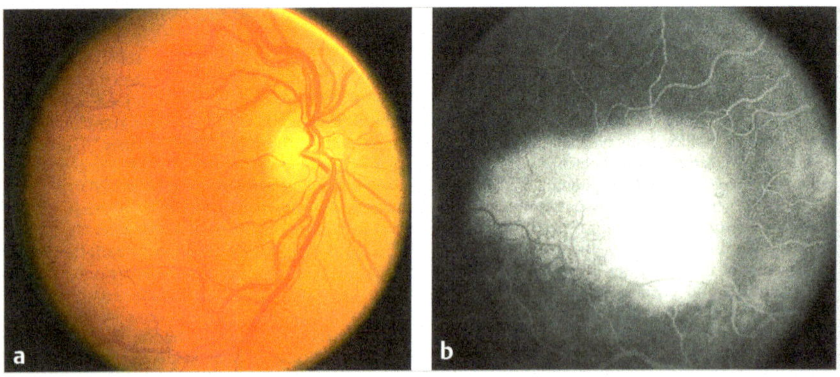

Fig. 24.12 (**a**) Syphilitic chorioretinitis in a patient with secondary lues: The yellowish orange color of an ill-defined area of retinal elevation is characteristic. (**b**) Corresponding fluorescein angiogram in the late venous stage shows extensive, deep leakage of dye.

year in a randomized, placebo-controlled trial.[79] The perceived response to antibiotics may be excellent in AIDS-related toxoplasmic chorioretinitis if there is minimal inflammation (▸ Fig. 24.11).

Prednisone in low doses of 30 to 40 mg for 2 to 3 weeks can be useful to reduce macular or optic nerve inflammation or dense vitreous reaction. When used for this brief period, the prednisone can be stopped abruptly without taper. Periocular or intravitreal corticosteroid injection risks fulminant retinitis, scleritis, or panophthalmitis.[80]

Pearls

- Other than topical corticosteroids for anterior segment inflammation, corticosteroids should not be given without antibiotic coverage for toxoplasmosis.

Pneumocystis Choroiditis

This rare choroidal infection occurs in the setting of HIV infection and other severe immunocompromised conditions. *Pneumocystis* choroiditis is interesting because of its distinctive appearance of patchy orange lesions in the posterior choroid and because vision is preserved over the lesions, either because of the low pathogenicity of the organism or the deep choroidal location, which preserves the choriocapillaris and outer retinal function. Pneumocystic lesions undergo only a mild evolution from creamy, slightly elevated lesions to flat orange macules during treatment. The relatively large size and homogeneous appearance of the lesions without secondary reactive pigmentation is another important characteristic.

24.3.3 Bacterial Infections

Syphilitic Chorioretinitis

The incidence of primary and secondary syphilis infections in the United States in 2013 compared to 2000 was 5.3 cases versus 2.1 per 100,000 population.[81] In the United Kingdom, incident ocular syphilis occurred in 41 persons (63 eyes) from 2009 to 2011, equivalent to 0.3 cases per million adult population.[82] Mean patient age was 49 years and 90% were men. HIV-positive patients were more likely to have panuveitis and less than 10% of patients overall had isolated anterior uveitis. Posterior segment manifestations can include choroiditis, retinitis, retinal vasculitis, and optic neuritis or neuroretinitis. Chorioretinal atrophy and pigmentation with or without vascular narrowing and optic atrophy are common sequelae.[83] A specific pattern of syphilitic posterior uveitis is acute posterior placoid chorioretinitis,[2] characterized by yellow, deep infiltrates in the temporal macula. Fluorescein angiography shows multiple pinpoint leaks, usually alternating with blockage caused by focal areas of pigment epithelial hyperplasia. A second specific pattern is the presence of superficial retinal precipitates.[84] Spectral domain optical coherence tomography demonstrates disruption of the ellipsoid zones and nodular hyperreflectivity of the RPE with occasional subretinal fluid (▸ Fig. 24.12).[85]

Because of variable presentations, serology is key to diagnosis. Most cases of syphilitic uveitis are associated with a positive RPR or Venereal Disease Research Laboratory (VDRL) test result and occur in the second stage of syphilis. HIV-infected persons are an exception, as they may have syphilis without a positive RPR or VDRL result; PCR testing provides greater sensitivity.[86] Enzyme or chemiluminescent immunoassays (EIA or CIA) for syphilis antibody are also more sensitive and the Centers for Disease Control and Prevention (CDC) now recommends them

Table 24.4 Treatment regimens for ocular syphilis

Drug	Dose	Route	Comment
Aqueous procaine penicillin G - plus -	2.4 million units daily for 10 d	Intramuscular	Dose divided between two separate sites
Probenecid - or -	500 mg four times daily for 10 d	Oral	Needed to raise blood levels of penicillin
Penicillin G	2–4 million units every 6 h for 10–14 d	Intravenous	Up to 21–28 d of treatment, or followed by three weekly benzathine shots may be more efficacious. Recommended for HIV-positive patients

Source: Adapted from Bonfioli and Eller.[53]

for initial screening followed by a quantitative RPR or VDRL (www.cdc.gov/STD/syphilis/RSSS-webinar/Reverse-Sequence-Syphilis-Screening-webinar.mp4; accessed December 29, 2014). Patients with late syphilis, defined as disease lasting more than 1 year after infection, who have ocular inflammation or neuro-ophthalmologic findings should be considered to have neurosyphilis and receive a lumbar puncture with cell counts and quantitative VDRL to help guide therapy. Only neurosyphilis regimens are recommended for treatment of ocular syphilis.

The CDC recommends that ocular syphilis be treated in the same way as neurosyphilis (▶ Table 24.4). It is possible that secondary syphilis associated with intraocular inflammation could be treated with a simpler regimen, such as benzathine penicillin intramuscular injections, as the ocular inflammation produces breakdown of the blood–aqueous barrier and allows higher intraocular levels of penicillin than can usually be achieved. Relapse of neurosyphilis after benzathine treatment has been reported.[87]

Topical corticosteroids can be combined with antibiotic treatment. Rarely, oral prednisone combined with antibiotics could be used to mitigate posterior segment inflammation.

Tuberculosis

Tuberculous uveitis has recognizable posterior patterns of choroidal granulomas, serpiginous-like choroidopathy, multifocal choroiditis, and retinal vasculitis.[88] Of these, retinal vasculitis or serpiginous-like choroidopathy, originally described in India,[89] are the most common in nonendemic areas.[90] Either tuberculin skin test or interferon-gamma release tests have adequate sensitivity and specificity to confirm prior exposure, but can give discordant results and are not in themselves diagnostic.[91] Interferon-gamma release assays have the advantage of not reacting with prior vaccination with Bacillus-Calmetté-Guerin (BCG), although reactions greater than 20 mm rarely occur after BCG vaccination. Fludeoxyglucose positron emission tomography (FDG-PET) can improve detection of small foci of tuberculous infection in the lungs amenable to biopsy and culture.[92] Often the diagnosis is unconfirmed and stated as tuberculosis-related uveitis or presumed tuberculous uveitis, requiring multidisciplinary decision making regarding antimycobacterial treatment.[88] Overlap with sarcoidosis occurs in patients with positive interferon-gamma release assays.[90]

The rate of true positive diagnoses of tuberculosis resulting from PPD screening of uveitis patients in the United States was formerly so low that it was recommended that routine PPD tests not be performed in the evaluation of uveitis patients.[93] More recently, interferon-gamma release assays were positive in 80 of 343 German uveitis patients of whom 43 were given a diagnosis of presumed tuberculosis, and 16 of who received full treatment.[94] True positives are difficult to ascertain before observing the response to treatment which, in many cases, will require concomitant corticosteroids.

Although interpretation of tests for tuberculosis in uveitis remains difficult, the CDC recommends treatment of latent tuberculosis in high-risk groups, such as immigrants; HIV-infected, homeless, or incarcerated persons; and those living in group homes regardless of whether tuberculous uveitis is suspected. There is also an increased risk in patients receiving more than 15 mg corticosteroids for more than 2 to 4 weeks or anti-tumor necrosis factor agents (http://www.cdc.gov/tb/default.htm; accessed December 29, 2014). Testing for tuberculosis prior to beginning immunosuppressive therapy for uveitis is, therefore, warranted even if the suspicion for tuberculous uveitis is low.

Atypical mycobacteria produced clinically inapparent, small choroidal granulomas in HIV-infected patients that were generally diagnosed only at autopsy.[95] Immune recovery may permit the development of large granulomatous lesions.[96] Culture of focal ocular lesions on Löwenstein–Jensen medium with PCR confirmation is the gold standard for diagnosis of tuberculosis uveitis. PCR determinations from ocular fluid are used successfully in endemic areas.[97,98]

Nocardiosis

In the posterior segment, *Nocardia* typically grows in the subretinal space (▶ Fig. 24.13). Results of vitreous cultures are, therefore, likely to be negative. Patients generally have evidence of *Nocardia* in other sites. Treatment is with maximum doses of trimethoprim–sulfamethoxazole, four double-strength tablets daily, for several weeks. Imipenem is an alternate intravenous antibiotic with good activity against *Nocardia* and good ocular penetration.

Bartonella Henselae Infection

Posterior segment manifestations of *Bartonella henselae* infection (cat-scratch disease) include neuroretinitis, as well as white retinal or choroidal lesions.[99] When the retinal infiltrates

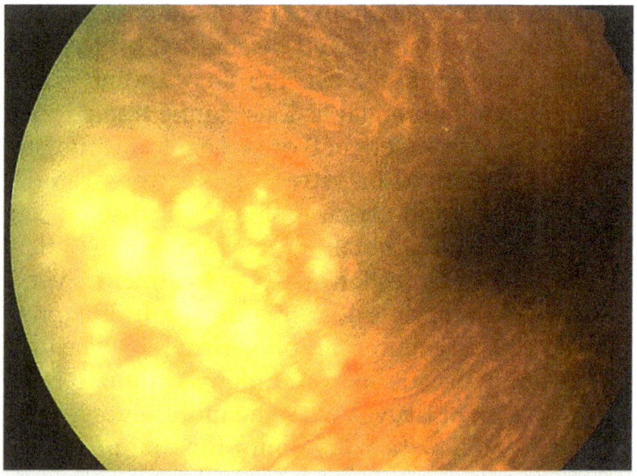

Fig. 24.13 Presumed nocardial endophthalmitis: Confinement to the subretinal pigment epithelial space is characteristic. In cases with little infiltration of the vitreous, vitreous culture is likely to be negative. A history of systemic nocardiosis may be helpful in suggesting the diagnosis and directing therapy with effective antibiotics. Clinical response to antibiotics confirms the diagnosis.

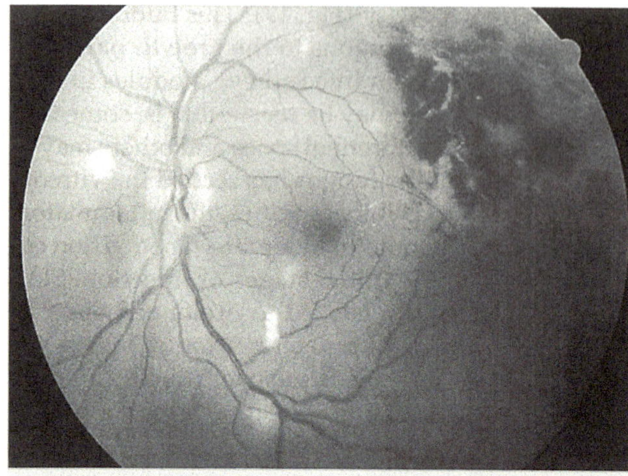

Fig. 24.14 This 36-year-old woman with fever, headache, and blurred vision had multiple retinal infiltrates in both eyes. A venous occlusion is seen along the superotemporal arcade. The retinal infiltrates enlarged and ultimately produced branch retinal arterial occlusions. She was treated with oral antibiotics with resolution of the lesions and had minimal residual scotomas. The *Bartonella henselae* IgG titer was reactive at the lowest level of positivity and there was a history of cat scratch preceding the fever.

overlap retinal blood vessels, arterial or venous occlusion may occur (▶ Fig. 24.14). Retinal and optic nerve neovascularization is reported. Antibiotics that produce high intracellular concentrations, such as erythromycin, clarithromycin, azithromycin, rifampicin, doxycycline, and gentamicin, appear to be the most effective for cat-scratch disease. Ciprofloxacin at a dosage of 750 mg orally twice daily for 3 weeks has also been used successfully. Diagnosis relies on a history of exposure and serology, although antibody titers are often unimpressive. It is possible that other organisms can produce the same type of retinal infection and would respond to similar antibiotics.

Other Bacterial Infections

Intermediate uveitis has been associated with late infection with *Borrelia burgdorferi*. Serologic testing is neither sensitive nor specific and a patient with posterior uveitis who does not have systemic Lyme disease and resides outside an endemic area will probably not benefit from testing. PCR testing of ocular fluid may improve the ability to confirm diagnoses.[100]

Rickettsial organisms and *Brucella* are among other exotic bacterial causes of infections that may occasionally produce retinal vasculitis. Febrile illness remains a good indicator that disseminated bacterial infection is associated with the eye disease. In some countries, there is gender specificity in brucellosis related to economic roles: *Brucella abortus* in men handling bovine meat and *Brucella suis* in women processing dairy products from sheep.[101]

24.3.4 Fungal Infections

Overall, endogenous fungal endophthalmitis accounts for less than 10% of all fungal endophthalmitis.[102] A large single-institution case series of endogenous fungal endophthalmitis from 1990 to 2011 identified 51 eyes of 39 patients with positive cultures for yeast and 16 eyes of 14 patients with molds.[21] Infections with molds were significantly more common in patients with iatrogenic immunosuppression, organ transplantation, and hypopyon and were associated with worse visual outcomes; 4 of 16 eyes with mold endophthalmitis underwent enucleation versus none of the eyes with yeast endophthalmitis.[21]

Candidal Endophthalmitis

The majority of endogenous endophthalmitis is due to *Candida* species. Candidal infection follows a typical growth pattern. Choroidal infiltrates enlarge into a small, subretinal white nodule that penetrates through the retina as a small, mushroom-shaped projection and then extends into the vitreous cavity (▶ Fig. 24.15).[10] This budding, contained growth is analogous to the growth pattern of the fungus itself. In an infected eye, nodules in various states of growth may be seen—that is, some may be confined to the subretinal space and others may be preretinal. Early cases with colonies confined to the retina and choroid are commonly treated with systemic antifungals with and without intravitreal treatment.[103] Unless the fungus has seeded the vitreous with multiple focal white opacities, the inflammatory reaction is usually mild to moderate. Good vision can be preserved in the initial stages of infection. Slow growth of the fungus has led to prolonged observation in some cases, with deterioration of vision and poor outcomes. Failure to suspect fungal infection and use of corticosteroids as treatment have also been associated with poor outcomes.

Because the organisms tend to cluster together in compact groups, a small, random sampling of vitreous and not an actual fungus ball may lead to a negative culture result. For this reason, pars plana vitrectomy with filtration of the vitreous wash material to trap as many organisms as possible is preferred as a diagnostic technique, as opposed to a simple vitreous tap. Debulking of the preretinal component of choroid-based lesions can usually be accomplished without creating retinal holes.

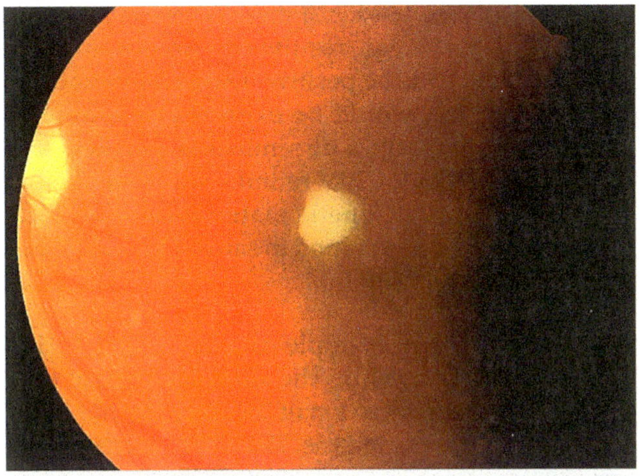

Fig. 24.15 Cytomegalovirus retinitis had been diagnosed elsewhere in this HIV-positive man, and he was being treated with ganciclovir. A small, white, raised, full-thickness nodule involved the macula. There was minimal vitritis. At the request of his infectious disease specialist, vitrectomy and culture were performed. Material scraped from the lesion grew *Candida albicans*. The white color, round shape, penetration from choroid through retina, relative paucity of inflammation, and slow progression are typical of candidal endophthalmitis. More fulminant disease occurs with chronicity, with corticosteroid rather than antifungal treatment, and with multiple lesions.

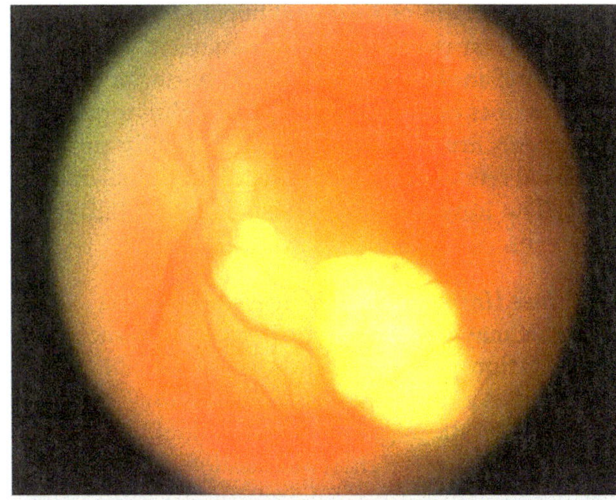

Fig. 24.16 Culture-proven *Aspergillus* endophthalmitis in a woman with chronic bronchitis and a history of drug abuse: No definite systemic source for the aspergillosis was ever found. Most candidal lesions this size would have already broken through the retina; *Aspergillus* tends to remain loculated. Despite this, the infection is tolerated poorly, and more inflammation relative to the size of the lesion and worse vision are noted than with *Candida*. The hand motion vision in this eye is possibly explainable by the propensity of *Aspergillus* to infect vascular channels; however, definite vascular occlusions were not identified.

Surgical management with silicone oil may also play a role in compartmentalizing the eye and preventing phthisis by analogy to its success in bacterial endogenous endophthalmitis.[104]

Access of antibiotics to the infected site must also be taken into account in planning treatment. Amphotericin B penetrates the blood–retinal barrier poorly.[105] The inflammatory reaction is usually mild enough that significant breakdown of the blood–aqueous and other ocular barriers cannot be counted on to facilitate drug entry into the eye. A rule of thumb is that choroidal and subretinal lesions can be treated with oral fluconazole or oral voriconazole,[106] but preretinal or vitreous infections require intravitreal amphotericin B 5 µg/0.1 mL or intravitreal voriconazole 50 to 100 µg/0.1 mL. Posaconazole and the echinocandins achieve poor intraocular concentrations.[105] Infectious disease consultation is usually obtained to evaluate the patient for other sites of infection and plan treatment. Often, the more involved eye can be treated with vitrectomy for diagnosis and lavage purposes and the less involved eye can be treated with intravitreal medication injection plus systemic treatment.

Pearls

- The route of administration of an antifungal agent should be matched to the site of infection: intravitreal for vitreous seeding, intravenous or oral for isolated choroidal infiltrates.

Aspergillus Endophthalmitis

The classic picture of *Aspergillus* endophthalmitis is one of a diffuse yellow chorioretinal plaque, which typically involves the macula and abundant vitritis (▶ Fig. 24.16). *Aspergillus* does not bud; it branches, and the fungal lesions it produces tend to be much larger subretinal nodules than those found with *Candida*. The ability of *Aspergillus* to propagate intravascularly may result in dissemination via the retinal blood vessels and account for many outcomes of extremely poor vision. The infections are less well tolerated by the eye and patients become symptomatic sooner than with candidal endophthalmitis, which may often be present for weeks or months before symptoms develop, compared with days for *Aspergillus* infection.[107] Either the rapid growth and early presentation or some inherent difference in growth pattern results in a much lower frequency of vitreous seeding. The nodules are denser than those associated with *Candida* and appear to be surrounded by a pseudocapsule. Bronchopulmonary aspergillosis and intravenous drug abuse are common historical features. Treatment is as for candidal endophthalmitis; itraconazole may be used for extraocular *Aspergillus* infections, but intraocular penetration appears to be poor.

Cryptococcosis

Endogenous retinochoroiditis with *Cryptococcus neoformans* is rare since improved treatment of HIV infection. The classic scenario in HIV with severe immunosuppression was meningeal symptoms and signs presenting with papilledema or cranial nerve palsy. Cryptococcal torulomas and choroiditis have been reported.[108]

Other Fungal Infections

Coccidioidomycosis is endemic to the American Southwest and can produce a disseminated chorioretinitis consisting of scattered, poorly defined, white subretinal lesions. Extension into the retina or vitreous is uncommon. The rather nonspecific features of posterior segment disease can lead to significant delays in diagnosis and treatment with poor outcomes, although aggressive management with intravitreal therapy and surgical debridement may be helpful.[109,110] Chronic cough and fever in an endemic area or in someone who has traveled to arid regions of California or Arizona should lead the clinician to suspect coccidioidomycosis.

Other than the indolent or healed lesions of the presumed ocular histoplasmosis syndrome (POHS), endogenous endophthalmitis from *Histoplasma* is uncommon,[111] as are infections caused by other organisms such as *Fusarium*, *Paecilomyces*, and *Pseudallescheria* species.[21,102,112]

24.3.5 Helminthic Infections

Nematode (Intestinal Roundworm) Infections

Toxocariasis

Three basic forms of toxocaral infection of the posterior segment are recognized: posterior granuloma, peripheral granuloma, and endophthalmitis. Although visceral larval migrans (VLM) with eosinophilia, fever, and malaise as well as more serious systemic manifestations is a well-recognized clinical entity, most children with ocular toxocariasis do not have histories or current signs of VLM. Both *T. canis* and *T. catis* as well as *Baylisascaris procyonis* are implicated in eye disease.[113]

Death of the nematode may precipitate an inflammatory crisis. Because of a tendency for scar formation, including cicatricial retinal detachments and cyclitic membranes, intensive local and systemic corticosteroid treatment as well as surgical management should be considered for this form of the disease to remove inflamed vitreous and prevent secondary complications. Because the nematode is presumed already to have died, antihelminthic medications play no role in treatment. It is possible that antihelminthic treatment could precipitate an inflammatory crisis in an infected eye, but that has not been described for small nematodes such as *Toxocara*.

Some eyes with intense inflammation will eventually quieten, and the clearer vitreous then permits a view of the peripheral granuloma that has formed at the site of the dead nematode. Fibrocellular stalks extending to the disc are the most classic manifestation (▶ Fig. 24.17). If retinal detachment occurs, retinotomy to relieve traction emanating from the granuloma may be used to permit retinal reattachment.

Incomplete bands and dense white inflammatory masses peripherally can be mistaken for pars planitis. Examination of the other eye may be critically important in distinguishing the two diseases, as bilateral toxocaral infection should not occur. Other important entities in the differential diagnosis include retinoblastoma, retinopathy of prematurity, persistent hyperplastic primary vitreous, and Coats' disease. Positive serology for *Toxocara* is helpful when present, but some cases have been reported in which only the intraocular fluid was found to contain antitoxocaral antibodies. A report published by the CDC reported 68 incident cases between September 2009 and 2010 in the United States based on a survey of ophthalmologists. Only 14 of 20 cases were serologically positive.[114] Median patient age was 8.5 years.

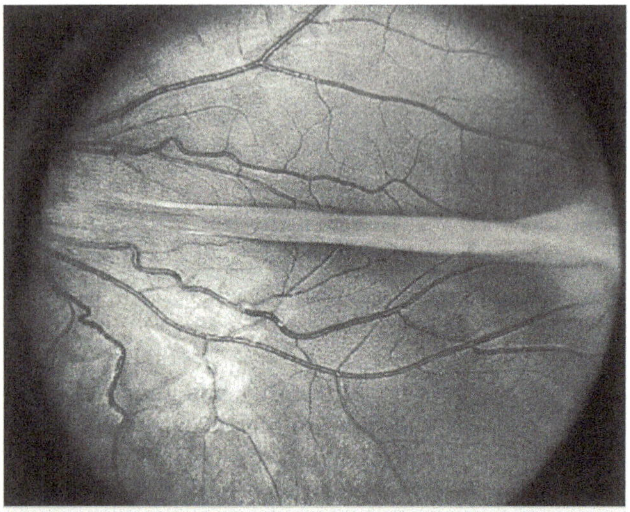

Fig. 24.17 Typical fibrocellular stalk bridging between the disc and a peripheral healed toxocaral granuloma in a 12-year-old. Visual prognosis can be good in these cases if retinal detachment does not occur. (Image courtesy of Dr. Harry Flynn, used with permission.)

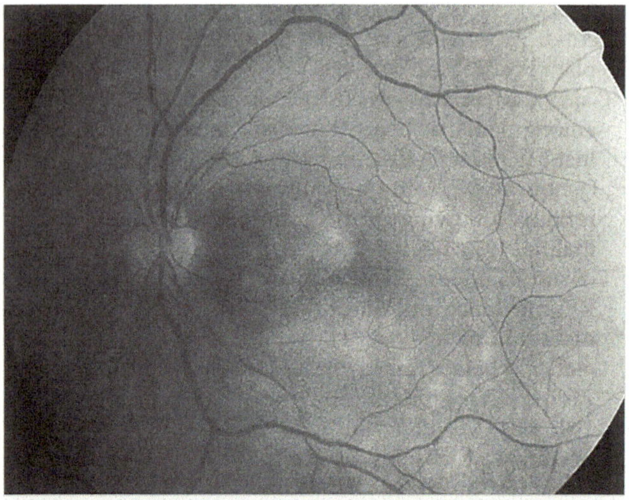

Fig. 24.18 Clusters of deep retinal lesions are typical of diffuse unilateral subacute neuroretinitis. The nematode is seen as a small circle 1 disc diameter from the center of the macula along the 11:00 meridian. Because of the small size of the nematode and a 10-year history of visual complaints, the diagnosis was not initially suspected but became obvious as new crops of lesions appeared in other sites. The nematode was eventually photocoagulated successfully. Vision remained hand motions despite the overall excellent appearance of the disc and macula.

Diffuse Unilateral Subacute Neuroretinitis

Toxocara canis may produce the characteristic constellation of ocular findings of DUSN,[115] but heterogeneous agents are more likely.[116,117] First described as a unilateral loss or "wipe-out" of vision, the characteristic migratory chorioretinal lesions, pigmentary changes, vascular attenuation, optic atrophy, and vitreous inflammation can be highly variable among patients and depend on the stage of the disease.[118] Identification of the intraocular nematode is the gold standard for diagnosis and laser photocoagulation is the definitive treatment. Successive crops of small clusters of yellow-white, focal chorioretinal inflammatory lesions (▶ Fig. 24.18) are useful to indicate the location of the live nematode. Both photographic and contact lens examination may reveal the location of the nematode. Frequent visits at short intervals until the worm is located are reasonable, as vision rarely improves after the nematode is killed, although further visual loss seems to be stopped.

In one large series, a motile nematode was identified and coagulated in 48 of 121 patients (39.7%).[118] Patients suspected of DUSN in whom a nematode cannot be visualized can be treated with albendazole, conventionally for 30 days.[119,120] In some eyes, visible nematodes were immobilized by treatment with albendazole.[119]

Spectral domain optical coherence tomography indicates mainly inner retinal volume loss and nerve fiber layer damage,[121] possibly because the nematode migrates within the retina[114] rather than preferentially in the subretinal space as is conventionally thought. Electroretinography indicates more dysfunction of the inner retina than the outer retina.[120]

Onchocerciasis is responding to ivermectin treatment programs. Established chorioretinitis and optic neuropathies tend to progress, indicating an inflammatory component that persists after eradication of the parasite.[122]

Pearls

- The diagnosis of DUSN is easily missed and should be considered in all cases of unilateral posterior uveitis, especially in children.

Other Zoonotic Infections—Cestodes and Trematodes

Cestodal and other flatworm infections of the eye are typically food borne and are easy to detect because of the large size of the organisms. Translucent, fluid-filled cystic structures in the vitreous or subretinal space can be stimulated with light to produce movement of the protoscolex and confirm viability. Ultrasound examination shows a vesicle with a highly reflective spot indicating the scolex.[123] Surgical removal prior to medical treatment for systemic cysticercosis prevents severe ocular inflammation that may ensue if the parasite dies in situ. Echinococcus is another cestode that can localize to the intraocular compartment.[113]

Large trematodes (flukes) have been reported to infest the eye in two individuals consuming undercooked frog legs in the United States.[124] The lesions were clearly visible on ophthalmoscopy. Ophthalmomyiasis interna is caused by segmented larvae of flies and results from penetrative laying of eggs directly into the conjunctival sac or skin followed by migration into the eye. Characteristic crisscrossing tracks in the pigment epithelium suggest the diagnosis, but the larvae cannot always be identified. Similar tracks occur in the pigmentary epitheliopathy of Guamanian natives, yet maggots have not been retrieved from these eyes.[125]

Key Points

- All common classes of human pathogens can infect chorioretinal tissues.
- Systemic infection that precedes retinochoroidal infection may be inapparent but is usually medically significant.
- Individuals who are immunocompromised from any cause are more likely to develop chorioretinal infections.
- Appreciation of the distinctive patterns of retinochoroidal infections of different etiologies enables provisional diagnoses and prompt empiric therapy pending definitive testing.

References

[1] Davis JL. Diagnostic dilemmas in retinitis and endophthalmitis. Eye (Lond). 2012; 26(2):194–201

[2] Eandi CM, Neri P, Adelman RA, Yannuzzi LA, Cunningham ET, Jr, International Syphilis Study Group. Acute syphilitic posterior placoid chorioretinitis: report of a case series and comprehensive review of the literature. Retina. 2012; 32(9):1915–1941

[3] Gupta A, Bansal R, Gupta V, Sharma A, Bambery P. Ocular signs predictive of tubercular uveitis. Am J Ophthalmol. 2010; 149(4):562–570

[4] Abu El-Asrar AM, Abouammoh M, Al-Mezaine HS. Tuberculous uveitis. Int Ophthalmol Clin. 2010; 50(2):19–39

[5] Empeslidis T, Tsaousis KT, Konidaris V, Pradeep A, Deane J. Multifocal chorioretinitis caused by Bartonella henselae: imaging findings of spectral domain optical coherence tomography during treatment with trimethoprim-sulfamethoxazole. Eye (Lond). 2014; 28(7):907–909

[6] Rubinov A, Blumenthal EZ, Beiran I. Cat scratch disease associated with retinal vein occlusion. Isr Med Assoc J. 2014; 16(8):522–523

[7] Chi SL, Stinnett S, Eggenberger E, et al. Clinical characteristics in 53 patients with cat scratch optic neuropathy. Ophthalmology. 2012; 119(1):183–187

[8] Holland GN, Executive Committee of the American Uveitis Society. Standard diagnostic criteria for the acute retinal necrosis syndrome. Am J Ophthalmol. 1994; 117(5):663–667

[9] Moshfeghi DM, Dodds EM, Couto CA, et al. Diagnostic approaches to severe, atypical toxoplasmosis mimicking acute retinal necrosis. Ophthalmology. 2004; 111(4):716–725

[10] Mahendradas P, Avadhani K, Yadav NK, et al. Role of Spectralis HRA+OCT spectral domain optical coherence tomography in the diagnosis and management of fungal choroidal granuloma. Ocul Immunol Inflamm. 2010; 18 (5):408–410

[11] Farber BP, Weinbaum DL, Dummer JS. Metastatic bacterial endophthalmitis. Arch Intern Med. 1985; 145(1):62–64

[12] Greenwald MJ, Wohl LG, Sell CH. Metastatic bacterial endophthalmitis: a contemporary reappraisal. Surv Ophthalmol. 1986; 31(2):81–101

[13] Okada AA, Johnson RP, Liles WC, D'Amico DJ, Baker AS. Endogenous bacterial endophthalmitis. Report of a ten-year retrospective study. Ophthalmology. 1994; 101(5):832–838

[14] Schiedler V, Scott IU, Flynn HW, Jr, Davis JL, Benz MS, Miller D. Culture-proven endogenous endophthalmitis: clinical features and visual acuity outcomes. Am J Ophthalmol. 2004; 137(4):725–731

[15] Kashani AH, Eliott D. The emergence of Klebsiella pneumoniae endogenous endophthalmitis in the USA: basic and clinical advances. J Ophthalmic Inflamm Infect. 2013; 3(1):28

[16] Dozier CC, Tarantola RM, Jiramongkolchai K, Donahue SP. Fungal eye disease at a tertiary care center: the utility of routine inpatient consultation. Ophthalmology. 2011; 118(8):1671–1676

[17] Donahue SP, Greven CM, Zuravleff JJ, et al. Intraocular candidiasis in patients with candidemia. Clinical implications derived from a prospective multicenter study. Ophthalmology. 1994; 101(7):1302–1309

[18] Meyers SM. The incidence of fundus lesions in septicemia. Am J Ophthalmol. 1979; 88(4):661–667

[19] Herschorn BJ, Brucker AJ. Embolic retinopathy due to Corynebacterium minutissimum endocarditis. Br J Ophthalmol. 1985; 69(1):29–31

[20] Davis JL, Nussenblatt RB, Bachman DM, Chan CC, Palestine AG. Endogenous bacterial retinitis in AIDS. Am J Ophthalmol. 1989; 107(6):613–623

[21] Sridhar J, Flynn HW, Jr, Kuriyan AE, Miller D, Albini T. Endogenous fungal endophthalmitis: risk factors, clinical features, and treatment outcomes in mold and yeast infections. J Ophthalmic Inflamm Infect. 2013; 3(1):60

[22] Vann VR, Atherton SS. Neural spread of herpes simplex virus after anterior chamber inoculation. Invest Ophthalmol Vis Sci. 1991; 32(9):2462–2472

[23] Miller D, Davis J, Rosa R, Diaz M, Perez E. Utility of tissue culture for detection of Toxoplasma gondii in vitreous humor of patients diagnosed with toxoplasmic retinochoroiditis. J Clin Microbiol. 2000; 38(10):3840–3842

[24] Harper TW, Miller D, Schiffman JC, Davis JL. Polymerase chain reaction analysis of aqueous and vitreous specimens in the diagnosis of posterior segment infectious uveitis. Am J Ophthalmol. 2009; 147(1):140–147.e2

[25] Rothova A, de Boer JH, Ten Dam-van Loon NH, et al. Usefulness of aqueous humor analysis for the diagnosis of posterior uveitis. Ophthalmology. 2008; 115(2):306–311

[26] Cornut PL, Sobas CR, Perard L, et al. Detection of Treponema pallidum in aqueous humor by real-time polymerase chain reaction. Ocul Immunol Inflamm. 2011; 19(2):127–128

[27] Gordon SM, Eaton ME, George R, et al. The response of symptomatic neurosyphilis to high-dose intravenous penicillin G in patients with human immunodeficiency virus infection. N Engl J Med. 1994; 331(22):1469–1473

[28] Halperin LS. Neuroretinitis due to seronegative syphilis associated with human immunodeficiency virus. J Clin Neuroophthalmol. 1992; 12(3):171–172

[29] Kuppermann BD, Petty JG, Richman DD, et al. Correlation between CD4+ counts and prevalence of cytomegalovirus retinitis and human immunodeficiency virus-related noninfectious retinal vasculopathy in patients with acquired immunodeficiency syndrome. Am J Ophthalmol. 1993; 115(5):575–582

[30] Jacobson MA, Tan QX, Girling V, et al. Studies of Ocular Complications of AIDS Research Group. Poor predictive value of cytomegalovirus (CMV)-specific T cell assays for the development of CMV retinitis in patients with AIDS. Clin Infect Dis. 2008; 46(3):458–466

[31] Sinclair E, Tan QX, Sharp M, et al. Studies of Ocular Complications of AIDS Research Group. Protective immunity to cytomegalovirus (CMV) retinitis in AIDS is associated with CMV-specific T cells that express interferon- gamma and interleukin-2 and have a CD8+cell early maturational phenotype. J Infect Dis. 2006; 194(11):1537–1546

[32] Holbrook JT, Colvin R, van Natta ML, Thorne JE, Bardsley M, Jabs DA, Studies of Ocular Complications of AIDS (SOCA) Research Group. Evaluation of the United States public health service guidelines for discontinuation of anticytomegalovirus therapy after immune recovery in patients with cytomegalovirus retinitis. Am J Ophthalmol. 2011; 152(4):628–637.e1

[33] Rao NA, Zhang J, Ishimoto S. Role of retinal vascular endothelial cells in development of CMV retinitis. Trans Am Ophthalmol Soc. 1998; 96:111–123, discussion 124–126

[34] Chung H, Kim KH, Kim JG, Lee SY, Yoon YH. Retinal complications in patients with solid organ or bone marrow transplantations. Transplantation. 2007; 83(6):694–699

[35] Sugar EA, Jabs DA, Ahuja A, Thorne JE, Danis RP, Meinert CL, Studies of the Ocular Complications of AIDS Research Group. Incidence of cytomegalovirus retinitis in the era of highly active antiretroviral therapy. Am J Ophthalmol. 2012; 153(6):1016–24.e5

[36] Foscarnet-Ganciclovir Cytomegalovirus Retinitis Trial: 5. Clinical features of cytomegalovirus retinitis at diagnosis. Studies of ocular complications of AIDS Research Group in collaboration with the AIDS Clinical Trials Group. Am J Ophthalmol. 1997; 124(2):141–157

[37] Jabs DA, Ahuja A, Van Natta M, Lyon A, Srivastava S, Gangaputra S, Studies of the Ocular Complications of AIDS Research Group. Course of cytomegalovirus retinitis in the era of highly active antiretroviral therapy: five-year outcomes. Ophthalmology. 2010; 117(11):2152–61.e1, 2

[38] Davis JL, Serfass MS, Lai MY, Trask DK, Azen SP. Silicone oil in repair of retinal detachments caused by necrotizing retinitis in HIV infection. Arch Ophthalmol. 1995; 113(11):1401–1409

[39] Mortality in patients with the acquired immunodeficiency syndrome treated with either foscarnet or ganciclovir for cytomegalovirus retinitis. Studies of Ocular Complications of AIDS Research Group, in collaboration with the AIDS Clinical Trials Group. N Engl J Med. 1992; 326(4):213–220

[40] Martin DF, Parks DJ, Mellow SD, et al. Treatment of cytomegalovirus retinitis with an intraocular sustained-release ganciclovir implant. A randomized controlled clinical trial. Arch Ophthalmol. 1994; 112(12):1531–1539

[41] Young SH, Morlet N, Heery S, Hollows FC, Coroneo MT. High dose intravitreal ganciclovir in the treatment of cytomegalovirus retinitis. Med J Aust. 1992; 157(6):370–373

[42] Staras SA, Dollard SC, Radford KW, Flanders WD, Pass RF, Cannon MJ. Seroprevalence of cytomegalovirus infection in the United States, 1988–1994. Clin Infect Dis. 2006; 43(9):1143–1151

[43] Davis JL, Haft P, Hartley K. Retinal arteriolar occlusions due to cytomegalovirus retinitis in elderly patients without HIV. J Ophthalmic Inflamm Infect. 2013; 3(1):17

[44] Schneider EW, Elner SG, van Kuijk FJ, et al. Chronic retinal necrosis: cytomegalovirus necrotizing retinitis associated with panretinal vasculopathy in non-HIV patients. Retina. 2013; 33(9):1791–1799

[45] Eid AJ, Bakri SJ, Kijpittayarit S, Razonable RR. Clinical features and outcomes of cytomegalovirus retinitis after transplantation. Transpl Infect Dis. 2008; 10(1):13–18

[46] Saidel MA, Berreen J, Margolis TP. Cytomegalovirus retinitis after intravitreous triamcinolone in an immunocompetent patient. Am J Ophthalmol. 2005; 140(6):1141–1143

[47] Culbertson WW, Blumenkranz MS, Pepose JS, Stewart JA, Curtin VT. Varicella zoster virus is a cause of the acute retinal necrosis syndrome. Ophthalmology. 1986; 93(5):559–569

[48] Thompson WS, Culbertson WW, Smiddy WE, Robertson JE, Rosenbaum JT. Acute retinal necrosis caused by reactivation of herpes simplex virus type 2. Am J Ophthalmol. 1994; 118(2):205–211

[49] Lewis ML, Culbertson WW, Post JD, Miller D, Kokame GT, Dix RD. Herpes simplex virus type 1. A cause of the acute retinal necrosis syndrome. Ophthalmology. 1989; 96(6):875–878

[50] Silva RA, Berrocal AM, Moshfeghi DM, Blumenkranz MS, Sanislo S, Davis JL. Herpes simplex virus type 2 mediated acute retinal necrosis in a pediatric population: case series and review. Graefes Arch Clin Exp Ophthalmol. 2013; 251(2):559–566

[51] Regillo CD, Sergott RC, Ho AC, Belmont JB, Fischer DH. Hemodynamic alterations in the acute retinal necrosis syndrome. Ophthalmology. 1993; 100(8):1171–1176

[52] Yeh S, Suhler EB, Smith JR, et al. Combination systemic and intravitreal antiviral therapy in the management of acute retinal necrosis syndrome. Ophthalmic Surg Lasers Imaging Retina. 2014; 45(5):399–407

[53] Bonfioli AA, Eller AW. Acute retinal necrosis. Semin Ophthalmol. 2005; 20(3):155–160

[54] Palay DA, Sternberg P, Jr, Davis J, et al. Decrease in the risk of bilateral acute retinal necrosis by acyclovir therapy. Am J Ophthalmol. 1991; 112(3):250–255

[55] Matsuo T, Morimoto K, Matsuo N. Factors associated with poor visual outcome in acute retinal necrosis. Br J Ophthalmol. 1991; 75(8):450–454

[56] Sternberg P, Jr, Han DP, Yeo JH, et al. Photocoagulation to prevent retinal detachment in acute retinal necrosis. Ophthalmology. 1988; 95(10):1389–1393

[57] Sellitti TP, Huang AJ, Schiffman J, Davis JL. Association of herpes zoster ophthalmicus with acquired immunodeficiency syndrome and acute retinal necrosis. Am J Ophthalmol. 1993; 116(3):297–301

[58] Engstrom RE, Jr, Holland GN, Margolis TP, et al. The progressive outer retinal necrosis syndrome. A variant of necrotizing herpetic retinopathy in patients with AIDS. Ophthalmology. 1994; 101(9):1488–1502

[59] Rostad SW, Olson K, McDougall J, Shaw CM, Alvord EC, Jr. Transsynaptic spread of varicella zoster virus through the visual system: a mechanism of viral dissemination in the central nervous system. Hum Pathol. 1989; 20(2):174–179

[60] Johnston WH, Holland GN, Engstrom RE, Jr, Rimmer S. Recurrence of presumed varicella-zoster virus retinopathy in patients with acquired immunodeficiency syndrome. Am J Ophthalmol. 1993; 116(1):42–50

[61] de Boer JH, Verhagen C, Bruinenberg M, et al. Serologic and polymerase chain reaction analysis of intraocular fluids in the diagnosis of infectious uveitis. Am J Ophthalmol. 1996; 121(6):650–658

[62] Matoba AY. Ocular disease associated with Epstein-Barr virus infection. Surv Ophthalmol. 1990; 35(2):145–150

[63] Haltia M, Tarkkanen A, Vaheri A, Paetau A, Kaakinen K, Erkkilä H. Measles retinopathy during immunosuppression. Br J Ophthalmol. 1978; 62(6):356–360

[64] Khandekar R, Al Awaidy S, Ganesh A, Bawikar S. An epidemiological and clinical study of ocular manifestations of congenital rubella syndrome in Omani children. Arch Ophthalmol. 2004; 122(4):541–545
[65] Sugita S, Shimizu N, Watanabe K, et al. Virological analysis in patients with human herpes virus 6-associated ocular inflammatory disorders. Invest Ophthalmol Vis Sci. 2012; 53(8):4692–4698
[66] Villena I, Ancelle T, Delmas C, et al. Toxosurv network and National Reference Centre for Toxoplasmosis. Congenital toxoplasmosis in France in 2007: first results from a national surveillance system. Euro Surveill. 2010; 15(25)
[67] Phan L, Kasza K, Jalbrzikowski J, et al. Toxoplasmosis Study Group. Longitudinal study of new eye lesions in children with toxoplasmosis who were not treated during the first year of life. Am J Ophthalmol. 2008; 146(3):375–384
[68] Phan L, Kasza K, Jalbrzikowski J, et al. Toxoplasmosis Study Group. Longitudinal study of new eye lesions in treated congenital toxoplasmosis. Ophthalmology. 2008; 115(3):553–559.e8
[69] Johnson MW, Greven GM, Jaffe GJ, Sudhalkar H, Vine AK. Atypical, severe toxoplasmic retinochoroiditis in elderly patients. Ophthalmology. 1997; 104 (1):48–57
[70] Cochereau-Massin I, LeHoang P, Lautier-Frau M, et al. Ocular toxoplasmosis in human immunodeficiency virus-infected patients. Am J Ophthalmol. 1992; 114(2):130–135
[71] Engstrom RE, Jr, Holland GN, Nussenblatt RB, Jabs DA. Current practices in the management of ocular toxoplasmosis. Am J Ophthalmol. 1991; 111 (5):601–610
[72] Opremcak EM, Scales DK, Sharpe MR. Trimethoprim-sulfamethoxazole therapy for ocular toxoplasmosis. Ophthalmology. 1992; 99(6):920–925
[73] Rajapakse S, Chrishan Shivanthan M, Samaranayake N, Rodrigo C, Deepika Fernando S. Antibiotics for human toxoplasmosis: a systematic review of randomized trials. Pathog Glob Health. 2013; 107(4):162–169
[74] Balaskas K, Vaudaux J, Boillat-Blanco N, Guex-Crosier Y. Azithromycin versus Sulfadiazine and Pyrimethamine for non-vision-threatening toxoplasmic retinochoroiditis: a pilot study. Med Sci Monit. 2012; 18(5):CR296–CR302
[75] Winterhalter S, Severing K, Stammen J, Maier AK, Godehardt E, Joussen AM. Does atovaquone prolong the disease-free interval of toxoplasmic retinochoroiditis? Graefes Arch Clin Exp Ophthalmol. 2010; 248(8):1187–1192
[76] Baharivand N, Mahdavifard A, Fouladi RF. Intravitreal clindamycin plus dexamethasone versus classic oral therapy in toxoplasmic retinochoroiditis: a prospective randomized clinical trial. Int Ophthalmol. 2013; 33(1):39–46
[77] Soheilian M, Ramezani A, Azimzadeh A, et al. Randomized trial of intravitreal clindamycin and dexamethasone versus pyrimethamine, sulfadiazine, and prednisolone in treatment of ocular toxoplasmosis. Ophthalmology. 2011; 118(1):134–141
[78] Lasave AF, Díaz-Llopis M, Muccioli C, Belfort R, Jr, Arevalo JF. Intravitreal clindamycin and dexamethasone for zone 1 toxoplasmic retinochoroiditis at twenty-four months. Ophthalmology. 2010; 117(9):1831–1838
[79] Felix JP, Lira RP, Zacchia RS, Toribio JM, Nascimento MA, Arieta CE. Trimethoprim-sulfamethoxazole versus placebo to reduce the risk of recurrences of Toxoplasma gondii retinochoroiditis: randomized controlled clinical trial. Am J Ophthalmol. 2014; 157(4):762–766.e1
[80] Rush R, Sheth S. Fulminant toxoplasmic retinochoroiditis following intravitreal triamcinolone administration. Indian J Ophthalmol. 2012; 60(2):141–143
[81] Patton ME, Su JR, Nelson R, Weinstock H, Centers for Disease Control and Prevention (CDC). Primary and secondary syphilis—United States, 2005-2013. MMWR Morb Mortal Wkly Rep. 2014; 63(18):402–406
[82] Mathew RG, Goh BT, Westcott MC. British Ocular Syphilis Study (BOSS): 2-year national surveillance study of intraocular inflammation secondary to ocular syphilis. Invest Ophthalmol Vis Sci. 2014; 55(8):5394–5400
[83] Davis JL. Ocular syphilis. Curr Opin Ophthalmol. 2014; 25(6):513–518
[84] Fu EX, Geraets RL, Dodds EM, et al. Superficial retinal precipitates in patients with syphilitic retinitis. Retina. 2010; 30(7):1135–1143
[85] Pichi F, Ciardella AP, Cunningham ET, Jr, et al. Spectral domain optical coherence tomography findings in patients with acute syphilitic posterior placoid chorioretinopathy. Retina. 2014; 34(2):373–384
[86] Shields M, Guy RJ, Jeoffreys NJ, Finlayson RJ, Donovan B. A longitudinal evaluation of Treponema pallidum PCR testing in early syphilis. BMC Infect Dis. 2012; 12:353
[87] Walter T, Lebouche B, Miailhes P, et al. Symptomatic relapse of neurologic syphilis after benzathine penicillin G therapy for primary or secondary syphilis in HIV-infected patients. Clin Infect Dis. 2006; 43(6):787–790
[88] Sudharshan S, Ganesh SK, Balu G, et al. Utility of QuantiFERON®-TB Gold test in diagnosis and management of suspected tubercular uveitis in India. Int Ophthalmol. 2012; 32(3):217–223
[89] Bansal R, Gupta A, Gupta V, Dogra MR, Sharma A, Bambery P. Tubercular serpiginous-like choroiditis presenting as multifocal serpiginoid choroiditis. Ophthalmology. 2012; 119(11):2334–2342
[90] La Distia Nora R, van Velthoven ME, Ten Dam-van Loon NH, et al. Clinical manifestations of patients with intraocular inflammation and positive QuantiFERON-TB gold in-tube test in a country nonendemic for tuberculosis. Am J Ophthalmol. 2014; 157(4):754–761
[91] Ang M, Kiew SY, Wong WL, Chee SP. Discordance of two interferon-? release assays and tuberculin skin test in patients with uveitis. Br J Ophthalmol. 2014; 98(12):1649–1653
[92] Doycheva D, Deuter C, Hetzel J, et al. The use of positron emission tomography/CT in the diagnosis of tuberculosis-associated uveitis. Br J Ophthalmol. 2011; 95(9):1290–1294
[93] Rosenbaum JT, Wernick R. The utility of routine screening of patients with uveitis for systemic lupus erythematosus or tuberculosis. A Bayesian analysis. Arch Ophthalmol. 1990; 108(9):1291–1293
[94] Jakob E, Max R, Zimmermann S, et al. Three years of experience with QuantiFERON-TB gold testing in patients with uveitis. Ocul Immunol Inflamm. 2014; 22(6):478–484
[95] Pepose JS, Holland GN, Nestor MS, Cochran AJ, Foos RY. Acquired immune deficiency syndrome. Pathogenic mechanisms of ocular disease. Ophthalmology. 1985; 92(4):472–484
[96] Zamir E, Hudson H, Ober RR, et al. Massive mycobacterial choroiditis during highly active antiretroviral therapy: another immune-recovery uveitis? Ophthalmology. 2002; 109(11):2144–2148
[97] Ortega-Larrocea G, Bobadilla-del-Valle M, Ponce-de-León A, Sifuentes-Osornio J. Nested polymerase chain reaction for Mycobacterium tuberculosis DNA detection in aqueous and vitreous of patients with uveitis. Arch Med Res. 2003; 34(2):116–119
[98] Sharma K, Gupta V, Bansal R, Sharma A, Sharma M, Gupta A. Novel multi-targeted polymerase chain reaction for diagnosis of presumed tubercular uveitis. J Ophthalmic Inflamm Infect. 2013; 3(1):25
[99] Solley WA, Martin DF, Newman NJ, et al. Cat scratch disease: posterior segment manifestations. Ophthalmology. 1999; 106(8):1546–1553
[100] Bodaghi B. [Ocular manifestations of Lyme disease]. Med Mal Infect. 2007; 37(7–8):518–522
[101] Davis JL. Sex and reproduction in the transmission of infectious uveitis. J Ophthalmol. 2014; 2014:683246
[102] Chakrabarti A, Shivaprakash MR, Singh R, et al. Fungal endophthalmitis: fourteen years' experience from a center in India. Retina. 2008; 28 (10):1400–1407
[103] Hamada Y, Okuma R, Katori Y, et al. Bibliographical investigation (domestic and overseas) on the treatment of endogenous Candida endophthalmitis over an 11-year period. Med Mycol J. 2013; 54(1):53–67
[104] Do T, Hon N, Aung T, Hien ND, Cowan CL, Jr. Bacterial endogenous endophthalmitis in Vietnam: a randomized controlled trial comparing vitrectomy with silicone oil versus vitrectomy alone. Clin Ophthalmol. 2014; 8:1633–1640
[105] Riddell J, IV, Comer GM, Kauffman CA. Treatment of endogenous fungal endophthalmitis: focus on new antifungal agents. Clin Infect Dis. 2011; 52 (5):648–653
[106] Hariprasad SM, Mieler WF, Lin TK, Sponsel WE, Graybill JR. Voriconazole in the treatment of fungal eye infections: a review of current literature. Br J Ophthalmol. 2008; 92(7):871–878
[107] Weishaar PD, Flynn HW, Jr, Murray TG, et al. Endogenous Aspergillus endophthalmitis. Clinical features and treatment outcomes. Ophthalmology. 1998; 105(1):57–65
[108] Wykoff CC, Albini TA, Couvillion SS, Dubovy SR, Davis JL. Intraocular cryptococcoma. Arch Ophthalmol. 2009; 127(5):700–702
[109] Reed DC, Shah KH, Hubschman JP. Resolution of Coccidioides immitis endophthalmitis with an aggressive surgical and medical therapeutic approach. Semin Ophthalmol. 2013; 28(4):251–252
[110] Vasconcelos-Santos DV, Lim JI, Rao NA. Chronic coccidioidomycosis endophthalmitis without concomitant systemic involvement: a clinicopathological case report. Ophthalmology. 2010; 117(9):1839–1842
[111] Gonzales CA, Scott IU, Chaudhry NA, et al. Endogenous endophthalmitis caused by Histoplasma capsulatum var. capsulatum: a case report and literature review. Ophthalmology. 2000; 107(4):725–729
[112] Moloney TP, Park J. Pseudallescheria endophthalmitis: four cases over 15 years in Queensland, Australia, and a review of the literature. Retina. 2014; 34(8):1683–1701
[113] Otranto D, Eberhard ML. Zoonotic helminths affecting the human eye. Parasit Vectors. 2011; 4:41

[114] Centers for Disease Control and Prevention (CDC). Ocular toxocariasis—United States, 2009–2010. MMWR Morb Mortal Wkly Rep. 2011; 60 (22):734–736

[115] De Souza EC, Raskin E, Castro L, Muralha L, Souza O, Pena R. Migrating behavior of presumed Toxocara presenting as punctate inner choroidopathy, idiopathic choroidal neovascularization, and diffuse unilateral subacute neuroretinitis. Retin Cases Brief Rep. 2012; 6(4):430–434

[116] Kunavisarut P, Patikulsila D, Somboon P, Pathanapitoon K, Rothova A. Subretinal Thelazia-induced diffuse unilateral subacute neuroretinitis. JAMA Ophthalmol. 2014; 132(7):896–898

[117] Arevalo JF, Arevalo FA, Garcia RA, de Amorim Garcia Filho CA, de Amorim Garcia CA. Diffuse unilateral subacute neuroretinitis. J Pediatr Ophthalmol Strabismus. 2013; 50(4):204–212

[118] de Amorim Garcia Filho CA, Gomes AH, de A Garcia Soares AC, de Amorim Garcia CA. Clinical features of 121 patients with diffuse unilateral subacute neuroretinitis. Am J Ophthalmol. 2012; 153(4):743–749

[119] Souza EC, Casella AM, Nakashima Y, Monteiro ML. Clinical features and outcomes of patients with diffuse unilateral subacute neuroretinitis treated with oral albendazole. Am J Ophthalmol. 2005; 140(3):437–445

[120] Vezzola D, Kisma N, Robson AG, Holder GE, Pavesio C. Structural and functional retinal changes in eyes with DUSN. Retina. 2014; 34(8):1675–1682

[121] Berbel RF, Casella AM, de Souza EC, Farah ME. Evaluation of patients with diffuse unilateral subacute neuroretinitis by spectral domain optical coherence tomography with enhanced depth imaging. Clin Ophthalmol. 2014; 8:1081–1087

[122] Banla M, Tchalim S, Karabou PK, et al. Sustainable control of onchocerciasis: ocular pathology in onchocerciasis patients treated annually with ivermectin for 23 years: a cohort study. PLoS ONE. 2014; 9(6):e98411

[123] Li JJ, Zhang LW, Li H, Hu ZL. Clinical and pathological characteristics of intraocular cysticercosis. Korean J Parasitol. 2013; 51(2):223–229

[124] McDonald HR, Kazacos KR, Schatz H, Johnson RN. Two cases of intraocular infection with Alaria mesocercaria (Trematoda). Am J Ophthalmol. 1994; 117(4):447–455

[125] Campbell RJ, Steele JC, Cox TA, et al. Pathologic findings in the retinal pigment epitheliopathy associated with the amyotrophic lateral sclerosis/parkinsonism-dementia complex of Guam. Ophthalmology. 1993; 100 (1):37–42

25 Noninfectious Chorioretinal Inflammatory Conditions

Mariana Cabrera, Nidhi Relhan, and Thomas A. Albini

25.1 Introduction

Numerous types of noninfectious posterior segment ocular inflammation exist. Most are thought to be autoimmune in nature. Infectious uveitis, toxicity reactions, and cancer, especially primary intraocular lymphoma, can masquerade as noninfectious uveitis and are essential to identify early because specific treatment of these diseases is critical to optimize outcomes. The remaining noninfectious, non-neoplastic causes are all treated with systemic and/or local inhibition of the immune response. This chapter outlines commonly used treatment approaches for posterior segment ocular inflammatory disease, starting with intermediate uveitis and then examining approaches to self-limiting, acute, and chronic posterior segment inflammation. Although beyond the scope of this chapter, a broad familiarity with the many types of noninfectious posterior segment uveitides is required to avoid improper treatment of masquerading conditions and to treat with therapy that is adequate while avoiding unnecessary side effects. Our goal is to provide an outline of the most commonly used treatment modalities.

The mainstay of therapy for uveitis remains corticosteroids.[1] Topical steroids are the first-line approach to anterior uveitis, but are better used as adjunctive therapy for intermediate or posterior inflammation. Periocular corticosteroids are useful in the treatment of intermediate uveitis and uveitic macular edema. Many patients will require systemic immunosuppression to control their inflammation. This can be a short course of high-dose corticosteroids to control acute, severe inflammation or, in patients with chronic inflammation, systemic corticosteroids may be required initially to control the symptoms followed by long-term corticoid-sparing immunosuppression. As a general rule, systemic corticosteroids must be used in limited amounts, if they are to be used chronically, due to systemic side effects. The American College of Rheumatology, for example, recommends that prednisone not be used at doses higher than 10 mg/day for over 2 months.[2,3] In patients in whom systemic immunosuppression is relatively contraindicated (unilateral disease, patient intolerance to immunosuppressants), sustained release corticosteroid implants are available. These therapeutic options are discussed in detail later.

25.2 Intermediate Uveitis

Intermediate uveitis is a noninfectious entity of unknown etiology that affects otherwise young, healthy individuals, typically between the ages of 5 and 65 years.[4] Most patients with intermediate uveitis present with reduced visual acuity and floaters. Reduced visual acuity may be caused by cystoid macular edema (CME), cataract, vitreous opacities, and rarely vitreous hemorrhage and rhegmatogenous retinal detachment. Most cases tend to be asymmetric at presentation but often become symptomatically bilateral with time. Men and women are affected equally. There is no racial predilection. Intermediate uveitis is associated with multiple sclerosis.[5,6] Up to one-fourth of patients with multiple sclerosis may have intermediate uveitis with retinal venous sheathing. However, among patients with intermediate uveitis, fewer than 15% have a demyelinating disorder resembling multiple sclerosis.[6,7] Diagnosis is based on clinical manifestations of vitritis, CME, and pars plana snowbank, the pathognomonic sign of intermediate uveitis (▶ Fig. 25.1 and ▶ Fig. 25.2). The main findings on optical coherence tomography (OCT) are related to uveitic CME, consisting of retinal thickening, intraretinal fluid, and subretinal fluid (the latter appearing especially in the initial phases of

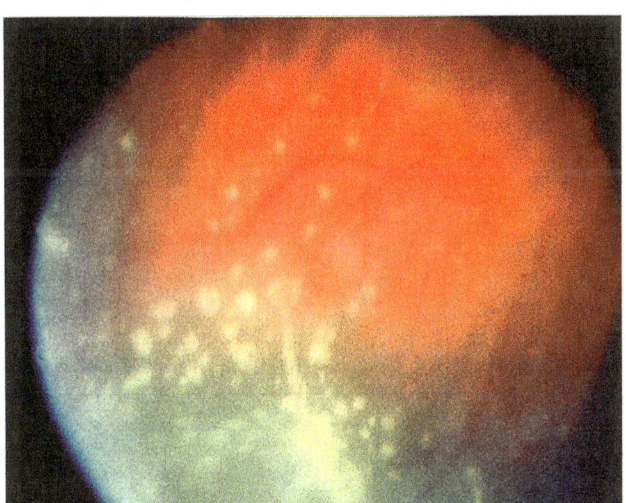

Fig. 25.1 Pars planitis: Vitreous cellular clumps or "snowballs" in the inferior fundus.

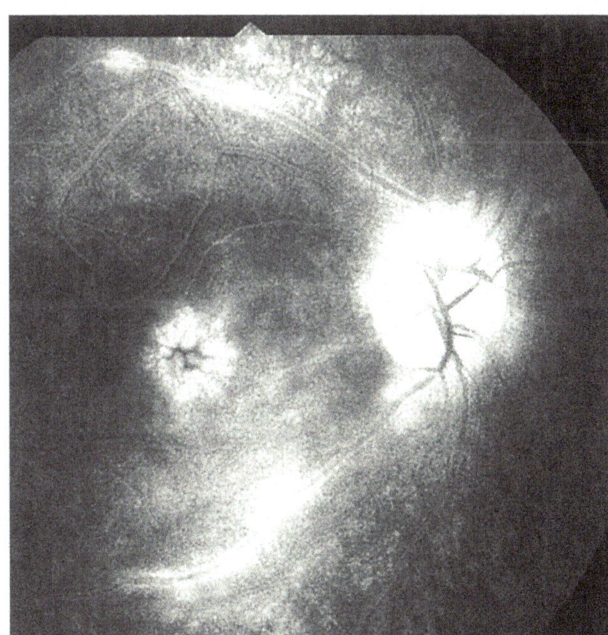

Fig. 25.2 Pars planitis: Fluorescein angiogram shows cystoid macular edema and staining of the major retinal vessels.

inflammation).[8,9,10] Anterior segment manifestations may include variable amounts of anterior chamber flare and cell. Children with intermediate uveitis may have episodes of acute fibrinous iridocyclitis. There may be evidence of posterior synechiae, particularly in children. End-stage cases of intermediate uveitis may be associated with rubeosis. Posterior subcapsular cataracts are the most common anterior segment complication of intermediate uveitis. Glaucoma can occur but is uncommon.[11]

Intermediate uveitis is a chronic disease and occasionally may have a mild course. Therefore, to optimize the risk–benefit ratio of the various treatments, therapy has traditionally been approached in a logical, stepwise fashion and initiated when the visual acuity drops to 20/40 level or worse. Corticosteroids are the treatment of choice for intermediate uveitis. They may be used in a periocular fashion or systemically. Topical corticosteroids can help control anterior segment inflammation, but alone will not typically have any significant effect on vitritis or CME. Periocular injections of 40 mg of triamcinolone given up to every 2 weeks and repeated four times in each eye may be an adequate first course to control intraocular inflammation. This is the preferred route of treatment for children with intermediate uveitis. Systemic corticosteroids may be utilized at 1 mg/kg daily with a taper based on response for intraocular inflammation and CME. Treatment with systemic corticosteroids may be required for 6 or more months. The side effects of both oral and periocular corticosteroids are well known and are not discussed here.[1]

If corticosteroids do not control inflammation or are not tolerated by the patient, cryoretinopexy of the snowbank may be performed. Cryopexy using a double freeze–thaw technique over the snowbank with one freeze width of treatment extension into normal retina and uninvolved ciliary body may be performed. Complications may include progressive inflammation posterior to the area of cryopexy, vitreous hemorrhage, tractional retinal detachments, and hypotony.[4,12]

In cases of recalcitrant intraocular inflammation or inability to lower steroid dose to an acceptable level, systemic steroid-sparing immunosuppressive therapy may be utilized. Systemic methotrexate, cyclosporine, azathioprine, or anti–tumor necrosis factor (TNF) biologics in low doses may be utilized in conjunction with systemic corticosteroids to gain control of chronic intraocular inflammation and chronic CME. Intravitreal injections with triamcinolone, sustained-release dexamethasone, or anchored fluocinolone implant in severe cases are often successful in treating CME, but almost always result in cataract and often in ocular hypertension or even glaucoma.[13,14]

The retinal complications of intermediate uveitis can be difficult to manage. Panretinal laser photocoagulation is typically used to promote regression of retinal or disc neovascularization.[12] Traction retinal detachments that do not involve the macula may be followed up closely for signs of progression. If macular involvement does occur, pars plana vitrectomy surgery (combined with scleral buckling surgery if a rhegmatogenous component is present) should be considered. The presence of active intraocular inflammation increases the risk for proliferative vitreoretinopathy in these patients.[15]

Pars plana vitrectomy and lensectomy are often preferred as a treatment for chronic, recalcitrant, intermediate uveitis associated with cataract and CME. The anterior and posterior hyaloid and epiretinal membranes should be removed to relieve retinal traction, and peripheral neovascularization should be treated with intraoperative scatter laser photocoagulation or cryotherapy. This aggressive approach appears to be associated with visual improvement and good long-term visual prognosis, but controlled, prospective data are not available.

Intermediate uveitis has a highly variable course and outcome. Some patients have benign disease that requires little or no treatment. In other patients, particularly children, severe disease develops that can result in blindness and phthisis in one or both eyes. Patients with a benign course and no significant exacerbations are uncommon and account for 10 to 15% of cases. The vast majority, representing about 50% of patients, have a chronic, smoldering course without significant exacerbations. Approximately one-third of cases have a chronic, smoldering course with occasional severe exacerbations.[4,16,17]

The long-term prognosis of untreated intermediate uveitis is not well known. The severity rather than the duration of inflammation appears to be the stronger prognostic indicator of visual outcome. The development of macular complications is associated with a poorer visual prognosis. CME develops more commonly in those patients who have definite pars plana exudates and vitritis.[4,16,17]

25.3 Self-Limiting Posterior Uveitis Often Not Requiring Treatment

Some posterior segment inflammatory disorders such as multiple evanescent white dot syndrome (MEWDS), acute posterior multifocal placoid pigment epitheliopathy (APMPPE), or punctate inner choroiditis (PIC) may not require any treatment. All these entities fall into a group of diseases grouped together as white dot syndromes (▶ Table 25.1 and ▶ Table 25.2).

25.3.1 Multiple Evanescent White Dot Syndrome

MEWDS is a well-defined posterior segment inflammatory disease typically presenting with unilateral photopsias and vision loss in young patients with a female predilection. Numerous small white dots are always seen throughout the peripheral retina. Subfoveal retinal pigment epithelium (RPE) changes in the involved eye may lead to central macular stippling, often termed *peau d'orange changes.* The diagnosis of MEWDS is confirmed by fluorescein angiography (FA) findings of late-phase hyperfluorescent lesions with central hypofluorescence. Indocyanine green angiography (ICG) shows multifocal hypofluorescent lesions (▶ Fig. 25.3). OCT shows focal defects in the ellipsoid zone and RPE alterations in the fovea.[25] This is a self-limited condition that resolves in 4 to 8 weeks and does not require treatment. Rare cases may be recurrent or have features of more aggressive, vision-threatening disease, such as multifocal choroiditis, and require prednisone treatment.[25,26,27,28,29,30,31]

25.3.2 Acute Posterior Multifocal Placoid Pigment Epitheliopathy

Acute posterior multifocal placoid pigment epitheliopathy (APMPPE) is a bilateral inflammatory disease that affects the

Table 25.1 Inflammatory chorioretinopathies (white dot syndromes)

	Age (decades)	Sex	Viral prodrome	Unilateral or bilateral	Other systemic findings	Symptoms
APMPPE	2nd–3rd	M = F	Y	Bilateral	Meningoencephalitis Acute nephritis	Blurred vision
MEWDS	2nd–5th	F	Y (50%)	Unilateral Bilateral (rare)	none	Scotoma Temporal Photopsias
Serpiginous choroidopathy	2nd–7th	M = F	N	Bilateral (eventually)	none	Scotoma Decreased vision
Birdshot retinochoroidopathy	3rd–6th	F > M	N	Bilateral	HLA-A29 positive (90%)	Floaters Blurred vision Photopsias Nyctalopia (late) Color blindness (late)
SFU[18,19]	2nd–3rd	F	N	Bilateral	none	Decreased vision Floaters
MFC and panuveitis	2nd–6th	F	N	Bilateral	EBV association (controversial)	Decreased vision Photopsias Enlarged Blind Spot
PIC[20]	2nd–4th	F	N	Unilateral	Myopia	Blurred vision Photopsias Scotoma
Acute retinal pigment epitheliitis[21]	2nd–4th	M = F	N	Unilateral Bilateral (rare)	none	Visual loss (variable)
AMN[22]	2nd–4th	F	Y (rare)	Unilateral Bilateral (rare)	none	Paracentral scotoma
UAIM[23]	2nd–4th	M = F	Y	Unilateral	none	Severe vision loss
AZOOR[24]	2nd–4th	F	N	either	none	Visual field loss Photopsias

Abbreviations: AMN, acute macular neuroretinopathy; APMPPE, acute posterior multifocal placoid pigment epitheliopathy; AZOOR, acute zonal occult outer retinopathy; CME, cystoid macular edema; CNVM, choroidal neovascular membrane; EBV, Epstein–Barr virus; Immun, cytotoxic or cytostatic immunosuppressives; MEWDS, multiple evanescent white dot syndrome; MFC and panuveitis, multifocal choroiditis and panuveitis; PIC, punctate inner choroidopathy; RPE, retinal pigment epithelium; SFU, subretinal fibrosis and uveitis; UAIM, unilateral acute idiopathic maculopathy.

choriocapillaris, RPE, and outer retina. It occurs in otherwise healthy, young adults in the second to third decades of life. There is no gender predilection. A flulike syndrome precedes the onset of ocular disease in about one-third of patients.[32,33] Symptoms of myelomeningeal encephalitis, such as meningismus, headaches, and hearing loss, may be seen after the viral prodrome in some patients.[34,35] Most patients present with sudden onset of painless visual loss in both eyes. Retinal examination reveals few, if any, vitreous cells and multiple yellow or gray, flat placoid lesions of variable size in the posterior pole.[32] Episcleritis, disc hyperemia, and, rarely, exudative retinal detachment have been reported.[34,36] FA demonstrates early hypofluorescence and late hyperfluorescence of the active lesions[32,33] (▶ Fig. 25.4). OCT findings include early elevation and disruption in the ellipsoid layer with accumulation of hyperreflective material and subretinal fluid. The ellipsoid layer becomes separated from the RPE with concomitant thickening of the outer nuclear layer. These findings resolve as visual acuity improves.[37]

25.3.3 Punctate Inner Choroiditis

Punctate inner choroiditis (PIC) is a rare inflammatory condition affecting the choroid and RPE. It presents in young (median age: 30 years) women (> 90% of the cases) who are myopic (mean refraction: -4.6D). Patients present with photopsias, scotomata, and blurred vision. It is bilateral in 50 to 88% of cases. There is an absence of intraocular inflammation, and fundus examination reveals multiple, small (100–300 µm), white or yellow lesions in the posterior pole (▶ Fig. 25.5). The lesions resolve in a few weeks, progressing into atrophic or hyperpigmented chorioretinal scars. The main vision threatening complication is choroidal neovascularization which has been reported to occur in 69 to 75% of patients, leading to subretinal fibrosis in up to 56% of patients. Acute lesions show disturbances in the sub-RPE space and ellipsoid zone.[38] A study of OCT findings in 35 eyes with inactive PIC demonstrated that half of PIC lesions consisted of focal atrophy of the outer retina and RPE, a third of lesions consisted of sub-RPE hyperreflective

Table 25.2 Inflammatory chorioretinopathies

	Clinical features	Duration	Etiology	Treatment	Visual prognosis	Recurrences	CNVM
APMPPE	Creamy, placoid, RPE level lesions	2–6 wk	Unknown	None	Good (> 20/40)	Very rare	Y (rare)
MEWDS	Vitritis Disc edema Deep retinal white dots	2–6 wk	Unknown	None	Good (> 20/40)	Uncommon	Y (rare)
Serpiginous choroidopathy	Peripapillary choroiditis Variable vitritis	Chronic	Unknown	Steroids Immun	Poor (< 20/400), progressive	Common	Y (common)
Birdshot retinochoroidopathy	Vitritis Disc edema CME Retinal vascular Sheathing	Chronic	Unknown	Steroids Immun	Guarded to poor	Chronic	Not reported
SFU[18,19]	Vitritis Subretinal fibrosis	Chronic	Unknown	Steroids	Poor	Chronic	Y
MFC and panuveitis	Iridocyclitis and vitritis Peripapillary RPE disturbed	Chronic	?EBV	Steroids Immun	Guarded to poor	Chronic	Y
PIC[20]	Small, yellow lesions at level of RPE or choroid Serous retinal detachment Atrophic scars when healed	2–6 wk	Unknown	None	Good to poor	Common	Y (common)
Acute retinal pigment epitheliitis[21]	Small, brown or gray spots	6–12 wk	Unknown	None	Good	Rare	Not reported
AMN[22]	Parafoveal petaloid lesions darker than macula	> 6 wk	Unknown	None	Good but scotoma may persist	Occasional	Not reported
UAIM[23]	Exudative detachment of macula "Wedge" retinal elevation White-gray RPE thickening Overlying vitritis	4–6 wk	Unknown	None	Good	Not reported	Not reported
AZOOR[24]	Narrowed retinal vessels Variable vitritis Depigmentation of RPE in zones	Chronic	Unknown	None	Guarded	Possible	Not reported

Abbreviations: AMN, acute macular neuroretinopathy; APMPPE, acute posterior multifocal placoid pigment epitheliopathy; AZOOR, acute zonal occult outer retinopathy; CME, cystoid macular edema; CNVM, choroidal neovascular membrane; EBV, Epstein–Barr virus; Immun, cytotoxic or cytostatic immunosuppressives; MEWDS, multiple evanescent white dot syndrome; MFC, multifocal choroiditis; PIC, punctate inner choroidopathy; RPE, retinal pigment epithelium; SFU, subretinal fibrosis and uveitis; UAIM, unilateral acute idiopathic maculopathy.

deposits, and the remainder consisted of focal RPE elevations with underlying hyporeflective space.[39] Treatment for the inflammatory lesions (mainly with systemic steroids) can be considered if they are very close to fixation, but most lesions resolve with a good visual prognosis. Treatment with intravitreal anti-vascular endothelial growth factor (anti-VEGF) injections is recommended for choroidal neovascularization.[40]

25.3.4 Acute Posterior Uveitis

Many patients suffer from acute inflammation of the posterior segment. When the pattern of inflammation can be differentiated, often a diagnosis of an acute exacerbation of a chronic disease can be made, for example, a bout of retinitis and vitritis in Behçet's disease, or a bout of vasculitis in sarcoidosis. The acute exacerbations of the condition are treated as described below and then followed by chronic steroid-sparing treatment as outlined in the next section. Alternatively, some patients may not need chronic immunosuppression and may need only a short course of treatment as detailed in this section.

Corticosteroids remain the mainstay for the treatment of acute uveitis because of their rapid potent effect. Prednisone is the most frequently used oral corticosteroid. Prednisolone, which is the active form of prednisone, can be prescribed in patients with liver dysfunction. Initial therapy is typically 0.5 to 1 mg/kg/day of prednisone followed by a slow taper when the inflammation has been controlled. Corticosteroids should be tapered slowly (over the course of at least 3–4 weeks) to

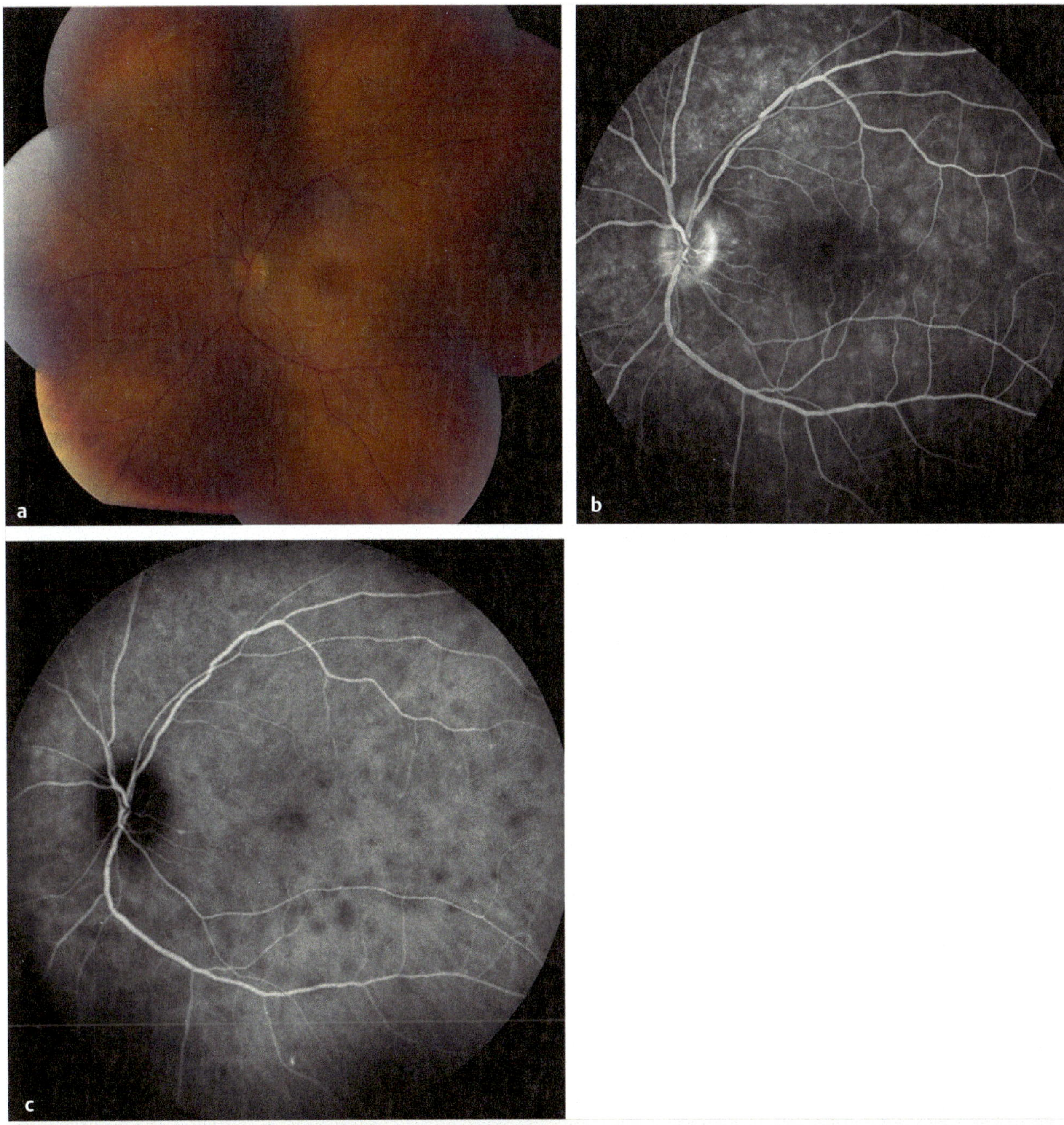

Fig. 25.3 A 19-year-old woman with loss of vision in the left eye from multiple evanescent white dot syndrome. (**a**) Fundus photograph showing multifocal white lesions throughout posterior pole. (**b**) Multifocal hyperfluorescence in a late-phase fluorescein angiogram with central hypofluorescence forming a reef. (**c**) Late phase of an indocyanine green angiogram showing multifocal hypofluorescence in the middle phase.

prevent rebound inflammation, except in short 1-week courses used for anterior uveitis. If the disease recurs, a higher dose should be used for another month and slowly tapered again. Initial treatment must be aggressive. In cases of acute vision-threatening inflammation (such as bilateral serous retinal detachment), intravenous methylprednisolone at a dose of 500 to 1,000 mg/day for 3 days may be used, followed by oral corticosteroid therapy. An immunosuppressive drug should be considered if an adequate response in not seen with 2 to 4 weeks of high-dose corticosteroids or if, after 3 months of adequate treatment and taper, the disease in not controlled on less than 10 mg of prednisone a day.

Complications of systemic steroids include altered mood (and, in severe cases, psychosis), systemic hypertension, elevated blood glucose, leukocytosis, hypokalemia, acne, osteoporosis, avascular necrosis of the hip, weight gain, and pancreatitis. Prolonged use in children should be avoided, as delayed growth can be observed even with 0.4 mg/kg of prednisone[41] and may be irreversible.[42] Cataract formation with systemic steroids is dose and duration dependent; 83% of patients

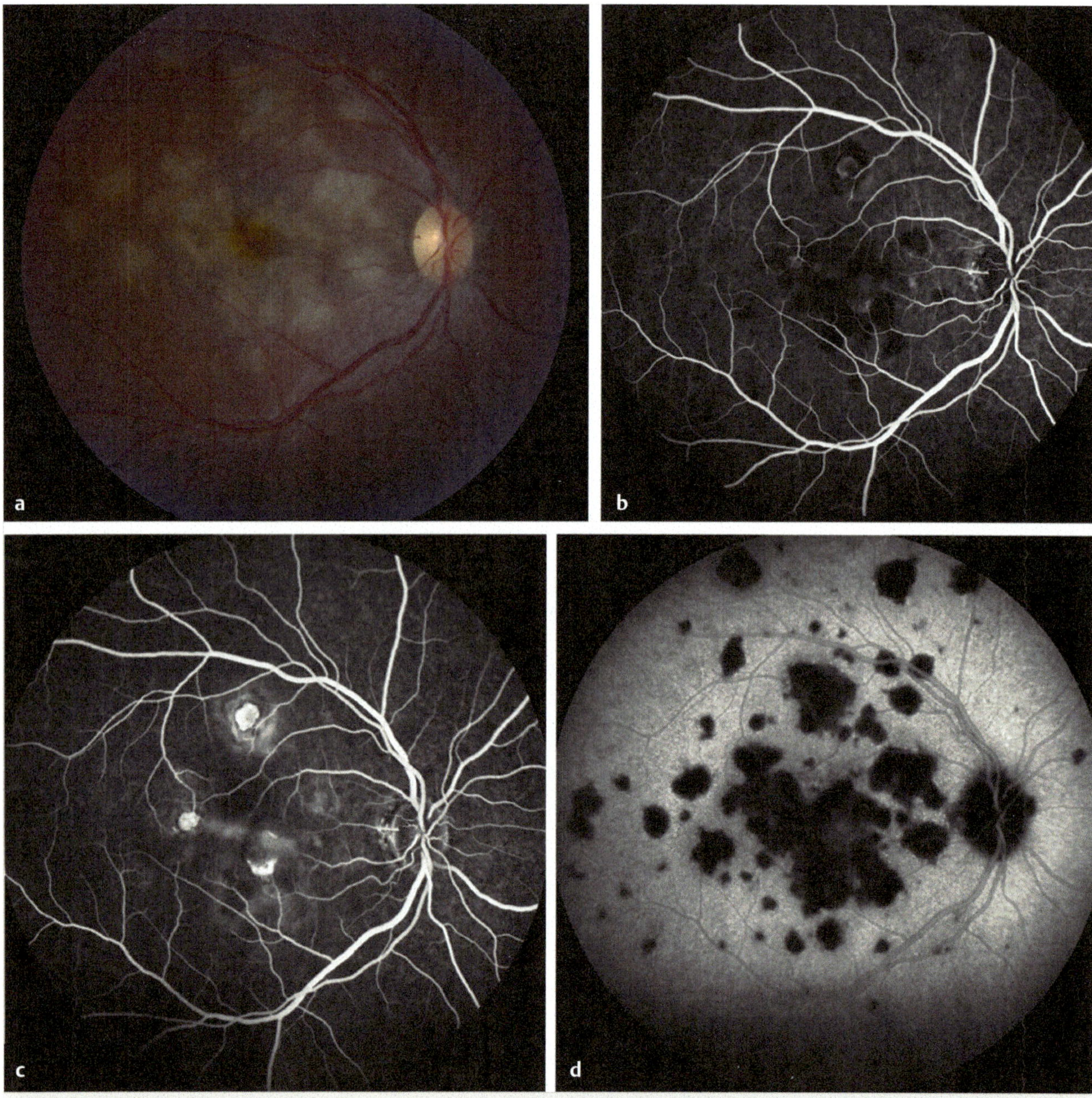

Fig. 25.4 A 13-year-old boy with acute posterior multifocal placoid pigment epitheliopathy presents with sudden painless vision loss following a viral prodrome. (**a**) Multifocal creamy lesions in both posterior poles. (**b**) Multifocal hypofluorescence on fluorescein angiography. (**c**) Hyperfluorescence in late frames on angiography. (**d**) Multifocal hypofluorescence on indocyanine green angiography midphase.

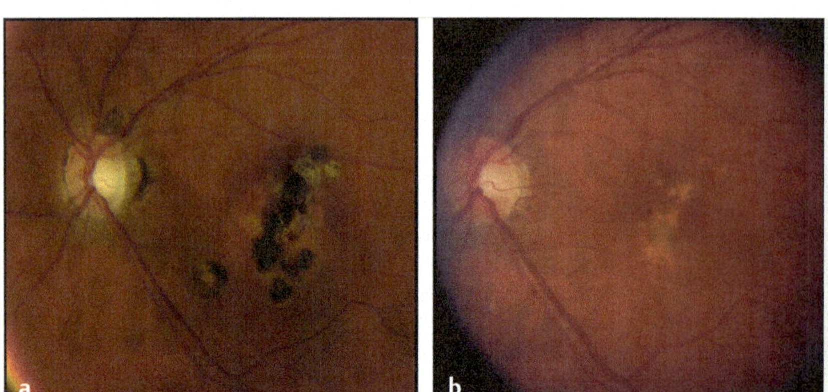

Fig. 25.5 A 21-year-old patient with punctate inner choroidopathy. (a) Shows multiple punched-out, clustered lesions in the posterior pole. (b) Shows extensive scarring and progression at 2 years of follow-up.

will develop cataract if taking corticosteroids (even maintenance doses) for more than 4 years.[43] Blood pressure and blood glucose should be monitored every 3 months, and bone density and cholesterol levels should be checked on an annual basis. Calcium and vitamin D supplementation is advised, as well as weight-bearing exercises.

25.4 Posterior Uveitis Requiring Chronic Treatment

Immunosuppressive drugs should be considered when an unacceptably high dose of corticosteroids is required to control inflammation (i.e., >10 mg/day of corticosteroids after 3 months) or if there is an inadequate response to high-dose corticosteroids. Additionally, in some diseases, immunosuppressive drugs are indicated at presentation because of poor prognosis when treated with appropriate dose of corticosteroid alone. These include Behçet's disease with posterior involvement, serpiginous choroidopathy, sympathetic ophthalmia, and birdshot chorioretinopathy. Some authors recommend early treatment with immunosuppressive drugs in multifocal choroiditis with panuveitis and Vogt-Koyanagi-Harada's (VKH) syndrome.[44]

25.4.1 Behçet's Disease

Behçet's disease is a systemic disorder that produces occlusive vasculitis in the skin, circulatory system, and central nervous system, including the eyes.[45] Diagnosis of Behçet's disease is based on the involvement of one or more of these organ systems. The etiology of this disorder is unknown. It tends to affect men more commonly than women. It is particularly common in Japan, Southeast Asia, the Middle East, and the Mediterranean region.[45] Behçet's disease is associated with panuveitis. The nonocular features of Behçet's disease can dominate and precede the ocular involvement. Oral aphthous ulcers occur in up to 98% of patients. They typically heal within 1 week and are recurrent. Genital lesions may occur in 80% of patients. Cutaneous lesions occur in up to 90% of patients. Central nervous system involvement is seen in more than 50% of patients. These patients often have no ocular involvement.[46]

Patients with ocular manifestations of Behçet's disease may present with pain, photophobia, redness, and reduced vision. Ocular manifestations occur in up to 70% of patients with Behçet's disease, but fewer than 25% of patients complain about the manifestation.[46] Hypopyon iridocyclitis is seen in one-third of patients with ocular manifestations.[45,46] It is usually transient and is associated with pain, photophobia, and reduced vision. Posterior segment inflammation is marked by retinal vascular sheathing and retinal venous and arteriolar occlusions. Branch retinal vein occlusions with intraretinal hemorrhages, retinal venous sheathing, and associated macular edema are typical and characteristic. However, vision may be more severely affected if concomitant retinal arteriolar involvement is present. In these cases, white necrotic infiltrates of the inner retina may be seen along with intraretinal hemorrhages (▶ Fig. 25.6). Vitritis is variable but can be severe. Recurrent attacks of retinal vasculitis can result in severe ischemia and retinal neovascularization. Ischemic changes and recurrent ocular inflammation causes thinning of the outer retinal layers and loss of the ellipsoid layer in the fovea and throughout the macula on OCT.[47,48] Like the nonocular manifestations, the ocular manifestations of Behçet's disease follow a cyclical course punctuated by exacerbations of uveitis.[45,46]

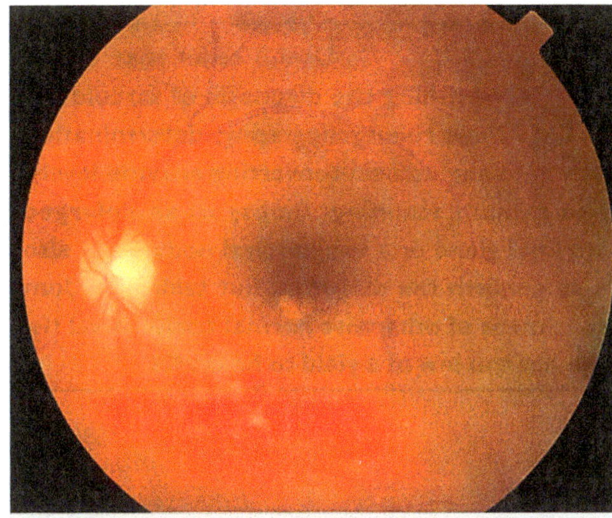

Fig. 25.6 Bechet's disease: Localized patch of occlusive vasculitis along the inferotemporal arcade.

25.4.2 Sympathetic Ophthalmia

Sympathetic ophthalmia is a rare, bilateral granulomatous panuveitis that occurs only after penetrating ocular injury or ocular surgery, especially full-thickness, glaucoma-filtering procedures. It occurs in fewer than 1% of patients with penetrating ocular injuries and in 0.01% of patients who have undergone intraocular surgery.[49,50,51]

Sympathetic ophthalmia affects individuals of all ages.[49,50,51] Ocular trauma is more common in men, but there is no gender predilection in sympathetic ophthalmia.

Inflammation characteristically occurs as early as 4 to 8 weeks following the ocular insult. The interval between the injury and the onset of intraocular inflammation varies. It may be as short as 5 days or as long as 42 years.[49,50,51] When inflammation develops in the sympathizing eye, patients often present with pain, photophobia, and decreased vision in that eye. The granulomatous anterior segment inflammation manifests with mutton fat keratic precipitates, iris nodules, and anterior chamber cell and flare. In the acute phases of the illness, optic disc edema is present. In the retina, multiple, deep, yellow lesions (Dalen-Fuchs's nodules) can be seen, particularly in the inferior periphery of the fundus (Chapter 32, Fig. 32.23) (▶ Fig. 25.7). These nodules represent aggregates of epithelioid cells at the level of Bruch's membrane. Serous retinal detachments may also be present. Serous retinal detachments, cystoid intraretinal fluid with retinal thickening, and irregularity of the ellipsoid layer are common spectral domain optical coherence tomography (SD-OCT) findings.[52] The choroid is greatly thickened and there is RPE undulation proportional to the degree of inflammation, which improves with treatment.[53] Dalen-Fuchs's nodules are seen as hyperreflective lesions at the level of the RPE with disruption of the ellipsoid layer.[54] Diffuse choroidal

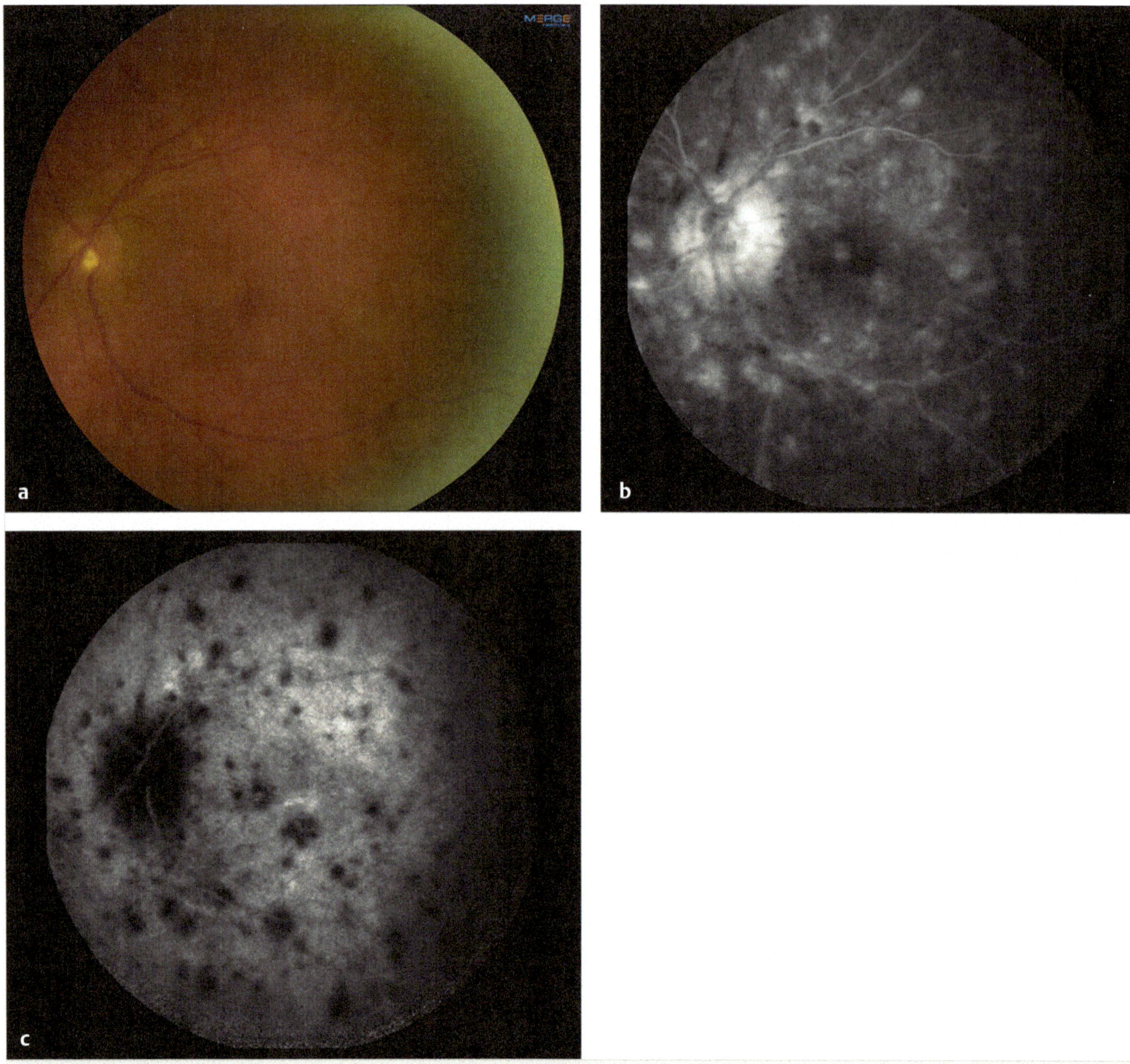

Fig. 25.7 (a) A 52-year-old man with a history of multiple vitrectomies for retinal detachment in right eye, now with new vision loss in the left eye secondary to sympathetic ophthalmia. Fundus examination shows vitritis, loss of optic disc borders, areas of subretinal fluid, and deep creamy lesions through posterior pole. Optical coherence tomography reveals intraretinal and subretinal fluid. (b) Late-stage fluorescein angiogram with multifocal hyperfluorescence. (c) Multifocal hypofluorescence in the late-stage indocyanine green angiogram.

thickening from inflammatory infiltrates is a consistent finding, best demonstrated by ultrasonography (see later). Occasionally, cutaneous and neurologic manifestations similar to those of VKH syndrome occur.[50]

25.4.3 Vogt-Koyanagi-Harada's Syndrome

Vogt-Koyanagi-Harada's (VKH) syndrome is a bilateral granulomatous panuveitis associated with dermatologic and neurologic extraocular manifestations.[55] VKH syndrome affects darkly pigmented races, including Asians, Hispanics, American Indians, Asian Indians, and blacks.[50,55,56] Female patients predominate, particularly in the Hispanic population, where the female–male ratio is 3:1.[55] The patients are typically between the ages of 20 and 50 when affected, although patients of younger age have been reported with the disease. The extraocular manifestations appear to vary widely between Japanese and Hispanic patients. Hispanic patients do not typically tend to have extraocular manifestations of vitiligo, alopecia, and poliosis. However, they do tend more commonly to have meningismus and cerebrospinal fluid pleocytosis, the neurologic manifestations of the disease.[55,56]

VKH syndrome can be divided into four distinct phases.[55] The prodromal phase is characterized by a flulike illness associated with meningismus, headache, tinnitus, and dysacusis. Cerebrospinal fluid pleocytosis can occur in this phase. The second, or uveitic, phase is associated with an acute onset of bilateral granulomatous iridocyclitis, vitritis, optic disc edema, and multiple

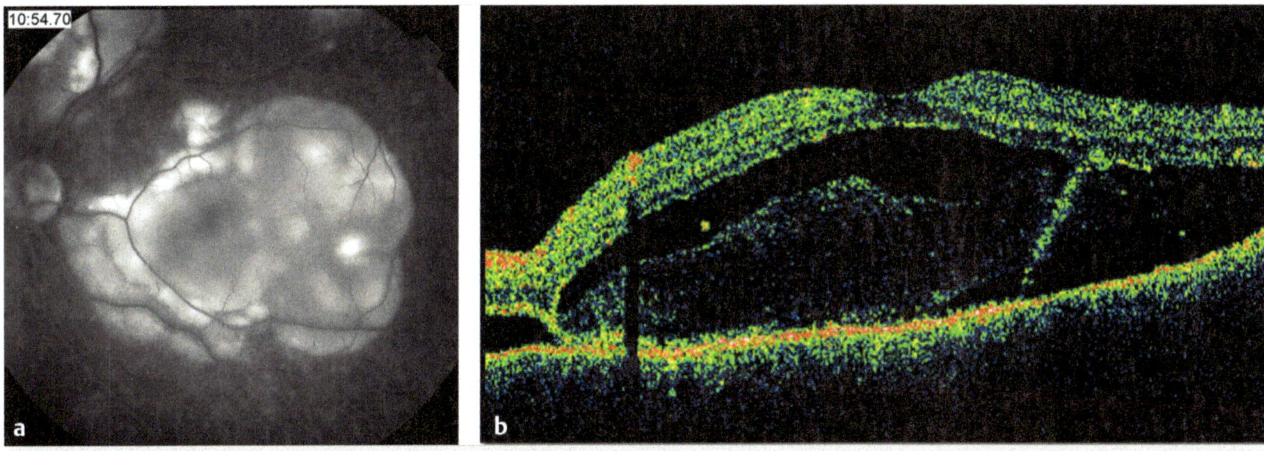

Fig. 25.8 A 35-year old man with sudden loss of vision in both eyes from VKH. (**a**) Diffuse pooling of fluorescein in late frame. (**b**) Multilobular neurosensory detachments on time-domain OCT.

serous retinal detachments. OCT will show the characteristic serous retinal detachments of VKH (▶ Fig. 25.8). These detachments are not continuous, but are made of multilobular pools of subretinal fluid, separated by septa that seem to arise from splitting off of the outer segments of photoreceptors from the inner segments and binding of inflammatory products.[57] Choroidal thickness increases markedly in the acute phase of VKH and decreases quickly after systemic corticosteroid therapy.[58] In long-standing VKH, the choroid is significantly thinner and thickness is inversely correlated with disease duration.[59] Pain, photophobia, and sudden vision loss are common symptoms. This phase lasts for 2 to 6 weeks. The third, convalescent phase, is associated with subsiding uveitis but depigmentation of skin and uveal structures. These manifestations can include vitiligo, poliosis, and diffuse depigmentation of the choroid. Perilimbal vitiligo is called *Sugiura's sign* and is often seen along with the development of a "sunset glow" appearance to the fundus. In the absence of depigmentation, the structure of the retina and choroid are preserved. In contrast, eyes with severe depigmentation have significantly thinner choroids on OCT.[60] In the inferior far periphery of the retina, well-circumscribed, white-yellow, punched-out chorioretinal scars, representing resolved Dalen-Fuchs's nodules, are usually present. This appearance is very similar to that of sympathetic ophthalmia. The final phase is the chronic, recurrent inflammatory phase. This is characterized by recurrent anterior segment inflammation and is associated with the major ophthalmic complications of VKH syndrome, including cataracts, glaucoma, and choroid neovascularization.[55]

25.4.4 Serpiginous Choroiditis

Serpiginous choroiditis has also been called *helicoid* and *geographic choroidopathy*. It is an acute and chronic recurrent inflammatory disease affecting the RPE, choriocapillaris, and choroid. The name of the disease is derived from the serpentine progression of the choroiditis in the posterior pole. The disease tends to affect men and women equally and manifests between the second and seventh decades of life. It is unilateral or very asymmetric at presentation, but significant involvement of both eyes eventually ensues.[61,62,63,64,65]

Patients with serpiginous choroiditis usually present with some degree of vision loss and associated central or paracentral scotomas in one or both eyes. There is variable anterior chamber and vitreous cellular reaction, the latter of which is present in about one-third of cases. Active choroiditis appears ophthalmoscopically as well-circumscribed, gray-white, geographically shaped lesions at the level of the RPE and choriocapillaris that involve the peripapillary region or macula of both eyes[61,62,65,66] (▶ Fig. 25.9). Some sensory retinal thickening can usually be appreciated overlying these areas of active choroiditis. OCT typically demonstrates retinal atrophy, subretinal fibrosis, varying degrees of intraretinal fluid, and marked attenuation of the ellipsoid layer.[67]

The lesions enlarge over a period of months with progression in a characteristic serpentine fashion from their origin. Activity classically resides at the leading edge of the lesion, and with enlargement, an increasing area of chorioretinal atrophy is left in its wake. With recurrences, the process eventually ends up involving the entire posterior pole. Furthermore, choroid neovascularization can develop in eyes with serpiginous choroiditis at some point in the course of disease, potentially causing further vision loss from the associated exudative changes and subsequent subretinal fibrosis.[61,62,65]

25.4.5 Birdshot Retinochoroidopathy

Birdshot retinochoroidopathy has also been called *vitiliginous chorioretinitis*. It is a bilateral condition that affects women more commonly than men and typically is seen in the third to sixth decades of life.[68,69] Nearly 90% of patients with birdshot retinochoroidopathy are HLA-A29 positive, which represents the highest association of any HLA antigen to human disease.[70]

Pearls

- Nearly 90% of patients with birdshot retinochoroidopathy are HLA-A29 positive, which represents the highest association of any HLA antigen to human disease.

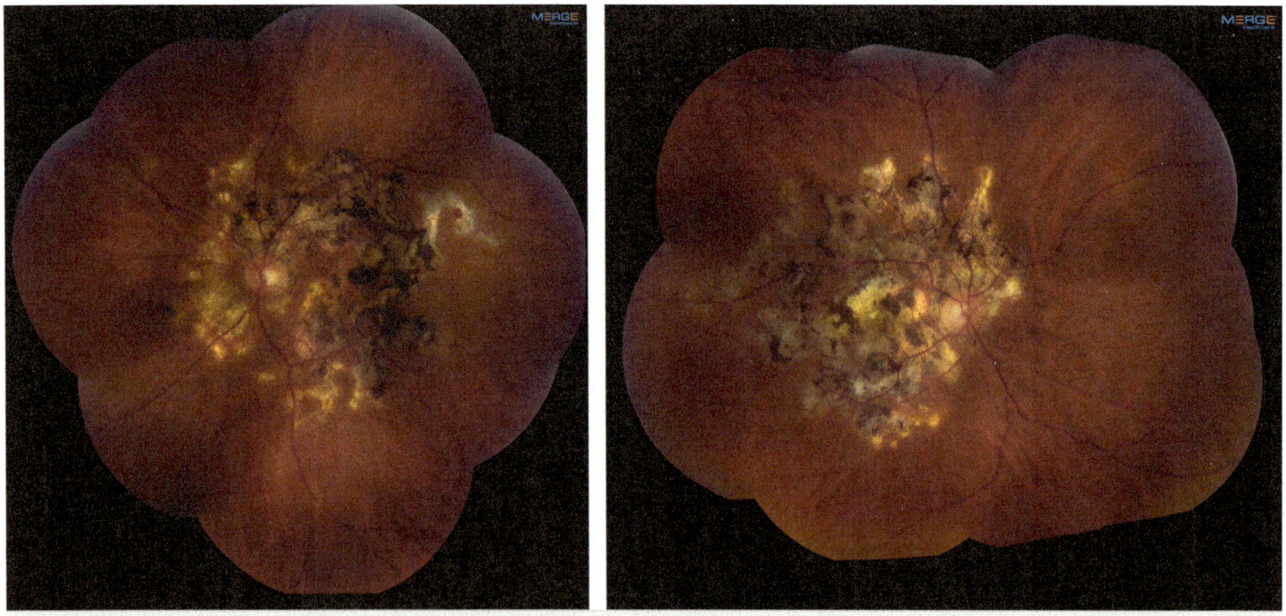

Fig. 25.9 Fundus photo of serpiginous choroiditis in a 52-year-old man, showing predominantly inactive lesion with newer satellite lesions and a small extrafoveal choroidal neovascular membrane with subretinal hemorrhage in the superotemporal macula of the left eye.

Patients often present with blurred vision, floaters, and peripheral photopsias. Later manifestations can include nyctalopia and color blindness.[68,69] Vitreous inflammation is present. The characteristic lesions are the multiple depigmented patches that are scattered throughout the fundus, hence the name *birdshot retinochoroidopathy*. They have a somewhat creamy appearance, are typically less than 1 disc diameter in size, and have a predilection for the nasal retina[68] (▶ Fig. 25.10). Disc edema, retinal vascular narrowing, and CME can also occur. The most common cause of decreased visual acuity and visual blurring in these patients is CME.[68,69] Diagnosis is based on the characteristic ocular findings in combination with the presence of HLA-A29 antigen. FA reveals disc leakage, vascular leakage, and late CME. Hypopigmented patches are not visible in the early phases of the angiogram but demonstrate late staining. Other than CME, SD-OCT is characterized by generalized loss of ellipsoid zone, and generalized loss and thinning of retinal architecture. Enhanced-depth imaging OCT often shows thinning or absence of the Sattler layer, but not discrete choroidal lesions.[71] Electrophysiologic testing demonstrates moderate to severely depressed photoreceptor function.[68,69]

25.4.6 Multifocal Choroiditis and Panuveitis

Multifocal choroiditis and panuveitis is a relatively common inflammatory disease entity that primarily affects women between the second and sixth decades of life. Most cases are bilateral at presentation or eventually become bilateral.[72,73]

Patients present with decreased visual acuity, photopsias, floaters, and various visual field defects, including scotomas and an enlarged blind spot. There is very little anterior segment inflammation and vitritis. The optic discs are normal, but the peripapillary RPE is disrupted. A napkin holder–shaped area of fibrosis can surround the disc, and peripapillary and macular choroidal neovascularization can occur.[73] In the acute phase of the disease, the lesions are yellow to gray in color and are at the level of the RPE.[74] Numerous acute choroidal lesions may occur in the active phases of the disease; they eventually evolve into chorioretinal scars that look much like the punched-out lesions of ocular histoplasmosis (▶ Fig. 25.11 and Fig. ▶ Fig. 25.12). There can be hundreds of these scars, located primarily in the posterior pole and midperiphery.[74]

Diagnosis is based on clinical examination. As noted earlier, the ocular findings are reminiscent of changes seen in the presumed ocular histoplasmosis syndrome, except that both anterior segment and vitreous inflammation are present, neither of which is seen in presumed ocular histoplasmosis syndrome. Furthermore, extensive fibrosis and RPE clumping are more common in multifocal choroiditis than in presumed ocular histoplasmosis syndrome (▶ Fig. 25.11). FA may be helpful in the diagnosis; the active yellow lesions show early blocked fluorescence and late staining, similar to other acute inflammatory choroidal infiltrates.[73] With progression into chorioretinal atrophy, typical scar-like angiographic changes are evident, with early hyperfluorescence and discrete late staining. Choroidal neovascularization is usually well delineated and angiographically demonstrates the classic early lacy hyperfluorescence and late leakage of dye. ICG should be expected to show the lesions, both active and inactive, to be primarily hypofluorescent, and the test may be helpful to distinguish an active inflammatory focus from choroid neovascularization, which is hyperfluorescent. ICG may also show some peripapillary hypofluorescence, as in MEWDS, a finding that may explain the enlarged blind spot in these conditions. OCT is characterized by disturbances in the sub-RPE space and ellipsoid zone, indistinguishable from PIC.[38]

Treatment

In all these conditions, chronic steroid-sparing immunosuppressive drugs are essential in treating patients for long periods

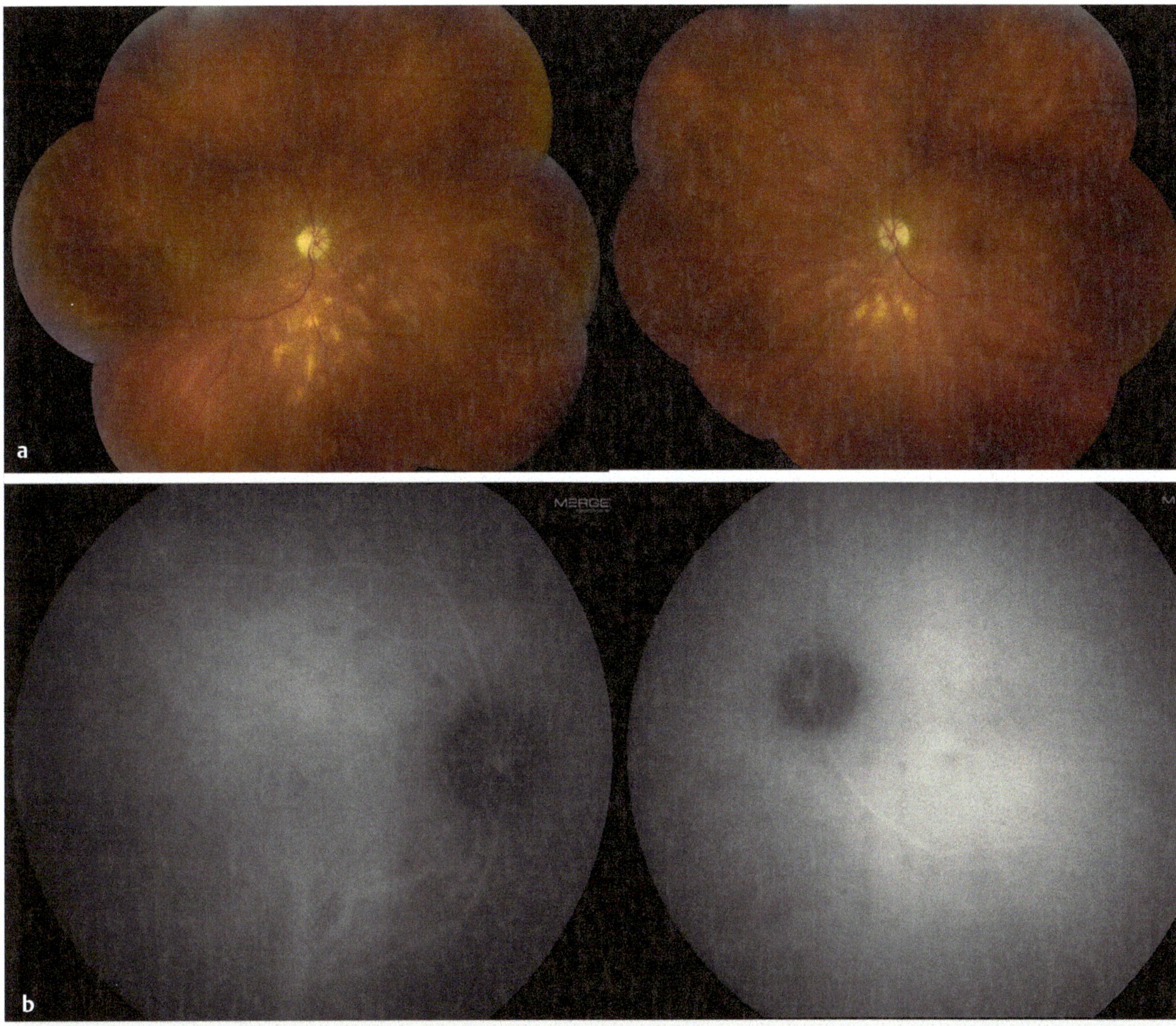

Fig. 25.10 A 54-year-old man with decreased vision in both eyes with mild vitritis. Fundus examination reveals radially oriented cream-colored lesions predominantly inferonasally around both optic nerves. (a) Fundus photography of both eyes. (b) Multifocal hypofluorescent spots on indocyanine green angiography.

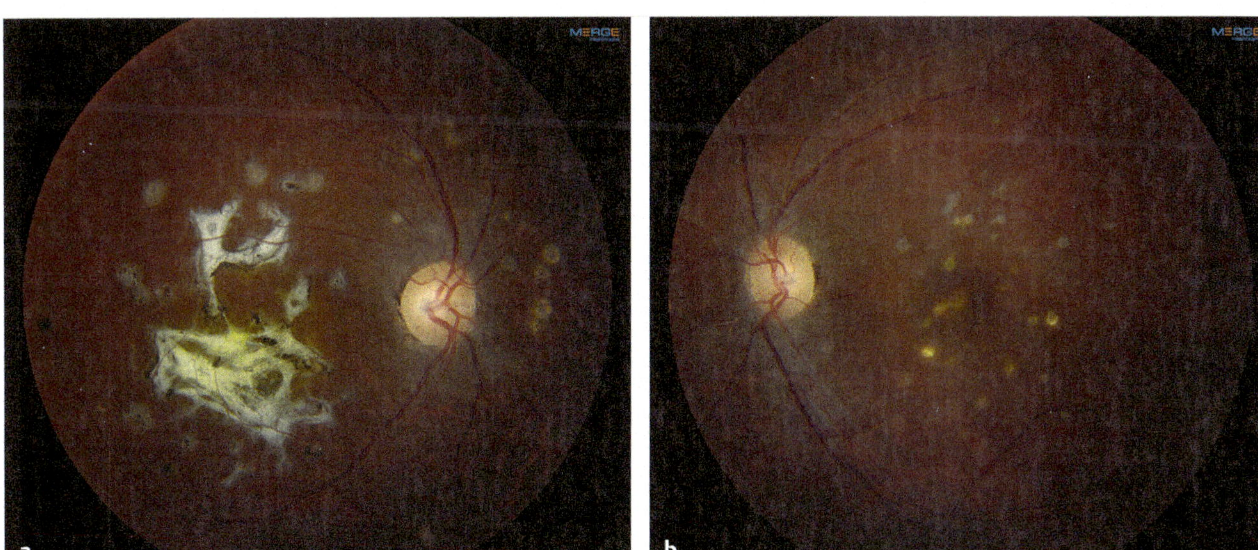

Fig. 25.11 Multifocal choroiditis: (a) right eye, (b) left eye. Fundus picture of both eyes of a 30-year-old female showing multiple yellow-white focal punched-out lesions at the posterior pole (right eye > left eye) with scar formation in the right eye.

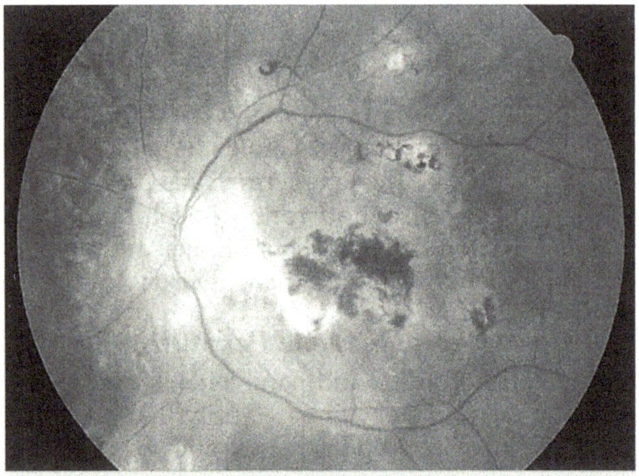

Fig. 25.12 Multifocal choroiditis: Inactive disease with peripapillary and scattered punched-out chorioretinal scarring along with significant subretinal fibrosis in the central macular region.

of time with reduced side effects, as compared to chronic high-dose systemic steroids. Immunosuppressive drugs can be divided into antimetabolites (methotrexate, azathioprine, mycophenolate mofetil), calcineurin inhibitors (cyclosporine, tacrolimus), and alkylating agents (cyclophosphamide and chlorambucil). Antimetabolites take at least 8 weeks to reach their full effect, so it is important to taper steroids slowly to coincide with the effect of the chosen immunosuppressive. In general, therapy should be continued for 1 to 2 years after control of the inflammation to obtain a durable remission.

The Systemic Immunosuppressive Therapy for Eye Diseases (SITE) study is a retrospective cohort study conducted at five university-affiliated ocular inflammatory disease subspecialty practices in the United States. Data including the use of immunosuppressive therapies for inflammatory eye diseases were obtained by review of original medical records of approximately 8,560 ocular inflammation patients over up to 30 years.[75] It has provided the most robust evidence of effectiveness and adverse events for commonly used immunosuppressants. The results of the SITE study are summarized in ▶ Table 25.1 and ▶ Table 25.2.

25.5 Antimetabolites

25.5.1 Methotrexate

Indications

Methotrexate is used in corticoid-sparing therapy in all forms of chronic, sight-threatening uveitis. It is the first-line treatment in chronic uveitis in children because it is well tolerated and has a good safety profile. In a survey of uveitis specialists in the United States, methotrexate was the most commonly used initial therapy for anterior, intermediate, and posterior/panuveitis.[76]

Mechanism of Action

It acts as a folic acid analog and irreversible inhibitor of dihydrofolate reductase. It inhibits the production of thymidylate which is required for DNA replication. It decreases lymphocyte proliferation, induces T-cell apoptosis, alters B-cell response, and inhibits cytokine production and angiogenesis. Primary mechanism of action may be through apoptosis. The drug has also been shown to exert much of its anti-inflammatory effect though the release of adenosine,[77] and much of its effect may not be limited to its antiproliferative properties, explaining why minimal efficacy may be lost when coadministered with folic acid to reduce side effects.

Dose

It is administered at a dose of 15 to 25 mg once weekly, oral or subcutaneous injection. It can be started at 7.5 mg and gradually increased to improve tolerance. Patients should take 1 mg of folate per day to minimize nausea. When given orally, up to 35% may be metabolized by the intestinal flora before being absorbed. Subcutaneously, 100% is absorbed and gastrointestinal side effects are minimized. It takes 6 to 8 weeks to see the full effect.

Adverse Effects

Adverse effects include hepatotoxicity (abnormal liver function in 15% and cirrhosis in 0.1%), cytopenias, and interstitial pneumonia. Five percent to 25% of patients have gastrointestinal symptoms (mainly stomach upset and nausea). Alopecia and rash may occur. Methotrexate is contraindicated in pregnancy. Unlike other immunosuppressants, it does not seem to increase the risk of cancer. Before starting therapy, the clinician should obtain a complete blood cell count (CBC), hepatitis B surface antigen and hepatitis C antibody, and complete liver function tests. CBC and liver function should be checked every 1 to 2 months.

Evidence

The results of the SITE cohort study for methotrexate are summarized in ▶ Table 25.3.[78] At 12 months, 66% of patients had no inflammation, and 58.4% were able to maintain a dose of 10 mg/day of prednisone or less (18.8% were able to discontinue steroids completely). Control of inflammation was achieved more often in patients with anterior uveitis than in patients with posterior uveitis or panuveitis. One meta-analysis showed that the probability of improvement of intraocular inflammation in children treated with methotrexate is 73%.[79]

25.5.2 Mycophenolate Mofetil

Indications

Mycophenolate mofetil is used in corticoid-sparing therapy in all forms of chronic, sight-threatening uveitis. It is safe and effective for use in children. A survey of uveitis specialists[76] showed that mycophenolate mofetil was the preferred treatment for intermediate and posterior/panuveitis compared to other immunosuppressants (although its cost limited its actual use).

Mechanism of Action

It acts as a selective inhibitor of inosine monophosphate dehydrogenase (IMPDH) which interferes with guanosine nucleotide synthesis (essential in the proliferation of B and T lymphocytes).

Table 25.3 Summary of results from the Systemic Immunosuppressive Therapy for Eye Diseases (SITE) study

Immunosuppressant					
	Methotrexate	**Mycophenolate mofetil**	**Azathioprine**	**Cyclosporine**	**Cyclophosphamide**
Reference	Gangaputra et al (2009)[78]	Daniel et al (2010)[80]	Pasadhika et al (2009)[20]	Kaçmaz et al (2010)[81]	Pujari et al (2010)[82]
Number of patients (number of eyes)	384 (639)	236 (397)	145 (255)	373 (681)	215 (381)
Type/location of inflammation					
Anterior	32.8%	20.3%	14.5%	20.1%	N/A
Intermediate	9.8%	11.9%	12.4%	26.5%	N/A
Posterior	21.4%	39.8%	35.9%	46.0%	20.4% (all forms)[a]
Others (mucous membrane pemphigoid, scleritis)	35.9%	28.0%	37.2%	7.5%	79.8%
Follow-up at 6 mo					
No activity	49.4%	53.1%	40.8%	33.3%	49.2%
% of patients with maintenance dose =10 mg prednisone	37.7%	40.7%	32.2%	22.1%	30.1%
% of patients who discounted steroids	5.1%	4.4%	5.2%	3.6%	3.3%
Follow-up at 12 mo					
No activity	66.0%	73.1%	62.2%	51.9%	76.4%
% of patients with maintenance dose =10 mg prednisone	58.4%	55.0%	46.9%	36.1%	61.2%
% of patients with discontinued steroids	18.8%	12.1%	9.1%	8.2%	12.6%
% of patients who discontinued due to side effects[b]	18.3%	12–23.3%	24–28.4%	10.7–23.1%	35.5–44.3%
% of patients who required a second immunosuppressant	15.6%	17.4%	9.0%	17.0%	9.7%[c]

[a]Location of uveitis not reported.

[b]Range of values includes patients who discontinued the drug due to unknown reasons.

[c]Cyclophosphamide was discontinued due to uncontrolled inflammation.

It also suppresses antibody synthesis, interferes with cellular adhesion to vascular endothelium, and decreases recruitment of lymphocytes.[83]

Dose

It is administered at a dose of 1 to 1.5 g taken orally twice daily. Clinical effect is seen after 6 weeks.

Adverse Effects

Adverse effects include gastrointestinal (pain, nausea, vomiting, and diarrhea), leukopenia (up to 19%), lymphoma (1%), and opportunistic infections (up to 46%, the majority being cytomegalovirus and herpes simplex infections, with less than 2% being fatal). Although not conclusive, a review of the evidence has shown that mycophenolate mofetil does not significantly increase the risk of cancer.[84] CBCs should be obtained monthly and liver function tests should be obtained every 3 months.

Evidence

The results of the SITE cohort study for mycophenolate mofetil are summarized in ▶ Table 25.3 and ▶ Fig. 25.2.[80] At 12 months, 73.1% of patients had no inflammation, and 55% were able to maintain a dose of 10 mg/day of prednisone or less (12.1% were able to discontinue steroids completely). Another large study[85] of 60 patients (most with intermediate uveitis) reported controlled inflammation in 77% of patients treated with =7.5 mg/day of prednisone after one year and 94% after 2 years. A retrospective study of 52 pediatric patients with uveitis showed 73.1% improved on mycophenolate mofetil monotherapy, and 48.1% were quiescent or had no more than two flare-ups in at least 2 years.[86]

25.5.3 Azathioprine

Indications

Azathioprine is used in corticoid-sparing therapy in all forms of chronic, sight-threatening uveitis, particularly posterior uveitis.

Mechanism of Action

Purine nucleoside analog: It acts as a false precursor for the formation of purine nucleotides such as adenine and guanine, interfering with DNA replication and RNA transcription. It decreases the numbers of peripheral T and B lymphocytes, reduces mixed lymphocyte reactivity, reduces interleukin-2 (IL-2) synthesis and IgM production.[18]

Dose

Initial dose is 2 to 3 mg/kg/day orally and then adjusted based on clinical response. Some authors advocate a quantitative testing for thiopurine methyltransferase enzyme activity, as it will not be effective in patients with low or no enzyme activity.

Adverse Effects

Adverse effects include gastrointestinal intolerance (up to 25% of patients) and hepatotoxicity (rare). There is a risk of reversible bone marrow suppression, so all patients should have a CBC every 4 to 6 weeks, and liver function should be checked every 3 months. In transplant patient cohorts, azathioprine has shown an increased risk of malignancy, but this has not been seen in patients treated for rheumatologic conditions.[84]

Evidence

Azathioprine has been used for ocular inflammatory conditions since 1967,[19] but randomized trials evaluating it for uveitis are lacking. ▶ Table 25.3 show the SITE cohort study evaluation of azathioprine.[20] At 12 months, 62.2% had no inflammation and 46.9% were able to maintain a dose of 10 mg/day of prednisone or less (9.1% were able to discontinue steroids completely). Azathioprine does not seem to increase the risk of cancer.[84]

25.5.4 Comparative Results of Antimetabolites

Control of inflammation and side effects were compared between methotrexate, mycophenolate mofetil, and azathioprine in a retrospective cohort study[21] of 257 patients. The time to control ocular inflammation with = 10 mg of prednisone a day was significantly longer with methotrexate compared to the other two. Corticosteroid-sparing success was achieved in 79% with mycophenolate mofetil, in 58% with azathioprine, and in 42% with methotrexate. Discontinuation of therapy because of side effects was higher in patients with azathioprine compared to methotrexate or mycophenolate mofetil. A prospective study[22] compared methotrexate versus mycophenolate mofetil in 80 patients. Corticosteroid-sparing success was achieved in 69% of patients with methotrexate versus 47% of patients with mycophenolate mofetil. Time to success and side effects were similar between the two groups. Few randomized clinical trials exist comparing antimetabolites, hence the conflicting results. A prospective randomized trial of methotrexate versus mycophenolate mofetil in noninfectious uveitis failed to show a difference in efficacy.[22]

25.6 Calcineurin Inhibitors

25.6.1 Cyclosporine

Indications

Cyclosporine is used in second-line, corticoid-sparing therapy in all forms of chronic, sight-threatening uveitis. Cyclosporine may be used in combination with an antimetabolite, as they have different mechanisms of action and side effects.

Mechanism of Action

Cyclosporine A is a natural product of the fungi Tolypocladium inflatum. It affects immunocompetent T lymphocytes that are in the G0 and G1 phase of their cell cycle, inhibiting transcription in these cells. This blocks their replication and lymphokine production. It inhibits the calcium (Ca^{++})-dependent pathway involved in producing proinflammatory factors. In the end, cyclosporine A acts to inhibit T-helper cells while leaving T-suppressor cells active.

Dose

When administered orally, its gastrointestinal absorption is variable. The bioavailability is 30% of the original dose.[23] Dose is 2.5 to 5 mg/kg/day, always making sure the serum creatinine remains within 30% of its baseline value to prevent renal impairment (which occurs in 100% with a dose of 10 mg/kg/day).

Adverse Effects

Fifteen percent to 27% of patients will develop hypertension.[24] Patients may exhibit a normocytic anemia and increased erythrocyte sedimentation rate. Other side effects include paresthesias, fatigue, headache, nausea, hirsutism, and gingival hyperplasia. Cyclosporine seems to increase the risk of nonmelanoma skin cancers.[84] Renal function should be checked every 2 weeks while adjusting the dose, and then CBC and renal function tests should be performed every 4 to 6 weeks as well as blood pressure measurements.

Evidence

Cyclosporine has been used for uveitis since 1983.[87] Initial studies showed it to be an effective anti-inflammatory in uveitis, but these studies used 10 mg/kg/day which proved to be nephrotoxic. Results of the SITE cohort study are shown in ▶ Table 25.3.[81] At 12 months, 51.9% had no inflammation and 36.1% were able to maintain a dose of 10 mg/day of prednisone or less (8.2% were able to discontinue steroids completely). Patients older than 55 years were more than threefold more likely to discontinue therapy because of toxicity than younger patients.

25.6.2 Tacrolimus

Indications

Tacrolimus is used as second-line, corticoid-sparing therapy in all forms of chronic, sight-threatening uveitis.

Mechanism of Action

It is a macrolide antibiotic produced by *Streptomyces tsukubaensis*. It inhibits T lymphocytes by a mechanism similar to cyclosporine.[88]

Dose

Dose is not well established, but frequently dosed at 0.05 mg/kg/day orally for uveitis.

Adverse Effects

Adverse effects include renal impairment, neurologic symptoms, gastrointestinal symptoms, and hyperglycemia. Liver function should be monitored closely. Monitoring of blood concentrations may be necessary as absorption is variable.[3]

Evidence

The SITE study is not available for tacrolimus because experience with this in uveitis is insufficient. The largest long-term study of tacrolimus for uveitis included 62 patients[89] and reported an 85% probability of a successful prednisone taper to 10 mg after 1 year and 2 months of treatment. Intolerance to the drug led to discontinuation of therapy in 23.3% of patients. A small randomized study by Murphy et al[90] showed a similar efficacy but a lower incidence of reported adverse events, especially fatigue, compared to cyclosporine.

T-cell inhibitors such as everolimus (given orally) have shown promise in some case reports. A local preparation of sirolimus has been developed for intravitreal or subconjunctival administration, and phase II (SAVE-2) and phase III (SAKURA) studies are underway.

25.7 Alkylating Agents

25.7.1 Cyclophosphamide

Indications

Cyclophosphamide is used in the treatment of patients with severe inflammatory eye disease who have failed other immunosuppressive therapy or in whom there is a need for rapid disease control where other treatments are not available or are contraindicated. It is most frequently used in ocular cicatricial pemphigoid[91] and systemic vasculitis.

Mechanism of Action

It is a nitrogen mustard-alkylating agent of DNA and RNA, resulting in cross-linking, aberrant base pairing and breaks in DNA strands, causing a cytotoxic effect on proliferating cells such as lymphocytes. With short-term administration of high doses, it targets B cells,[92] but when administered chronically at lower doses it targets both B and T cells[93] and suppresses both primary and secondary antibody responses.

Dose

Oral cyclophosphamide is dosed at 1 to 3 mg/kg/day. It is recommended to start at 2 mg/kg/day and adjust the dose.[3] Patients should be instructed to consume 3 to 4 L of fluids to decrease urinary complications such as hemorrhagic cystitis and bladder cancer. Cyclophosphamide may be administered in intravenous pulses which decreases the risk of bladder complications, but limited data have shown that oral cyclophosphamide may be more effective at maintaining remission.[94]

Adverse Effects

The most common side effect is bone marrow suppression which is dose dependent, reversible, and more common in individuals older than 65 years. It is contraindicated in pregnancy because of its teratogenic effects. Other side effects include alopecia, nausea, and vomiting. Cyclophosphamide has been associated with an increase in cancer-related mortality in the SITE study[82] (especially acute myelocytic leukemia, bladder cancer, and skin cancer), but larger studies are lacking. Additionally, gonadal dysfunction has been observed in 60% of patients after 6 months of treatment.[95] CBC and urinalysis should be obtained every 2 weeks. Prophylaxis for *Pneumocystis jirovecii* prophylaxis (trimethoprim–sulfamethoxazole, given orally) is recommended.

Evidence

The results from the SITE cohort study are shown in ▶ Table 25.1 and ▶ Table 25.3.[82] It is important to note that only 20.4% had uveitis, 45.6% had mucous membrane pemphigoid, and 22.3% had scleritis. Hence, there was a selection bias for more complicated and recalcitrant cases treated with cyclophosphamide. At 12 months, 76.4% had no inflammation (81.3% of patients with uveitis) and 61.2% were able to maintain a dose of 10 mg/day or less of prednisone (12.6% were able to discontinue steroids completely).

25.7.2 Chlorambucil

Indications

Chlorambucil is rarely used for uveitis, with indications similar to cyclophosphamide.

Mechanism of Action

An alkylating agent, its mechanism is similar to that of cyclophosphamide, inhibiting DNA and RNA replication. Like cyclophosphamide, it is a prodrug that is metabolized into its active form (phenylacetic acid) in the liver and excreted through the kidney.

Dose

Chlorambucil is administered at a dose of 0.1 to 0.2 mg/kg/day as a single daily dose for 1 year after quiescence to induce remission. It can also be given as a short-term, high-dose therapy, starting at 2 mg/daily for 1 week and increasing 2 mg/day each week until the inflammation is completely suppressed up to 3 to 6 months.[3]

Adverse Effects

The effect profile of chlorambucil is similar to cyclophosphamide. The main adverse effect is bone marrow suppression, which is reversible but may be prolonged. *P. jirovecii* prophylaxis (trimethoprim–sulfamethoxazole, given orally) is recommended. Alopecia and bladder toxicity do not occur with chlorambucil, but the drug produces infertility and is contraindicated in pregnancy. A CBC should be performed weekly until the dose is stabilized and then at least monthly.

Evidence

No large multicenter studies have been published on the use of chlorambucil for uveitis. A few studies have shown it to be effective in controlling inflammation in patients with Behçet's disease, including long-term remission of this disease.[96]

25.7.3 Biologics

Biologics are medications manufactured with recombinant DNA, designed to target specific inflammatory pathways based on disease pathogenesis. They include monoclonal antibodies to proteins such as cytokines (TNF-a), cell adhesion molecules, and cytokine receptors.

25.7.4 Tumor Necrosis Factor - a Inhibitors

Infliximab

Indications

Infliximab is used to treat chronic and severe disease in patients intolerant or unresponsive to traditional immunosuppressor therapies. It may be considered as first-line, corticosteroid-sparing therapy for patients with ophthalmic manifestations of Behçet's disease, and acute exacerbations of preexisting Behçet's disease.[97]

Mechanism of Action

Infliximab is a chimeric monoclonal antibody that binds circulating and membrane-bound TNF-a. TNF- a is a proinflammatory cytokine involved in systemic inflammation and acute phase reaction. It activates other cytokines, upregulates endothelial adhesion molecules, and increases cell-mediated immunity. It has been found to be elevated in animal models of uveitis and in ocular fluids of patients with uveitis.[98,99]

Dose

Infliximab is dosed 3 mg/kg as an intravenous infusion at weeks 0, 2, and 6, and then every 8 weeks. It is recommended as a combination therapy with methotrexate to prevent formation of antibodies to the drug.

Adverse Effects

Increased risk of infection, reactivation of tuberculosis, and invasive, opportunistic fungal infections, in particular, have been documented. Anti-TNF agents have also been related to the development or worsening of demyelinating disorders. Patients can develop lupus-like symptoms with a 1% risk of severe lupus-like disease. A subset of patients develops positive ANAs and anti-DNA titers. Some evidence exists that there is an increased risk of lymphoma, but larger retrospective studies have failed to confirm this. Two large observational studies detected no increased risk of malignancy, except for nonmelanotic skin cancer in one study (odds ratio: 1.5).[100,101] A large meta-analysis of more than 2,900 patients treated for rheumatoid arthritis found no evidence of increased malignancy with any of the biologic agents.[102] Baseline tuberculin skin test is required and repeated annually during the duration of therapy and CBCs and liver function tests should be done every 4 to 6 weeks. Given the relationship between intermediate uveitis and demyelinating disease, the latter must be excluded before starting therapy.

Evidence

Infliximab has been shown to be rapid and effective in Behçet's disease–related panuveitis and retinal vasculitis.[103] It has been shown to be more effective than conventional immunosuppression for Behçet's disease vasculitis.[104] A recent meta-analysis[105] of infliximab for systemic Behçet's disease suggested very high response rates (> 90%) in patients with disease inadequately controlled by conventional immunosuppression. TNF-a inhibitors have shown to be effective in small studies of sarcoid posterior uveitis.[106] However, there are multiple reports that infliximab (and TNF-a inhibitors in general) may cause sarcoid-like conditions.[107,108] Small studies have suggested the efficacy of infliximab for the treatment of several types of uveitis, including refractory birdshot chorioretinopathy[109] (control of inflammation in 89% of patients) and VKH disease.[110,111] Some reports also show efficacy in serpiginous choroidopathy.[112] However, infliximab should be used with caution, as serpiginous choroidopathy has been related to tuberculosis in countries such as India and Germany[113,114] and disseminated tuberculosis is a significant risk in patients using anti-TNF therapy.

Adalimumab

Indications

Adalimumab is used as a second-line, corticosteroid-sparing therapy for patients with ophthalmic manifestations/acute exacerbations of Behçet's disease. It may be considered in patients with vision-threatening, corticosteroid-dependent disease who have failed first-line immunosuppressive therapies.

Mechanism of Action

Adalimumab is a fully human monoclonal antibody against TNF-a.

Dose

It is administered at a dose of 40 mg subcutaneous every other week, and can be increased to every week if additional control is necessary. It can be used in conjunction with other agents such as methotrexate and mycophenolate mofetil.

Adverse Effects

Adverse effects are similar to other TNF-a inhibitors (discussed earlier). Low titers of antibodies have been detected with adalimumab, which itself is a fully humanized antibody.

Evidence

It has been shown to be effective in noninfectious uveitis of various etiologies. A prospective study of 131 patients (48% with posterior/panuveitis) with refractory uveitis showed a significant improvement in vision, inflammation, and macular edema with the use of adalimumab.[115]

A more recent prospective trial of 31 patients with refractory uveitis described a favorable clinical response in 68% of patients at 10 weeks.[116] For Behçet's disease–related uveitis, adalimumab could be an effective alternative to infliximab for well-controlled patients on infliximab wishing to avoid infusions.[117]

Etanercept

Indications

Etanercept may be useful in the treatment of some forms of ocular inflammatory disease, but it has been associated with the development of uveitis and sarcoid-like disease. Use of infliximab or adalimumab should be considered before etanercept, and patients taking etanercept previously should consider switching to infliximab or adalimumab if they have uncontrolled ocular inflammation.

Evidence

Studies have shown that etanercept is less effective at controlling uveitis than other TNF-a inhibitors.[118,119] A retrospective study published in 2006 showed etanercept to be less effective than infliximab for recalcitrant uveitis.[120]

Golimumab is another anti-TNF- a agent which is administered as a subcutaneous injection every month. A few reports available support its efficacy for uveitis.[121,122] Certolizumab contains the fab fragment bound to polyethylene glycol to increase its half-life, but there are no reports on its use for uveitis.

25.7.5 Other Biologic Agents

Rituximab

Indications

Rituximab is currently being studied for use in patients with scleritis, but results are lacking for other forms of uveitis.

Mechanism of Action

It is a murine/human chimeric monoclonal immunoglobulin (Ig) G cytolytic antibody against the CD20 antigen in B lymphocytes. It is given by intravenous infusions of 375 mg/m^2 every week for 4 weeks.

Adverse Effects

Adverse effects include flulike symptoms, headache, nausea, fatigue, and skin rash.

Evidence

Rituximab has been used in Behçet's disease with good results.[123,124] Abatacept is another lymphocyte inhibitor which has been shown to be effective in uveitis secondary to juvenile idiopathic arthritis.

25.8 Specific Receptor Antagonists

25.8.1 Anakinra

Anakinra is a competitive IL-1 receptor antagonist that prevents the activation of IL-1-mediated immune response. Only one report of its use in uveitis exists, but a clinical trial for patients with Behçet's disease is underway.

25.8.2 Canakinumab

Canakinumab is a IL-1ß blocker administered by subcutaneous injection every 4 to 8 weeks. Two reports of success with its use have been published.[125,126]

25.8.3 Gevokizumab

Gevokizumab is a humanized monoclonal antibody that binds to IL-1ß. Phase III, multicenter clinical trials (EYEGUARD) are underway to evaluate its efficacy and safety in active or controlled noninfectious uveitis and Behçet's disease–associated uveitis.

25.8.4 Tocilizumab

Tocilizumab is an anti-IL-6 receptor monoclonal antibody. Doses vary from 4 to 12 mg/kg intravenously every 2 to 4 weeks. Initial evidence for its efficacy in uveitis has been promising, especially regarding uveitic macular edema.[127] Clinical studies are underway.

Alemtuzumab (a CD52-directed cytolytic antibody) is another antibody which was used in a series of six patients with posterior uveitis with five demonstrating clinical improvement.[128] Daclizumab is a monoclonal antibody which binds the IL-2a receptor subunit expressed by B lymphocytes and natural killer cells. Although promising for the treatment of numerous ocular inflammatory conditions, it was discontinued in 2009.

25.8.5 Interferon

Indication

Interferon may be considered for treatment of Behçet's disease and uveitic CME not responsive to traditional immunosuppression.

Mechanism of Action

Interferon-a (IFN-a) is a naturally occurring cytokine, mainly produced by antigen presenting cells. It can lead to the induction of T-helper cells, but also the development of tolerance-promoting regulatory cells. It acts as a modulator of inflammation, exerting an antiproliferative and apoptotic effect on T cells.

Dose

Dosage is controversial, but most authors recommend 3 to 6 million IU per day. It is important to stop all other immunosuppressants and decrease steroids to less than 10 mg as soon as possible because it is believed that these drugs may antagonize the therapeutic effect of interferon.

Adverse Effects

Ninety percent of patients suffer from flulike symptoms, most of which resolve during the first weeks after initiation. Other adverse effects include mild leukopenia (30%), alopecia (10%), and depression (8%). In general, 4 to 7.5% of patients discontinue IFN because of side effects.[129,130]

Evidence

Kötter et al have reported that more than 90% of patients with Behçet's disease responded to treatment and achieved complete remission.[131,132] Interferon has also been found to be effective for CME in those studies.[133] Some authors have stated that using IFN-a induces remission even after discontinuing it (from 20 to 88.7%).[134,135,136] It has also been shown to be effective in uveitic CME not related to Behçet's disease. Uveitic CME frequently does not respond to systemic immunosuppression, so it is believed that interferon has an effect additional to just being an anti-inflammatory.[137] Unlike the Behçet's disease series, these patients did need to continue interferon indefinitely to control their macular edema. There was complete or partial resorption of chronic CME in 87.5% of patients.

25.9 Local Treatments

25.9.1 Topical

Topical steroids are used in the treatment of anterior uveitis and in combination with a nonsteroidal anti-inflammatory for CME.

25.9.2 Periocular Steroids

Indications

Periocular steroids are used in the treatment of posterior segment inflammation, uveitic CME, retinal, optic disc or choroidal neovascularization, chronic anterior chamber, or vitreous inflammation.[1] It is preferred in asymmetric or unilateral disease. It is particularly useful in intermediate uveitis.

Mechanism of Action

Periocular administration permits delivery of a high local concentration of medication minimizing systemic side effects. The duration of action depends on the substance used.

Dose

Doses are 40 mg of triamcinolone acetonide or 3 mg of betamethasone phosphate. Triamcinolone acetonide has an effect for 3 months or more, recommended for conditions such as macular edema. Betamethasone has an effect for about 7 to 10 days which may be useful to treat severe anterior uveitis.

Adverse Effects

Side effects include cataract, ocular hypertension (which can occur in 40% of patients),[138] glaucoma, retinal detachment, vitreous hemorrhage, and endophthalmitis. Other side effects include ptosis, cataracts, globe perforation, and intraocular injection.

Evidence

In a recent review of 914 patients who received periocular injections in the SITE cohort study,[139] the probability of obtaining complete resolution of inflammation was 72.1% (88.9% for anterior uveitis, 66.9% for intermediate uveitis, and 63.6% for posterior uveitis). Visual acuity improved to 20/40 or better in 49.7% of patients. An improvement of 0.2 log MAR or more was reported by 33.1% of patients who had decreased visual acuity because of macular edema. Intraocular pressure higher or equal to 24 mm Hg and higher than 30 mm Hg was experienced by 34 and 15% patients, respectively. Glaucoma surgery was required in 2.4% of patients. Multiple studies have shown that, for uveitic macular edema, repeated injections may be beneficial.[140]

25.9.3 Intraocular Steroids

Intravitreal Triamcinolone

Indications

Intravitreal triamcinolone is used for the treatment of uveitic CME.[141] It can be used to control inflammation in various forms of posterior uveitis.

Dose

It is administered at a dose of 4 mg of triamcinolone acetonide (0.1 mL of a 40 mg/mL suspension) via pars plana injection according to standard procedure. It has a duration of 2 to 4 months and may be repeated based on inflammation. However, as the risk of endophthalmitis increases with numerous injections, if repeated doses are required it is recommended to consider a sustained release corticosteroid implant (see later).

Adverse Effects

Adverse effects include cataract, ocular hypertension (40% of patients develop an IOP higher than 21 mm Hg), glaucoma, retinal detachment, vitreous hemorrhage, and endophthalmitis, which occurs at a rate of between 0.1 and 0.9%.

Evidence

Ample experience with intravitreal triamcinolone has shown its effectiveness in all types of macular edema. In a series of 54 patients with refractory uveitis CME, 83% of patients responded to intravitreal triamcinolone.[142] It has been shown to be effective in several types of uveitis, including Behçet's disease,[143] VKH syndrome,[144] and sympathetic ophthalmia,[145] among others.

25.10 Sustained-Release Corticosteroid Implants

Sustained-release corticosteroid implants are an available alternative to obtain a constant concentration of intraocular steroid without the need for frequent intraocular injections. There are currently three devices available.

25.10.1 Dexamethasone Drug Delivery System

Indications

Dexamethasone drug delivery system was approved by the Food and Drug Administration (FDA) for the treatment of noninfectious posterior uveitis. It is indicated in patients who cannot tolerate systemic immunosuppression and patients with uveitic macular edema or unilateral disease.

Mechanism of Action

Ozurdex (Allergan Inc) is a biodegradable polymer that dissolves completely in the vitreous.[146] The implant contains 700 µg of dexamethasone which is released to the vitreous cavity over a 6-month period. It is administered via a 22-gauge injecting applicator through the pars plana. The pharmacokinetic profile is similar between vitrectomized and nonvitrectomized eyes.[147]

Dose

The dexametasone implants administered through intravitreal injection. It may be repeated when required (4–6 months). The implant is contraindicated in patients with periocular infections, advanced glaucoma, and in patients whose posterior lens capsule is not intact (the latter because of the risk of implant migration into the anterior chamber).

Adverse Events

Adverse events include cataract (with repeated injections), ocular hypertension (15% of patients develop an IOP higher than 21 mm Hg), glaucoma, retinal detachment, vitreous hemorrhage, and endophthalmitis.

Evidence

The phase III trial for Ozurdex for the treatment of noninfectious intermediate or posterior uveitis was published by Lowder et al in 2011.[13] This study included 229 patients and compared two concentrations of dexamethasone versus sham. The group that received the implant had significantly less inflammation which persisted up to 26 weeks. Best corrected visual acuity was also significantly better in the dexamethasone-treated eyes compared to sham (▶ Fig. 25.13).

25.10.2 Fluocinolone Acetonide Implant

Indications

Fluocinolone acetonide implant was approved by the FDA for the treatment of noninfectious posterior uveitis. It is indicated in patients who cannot tolerate systemic immunosuppression and in patients with macular edema or unilateral disease.

Mechanism of Action

Retisert (Bausch & Lomb) contains a 0.59-mg pellet of fluocinolone acetonide in a non-biodegradable polyvinyl acetate/silicone laminate.

Dose

It is implanted in the operating room through a pars plana sclerotomy and secured by a suture in the sclera. The implant loses its effect after about 2.5 to 3 years, when it can be exchanged for a new implant if inflammation recurs.[148] Ocular drug levels are stable over a year with no evidence of systemic absorption.

Adverse Effects

At 3 years of follow-up, 93% of eyes underwent cataract surgery, 75% were treated with IOP-lowering medication, and 40% underwent glaucoma surgery. In some cases, the implant can

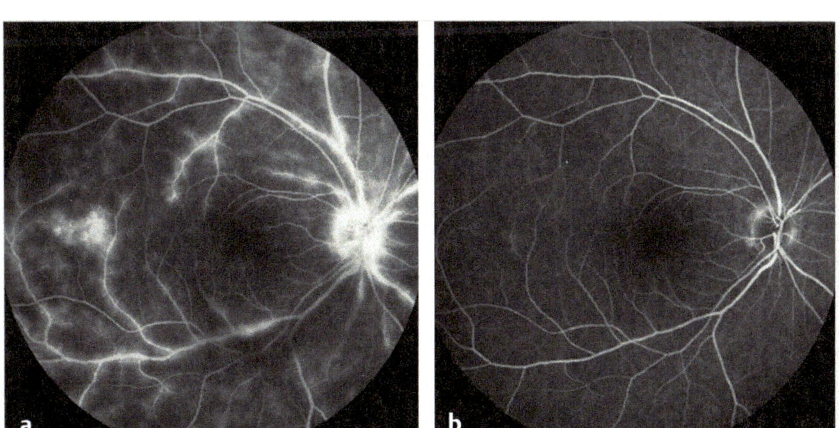

Fig. 25.13 Late-frame fluorescein angiograms of right eye of a 50-year-old woman with posterior segment retinal vasculitis on 2,500 mg of mycophenolate mofetil daily immediately (a) before and (b) 6 weeks after intravitreal injection of dexamethasone sustained delivery implant.

become dissociated from its strut during the removal/exchange procedure.[149,150]

Evidence

The fluocinolone acetonide implant has been shown to decrease recurrence rates of uveitis up to 3 years, increase visual acuity, and allow the tapering of systemic medications in various large prospective trials.[151,152,153] The MUST (Multicenter Uveitis Steroid Treatment) trial was a large prospective trial (255 patients, 479 eyes with uveitis) to compare the efficacy of the implant versus systemic immunosuppression with a follow-up of 24 months.[14] Visual acuity improvement was comparable between both groups, with a gain of 6 letters in the implant group and of 3.2 letters in the systemic therapy group at 24 months ($p = 0.16$). Control of uveitis was more frequent in the implant group (88 vs. 71%, $p = 0.0001$) and CME was significantly decreased up to 6 months. The implant group had a higher rate of cataract surgery (80 vs. 31% in the systemic treatment group) and glaucoma surgery (26.2 vs. 3.7% in the systemic treatment group). Systemic infection requiring prescription therapy was lower in the implant group (0.36 events/person-year in the implant group vs. 0.60 in the systemic therapy group, $p = 0.034$), but the risk of hospitalization was similar between both groups.

25.10.3 Fluocinolone Acetonide Insert

Indications

Pivotal trials are underway to evaluate its effect on noninfectious posterior uveitis.

Mechanism of Action and Dose

Iluvien (Alimera Science) is a small, non-biodegradable cylindrical tube with a central drug-polymer matrix that releases 0.19 mg of fluocinolone acetonide into the vitreous cavity. It is inserted intravitreally via a 25-gauge needle in the same manner as in intravitreal injection. It releases small doses of fluocinolone acetonide for at least 3 years. No systemic absorption has been documented.[154]

Adverse Effects

At 36 months, 81.7% of patients developed cataract, 37.1% had raised IOP, and 4.8% of patients underwent glaucoma surgery.

Evidence

As of the completion of this chapter, no data for its use in uveitis are available.

Special Considerations

- Treat with a steroid-sparing immunosuppressive drug if, after 3 months of adequate treatment and taper, the disease in not controlled on 10 mg of prednisone a day or less.
- Behçet's disease, Birdshot chorioretinitis, serpiginous choroiditis, and sympathetic ophthalmia need steroid-sparing immunosuppression, often in conjunction with steroids, as the initial treatment because the likelihood of control with tolerable doses of steroid is low.
- Multimodal imaging including widefield fundus imaging, OCT, fundus fluorescein angiography, and ICG helps distinguish macular pathology in various posterior segment uveitides.

References

[1] Cunningham ET, Jr, Wender JD. Practical approach to the use of corticosteroids in patients with uveitis. Can J Ophthalmol. 2010; 45(4):352–358

[2] Jabs DA, Nussenblatt RB, Rosenbaum JT, Standardization of Uveitis Nomenclature (SUN) Working Group. Standardization of uveitis nomenclature for reporting clinical data. Results of the First International Workshop. Am J Ophthalmol. 2005; 140(3):509–516

[3] Jabs DA, Rosenbaum JT, Foster CS, et al. Guidelines for the use of immunosuppressive drugs in patients with ocular inflammatory disorders: recommendations of an expert panel. Am J Ophthalmol. 2000; 130(4):492–513

[4] Aaberg TM. The enigma of pars planitis. Am J Ophthalmol. 1987; 103 (6):828–830

[5] Giles CL. Peripheral uveitis in patients with multiple sclerosis. Am J Ophthalmol. 1970; 70(1):17–19

[6] Lam S, Tessler HH. Quadruple therapy for ocular toxoplasmosis. Can J Ophthalmol. 1993; 28(2):58–61

[7] Malinowski SM, Pulido JS, Folk JC. Long-term visual outcome and complications associated with pars planitis. Ophthalmology. 1993; 100(6):818–824, discussion 825

[8] Iannetti L, Spinucci G, Abbouda A, De Geronimo D, Tortorella P, Accorinti M. Spectral-domain optical coherence tomography in uveitic macular edema: morphological features and prognostic factors. Ophthalmologica. 2012; 228 (1):13–18

[9] Castellano CG, Stinnett SS, Mettu PS, McCallum RM, Jaffe GJ. Retinal thickening in iridocyclitis. Am J Ophthalmol. 2009; 148(3):341–349

[10] Ossewaarde-van Norel J, Berg EM, Sijssens KM, Rothova A. Subfoveal serous retinal detachment in patients with uveitic macular edema. Arch Ophthalmol. 2011; 129(2):158–162

[11] Kimura SJ, Hogan MJ. CHRONIC CYCLITIS. Arch Ophthalmol. 1964; 71:193–201

[12] Park SE, Mieler WF, Pulido JS. 2 peripheral scatter photocoagulation for neovascularization associated with pars planitis. Arch Ophthalmol. 1995; 113 (10):1277–1280

[13] Lowder C, Belfort R, Jr, Lightman S, et al. Ozurdex HURON Study Group. Dexamethasone intravitreal implant for noninfectious intermediate or posterior uveitis. Arch Ophthalmol. 2011; 129(5):545–553

[14] Kempen JH, Altaweel MM, Holbrook JT, et al. Multicenter Uveitis Steroid Treatment (MUST) Trial Research Group. Randomized comparison of systemic anti-inflammatory therapy versus fluocinolone acetonide implant for intermediate, posterior, and panuveitis: the multicenter uveitis steroid treatment trial. Ophthalmology. 2011; 118(10):1916–1926

[15] Kaplan HJ. Surgical treatment of intermediate uveitis. Dev Ophthalmol. 1992; 23:185–189

[16] Smith RE, Godfrey WA, Kimura SJ. Chronic cyclitis. I. Course and visual prognosis. Trans Am Acad Ophthalmol Otolaryngol. 1973; 77(6):OP760–OP768

[17] Smith RE, Godfrey WA, Kimura SJ. Complications of chronic cyclitis. Am J Ophthalmol. 1976; 82(2):277–282

[18] Bacon PA, Salmon M. Modes of action of second-line agents. Scand J Rheumatol Suppl. 1987; 64:17–24

[19] Newell FW, Krill AE. Treatment of uveitis with azathioprine (Imuran). Trans Ophthalmol Soc U K. 1967; 87:499–511

[20] Pasadhika S, Kempen JH, Newcomb CW, et al. Azathioprine for ocular inflammatory diseases. Am J Ophthalmol. 2009; 148(4):500–509.e2

[21] Galor A, Jabs DA, Leder HA, et al. Comparison of antimetabolite drugs as corticosteroid-sparing therapy for noninfectious ocular inflammation. Ophthalmology. 2008; 115(10):1826–1832

[22] Rathinam SR, Babu M, Thundikandy R, et al. A randomized clinical trial comparing methotrexate and mycophenolate mofetil for noninfectious uveitis. Ophthalmology. 2014; 121(10):1863–1870

[23] Kruh J, Foster CS. Corticosteroid-sparing agents: conventional systemic immunosuppressants. Dev Ophthalmol. 2012; 51:29–46

[24] Mathews D, Mathews J, Jones NP. Low-dose cyclosporine treatment for sight-threatening uveitis: efficacy, toxicity, and tolerance. Indian J Ophthalmol. 2010; 58(1):55–58

[25] Thomas BJ, Albini TA, Flynn HW, Jr. Multiple evanescent white dot syndrome: multimodal imaging and correlation with proposed pathophysiology. Ophthalmic Surg Lasers Imaging Retina. 2013; 44(6):584–587

[26] dell'Omo R, Pavesio CE. Multiple evanescent white dot syndrome (MEWDS). Int Ophthalmol Clin. 2012; 52(4):221–228

[27] Gross NE, Yannuzzi LA, Freund KB, Spaide RF, Amato GP, Sigal R. Multiple evanescent white dot syndrome. Arch Ophthalmol. 2006; 124(4):493–500

[28] Bryan RG, Freund KB, Yannuzzi LA, Spaide RF, Huang SJ, Costa DL. Multiple evanescent white dot syndrome in patients with multifocal choroiditis. Retina. 2002; 22(3):317–322

[29] Tsai L, Jampol LM, Pollock SC, Olk J. Chronic recurrent multiple evanescent white dot syndrome. Retina. 1994; 14(2):160–163

[30] Callanan D, Gass JD. Multifocal choroiditis and choroidal neovascularization associated with the multiple evanescent white dot and acute idiopathic blind spot enlargement syndrome. Ophthalmology. 1992; 99(11):1678–1685

[31] Jampol LM, Sieving PA, Pugh D, Fishman GA, Gilbert H. Multiple evanescent white dot syndrome. I. Clinical findings. Arch Ophthalmol. 1984; 102 (5):671–674

[32] Gass JD. Acute posterior multifocal placoid pigment epitheliopathy. Arch Ophthalmol. 1968; 80(2):177–185

[33] Ryan SJ, Maumenee AE. Acute posterior multifocal placoid pigment epitheliopathy. Am J Ophthalmol. 1972; 74(6):1066–1074

[34] Savino PJ, Weinberg RJ, Yassin JG, Pilkerton AR. Diverse manifestations of acute posterior multifocal placoid pigment epitheliopathy. Am J Ophthalmol. 1974; 77(5):659–662

[35] Kersten DH, Lessell S, Carlow TJ. Acute posterior multifocal placoid pigment epitheliopathy and late-onset meningo-encephalitis. Ophthalmology. 1987; 94(4):393–396

[36] Wright BE, Bird AC, Hamilton AM. Placoid pigment epitheliopathy and Harada's disease. Br J Ophthalmol. 1978; 62(9):609–621

[37] Goldenberg D, Habot-Wilner Z, Loewenstein A, Goldstein M. Spectral domain optical coherence tomography classification of acute posterior multifocal placoid pigment epitheliopathy. Retina. 2012; 32(7):1403–1410

[38] Spaide RF, Goldberg N, Freund KB. Redefining multifocal choroiditis and panuveitis and punctate inner choroidopathy through multimodal imaging. Retina. 2013; 33(7):1315–1324

[39] Zarranz-Ventura J, Sim DA, Keane PA, et al. Characterization of punctate inner choroidopathy using enhanced depth imaging optical coherence tomography. Ophthalmology. 2014; 121(9):1790–1797

[40] Leung TG, Moradi A, Liu D, et al. Clinical features and incidence rate of ocular complications in punctate inner choroidopathy. Retina. 2014; 34(8):1666–1674

[41] Byron MA, Jackson J, Ansell BM. Effect of different corticosteroid regimens on hypothalamic-pituitary-adrenal axis and growth in juvenile chronic arthritis. J R Soc Med. 1983; 76(6):452–457

[42] Holland GN, Stiehm ER. Special considerations in the evaluation and management of uveitis in children. Am J Ophthalmol. 2003; 135(6):867–878

[43] Urban RC, Jr, Cotlier E. Corticosteroid-induced cataracts. Surv Ophthalmol. 1986; 31(2):102–110

[44] Foster CS, Vitale AT. Diagnosis and Treatment of Uveitis. New Delhi; London: Jaypee Brothers Medical; 2013

[45] Michelson JB, Chisari FV. Behçet's disease. Surv Ophthalmol. 1982; 26 (4):190–203

[46] Mishima S, Masuda K, Izawa Y, Mochizuki M, Namba K. The eighth Frederick H. Verhoeff Lecture. Presented by Saiichi Mishima, MD Behçet's disease in Japan: ophthalmologic aspects. Trans Am Ophthalmol Soc. 1979; 77:225–279

[47] Unoki N, Nishijima K, Kita M, Hayashi R, Yoshimura N. Structural changes of fovea during remission of Behçet's disease as imaged by spectral domain optical coherence tomography. Eye (Lond). 2010; 24(6):969–975

[48] Takeuchi M, Iwasaki T, Kezuka T, et al. Functional and morphological changes in the eyes of Behçet's patients with uveitis. Acta Ophthalmol (Copenh). 2010; 88(2):257–262

[49] Chan CC, Roberge RG, Whitcup SM, Nussenblatt RB. 32 cases of sympathetic ophthalmia. A retrospective study at the National Eye Institute, Bethesda, MD., from 1982 to 1992. Arch Ophthalmol. 1995; 113(5):597–600

[50] Goto H, Rao NA. Sympathetic ophthalmia and Vogt-Koyanagi-Harada syndrome. Int Ophthalmol Clin. 1990; 30(4):279–285

[51] Albert DM, Diaz-Rohena R. A historical review of sympathetic ophthalmia and its epidemiology. Surv Ophthalmol. 1989; 34(1):1–14

[52] Gupta V, Gupta A, Dogra MR, Singh I. Reversible retinal changes in the acute stage of sympathetic ophthalmia seen on spectral domain optical coherence tomography. Int Ophthalmol. 2011; 31(2):105–110

[53] Behdad B, Rahmani S, Montahaei T, Soheilian R, Soheilian M. Enhanced depth imaging OCT (EDI-OCT) findings in acute phase of sympathetic ophthalmia. Int Ophthalmol. 2015; 35(3):433–439

[54] Muakkassa NW, Witkin AJ. Spectral-domain optical coherence tomography of sympathetic ophthalmia with Dalen-Fuchs nodules. Ophthalmic Surg Lasers Imaging Retina. 2014; 45(6):610–612

[55] Moorthy RS, Inomata H, Rao NA. Vogt-Koyanagi-Harada syndrome. Surv Ophthalmol. 1995; 39(4):265–292

[56] Beniz J, Forster DJ, Lean JS, Smith RE, Rao NA. Variations in clinical features of the Vogt-Koyanagi-Harada syndrome. Retina. 1991; 11(3):275–280

[57] Ishihara K, Hangai M, Kita M, Yoshimura N. Acute Vogt-Koyanagi-Harada disease in enhanced spectral-domain optical coherence tomography. Ophthalmology. 2009; 116(9):1799–1807

[58] Nakayama M, Keino H, Okada AA, et al. Enhanced depth imaging optical coherence tomography of the choroid in Vogt-Koyanagi-Harada disease. Retina. 2012; 32(10):2061–2069

[59] da Silva FT, Sakata VM, Nakashima A, et al. Enhanced depth imaging optical coherence tomography in long-standing Vogt-Koyanagi-Harada disease. Br J Ophthalmol. 2013; 97(1):70–74

[60] Takahashi H, Takase H, Ishizuka A, et al. Choroidal thickness in convalescent Vogt-Koyanagi-Harada disease. Retina. 2014; 34(4):775–780

[61] Albert DM, Jakobiec FA. Principles and Practice of Ophthalmology: Clinical practice. Philadelphia, PA: W.B. Saunders; 1994

[62] Gass JDM. Stereoscopic Atlas of Macular Diseases: Diagnosis and Treatment. St. Louis, MO: Mosby; 1997

[63] Laatikainen L, Erkkilä H. A follow-up study on serpiginous choroiditis. Acta Ophthalmol (Copenh). 1981; 59(5):707–718

[64] Nussenblatt RB, Whitcup SM, Palestine AG. Uveitis: Fundamentals and Clinical Practice. Mosby; 1996

[65] Weiss H, Annesley WH, Jr, Shields JA, Tomer T, Christopherson K. The clinical course of serpiginous choroidopathy. Am J Ophthalmol. 1979; 87(2):133–142

[66] Mansour AM, Jampol LM, Packo KH, Hrisomalos NF. Macular serpiginous choroiditis. Retina. 1988; 8(2):125–131

[67] Punjabi OS, Rich R, Davis JL, et al. Imaging serpiginous choroidopathy with spectral domain optical coherence tomography. Ophthalmic Surg Lasers Imaging. 2008; 39(4) Suppl:S95–S98

[68] Ryan SJ, Maumenee AE. Birdshot retinochoroidopathy. Am J Ophthalmol. 1980; 89(1):31–45

[69] Gass JD. Vitiliginous chorioretinitis. Arch Ophthalmol. 1981; 99(10):1778–1787

[70] Nussenblatt RB, Mittal KK, Ryan S, Green WR, Maumenee AE. Birdshot retinochoroidopathy associated with HLA-A29 antigen and immune responsiveness to retinal S-antigen. Am J Ophthalmol. 1982; 94(2):147–158

[71] Keane PA, Allie M, Turner SJ, et al. Characterization of birdshot chorioretinopathy using extramacular enhanced depth optical coherence tomography. JAMA Ophthalmol. 2013; 131(3):341–350

[72] Dreyer RF, Gass DJ. Multifocal choroiditis and panuveitis. A syndrome that mimics ocular histoplasmosis. Arch Ophthalmol. 1984; 102(12):1776–1784

[73] Morgan CM, Schatz H. Recurrent multifocal choroiditis. Ophthalmology. 1986; 93(9):1138–1147

[74] Spaide RF, Yannuzzi LA, Freund KB. Linear streaks in multifocal choroiditis and panuveitis. Retina. 1991; 11(2):229–231

[75] Kempen JH, Daniel E, Gangaputra S, et al. Methods for identifying long-term adverse effects of treatment in patients with eye diseases: the Systemic Immunosuppressive Therapy for Eye Diseases (SITE) Cohort Study. Ophthalmic Epidemiol. 2008; 15(1):47–55

[76] Esterberg E, Acharya NR. Corticosteroid-sparing therapy: practice patterns among uveitis specialists. J Ophthalmic Inflamm Infect. 2012; 2(1):21–28

[77] Chan ES, Cronstein BN. Molecular action of methotrexate in inflammatory diseases. Arthritis Res. 2002; 4(4):266–273

[78] Gangaputra S, Newcomb CW, Liesegang TL, et al. Systemic Immunosuppressive Therapy for Eye Diseases Cohort Study. Methotrexate for ocular inflammatory diseases. Ophthalmology. 2009; 116(11):2188–98.e1

[79] Simonini G, Paudyal P, Jones GT, Cimaz R, Macfarlane GJ. Current evidence of methotrexate efficacy in childhood chronic uveitis: a systematic review and meta-analysis approach. Rheumatology (Oxford). 2013; 52(5):825–831

[80] Daniel E, Thorne JE, Newcomb CW, et al. Mycophenolate mofetil for ocular inflammation. Am J Ophthalmol. 2010; 149(3):423–32.e1, 2

[81] Kaçmaz RO, Kempen JH, Newcomb C, et al. Cyclosporine for ocular inflammatory diseases. Ophthalmology. 2010; 117(3):576–584

[82] Pujari SS, Kempen JH, Newcomb CW, et al. Cyclophosphamide for ocular inflammatory diseases. Ophthalmology. 2010; 117(2):356–365

[83] Allison AC. Mechanisms of action of mycophenolate mofetil. Lupus. 2005; 14 Suppl 1:s2–s8

[84] Kempen JH, Gangaputra S, Daniel E, et al. Long-term risk of malignancy among patients treated with immunosuppressive agents for ocular inflammation: a critical assessment of the evidence. Am J Ophthalmol. 2008; 146 (6):802–12.e1

[85] Doycheva D, Zierhut M, Blumenstock G, Stuebiger N, Deuter C. Mycophenolate mofetil in the therapy of uveitic macular edema—long-term results. Ocul Immunol Inflamm. 2012; 20(3):203–211

[86] Chang PY, Giuliari GP, Shaikh M, Thakuria P, Makhoul D, Foster CS. Mycophenolate mofetil monotherapy in the management of paediatric uveitis. Eye (Lond). 2011; 25(4):427–435

[87] Nussenblatt RB, Palestine AG, Rook AH, Scher I, Wacker WB, Gery I. Treatment of intraocular inflammatory disease with cyclosporin A. Lancet. 1983; 2(8344):235–238

[88] Suzuki N, Kaneko S, Ichino M, Mihara S, Wakisaka S, Sakane T. In vivo mechanisms for the inhibition of T lymphocyte activation by long-term therapy with tacrolimus (FK-506): experience in patients with Behçet's disease. Arthritis Rheum. 1997; 40(6):1157–1167

[89] Hogan AC, McAvoy CE, Dick AD, Lee RW. Long-term efficacy and tolerance of tacrolimus for the treatment of uveitis. Ophthalmology. 2007; 114(5):1000–1006

[90] Murphy CC, Greiner K, Plskova J, et al. Cyclosporine vs tacrolimus therapy for posterior and intermediate uveitis. Arch Ophthalmol. 2005; 123(5):634–641

[91] Foster CS. Cicatricial pemphigoid. Trans Am Ophthalmol Soc. 1986; 84:527–663

[92] Stockman GD, Heim LR, South MA, Trentin JJ. Differential effects of cyclophosphamide on the B and T cell compartments of adult mice. J Immunol. 1973; 110(1):277–282

[93] Clements PJ, Yu DT, Levy J, Paulus HE, Barnett EV. Effects of cyclophosphamide on B- and T-lymphocytes in rheumatoid arthritis. Arthritis Rheum. 1974; 17(4):347–353

[94] Guillevin L, Cordier JF, Lhote F, et al. A prospective, multicenter, randomized trial comparing steroids and pulse cyclophosphamide versus steroids and oral cyclophosphamide in the treatment of generalized Wegener's granulomatosis. Arthritis Rheum. 1997; 40(12):2187–2198

[95] Fairley KF, Barrie JU, Johnson W. Sterility and testicular atrophy related to cyclophosphamide therapy. Lancet. 1972; 1(7750):568–569

[96] Abdalla MI, el-D Bahoat N. Long-lasting remission of Behcet's disease after chlorambucil therapy. Br J Ophthalmol. 1973; 57(9):706–711

[97] Levy-Clarke G, Jabs DA, Read RW, Rosenbaum JT, Vitale A, Van Gelder RN. Expert panel recommendations for the use of anti-tumor necrosis factor biologic agents in patients with ocular inflammatory disorders. Ophthalmology. 2014; 121(3):785–96.e3

[98] de Vos AF, Klaren VN, Kijlstra A. Expression of multiple cytokines and IL-1RA in the uvea and retina during endotoxin-induced uveitis in the rat. Invest Ophthalmol Vis Sci. 1994; 35(11):3873–3883

[99] Pérez-Guijo V, Santos-Lacomba M, Sánchez-Hernández M, Castro-Villegas MdelC, Gallardo-Galera JM, Collantes-Estévez E. Tumour necrosis factor-alpha levels in aqueous humour and serum from patients with uveitis: the involvement of HLA-B27. Curr Med Res Opin. 2004; 20(2):155–157

[100] Wolfe F, Michaud K. The effect of methotrexate and anti-tumor necrosis factor therapy on the risk of lymphoma in rheumatoid arthritis in 19,562 patients during 89,710 person-years of observation. Arthritis Rheum. 2007; 56(5):1433–1439

[101] Chakravarty EF, Michaud K, Wolfe F. Skin cancer, rheumatoid arthritis, and tumor necrosis factor inhibitors. J Rheumatol. 2005; 32(11):2130–2135

[102] Lopez-Olivo MA, Tayar JH, Martinez-Lopez JA, et al. Risk of malignancies in patients with rheumatoid arthritis treated with biologic therapy: a meta-analysis. JAMA. 2012; 308(9):898–908

[103] Suhler EB, Smith JR, Wertheim MS, et al. A prospective trial of infliximab therapy for refractory uveitis: preliminary safety and efficacy outcomes. Arch Ophthalmol. 2005; 123(7):903–912

[104] Tabbara KF, Al-Hemidan AI. Infliximab effects compared to conventional therapy in the management of retinal vasculitis in Behçet disease. Am J Ophthalmol. 2008; 146(6):845–50.e1

[105] Arida A, Fragiadaki K, Giavri E, Sfikakis PP. Anti-TNF agents for Behçet's disease: analysis of published data on 369 patients. Semin Arthritis Rheum. 2011; 41(1):61–70

[106] Cruz BA, Reis DD, Araujo CA, Minas Gerais Vasculitis Study Group. Refractory retinal vasculitis due to sarcoidosis successfully treated with infliximab. Rheumatol Int. 2007; 27(12):1181–1183

[107] Clementine RR, Lyman J, Zakem J, Mallepalli J, Lindsey S, Quinet R. Tumor necrosis factor-alpha antagonist-induced sarcoidosis. J Clin Rheumatol. 2010; 16(6):274–279

[108] Daïen CI, Monnier A, Claudepierre P, et al. Club Rhumatismes et Inflammation (CRI). Sarcoid-like granulomatosis in patients treated with tumor necrosis factor blockers: 10 cases. Rheumatology (Oxford). 2009; 48(8):883–886

[109] Artornsombudh P, Gevorgyan O, Payal A, Siddique SS, Foster CS. Infliximab treatment of patients with birdshot retinochoroidopathy. Ophthalmology. 2013; 120(3):588–592

[110] Khalifa YM, Bailony MR, Acharya NR. Treatment of pediatric Vogt-Koyanagi-Harada syndrome with infliximab. Ocul Immunol Inflamm. 2010; 18 (3):218–222

[111] Zmuda M, Tiev KP, Knoeri J, Héron E. Successful use of infliximab therapy in sight-threatening corticosteroid-resistant Vogt-Koyanagi-Harada disease. Ocul Immunol Inflamm. 2013; 21(4):310–316

[112] Seve P, Mennesson E, Grange JD, Broussolle C, Kodjikian L. Infliximab in serpiginous choroiditis. Acta Ophthalmol (Copenh). 2010; 88(8):e342–e343

[113] Mackensen F, Becker MD, Wiehler U, Max R, Dalpke A, Zimmermann S. QuantiFERON TB-Gold—a new test strengthening long-suspected tuberculous involvement in serpiginous-like choroiditis. Am J Ophthalmol. 2008; 146(5):761–766

[114] Nazari Khanamiri H, Rao NA. Serpiginous choroiditis and infectious multifocal serpiginoid choroiditis. Surv Ophthalmol. 2013; 58(3):203–232

[115] Diaz-Llopis M, García-Delpech S, Salom D, et al. Adalimumab therapy for refractory uveitis: a pilot study. J Ocul Pharmacol Ther. 2008; 24(3):351–361

[116] Suhler EB, Lowder CY, Goldstein DA, et al. Adalimumab therapy for refractory uveitis: results of a multicentre, open-label, prospective trial. Br J Ophthalmol. 2013; 97(4):481–486

[117] Mushtaq B, Saeed T, Situnayake RD, Murray PI. Adalimumab for sight-threatening uveitis in Behçet's disease. Eye (Lond). 2007; 21(6):824–825

[118] Reiff A, Takei S, Sadeghi S, et al. Etanercept therapy in children with treatment-resistant uveitis. Arthritis Rheum. 2001; 44(6):1411–1415

[119] Smith JA, Thompson DJ, Whitcup SM, et al. A randomized, placebo-controlled, double-masked clinical trial of etanercept for the treatment of uveitis associated with juvenile idiopathic arthritis. Arthritis Rheum. 2005; 53 (1):18–23

[120] Galor A, Perez VL, Hammel JP, Lowder CY. Differential effectiveness of etanercept and infliximab in the treatment of ocular inflammation. Ophthalmology. 2006; 113(12):2317–2323

[121] Cordero-Coma M, Salom D, Díaz-Llopis M, López-Prats MJ, Calleja S. Golimumab for uveitis. Ophthalmology. 2011; 118(9):1892.e3–1892.e4

[122] Miserocchi E, Modorati G, Pontikaki I, Meroni P, Gerloni V. Golimumab treatment for complicated uveitis. Clin Exp Rheumatol. 2013; 31(2):320–321

[123] Davatchi F, Shams H, Rezaipoor M, et al. Rituximab in intractable ocular lesions of Behcet's disease; randomized single-blind control study (pilot study). Int J Rheum Dis. 2010; 13(3):246–252

[124] Sadreddini S, Noshad H, Molaeefard M, Noshad R. Treatment of retinal vasculitis in Behçet's disease with rituximab. Mod Rheumatol. 2008; 18 (3):306–308

[125] Ugurlu S, Ucar D, Seyahi E, Hatemi G, Yurdakul S. Canakinumab in a patient with juvenile Behcet's syndrome with refractory eye disease. Ann Rheum Dis. 2012; 71(9):1589–1591

[126] Simonini G, Xu Z, Caputo R, et al. Clinical and transcriptional response to the long-acting interleukin-1 blocker canakinumab in Blau syndrome-related uveitis. Arthritis Rheum. 2013; 65(2):513–518

[127] Adán A, Mesquida M, Llorenç V, et al. Tocilizumab treatment for refractory uveitis-related cystoid macular edema. Graefes Arch Clin Exp Ophthalmol. 2013; 251(11):2627–2632

[128] Dick AD, Meyer P, James T, et al. Campath-1H therapy in refractory ocular inflammatory disease. Br J Ophthalmol. 2000; 84(1):107–109

[129] Bodaghi B, Gendron G, Wechsler B, et al. Efficacy of interferon alpha in the treatment of refractory and sight threatening uveitis: a retrospective monocentric study of 45 patients. Br J Ophthalmol. 2007; 91(3):335–339

[130] Deuter C, Stübiger N, Zierhut M. Interferon-a therapy in noninfectious uveitis. Dev Ophthalmol. 2012; 51:90–97

[131] Kötter I, Günaydin I, Zierhut M, Stübiger N. The use of interferon alpha in Behçet disease: review of the literature. Semin Arthritis Rheum. 2004; 33 (5):320–335

[132] Kötter I, Zierhut M, Eckstein AK, et al. Human recombinant interferon alfa-2a for the treatment of Behçet's disease with sight threatening posterior or panuveitis. Br J Ophthalmol. 2003; 87(4):423–431

[133] Butler NJ, Suhler EB, Rosenbaum JT. Interferon alpha 2b in the treatment of uveitic cystoid macular edema. Ocul Immunol Inflamm. 2012; 20(2):86–90

[134] Gueudry J, Wechsler B, Terrada C, et al. Long-term efficacy and safety of low-dose interferon alpha2a therapy in severe uveitis associated with Behçet disease. Am J Ophthalmol. 2008; 146(6):837–44.e1

[135] Deuter CM, Zierhut M, Möhle A, Vonthein R, Stöbiger N, Kötter I. Long-term remission after cessation of interferon- a treatment in patients with severe uveitis due to Behçet's disease. Arthritis Rheum. 2010; 62(9):2796–2805

[136] Krause L, Altenburg A, Pleyer U, Köhler AK, Zouboulis CC, Foerster MH. Long term visual prognosis of patients with ocular Adamantiades-Behçet's disease treated with interferon-alpha-2a. J Rheumatol. 2008; 35(5):896–903

[137] Deuter CM, Kötter I, Günaydin I, Stübiger N, Doycheva DG, Zierhut M. Efficacy and tolerability of interferon alpha treatment in patients with chronic cystoid macular oedema due to non-infectious uveitis. Br J Ophthalmol. 2009; 93(7):906–913

[138] Jonas JB, Degenring RF, Kreissig I, Akkoyun I, Kamppeter BA. Intraocular pressure elevation after intravitreal triamcinolone acetonide injection. Ophthalmology. 2005; 112(4):593–598

[139] Sen HN, Vitale S, Gangaputra SS, et al. Periocular corticosteroid injections in uveitis: effects and complications. Ophthalmology. 2014; 121(11):2275–2286

[140] Leder HA, Jabs DA, Galor A, Dunn JP, Thorne JE. Periocular triamcinolone acetonide injections for cystoid macular edema complicating noninfectious uveitis. Am J Ophthalmol. 2011; 152(3):441–448.e2

[141] Cunningham MA, Edelman JL, Kaushal S. Intravitreal steroids for macular edema: the past, the present, and the future. Surv Ophthalmol. 2008; 53 (2):139–149

[142] Kok H, Lau C, Maycock N, McCluskey P, Lightman S. Outcome of intravitreal triamcinolone in uveitis. Ophthalmology. 2005; 112(11):1916.e1–1916.e7

[143] Kramer M, Ehrlich R, Snir M, et al. Intravitreal injections of triamcinolone acetonide for severe vitritis in patients with incomplete Behcet's disease. Am J Ophthalmol. 2004; 138(4):666–667

[144] Andrade RE, Muccioli C, Farah ME, Nussenblatt RB, Belfort R, Jr. Intravitreal triamcinolone in the treatment of serous retinal detachment in Vogt-Koyanagi-Harada syndrome. Am J Ophthalmol. 2004; 137(3):572–574

[145] Ozdemir H, Karacorlu M, Karacorlu S. Intravitreal triamcinolone acetonide in sympathetic ophthalmia. Graefes Arch Clin Exp Ophthalmol. 2005; 243 (7):734–736

[146] de Smet MD. Corticosteroid intravitreal implants. Dev Ophthalmol. 2012; 51:122–133

[147] Chang-Lin JE, Burke JA, Peng Q, et al. Pharmacokinetics of a sustained-release dexamethasone intravitreal implant in vitrectomized and nonvitrectomized eyes. Invest Ophthalmol Vis Sci. 2011; 52(7):4605–4609

[148] Driot JY, Novack GD, Rittenhouse KD, Milazzo C, Pearson PA. Ocular pharmacokinetics of fluocinolone acetonide after Retisert intravitreal implantation in rabbits over a 1-year period. J Ocul Pharmacol Ther. 2004; 20(3):269–275

[149] Yeh S, Cebulla CM, Witherspoon SR, et al. Management of fluocinolone implant dissociation during implant exchange. Arch Ophthalmol. 2009; 127 (9):1218–1221

[150] Nicholson BP, Singh RP, Sears JE, Lowder CY, Kaiser PK. Evaluation of fluocinolone acetonide sustained release implant (Retisert) dissociation during implant removal and exchange surgery. Am J Ophthalmol. 2012; 154 (6):969–973.e1

[151] Jaffe GJ, Martin D, Callanan D, Pearson PA, Levy B, Comstock T, Fluocinolone Acetonide Uveitis Study Group. Fluocinolone acetonide implant (Retisert) for noninfectious posterior uveitis: thirty-four-week results of a multicenter randomized clinical study. Ophthalmology. 2006; 113(6):1020–1027

[152] Callanan DG, Jaffe GJ, Martin DF, Pearson PA, Comstock TL. Treatment of posterior uveitis with a fluocinolone acetonide implant: three-year clinical trial results. Arch Ophthalmol. 2008; 126(9):1191–1201

[153] Pavesio C, Zierhut M, Bairi K, Comstock TL, Usner DW, Fluocinolone Acetonide Study Group. Evaluation of an intravitreal fluocinolone acetonide implant versus standard systemic therapy in noninfectious posterior uveitis. Ophthalmology. 2010; 117(3):567–575, 575.e1

[154] Sadiq MA, Agarwal A, Soliman MK, et al. Sustained-release fluocinolone acetonide intravitreal insert for macular edema: clinical pharmacology and safety evaluation. Expert Opin Drug Saf. 2015; 14(7):1147–1156

26 Choroidal Nevus and Melanoma

Carol L. Shields and Jerry A. Shields

26.1 Introduction

There are several melanocytic neoplasms that can occur in the uveal tract (iris, ciliary body, and choroid). The two most important are choroidal nevus and melanoma. It is speculated that benign choroidal nevus can evolve into malignant choroidal melanoma. In this chapter, we will describe the clinical features and management of each condition.

26.2 Choroidal Nevus

26.2.1 Demographics

Choroidal nevus is the most common fundus tumor. It arises from the melanocytes in the choroidal stroma.[1,2] According to a population-based study, the prevalence of choroidal nevus in United States persons older than 40 years is 5% or greater.[3] Although it may arise from a congenital nest of melanocytes, a choroidal nevus may not become pigmented or clinically evident until puberty or young adulthood. In some instances, a choroidal nevus can undergo transformation and develop into a malignant melanoma.[4,5,6,7]

26.2.2 Clinical Features

Choroidal nevus, which is generally visible ophthalmoscopically, can assume several clinical variations. The most common is a flat, homogeneous, slate gray lesion with a slightly ill-defined border. With time, a nevus can develop fine drusen on the surface (▶ Fig. 26.1 and ▶ Fig. 26.2). In some instances, a nevus may be entirely amelanotic. Most nevi are less than 2 mm in thickness. Findings that suggest a nevus could be evolving into a malignant melanoma include a thickness greater than 2 mm, presence of orange pigment on the surface of the lesion, and localized secondary retinal detachment (▶ Fig. 26.3).

The clinical features of choroidal nevus differ slightly depending on patient age. Young patients tend to show little overlying retinal pigment epithelial (RPE) changes or drusen. With increasing age, choroidal nevus demonstrates slightly increased thickness, greater chance for multifocality, and more obvious overlying drusen.[8]

Most choroidal nevi are asymptomatic, but 10to 11% of cases can become symptomatic with decreased visual acuity.[9] The

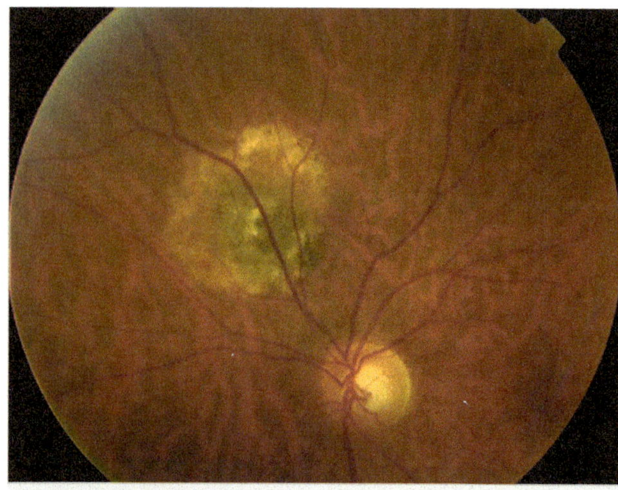

Fig. 26.1 Choroidal nevus with drusen.

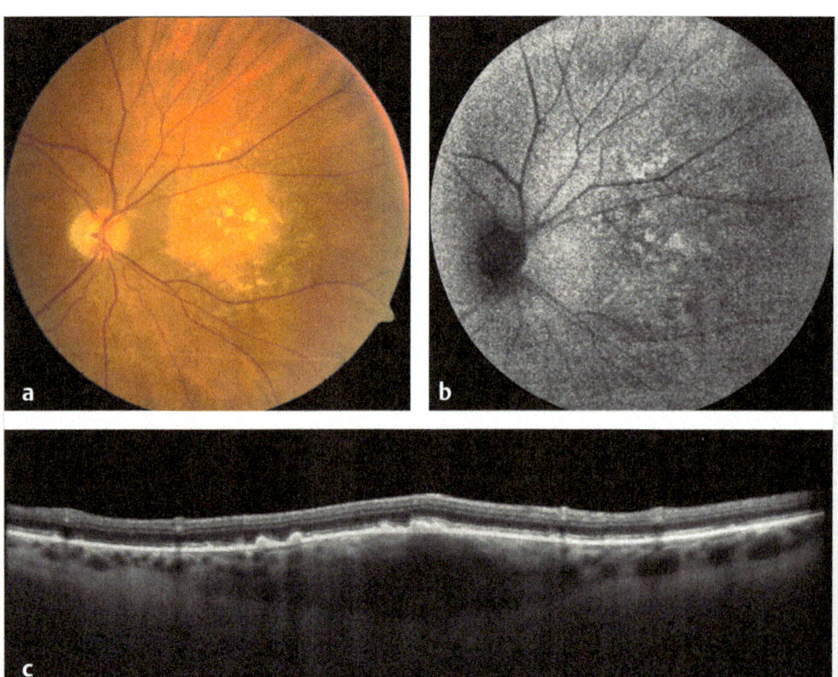

Fig. 26.2 Choroidal nevus showing low risk features. (**a**) Amelanotic nevus with drusen. (**b**) Slight hyperautofluorescence of drusen. (**c**) OCT showing choroidal mass with overlying drusen and outer retinal irregularity.

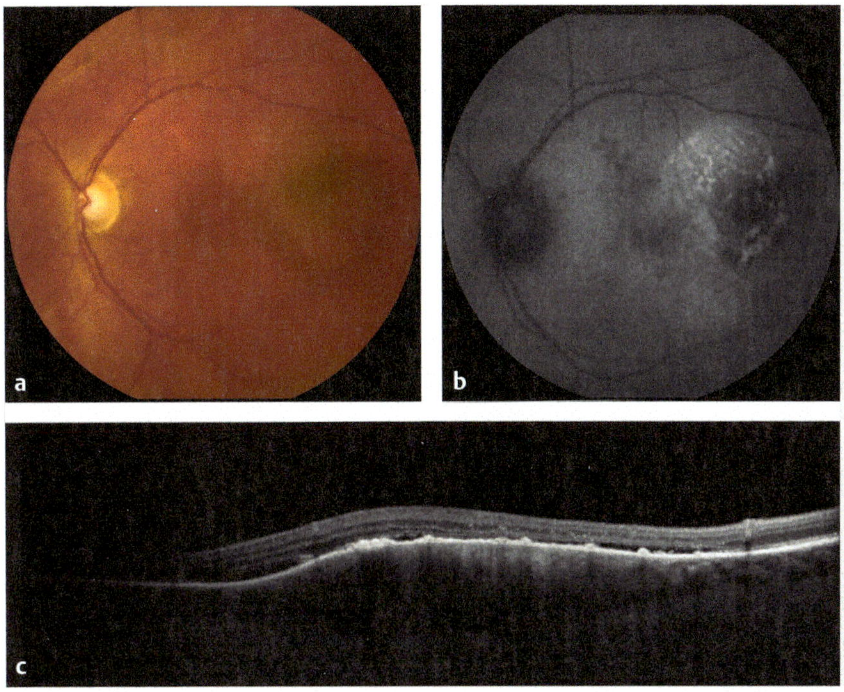

Fig. 26.3 Choroidal nevus with high risk features. (**a**) Nevus with subtle subretinal fluid. (**b**) Hyperautofluorescence of overlying lipofuscin and subretinal fluid. (**c**) OCT showing choroidal mass with overlying drusen, subretinal fluid, and photoreceptor loss.

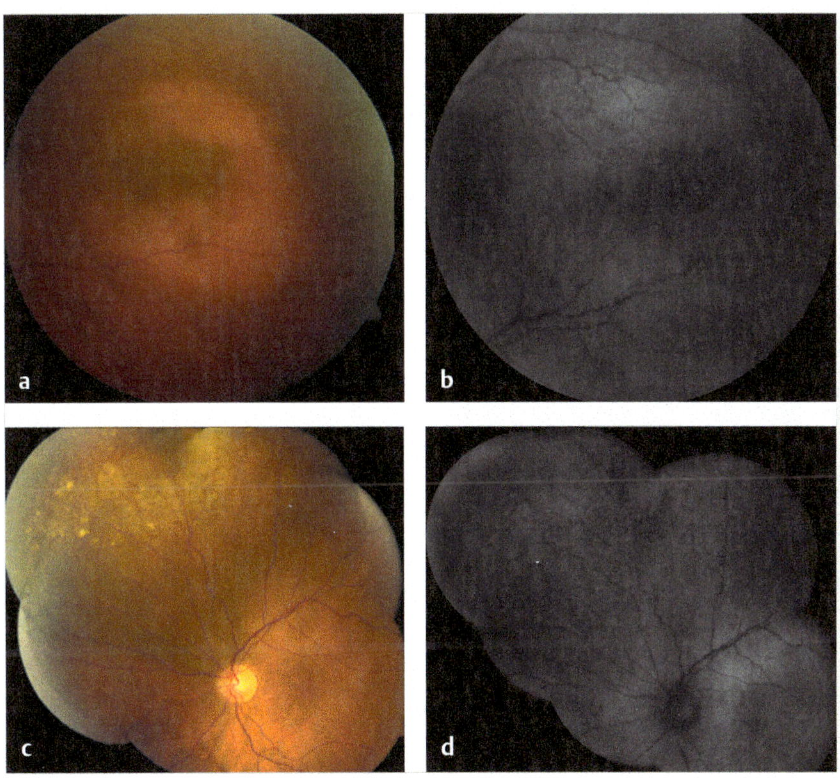

Fig. 26.4 Atypical choroidal nevus. (**a**) Halo nevus with yellow halo. (**b**) Slight hyperautofluorescence of the halo from scleral unmasking. (**c**) Giant nevus with drusen. (**d**) Slight hyperautofluorescence of the drusen.

causes of decreased visual acuity include secondary serous foveal detachment (50%), photoreceptor degeneration (42%), and subretinal choroidal neovascularization overlying the nevus (8%). Decreased visual acuity is more common in patients with subfoveolar nevus. Analysis of visual acuity in 3,422 eyes with choroidal nevi revealed the Kaplan–Meier estimates at 5, 10, and 15 years for vision loss of 3 or more logarithm of the minimum angle of resolution lines at < 1, 1, and 2% of eyes with extrafoveolar nevus compared to 15, 20, and 26% of eyes with subfoveolar nevus.[9]

Choroidal nevus can show minimal growth (< 1 mm base) over many years of follow-up. This does not indicate melanoma transformation. In one large study, about 40% of patients showed growth when comparing images over 7 to 10 years.[10] In about 5% of cases, choroidal nevus demonstrates a surrounding halo, termed "halo nevus" (▶ Fig. 26.4). Patients with halo

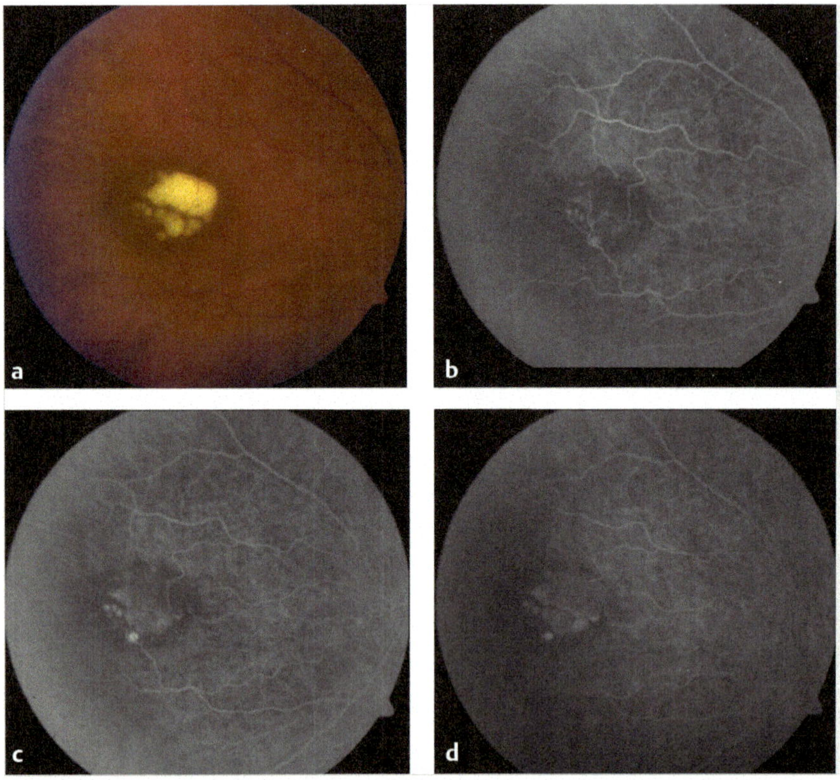

Fig. 26.5 (a) Fluorescein angiography of choroidal nevus (b–d) showing hypofluorescence with staining of overlying RPE detachment.

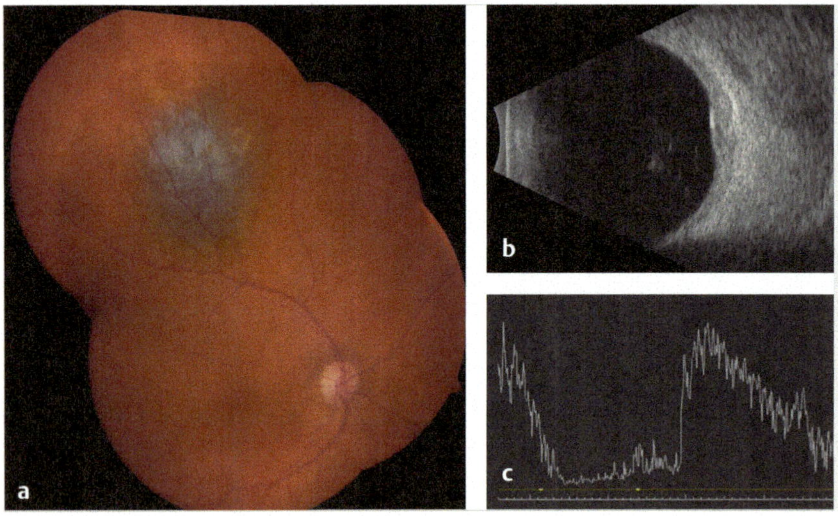

Fig. 26.6 (a) Ultrasonography of choroidal nevus showing (b) acoustically dense mass and (c) high internal reflectivity.

nevus show low risk for transformation to choroidal melanoma.[11] Occasionally, they give a history of skin melanoma and the halo is believed to be an autoimmune response. In about 5% of cases, choroidal nevus can be giant in basal diameter, occupying 10 mm or greater. The giant nevus often has overlying drusen and RPE abnormalities, but has an approximate 15% risk for transformation into melanoma.[12]

26.2.3 Diagnosis

The best way to diagnose a choroidal nevus is with indirect ophthalmoscopy, which reveals the typical ophthalmoscopic features described above. Certain ancillary studies can be employed to facilitate the diagnosis.

Fluorescein angiography of a typical choroidal nevus reveals hypofluorescence of the pigmented portion of the lesion in the vascular filling phases (▶ Fig. 26.5). Amelanotic nevus shows less hypofluorescence and even some hyperfluorescence in the late angiograms. This contrasts with choroidal melanoma, which is generally more hyperfluorescent. Drusen on the surface of a choroidal nevus usually show hyperfluorescence throughout the angiogram sequence as a result of transmission of fluorescence from the choroid. Indocyanine green angiography also generally demonstrates hypofluorescence of most choroidal nevi.

Ultrasonography is of little diagnostic value for choroidal nevus, except to document lesions that are greater than 1 mm in thickness (▶ Fig. 26.6). When a nevus measures greater than 2 mm in thickness on ultrasonography, it should be followed

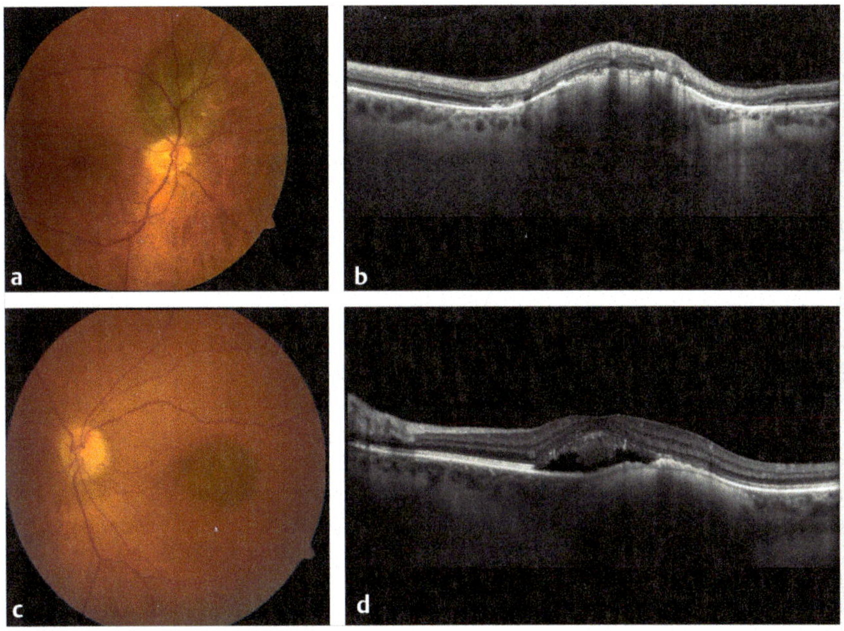

Fig. 26.7 Comparison of (a, b) OCT overlying nevus versus (c, d) small melanoma showing (b) the RPE alterations over the nevus and (d) the shaggy photoreceptors and subretinal fluid over the melanoma.

Table 26.1 Factors for detection of growth of choroidal nevus (=3 mm) into melanoma using the mnemonic "*To find small ocular melanoma using helpful hints daily*"

Initials	Mnemonic	Features	Hazard ratio[a]	Nevus growth into melanoma if feature present (%)	Nevus growth into melanoma if feature absent (%)
T	To	Thickness > 2 mm	2	19	5
F	Find	Fluid	3	27	5
S	Small	Symptoms	2	23	5
O	Ocular	Orange pigment	3	30	5
M	Melanoma	Margin =3 mm to disc	2	13	4
UH	Using helpful	Ultrasound hollow	3	25	4
H	Hints	Halo absent	6	7	2
D	Daily	Drusen absent	N/A	N/A	N/A

Abbreviation: TFSOM UHHD, To find small ocular melanoma using helpful hints daily.

Source: Data adapted from Shields et al.[7]

[a]Not applicable (N/A) as this factor "drusen absent" was identified in other studies to be significant, so it was included in this mnemonic for risk factors.

more closely for evolution into malignant melanoma. Optical coherence tomography (OCT) can assist in demonstrating the choroidal nevus arising in the outer choroid and compressing the choriocapillaris inward[13] (▶ Fig. 26.7). Occasionally there is overlying outer retinal atrophy with photoreceptor loss, subretinal fluid, subretinal cleft, RPE detachment, and retinal edema. On autofluorescence imaging, a choroidal nevus tends to be hypoautofluorescent and the overlying RPE is hypoautofluorescent from chronic atrophy.[14]

26.2.4 Management and Course

A choroidal nevus generally requires no treatment. A choroidal nevus that has produced visual loss through a serous detachment of the fovea can sometimes be managed by anti-vascular endothelial growth factor medications, delimiting photocoagulation, surface photocoagulation directed at leaks, or transpupillary thermotherapy (TT). The patient with a choroidal nevus should be followed periodically on an annual basis, and if growth of the lesion is documented, then evolution into early malignant melanoma should be suspected and the lesion managed accordingly.

The risk factors predictive of transformation of choroidal nevus into melanoma include greater thickness (> 2 mm), subretinal fluid, symptoms (decreased vision, visual field defect, flashes, floaters), orange pigment, margin near disc, ultrasonographic hollowness, and absence of halo or drusen.[4,5,7] A mnemonic (TFSOM UHHD) to recall risk factors of ocular melanoma is "*To find small ocular melanoma using helpful hints daily*," representing *t*hickness, *f*luid, *s*ymptoms, *o*range pigment, *m*argin, *u*ltrasonographic *h*ollowness, *h*alo absence, and *d*rusen absence[7] (▶ Table 26.1). Tumors that display one factor have a 38% chance for growth and those with two or more factors show growth in over 50% of cases at 5 years. The most dangerous combination of factors with a 69% risk for growth include thickness greater than 2 mm, symptoms, and tumor margin at disc. The median hazard ratio for choroidal nevus growth into melanoma for those with 1 to 2 risk factors is 3; for 3 or 4 risk factors is 5; for 5 to 6 risk factors is 9; and for all 7 risk factors is 21. Choroidal nevus with any of the above features should be followed every 6 months or sooner. Most of those tumors with two or more risk factors probably represent small choroidal melanoma and early treatment is indicated.

Controversial Points

- Detection of choroidal melanoma at the earliest point, when it might be as small as a nevus, can be achieved using clinical risk factors of thickness > 2 mm, subretinal fluid, symptoms, orange pigment, margin < 3 mm from optic disc, ultrasound hollow, drusen absent, and halo absent. This could improve patient life prognosis.

26.2.5 Differential Features of Choroidal Nevus versus Melanoma

It is important to differentiate choroidal nevus from a small choroidal melanoma. A small choroidal melanoma generally has a tumor thickness of =2 or 3 mm and exhibits signs of activity including subretinal fluid and/or orange pigment, while a choroidal nevus generally has a thickness < 2 mm and displays signs of chronicity (drusen, RPE atrophy, RPE hyperplasia, RPE detachment, or fibrous metaplasia). On ultrasonography, choroidal nevus exhibits high internal reflectivity and acoustic solidity in contrast to small choroidal melanoma that exhibits medium to low internal reflectivity and acoustic hollowness. Hot spots and leakage on fluorescein angiography are suggestive of growth and transformation of nevus to melanoma. The OCT features of small choroidal melanoma compared with choroidal nevus include increased tumor thickness, subretinal fluid, subretinal lipofuscin deposition, retinal irregularities, and shaggy photoreceptors[13,15] (► Fig. 26.8). The other differential diagnosis of pigmented choroidal nevus includes congenital hypertrophy of RPE, RPE hyperplasia, combined hamartoma of the retinal epithelium and RPE, and subretinal hemorrhage. The amelanotic choroidal nevus must be differentiated from choroidal metastasis, choroidal granuloma, and choroidal lymphoma. Careful fundus examination by an experienced clinician in conjunction with imaging techniques of OCT and fluorescein angiography can differentiate choroidal nevus from other simulating lesions.

26.2.6 Histopathology

Choroidal nevus is a tumor composed of benign uveal melanocytes. Several types of nevus cells have been recognized, but most are composed of spindle-shaped or round to oval cells with benign cytologic features. Choroidal nevi that are composed predominantly of large, ovoid to round cells with densely packed cytoplasmic melanosomes are called melanocytomas, and these cells are identical to cells that comprise the better-known melanocytomas of the optic disc.

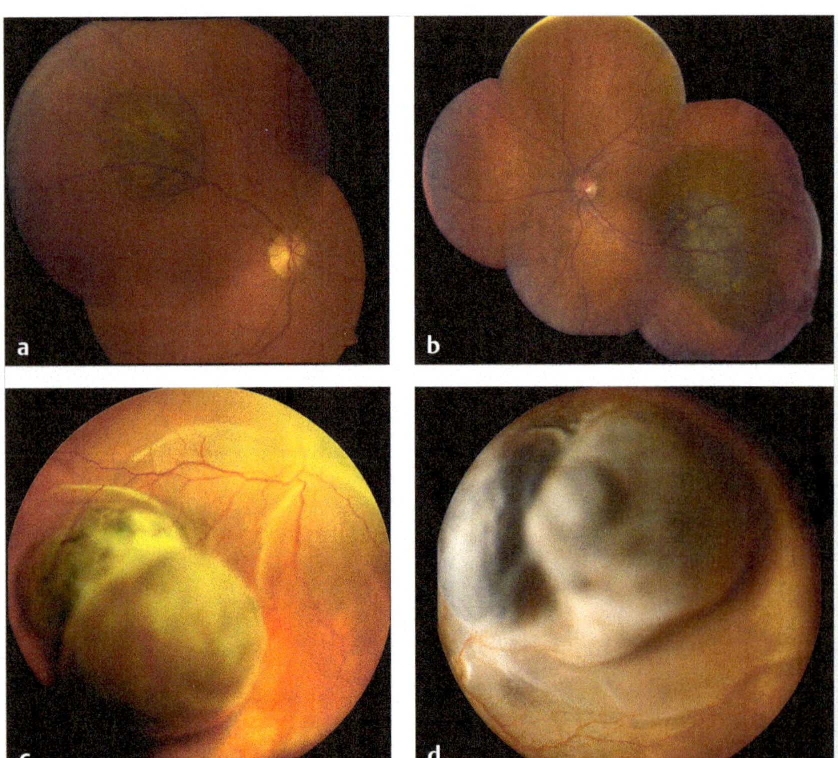

Fig. 26.8 Choroidal melanoma. (**a**) Small choroidal melanoma with orange pigment and subretinal fluid. (**b**) Medium choroidal melanoma with orange pigment and subretinal fluid. (**c**) Large choroidal melanoma with extensive subretinal fluid. (**d**) Extra-large choroidal melanoma with mushroom configuration and subretinal fluid.

Pearls

- Risk factors for choroidal nevus growth to melanoma can be remembered by the mnemonic "*T*o *f*ind *s*mall *o*cular *m*ela*n*oma *u*sing *h*elpful *h*ints *d*aily," representing *t*hickness, *f*luid, *s*ymptoms, *o*range pigment, *m*argin, *u*ltrasonographic *h*ollowness, *h*alo absence, and *d*rusen absence.

26.3 Choroidal Melanoma

26.3.1 Demographics

Choroidal melanoma is the most common primary intraocular malignant tumor among white patients.[16,17] In North America, it is estimated that approximately 2,500 persons develop uveal melanoma annually.[18] It is estimated that there are 7,095 new cases of uveal melanoma worldwide on an annual basis and 4,747 occur in White, 738 in Hispanic, 1,286 in Asian, and 316 in African patients.[18]

The mean age-adjusted incidence of uveal melanoma is 4.3 per million.[19] This figure has remained relatively stable over the past 5 decades. In an analysis of 2,493 cases of uveal melanoma from the National Cancer Institute's Surveillance, Epidemiology, and End Results (SEER) database, uveal melanoma at all ages was more common in men at 4.9 per million compared with women at 3.7 per million.[19] The mean age at presentation was 60 years and there was a range of 6 to 100 years. The age-specific incidence per million population (male/female) differs depending on age and includes 0 to 4 years (0/0), 10 to 14 years (0.2/0), 20 to 24 years (0.4/0.6), 30 to 34 years (1.7/1.7), 40 to 44 years (3.9/2.4), 50 to 54 years (10.5/6.5), 60 to 64 years (14.9/11.7), 70 to 74 years (24.5/17.8), and 80 to 84 years (23.2/16.1).

In an analysis of 8,033 patients with uveal melanoma from a single tertiary referral center over a 4-decade period, Shields and coworkers reported melanoma primarily involving the choroid (90%), ciliary body (6%), or iris (4%).[20] The tumor affected males (51%) or females (49%) and primarily occurred in Caucasians (98%) compared to African American (< 1%), Hispanic (1%), and Asian, Native American, Middle Eastern, and Asian Indian (each < 1%). In this clinic-based study, the mean patient age at detection was 58 years with a range from 3 to 99 years.[20] The tumor was detected in children 20 years or younger (1%), mid-adults 21 to 60 years (53%), and older adults over 60 years (45%).

26.3.2 Symptoms

Choroidal melanoma usually manifests with symptoms of photopsia (flashes), floaters, visual field loss, or visual acuity loss.[20] Some patients have no symptoms. If the tumor involves the ciliary body, sentinel vessels can be noted. Rarely this tumor can cause pain from secondary glaucoma or tumor-related inflammation or necrosis.[21] The importance of annual eye examination is underscored by the fact that uveal melanoma can be asymptomatic and detected on routine eye examination.

26.3.3 Predisposing Factors

Factors related to the development of uveal melanoma involve both host and environmental factors. Weis and coworkers provided a meta-analysis of all published reports on host factors for uveal melanoma and found that light eye color, fair skin color, and inability to tan were risk factors for development of uveal melanoma.[22] Shah and colleagues investigated environmental factors and found that intermittent ultraviolet exposure to arc welding was a significant risk factor.[23] Chronic ultraviolet exposure and occupational sunlight exposure were borderline factors. Factors such as geographic birth latitude and outdoor leisure sunlight exposure were not significantly related to the development of uveal melanoma.

Two important factors for development of uveal melanoma are the presence of a preexisting choroidal nevus and the presence of congenital ocular/oculodermal melanocytosis, also termed "Nevus of Ota." Oculodermal melanocytosis manifests as gray episcleral and cutaneous pigmentation, often with related uveal hyperpigmentation. This condition carries a 1 in 400 lifetime risk for uveal melanoma in Caucasians.[24] The other risk, choroidal nevus, is generally detected in pre-teenage or teenage patients as a pigmented choroidal mass that gradually acquires chronic overlying drusen. In a population-based study, the prevalence of choroidal nevus was 4% in Caucasians, 1% in Hispanics, < 1% in Blacks, and < 1% in Chinese.[25] Singh and associates estimated transformation in 1 in 8,845 in the white population.[6]

Shields and coworkers further investigated the clinical risk factors for transformation of choroidal nevus into melanoma.[4,5,7] They identified eight clinical features that predicted transformation including thickness over 2 mm, subretinal fluid, symptoms, orange pigment, tumor proximity within 3 mm of the optic disc, ultrasound hollowness, halo absent, and drusen absent.[7] Each feature imparted approximately three times greater risk for transformation compared to a tumor without the feature.

26.3.4 Clinical Features

Choroidal melanoma is pigmented in 55%, nonpigmented in 15%, and mixed pigmented/nonpigmented in 30%.[20,26] Choroidal melanoma appears in one of three configurations including dome (75%), mushroom (20%), or diffuse (5%). The mean basal dimension is 11.3 mm and mean thickness is 5.5 mm.[27] Mushroom-shaped choroidal melanoma develops when the tumor breaks through Bruch's membrane and herniates into the subretinal space, giving a bilobed appearance to the tumor. Diffuse melanoma is flat and is often mistaken for a choroidal nevus.[28]

Choroidal melanoma appears as a mass deep to the retina, without retinal feeder vessels, and often produces overlying retinal detachment (▶ Fig. 26.8). Occasionally subretinal hemorrhage is present from rupture in Bruch's membrane and occasionally vitreous hemorrhage is present from retinal invasion. Both can obscure a view of the tumor. In these cases, the tumor can be visible on ocular ultrasonography or magnetic resonance imaging. Rarely, secondary glaucoma can develop.

Special Considerations

- A melanoma or other neoplasm should be suspected in any eye that has unexplained hazy or opaque ocular media. Ultrasonography should be performed in such cases to rule out an intraocular tumor.

Choroidal melanoma is clinically grouped into three sizes based on tumor thickness including small (0–3.0 mm), medium (3.1–8.0 mm), and large (8.1 mm or greater) (▶ Fig. 26.8). In the 1970s, the average melanoma thickness at diagnosis was 5.5 mm. This decreased to approximately 4.5 mm in the 1990s and is currently approximately 4.0 mm. There is hope that efforts at early detection using the mnemonic "*T*o *f*ind *s*mall *o*cular *m*elanoma *u*sing *h*elpful *h*ints *d*aily" will assist in earlier recognition of melanoma and differentiation from nevus[7] (▶ Table 26.1).

26.3.5 Classification

The American Joint Committee on Cancer (AJCC) staging manual, 7th edition, provides a detailed classification for anterior (iris) and posterior (ciliary body [CB] and choroid) uveal melanoma for prognostication. The AJCC classification for posterior uveal melanoma involves grading according to size category based on a combination of basal diameter and thickness, labeled as T1, T2, T3, and T4 with increasing category[29,30] (▶ Table 26.2). Subclassification of each category is judged by absence of CB involvement and extraocular extension (EOE) (a), presence of CB involvement (b), presence of EOE =5 mm (c), and presence of both CB involvement and EOE (d). Of 7,731 patients with posterior uveal melanoma, the AJCC classification based category T1 in 3,557 (46%), T2 in 2,082 (27%), T3 in 1,599 (21%), and T4 in 493 (6%)[29] (▶ Table 26.3). Based on tumor category T1, T2, T3, and T4, respectively, features that showed significant increase with tumor category include patient age at presentation (57, 58, 58, and 61 years) ($p < 0.001$), tumor base (mm) (8, 12, 15, and 20) ($p < 0.001$), tumor thickness (mm) (3.5, 5.2, 8.9, and 11.4) ($p < 0.001$), mushroom configuration (8, 20, 38, and 39%) ($p < 0.001$), associated subretinal fluid (64, 80, 82, and 83%) ($p < 0.001$), intraocular hemorrhage (5, 12, 17, and 18%) ($p < 0.001$), rupture of Bruch's membrane (9, 24, 40, and 40%) ($p < 0.001$), and EOE (1, < 1, 4, and 12%) ($p < 0.001$).[28] Kaplan Meier estimates of metastasis at 10 years were 15% for T1, 25% for T2, 49% for T3, and 63% for T4.[29] Compared with uveal melanoma classified as T1, the rate of metastasis and death was 2 times greater for T2, 4 times greater for T3, and 8 times greater for T4.[29]

26.3.6 Diagnostic Testing

The most reliable way to establish the diagnosis of choroidal melanoma is based on clinical examination in the hands of an experienced observer. Ancillary testing using transillumination, fluorescein angiography, indocyanine green angiography, ultrasonography, enhanced depth imaging OCT, autofluorescence, and fine needle aspiration biopsy can also be helpful.[13,14,15]

Table 26.2 Classification of posterior uveal melanoma using the American Joint Commission on Cancer Classification (7th ed): Tumor category

Melanoma thickness (mm)	Category						
> 15	4	4	4	4	4	4	4
12.1–15	3	3	3	3	3	4	4
9.1–12	3	3	3	3	3	3	4
6.1–9	2	2	2	2	3	3	4
3.1–6	1	1	1	2	2	3	4
=3	1	1	1	1	2	2	4
	=3	3.1–6	6.1–9	9.1–12	12.1–15	15.1–18	> 18
	Melanoma basal diameter (mm)						

Source: Adapted from Shields et al.[29]

Table 26.3 Metastasis of choroidal melanoma based on the American Joint Commission on Cancer Classification (7th ed) in 7,731 patients

Metastasis by category	% at 1 y	% at 3 y	% at 5 y	% at 10 y	% at 15 years	% at 20 y
T1	1	4	8	15	20	25
T2	1	7	14	25	32	40
T3	3	19	31	49	60	62
T4	11	32	51	63	68	68

Source: Data adapted from Shields et al.[29]

Transillumination techniques can be used to document the shadow caused by uveal melanoma. The size of the shadow is helpful in determining what type of treatment can be employed. With fluorescein angiography, choroidal melanoma typically shows initial mottled hyperfluorescence in the venous phase and progressive hyperfluorescence into the recirculation phase. A larger choroidal melanoma can show early hyperfluorescence, representing tumor vessels deep within the mass. Clearly visible intratumoral vessels underlying the elevated retinal vessels on fluorescein angiography are referred to as the "double circulation" sign. In contrast, a subretinal hematoma, which can simulate a melanoma, is generally hypofluorescent throughout the fluorescein angiogram. In some instances, indocyanine green angiography can better delineate typical intratumoral blood vessels that may not be evident with ophthalmoscopy or standard fluorescein angiography.

B-scan ultrasonography usually shows a choroidal melanoma to have acoustic hollowness, choroidal excavation, and orbital shadowing. A-scan ultrasonography shows relatively low internal reflectivity within the tumor. A characteristic feature of choroidal melanoma is spontaneous vascular pulsation that can be best visualized with dynamic standardized A-scan ultrasonography. A typical mushroom-shaped mass with B-scan ultrasonography is highly suggestive of choroidal melanoma. OCT depicts small melanoma within the choroid as dome shaped and often with overlying subretinal fluid that shows shaggy photoreceptors. Larger tumors are not well imaged with OCT, but shallow subretinal fluid can be seen. Small to medium melanoma tend to show hyperautofluorescence form the overlying orange pigment, representing lipofuscin. In the occasional case that is atypical and defies diagnosis with less invasive measures, fine-needle aspiration biopsy can be employed to establish the diagnosis.[31]

Pearls

Characteristic ultrasonographic features of a choroidal melanoma include the following:

- A scan: low-to-medium internal reflectivity and spontaneous vascular pulsations
- B scan: dome- or mushroom-shape, acoustic hollowness, choroidal excavation

26.3.7 Management

The management of melanoma depends on tumor size, tumor location, associated features, status of the opposite eye, patient systemic status, and patient desire. Management choices for choroidal melanoma include TT, plaque radiotherapy, charged particle irradiation, local resection, enucleation, or orbital exenteration.[16,17] The two most frequently employed treatments for choroidal melanoma include enucleation or focal radiotherapy, using plaque radiotherapy or proton beam radiotherapy. The goal of treatment is to eradicate or inactivate the tumor before metastasis occurs. A patient with a suspected uveal melanoma should have a physical examination, blood studies for liver enzymes, chest X-ray, and magnetic resonance imaging (MRI) of the liver. The great majority of affected patients have a negative initial systemic evaluation. However, metastatic disease can occur later in the course of disease at an interval of 3 to 10 years and rarely after 17 years.[32]

Laser photocoagulation was employed in the past for treatment of small choroidal melanoma, but late recurrences were a problem so this method has been replaced by TT, with deeper choroidal effect, and custom plaque radiotherapy.

TTT is a method of treatment for small, pigmented choroidal melanomas that are less than 3 mm in thickness, outside the macular and juxtapapillary region, and with minimal related subretinal fluid. Focused heat is delivered to the tumor with a diode laser delivery system in the infrared range. A large spot size of 3.0 mm and long exposure of 1 minute per spot are employed to provide deep slow burns to the choroid, leading to focal choroidal atrophy. TTT is also used as a consolidation therapy follow plaque radiotherapy to minimize tumor recurrence and to eradicate residual scar that could lead to "toxic tumor syndrome," in which the tumor exudes factors into the vitreous cavity that could lead to retinal degeneration and vision loss.

Photodynamic therapy with verteporfin dye is occasionally used as a primary or secondary treatment for amelanotic melanoma.

Radiotherapy is effective for treatment of melanoma using a radioactive plaque (brachytherapy) or charged particles (proton bream or helium ion). The most widely employed method of radiotherapy is application of a radioactive plaque on the sclera over the base of the tumor. Iodine 125 and Ruthenium 106 are the most commonly employed isotopes. In most cases, melanoma can be controlled with radiotherapy.[32,33,34,35,36,37] The Collaborative Ocular Melanoma Study (COMS) showed prospectively that plaque radiotherapy provided equivalent life prognosis compared to enucleation for medium-sized melanoma.[34] For melanoma near the optic nerve, special notched radioactive plaques are used. Combined plaque radiotherapy and thermotherapy has been shown to improve tumor control to approximately 98%.

Local resection is a surgical method to excise melanoma and salvage the eye, particularly for those tumors located in the ciliary body or peripheral choroid. This technique, termed partial lamellar sclerouvectomy, allows removal of the tumor with a thin scleral base, leaving intact the outer sclera and the retina. It is a difficult surgical procedure and is best performed by ophthalmic oncologists who are experienced with such surgery.

Enucleation is employed for large melanoma or those where no useful vision can be expected with conservative methods. Enucleation is performed with a gentle, minimal manipulation technique to minimize the theoretical possibility of tumor dissemination from surgical trauma. Most surgeons who perform enucleation prefer to use one of the newer integrated orbital implants, such as the hydroxyapatite implant. When a melanoma demonstrates transscleral extension with massive orbital involvement, an eyelid-sparing orbital exenteration is warranted.

26.3.8 Prognosis

Patients with uveal melanoma are at risk for metastatic disease to the liver, lung, and skin. Systemic monitoring with physical examination and liver function tests twice yearly and chest radiograph and liver imaging using MRI or ultrasonography annually is advised.

Table 26.4 Metastasis of choroidal melanoma based on millimeters in tumor thickness in 7,354 patients

Choroidal melanoma		Kaplan–Meier estimates for metastasis		
Tumor thickness (mm)	Number of patients	% at 3 y	% at 5 y	% at 10 y
0–1.0	68	2	4	7
1.1–2.0	535	3	6	13
2.1–3.0	1,467	2	4	10
3.1–4.0	1,247	3	7	16
4.1–5.0	809	7	12	24
5.1–6.0	611	8	14	27
6.1–7.0	513	8	13	27
7.1–8.0	512	12	20	39
8.1–9.0	403	16	26	49
9.1–10.0	381	16	28	53
> 10.0	808	23	35	58
Total	7,354	8	13	25

Source: Data adapted from Shields et al.[27]

Poor prognosis with uveal melanoma depends on several factors, such as tumor location in the ciliary body, large tumor size, diffuse (flat) configuration, and EOE. Additionally, histopathologic and cytogenetic factors including epithelioid cell type, increased mitotic activity, infiltrating lymphocytes, tumor vascular networks, and chromosomal mutations including monosomy 3 and 8q addition can indicate poor outcome. Shields and coworkers provided a comprehensive overview of metastasis of uveal melanoma by millimeter size in 8,033 patients and found that each millimeter increase in thickness was associated with a 5% increased rate of metastasis[27] (▶ Table 26.4). Thus, the rate of metastasis for choroidal melanomas measuring 4 or 8 mm in thickness would be estimated at 20 or 40%, respectively. Clinical factors predictive of metastasis by multivariate analysis include increasing patient age, ciliary body location, increasing tumor diameter, increasing tumor thickness, pigmented melanoma, and the presence of subretinal fluid, intraocular hemorrhage, or EOE.[27]

Diffuse melanoma has a clinically distinct, relatively flat melanoma growth pattern, with tumor thickness of 3 mm or less and thickness to base ratio less than 20%.[28] This tumor is often mistaken for benign choroidal nevus. In an analysis of 8,033 patients with uveal melanoma, diffuse melanoma represented 3% of all cases and imparted a 3.84 relative risk for metastasis compared to nondiffuse melanoma. Recent analysis of 1,751 cases of diffuse choroidal melanoma disclosed melanoma-related metastasis (diffuse vs. nondiffuse) was 17% versus 10% at 10 years.[28] Even in the thinnest tumors of 2 mm or less, diffuse configuration has worse prognosis with melanoma-related death (diffuse versus nondiffuse) of 10% versus 2% at 10 years.

Ocular melanocytosis imparts an increased risk for melanoma and is associated with a higher risk for metastatic disease. In an assessment of 7,872 patients with uveal melanoma, metastasis was 2.6 times higher in patients with choroidal melanocytosis ($p = 0.021$), and 1.9 times higher in patients with scleral melanocytosis ($p < 0.001$).[38] By Kaplan–Meier estimates, metastasis in patients with ocular melanocytosis versus no melanocytosis was 48% Kaplan–Meier versus 24% at 10 years.[38]

It is unclear at what size choroidal melanoma poses a risk for metastasis. Based on clinical studies, small melanoma, at approximately 1 mm in thickness, has occasionally shown metastasis.[27] Based on mathematical studies of tumor doubling time of choroidal melanoma and related metastasis, some authors have estimated that 30 doubling times of a metastatic tumor will occur before a metastasis is clinically detectable, at 1,000 mm3 in size.[39,40] These authors theorized that the average volume of a uveal melanoma at the time that tumor metastasis occurs to other organs, is approximately 7 mm3 size or 3 mm in base and 1.5 mm in thickness. Hence, metastases from choroidal melanoma generally occur when melanoma is small and easily confused with a benign choroidal nevus.

The COMS was designed to evaluate management of choroidal melanoma in a prospective fashion. The COMS comprised three substudies including the large, medium, and small choroidal melanoma trials. The large tumor trial showed no difference in patient survival when comparing enucleation versus preenucleation radiation groups.[33] Five-year Kaplan–Meier estimates for survival were 57% for the enucleation group and 62% for the preenucleation radiation group. The medium tumor trial showed no difference in patient survival when comparing enucleation versus plaque radiotherapy.[34] The cumulative all-cause mortality at 12 years was 43% for patients in the plaque radiotherapy group versus 41% for those in the enucleation group. The small tumor trial showed that small choroidal melanomas managed by observation showed tumor growth in 21% of patients by 2 years and 31% by 5 years.

26.3.9 Histopathology and Cytogenetics

Posterior uveal melanoma probably develops most often from malignant transformation of a preexisting benign nevus, and less often it seems to arise de novo, without evidence of a preexisting lesion. The stimulus for evolution into melanoma is unknown.

On gross examination following enucleation or surgical resection, posterior uveal melanoma has a characteristic appearance. It can be dome-shaped, mushroom-shaped, or diffuse. Microscopically, it can be composed of less malignant spindle cells, more malignant epithelioid cells, or a combination of both (mixed cell type). Pathologic findings that are associated with a worse systemic prognosis include more malignant cell type, larger basal tumor diameter, presence of extrascleral extension, and ciliary body involvement.

Cytogenetic analysis of melanoma using DNA or RNA methods can add to the prognostication of uveal melanoma. Regarding DNA evaluation, the original work from Prescher and colleagues in 1996 demonstrated that uveal melanoma in enucleated eyes often showed chromosome 3 monosomy, which imparted poor prognosis with metastatic disease in 50% by 3 years compared to no metastatic disease in those with disomy 3.[41] Kilic and colleagues found additional mutations in chromosome 8 (53%), chromosome 6 (46%), and chromosome 1 (24%).[42] They concluded that Damato monosomy 3 and largest tumor diameter were the most significant factors in patient survival. and associates evaluated 452 choroidal melanomas for DNA using multiplex ligation-dependent probe amplification (MLPA) and found a 10-year melanoma-related mortality rate of 0% for those with disomy compared to 55% for those with monosomy 3 and 71% for those with monosomy 3 plus 8q gain.[43] Shields and coworkers reported on 500 consecutive eyes with melanoma sampled by fine needle aspiration biopsy at the time of plaque radiotherapy. They concluded that tumors with complete monosomy 3 showed a cumulative probability of metastasis of 0% for small, 24% for medium, and 58% for large melanomas at 3 year follow-up and speculated that the risk increased with longer follow-up.[44]

Regarding RNA evaluation, gene expression profiling (GEP) has been employed. In 2003, GEP was explored by Tschentscher and colleagues, who identified two groups of melanoma that correlated with monosomy 3 and disomy 3 tumors.[45] In 2004, Onken and colleagues used GEP to confirm the presence of 2 classes of melanoma in which class 1 (low grade) was associated with 95% survival and class 2 (high grade) was associated with only 31% survival at 8 years.[46]

26.3.10 Pseudomelanoma

There are conditions that can simulate melanoma clinically, leading to diagnostic ambiguity. In an analysis of 12,000 patients referred for uveal melanoma over a 25-year period, 1,739 were found to have pseudomelanoma.[47] The lesions misdiagnosed as uveal melanoma most frequently include choroidal nevus ($n = 851$, 49%), peripheral exudative hemorrhagic chorioretinopathy (PEHCR) ($n = 139$, 8%), congenital hypertrophy of the RPE (CHRPE) ($n = 108$ cases, 6%), idiopathic hemorrhagic detachment of the retina or RPE ($n = 86$, 5%), circumscribed choroidal hemangioma ($n = 79$ cases, 5%) and age-related macular degeneration ($n = 76$ cases, 4%) (▶ Fig. 26.9; ▶ Table 26.5).

The most common pseudomelanoma, choroidal nevus, can appear remarkably similar to small choroidal melanoma. Melanoma typically shows growth over time whereas nevus is usually stable. Using the aforementioned clinical risk factors (▶ Table 26.1), melanoma can generally be differentiated from nevus.

Peripheral exudative hemorrhagic chorioretinopathy (PEHCR) is a peripheral retinal degeneration of the elderly manifesting

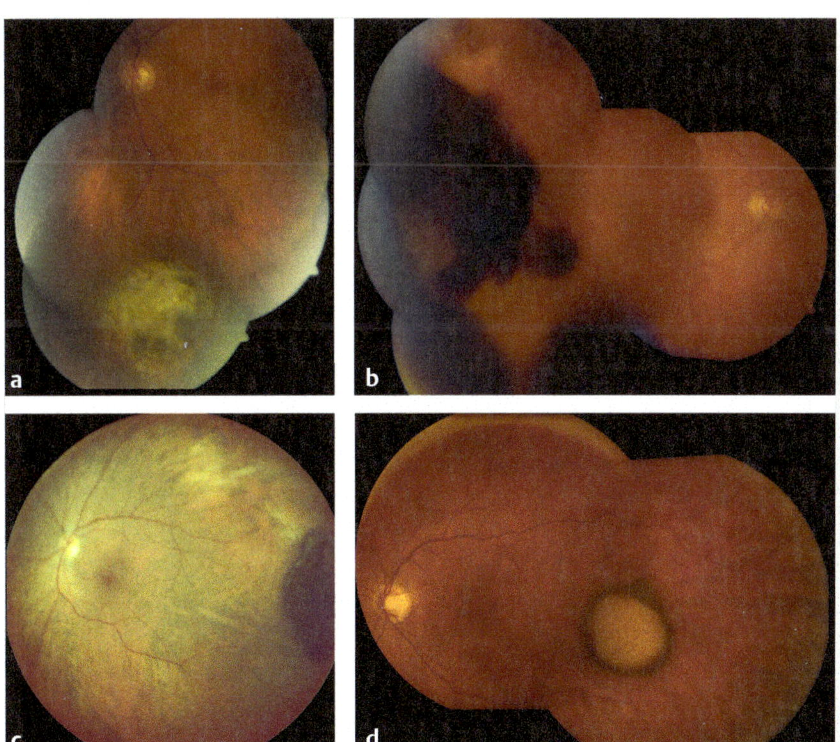

Fig. 26.9 Choroid pseudomelanoma. (**a**) Choroid nevus with overlying drusen. (**b**) Peripheral exudative hemorrhagic chorioretinopathy with extensive subretinal hemorrhage. (**c**) Congenital hypertrophy of the retinal pigment epithelium with crisp margin. (**d**) Retinal pigment epithelial hemorrhagic detachment with partial resolution of blood.

Table 26.5 Choroidal pseudomelanomas in 1,739 cases (most common diagnoses)

Rank	Diagnosis	Number	%
1	Choroidal nevus	851	49
2	Peripheral exudative hemorrhagic chorioretinopathy	139	8
3	Congenital hypertrophy of retinal pigment epithelium	108	6
4	Idiopathic hemorrhagic detachment retina or pigment epithelium	86	5
5	Circumscribed choroidal hemangioma	79	5
6	Age-related macular degeneration	76	4
7	Hyperplasia or RPE	42	2
8	Optic disc melanocytoma	37	2
9	Choroidal metastasis	34	2
10	Hemorrhagic choroidal detachment	29	2
11	Vasoproliferative tumor	20	1
12	Rhegmatogenous retinal detachment	18	1
13	Choroidal detachment	17	1
14	Uveal effusion syndrome	17	1
15	Choroidal or disc granuloma	14	1
16	Adenoma RPE or CPE	13	< 1
17	Sclerochoroidal calcification	12	1
18	Staphyloma	12	1
19	Cataract	10	1
20	Retinal capillary hemangioma (capillary or cavernous)	10	1
21	Adenoma of nonpigmented ciliary body epithelium	10	< 1
22	Leiomyoma, ciliary body	10	< 1
23	Degenerative retinoschisis	8	< 1
24	Retinal cavernous hemangioma	7	< 1
25	Chorioretinal scar	7	< 1
26	Vortex vein varix	7	< 1
27	Vitreous hemorrhage	7	< 1
28	Choroidal osteoma	5	< 1
29	Preretinal macular gliosis	5	< 1
30	Scleritis	5	< 1

Abbreviations: CPE, ciliary pigment epithelium; RPE, retinal pigment epithelial.

Source: Data adapted from Shields et al.[47]

with exudative and hemorrhagic changes. This condition can simulate melanoma closely as a homogenous deep brown mass in the periphery. However, PEHCR shows blockage on fluorescein angiography, echodensity with retraction cleft on ultrasonography, and spontaneous resolution. In an analysis of 173 eyes with PEHCR, the hemorrhagic pseudomelanoma showed a mean diameter of 10 mm and a mean thickness of 3 mm. Spontaneous resolution occurred in 89% of cases.

26.4 Conclusion

Choroidal nevus is the most common benign tumor of the choroid. It generally remains asymptomatic, unless the tumor is located under the foveola, in which case visual loss can ensue. Periodic observation is recommended for all patients with choroidal nevus. The ophthalmologist should be aware of the risk features predictive of growth of choroidal nevus into melanoma. The risk factors can be recalled using the mnemonic "*To find small ocular melanoma using helpful hints daily*," representing *t*hickness > 2 mm, *f*luid, *s*ymptoms, *o*range pigment, *m*argin near disc, *u*ltrasonographic *h*ollowness, *h*alo absence, and *d*rusen absence.

Choroidal melanoma is a malignant tumor with a 30 to 40% risk for metastasis and death. Some melanomas are tiny, as small as choroidal nevi. Patients with suspicious nevi should be examined by an ocular oncologist to ascertain the possibility for melanoma. Early detection is important, particularly when the tumor is small, to minimize risk for metastasis. Patients with suspected choroidal melanoma should have prompt ocular treatment.

26.5 Acknowledgments

The authors thank the Ocular Oncology Service, Wills Eye Hospital, Thomas Jefferson University, Philadelphia, PA. The authors also received support from the Eye Tumor Research Foundation, Philadelphia, PA, and Lift for a Cure, Morrisville, PA.

References

[1] Shields JA, Shields CL. Choroidal nevus. In: Shields JA, Shields CL. An Atlas and Textbook. 3rd edition. Philadelphia, Lippincott Wolters Kluwers; 2016; 69-212.

[2] Shields JA, Shields CL. Choroidal Nevus. Intraocular Tumors. An Atlas and Textbook. 2nd ed. Philadelphia: Lippincott Williams and Wilkins; 2008;59-68

[3] Qiu M, Shields CL. Choroidal Nevus in the United States Adult Population: Racial Disparities and Associated Factors in the National Health and Nutrition Examination Survey. Ophthalmology. 2015 Oct; 122(10):2071–83

[4] Shields CL, Shields JA, Kiratli H, De Potter P, Cater JR. Risk factors for growth and metastasis of small choroidal melanocytic lesions. Ophthalmology. 1995; 102(9):1351–1361

[5] Shields CL, Cater J, Shields JA, Singh AD, Santos MC, Carvalho C. Combination of clinical factors predictive of growth of small choroidal melanocytic tumors. Arch Ophthalmol. 2000; 118(3):360–364

[6] Singh AD, Kalyani P, Topham A. Estimating the risk of malignant transformation of a choroidal nevus. Ophthalmology. 2005; 112(10):1784–1789

[7] Shields CL, Furuta M, Berman EL, et al. Choroidal nevus transformation into melanoma: analysis of 2514 consecutive cases. Arch Ophthalmol. 2009; 127 (8):981–987
[8] Shields CL, Furuta M, Mashayekhi A, et al. Clinical spectrum of choroidal nevi based on age at presentation in 3422 consecutive eyes. Ophthalmology. 2008; 115(3):546–552.e2
[9] Shields CL, Furuta M, Mashayekhi A, et al. Visual acuity in 3422 consecutive eyes with choroidal nevus. Arch Ophthalmol. 2007; 125(11):1501–1507
[10] Mashayekhi A, Siu S, Shields CL, Shields JA. Slow enlargement of choroidal nevi: a long-term follow-up study. Ophthalmology. 2011; 118(2):382–388
[11] Shields CL, Maktabi AM, Jahnle E, Mashayekhi A, Lally SE, Shields JA. Halo nevus of the choroid in 150 patients: the 2010 Henry van Dyke Lecture. Arch Ophthalmol. 2010; 128(7):859–864
[12] Li HK, Shields CL, Mashayekhi A, et al. Giant choroidal nevus clinical features and natural course in 322 cases. Ophthalmology. 2010; 117(2):324–333
[13] Shah SU, Kaliki S, Shields CL, Ferenczy SR, Harmon SA, Shields JA. Enhanced depth imaging optical coherence tomography of choroidal nevus in 104 cases. Ophthalmology. 2012; 119(5):1066–1072
[14] Almeida A, Kaliki S, Shields CL. Autofluorescence of intraocular tumours. Curr Opin Ophthalmol. 2013; 24(3):222–232
[15] Shields CL, Kaliki S, Rojanaporn D, Ferenczy SR, Shields JA. Enhanced depth imaging optical coherence tomography of small choroidal melanoma: comparison with choroidal nevus. Arch Ophthalmol. 2012; 130(7):850–856
[16] Shields JA, Shields CL. Management of posterior uveal melanoma. In: Shields JA, Shields CL, eds. Intraocular Tumors. A Text and Atlas. Philadelphia, PA: WB Saunders; 1992;171–205
[17] Shields JA, Shields CL. Intraocular Tumors. An Atlas and Textbook. 2nd ed. Philadelphia, PA: Lippincott Williams and Wilkins; 2008;85–176
[18] Kivelä T. The epidemiological challenge of the most frequent eye cancer: retinoblastoma, an issue of birth and death. Br J Ophthalmol. 2009; 93(9):1129–1131
[19] Singh AD, Topham A. Incidence of uveal melanoma in the United States: 1973–1997. Ophthalmology. 2003; 110(5):956–961
[20] Shields CL, Kaliki S, Furuta M, Mashayekhi A, Shields JA. Clinical spectrum and prognosis of uveal melanoma based on age at presentation in 8,033 cases. Retina. 2012; 32(7):1363–1372
[21] Rishi P, Shields CL, Khan MA, Patrick K, Shields JA. Headache or eye pain as the presenting feature of uveal melanoma. Ophthalmology. 2013; 120 (9):1946–7.e2
[22] Weis E, Shah CP, Lajous M, Shields JA, Shields CL. The association between host susceptibility factors and uveal melanoma: a meta-analysis. Arch Ophthalmol. 2006; 124(1):54–60
[23] Shah CP, Weis E, Lajous M, Shields JA, Shields CL. Intermittent and chronic ultraviolet light exposure and uveal melanoma: a meta-analysis. Ophthalmology. 2005; 112(9):1599–1607
[24] Singh AD, De Potter P, Fijal BA, Shields CL, Shields JA, Elston RC. Lifetime prevalence of uveal melanoma in white patients with oculo(dermal) melanocytosis. Ophthalmology. 1998; 105(1):195–198
[25] Greenstein MB, Myers CE, Meuer SM, et al. Prevalence and characteristics of choroidal nevi: the multi-ethnic study of atherosclerosis. Ophthalmology. 2011; 118(12):2468–2473
[26] Shields CL, Manalac J, Das C, Ferguson K, Shields JA. Choroidal melanoma: clinical features, classification, and top 10 pseudomelanomas. Curr Opin Ophthalmol. 2014; 25(3):177–185
[27] Shields CL, Furuta M, Thangappan A, et al. Metastasis of uveal melanoma millimeter-by-millimeter in 8033 consecutive eyes. Arch Ophthalmol. 2009; 127(8):989–998
[28] Shields CL, Kaliki S, Furuta M, Shields JA. Diffuse versus nondiffuse small (= 3 MM thickness) choroidal melanoma: comparative analysis in 1,751 cases. The 2012 F. Phinizy Calhoun lecture. Retina. 2013; 33(9):1763–1776
[29] Shields CL, Kaliki S, Furuta M, Fulco E, Alarcon C, Shields JA. American Joint Committee on Cancer classification of posterior uveal melanoma (tumor size category) predicts prognosis in 7731 patients. Ophthalmology. 2013; 120 (10):2066–2071
[30] Kujala E, Damato B, Coupland SE, et al. Staging of ciliary body and choroidal melanomas based on anatomic extent. J Clin Oncol. 2013; 31(22):2825–2831
[31] Shields JA, Shields CL, Ehya H, Eagle RC, Jr, De Potter P. Fine-needle aspiration biopsy of suspected intraocular tumors. The 1992 Urwick Lecture. Ophthalmology. 1993; 100(11):1677–1684
[32] Shields CL, Shields JA, Cater J, et al. Plaque radiotherapy for uveal melanoma: long-term visual outcome in 1106 consecutive patients. Arch Ophthalmol. 2000; 118(9):1219–1228
[33] The Collaborative Ocular Melanoma Study Group. The Collaborative Ocular Melanoma Study (COMS) randomized trial of pre-enucleation radiation of large choroidal melanoma II: initial mortality findings. COMS report no. 10. Am J Ophthalmol. 1998; 125(6):779–796
[34] Diener-West M, Earle JD, Fine SL, et al. Collaborative Ocular Melanoma Study Group. The COMS randomized trial of iodine 125 brachytherapy for choroidal melanoma, III: initial mortality findings. COMS Report No. 18. Arch Ophthalmol. 2001; 119(7):969–982
[35] Sagoo MS, Shields CL, Mashayekhi A, et al. Plaque radiotherapy for choroidal melanoma encircling the optic disc (circumpapillary choroidal melanoma). Arch Ophthalmol. 2007; 125(9):1202–1209
[36] Sagoo MS, Shields CL, Mashayekhi A, et al. Plaque radiotherapy for juxtapapillary choroidal melanoma overhanging the optic disc in 141 consecutive patients. Arch Ophthalmol. 2008; 126(11):1515–1522
[37] Sagoo MS, Shields CL, Mashayekhi A, et al. Plaque radiotherapy for juxtapapillary choroidal melanoma: tumor control in 650 consecutive cases. Ophthalmology. 2011; 118(2):402–407
[38] Shields CL, Kaliki S, Livesey M, et al. Association of ocular and oculodermal melanocytosis with the rate of uveal melanoma metastasis: analysis of 7872 consecutive eyes. JAMA Ophthalmol. 2013; 131(8):993–1003
[39] Eskelin S, Pyrhönen S, Summanen P, Hahka-Kemppinen M, Kivelä T. Tumor doubling times in metastatic malignant melanoma of the uvea: tumor progression before and after treatment. Ophthalmology. 2000; 107(8):1443–1449
[40] Eskelin S, Kivela T. Uveal melanoma: Implications of tumor doubling time. (Author's reply). Ophthalmology. 2001; 108:830–831
[41] Prescher G, Bornfeld N, Hirche H, Horsthemke B, Jöckel KH, Becher R. Prognostic implications of monosomy 3 in uveal melanoma. Lancet. 1996; 347 (9010):1222–1225
[42] Kilic E, van Gils W, Lodder E, et al. Clinical and cytogenetic analyses in uveal melanoma. Invest Ophthalmol Vis Sci. 2006; 47(9):3703–3707
[43] Damato B, Dopierala JA, Coupland SE. Genotypic profiling of 452 choroidal melanomas with multiplex ligation-dependent probe amplification. Clin Cancer Res. 2010; 16(24):6083–6092
[44] Shields CL, Ganguly A, Bianciotto CG, Turaka K, Tavallali A, Shields JA. Prognosis of uveal melanoma in 500 cases using genetic testing of fine-needle aspiration biopsy specimens. Ophthalmology. 2011; 118(2):396–401
[45] Tschentscher F, Hüsing J, Hölter T, et al. Tumor classification based on gene expression profiling shows that uveal melanomas with and without monosomy 3 represent two distinct entities. Cancer Res. 2003; 63(10):2578–2584
[46] Onken MD, Worley LA, Ehlers JP, Harbour JW. Gene expression profiling in uveal melanoma reveals two molecular classes and predicts metastatic death. Cancer Res. 2004; 64(20):7205–7209
[47] Shields JA, Mashayekhi A, Ra S, Shields CL. Pseudomelanomas of the posterior uveal tract: the 2006 Taylor R. Smith Lecture. Retina. 2005; 25(6):767–771

27 Retinoblastoma

Carol L. Shields and Jerry A. Shields

27.1 Introduction

Retinoblastoma is the most common intraocular cancer of childhood.[1,2,3,4] It represents approximately 4% of all pediatric malignancies. It is estimated that 250 to 300 new cases of retinoblastoma are diagnosed in the United States each year and 7,000 cases are diagnosed annually worldwide. This serious ocular malignancy can manifest covertly with painless leukocoria and can threaten survival of the patient.[2,3] If untreated, retinoblastoma can lead to death within 1 to 2 years. Advanced disease with massive tumor, invasive into surrounding structures, has the greatest risk for metastasis. Worldwide, survival parallels economic development as retinoblastoma survival is approximately 30% in Africa, 60% in Asia, 80% in Latin American, and 95 to 97% in Europe and North America.[4]

Large continents like Asia manage approximately 4,000 patients with retinoblastoma yearly and Africa has approximately 2,000 patients annually.[4] Reasons for the poor survival associated with retinoblastoma in undeveloped nations relate to late detection of advanced retinoblastoma, often presenting with orbital invasion or metastatic disease, and the lack of chemotherapy. In Brazil, the mean age at presentation for retinoblastoma is approximately 25 months, compared to 18 months or less in the United States.[5] It has been reported that Brazilian families delay seeking medical care for a mean of 6 months, and the delay was longer if the symptom was only strabismus of an eye with retinoblastoma (lag time: 9 mo) compared to if the symptom was leukocoria (lagtime: 6 mo) or tumor mass (lag time: 2 mo).[5]

27.2 Basic Genetics

Retinoblastoma affects approximately 1 infant in 15,000 to 20,000 live births in the United States each year.[1,2,4] Most studies indicate that the incidence of retinoblastoma among the various geographic populations is relatively constant. The role of environmental influences in the development of this malignant intraocular tumor remains unclear. Prior to the 1860s, before the role of enucleation in the management of retinoblastoma was known, most cases of retinoblastoma proved fatal. At that time, little was suspected about the inheritance patterns of this tumor because few patients survived to reproductive age. Later, as more patients survived and had children of their own, more evidence arose suggesting the hereditary nature of retinoblastoma. It is now known that retinoblastoma can be inherited as a familial tumor, in which the affected child has a positive family history of retinoblastoma, or as a nonfamilial (sporadic) tumor in which the family history is negative for retinoblastoma. All patients with familial retinoblastoma are at risk to pass the trait to their offspring.

Retinoblastoma is classified in four different ways: familial or sporadic, bilateral or unilateral, heritable or nonheritable, and germline or somatic. Our preference is germline or somatic. It is recognized that bilateral and familial retinoblastoma are caused by a germline mutation and are, thus, a heritable tumor. Unilateral sporadic retinoblastoma is usually not heritable, but approximately 10 to 15% of children with unilateral sporadic retinoblastoma have a germline mutation. Genetic testing of the patient's tumor and peripheral blood can help identify those with a germline mutation.

The retinoblastoma gene is located on the long arm of chromosome 13 (13q14). It is a large 4.73 kilobase message. An intact gene protects against expression of retinoblastoma. It is believed that the gene is a recessive suppressor gene and may play a role in cell growth and development. In order for retinoblastoma to develop, both copies of the gene at the 13q14 locus must be lost, deleted, mutated, or inactivated. If either the maternal or the paternal copy of the gene that is inherited by an individual is defective, then that individual is heterozygous for the mutant allele. Tumor formation requires both alleles of the gene to be mutant or inactive. These two mutations correlate to the two "hits" (two-hit hypothesis) theorized by Knudson in 1971.[6] Knudson proposed that the development of retinoblastoma was caused by two complementary chromosomal mutations. Each genetic event could occur randomly with a frequency of 2×10^{-7} per year. Therefore, in familial cases of retinoblastoma, all cells in the body are predisposed to possible tumor development since a germline mutation ("first hit") has been inherited in all cells of the body, including the ovaries and testes. This explains the high incidence of second nonocular tumors, such as osteosarcoma, soft tissue sarcoma, and cutaneous melanoma seen in patients with familial retinoblastoma or bilateral sporadic retinoblastoma. The offspring in cases of familial retinoblastoma are likewise predisposed because their germinal mutation will be passed on. In contrast, in most cases of unilateral sporadic retinoblastoma, the "two hits" occur during development of the retina and both "hits" are somatic mutations. The rest of the body theoretically carries no higher risk to develop other tumors because these patients presumably have normal chromosomal structure elsewhere in the body.

27.2.1 Genetics: 13q Deletion Syndrome

The 13q deletion syndrome can manifest by several phenotypic abnormalities. Many patients have minimal or no visible abnormality. The characteristic findings include some degree of the following dysmorphic features: microcephaly, broad prominent nasal bridge, hypertelorism, microphthalmos, epicanthus, ptosis, protruding upper incisors, micrognathia, short neck with lateral folds, large prominent low-set ears, facial asymmetry, imperforate anus, genital malformations, perineal fistula, hypoplastic or absent thumbs, toe abnormalities, and psychomotor and mental retardation. The midface of patients with 13q deletion is notable for prominent eyebrows, broad nasal bridge, bulbous tipped nose, large mouth, and thin upper lip.

27.2.2 Genetic Counseling Regarding Future Offspring

When counseling the patient and family about the possibility of future children developing retinoblastoma, it is critical to know if the child or family carries a germline mutation for the retinoblastoma gene. Those patients with bilateral retinoblastoma and those with a family history of retinoblastoma can be assumed to have a germline mutation. These children are at a 50% risk of passing this gene to future children. The retinoblastoma gene is about 80% penetrant so that only 40% of their offspring will manifest the clinical findings of the gene and some offspring may only be carriers of the gene without developing retinoblastoma. All children with retinoblastoma should be offered genetic counseling and testing. A recommended screening protocol for newborn children with family history of retinoblastoma is listed in ▶ Table 27.1.[7]

27.3 Life-Threatening Problems

Children with retinoblastoma are at risk for three important life-threatening problems including metastasis from retinoblastoma, intracranial neuroblastic malignancy (trilateral retinoblastoma), and second primary tumors.

27.3.1 At Risk for Metastases

Retinoblastoma metastasis, when it occurs, generally develops within 1 year of the diagnosis of the intraocular tumor. Those at greatest risk for metastasis show features of retinoblastoma invasion beyond the lamina cribrosa in the optic nerve, in the choroid (> 2 mm dimension), in the sclera, in the orbit, or in the anterior chamber.[8,9,10] Eyes with invasion of the optic nerve or choroid generally demonstrate large retinoblastoma (over 15 mm greatest dimension) along with elevated intraocular pressure and total retinal detachment.[11,12] Patients with evidence of invasive retinoblastoma should be treated with chemotherapy for 6 months to prevent metastases. Honavar et al demonstrated that high-risk eyes showed reduction in metastases from 24% in those without preventative chemotherapy to 4% in those treated with chemotherapy.[8] Kaliki et al demonstrated that the use of vincristine, etoposide, and carboplatin for high-risk eyes was nearly uniformly effective.[9]

Table 27.1 Screening protocol for newborn children with family history of retinoblastoma

Age of baby	Examination period
Birth	First examination by 2 wk of age
Birth–3 mo	Every 1 mo
3 mo–1 y	Every 2 mo
1–2 y	Every 3 mo
2–3 y	Every 4 mo
3–4 y	Every 6 mo

Source: Data based on Moll et al.[7]

Note: Using this protocol, familial retinoblastoma can be detected in 50% of cases by 2 months of age, 85% by 6 months, and nearly 100% by 12 months.

Pearls

Eyes at high risk for retinoblastoma are those with
- postlaminar optic nerve invasion.
- choroidal invasion > 3 mm.
- any combination of optic nerve and choroidal invasion.
- anterior segment invasion (possible risk).

Affected patients need six cycles of additional chemotherapy to prevent metastasis.

27.3.2 At Risk for Neuroblastic Intracranial Malignancy (Trilateral Retinoblastoma)

There is an association of neuroblastic intracranial malignancy in patients with the hereditary form of retinoblastoma, most often manifesting as pineoblastoma or other parasellar tumors.[13,14,15,16,17] The pineoblastoma is identical to retinoblastoma from an embryologic and pathologic standpoint. This association of midline intracranial pineal tumors and suprasellar/parasellar neuroblastic tumors with bilateral retinoblastoma has been termed "trilateral" retinoblastoma.[13] Loss of function of the retinoblastoma gene is believed to confer an increased susceptibility to developing these intracranial tumors. Trilateral retinoblastoma is found in approximately 3% of all children with retinoblastoma.[16] Those patients with bilateral or familial disease are at greatest risk, with 5 to 15% developing this finding.[16] Hence, patients with bilateral or familial retinoblastoma are advised to undergo screening for pineoblastoma using magnetic resonance imaging (MRI) twice yearly for the first 5 years of life. In some cases, the intracranial tumor precedes the diagnosis of retinoblastoma. Unlike other second tumors, the pineoblastoma usually occurs during the first 5 years of life, whereas second tumors often take many decades to develop. Unfortunately, pineoblastoma is often fatal.

Systemic chemoreduction for retinoblastoma can prevent trilateral retinoblastoma.[18,19,20] In a study of 100 patients with hereditary retinoblastoma, trilateral retinoblastoma was found in no patient who received chemoreduction, and it would have been expected in 5 to 15 patients.[18] Additional evidence in the chemoreduction era indicates that pineoblastoma is rare and that chemoreduction might be preventing incipient malignancy.[20] Others believe that the avoidance of external beam radiotherapy is the main reason for reduction in the frequency of trilateral retinoblastoma.[21,22] It should also be recognized that pineal gland enlargement might not be a solid tumor and may represent a benign cyst.[20,23]

27.3.3 At Risk for Second Primary Cancers

Another important aspect of genetic counseling concerns the development of new genetically related cancers in survivors of bilateral or heritable retinoblastoma. Children with retinoblastoma have approximately a 5% chance of developing another malignancy during the first 10 years of follow-up, 18% during the first 20 years, and 26% within 30 years.[24] The 30-year cumulative incidence is about 35% or even higher for those patients who received radiation therapy (external beam therapy) compared to an incidence rate of 6% for those patients who avoided radiation. Osteogenic sarcoma, often involving the femur, is most common, but other tumors such as spindle cell sarcoma, chondrosarcoma, rhabdomyosarcoma, neuroblastoma, glioma, leukemia, sebaceous carcinoma, squamous cell carcinoma, and malignant melanoma have also been recognized. Patients who survive a second tumor are at risk for a third, fourth, and even fifth nonocular tumors.[25]

27.4 Clinical Features of Retinoblastoma

The clinical features of retinoblastoma vary depending on the extent of tumor. In the United States, an evaluation of 1,265 patients revealed that the most common presenting signs included leukocoria (56%), strabismus (24%), and poor vision (8%).[26] Further study on a cohort of 1,196 eyes found a median age at presentation of 15 months with 51% male, 49% female, 53% unilateral, and 47% bilateral.[27] Zhao et al from China reviewed 470 eyes and found leukocoria (47%) as the most common presenting sign.[28] Presentations of retinoblastoma differ. In a report from Sudan,[29] buphthalmos (56%) and leukocoria (32%) were the most common presenting signs; in a study from Mali,[30] proptosis (55%), leukocoria (38%), strabismus (6%), and buphthalmos (2%) were reported. Efforts are underway internationally to educate clinicians, nurses, patients, and entire populations for improvement in retinoblastoma detection.

The clinical manifestations of retinoblastoma vary with the stage of the disease at the time of recognition. In its earliest clinical stage, a small retinoblastoma under 2 mm in basal dimension appears ophthalmoscopically as a subtle, transparent, or slightly translucent lesion in the sensory retina.[2,3,31] Slightly larger tumors lead to dilated retinal blood vessels that feed and drain the tumor. Some larger tumors show foci of chalk-like calcification that resemble cottage cheese. A retinoblastoma of any size can produce leukocoria. The larger tumors more often present with leukocoria. This white pupillary reflex is a result of reflection of light from the white mass in the retrolental area.

Retinoblastoma growth patterns are divided into intraretinal, endophytic, and exophytic. Intraretinal tumors are limited to the substance of the retina. Endophytic retinoblastoma grows from the retina inward toward the vitreous cavity. Hence, it is characterized by a white hazy mass with obscuration of the retinal blood vessels. Because of its friable nature, an endophytic tumor can seed the vitreous cavity and anterior chamber and simulate endophthalmitis. An exophytic retinoblastoma grows from the retina outward into the subretinal space. Such tumors produce a progressive retinal detachment, with the retina often displaced anteriorly behind a clear lens. An exophytic retinoblastoma can clinically resemble Coats' disease or other forms of exudative retinal detachment. Occasionally, a retinoblastoma can assume a diffuse infiltrating pattern, characterized by a relatively flat infiltration of the retina by tumor cells without an obvious mass.[32] In such cases, the diagnosis can be more difficult and simulate uveitis or endophthalmitis. Less frequently, the presenting feature can be pseudohypopyon due to tumor seeding in the anterior chamber, hyphema secondary to iris neovascularization, vitreous hemorrhage, or signs of orbital cellulitis.

27.5 Classification of Retinoblastoma

There have been several classifications[33,34,35,36,37,38] proposed for intraocular retinoblastoma including the Reese-Ellsworth Classification,[34] Essen Classification,[35] and Philadelphia Classification.[36] The most commonly used current classification is the International Classification of Retinoblastoma[16,17] designed in Paris in 2003 and based predominantly on the presence and extent of subretinal and vitreous tumors seeds (▶ Table 27.2). The International Classification of Retinoblastoma is practical and applicable specifically for chemotherapy outcomes as it has been found predictive of treatment success following intravenous chemotherapy (IVitC).

27.6 Leading Simulators of Retinoblastoma

The diagnosis of retinoblastoma is based on characteristic clinical features of a yellow-white retinal mass often with surrounding subretinal fluid, subretinal seeding, and vitreous seeding. Ancillary testing can confirm the diagnosis. Fine needle aspiration biopsy or open biopsy of retinoblastoma is not performed due to risk for local tumor dissemination. The diagnosis is established based on clinical features alone. Despite classic manifestations, retinoblastoma can display a spectrum of unusual features that overlap with other conditions (pseudoretinoblastomas) and can lead to diagnostic confusion.[39]

Accurate clinical diagnosis is important to avoid mistreatment, particularly with chemotherapy. In a large series of 2,775 eyes referred with possible retinoblastoma, retinoblastoma was confirmed in 2,171 (78%) eyes and a simulating lesion (pseudoretinoblastoma) in 604 (22%).[39] Overall, the leading pseudoretinoblastoma lesions included Coats' disease (40%), persistent fetal vasculature (PFV) (26%), and vitreous hemorrhage (5%) (▶ Table 27.3). The pseudoretinoblastomas differed based on age at presentation. Of patients age =1 year, PFV (49%) was the most common pseudoretinoblastoma, whereas in children > 2 years, Coats' disease (60%) was most common (▶ Table 27.3 and ▶ Table 27.4).

27.7 Diagnostic Testing

Accurate diagnosis in a child with suspected retinoblastoma is accomplished by taking a detailed history and performing a detailed physical evaluation, external ocular examination, slit-lamp biomicroscopy, and binocular indirect ophthalmoscopy with scleral depression. This is generally performed either in the office or under anesthesia in order to determine precisely the number and location of all tumors. The diagnosis is

Table 27.2 The International Classification of Retinoblastoma

Group	Quick reference	Philadelphia version	Los Angeles version
A	Small Rb	Rb = 3 mm	Rb = 3 mm, at least 3 mm from the foveola and 1.5 mm from optic nerve. No seeding
B	Bigger Rb Macular Rb Juxtapapillary Rb Subretinal fluid	Rb > 3 mm or • Macular location or • Juxtapapillary location (< 1.5 mm to disc) or • SRF present	Eyes with no vitreous or subretinal seeding and retinal tumors of any size or location not included in group A. Small cuff of subretinal fluid = 5 mm from tumor margin
C	Contained (focal) seeds	Rb with • SRS =3 mm from Rb or • VS -3 mm from Rb	Eyes with focal vitreous or subretinal seeding and discrete tumor of any size or location. Seeding must be local, fine, and limited so as to be theoretically treatable with a radioactive plaque. Up to one quadrant subretinal fluid may be present
D	Diffuse seeds	Rb with • SRS > 3 mm from Rb or • VS > 3 mm from Rb	Eyes with diffuse vitreous or subretinal seeding and/or massive, nondiscrete endophytic or exophytic disease. Seeding more extensive than group C. Retinal detachment > 1 quadrant
E	Extensive Rb	Rb with • Size > 50% of globe or • Neovascular glaucoma or • Opaque media or • Invasion of optic nerve, choroid, sclera, orbit, anterior chamber	Massive Rb with anatomic or functional destruction of the eye with one or more of the following: • Neovascular glaucoma • Massive intraocular hemorrhage • Aseptic orbital cellulitis • Tumor anterior to anterior vitreous face • Tumor touching lens • Diffuse infiltrating tumor • Phthisis or prephthisis

Abbreviations: Rb, retinoblastoma; SRF, subretinal fluid; SRS, subretinal seeds; VS, vitreous seeds.

Table 27.3 Lesions referred with the diagnosis of possible retinoblastoma but proved to be other condition (pseudoretinoblastoma) in 604 consecutive patients based on age at presentation

	Patient age **Number (% per diagnosis) [% per age group]**					
Pseudoretinoblastoma diagnosis	**Mean, median [range] in y**	**0–1 y** n = 283	**>1 to 2 y** n = 57	**>2 to 5 y** n = 89	**>5 y** n = 175	**All ages** n = 604
Coats' disease	6, 4 [0.2–30]	58 (24) [20]	33 (14) [58]	54 (22) [61]	99 (41) [57]	244 (100) [40]
Persistent fetal vasculature	2, 1 [0.2–24]	138 (87) [49]	6 (4) [11]	6 (4) [7]	8 (5) [5]	158 (100) [26]
Vitreous hemorrhage	1, 1 [0.5–8]	21 (78) [7]	3 (11) [5]	1 (4) [1]	2 (7) [1]	27 (100) [5]
Toxocariasis	8, 8 [1–18]	1 (5) [< 1]	0 (0) [0]	7 (32) [8]	14 (64) [8]	22 (100) [4]
Familial exudative vitreoretinopathy	7, 7 [0.6–16]	5 (28) [2]	1 (6) [2]	1 (6) [1]	11 (61) [6]	18 (100) [3]
Rhegmatogenous retinal detachment	5, 1 [0.5–24]	10 (56) [4]	0 (0) [0]	3 (17) [3]	5 (28) [3]	18 (100) [3]
Coloboma	3,1 [0.3–11]	9 (53) [3]	1 (6) [2]	3 (18) [3]	4 (24) [2]	17 (100) [3]
Astrocytic hamartoma	8, 6 [0.5–28]	3 (20) [1]	1 (7) [2]	3 (20) [3]	8 (53) [5]	15 (100) [2]
Combined hamartoma	4, 2 [0.5–16]	4 (27) [1]	5 (33) [9]	1 (7) [1]	5 (33) [3]	15 (100) [2]
Endogenous endophthalmitis	5, 5 [0.2–11]	2 (20) [< 1]	0 (0) [0]	2 (20) [2]	6 (60) [3]	10 (100) [2]

Table 27.3 continued

	Patient age Number (% per diagnosis) [% per age group]					
Pseudoretinoblastoma diagnosis	**Mean, median [range] in y**	**0–1 y** *n* = 283	**>1 to 2 y** *n* = 57	**>2 to 5 y** *n* = 89	**>5 y** *n* = 175	**All ages** *n* = 604
Myelinated nerve fibers	4, 4 [0.5–11]	3 (33) [1]	0 (0) [0]	2 (22) [2]	4 (44) [2]	9 (100) [1]
Congenital cataract	3, 1 [0.2–12]	5 (63) [2]	1 (13) [2]	0 (0) [0]	2 (25) [1]	8 (100) [1]
Peripheral uveoretinitis	3, 2 [0.5 to 6]	3 (43) [1]	1 (14) [2]	0 (0) [0]	3 (43) [2]	7 (100) [1]
Retinopathy of prematurity	2, 2 [0.8–7]	3 (43) [1]	2 (29) [4]	1 (14) [1]	1 (14) [<1]	7 (100) [1]
Nonrhegmatogenous retinal detachment	1, 1 [0.6–4]	4 (80) [1]	0 (0) [0]	1 (20) [1]	0 (0) [0]	5 (100) [<1]
Medulloepithelioma	4, 4 [2–5]	0 (0) [0]	1 (25) [2]	3 (75) [3]	0 (0) [0]	4 (100) [<1]
X-linked retinoschisis	2, 1 [0.6–7]	3 (75) [1]	0 (0) [0]	0 (0) [0]	1 (25) [<1]	4 (100) [<1]
Vitreoretinal tuft	3, 1 [0.6–8]	2 (67) [<1]	0 (0) [0]	0 (0) [0]	1 (33) [<1]	3 (100) [<1]
Incontinentia pigmenti	4, 4 [2–6]	0 (0) [0]	1 (50) [2]	0 (0) [0]	1 (50) [<1]	2 (100) [<1]
Juvenile xanthogranuloma	1, 1 [0.7–0.8]	2 (100) [<1]	0 (0) [0]	0 (0) [0]	0 (0) [0]	2 (100) [<1]
Norrie's disease	1, 1 [0.7–0.8]	2 (100) [<1]	0 (0) [0]	0 (0) [0]	0 (0) [0]	2 (100) [<1]
Vasoproliferative tumor	10, 10 [3–17]	2 (100) [<1]	0 (0) [0]	0 (0) [0]	0 (0) [0]	2 (100) [<1]
Choroidal osteoma	3	0 (0) [0]	0 (0) [0]	1 (100) [1]	0 (0) [0]	1 (100) [<1]
Morning glory disc anomaly	1	1 (100) [<1]	0 (0) [0]	0 (0) [0]	0 (0) [0]	1 (100) [<1]
Retinal capillary hemangioma	16	1 (100) [<1]	0 (0) [0]	0 (0) [0]	0 (0) [0]	1 (100) [<1]
Retrolental fibrosis	2	0 (0) [0]	1 (100) [2]	0 (0) [0]	0 (0) [0]	1 (100) [<1]
Toxoplasmosis	1	1 (100) [<1]	0 (0) [0]	0 (0) [0]	0 (0) [0]	1 (100) [<1]

Source: Data gathered from Shields et al.[39]

Note: (%) indicates percentage per diagnosis, by row.

[%] indicates percentage by age group, by column.

established by the classic appearance of the retinal tumors by an experienced examiner. Needle biopsy confirmation is rarely, if ever, necessary.

Ancillary diagnostic studies can be helpful in confirming the diagnosis of retinoblastoma.[2,3] Ultrasonography is the first test for detection of retinoblastoma and typically there is an intraocular mass with intrinsic calcification and orbital shadowing (▶ Fig. 27.1). About 5 to 10% of retinoblastomas show no intrinsic calcification. Fluorescein angiography shows early vascularity and late hyperfluorescence of the tumor (▶ Fig. 27.2). Computed tomography can demonstrate the intraocular tumor and particularly the calcification (▶ Fig. 27.3). MRI does not usually detect calcium but may be of most value in the assessment of the optic nerve, orbit, and brain. Optic coherence tomography (OCT) has been found useful in the detection of cavitary retinoblastoma that might show a less dramatic response to chemotherapy. OCT also demonstrates that retinoblastoma tends to arise in the middle to outer layers of the retina

Table 27.4 Differentiation of Coats' disease from retinoblastoma

Feature	Coats' disease	Retinoblastoma
Age of onset (mean)	5 y	1.5 y
Gender		
Male	76%	50%
Female	24%	50%
Laterality		
Unilateral	95%	60%
Bilateral	5%	40%
Family history of disease	0%	10%
Eye findings		
Anterior chamber	Rare cholesterol crystals	Rare white cells with hypopyon
Iris neovascularization	Present in 8%	Present in 17%
Cataract	Absent	Absent
Vitreous	Murky	White fluffy seeds
Retinal vessels	• Irregular dilation with telangiectasia • Remain visible throughout course • Most commonly seen temporally	• Tortuous, but regular dilation towards a mass • Disappear into tumor • Occur in quadrant of tumor
Retinal exudation	Present	Absent
Retinal mass	Absent	Present
Retinal gliosis	Present, forming subretinal scar	Absent
Retinoschisis/macrocyst	Present	Absent
Subretinal fluid	Present, with exudation and refractile cholesterol	Present, with white subretinal seeds
Diagnostic testing		
Ultrasonography	• Retinal detachment • Subretinal echoes minimal • Rare calcification at level of retinal pigment epithelium	• Retinal detachment • Subretinal echoes from seeds • Calcification within retinal tumor and shadowing
Optical coherence tomography	• Retinal detachment • Retinal edema • Subretinal deposits	• Retinal detachment • Solid intraretinal mass arising in middle to outer retina • Normal retina draped over mass.
Computed tomography	Retinal detachment	Retinal detachment with calcified retinal mass
Magnetic resonance tomography	Retinal detachment	Retinal detachment with enhancement of retinal mass

with normal adjacent retinal draping over the peripheral tumor surface. Additionally, OCT is useful in the follow-up of patients to assess macular anatomy.[40]

27.8 Management of Retinoblastoma

Management of a child with retinoblastoma involves a balance of patient life with globe salvage and ultimate visual potential.[2,3,31,33] Management of retinoblastoma is a practiced science and art that involves tumor recognition and differentiation from simulating conditions, decision-making regarding appropriate therapeutic approach, and meticulous follow-up for detection of tumor recurrence. There are numerous tools for management of retinoblastoma including enucleation, radiotherapy by teletherapy (external beam radiotherapy [EBRT]) or brachytherapy (plaque radiotherapy), chemotherapy using various delivery routes and chemotherapy protocols, and focal treatments with laser photocoagulation, transpupillary thermotherapy, cryotherapy, and plaque radiotherapy.[31,33,41] Chemotherapy remains the most common method for conservative globe salvage.

Chemotherapy with various agents and duration, usually combined with consolidation with thermotherapy, cryotherapy, or plaque radiotherapy, has been used for over 2 decades to

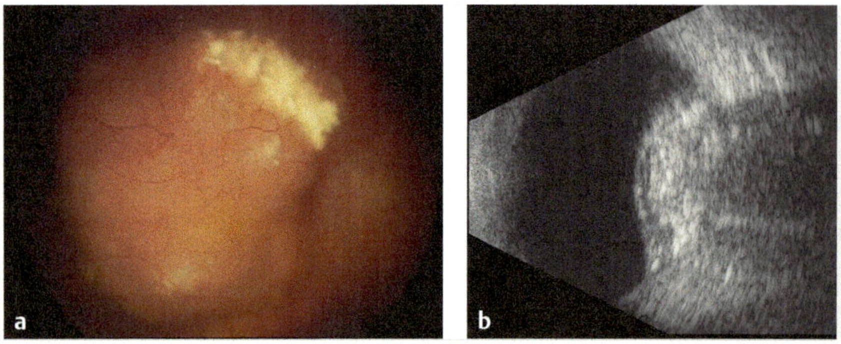

Fig. 27.1 (**a**) Retinoblastoma (**b**) appears acoustically dense on B-scan ultrasonography.

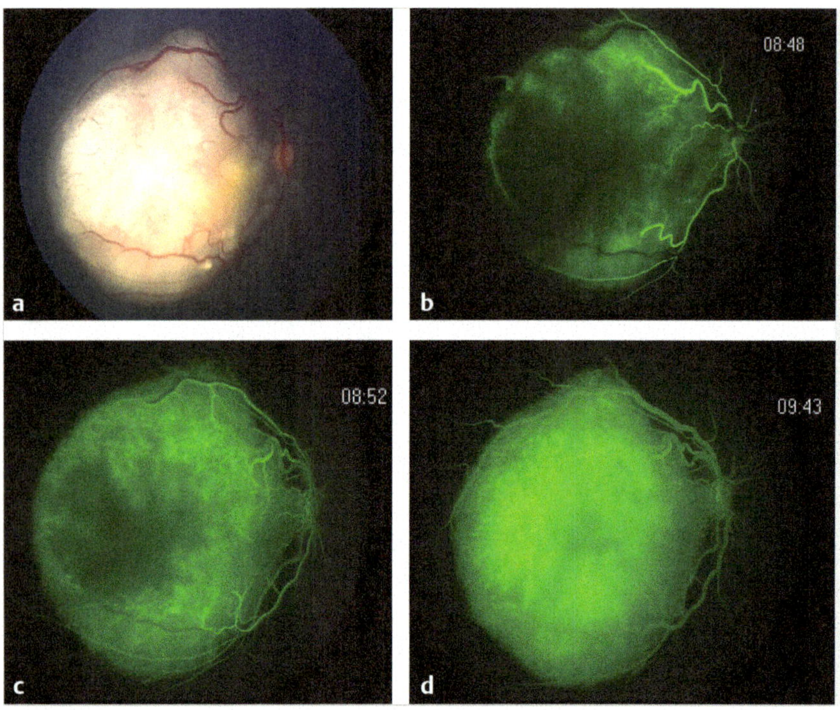

Fig. 27.2 (**a**) Retinoblastoma shows rapid hyperfluorescence in the (**b**) arterial, (**c**) laminar venous, and (**d**) late phases of fluorescein angiography.

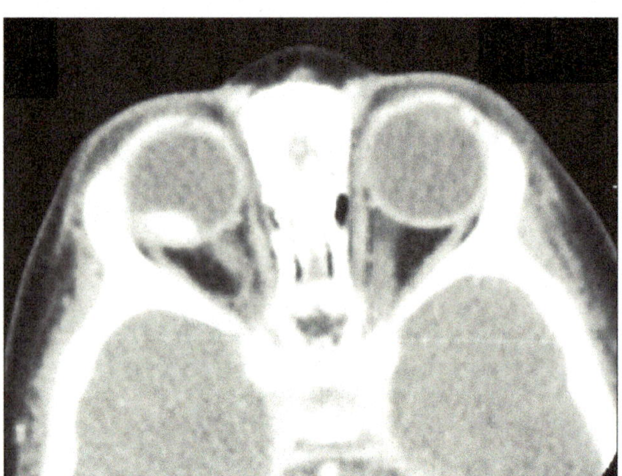

Fig. 27.3 Retinoblastoma appears calcified on computed tomography.

manage retinoblastoma. There are four major routes for chemotherapy delivery including IVitC, intra-arterial chemotherapy (IAC), sub-Tenon's fascia chemotherapy (STC), and intravitreal chemotherapy (IVitC).[31,42] Each requires certain medication, drug dosing, and preparations, and is associated with different indications and anticipated outcomes (▸ Table 27.5, ▸ Table 27.6, ▸ Table 27.7).

27.8.1 Intravenous Chemotherapy (Chemoreduction)

In the early 1990s, Kingston et al from London recognized that a specific protocol of IVitC, classically used for neuroblastoma was particularly effective for retinoblastoma.[41] If delivered prior to EBRT for advanced retinoblastoma, then classified as Reese-Ellsworth group V, IVitC increased tumor control with ocular salvage from 30 to 70%.[41] Others observed similar results.[43,44,45] These landmark observations began the IVitC era, otherwise termed "chemoreduction era," and this protocol continues to provide excellent tumor control (▸ Fig. 27.4 and ▸ Table 27.5).

The IVitC protocol is used with standard dose vincristine, etoposide, and carboplatin (VEC) based on patient weight

Table 27.5 Chemotherapy protocols for retinoblastoma

Chemotherapy drug	Dose	Schedule
Intravenous chemotherapy		
Carboplatin (C)	560 mg/m^2 in 120 cc/m^2 D51/4NS IVSS over 60 min	Day 0 of each cycle (18.6 mg/kg for patients < 36 mo of age)
Etoposide (E)	150 mg/m^2 in 150 cc/m^2 D51/4NS IVSS over 60 min	Days 0 and 1 of each course (5 mg/kg for patients < 36 mo of age)
Vincristine (V)	1.5 mg/m^2 IVSS over 15 min	Day 0 of each cycle (0.05 mg/kg for patients < 36 mo of age). Maximum vincristine dose not to exceed 2 mg
Antiemetic drug		
Ondansetron	0.45 mg/kg IVSS (maximum dose 24 mg) prior to therapy	Days 0 and 1 of each cycle, with dexamethasone 0.25 mg/kg IVSS prior to therapy days 0 and 1 of each cycle
Phenergen	0.5 mg/kg orally at bedtime	Day 0 and then every 6 h as needed with emesis
Diphenhydramine	1 mg/kg p.o. h.s. orally at bedtime	Day 0 and then every 6 h
Therapy continues every 4 wk for a total of six cycles. Prior to institution of each subsequent cycle, the absolute neutrophil count must be > 750 cells/uL and platelets must be > 75,000 cells/uL		
Intra-arterial chemotherapy		
Melphalan		
0–2 y old	3 mg/30 cc	Slow pulsatile infusion over 30 min
2–5 y old	5 mg/30 cc	
> 5 y old	7.5 mg/30 cc	
Carboplatin	30 mg/30 cc	Slow pulsatile infusion over 30 min
Topotecan		
0–2 y old	0.5 mg/30 cc	Slow pulsatile infusion over 30 min
> 2 y old	1.0 mg/30 cc	
Sub-Tenon's chemotherapy		
Carboplatin	20 mg/2 cc	Inject into sub-Tenon's space directly over sclera in area of tumor
Intravitreal chemotherapy		
Melphalan	20–30 ug/0.1 cc	Inject intravitreally through pars plana or clear corneal approach, cryotherapy to injection site, jiggle eye to mix chemotherapy. Deliver monthly
Methotrexate	400–800 ug/0.1 cc	Inject intravitreally through pars plana or clear corneal approach, cryotherapy to injection site. Deliver twice weekly for 1 month, then weekly for 1 month, then monthly for 1 y
Topotecan	20 ug/0.1 cc	Inject intravitreally through pars plana or clear corneal approach, cryotherapy to injection site, jiggle eye to mix chemotherapy. Deliver monthly

(▸ Table 27.5) and escalated to higher dose if there are bilateral tumors in groups D and/or E. This chemotherapy, usually delivered with consolidation treatment, is used worldwide and is effective for intraocular retinoblastoma control as well as prevention of metastasis, pinealoblastoma, and second cancers.

Chemoreduction Control of Intraocular Retinoblastoma

There have been several reports to provide evidence that three-agent IVitC for 6 to 9 consecutive months is remarkably

Table 27.6 Indications for various chemotherapy methods for retinoblastoma

Feature	Intravenous chemotherapy	Intra-arterial chemotherapy	Periocular chemotherapy	Intravitreal chemotherapy
Primary therapy				
Bilateral retinoblastoma	+ + +	+	+	~
Unilateral retinoblastoma	+ +	+ + +	+	~
Secondary therapy for recurrent/persistent tumor				
Retinoblastoma	+ +	+ + +	+	~
Subretinal seeds	+ +	+ + +	+	~
Vitreous seeds	+ +	+ +	+	+ + +

Note: + + +, marked; + +, intermediate; +, minimal; ~, little to none.

Sub-Tenon's chemotherapy as primary therapy is used in conjunction with intravenous chemotherapy for groups D and E.

If intravenous chemotherapy is used as primary and secondary therapy, the regimen is changed to different agents in secondary therapy.

Table 27.7 Outcomes of various chemotherapy methods for retinoblastoma

Feature	Intravenous chemotherapy	Intra-arterial chemotherapy	Periocular chemotherapy	Intravitreal chemotherapy
Tumor control of				
• Retinoblastoma	+ + +	+ + +	+	~
• Subretinal seeds	+ + +	+ + +	+ +	~
• Vitreous seeds	+ +	+ +	+	+ + +
Resolution of retinal detachment	+ + +	+ + +	~	~
Prevention of pinealoblastoma	+ + +	~	~	~
Reduction in long-term second cancers	+ +	~	~	~
Complications ocular				
Ptosis	~	+ +	+	~
Eyelid edema	~	+	+ +	~
Forehead redness	~	+	~	~
Dysmotility	~	+	+	~
Ophthalmic artery obstruction	~	+	~	~
Retinal artery obstruction	~	+ +	~	~
Choroidal vascular attenuation	~	+	~	~
Vitreous hemorrhage	~	+	~	~
Retinal vasculitis	~	+	~	+
Optic neuropathy	~	+ +	+	+
Phthisis	~	+	~	+ +
Complications brain				
Carotid spasm	~	+	~	~
Stroke	~	+	~	~
Brain hemorrhage	~	~	~	~
Brain vascular perfusion defects	~	+	~	~

Table 27.7 continued

Feature	Intravenous chemotherapy	Intra-arterial chemotherapy	Periocular chemotherapy	Intravitreal chemotherapy
Complications systemic				
Transient pancytopenia	+ +	+	~	~
Ototoxicity	+	~	~	~
Renal toxicity	+	~	~	~
Leukemia	+	+	~	~

Note: Outcome indicates as: + + +, marked; + +, intermediate; +, minimal; ~, little to none.

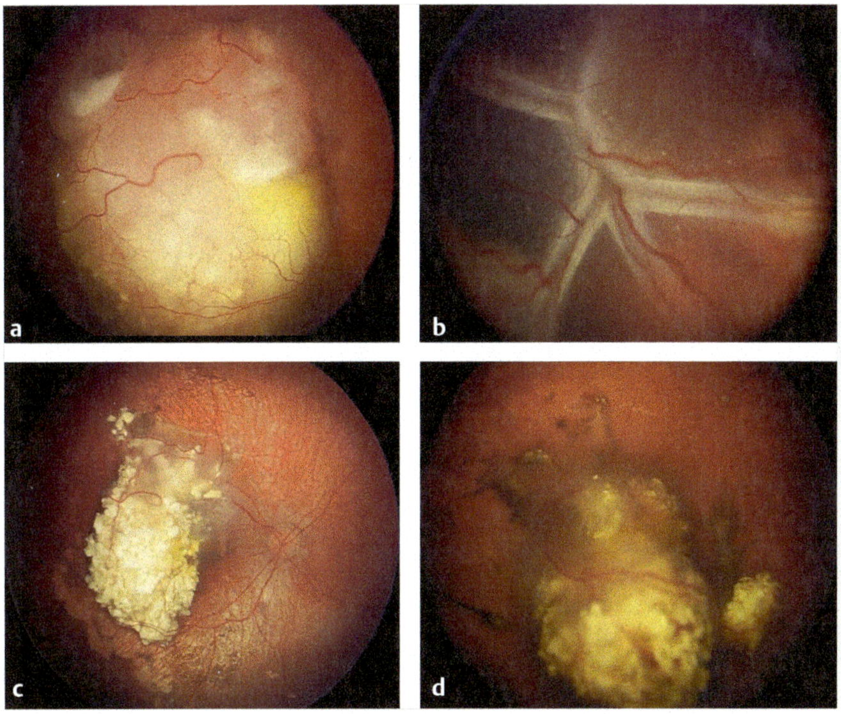

Fig. 27.4 Bilateral retinoblastoma (**a**, **b**) before and (**c**, **d**) after chemoreduction.

effective for retinoblastoma.[42] According to the International Classification of Retinoblastoma in 249 consecutive eyes, globe salvage was achieved in 100% of group A eyes, 93% of group B, 90% of group C, 47% of group D, and 25% of group E eyes.[46] Currently, groups D and E eyes show improved control with additional sub-Tenon's carboplatin or additional IAC.

Long-term systemic toxicity related to IVitC is minimal. Transient pancytopenia and fever can be encountered, as with most systemic chemotherapy. Long-term hearing and renal toxicity are rare, particularly if medications are prescribed accurately.[47] Furthermore, despite inaccurate comments about fertility issues,[48] there is no evidence that current VEC regimen causes infertility.[47] Our experience in Philadelphia over 25 years has resulted in excellent tumor control with minimal toxicities and no fertility issues. Results from India indicate that VEC has improved survival in patients with retinoblastoma up to 95%, similar to the United States and Europe (presentation by Honavar S. at the 25th Jubilee Anniversary Meeting of LV Prasad Eye Institute, Hyderabad, India, June 1, 2012).

Chemoreduction Control of Retinal Detachment

Using IVitC for retinoblastoma with total retinal detachment, complete resolution of subretinal fluid was documented in 76% eyes following therapy.[31] The presence of retinal detachment does not preclude use of IVitC, but caution is advised to withhold consolidation therapy with thermotherapy until the subretinal fluid resolves.

Chemoreduction Saving Advanced Group D or E Eyes

Most children with advanced groups D or E retinoblastoma are managed with enucleation because of large tumor, poor visual potential, and risk for metastatic disease. However, if globe salvage is considered, particularly if the opposite eye has been enucleated, then IVitC is employed to control the intraocular malignancy as well as prevent systemic metastasis. The

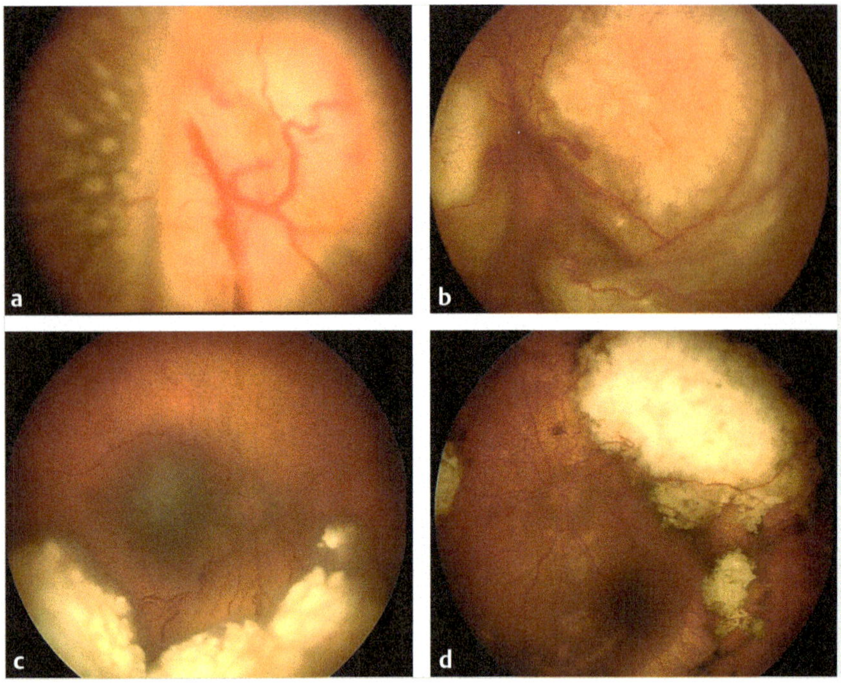

Fig. 27.5 Bilateral advanced retinoblastoma (**a, b**) before and (**c, d**) after chemoreduction plus sub-Tenon's fascia carboplatin.

chemotherapy protocol for IVitC is similar to that used for prevention of metastasis in high-risk retinoblastoma. Unfortunately, IVitC alone might not completely control advanced retinoblastoma. In one analysis, globe salvage was achieved using IVitC followed by IAC in 57% of eyes classified as group D or E.[49]

Chemoreduction Preservation of Visual Acuity

Demirci et al studied long-term visual acuity outcome in eyes treated with IVitC.[50] If treatment was successful and enucleation and/or external beam radiotherapy was avoided, mean 5-year visual outcome was 20/20 to 20/40 in 50% of patients and 20/200 or better in 67%. The main factor predictive of poor vision was foveal involvement with initial tumor or subretinal fluid. There was no local toxicity of IVitC on the eye or visual outcome. Narang et al reported a visual acuity of 20/200 in 71% eyes and 20/40 or better in 37% at 6 years following IVitC.[51]

Chemoreduction Prevention of Pinealoblastoma

In 2000, Shields et al noted that the incidence of fatal pinealoblastoma had dropped dramatically in children who received IVitC, likely related to the neoadjuvant use of chemotherapy in providing tumor control.[19] Others believed that this finding might be related to the avoidance of EBRT.[21] Analysis of 100 consecutive children with germline-mutation retinoblastoma on IVitC disclosed no case of pinealoblastoma, despite the fact that it was estimated that 8 to 10% should have manifested pinealoblastoma.[19] Ramasubramanian restudied the incidence of pinealoblastoma during the chemoreduction era and found this malignancy was detected in only 0.4% of cases, far fewer than reported in the past (3% overall and 8 to 10% for germline mutation patients).[20]

Chemoreduction Prevention of Systemic Metastasis in High-Risk Retinoblastoma

Patients at greatest danger for metastasis from retinoblastoma are those that display high-risk retinoblastoma, defined histopathologically as retinoblastoma with tumor invasion into the optic nerve, uvea, or a combination of both.[8,9,10] High-risk retinoblastoma leads to metastasis in 24% of patients if not treated with systemic chemotherapy compared to 4% of those who receive IVitC.[8]

The International Classification of Retinoblastoma can predict those eyes with high-risk retinoblastoma. It is presumed that groups A, B, and C rarely show high-risk features, but they rarely come to enucleation for histopathologic inspection. However, eyes with group D retinoblastoma show high-risk features in 15 to 17% and eyes with group E retinoblastoma show high-risk features in 24 to 50% cases.[10,52] It appears that patients with high-risk retinoblastoma should receive systemic IVitC for prevention of metastatic disease as well as for control of the intraocular tumor. Kaliki et al found that the standard IVitC protocol using vincristine, etoposide, and carboplatin resulted in complete tumor control in all (100%) high-risk cases with no evident metastasis.[9]

One concern with the current IVitC protocol was the induction of secondary leukemia from etoposide, usually within 5 years after exposure. Gombos et al identified several cases worldwide, but high and prolonged dosing could have been a factor in those cases.[53] In our extensive experience with over 500 patients treated with IVitC, there has been no case of leukemia to develop in any child treated with chemotherapy alone.[54] Furthermore, evidence from the Surveillance, Epidemiology, and End Results (SEER) database confirmed the lack of secondary leukemia in this population.[54]

Children with germline mutation retinoblastoma are at risk for long-term second malignant neoplasms. Turaka et al recently reported that fewer than expected second cancers were found in children treated with IVitC using standard six-cycle chemotherapy.[54] In that report, only 4% of children with germline mutation retinoblastoma treated with IVitC as front-line therapy developed second cancers with a mean follow-up of 11 years and no patient with nongermline mutation showed second cancer.[54] Based on those observations, the authors concluded that IVitC might reduce the risk for second cancer.

27.8.2 Intra-arterial Chemotherapy

Intra-arterial chemotherapy (IAC) is an exciting new option for management of eyes with retinoblastoma, particularly unilateral cases. The method of IAC has been described by Yamane et al and later refined by Abramson et al and Gobin et al.[55,56,57] Shields and Shields published a 4-decade perspective of retinoblastoma therapy on various treatments that have been popular and later abandoned, issuing caution with new therapies until proper assessment of limitations are realized.[58] In a 4-year review, Gobin et al found IAC safe and effective for treatment of retinoblastoma with successful catheterization in most cases with ocular survival at 2 years in 82% if IAC was primary treatment and 58% if IAC was secondary treatment.[57] Shields et al found preliminary evidence that primary therapy with IAC was successful in 100% of group C, 100% of group D, and 33% of group E eyes.[59] Later, Shields et al pursued longer follow-up and found success with primary IAC in 72% and secondary IAC in 62%[60] (▶ Fig. 27.6 and ▶ Fig. 27.7). Specifically, in those 70 cases, globe salvage was achieved in 100% of group B, 100% of group C, 94% of group D, and 36% of group E eyes.[60] Muen et al reported secondary IAC for eyes that failed previous systemic IVitC or

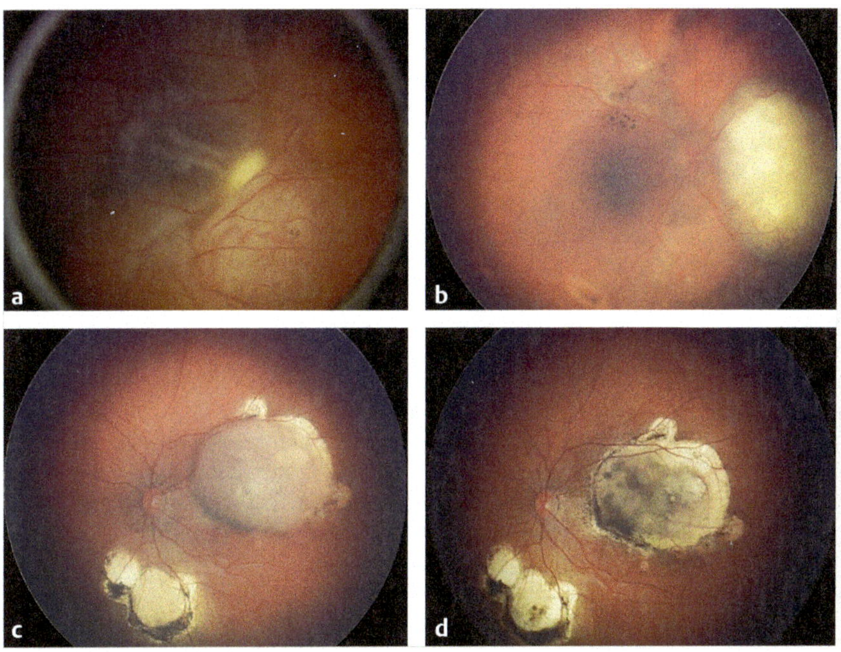

Fig. 27.6 Intra-arterial chemotherapy as primary treatment of retinoblastoma (**a**) before and (**b**) after completion of therapy. Intra-arterial chemotherapy as secondary treatment of retinoblastoma after failure of chemoreduction (**c**) before and (**d**) after completion of therapy.

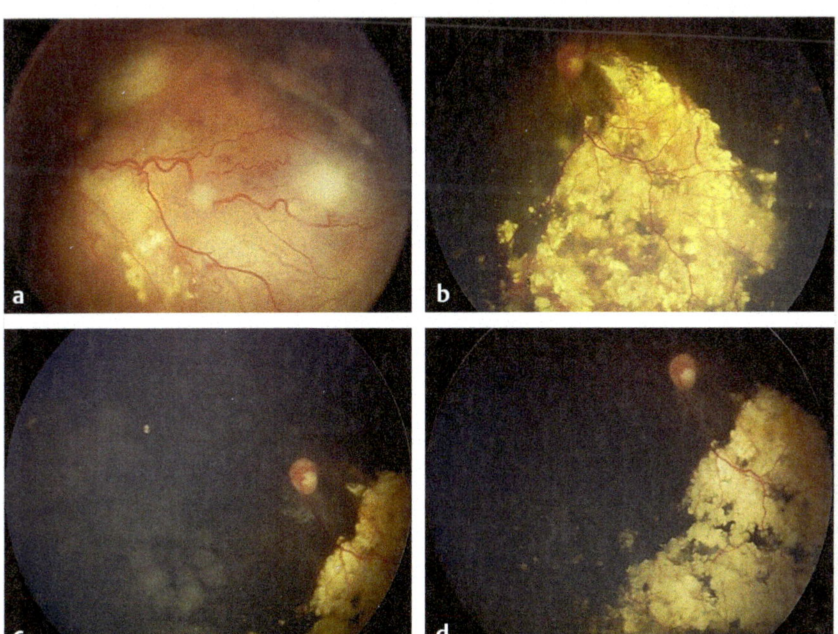

Fig. 27.7 (**a**) Chemoreduction for advanced retinoblastoma (**b**) showed satisfactory regression, (**c**) but recurrence of subretinal seeds (**d**) necessitated intra-arterial chemotherapy with tumor control.

local therapy and found 80% control.[61] Shields et al found "minimal exposure IAC," using only one or two doses of IAC, remarkably effective for select group C and less advanced group D eyes.[62] Eyes with retinal detachment from retinoblastoma show complete resolution of detachment following IAC if the detachment is partial and complete reattachment in most eyes with total detachment.

Pearls

IAC can control retinoblastoma. Complete tumor control is achieved in

- hundred percent of group B.
- hundred percent of group C.
- ninety-four percent of group D.
- thirty-six percent of group E.

There are few systemic complications of IAC, including hematoma at the groin entry site and transient pancytopenia from bone marrow suppression. Brain complications have been rarely encountered with carotid vascular spasm, stroke, and MRI displaying focal perfusion defects. Local ocular toxicities of IAC relate mostly to vascular compromise of the ophthalmic artery, central or branch retinal artery, or choroidal vessels. Muen found that 80% of eyes treated with IAC showed ocular side effects including cranial nerve palsy (40%), orbit/eyelid edema (20%), retinal detachment (7%), vitreous hemorrhage (27%), and retinal pigment epithelial (RPE) changes (47%).[61] The RPE changes could be related to previous retinal detachment or choroidal vascular compromise from chemotherapy toxicity. Both Munier et al and Shields et al observed this finding.[63,64] Ocular vascular compromise likely leads to poor visual outcome, but long-term assessment of visual acuity in eyes treated with IAC has not yet been analyzed. New approaches with delivery of chemotherapy into the ostium of the ophthalmic artery, to avoid wedging of blood flow and intimal trauma, have been advised. Additionally, greater facility with technique and short time of surgery can reduce vascular events. Fortunately, in our series, there was no incident of stroke, metastasis, or death.

Studies of the effects of IAC in animals has been pursued by Wilson et al.[65,66] They showed in a monkey model with real-time imaging that IAC with melphalan caused whitening of the retinal vessels at optic disc, choroidal blanching, retinal arterial narrowing, and retinal edema in all cases at the time of injection. They additionally showed in vitro that IAC with melphalan could be toxic to the vascular endothelium, leading to factors that might cause endothelial changes and fibrosis.

27.8.3 Sub-Tenon's Fascia Chemotherapy

Periocular injection of carboplatin has been used for retinoblastoma control over 2 decades, often as an adjunct to systemic chemotherapy. Periocular chemotherapy achieves rapid levels within the vitreous in 30 minutes, achieves doses that are 6 to 10 times that achieved by the intravenous route, and can last for hours. The method of injection as a plain liquid injection or injection with a vehicle such as a Lincoff balloon, iontophoresis, long-acting fibrin sealant, or nanoparticles has been explored. Initial reports suggested some success with sub-Tenon's carboplatin as primary therapy.[67] Because of later recurrences, however, this therapy was used more often in conjunction with systemic chemotherapy to boost the local dose of chemotherapy in the vitreous.

Complications of periocular chemotherapy include orbital and eyelid edema and ecchymosis, orbital fat atrophy, muscle fibrosis leading to strabismus, and optic atrophy. Long-term observations on complications have not been published.

27.8.4 Intravitreal Chemotherapy

Intravitrial chemotherapy (IVC) for retinoblastoma was explored initially in the 1960s using thiotepa. Ocular toxicity was established in rabbit eyes. Inomata and Kaneko and Ueda et al found melphalan to be the most effective chemotherapeutic agent against retinoblastoma based on in vitro testing of 12 agents, and a dose of 4 ug/ml achieved complete tumor suppression.[68,69] In their rabbit model, a concentration of 5.9 µg/ml showed no retinal toxicity, and this correlates to human vitreous doses of 20 to 30 ug, depending on globe size. Kaneko performed intravitreal injection of 8 to 30 µg melphalan combined with ocular hyperthermia for vitreous tumor seeding in 41 eyes, and unpublished results revealed eye-preservation rate of nearly 51% (presentation at the International Society of Ocular Oncology, Buenos Aires, Argentina, on November 16, 2011). Munier studied 23 patients with heavily treated retinoblastoma with recurrent vitreous seeds, treated with 20- to 30-µg melphalan on a weekly basis, and noted 83% success with avoidance of enucleation and/or external beam radiotherapy at 15 months.[70] Kivelä et al found success with intravitreal methotrexate, but this included numerous injections into the eye of a child over a 1-year period.[71]

Ghassemi and Shields evaluated 12 eyes treated with intravitreal melphalan for recurrent vitreous seeds following previous therapies of IVitC and IAC.[72] Eyes treated with low-dose melphalan (8–10 µg) showed less tumor control and minimal side effects, whereas those treated with higher doses (30–50 µg) showed excellent tumor control, but the 50-µg dose was toxic with persistent globe hypotonia and phthisis bulbi. There was no extraocular tumor seeding. Later, Shields et al reviewed an additional 11 eyes treated with 20- to 30-ug dose melphalan IVitC and found 100% control with minimal toxicity[73] (▶ Fig. 27.8). Ghassemi et al reported the combination of IVitC melphalan and topotecan to be especially useful for those patients who have recurrence after melphalan alone.[74]

The role of IVitC has yet to be defined, but it could be important as second-line therapy for recurrent vitreous seeding. In addition, it might be considered with systemic IVitC during first-line therapy if vitreous seeding persists while on IVitC.

Controversial Points

- IVitC has changed the frontier in the management of retinoblastoma, allowing salvage of eyes that would have otherwise been enucleated for vitreous seeds.

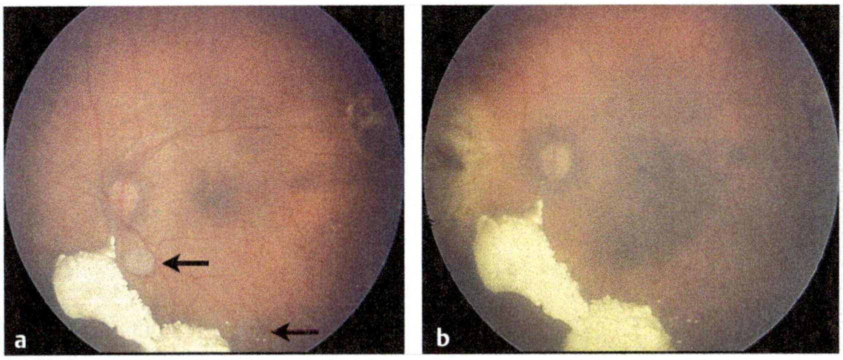

Fig. 27.8 (a) Intravitreal chemotherapy for recurrent vitreous seeds (arrows) (b) from retinoblastoma, showing seed regression.

27.8.5 Other Therapies

Other therapies for retinoblastoma management include focal therapies (thermotherapy, cryotherapy, laser photocoagulation, plaque radiotherapy) or whole-eye therapies (external beam radiotherapy, enucleation, orbital exenteration).[31,42]

Focal therapies are employed for small tumors, especially those that have been reduced by chemoreduction. Commonly, focal therapies are applied to an eye while the child is receiving chemoreduction, and they are repeated to each tumor at each chemotherapy session. Plaque radiotherapy is generally reserved for tumors that fail other focal therapies, even those that reach a moderate size, up to 8 or 10 mm in thickness. The remainder of the focal therapies is reserved for small tumors, generally those under 3 mm in greatest dimension.

Laser Photocoagulation

Laser photocoagulation is usually employed for small retinoblastomas posterior to the equator of the eye. In the era of chemoreduction, laser photocoagulation is rarely employed as its success depends on vascular coagulation and tumor ischemia, whereas the opposite applies to chemoreduction. Thus, it is not employed in eyes receiving chemoreduction. Laser photocoagulation is performed using the indirect ophthalmoscopic argon or green diode laser with two rows of photocoagulation surrounding the tumor base and special effort to avoid direct treatment to the tumor as that could lead to vitreous seeding. This technique requires multiple sessions for complete control.

Thermotherapy

Thermotherapy is a method of tumor heating using a diode infrared laser system. It is usually performed in conjunction with chemoreduction or carboplatin alone so that the two techniques work in synergy to treat the tumor. The goal is to deliver a temperature of 42–60 °C, a temperature that is below the coagulative threshold, therefore sparing the retinal vessels of photocoagulation. The combination of heat and chemotherapy is termed chemothermotherapy and the combination of heat and radiation is termed thermoradiotherapy. Heat has been found to have a synergistic effect with both chemotherapy and radiation therapy for the treatment of systemic and ocular cancers.[70] We employ thermotherapy as the main focal treatment to tumors following chemoreduction. The goal of this treatment is to heat the tumor to a gray-white scar. In general, small tumors require approximately 300 mW power for 10 minutes or less and large tumors require up to 800 mW power for 10 minutes, each delivered over three sessions at 1-month intervals. Thermotherapy coupled with chemoreduction is especially suited for tumors adjacent to the fovea and optic nerve where radiation or laser photocoagulation would possibly induce more visual loss. It is a time-consuming, tedious process that requires careful delivery of heat.

Cryotherapy

Cryotherapy is a useful method for treatment of equatorial and peripheral small retinoblastomas.[71] Tumor destruction is usually achieved with one or two sessions of triple freeze-thaw cryotherapy delivered at 1-month intervals. It is important to recognize that cryotherapy will usually fail if there is overlying vitreous seeds. In these failed cases, plaque radiotherapy is usually employed. Cryotherapy remains an important method for tumor consolidation following chemoreduction. It is a critical modality for management of recurrent subretinal seeds near the ora serrata.

Plaque Radiotherapy

Plaque radiotherapy is a method of brachytherapy in which a radioactive implant is placed on the sclera over the base of a retinoblastoma to irradiate the tumor transclerally. Generally, it is limited to tumors less than 16 mm in base and 8 mm in thickness. It requires an average of 4 days of treatment time to deliver the total dose of 4,000 cGy to the apex of the tumor. Plaque radiotherapy can be used as a primary treatment or as a secondary treatment.[75,76,77] In fact, in 70% of cases, plaque radiotherapy is used as a secondary treatment to salvage a globe after prior failed treatment, usually failed chemoreduction.[77]

Overall, using Kaplan–Meier estimates, there is approximately 80% tumor control rate at 4 years with one application of plaque radiotherapy.[77] Carefully selected retinoblastoma, even juxtapapillary and macular tumors, can be treated successfully with plaque radiotherapy. Retinoblastomas that are treated with plaque as a primary treatment show tumor control in 88% and those treated with plaque following chemoreduction show 92% control.[77] Tumor control is poorer following plaque for previous failed external beam radiotherapy (75%). The visual outcome varies with tumor size and location as well as radiation problems of retinopathy and papillopathy. The visual outcome has been reported to be good in 62% and the measured vision was 20/20 to 20/30 in over 50% of cases.[77] Radiation maculopathy is found in 25% of treated eyes and papillopathy in 26% of eyes by 5 years. A more recent report on the results of plaque radiotherapy following failure of chemoreduction continues to show favorable results with tumor control of 95% at 10 years, and recurrence was generally detected within 1 year of plaque treatment.[77] Plaque radiotherapy has not been associated with induction of second cancers.

External Beam Radiotherapy

Retinoblastoma is generally a radiosensitive tumor. External beam radiotherapy is a method of delivering whole-eye irradiation to treat advanced retinoblastoma, particularly following failure of previous chemotherapy methods. This technique is not commonly used currently due to the risk for related second cancers. The 30-year cumulative incidence for a second cancer in patients with bilateral retinoblastoma has been reported at 35% for patients who received radiation therapy compared with 6% for those who did not receive radiation.[78] Abramson and Frank found that external beam radiotherapy increased the incidence of second cancers in the field of radiation but did not stimulate second cancers outside the field of irradiation.[79] Importantly, the risk for radiation-induced cancers has been found to be dependent on patient age at the time of irradiation as well as other factors. Patients treated with external beam radiotherapy at an age younger than 12 months have a greater risk for second cancers than patients older than 12 months.

Enucleation

Enucleation is a frequently used and important method for managing retinoblastoma. With advanced disease and no hope for useful vision in the affected eye or if there is a concern for invasion of the tumor into the optic nerve, choroid, or orbit, then enucleation is appropriate. Those eyes with secondary glaucoma, pars plana seeding, or anterior chamber invasion are also generally best managed with enucleation.

The technique of enucleation is to gently remove the eye intact without seeding the malignancy into the orbit.[31] After the globe is removed, it is placed on a separate tray and fresh tissue is harvested in the operating room for DNA analysis, using a specific technique.[80] The surgeon must change sterile gloves after this step to avoid the risk of tumor contamination into the child's orbit.

Many years ago, an orbital implant was usually not placed after enucleation for retinoblastoma because it interfered with palpation of the socket and clinical detection of orbital tumor recurrence. More recently, with improved knowledge of the behavior of retinoblastoma and its low risks for local orbital recurrence, there is less hesitation for placing an orbital implant. In addition, available orbital imaging modalities of computed tomography and MRI allow detailed orbital evaluation, despite the presence of an implant. The orbital implant provides a more natural cosmetic appearance of the patient's artificial eye, minimizing sinking of the prosthesis and enabling motility of the prosthesis. There are several available orbital implants including polymethyl methacrylate sphere, coralline hydroxyapatite, polyethylene, and others. Currently, we use the coated hydroxyapatite implant. There are few problems with this implant if placed properly and there is no need for scleral wrap as the implant is wrapped in an inert polymer. Shah et al studied hydroxyapatite orbital implant following enucleation in 531 children and noted excellent long-term outcomes with low rates of conjunctival thinning (2%), implant infection (1%), implant exposure (3%), and favorable motility and cosmesis over a mean follow-up of 5 years.[81]

27.9 Histopathology

On gross examination of the enucleated specimen, retinoblastoma appears as a chalky white, friable tumor with dense foci of calcification. An endophytic retinoblastoma usually produces seeding into the vitreous cavity. An exophytic tumor tends to push the retina anteriorly and occupy the subretinal space. Cytologically, retinoblastomas make up a spectrum ranging from poorly differentiated to well-differentiated tumors. The poorly differentiated tumor consists of small to medium-sized round neuroblastic cells with large hyperchromatic nuclei and scanty cytoplasm. The well-differentiated retinoblastoma is characterized by the presence of rosettes and fleurettes. The Flexner–Wintersteiner rosette consists of columnar cells arranged around a clear central lumen. Some well-differentiated retinoblastomas and retinocytomas are also characterized by the presence of fleurettes. A fleurette is a lightly eosinophilic structure composed of groups of tumor cells that contain pear-shaped eosinophilic processes that project through the fenestrated membrane.

27.10 Conclusion

In summary, the management of retinoblastoma begins with establishing the correct diagnosis and choosing appropriate therapy. There are several pediatric conditions that can simulate retinoblastoma. Chemotherapy is the most common conservative treatment for retinoblastoma using intravenous, intra-arterial, sub-Tenon's fascia, or intravitreal routes. In general, most children with bilateral retinoblastoma receive IVitC (chemoreduction) for ocular tumor control and prevention of metastasis, pinealoblastoma, and long-term second cancers. For unilateral retinoblastoma, IAC provides excellent control with minimal systemic effect. STC is used in conjunction with chemoreduction to enhance dose at the eye in advanced cases. IVitC is currently reserved for those eyes with recurrent vitreous seeds following incomplete control with other methods. Plaque radiotherapy is an excellent salvage method for recurrence following chemotherapy. Eyes with advanced retinoblastoma, particularly if unilateral or considered high-risk for metastasis, should be managed with enucleation.

27.11 Acknowledgments

We thank the Ocular Oncology Service, Wills Eye Hospital, Thomas Jefferson University, Philadelphia, PA. Support was provided by the Eye Tumor Research Foundation, Philadelphia, PA, Lucille Wiedman Fund for Pediatric Eye Cancer, and Lift for a Cure, Morrisville, PA.

References

[1] Ramasubramanian A, Shields CL. Epidemiology and magnitude of the problem. In: Ramasubramanian A, Shields CL, eds. Retinoblastoma. New Delhi: Jaypee Brothers Medical Publishers; 2012:10–5

[2] Shields JA, Shields CL. Retinoblastoma. In: Shields JA, Shields CL, eds. Intraocular Tumors. An Atlas and Textbook. 2nd ed. Philadelphia, PA: Lippincott Williams & Wilkins; 2008:293–365

[3] Shields JA, Shields CL. Intraocular Tumors. An Atlas and Textbook. 3rd edition. Philadelphia, PA: Lippincott Wolters Kluwers; 2016:335-387

[4] Kivelä T. The epidemiological challenge of the most frequent eye cancer: retinoblastoma, an issue of birth and death. Br J Ophthalmol. 2009; 93(9):1129–1131

[5] Rodrigues KE, Latorre MdoR, de Camargo B. Delayed diagnosis in retinoblastoma [in Portuguese]. J Pediatr (Rio J). 2004; 80(6):511–516

[6] Knudson AG, Jr, Meadows AT, Nichols WW, Hill R. Chromosomal deletion and retinoblastoma. N Engl J Med. 1976; 295(20):1120–1123

[7] Moll AC, Imhof SM, Meeteren AY, Boers M. At what age could screening for familial retinoblastoma be stopped? A register based study 1945–98. Br J Ophthalmol. 2000; 84(10):1170–1172

[8] Honavar SG, Singh AD, Shields CL, et al. Postenucleation adjuvant therapy in high-risk retinoblastoma. Arch Ophthalmol. 2002; 120(7):923–931

[9] Kaliki S, Shields CL, Shah SU, Eagle RC, Jr, Shields JA, Leahey A. Postenucleation adjuvant chemotherapy with vincristine, etoposide, and carboplatin for the treatment of high-risk retinoblastoma. Arch Ophthalmol. 2011; 129 (11):1422–1427

[10] Kaliki S, Shields CL, Rojanaporn D, et al. High-risk retinoblastoma based on international classification of retinoblastoma: analysis of 519 enucleated eyes. Ophthalmology. 2013; 120(5):997–1003

[11] Shields CL, Shields JA, Baez K, Cater JR, De Potter P. Optic nerve invasion of retinoblastoma. Metastatic potential and clinical risk factors. Cancer. 1994; 73(3):692–698

[12] Shields CL, Shields JA, Baez KA, Cater J, De Potter PV. Choroidal invasion of retinoblastoma: metastatic potential and clinical risk factors. Br J Ophthalmol. 1993; 77(9):544–548

[13] Bader JL, Miller RW, Meadows AT, Zimmerman LE, Champion LA, Voûte PA. Trilateral retinoblastoma. Lancet. 1980; 2(8194):582–583

[14] Donoso LA, Rorke LB, Shields JA, Augsburger JJ, Brownstein S, Lahoud S. S-antigen immunoreactivity in trilateral retinoblastoma. Am J Ophthalmol. 1987; 103(1):57–62

[15] Pesin SR, Shields JA. Seven cases of trilateral retinoblastoma. Am J Ophthalmol. 1989; 107(2):121–126

[16] De Potter P, Shields CL, Shields JA. Clinical variations of trilateral retinoblastoma: a report of 13 cases. J Pediatr Ophthalmol Strabismus. 1994; 31(1):26–31

[17] Kivelä T. Trilateral retinoblastoma: a meta-analysis of hereditary retinoblastoma associated with primary ectopic intracranial retinoblastoma. J Clin Oncol. 1999; 17(6):1829–1837

[18] Shields CL, Shields JA, Meadows AT. Chemoreduction for retinoblastoma may prevent trilateral retinoblastoma. J Clin Oncol. 2000; 18(1):236–237

[19] Shields CL, Meadows AT, Shields JA, Carvalho C, Smith AF. Chemoreduction for retinoblastoma may prevent intracranial neuroblastic malignancy (trilateral retinoblastoma). Arch Ophthalmol. 2001; 119(9):1269–1272

[20] Ramasubramanian A, Kytasty C, Meadows AT, Shields JA, Leahey A, Shields CL. Incidence of pineal gland cyst and pineoblastoma in children with retinoblastoma during the chemoreduction era. Am J Ophthalmol. 2013; 156 (4):825–829

[21] Moll AC, Imhof SM, Schouten-van Meeteren AY, Boers M, van Leeuwen F, Hofman P. Chemoreduction for retinoblastoma. Arch Ophthalmol. 2003; 121 (10):1513

[22] Meadows AT, Shields CL. Regarding chemoreduction for retinoblastoma and intracranial neoplasms. Arch Ophthalmol. 2004; 122(10):1570–1571, author reply 1571

[23] Karatza EC, Shields CL, Flanders AE, Gonzalez ME, Shields JA. Pineal cyst simulating pinealoblastoma in 11 children with retinoblastoma. Arch Ophthalmol. 2006; 124(4):595–597

[24] Abramson DH, Ronner HJ, Ellsworth RM. Nonocular cancer in nonirradiated retinoblastoma. Am J Ophthalmol. 1979; 87:624–627

[25] Abramson DH, Melson MR, Dunkel IJ, Frank CM. Third (fourth and fifth) nonocular tumors in survivors of retinoblastoma. Ophthalmology. 2001; 108 (10):1868–1876

[26] Abramson DH, Frank CM, Susman M, Whalen MP, Dunkel IJ, Boyd NW, III. Presenting signs of retinoblastoma. J Pediatr. 1998; 132(3)(,)(Pt 1):505–508

[27] Epstein JA, Shields CL, Shields JA. Trends in the management of retinoblastoma: evaluation of 1,196 consecutive eyes during 1974 to 2001. J Pediatr Ophthalmol Strabismus. 2003; 40(4):196–203, quiz 217–218

[28] Zhao J, Li S, Shi J, Wang N. Clinical presentation and group classification of newly diagnosed intraocular retinoblastoma in China. Br J Ophthalmol. 2011; 95(10):1372–1375

[29] Ali AA, Elsheikh SM, Elhaj A, et al. Clinical presentation and outcome of retinoblastoma among children treated at the National Cancer Institute (NCI) in Gezira, Sudan: a single Institution experience. Ophthalmic Genet. 2011; 32 (2):122–125

[30] Boubacar T, Fatou S, Fousseyni T, et al. A 30-month prospective study on the treatment of retinoblastoma in the Gabriel Toure Teaching Hospital, Bamako, Mali. Br J Ophthalmol. 2010; 94(4):467–469

[31] Shields CL, Shields JA. Retinoblastoma management: advances in enucleation, intravenous chemoreduction, and intra-arterial chemotherapy. Curr Opin Ophthalmol. 2010; 21(3):203–212

[32] Shields CL, Ghassemi F, Tuncer S, Thangappan A, Shields JA. Clinical spectrum of diffuse infiltrating retinoblastoma in 34 consecutive eyes. Ophthalmology. 2008; 115(12):2253–2258

[33] Ramasubramanian A, Shields CL. Staging and treatment strategies. In: Ramasubramanian A, Shields CL, eds. Retinoblastoma. New Delhi: Jaypee Brothers Medical Publishers; 2012:70–78

[34] Reese AB, Ellsworth RM. The evaluation and current concept of retinoblastoma therapy. Trans Am Acad Ophthalmol Otolaryngol. 1963; 67:164–172

[35] Hopping W. The new Essen prognosis classification for conservative sight-saving treatment of retinoblastoma. In: Lommatzsch PK, Blodi FC, eds. Intraocular Tumors: International Symposium under the Auspices of the European Ophthalmological Society. Berlin, Germany: Springer-Verlag; 1983:497–505

[36] Shields CL, Mashayekhi A, Demirci H, Meadows AT, Shields JA. Practical approach to management of retinoblastoma. Arch Ophthalmol. 2004; 122 (5):729–735

[37] Linn Murphree A. Intraocular retinoblastoma: the case for a new group classification. Ophthalmol Clin North Am. 2005; 18(1):41–53, viii

[38] Shields CL, Shields JA. Basic understanding of current classification and management of retinoblastoma. Curr Opin Ophthalmol. 2006; 17(3):228–234

[39] Shields CL, Schoenberg E, Kocher K, Shukla SY, Kaliki S, Shields JA. Lesions simulating retinoblastoma (pseudoretinoblastoma) in 604 cases: results based on age at presentation. Ophthalmology. 2013; 120(2):311–316

[40] Cao C, Markovitz M, Ferenczy S, Shields CL. Hand-held spectral-domain optical coherence tomography of small macular retinoblastoma in infants before and after chemotherapy. J Pediatr Ophthalmol Strabismus. 2014; 51(4):230–234

[41] Kingston JE, Hungerford JL, Madreperla SA, Plowman PN. Results of combined chemotherapy and radiotherapy for advanced intraocular retinoblastoma. Arch Ophthalmol. 1996; 114(11):1339–1343

[42] Shields CL, Fulco EM, Arias JD, et al. Retinoblastoma frontiers with intravenous, intra-arterial, periocular, and intravitreal chemotherapy. Eye (Lond). 2013; 27(2):253–264

[43] Gallie BL, Budning A, DeBoer G, et al. Chemotherapy with focal therapy can cure intraocular retinoblastoma without radiotherapy. Arch Ophthalmol. 1996; 114(11):1321–1328

[44] Murphree AL, Villablanca JG, Deegan WF, III, et al. Chemotherapy plus local treatment in the management of intraocular retinoblastoma. Arch Ophthalmol. 1996; 114(11):1348–1356

[45] Shields CL, De Potter P, Himelstein BP, Shields JA, Meadows AT, Maris JM. Chemoreduction in the initial management of intraocular retinoblastoma. Arch Ophthalmol. 1996; 114(11):1330–1338

[46] Shields CL, Mashayekhi A, Au AK, et al. The International Classification of Retinoblastoma predicts chemoreduction success. Ophthalmology. 2006; 113 (12):2276–2280

[47] Leahey A. A cautionary tale: dosing chemotherapy in infants with retinoblastoma. J Clin Oncol. 2012; 30(10):1023–1024

[48] Friedrich MJ. Retinoblastoma therapy delivers power of chemotherapy with surgical precision. JAMA. 2011; 305(22):2276–2278

[49] Shields CL, Kaliki S, Al-Dahmash S, et al. Management of advanced retinoblastoma with intravenous chemotherapy then intra-arterial chemotherapy as alternative to enucleation. Retina. 2013; 33(10):2103–2109

[50] Demirci H, Shields CL, Meadows AT, Shields JA. Long-term visual outcome following chemoreduction for retinoblastoma. Arch Ophthalmol. 2005; 123 (11):1525–1530

[51] Narang S, Mashayekhi A, Rudich D, Shields CL. Predictors of long-term visual outcome after chemoreduction for management of intraocular retinoblastoma. Clin Experiment Ophthalmol. 2012; 40(7):736–742
[52] Wilson MW, Qaddoumi I, Billups C, Haik BG, Rodriguez-Galindo C. A clinicopathological correlation of 67 eyes primarily enucleated for advanced intraocular retinoblastoma. Br J Ophthalmol. 2011; 95(4):553–558
[53] Gombos DS, Hungerford J, Abramson DH, et al. Secondary acute myelogenous leukemia in patients with retinoblastoma: is chemotherapy a factor? Ophthalmology. 2007; 114(7):1378–1383
[54] Turaka K, Shields CL, Leahey A, Meadows AT. Second malignant neoplasms following chemoreduction with carboplatin, etoposide, and vincristine in 245 patients with intraocular retinoblastoma. Pediatr Blood Cancer. 2012; 59:121–125
[55] Yamane T, Kaneko A, Mohri M. The technique of ophthalmic arterial infusion therapy for patients with intraocular retinoblastoma. Int J Clin Oncol. 2004; 9 (2):69–73
[56] Abramson DH, Dunkel IJ, Brodie SE, Kim JW, Gobin YP. A phase I/II study of direct intraarterial (ophthalmic artery) chemotherapy with melphalan for intraocular retinoblastoma initial results. Ophthalmology. 2008; 115 (8):1398–1404, 1404.e1
[57] Gobin YP, Dunkel IJ, Marr BP, Brodie SE, Abramson DH. Intra-arterial chemotherapy for the management of retinoblastoma: four-year experience. Arch Ophthalmol. 2011; 129(6):732–737
[58] Shields CL, Shields JA. Intra-arterial chemotherapy for retinoblastoma: the beginning of a long journey. Clin Experiment Ophthalmol. 2010; 38(6):638–643
[59] Shields CL, Bianciotto CG, Jabbour P, et al. Intra-arterial chemotherapy for retinoblastoma: report No. 1, control of retinal tumors, subretinal seeds, and vitreous seeds. Arch Ophthalmol. 2011; 129(11):1399–1406
[60] Shields CL, Manjandavida FP, Lally SE, et al. Intra-arterial chemotherapy for retinoblastoma in 70 eyes: outcomes based on the international classification of retinoblastoma. Ophthalmology. 2014; 121(7):1453–1460
[61] Muen WJ, Kingston JE, Robertson F, Brew S, Sagoo MS, Reddy MA. Efficacy and complications of super-selective intra-ophthalmic artery melphalan for the treatment of refractory retinoblastoma. Ophthalmology. 2012; 119 (3):611–616
[62] Shields CL, Kaliki S, Shah SU, et al. Minimal exposure (one or two cycles) of intra-arterial chemotherapy in the management of retinoblastoma. Ophthalmology. 2012; 119(1):188–192
[63] Munier FL, Beck-Popovic M, Balmer A, Gaillard MC, Bovey E, Binaghi S. Occurrence of sectoral choroidal occlusive vasculopathy and retinal arteriolar embolization after superselective ophthalmic artery chemotherapy for advanced intraocular retinoblastoma. Retina. 2011; 31(3):566–573
[64] Shields CL, Bianciotto CG, Jabbour P, et al. Intra-arterial chemotherapy for retinoblastoma: report No. 2, treatment complications. Arch Ophthalmol. 2011; 129(11):1407–1415
[65] Wilson MW, Jackson JS, Phillips BX, et al. Real-time ophthalmoscopic findings of superselective intraophthalmic artery chemotherapy in a nonhuman primate model. Arch Ophthalmol. 2011; 129(11):1458–1465
[66] Wilson MW, Haik BG, Dyer MA. Superselective intraophthalmic artery chemotherapy: what we do not know. Arch Ophthalmol. 2011; 129(11):1490–1491
[67] Abramson DH. Periocular chemotherapy for retinoblastoma: success with problems? Arch Ophthalmol. 2005; 123(1):128–129, author reply 129
[68] Inomata M, Kaneko A. Chemosensitivity profiles of primary and cultured human retinoblastoma cells in a human tumor clonogenic assay. Jpn J Cancer Res. 1987; 78(8):858–868
[69] Ueda M, Tanabe J, Inomata M, Kaneko A, Kimura T. Study on conservative treatment of retinoblastoma—effect of intravitreal injection of melphalan on the rabbit retina [in Japanese]. Nippon Ganka Gakkai Zasshi. 1995; 99 (11):1230–1235
[70] Munier FL, Gaillard MC, Balmer A, et al. Intravitreal chemotherapy for vitreous disease in retinoblastoma revisited: from prohibition to conditional indications. Br J Ophthalmol. 2012; 96(8):1078–1083
[71] Kivelä T, Eskelin S, Paloheimo M. Intravitreal methotrexate for retinoblastoma. Ophthalmology. 2011; 118(8):1689–, 1689.e1–1689.e6
[72] Ghassemi F, Shields CL. Intravitreal melphalan for refractory or recurrent vitreous seeding from retinoblastoma. Arch Ophthalmol. 2012; 130(10):1268–1271
[73] Shields CL, Manjandavida FP, Arepalli S, Kaliki S, Lally SE, Shields JA. Intravitreal melphalan for persistent or recurrent retinoblastoma vitreous seeds: preliminary results. JAMA Ophthalmol. 2014; 132(3):319–325
[74] Ghassemi F, Shields CL, Ghadimi H, Khodabandeh A, Roohipoor R. Combined intravitreal melphalan and topotecan for refractory or recurrent vitreous seeding from retinoblastoma. JAMA Ophthalmol. 2014; 132(8):936–941
[75] Shields CL, Shields JA, De Potter P, et al. Plaque radiotherapy in the management of retinoblastoma. Use as a primary and secondary treatment. Ophthalmology. 1993; 100(2):216–224
[76] Shields CL, Shields JA, Cater J, Othmane I, Singh AD, Micaily B. Plaque radiotherapy for retinoblastoma: long-term tumor control and treatment complications in 208 tumors. Ophthalmology. 2001; 108(11):2116–2121
[77] Shields CL, Mashayekhi A, Sun H, et al. Iodine 125 plaque radiotherapy as salvage treatment for retinoblastoma recurrence following chemoreduction. Tumor control and treatment complications in 84 tumors. The Ingrid Kreissig Award Lecture. Ophthalmology. 2006; 113(11):2087–2092
[78] Roarty JD, McLean IW, Zimmerman LE. Incidence of second neoplasms in patients with bilateral retinoblastoma. Ophthalmology. 1988; 95(11):1583–1587
[79] Abramson DH, Frank CM. Second nonocular tumors in survivors of bilateral retinoblastoma: a possible age effect on radiation-related risk. Ophthalmology. 1998; 105(4):573–579, discussion 579–580
[80] Shields JA, Shields CL, Lally SE, Eagle RC, Jr. Harvesting fresh tumor tissue from enucleated eyes: the 2008 Jack S. Guyton lecture. Arch Ophthalmol. 2010; 128(2):241–243
[81] Shah SU, Shields CL, Lally SE, Shields JA. Hydroxyapatite orbital implant in children following enucleation: analysis of 531 sockets. Ophthal Plast Reconstr Surg. 2015; 31(2):108–114

28 Other Retinal, Retinal Pigment Epithelial, and Choroidal Tumors

Carol L. Shields and Jerry A. Shields

28.1 Introduction

Several benign and malignant neoplasms can occur in the retina and choroid. The most important malignancies, retinoblastoma and choroidal melanoma, have been covered in other chapters. Herein, we review the clinical features, pathologic characteristics, diagnostic approaches, and management of other selected tumors of the retina and choroid.

28.2 Retinal Tumors

There are several benign and malignant neoplasms that can arise in the retina and retinal pigment epithelium (RPE). Tumors can arise from the neural elements (retinoblastoma), vascular elements (hemangioma/hemangioblastoma), and glial elements (astrocytic hamartoma/astrocytoma) of the retina. The most important of these tumors is retinoblastoma, a malignant neoplasm of childhood that arises from the neurons of the sensory retina. There are several distinct types of retinal vascular tumors and glial tumors that can arise in the sensory retina, some of which are associated with the oculoneurocutaneous syndromes, or phakomatoses. Therefore, the finding of a vascular or glial tumor should prompt the clinician to perform an appropriate systemic evaluation, looking for evidence of these syndromes. The RPE can spawn a number of tumors and pseudotumors, most of which are benign and should be differentiated from malignant choroidal melanoma.

It is important for the clinician to have a basic knowledge of the ophthalmoscopic features of retinal and RPE lesions to be able to advise the patient regarding the best approach to management or refer the patient to an ocular oncologist who manages ocular tumors routinely. We will review the more important tumors of the sensory retina and the RPE. When pertinent, the results of ancillary techniques, such as fluorescein angiography, ultrasonography, optical coherence tomography (OCT), and other studies, are described.

28.2.1 Retinoblastoma

Retinoblastoma is a malignant tumor that arises in the sensory retina in children. This malignancy is discussed in detail in Chapter 27.

28.2.2 Retinal Hemangioblastoma (Retinal Capillary Hemangioma)

Several benign vascular tumors can arise in the sensory retina. It is important to differentiate the various retinal vascular tumors as each has distinct ophthalmologic features, fluorescein angiographic characteristics, complications, associated systemic findings, and management.

Retinal hemangioblastoma is a vascular hamartoma that usually has its clinical onset in the first two decades of life. In the past, this tumor was termed "retinal capillary hemangioma," but currently it is termed "retinal hemangioblastoma." Unilateral solitary lesions can occur due to sporadic mutations and have no systemic associations, whereas bilateral or multiple lesions are more likely to be associated with the von Hippel–Lindau (VHL) syndrome (▶ Table 28.1).

Pearls

- Bilateral or multiple retinal hemangioblastomas are associated with VHL syndrome and patients should be evaluated for this condition with brain and renal imaging. Solitary retinal hemangioblastoma may or may not be associated with VHL syndrome. Genetic testing is advised.

Clinical Features

Retinal hemangioblastoma appears ophthalmoscopically as a reddish orange mass, located in the peripheral retina or near the macula or optic disc[1,2,3,4,5] (▶ Fig. 28.1 and ▶ Fig. 28.2). This tumor appears as a red-orange retinal mass with dilated retinal vessels that feed and drain the tumor. As the tumor enlarges, the vessels become more dilated and tortuous. This tumor may be associated with subretinal and intraretinal exudation, subretinal fluid, and vitreoretinal fibrosis. The exudation has a tendency to accumulate selectively in the macular area. When retinal hemangioblastoma is located at the optic disc, the dilated retinal vessels are often not visible. Regardless of tumor location, accumulation of subretinal fluid with exudation can lead to profound visual acuity loss.

Table 28.1 Diagnostic criteria for the diagnosis of von Hippel–Lindau syndrome

Family history[a]	Feature
Positive	Any one of the following: • Retinal hemangioblastoma • Brain hemangioblastoma • Visceral lesion
Negative	Any one of the following: • Two or more retinal hemangioblastomas • Two or more brain hemangioblastomas • Single retinal or brain hemangioblastoma with a visceral lesion

Note: Visceral lesions include renal cysts, renal carcinoma, pheochromocytoma, pancreatic cysts, islet cell tumors, epididymal cystadenoma, endolymphatic sac tumor, and adnexal papillary cystadenoma of probable mesonephric origin.

[a]Family history of retinal or brain hemangioma or visceral lesion.

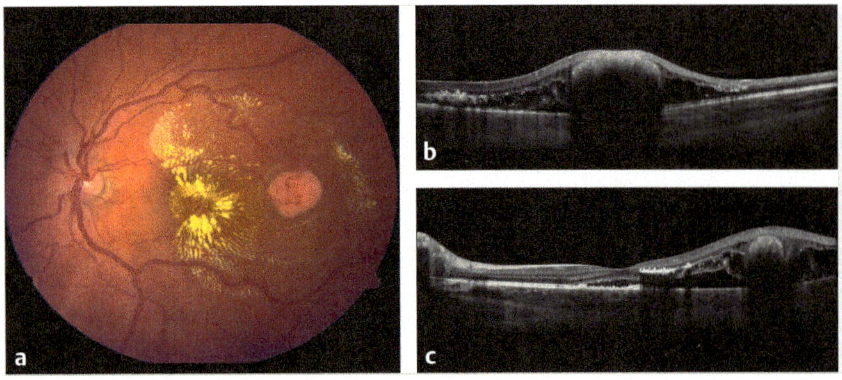

Fig. 28.1 (**a**) Retinal hemangioblastoma showing surrounding exudative retinopathy and (**b**) optical coherence tomography demonstrating the dense retinal mass and (**c**) subfoveal exudation and fluid with cystoid edema.

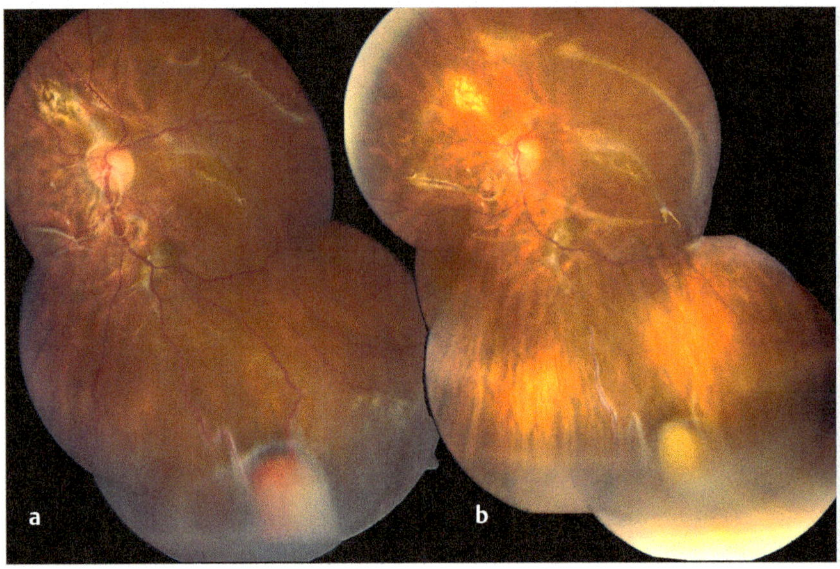

Fig. 28.2 Retinal hemangioblastoma (**a**) before and (**b**) after photodynamic therapy.

Genetics and Pathogenesis

In the VHL syndrome, the stromal cells have a mutation on chromosome 3p25–26, which leads to dysfunctional VHL protein.[6,7] These cells cannot degrade hypoxia-inducible factor 1a, so it accumulates and causes production of vascular endothelial growth factor (VEGF), platelet-derived growth factor, erythropoietin, and transforming growth factor alpha, all of which lead to proliferation and vascularization of the tumor.[7]

There are three types of mutations in the VHL gene: (1) type 1 with a deletion or nonsense mutation and manifesting mainly hemangioblastomas only; (2) type 2 with a missense mutation predisposing to hemangioblastomas and pheochromocytomas (type 2A), or also renal cell carcinoma (type 2B), or only pheochromocytoma (type 2C); and (3) type 3, which predisposes to polycythemia.[8]

Diagnosis

Retinal hemangioblastoma may be diagnosed with fluorescein angiography. This test characteristically shows rapid filling of the vascular tumor with fluorescein through the feeding artery into the tumor; fluorescein then exits rapidly through the draining vein. Larger tumors show leakage of fluorescein dye from the mass into the adjacent retina and vitreous cavity.

Ultrasonography can depict the intraocular mass as an acoustically solid mass and can also demonstrate surrounding subretinal fluid. OCT can show the intraretinal tumor occupying full-thickness retina as a dense mass, with related subretinal fluid, intraretinal edema, and epiretinal membrane.[9] OCT is very helpful in judging treatment response.

Magnetic resonance imaging (MRI) or computed tomography (CT) can provide some help for diagnosis as each will show an enhancing mass in the retina, often with overlying retinal detachment. MRI or CT is helpful to look for associated central nervous system and abdominal neoplasms.

Management and Course

Management of retinal hemangioblastoma consists of both a systemic and an ocular evaluation. The systemic evaluation includes testing for tumors associated with the VHL syndrome, such as cerebellar hemangioblastoma, pheochromocytoma, renal cell carcinoma, and other associated neoplasms and cysts. Brain and abdominal MRI or CT should be performed periodically in affected patients. In addition, close ophthalmic follow-up is important to detect early retinal tumors. If a small retinal capillary hemangioma is detected, early treatment is advisable, often using laser photocoagulation or thermotherapy.

The treatment of a retinal hemangioblastoma varies with the clinical situation.[4,10,11,12,13] Tumors associated with the VHL syndrome tend to be more aggressive; thus, all hemangioblastomas associated with this syndrome are considered for treatment. Laser photocoagulation or photodynamic therapy can be used for small tumors (< 3 mm), but photodynamic therapy or cryotherapy should be used for medium tumors (3–6 mm) (▶ Fig. 28.2). Large tumors may require plaque radiotherapy or internal resection via pars plana vitrectomy.

For retinal hemangioblastomas unassociated with the VHL syndrome, small asymptomatic lesions without subretinal fluid can be observed carefully, particularly if they are in the perimacular or juxtapapillary region where treatment could be detrimental to vision. If leakage ensues, then treatment is warranted. However, most retinal hemangioblastomas require treatment to prevent subretinal fluid or macular complications. Laser photocoagulation or photodynamic therapy is useful for tumors located posterior to the equator and cryotherapy is employed for those anterior to the equator. Plaque radiotherapy is reserved for larger tumors. Surgical repair of secondary retinal detachment or epiretinal membrane is often necessary. In the case of an aggressive tumor that does not respond to conventional treatment, external beam radiotherapy or plaque radiotherapy can be employed.

There have been anecdotal cases that have responded to oral propranolol, oral acetazolamide, and oral prednisone, but large studies have not been performed. Oral and intravitreal anti-VEGF have not been successful in inducing tumor regression, but intravitreal anti-VEGF can be useful for reduction of macular edema and occasionally subretinal fluid. Wong and Chew reviewed the role of anti-VEGF and emerging therapies for retinal hemangioblastoma.[4]

Controversial Points

- The management of retinal hemangioblastoma is controversial as there are no singular excellent therapies. Most patients respond to cryotherapy if the tumor is peripheral or to laser photocoagulation if the tumor is small and posterior to the equator. For larger postequatorial tumors, photodynamic therapy can be effective.

Histopathology

Histopathologically, retinal hemangioblastoma consists of a proliferation of retinal capillaries that usually replace full-thickness neurosensory retina. With light microscopy, there appears to be a benign proliferation of endothelial cells, pericytes, and stromal cells. In the end stage, total retinal detachment with massive retinal gliosis, cataract, and phthisis bulbi ensue.

28.2.3 Retinal Cavernous Hemangioma

Retinal cavernous hemangioma has clinical features, systemic implications, and complications that are distinctly different from those of other retinal vascular tumors, such as retinal hemangioblastoma, racemose hemangioma, and the vasoproliferative tumor. This vascular tumor is often associated with similar skin and central nervous system lesions and, therefore, should be classified with the oculoneurocutaneous syndromes, or phakomatoses.

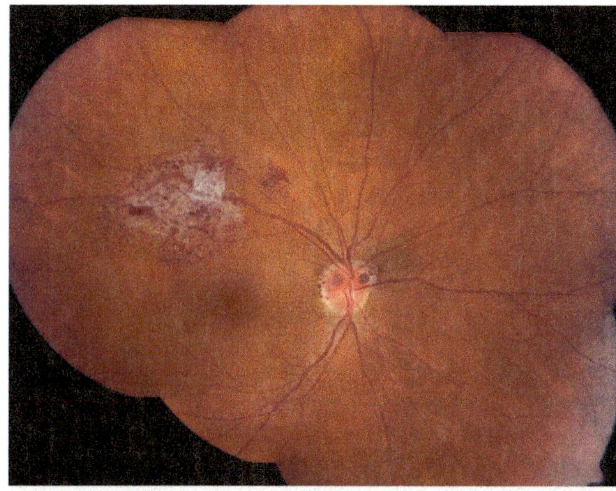

Fig. 28.3 Retinal cavernous hemangioma with "bunch of grapes" appearance and overlying fibrosis.

Clinical Features

Ophthalmoscopically, retinal cavernous hemangioma usually appears as a cluster of dark intraretinal venous aneurysms, sometimes referred to as a "bunch of concord grapes"[1,2,14,15,16,17,18,19,20] (▶ Fig. 28.3). This tumor can be asymptomatic or associated with moderate or severe visual impairment resulting from macular scarring, secondary retinal traction, or vitreous hemorrhage. Unlike retinal hemangioblastoma, cavernous hemangioma does not have a feeding artery and is typically located along the course of a retinal vein, but can be on the optic disc. Rarely is there exudation, but commonly there is overlying white fibroglial tissue on the tumor surface, suggesting previous vitreous or preretinal hemorrhage. Retinal cavernous hemangioma is usually nonprogressive but on rare occasions can show minimal enlargement over time. The main complication of retinal cavernous hemangioma is vitreous hemorrhage.

Pearls

- Retinal cavernous hemangioma is typically located along a retinal vein and can produce vitreous hemorrhage.

Genetics

Retinal cavernous hemangioma can occur with cerebral cavernous malformations as a sporadic or familial autosomal dominant disorder with incomplete penetrance. There are three cerebral cavernous malformation (CCM) genes, including CCM/KRIT1, CCM2/MGC4607, and CCM3/PDCD10.[18] CCM3 is associated with a higher risk for cerebral hemorrhage in childhood.

Diagnosis

In most instances, retinal cavernous hemangioma has a typical ophthalmoscopic appearance. The most helpful diagnostic ancillary test is fluorescein angiography, which produces nearly pathognomonic findings. During the arterial phase, the vascular channels are hypofluorescent; fluorescein enters slowly in the late phase of the angiogram. The fluorescein is contained within the venous aneurysms and occupies the superior portion of each cavernous space, while the red blood cells collect in the inferior portion of each aneurysm and there is no leakage of dye. This produces a "fluorescein–erythrocyte interface" in the late angiogram, a characteristic feature of cavernous hemangioma.

With large retinal cavernous hemangiomas, extensive vitreous hemorrhage can occur, obscuring the tumor which is then detectable by ultrasonography. With A-scan ultrasonography, there is a high initial spike and high internal reflectivity. With B-scan ultrasonography, the lesion shows an irregular but well-defined surface, acoustic solidity, and no choroidal excavation.

OCT demonstrates the numerous cavernous spaces within the retina which cause a markedly irregular retinal surface. In general, the retinal anatomy is disorganized from tumor compression.

Management and Course

Most cases of retinal cavernous hemangioma require no treatment. These tumors rarely progress or produce visual symptoms. Vitreous hemorrhage can occur and is managed with observation or vitrectomy. For repetitive hemorrhage, the tumor can be sclerosed with plaque radiotherapy, photodynamic therapy, or cryotherapy. It is important to perform brain MRI to evaluate for related cerebral cavernomas, and genetic testing for the CCM genes is advised, especially if there is a family history of cavernomas or the patient shows multiple cavernomas.

Histopathology

Histopathologically, retinal cavernous hemangioma appears as a mass of large-caliber vascular spaces in the inner retina, but potentially involving all layers of the retina. This tumor consists of endothelial-lined venous aneurysms interconnected by narrow channels.[20] There can be extensive cystic and fibrous degeneration of the retina.

28.2.4 Retinal Racemose Hemangioma

The retinal racemose hemangioma is not a true neoplasm but rather a simple or complex arteriovenous communication.[1,2] It can occur as a solitary unilateral lesion or it can be part of the Wyburn–Mason syndrome (also called Bonnet–Dechaume–Blanc syndrome), which is more anatomically termed retinoencephalofacial angiomatosis. This arteriovenous malformation can affect the retina, visual pathways, midbrain, and facial bones including the mandible and maxilla. There is no hereditary tendency.

Clinical Features

Ophthalmoscopically, the retinal racemose hemangioma is characterized by a large, dilated, tortuous retinal artery that passes from the optic disc for a variable distance into the fundus, where it then communicates directly with a similarly dilated retinal vein that passes back to the optic disc. In some cases, the vascular anomaly displays a complex array of blood vessels. This retinal malformation does not usually produce exudation or hemorrhage, unless branch retinal vein obstruction occurs. This retinal condition is classified by the Archer classification according to size and location of the malformation[21,22,23,24,25,26] (▶ Table 28.2).

Genetics

There is evidence that genetic or developmental factors early in gestation lead to dysgenesis of the embryologic vascular plexus.[26] The time of insult determines the location and extent of manifestations.

Diagnosis

The retinal racemose hemangioma is established with ophthalmoscopy and confirmed with fluorescein angiography, which shows rapid filling of the affected dilated artery and vein, usually with no intervening capillary channels and typically without leakage into surrounding tissues (▶ Fig. 28.4).

Management and Course

The management of a patient with a retinal racemose hemangioma consists of systemic and ophthalmic monitoring. The patient should be evaluated for the Wyburn–Mason syndrome with imaging studies investigating for the presence of vascular abnormalities in the brain and facial bones. The retinal lesion usually remains stable and treatment is rarely indicated.

Table 28.2 Archer classification for Wyburn–Mason syndrome

Group	Feature	Comments
I	Abnormal capillary plexus between the major vessels of the arteriovenous malformations	Such lesions tend to be small, patients asymptomatic, and intracranial involvement uncommon
II	Arteriovenous malformations lack any intervening capillary bed between the artery and vein	Risk of retinal decompensation resulting in retina edema, hemorrhage, and vision loss. Low risk for intracranial arteriovenous malformations
III	Extensive arteriovenous malformations with dilated and tortuous vessels and no distinction between artery and vein	High risk for visual loss due to retinal decompensation or retinal compression of nerve fiber layer, optic nerve, or other vessels. High risk for intracranial arteriovenous malformations

Source: Adapted from Archer et al.[21]

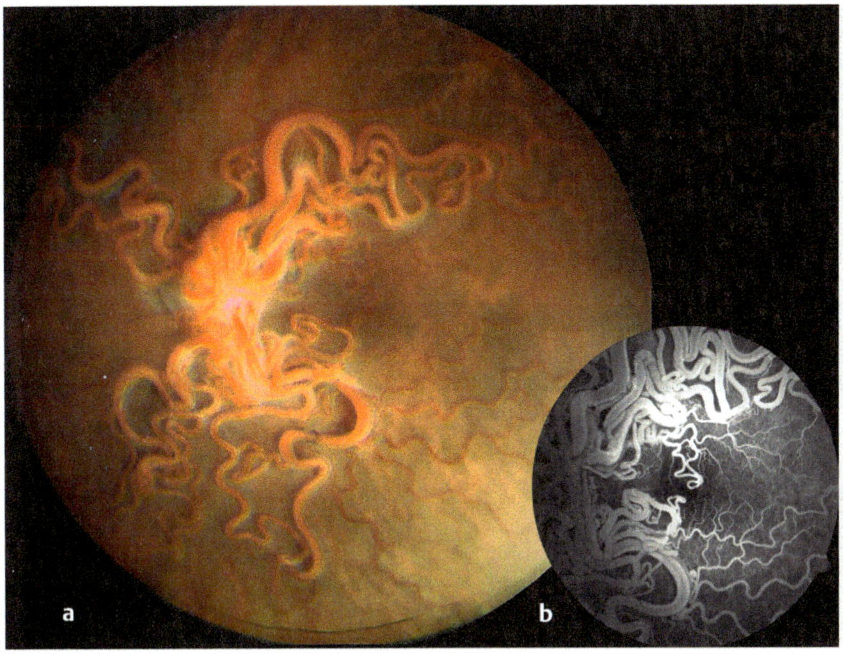

Fig. 28.4 (**a**) Retinal racemose hemangioma with dilated tortuous retinal vessels and (**b**) no leakage on fluorescein angiography.

Table 28.3 Associated ocular conditions in 67 eyes of 56 patients with secondary vasoproliferative tumor

Associated ocular condition	**Secondary VPT (*n* = 67 eyes), *n* (%)**	**Secondary VPT (*n* = 56 patients), *n* (%)**
Retinitis pigmentosa	15 (22)	10 (18)
Pars planitis	14 (21)	11 (20)
Coats' disease	11 (16)	11 (20)
Previous retinal detachment repair	8 (12)	8 (14)
Idiopathic peripheral retinal vasculitis	4 (6)	3 (5)
Familial exudative vitreoretinopathy	3 (4)	3 (5)
Toxoplasmosis	3 (4)	3 (5)
Aniridia	2 (3)	1 (2)
Congenital hypertrophy of retinal pigment epithelium	2 (3)	2 (4)
Idiopathic choroiditis	2 (3)	1 (2)
Retinopathy of prematurity	2 (3)	2 (4)
Histoplasmosis	1 (1)	1 (2)
Total	67	56

Abbreviation: VPT, vasoproliferative retinal tumor.

Source: Data adapted from Shields et al.[29]

Histopathology

Little histopathologic information is available on retinal racemose hemangioma. The large, dilated retinal vessels appear to have an acellular adventitial covering. The retina is thin and may show extensive degeneration.

28.2.5 Acquired Vasoproliferative Tumor

The acquired vasoproliferative tumor of the ocular fundus is a vascular mass that can occur as a primary or secondary condition, from predisposing intermediate uveitis, retinitis pigmentosa, Coats' disease, or chronic retinal detachment[27,28,29,30,31,32,33,34] (▶ Table 28.3). There are generally no systemic associations, but some patients have underlying hypertension or hyperlipidemia.

Clinical Features

Ophthalmoscopically, the acquired vasoproliferative tumor appears as an elevated sessile or dome-shaped mass that is usually located in the equatorial inferotemporal region (▶ Fig. 28.5 and ▶ Fig. 28.6). This mass can be circumscribed or ill-defined. An associated retinal feeding artery and draining vein can be minimally dilated, but not as markedly dilated or tortuous as seen with retinal hemangioblastoma. The tumor may be associated with complications including intraretinal and subretinal exudation, subretinal fluid, remote epiretinal membrane, cystoid macular edema, retinal hemorrhage, and vitreous hemorrhage. The retinal exudation generally begins at the tumor margin and gradually accumulates posteriorly into the macula, with ensuing visual loss.

Genetics

There are no genetic abnormalities associated with this condition, but for those tumors that are secondary, evaluation for underlying retinitis pigmentosa or other mutations can be performed.

Diagnosis

Fluorescein angiography demonstrates filling of the mass through a feeding, slightly dilated and minimally tortuous

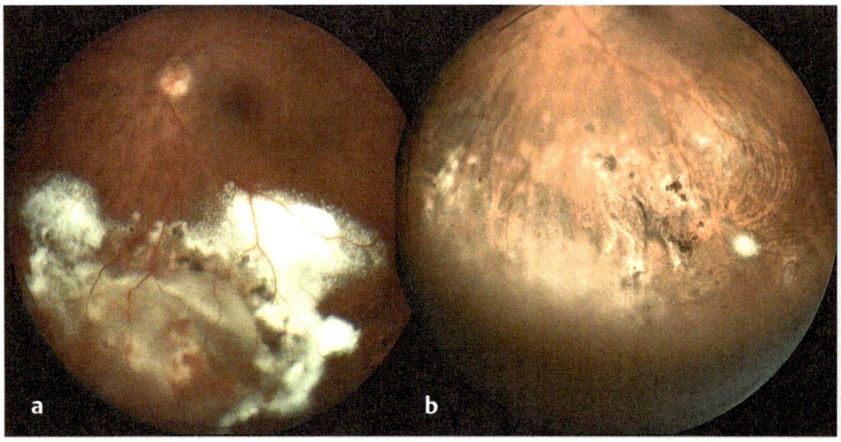

Fig. 28.5 (**a**) Retinal vasoproliferative tumor with ill-defined retinal mass and (**b**) exudative retinopathy showing complete response to single-session photodynamic therapy.

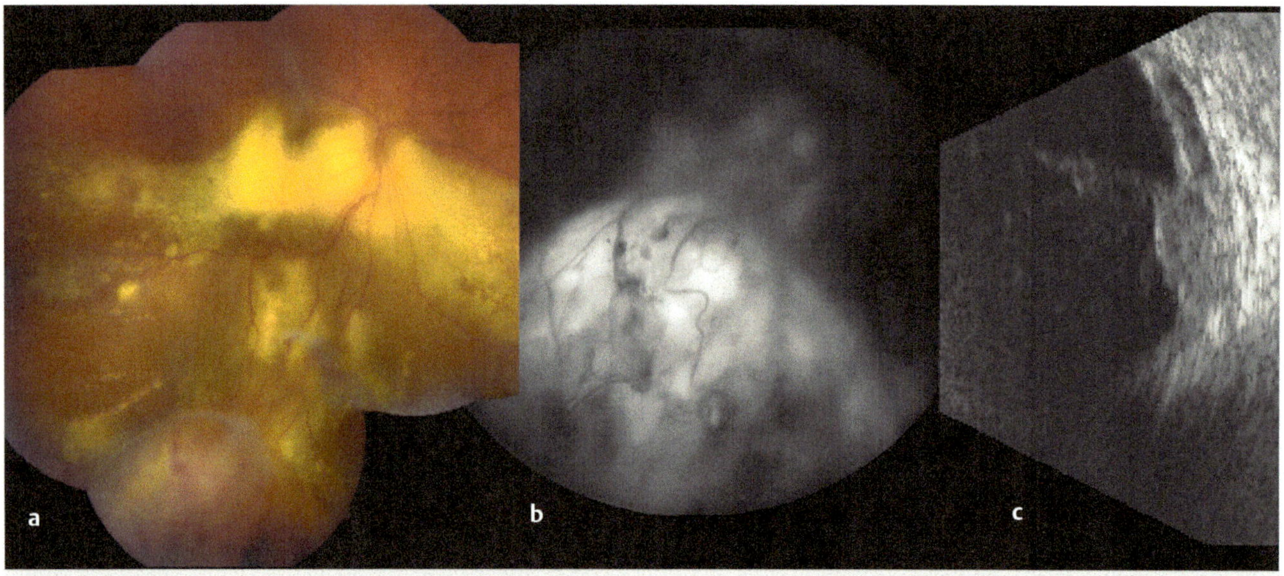

Fig. 28.6 (**a**) Retinal vasoproliferative tumor with well-defined retinal mass and (**b**) exudative retinopathy showing diffuse enhancement on fluorescein angiography and (**c**) echodensity on ultrasonography.

retinal artery and draining vein. There is frequently leakage from the vasoproliferative tumor into the surrounding retina and vitreous cavity. Remote macular edema is seen on fluorescein angiography and confirmed on OCT.

Management and Course

Small peripheral tumors may be observed carefully if there is no leakage. Those with active leakage require therapy including laser photocoagulation, thermotherapy, indocyanine green–enhanced thermoablation, photodynamic therapy, or plaque radiotherapy.[28,29,30,31,32,33] Intravitreal anti-VEGF therapy can assist in reducing remote macular edema, and sub-Tenon's fascia triamcinolone can minimize the inflammatory response associated with treatment.

Histopathology

Histopathology of the acquired vasoproliferative tumor in the early phases, when the tumor is mostly vascular, has not been clearly established. It is believed to represent a proliferation of blood vessels, glial tissue, and RPE, often in response to previous insults. Later, as the tumor becomes clinically fibrotic, a more reactive astrocytic appearance is documented.[34]

28.2.6 Astrocytic Hamartoma

Although reactive gliosis can occur in the retina after trauma or inflammation, true tumors arising from the glial elements of the retina are relatively uncommon. The most important retinal glial tumors are astrocytic hamartoma and acquired astrocytoma.[1,2,35,36,37,38,39,40,41,42,43] Although these two lesions appear different in most cases, there are some instances in which the clinical features overlap.

Astrocytic hamartoma of the retina (and optic disc) is a benign glial tumor that can occur as a manifestation of tuberous sclerosis. The general systemic manifestations of tuberous sclerosis include cutaneous sebaceous adenoma, cardiac rhabdomyoma, renal angiomyolipoma, and others. Detection of a retinal astrocytic hamartoma should alert the clinician

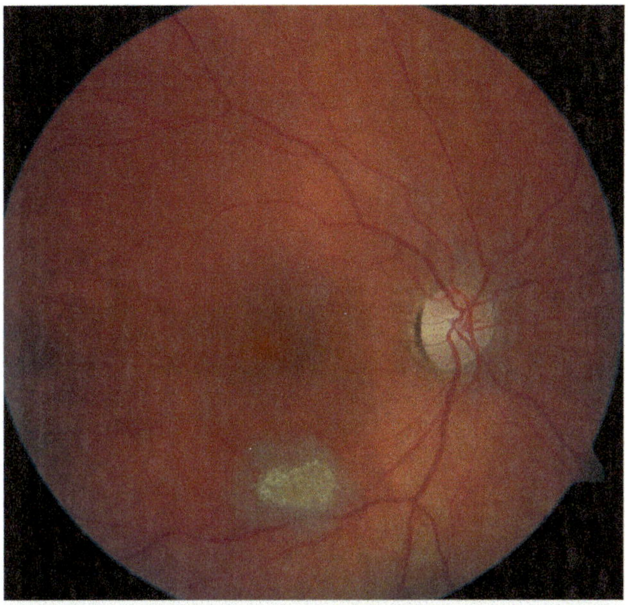

Fig. 28.7 Retinal astrocytic hamartoma with intralesional glistening calcification.

to the possibility of tuberous sclerosis or, less commonly, neurofibromatosis.

Clinical Features

Small retinal astrocytic hamartoma can be subtle, appearing as an ill-defined translucent thickening of the nerve fiber layer, sometimes with slight retinal traction (▶ Fig. 28.7). Larger tumors assume a more opaque appearance but typically remain sessile and yellow-white, located in the nerve fiber layer and overlying the retinal vessels. There are usually no dilated vessels leading to this tumor, but mild retinal traction may be observed. Astrocytic hamartoma can manifest intrinsic calcification that appears round, refractile, and yellow, resembling fish eggs, tapioca, or a yellow mulberry.[35,36,37,38,39,40] This tumor is generally stable and without complications, but vitreous or subretinal hemorrhage and retinal detachment can occur. Rarely does this tumor show uncontrolled growth. If related to tuberous sclerosis complex (TSC), there might be depigmented "punched-out" spots in the RPE.[38]

Genetics

An isolated, solitary astrocytic hamartoma may or may not be associated with TSC. Patients with multiple astrocytic hamartomas likely have TSC. TSC is a multisystem disorder that can occur in multiple tissues but primarily the skin, brain, and eye. This autosomal dominant condition displays two genetic loci, including 9q34 (TSC1) and 16p13 (TSC2). These two sites control products of hamartin (TSC1) and tuberin (TSC2) that act synergistically to regulate cellular growth and differentiation.[40,41] Deregulation of these products leads to hamartomatous tumors.

Table 28.4 Diagnostic criteria (revised) for establishing the diagnosis of tuberous sclerosis complex (TSC)

Category	Feature
Major feature	• Facial angiofibromas or forehead plaque • Ungual or periungual fibroma • Hypomelanotic macules (> 3) (ash-leaf macule) • Shagreen patch (connective tissue nevus) • Multiple retinal nodular hamartomas • Cortical tuber • Subependymal nodule • Subependymal giant cell astrocytoma • Cardiac rhabdomyoma • Lymphangiomyomatosis • Renal angiomyolipoma
Minor features	• Multiple pits in dental enamel • Hamartomatous rectal polyps • Bone cysts • Cerebral white matter migration lines • Gingival fibromas • Nonrenal hamartoma • Retinal achromic patch • Confetti skin lesions • Multiple renal cysts

Note on classification:

- Definite TSC: either two major or one major with two minor features
- Probable TSC: one major and one minor feature
- Possible TSC: either one major or two or more minor features

There are diagnostic criteria for TSC that were established by the Tuberous Sclerosis Consensus Conference in 1998[41,42] (▶ Table 28.4). A definite diagnosis of TSC is established by the presence of two major or one major plus two minor features. Probable TSC requires one major and one minor feature, and possible TSC requires either one major or two or more minor features.

Diagnosis

The diagnosis of retinal astrocytic hamartoma is usually made with indirect ophthalmoscopy and subsequent physical evaluation for signs of tuberous sclerosis or neurofibromatosis. Ancillary studies can be confirmatory, including fluorescein angiography, ultrasonography, and OCT. On fluorescein angiography, the tumor shows slow and incomplete filling in the late arterial or midvenous phases. There is a classic corkscrew or "hairpin" looping to the intrinsic vessels, suggestive of the diagnosis. These fine blood vessels can leak in the late phases.

Ultrasonography is of some diagnostic value to document the intrinsic calcification. With B-scan, medium and large astrocytic hamartomas appear as well-demarcated, oval masses with a sharp anterior border, acoustic solidity, and acoustic shadowing of the orbital fat posterior to the tumors. Persistent focal echoes at reduced sensitivities suggest calcification within the mass. A-scan ultrasonography shows a sharp anterior border, high internal reflectivity, and attenuation of orbital echoes posterior to the tumor.

OCT demonstrates the tumor, with sharp borders, arising in the nerve fiber layer or full-thickness retina. The intrinsic calcification can give a "moth-eaten" lucent appearance with posterior shadowing.[43] Fine-needle aspiration biopsy is rarely necessary.

Management and Course

Most retinal astrocytic hamartomas are asymptomatic and nonprogressive and, thus, do not require treatment. Ocular examination should be performed yearly. If there is associated serous retinal detachment, then photodynamic therapy may be employed. All patients with retinal astrocytic hamartoma should be evaluated for TSC, particularly if they display multiple lesions.

Histopathology

Histopathologically, the typical noncalcified retinal astrocytic hamartoma is a lightly eosinophilic lesion arising from the nerve fiber layer of the retina. It is composed of well-differentiated elongated fibrous astrocytes with lightly eosinophilic cytoplasm and round to oval nuclei. Mitotic figures are extremely rare. The more calcified tumors show fossilization and round, basophilic, laminated structures resembling corpora arenacea.[34]

28.2.7 Acquired Retinal Astrocytoma

The acquired retinal astrocytoma is a rare tumor, unrelated to TSC and showing features different from astrocytic hamartoma. Unlike astrocytic hamartoma that is usually found in children, the acquired astrocytoma develops at any age, demonstrates growth and exudative retinopathy, and is unassociated with systemic syndromes.

Clinical Features

The acquired retinal astrocytoma occurs as a solitary, pink-yellow retinal mass, usually in the posterior retina near the optic disc.[1,2,44] The retinal blood vessels can be slightly dilated and ramify over and into the lesion. Unlike the congenital astrocytic hamartoma, the acquired astrocytoma can show progressive growth and produce a secondary serous/exudative retinal detachment. A large, elevated astrocytoma can be pedunculated and have numerous superficial blood vessels, resembling an amelanotic choroidal melanoma. In contrast to a similar-sized melanoma, however, the astrocytoma is more likely to involve the sensory retina and be associated with retinal exudation, retinal detachment, and vitreous hemorrhage.

Genetics

There are no genetic abnormalities associated with this condition.

Diagnosis

Fluorescein angiography of an acquired retinal astrocytoma shows rapid filling of the tumor vessels through the retinal circulation in the early arterial phase. There is progressive leakage of dye from the retinal vessels and intense late staining of the mass. A-scan ultrasonography shows high internal reflectivity within the mass, and B-scan shows a rounded or dome-shaped mass that demonstrates acoustic solidity and lack of choroidal excavation. OCT documents the tumor within the retina with complete loss of retinal anatomic structure and with surrounding subretinal fluid or intraretinal edema.

Management and Course

The management of acquired retinal astrocytoma involves laser photocoagulation or photodynamic therapy to reduce associated subretinal fluid or edema.[45] In some instances, plaque radiotherapy is necessary for tumor control and to sclerose leaking vessels. Some eyes have been enucleated, misdiagnosed as uveal melanoma or retinoblastoma. For small astrocytomas with stable features and no leakage, management may consist of careful observation.

Histopathology

Low-power microscopy of acquired retinal astrocytoma shows a lightly eosinophilic mass arising from the sensory retina. Most cases seem to originate near the optic nerve, but there is generally no intraneural component. In some cases, the cells are spindle-shaped fibrillary astrocytes forming whorls and fascicles with minimal mitotic activity. Others contain more rounded astrocytic giant cells with abundant eosinophilic cytoplasm, vesicular nuclei, and prominent nucleoli.

28.3 Retinal Pigment Epithelial Tumors

Several tumors and related lesions arise in the retinal pigment epithelium (RPE). Most of these lesions are benign, and should be differentiated from choroidal melanoma.

28.3.1 Congenital Hypertrophy of the Retinal Pigment Epithelium

Congenital hypertrophy of the RPE (CHRPE) is a benign condition that can occur as a solitary lesion or as multifocal lesions, known as congenital grouped pigmentation of the RPE or "bear tracks."

Clinical Features

Ophthalmoscopically, solitary CHRPE is characteristically a unilateral, deeply pigmented, flat lesion with a sharply demarcated margin[46,47,48,49,50,51] (▶ Fig. 28.8). Although the size is variable, it usually ranges from 1 to 6 mm in diameter. Some lesions have a well-delineated surrounding pigmented and/or depigmented halo at their margin. CHRPE is a fairly stationary lesion, but it can show slowly progressive subtle flat enlargement over several years. In rare instances, a nodular proliferation can occur, representing RPE hyperplasia or RPE adenoma or adenocarcinoma.

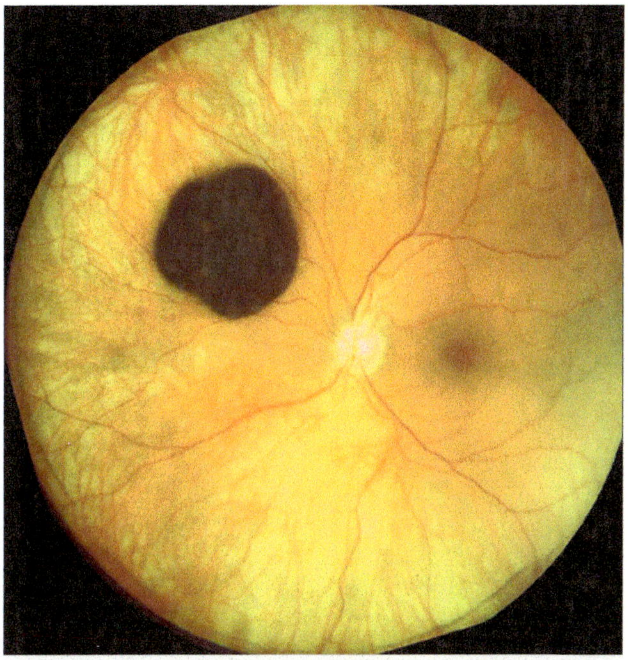

Fig. 28.8 Congenital hypertrophy of the retinal pigment epithelium (solitary type) showing black flat mass with sharp margins.

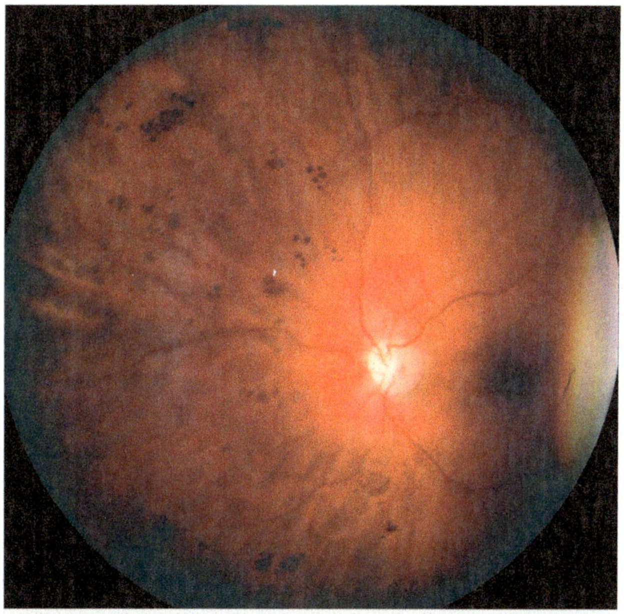

Fig. 28.9 Congenital hypertrophy of the retinal pigment epithelium (multifocal type) showing numerous round black spots at the level of the retinal pigment epithelium.

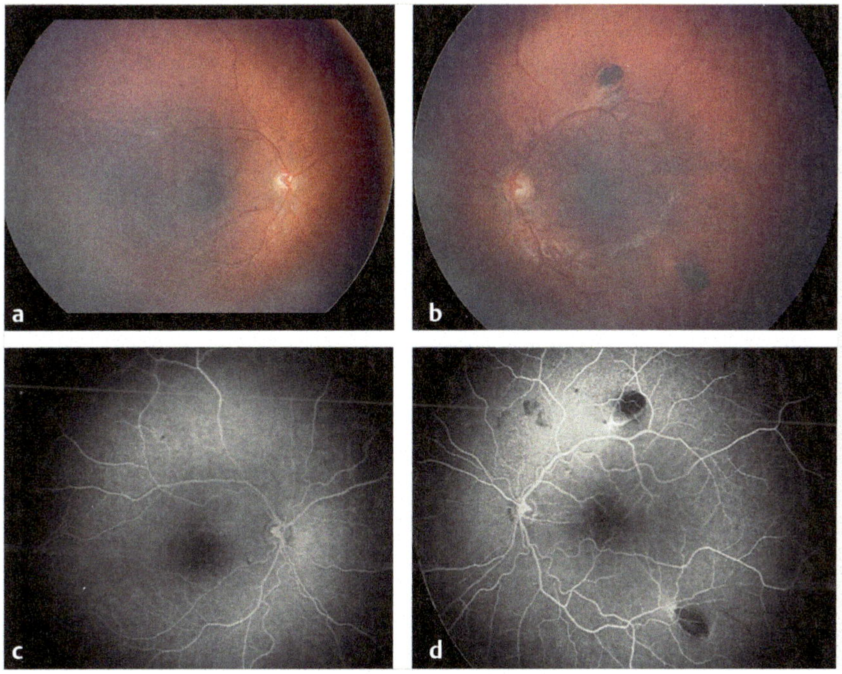

Fig. 28.10 (**a, b**) Pigmented ocular fundus lesions (POFLs) (**c, d**) with angiographic blockage of dye to demonstrate the lesions. These lesions are associated with familial adenomatous polyposis.

Pearls

- CHRPE is a fairly stationary lesion, but it can show slowly progressive subtle flat enlargement over several years.

Multifocal CHRPE is characterized by several groups of well-delineated, flat, slate gray lesions that can assume a sector distribution in the fundus (▶ Fig. 28.9). Each group consists of 3 to 30 individual pigmented lesions that can vary from 0.1 to 3.0 mm in diameter. Each individual lesion is similar to unifocal CHRPE but is usually smaller than the unifocal type and does not show the lacunae or haloes of depigmentation.

Multiple small pigmented ocular fundus lesions (POFLs) may be associated with familial adenomatous polyposis and Gardner's syndrome, conditions associated with familial colonic cancer. These fundus lesions were originally mislabeled as CHRPE, but they are actually different from multifocal CHRPE in that they are bilateral, have a more haphazard distribution, with more irregular or jagged borders, and assume a housiform (fish-like) appearance[52,53,54,55,56,57,58,59,60] (▶ Fig. 28.10). There is no association of the typical CHRPE with cancer syndromes.

Genetics

There are no genetic abnormalities associated with CHRPE. However, POFLs associated with familial adenomatous polyposis and Gardner's syndrome are caused by a mutation in the APC gene or the MUTYH gene. The APC gene mutation leads to cell overgrowth manifesting as colonic polyps and later carcinoma. The MUTYH gene mutation prevents DNA repair and leads to cell overgrowth, colon polyps, and colon cancer.

Special Considerations

- Multiple small pigmented fundus lesions are commonly found in patients with familial adenomatous polyposis and Gardner's syndrome. These lesions, however, differ from CHRPE or congenital grouped pigmentation ("bear tracks") in that they are bilateral, have a more haphazard distribution, and often have more irregular or jagged borders. Typical CHRPE and "bear tracks" are not associated with these cancer syndromes.

Diagnosis

The distinctive ophthalmoscopic appearance of CHRPE is sufficient for diagnosis. Sometimes a peripheral CHRPE might erroneously appear elevated, simulating melanoma. B-scan ultrasonography can demonstrate lack of elevation. Fluorescein angiography reveals marked hypofluorescence throughout all phases of the angiogram, and the nonpigmented halo and depigmented lacunae can show "window defect" hyperfluorescence. Autofluorescence shows marked hypoautofluorescence due to lack of lipofuscin in RPE. The lacunae unmask underlying scleral autofluorescence. OCT demonstrates the flat lesion as minimally thickened RPE with overlying photoreceptor atrophy.[50,51]

Management and Course

Treatment is not indicated for CHRPE. The lesion is usually asymptomatic and should be observed annually. Occasionally, slight enlargement can be noted over a long period of time and, rarely, this tumor develops a nodular growth into RPE hyperplasia or adenoma that might require surgical resection.

Histopathology

Only a few cases of CHRPE have been studied histopathologically. CHRPE consists of a focal area in which the RPE cells are abnormally tall and densely packed with melanosomes that obscure their nuclei, and the cells lack lipofuscin. The individual melanosomes are larger and oval or spherical compared with those of the normal RPE, which are smaller and rod-shaped or elliptical. Areas within the lesion where the pigment granules are very sparse correspond to the depigmented lacunae and haloes seen clinically in some cases. The general histopathologic features of the solitary and multifocal variants are similar.

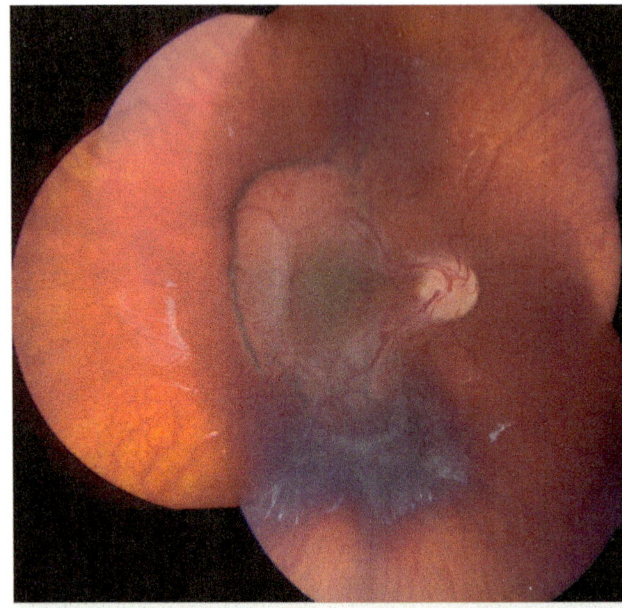

Fig. 28.11 Combined hamartoma of the retina and retinal pigment epithelium showing retinal fibrosis with dragging and mild pigmentation.

28.3.2 Combined Hamartoma of the Retina and Retinal Pigment Epithelium

Combined hamartoma of the retina and RPE is an unusual fundus lesion classified with RPE tumors due to its RPE component. Some investigators consider this lesion to be a hamartoma, but the pathogenesis is not clearly established. The lesion may result from vitreoretinal traction, inflammation, or trauma. Most cases are diagnosed in children, suggesting that the lesion is congenital.

Clinical Features

Combined hamartoma can occur as a juxtapapillary or a peripheral lesion.[61,62,63,64,65,66,67] The juxtapapillary lesion appears as a solitary mass adjacent to or overlying a portion of the optic disc, with variable amounts of pigmentation, vascularity, and typical gray-white tissue (▶ Fig. 28.11). The retinal vessels within and overlying the lesion show tractional stretching and tortuosity, often obscured by overlying fibroglial tissue at the vitreoretinal interface. This surface glial tissue tends to contract gradually, leading to further stretching of the blood vessels and retinal striae, which can distort the fovea. Chronic vitreoretinal traction can lead to accumulation of subfoveal exudation, secondary retinoschisis, and retinal hole. The peripheral lesion can be located in any portion of the fundus, appears as an elevated ridge, and characteristically manifests obvious dragging of large retinal vessels toward the lesion. Peripheral to the lesion, however, there is often minimal vascularity.

Genetics

The combined hamartoma can occur as a sporadic condition or it can be associated with neurofibromatosis type 2 (NF2). Multifocal tumors are highly associated with NF2[65,66] Some authorities have found that combined hamartoma in young patients should be considered part of the diagnostic criteria for NF2. The NF2 gene encodes the cytoskeletal protein called Merlin or neurofibromin 2 and is located on chromosome 22. Defects in this tumor suppressor gene lead to NF2-related tumors including schwannomas, meningiomas, and ependymomas.

Diagnostic criteria for neurofibromatosis type 2 (NF2)

Feature

- Bilateral eighth cranial nerve tumors confirmed on magnetic resonance imaging or computed tomography
- Unilateral eighth cranial nerve tumor
- Plus
- Relative (first degree) with NF2
- Two of following:
  - Meningioma
  - Glioma
  - Schwannoma
  - Juvenile posterior subcapsular lens opacity
- Plus
- Relative (first degree) with NF2

Source: Adapted from Stumpf DA et al[42] and Gutmann et al.[65]
Note: Diagnosis is established with at least one of the three situations listed above.

Diagnosis

The diagnosis of combined hamartoma is made on the basis of ophthalmoscopic findings. Fluorescein angiography shows relative hypofluorescence in the arterial phase, numerous fine blood vessels in the early venous phase, and gradual staining and leakage in the late angiogram. OCT demonstrates vitreoretinal traction causing the retinal surface to have a peaked or rounded appearance like the surface of a mountain.[67,68]

Management and Course

Most cases of combined hamartoma are observed, particularly if there is no visual loss. In those with visual loss from retinal traction and amblyopia, membrane peeling has been employed, but visual results are variable.

Histopathology

Combined hamartoma represents a thickening of the sensory retina and optic nerve with glial cells, vascular tissue, and strands and sheets of RPE cells. There can be thickening and reduplication of the RPE at the base and margins. The central, thicker portion of the mass shows proliferation of glial cells and fibrous tissue. The shrinkage of the fibroglial tissue accounts for the apparent preretinal membrane and tortuosity of the retinal vessels seen clinically.

28.3.3 Adenoma and Adenocarcinoma

The RPE has a tendency to undergo reactive hyperplasia but little tendency for true neoplasia. Rarely, benign adenoma or malignant adenocarcinoma can develop. Both show similar clinical behavior, with local growth and no tendency to metastasize.

Clinical Features

The RPE adenoma/adenocarcinoma appears as an oval-shaped, abruptly elevated, deeply pigmented mass[1,2,69,70,71,72] (▶ Fig. 28.12). Unlike a choroidal melanoma, it does not have a surrounding nevoid base, but rather arises abruptly from the adjacent RPE. The tumor is usually situated in the peripheral retina but can occur near the optic disc. In some instances, this tumor can assume a retinal blood supply, with dilated, tortuous feeding artery and draining vein.

Clinical Features

There are no genetic abnormalities associated with this tumor.

Diagnosis

Fluorescein angiography of RPE adenoma demonstrates early hypofluorescence and mild late staining. In some cases, a dilated retinal artery and vein can be demonstrated. The tumor does not show the "double circulation" that characterizes choroidal melanoma. A-scan ultrasonography shows high internal reflectivity, and B-scan demonstrates an abruptly elevated mass with a "derby hat" configuration and acoustic solidity. In uncertain cases, transocular fine-needle biopsy can be helpful.

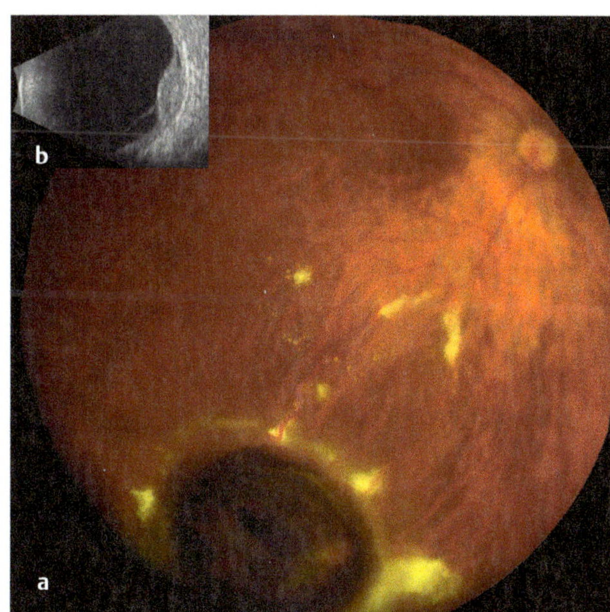

Fig. 28.12 (a) Retinal pigment epithelial adenoma with (b) feeder vessel and surrounding exudation and echodensity on ultrasonography.

Management and Course

Small suspected adenomas of the ciliary and RPE can be observed until growth is documented. Larger tumors can be managed by local resection with partial lamellar iridocyclectomy. Plaque radiotherapy has been attempted, but the results are not uniform. A progressively enlarging lesion might require enucleation.

Histopathology

RPE adenoma and adenocarcinoma can show vacuolated, tubular, or mixed histopathology. Those located in the ciliary body region tend to be more vacuolated. The clear vacuoles are intracellular structures within the cytoplasm of the pigmented tumor cells. The more posteriorly situated RPE tumors tend to have a tubular arrangement. Bleached preparations demonstrate the tumor cells to be large and polyhedral with eccentric round to oval nuclei and abundant granular cytoplasm. Adenocarcinoma of the RPE exhibits similar patterns but demonstrates more pleomorphic cells with apical concentration of pigment.

28.4 Choroidal Tumors

There are several benign and malignant neoplasms that can arise in the choroid. These include melanocytic, vascular, metastatic, osseous, neural, lymphomatous, and others.

28.4.1 Choroidal Nevus

Choroidal nevus is a common melanocytic tumor with benign features and carries the risk for transformation into melanoma. This tumor is described in detail in Chapter 26.

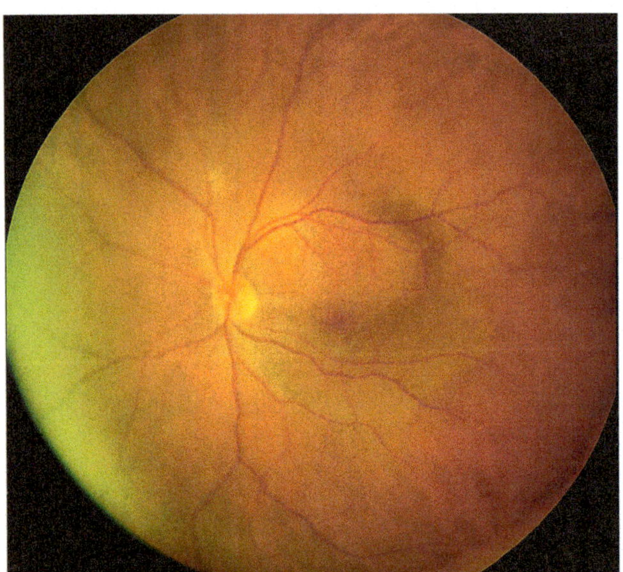

Fig. 28.13 Subtle circumscribed choroidal hemangioma with serous retinal detachment in macula.

28.4.2 Choroidal Melanoma

Choroidal melanoma is a malignant melanocytic tumor with a risk for metastasis and patient death. This tumor is described in detail in Chapter 26.

28.4.3 Choroidal Hemangioma

Although vascular tumors can occasionally affect the iris and rarely the ciliary body, most uveal vascular tumors occur in the choroid. Choroidal hemangioma is a benign tumor, composed of large, dilated choroidal blood vessels.[1,2,73,74,75,76,77,78,79] It can occur as a circumscribed or diffuse type. The diffuse hemangioma is associated with facial nevus flammeus or variations of Sturge–Weber syndrome. These two types have similarities and are discussed together.

The circumscribed type is usually diagnosed in patients between 20 and 40 years of age. Although it is occasionally confused clinically with choroidal melanoma or other tumors, in most cases it has distinctive clinical features.[74] The diffuse choroidal hemangioma is generally diagnosed at a much earlier age because the congenital nevus flammeus on the ipsilateral side of the face prompts an early fundus examination.

Clinical Features

Ophthalmoscopically, circumscribed choroidal hemangioma appears as a fairly well-defined, elevated, red-orange tumor deep to the retina (▶ Fig. 28.13 and ▶ Fig. 28.14). This tumor can show overlying RPE alterations or fibrous metaplasia. The diffuse choroidal hemangioma has a similar color, but is less well defined and involves a greater area of the fundus (▶ Fig. 28.15, ▶ Fig. 28.16, and ▶ Fig. 28.17). With time, both can produce visual impairment with secondary exudative retinal detachment, macular edema, or even amblyopia from induced hyperopia in children. In some instances, the retinal detachment can progress to involve the entire retina, predisposing to neovascular glaucoma.

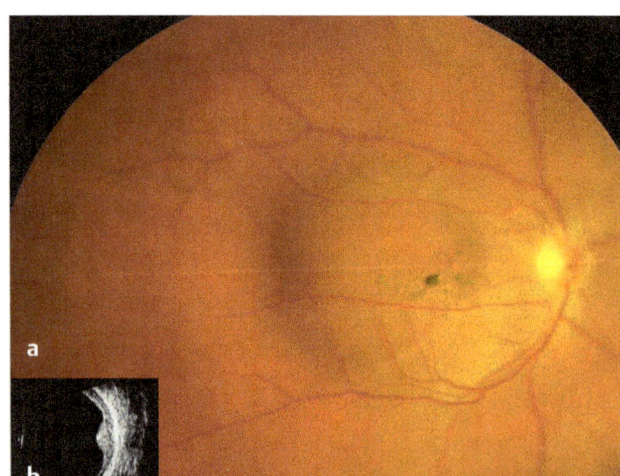

Fig. 28.14 (a) Subtle circumscribed choroidal hemangioma with (b) overlying retinal pigment epithelial clumping and ultrasound echodensity.

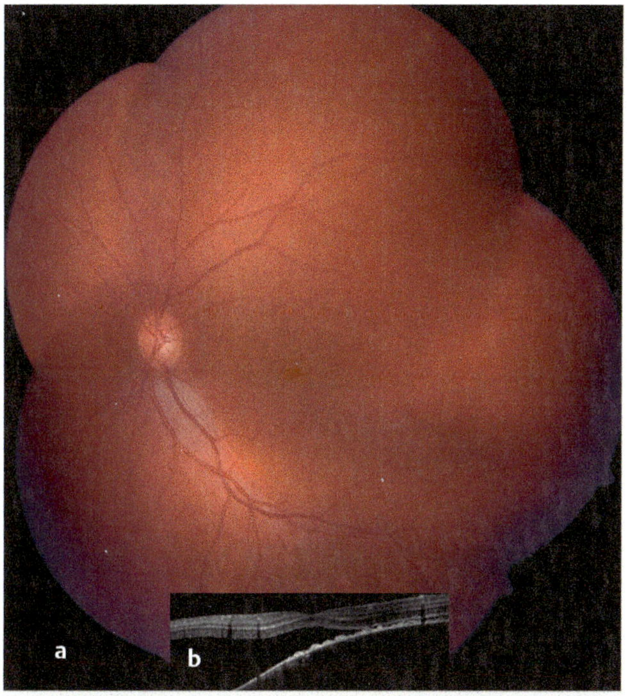

Fig. 28.15 (a) Subtle diffuse choroidal hemangioma with "tomato catsup" fundus and (b) ultrasound optical coherence tomography showing subretinal fluid and choroidal mass.

Pearls

- Choroidal hemangioma can produce visual impairment with secondary exudative retinal detachment, macular edema, or even amblyopia from induced hyperopia in children. In some instances, total retinal detachment can occur and lead to neovascular glaucoma.

Genetics

Circumscribed choroidal hemangioma has no known genetic defects. Diffuse choroidal hemangioma is associated with Sturge–Weber syndrome (▶ Table 28.5). This syndrome is an embryonal developmental anomaly resulting from a somatic activating mutation in the GNAQ gene.

Diagnosis

Choroidal hemangioma is diagnosed through characteristic features on indirect ophthalmoscopy. Ancillary studies can confirm the diagnosis. Fluorescein angiography shows lacey areas of hyperfluorescence in the prearterial or early arterial phase and progressive late hyperfluorescence. In the circumscribed type, indocyanine green angiography shows early hyperfluorescence by 1 minute and late "washout" of

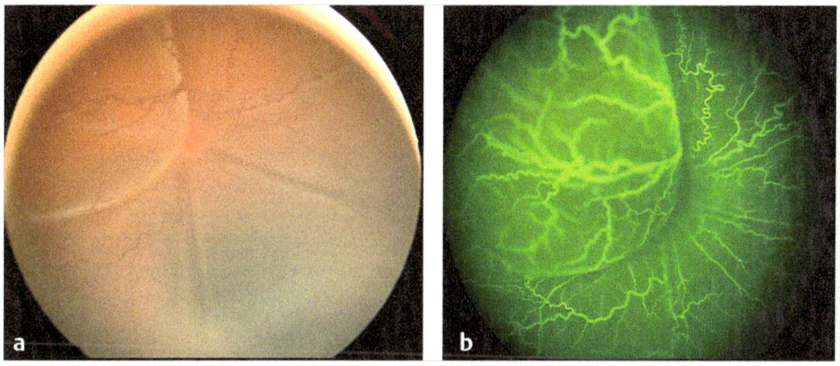

Fig. 28.16 (a) Extensive retinal detachment overlying choroidal hemangioma (b) with fluorescein angiographic demonstration of subretinal fluid.

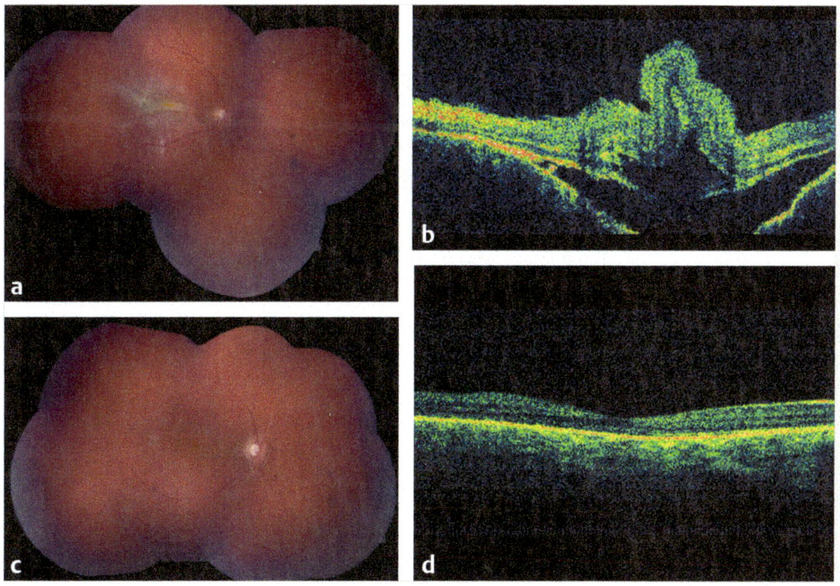

Fig. 28.17 (a) Subtle diffuse choroidal hemangioma (b) with retinal fold (c) before and (d) after external beam radiotherapy showing regression in the fundus and on optical coherence tomography.

Table 28.5 Roach diagnostic scale for classification of encephalotrigeminal angiomatosis (Sturge–Weber syndrome)

Type	Title	Involvement of skin, eye, and brain
Type I	Classic Sturge–Weber syndrome	Leptomeningeal angioma present
		Cutaneous facial angioma present
		Glaucoma likely present
Type II	Sturge–Weber syndrome	Leptomeningeal angioma absent
		Cutaneous facial angioma present
		Glaucoma possibly present
Type III	Sturge–Weber syndrome forme fruste	Leptomeningeal angioma present
		Cutaneous facial angioma absent
		Glaucoma absent

Source: Adapted from Roach ES. Neurocutaneous syndromes. Pediatr Clin North Am 1992;39(4):591–620.

hyperfluorescence, leaving a surrounding ring of hyperfluorescence.[75] Ultrasonography reveals the tumor to have acoustic solidity, similar to surrounding choroid. On B-scan, there is acoustic solidity, and on A-scan there is high internal reflectivity.

OCT can depict the mass as a smooth, dome-shaped choroidal mass with enlargement of the vascular lumens and often with overlying subretinal fluid and edema.[76] MRI can demonstrate larger tumors with bright signal on T1- and T2-weighted imaging and uniform enhancement with gadolinium contrast.

Management and Course

Choroidal hemangioma, if asymptomatic and without subretinal fluid, can be managed by observation. Those with subretinal fluid or macular edema can be treated with photodynamic therapy.[78,79] Larger tumors with extensive retinal detachment can be controlled with low-dose plaque radiotherapy or external beam radiotherapy. Following treatment, visual recovery can sometimes be achieved.

Histopathology

Choroidal hemangioma represents a thickening of the choroid from large dilated choroidal blood vessels. It is often associated with secondary fibrous or osseous metaplasia of the overlying RPE and sensory retinal detachment and edema. The circumscribed and diffuse types of choroidal hemangioma have similar histopathologic features.

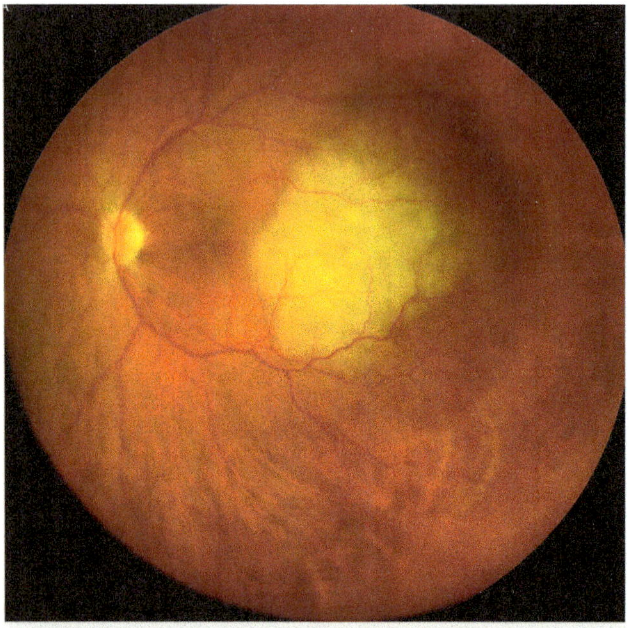

Fig. 28.18 Choroidal metastasis appearing yellow in color.

28.4.4 Choroidal Metastasis

Choroidal metastasis is a neoplasm that has spread hematogenously to the choroid from a distant primary malignancy. The most common neoplasms to exhibit choroidal metastasis are breast cancer and lung cancer, although other malignancies can occasionally be found.[1,2,80,81,82] About 25% of patients who present to the ophthalmologist with choroidal metastases have no known primary malignancy, and a systemic evaluation is necessary to detect the primary site.[82,83,84,85] Most patients with breast cancer metastatic to the choroid have a history of a primary malignancy. In contrast, many patients with lung cancer metastatic to the choroid have no history of the primary malignancy when they present to the ophthalmologist. Hence, it is important for the ophthalmologist to be familiar with the clinical manifestations of uveal metastasis.

Pearls

- One-fourth or more of patients who present with choroidal metastases have no prior history of a primary malignancy.

Clinical Features

Ophthalmoscopically, a choroidal metastasis usually appears as a sessile or dome-shaped, soft yellow mass, often with a secondary serous retinal detachment (▶ Fig. 28.17, ▶ Fig. 28.18, and ▶ Fig. 28.19). In contrast to an amelanotic melanoma, it rarely assumes a mushroom shape, is more likely to be bilateral or multifocal, and rarely produces overlying drusen.

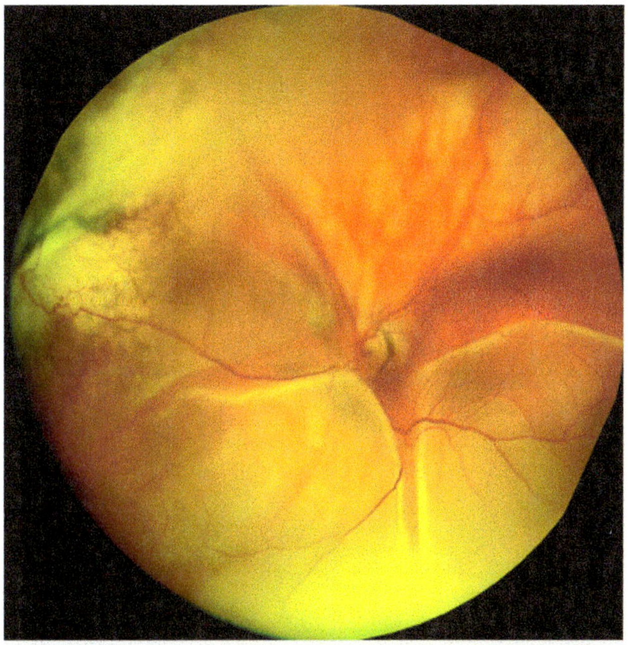

Fig. 28.19 Choroidal metastasis hidden under retinal detachment.

Genetics

There are no genetic abnormalities specifically related to the choroidal metastasis, but there are known mutations to occur with many systemic cancers that spread to the eye.

Diagnosis

Choroidal metastasis is diagnosed by recognition of its characteristic features on indirect ophthalmoscopy. In cases without a known primary malignancy, complete medical history and systemic evaluation can help detect the primary site, thus supporting the suspected ocular diagnosis (▶ Table 28.6).

Fluorescein angiography shows a pattern similar to that of melanoma, except that the progressive hyperfluorescence of the metastatic lesion starts in the late venous phase, slightly later than what is seen with a typical melanoma. Ultrasonography reveals findings similar to those seen with choroidal hemangioma, showing medium-to-high internal reflectivity on A-scan and acoustic solidity on B-scan. Unlike choroidal melanoma, choroidal metastasis shows no choroidal excavation. OCT depicts the choroidal mass with choriocapillaris compression, a slightly "lumpy bumpy" surface, and subretinal fluid.[86,87] On autofluorescence, there is overlying lipofuscin-related hyperautofluorescence and slight hyperautofluorescence of free fluorophores in the subretinal fluid.

Pearls

- Choroidal metastases shows a slightly "lumpy bumpy" surface on OCT, with choriocapillaris compression and subretinal fluid.

Table 28.6 Choroidal metastases: O, features, and therapy. Primary tumor origins

Primary tumor location ($n = 479$)	Number (%)
Breast	252 (53)
Lung	98 (20)
Gastrointestinal	18 (4)
Kidney	8 (2)
Prostate	10 (2)
Skin	5 (1)
Other	17 (4)
Unknown	71 (15)

Source: Adapted from a clinic-based study, Shields et al.[82]

Management and Course

The treatment of choroidal metastasis varies with the clinical situation.[88,89,90] A small, asymptomatic lesion can sometimes be observed closely. Others respond to intravenous chemotherapy that is being administered for the systemic malignancy. Patients who have visual loss despite chemotherapy are often managed with photodynamic therapy if the tumor is small or plaque radiotherapy if the tumor is larger or associated with subretinal fluid. External beam radiotherapy is reserved for advanced cases with extensive tumor and retinal detachment. The prognosis for recovery of vision is generally good, but some patients have visual loss as a result of retinal detachment involving the fovea. Occasionally, a choroidal metastasis does not respond to conventional treatment and neovascular glaucoma develops, requiring enucleation. Most patients with choroidal metastasis have a guarded systemic prognosis because the primary neoplasm has produced systemic metastasis.

Histopathology

The histopathology of choroidal metastasis varies with the primary tumor. A well-differentiated tumor will show features of the primary tumor, such as breast, lung, gastrointestinal, renal, or thyroid cancers, or cutaneous melanoma. In some instances, the uveal metastasis is poorly differentiated, so that immunohistochemistry or electron microscopy may be necessary to help determine its origin.

28.4.5 Choroidal Osteoma

Choroidal osteoma is an unusual choroidal tumor that can be unilateral or bilateral and usually occurs in young adult women.[91,92,93,94,95,96,97,98,99,100] The pathogenesis of choroidal osteoma is unknown.

Clinical Features

Choroidal osteoma is characteristically a well-defined, yellow-orange placoid mass, usually in the optic disc or macular regions (▶ Fig. 28.20). This tumor has distinct geographic

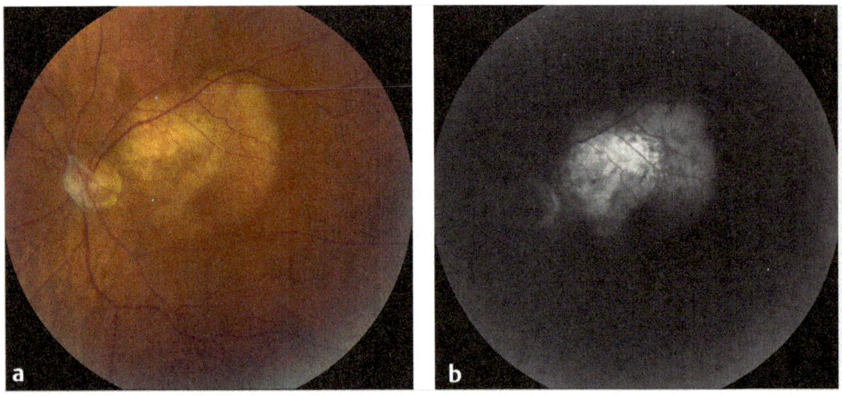

Fig. 28.20 (**a**) Choroidal osteoma with yellow mass and crisp margins showing (**b**) diffuse enhancement on fluorescein angiography.

margins with small pseudopodia-like projections. Choroidal osteoma can cause visual loss by producing overlying photoreceptor degeneration, subretinal fluid, or choroidal neovascularization with subretinal hemorrhage.

Genetics

There are no known genetic abnormalities associated with this condition.

Diagnosis

Choroidal osteoma has typical features, and the diagnosis is made with ophthalmoscopy. Ancillary studies are helpful in confirming the diagnosis. Fluorescein angiography shows gradual fluorescence and progressive late staining. In some cases, spider-like blood vessels that emerge from the bone beneath the RPE, presumed to represent haversian canals, can be seen. Choroidal neovascularization might be observed. Ultrasonography and CT are helpful in confirming the calcified bone within the choroid. OCT shows thickening of the choroid, with linear lines representing bone lamella and linear tubules representing haversian and Volkmann canals.[96,97] Overlying photoreceptor degeneration is common.

Management and Course

Choroidal osteoma can be classified into subfoveal and extrafoveal tumors. The subfoveal tumors do not require treatment as therapy can lead to decalcification, which subsequently causes photoreceptor atrophy. Extrafoveal osteoma can be treated with photodynamic therapy to decalcify and eradicate the tumor, leaving choroidal atrophy and reducing the risk for osteoma to grow toward the foveola.[99,100] Secondary choroidal neovascularization can be managed with anti-VEGF medication or, if extrafoveal, photodynamic therapy.

Histopathology

The cause of choroidal osteoma is unknown. Despite the fact that it represents an abnormal deposition of bone, affected patients generally have normal serum calcium and phosphorus levels. Pathologically, choroidal osteoma is a full-thickness replacement of the choroid in the affected area by mature bone. The overlying RPE and photoreceptors can be intact or degenerated.

28.4.6 Choroidal Leiomyoma

Leiomyoma is a benign tumor of smooth muscle, known to occur in the uterus as a uterine fibroid tumor. This tumor can rarely occur in the eye, where it has a predilection for the iris, ciliary body, and peripheral choroid. There is a distinct tendency for this tumor to occur in young adult women.

Clinical Features

Ciliochoroidal leiomyoma appears as a smooth, dome-shaped orange-colored mass in the periphery of the fundus.[101,102,103,104,105,106] Although the tumor is nonpigmented, it can often give the false impression of pigmentation because of overlying gray pigment epithelium. Leiomyoma can produce a secondary cataract, lens subluxation, retinal detachment, and scleral perforation.

Diagnosis

The most important aspect of the diagnostic evaluation is that the ophthalmologist must be familiar with the clinical features and clinical variations of leiomyoma. Unlike melanoma, which arises in the uveal stroma, uveal leiomyoma frequently grows in the suprauveal space between the uveal stroma and the sclera.[103] Therefore, fluorescein angiography may show a relatively normal choroidal vascular pattern over the tumor, whereas with melanoma, fluorescein angiography is more likely to demonstrate sinuous blood vessels within the tumor. Carefully performed ultrasonography may suggest an intact uveal tract over the tumor surface. However, these are subtle features, and most cases are somewhat difficult to differentiate clinically from melanoma.

Management and Course

Management of ciliochoroidal leiomyoma is usually by local resection using partial lamellar sclerouvectomy. The results of local resection are generally favorable.[103] Larger tumors may require enucleation. Observation is not usually advisable except when the tumor is very small and asymptomatic or when it occurs in a medically unstable patient.

Histopathology

On gross pathologic examination, leiomyoma can occupy the suprauveal space and spare the uveal stroma or it can be found within in the uveal stroma. Microscopically, leiomyoma is composed of a proliferation of benign spindle cells with features of smooth muscle.[101,102] Immunohistochemistry and electron microscopy are usually necessary to confirm the smooth-muscle derivation of the tumor.

28.4.7 Choroidal Neurilemoma

Neurilemoma is a benign tumor composed of Schwann's cells. When it occurs in the uveal tract, it arises from Schwann's cells of the ciliary nerves. This tumor can be associated with NF1 in some instances.

Clinical Features

In most cases, choroidal neurilemoma is clinically indistinguishable from amelanotic melanoma, leiomyoma, or metastatic carcinoma.[107,108] This smooth-surfaced, amelanotic mass usually occupies the uveal stroma or it can be found in the suprauveal space or even have a transscleral or episcleral component. Although it is a benign tumor, it tends to enlarge slowly and can produce secondary retinal detachment or cataract.

Diagnosis

This tumor is exceedingly rare, and there is little experience with ancillary testing. Fluorescein angiography and ultrasonography generally show features that are similar to uveal melanoma. The diagnosis is typically established following enucleation or resection.

Management and Course

The diagnosis of neurilemoma is difficult to establish clinically, so most tumors are managed as melanoma, with the therapeutic modality determined by the same criteria mentioned previously for uveal melanoma.

Histopathology

Choroidal neurilemoma is composed of spindle-shaped cells that usually have a neuroid appearance. The cell membranes are ill-defined, and there is abundant extracellular collagen. Immunohistochemistry may be necessary to exclude the diagnosis of melanoma or leiomyoma, and electron microscopy can demonstrate the Schwann's cells with the wide-spacing collagen that characterizes these cells.

28.5 Other Tumors

Several miscellaneous tumors can involve both the retina and choroid. Those included here are melanocytoma, lymphoma, and leukemia.

28.5.1 Optic Disc Melanocytoma

Melanocytoma is a name that was originally used to describe a deeply pigmented benign lesion that characteristically occurs within the optic disc[109,110,111,112,113,114] (▶ Fig. 28.21). This tumor is believed to be a congenital nevus that involves the peripapillary choroid, with extension around the termination of Bruch's membrane into the epipapillary tissues and juxtapapillary retina. A similar tumor can occur anywhere in the uveal tract, in the iris, ciliary body, and choroid. Unlike uveal melanoma, which occurs predominantly in whites, melanocytoma appears to have an equal incidence in whites, blacks, and Asians.

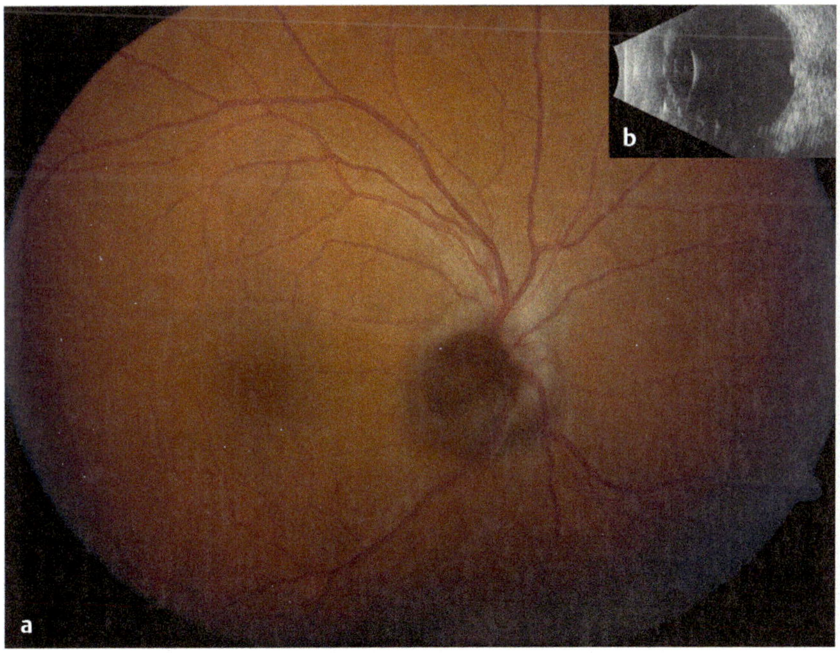

Fig. 28.21 (**a**) Optic disc melanocytoma with slight disc edema and (**b**) echodensity on ultrasonography.

Clinical Features

Melanocytoma of the optic disc is a dark brown to black mass that covers all or part of the optic disc. This tumor often has a retinal or choroidal component that is in continuity with the papillary component. The retinal component of the lesion shows feathery margins and the choroidal component resembles a nevus. Although benign, melanocytoma can produce an afferent pupillary defect (Marcus Gunn pupil) and a visual field defect, either an enlarged blind spot or an arcuate scotoma.

Diagnosis

The diagnosis is established with classic features on ophthalmoscopy. With fluorescein angiography, melanocytoma shows hypofluorescence throughout the angiogram. Larger tumors can sometimes show mild leakage of dye and late staining, but the characteristic double circulation of a choroidal melanoma is not present. OCT shows the anterior border layer of the mass as dome-shaped and relatively smooth, but overlying vitreous seeds can be found.[114] Deeper aspects are not visible on OCT due to dense shadowing.

Management and Course

There is no treatment for optic disc melanocytoma. When the optic disc melanocytomas are small and asymptomatic, periodic observation is advised. Occasionally, melanocytoma undergoes spontaneous necrosis and causes visual impairment, necessitating oral prednisone. Marked progressive enlargement and severe visual loss should suggest evolution into melanoma, and enucleation is recommended. Although melanocytoma usually remains stationary, minimal growth can be documented in about 15% of cases, but such mild change should not be misinterpreted as malignant transformation.[55]

Histopathology

Melanocytoma is a deeply pigmented lesion with round to ovoid cells that have intense cytoplasmic pigmentation. Bleached sections reveal that the cells have rather uniform small nuclei with prominent nucleoli. These benign features should suggest the diagnosis and help exclude the possibility of an epithelioid cell malignant melanoma.

28.5.2 Lymphoma

Benign or malignant lymphoma can occur in the retina, optic nerve, vitreous, or choroid.[115,116,117,118,119,120,121,122,123,124] The choroidal variant is more likely to be seen in patients with systemic or visceral lymphoma, and the vitreoretinal variant is more likely to be seen in patients who have central nervous system lymphoma. All patients with findings of intraocular lymphoma should be evaluated for systemic lymphoma.

Clinical Features

The choroidal form of intraocular lymphoma appears as a yellow infiltration in the choroid, usually with no involvement of the retina or vitreous[115,116,117,118,119,120,121,122] (▶ Fig. 28.22). This form can resemble choroidal metastasis. The vitreoretinal form of intraocular lymphoma presents in older patients with cells in the vitreous and areas of yellow-white retinal infiltration and sub-RPE greasy-appearing deposits (▶ Fig. 28.23). Often this is mistaken as uveitis.[123,124] In advanced cases, all of the ocular structures can be involved in either the choroidal form or the vitreoretinal form. These variants of intraocular lymphoma are not always distinct, and there may be overlap.

Diagnosis

If the diagnosis of intraocular lymphoma is suspected clinically, the patient should have a thorough physical examination, lumbar puncture, and MRI of the brain twice yearly to investigate for involvement of other sites. The features of clumped vitreous seeds and yellow sub-RPE infiltrates are suggestive. OCT confirms the sub-RPE debris with RPE detachment. In the vitreoretinal form, the ocular diagnosis can be established by vitreous biopsy and cytologic examination. Because the material

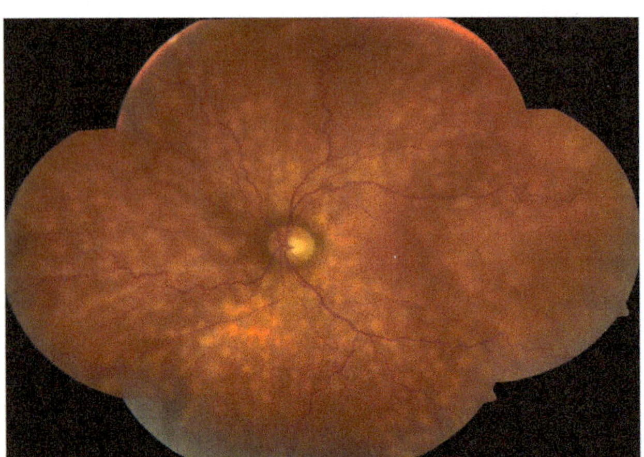

Fig. 28.22 Choroidal lymphoma with numerous yellow infiltrates.

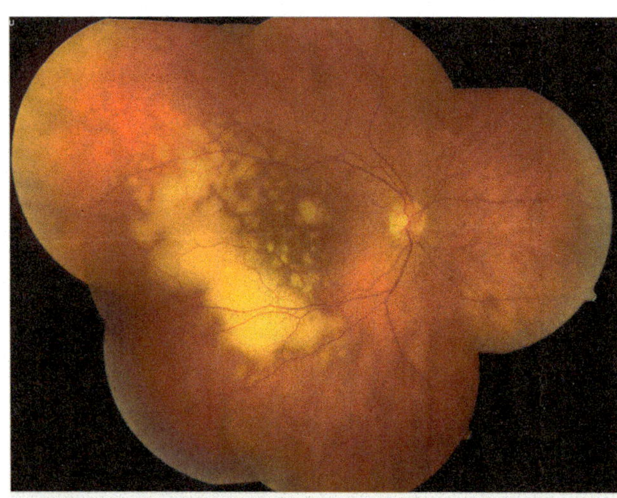

Fig. 28.23 Vitreoretinal lymphoma with numerous yellow retinal pigment epithelial detachments with yellow lymphomatous debris.

obtained by vitrectomy can be scanty, the results are occasionally negative and it sometimes necessitates repeat biopsy.

If the choroidal variant is found, the patient should be evaluated for systemic lymphoma and a search made for enlarged lymph nodes and abdominal or chest involvement. In this form, thorough inspection of the conjunctival fornices for subepithelial tumor, often found with the choroidal tumor, should lend support to the diagnosis of choroidal lymphoma. OCT shows thickened choroid with surface irregularity ranging from smooth if infiltration is thin, rippled if thicker, and "seasick" or undulating if thickest.[122]

Management and Course

If the diagnosis of choroidal lymphoma is confirmed, management depends on the features. If there is systemic involvement, then systemic chemotherapy or Rituxan could help, but if there is involvement of only the eye, then observation for asymptomatic patients and irradiation for symptomatic patients is advised.

If the diagnosis of vitreoretinal lymphoma is confirmed, the management is generally systemic with intrathecal chemotherapy for brain and eye involvement. However, if there is only eye involvement, then irradiation to the eye or intravitreal injection of methotrexate and/or Rituxan is advised. This could result in reduction of tumor and improvement in visual acuity.

Histopathology

The tissues affected by intraocular lymphoma are infiltrated by malignant B-cell lymphocytes. Depending on the degree of involvement, tumor cells can be identified in the retina, vitreous, optic nerve, and uveal tract.

28.5.3 Leukemia

The eye can be affected in patients with systemic leukemia, most often with retinal hemorrhage and white-centered hemorrhages, as a manifestation of underlying anemia and thrombocytopenia.[125] Microaneurysms and peripheral retinal neovascularization may develop. In addition, any form of leukemia in children or adults may be associated with intraocular infiltration of neoplastic cells into the eye.

Clinical Features

Leukemic infiltration of the fundus characteristically appears as a yellow thickening of the retina and choroid, often with hemorrhage and optic disc edema in patients with known leukemia. It is important to differentiate leukemic infiltration from an opportunistic infection, such as cytomegalovirus or fungus retinopathy, that can occur as a result of immunosuppressive treatment for leukemia.

Diagnosis

In cases in which the differential diagnosis is uncertain, a fine-needle aspiration biopsy can be helpful to establish the diagnosis.

Management and Course

The treatment of intraocular leukemia is generally chemotherapy and ocular radiotherapy, which should be performed promptly if swelling of the optic disc is causing visual impairment.

Histopathology

The choroid, optic nerve, and retina are typically infiltrated with leukemic blast cells. There is often hemorrhage intermixed with the tumor cells.

28.6 Conclusion

In summary, a number of benign and malignant neoplasms can affect the retina, RPE, and choroid. Recognition of the clinical and imaging features and understanding of therapeutic alternatives are important for patient care.

28.7 Acknowledgments

We thank the Ocular Oncology Service, Wills Eye Hospital, Thomas Jefferson University, Philadelphia, PA. Support was provided by the Eye Tumor Research Foundation, Philadelphia, PA (C. L. S., J. A. S.), and Lift for a Cure, Morrisville, PA (C. L. S., J. A. S.).

References

[1] Shields JA, Shields CL. Intraocular Tumors. An Atlas and Textbook. 3rd edition. Philadelphia, Lippincott Wolters Kluwers, 2016.
[2] Shields JA, Shields CL. Intraocular Tumors. An Atlas and Textbook. Philadelphia, PA: WB Saunders; 2008
[3] Singh AD, Shields CL, Shields JA. von Hippel-Lindau disease. Surv Ophthalmol. 2001; 46(2):117–142
[4] Wong WT, Chew EY. Ocular von Hippel-Lindau disease: clinical update and emerging treatments. Curr Opin Ophthalmol. 2008; 19(3):213–217
[5] Maher ER, Neumann HP, Richard S. von Hippel-Lindau disease: a clinical and scientific review. Eur J Hum Genet. 2011; 19(6):617–623
[6] Chan CC, Vortmeyer AO, Chew EY, et al. VHL gene deletion and enhanced VEGF gene expression detected in the stromal cells of retinal angioma. Arch Ophthalmol. 1999; 117(5):625–630
[7] Kaelin WG. Von Hippel-Lindau associated malignancies: mechanisms and therapeutic opportunities. Drug Discov Today Dis Mech. 2005; 2:225–231
[8] Calzada MJ. Von Hippel-Lindau syndrome: molecular mechanisms of the disease. Clin Transl Oncol. 2010; 12(3):160–165
[9] Shields CL, Pellegrini M, Ferenczy SR, Shields JA. Enhanced depth imaging optical coherence tomography of intraocular tumors: from placid to seasick to rock and rolling topography—the 2013 Francesco Orzalesi Lecture. Retina. 2014; 34(8):1495–1512
[10] Singh AD, Nouri M, Shields CL, Shields JA, Perez N. Treatment of retinal capillary hemangioma. Ophthalmology. 2002; 109(10):1799–1806
[11] Kreusel KM, Bornfeld N, Lommatzsch A, Wessing A, Foerster MH. Ruthenium-106 brachytherapy for peripheral retinal capillary hemangioma. Ophthalmology. 1998; 105(8):1386–1392
[12] Raja D, Benz MS, Murray TG, Escalona-Benz EM, Markoe A. Salvage external beam radiotherapy of retinal capillary hemangiomas secondary to von Hippel-Lindau disease: visual and anatomic outcomes. Ophthalmology. 2004; 111(1):150–153
[13] Ach T, Thiemeyer D, Hoeh AE, Schaal KB, Dithmar S. Intravitreal bevacizumab for retinal capillary haemangioma: longterm results. Acta Ophthalmol. 2010; 88(4):e137–e138
[14] Gass JDM. Cavernous hemangioma of the retina. A neuro-oculo-cutaneous syndrome. Am J Ophthalmol. 1971; 71(4):799–814

[15] Goldberg RE, Pheasant TR, Shields JA. Cavernous hemangioma of the retina. A four-generation pedigree with neuro-oculocutaneous involvement and an example of bilateral retinal involvement. Arch Ophthalmol. 1979; 97:2321–2324

[16] Sarraf D, Payne AM, Kitchen ND, Sehmi KS, Downes SM, Bird AC. Familial cavernous hemangioma: an expanding ocular spectrum. Arch Ophthalmol. 2000; 118(7):969–973

[17] Messmer E, Laqua H, Wessing A, et al. Nine cases of cavernous hemangioma of the retina. Am J Ophthalmol. 1983; 95(3):383–390

[18] Labauge P, Denier C, Bergametti F, Tournier-Lasserve E. Genetics of cavernous angiomas. Lancet Neurol. 2007; 6(3):237–244

[19] Reddy S, Gorin MB, McCannel TA, Tsui I, Straatsma BR. Novel KRIT1/CCM1 mutation in a patient with retinal cavernous hemangioma and cerebral cavernous malformation. Graefes Arch Clin Exp Ophthalmol. 2010; 248 (9):1359–1361

[20] Shields JA, Eagle RC, Jr, Ewing MQ, Lally SE, Shields CL. Retinal cavernous hemangioma: fifty-two years of clinical follow-up with clinicopathologic correlation. Retina. 2014; 34(6):1253–1257

[21] Archer DB, Deutman A, Ernest JT, Krill AE. Arteriovenous communications of the retina. Am J Ophthalmol. 1973; 75(2):224–241

[22] Bernth-Petersen P. Racemose haemangioma of the retina. Report of three cases with long term follow-up. Acta Ophthalmol (Copenh). 1979; 57 (4):669–678

[23] Shah GK, Shields JA, Lanning RC. Branch retinal vein obstruction secondary to retinal arteriovenous communication. Am J Ophthalmol. 1998; 126 (3):446–448

[24] Materin MA, Shields CL, Marr BP, Demirci H, Shields JA. Retinal racemose hemangioma. Retina. 2005; 25(7):936–937

[25] Papageorgiou KI, Ghazi-Nouri SM, Andreou PS. Vitreous and subretinal haemorrhage: an unusual complication of retinal racemose haemangioma. Clin Experiment Ophthalmol. 2006; 34(2):176–177

[26] Ponce FA, Han PP, Spetzler RF, Canady A, Feiz-Erfan I. Associated arteriovenous malformation of the orbit and brain: a case of Wyburn-Mason syndrome without retinal involvement. Case report. J Neurosurg. 2001; 95(2):346–349

[27] Shields JA, Decker WL, Sanborn GE, Augsburger JJ, Goldberg RE. Presumed acquired retinal hemangiomas. Ophthalmology. 1983; 90(11):1292–1300

[28] Shields CL, Shields JA, Barrett J, De Potter P. Vasoproliferative tumors of the ocular fundus. Classification and clinical manifestations in 103 patients. Arch Ophthalmol. 1995; 113(5):615–623

[29] Shields CL, Kaliki S, Al-Dahmash S, et al. Retinal vasoproliferative tumors: comparative clinical features of primary vs secondary tumors in 334 cases. JAMA Ophthalmol. 2013; 131(3):328–334

[30] Shields JA, Pellegrini M, Kaliki S, Mashayekhi A, Shields CL. Retinal vasoproliferative tumors in 6 patients with neurofibromatosis type 1. JAMA Ophthalmol. 2014; 132(2):190–196

[31] Anastassiou G, Bornfeld N, Schueler AO, et al. Ruthenium-106 plaque brachytherapy for symptomatic vasoproliferative tumours of the retina. Br J Ophthalmol. 2006; 90(4):447–450

[32] Heimann H, Bornfeld N, Vij O, et al. Vasoproliferative tumours of the retina. Br J Ophthalmol. 2000; 84(10):1162–1169

[33] Cohen VM, Shields CL, Demirci H, Shields JA. Iodine I 125 plaque radiotherapy for vasoproliferative tumors of the retina in 30 eyes. Arch Ophthalmol. 2008; 126(9):1245–1251

[34] Poole Perry LJ, Jakobiec FA, Zakka FR, et al. Reactive retinal astrocytic tumors (so-called vasoproliferative tumors): histopathologic, immunohistochemical, and genetic studies of four cases. Am J Ophthalmol. 2013; 155(3):593–608.e1

[35] Nyboer JH, Robertson DM, Gomez MR. Retinal lesions in tuberous sclerosis. Arch Ophthalmol. 1976; 94(8):1277–1280

[36] Williams R, Taylor D. Tuberous sclerosis. Surv Ophthalmol. 1985; 30(3):143–154

[37] Zimmer-Galler IE, Robertson DM. Long-term observation of retinal lesions in tuberous sclerosis. Am J Ophthalmol. 1995; 119(3):318–324

[38] Shields CL, Reichstein DA, Bianciotto C, Shields JA. Retinal pigment epithelial depigmented lesions associated with tuberous sclerosis complex. Arch Ophthalmol. 2012; 130(3):387–390

[39] Aronow ME, Nakagawa JA, Gupta A, Traboulsi EI, Singh AD. Tuberous sclerosis complex: genotype/phenotype correlation of retinal findings. Ophthalmology. 2012; 119(9):1917–1923

[40] Roach ES, DiMario FJ, Kandt RS, Northrup H, National Tuberous Sclerosis Association. Tuberous Sclerosis Consensus Conference: recommendations for diagnostic evaluation. J Child Neurol. 1999; 14(6):401–407

[41] Roach ES, Gomez MR, Northrup H. Tuberous sclerosis complex consensus conference: revised clinical diagnostic criteria. J Child Neurol. 1998; 13 (12):624–628

[42] Stumpf DA, Alksne JF, Annegers JF, National Institutes of Health Consensus Development Conference. Neurofibromatosis. Conference statement. Arch Neurol. 1988; 45(5):575–578

[43] Shields CL, Benevides R, Materin MA, Shields JA. Optical coherence tomography of retinal astrocytic hamartoma in 15 cases. Ophthalmology. 2006; 113 (9):1553–1557

[44] Shields CL, Shields JA, Eagle RC, Jr, Cangemi F. Progressive enlargement of acquired retinal astrocytoma in 2 cases. Ophthalmology. 2004; 111(2):363–368

[45] Shields CL, Materin MA, Marr BP, Krepostman J, Shields JA. Resolution of exudative retinal detachment from retinal astrocytoma following photodynamic therapy. Arch Ophthalmol. 2008; 126(2):273–274

[46] Buettner H. Congenital hypertrophy of the retinal pigment epithelium. Am J Ophthalmol. 1975; 79(2):177–189

[47] Chamot L, Zografos L, Klainguti G. Fundus changes associated with congenital hypertrophy of the retinal pigment epithelium. Am J Ophthalmol. 1993; 115(2):154–161

[48] Shields CL, Mashayekhi A, Ho T, Cater J, Shields JA. Solitary congenital hypertrophy of the retinal pigment epithelium: clinical features and frequency of enlargement in 330 patients. Ophthalmology. 2003; 110(10):1968–1976

[49] Shields JA, Shields CL, Shah P, Pastore DJ, Imperiale SM. Lack of association between typical congenital hypertrophy of the retinal pigment epithelium adenomatous polyposis, and Gardner syndrome. Ophthalmology. 1992; 99:1709–1713

[50] Shields CL, Materin MA, Walker C, Marr BP, Shields JA. Photoreceptor loss overlying congenital hypertrophy of the retinal pigment epithelium by optical coherence tomography. Ophthalmology. 2006; 113(4):661–665

[51] Fung AT, Pellegrini M, Shields CL. Congenital hypertrophy of the retinal pigment epithelium: enhanced-depth imaging optical coherence tomography in 18 cases. Ophthalmology. 2014; 121(1):251–256

[52] Blair NP, Trempe CL. Hypertrophy of the retinal pigment epithelium associated with Gardner's syndrome. Am J Ophthalmol. 1980; 90(5):661–667

[53] Gardner EJ, Richards RC. Multiple cutaneous and subcutaneous lesions occurring simultaneously with hereditary polyposis and osteomatosis. Am J Hum Genet. 1953; 5(2):139–147

[54] Traboulsi EI. Pigmented and depigmented lesions of the ocular fundus. Curr Opin Ophthalmol. 2012; 23(5):337–343

[55] Kasner L, Traboulsi EI, Delacruz Z, Green WR. A histopathologic study of the pigmented fundus lesions in familial adenomatous polyposis. Retina. 1992; 12(1):35–42

[56] Traboulsi EI, Maumenee IH, Krush AJ, Giardiello FM, Levin LS, Hamilton SR. Pigmented ocular fundus lesions in the inherited gastrointestinal polyposis syndromes and in hereditary nonpolyposis colorectal cancer. Ophthalmology. 1988; 95(7):964–969

[57] Burger B, Cattani N, Trueb S, et al. Prevalence of skin lesions in familial adenomatous polyposis: a marker for presymptomatic diagnosis? Oncologist. 2011; 16(12):1698–1705

[58] Agrawal D, Newaskar V, Shrivastava S, Nayak PA. External manifestations of Gardner's syndrome as the presenting clinical entity. BMJ Case Rep. 2014. DOI: 10.1136/bcr-2013-200293

[59] Traboulsi EI, Maumenee IH, Krush AJ, et al. Congenital hypertrophy of the retinal pigment epithelium predicts colorectal polyposis in Gardner's syndrome. Arch Ophthalmol. 1990; 108(4):525–526

[60] Traboulsi EI. Ocular manifestations of familial adenomatous polyposis (Gardner syndrome). Ophthalmol Clin North Am. 2005; 18(1):163–166, x

[61] Gass JDM. An unusual hamartoma of the pigment epithelium and retina simulating choroidal melanoma and retinoblastoma. Trans Am Ophthalmol Soc. 1973; 71:171–183, 184–185

[62] Destro M, D'Amico DJ, Gragoudas ES, et al. Retinal manifestations of neurofibromatosis. Diagnosis and management. Arch Ophthalmol. 1991; 109 (5):662–666

[63] Schachat AP, Shields JA, Fine SL, et al. Combined hamartomas of the retina and retinal pigment epithelium. Ophthalmology. 1984; 91(12):1609–1615

[64] Shields CL, Thangappan A, Hartzell K, Valente P, Pirondini C, Shields JA. Combined hamartoma of the retina and retinal pigment epithelium in 77 consecutive patients visual outcome based on macular versus extramacular tumor location. Ophthalmology. 2008; 115(12):2246–2252.e3

[65] Gutmann DH, Aylsworth A, Carey JC, et al. The diagnostic evaluation and multidisciplinary management of neurofibromatosis 1 and neurofibromatosis 2. JAMA. 1997; 278(1):51–57

[66] Kaye LD, Rothner AD, Beauchamp GR, Meyers SM, Estes ML. Ocular findings associated with neurofibromatosis type II. Ophthalmology. 1992; 99 (9):1424–1429
[67] Shields CL, Mashayekhi A, Dai VV, Materin MA, Shields JA. Optical coherence tomographic findings of combined hamartoma of the retina and retinal pigment epithelium in 11 patients. Arch Ophthalmol. 2005; 123(12):1746–1750
[68] Arepalli S, Pellegrini M, Ferenczy SR, Shields CL. Combined hamartoma of the retina and retinal pigment epithelium: findings on enhanced depth imaging optical coherence tomography in eight eyes. Retina. 2014; 34 (11):2202–2207
[69] Font RL, Zimmerman LE, Fine BS. Adenoma of the retinal pigment epithelium: histochemical and electron microscopic observations. Am J Ophthalmol. 1972; 73(4):544–554
[70] Shields JA, Shields CL, Eagle RC, Jr, Singh AD. Adenocarcinoma arising from congenital hypertrophy of retinal pigment epithelium. Arch Ophthalmol. 2001; 119(4):597–602
[71] Shields JA, Shields CL, Gündüz K, Eagle RC, Jr. Neoplasms of the retinal pigment epithelium: the 1998 Albert Ruedemann, Sr, memorial lecture, Part 2. Arch Ophthalmol. 1999; 117(5):601–608
[72] Shields JA, Shields CL, Singh AD. Acquired tumors arising from congenital hypertrophy of the retinal pigment epithelium. Arch Ophthalmol. 2000; 118 (5):637–641
[73] Witschel H, Font RL. Hemangioma of the choroid. A clinicopathologic study of 71 cases and a review of the literature. Surv Ophthalmol. 1976; 20 (6):415–431
[74] Shields CL, Honavar SG, Shields JA, Cater J, Demirci H. Circumscribed choroidal hemangioma: clinical manifestations and factors predictive of visual outcome in 200 consecutive cases. Ophthalmology. 2001; 108(12):2237–2248
[75] Arevalo JF, Shields CL, Shields JA, Hykin PG, De Potter P. Circumscribed choroidal hemangioma: characteristic features with indocyanine green videoangiography. Ophthalmology. 2000; 107(2):344–350
[76] Arepalli S, Shields CL, Kaliki S, Emrich J, Komarnicky L, Shields JA. Diffuse choroidal hemangioma management with plaque radiotherapy in 5 cases. Ophthalmology. 2013; 120(11):2358–2359, 2359.e1–2359.e2
[77] Mashayekhi A, Shields CL. Circumscribed choroidal hemangioma. Curr Opin Ophthalmol. 2003; 14(3):142–149
[78] Schmidt-Erfurth UM, Michels S, Kusserow C, Jurklies B, Augustin AJ. Photodynamic therapy for symptomatic choroidal hemangioma: visual and anatomic results. Ophthalmology. 2002; 109(12):2284–2294
[79] Blasi MA, Tiberti AC, Scupola A, et al. Photodynamic therapy with verteporfin for symptomatic circumscribed choroidal hemangioma: five-year outcomes. Ophthalmology. 2010; 117(8):1630–1637
[80] Ferry AP, Font RL. Carcinoma metastatic to the eye and orbit. I. A clinicopathologic study of 227 cases. Arch Ophthalmol. 1974; 92(4):276–286
[81] Stephens RF, Shields JA. Diagnosis and management of cancer metastatic to the uvea: a study of 70 cases. Ophthalmology. 1979; 86(7):1336–1349
[82] Shields CL, Shields JA, Gross NE, Schwartz GP, Lally SE. Survey of 520 eyes with uveal metastases. Ophthalmology. 1997; 104(8):1265–1276
[83] Demirci H, Shields CL, Chao AN, Shields JA. Uveal metastasis from breast cancer in 264 patients. Am J Ophthalmol. 2003; 136(2):264–271
[84] Shah SU, Mashayekhi A, Shields CL, et al. Uveal metastasis from lung cancer: clinical features, treatment, and outcome in 194 patients. Ophthalmology. 2014; 121(1):352–357
[85] De Potter P, Shields CL, Shields JA, Tardio DJ. Uveal metastasis from prostate carcinoma. Cancer. 1993; 71(9):2791–2796
[86] Arevalo JF, Fernandez CF, Garcia RA. Optical coherence tomography characteristics of choroidal metastasis. Ophthalmology. 2005; 112(9):1612–1619
[87] Al-Dahmash SA, Shields CL, Kaliki S, Johnson T, Shields JA. Enhanced depth imaging optical coherence tomography of choroidal metastasis in 14 eyes. Retina. 2014; 34(8):1588–1593
[88] Shields JA, Shields CL, Ehya H, Eagle RC, Jr, De Potter P. Fine-needle aspiration biopsy of suspected intraocular tumors. The 1992 Urwick Lecture. Ophthalmology. 1993; 100(11):1677–1684
[89] Shields CL, Shields JA, De Potter P, et al. Plaque radiotherapy for the management of uveal metastasis. Arch Ophthalmol. 1997; 115(2):203–209
[90] Kaliki S, Shields CL, Al-Dahmash SA, Mashayekhi A, Shields JA. Photodynamic therapy for choroidal metastasis in 8 cases. Ophthalmology. 2012; 119 (6):1218–1222
[91] Gass JD, Guerry RK, Jack RL, Harris G. Choroidal Osteoma. Arch Ophthalmol. 1978; 96(3):428–435
[92] Gass JD. New observations concerning choroidal osteomas. Int Ophthalmol. 1979; 1(2):71–84
[93] Aylward GW, Chang TS, Pautler SE, Gass JD. A long-term follow-up of choroidal osteoma. Arch Ophthalmol. 1998; 116(10):1337–1341
[94] Shields CL, Shields JA, Augsburger JJ. Choroidal osteoma. Surv Ophthalmol. 1988; 33(1):17–27
[95] Shields CL, Sun H, Demirci H, Shields JA. Factors predictive of tumor growth, tumor decalcification, choroidal neovascularization, and visual outcome in 74 eyes with choroidal osteoma. Arch Ophthalmol. 2005; 123(12):1658–1666
[96] Shields CL, Perez B, Materin MA, Mehta S, Shields JA. Optical coherence tomography of choroidal osteoma in 22 cases: evidence for photoreceptor atrophy over the decalcified portion of the tumor. Ophthalmology. 2007; 114(12):e53–e58
[97] Pellegrini M, Invernizzi A, Giani A, Staurenghi G. Enhanced depth imaging optical coherence tomography features of choroidal osteoma. Retina. 2014; 34(5):958–963
[98] Shields CL, Arepalli S, Atalay HT, Ferenczy SR, Fulco E, Shields JA. Choroidal osteoma shows bone lamella and vascular channels on enhanced depth imaging optical coherence tomography in 15 eyes. Retina. 2015; 35(4):750–757
[99] Shields CL, Materin MA, Mehta S, Foxman BT, Shields JA. Regression of extrafoveal choroidal osteoma following photodynamic therapy. Arch Ophthalmol. 2008; 126(1):135–137
[100] Khan MA, DeCroos FC, Storey PP, Shields JA, Garg SJ, Shields CL. Outcomes of anti-vascular endothelial growth factor therapy in the management of choroidal neovascularization associated with choroidal osteoma. Retina. 2014; 34(9):1750–1756
[101] Jakobiec FA, Witschel H, Zimmerman LE. Choroidal leiomyoma of vascular origin. Am J Ophthalmol. 1976; 82(2):205–212
[102] Jakobiec FA, Font RL, Tso MO, Zimmerman LE. Mesectodermal leiomyoma of the ciliary body: a tumor of presumed neural crest origin. Cancer. 1977; 39 (5):2102–2113
[103] Shields JA, Shields CL, Eagle RC, Jr, De Potter P. Observations on seven cases of intraocular leiomyoma. The 1993 Byron Demorest Lecture. Arch Ophthalmol. 1994; 112(4):521–528
[104] Heegaard S, Jensen PK, Scherfig E, Prause JU. Leiomyoma of the ciliary body. Report of 2 cases. Acta Ophthalmol Scand. 1999; 77(6):709–712
[105] Oh KJ, Kwon BJ, Han MH, et al. MR imaging findings of uveal leiomyoma: three cases. AJNR Am J Neuroradiol. 2005; 26(1):100–103
[106] Richter MN, Bechrakis NE, Stoltenburg-Didinger G, Foerster MH. Transscleral resection of a ciliary body leiomyoma in a child: case report and review of the literature. Graefes Arch Clin Exp Ophthalmol. 2003; 241(11):953–957
[107] Shields JA, Hamada A, Shields CL, De Potter P, Eagle RC, Jr. Ciliochoroidal nerve sheath tumor simulating a malignant melanoma. Retina. 1997; 17 (5):459–460
[108] Huang Y, Wei W. Choroidal schwannoma presenting as nonpigmented intraocular mass. J Clin Oncol. 2012; 30(31):e315–e317
[109] Zimmerman LE. Melanocytes, melanocytic nevi, and melanocytomas: The Jonas S. Friedenwald Memorial Lecture. Invest Ophthalmol. 1965; 4:11–41
[110] Reidy JJ, Apple DJ, Steinmetz RL, et al. Melanocytoma: nomenclature, pathogenesis, natural history and treatment. Surv Ophthalmol. 1985; 29(5):319–327
[111] Shields JA, Demirci H, Mashayekhi A, Shields CL. Melanocytoma of optic disc in 115 cases: the 2004 Samuel Johnson Memorial Lecture, part 1. Ophthalmology. 2004; 111(9):1739–1746
[112] Shields JA, Demirci H, Mashayekhi A, Eagle RC, Jr, Shields CL. Melanocytoma of the optic disk: a review. Surv Ophthalmol. 2006; 51(2):93–104
[113] Shields JA, Shields CL, Eagle RC, Jr. Melanocytoma (hyperpigmented magnocellular nevus) of the uveal tract: the 34th G. Victor Simpson lecture. Retina. 2007; 27(6):730–739
[114] Shields CL, Perez B, Benavides R, Materin MA, Shields JA. Optical coherence tomography of optic disk melanocytoma in 15 cases. Retina. 2008; 28 (3):441–446
[115] Chan CC, Buggage RR, Nussenblatt RB. Intraocular lymphoma. Curr Opin Ophthalmol. 2002; 13(6):411–418
[116] Coupland SE, Heimann H. Primary intraocular lymphoma [in German]. Ophthalmologe. 2004; 101(1):87–98
[117] Cockerham GC, Hidayat AA, Bijwaard KE, Sheng ZM. Re-evaluation of "reactive lymphoid hyperplasia of the uvea": an immunohistochemical and molecular analysis of 10 cases. Ophthalmology. 2000; 107(1):151–158
[118] Coupland SE, Foss HD, Hidayat AA, Cockerham GC, Hummel M, Stein H. Extranodal marginal zone B cell lymphomas of the uvea: an analysis of 13 cases. J Pathol. 2002; 197(3):333–340

[119] Grossniklaus HE, Martin DF, Avery R, et al. Uveal lymphoid infiltration. Report of four cases and clinicopathologic review. Ophthalmology. 1998; 105(7):1265–1273
[120] Mashayekhi A, Shukla SY, Shields JA, Shields CL. Choroidal lymphoma: clinical features and association with systemic lymphoma. Ophthalmology. 2014; 121(1):342–351
[121] Aronow ME, Portell CA, Sweetenham JW, Singh AD. Uveal lymphoma: clinical features, diagnostic studies, treatment selection, and outcomes. Ophthalmology. 2014; 121(1):334–341
[122] Shields CL, Arepalli S, Pellegrini M, Mashayekhi A, Shields JA. Choroidal lymphoma shows calm, rippled, or undulating topography on enhanced depth imaging optical coherence tomography in 14 eyes. Retina. 2014; 34 (7):1347–1353
[123] Ridley ME, McDonald HR, Sternberg P, Jr, Blumenkranz MS, Zarbin MA, Schachat AP. Retinal manifestations of ocular lymphoma (reticulum cell sarcoma). Ophthalmology. 1992; 99(7):1153–1160, discussion 1160–1161
[124] Nussenblatt RB, Chan CC, Wilson WH, Hochman J, Gottesman M, CNS and Ocular Lymphoma Workshop Group. International Central Nervous System and Ocular Lymphoma Workshop: recommendations for the future. Ocul Immunol Inflamm. 2006; 14(3):139–144
[125] Schachat AP, Markowitz JA, Guyer DR, Burke PJ, Karp JE, Graham ML. Ophthalmic manifestations of leukemia. Arch Ophthalmol. 1989; 107(5):697–700

29 Retinal Tears and Rhegmatogenous Retinal Detachments

Stephen G. Schwartz, Harry W. Flynn Jr., William F. Mieler, and James S. Tiedeman

Rhegmatogenous retinal detachment is caused by one or more retinal breaks ("rhegma" is a Greek word, meaning breach, cleft, or fissure). Most, but not all, retinal breaks occur in association with posterior vitreous detachment (PVD), a common aging change.

29.1 Posterior Vitreous Detachment

PVD is common with advancing age. Using B-scan echography, the incidence of complete PVD has been reported to increase from 11% in patients aged 65 to 69 years to 46% in patients aged 80 to 89 years.[1] The incidence of PVD is further increased by pseudophakia, myopia, trauma, and intraocular inflammation. PVD and associated vitreous floaters may cause troublesome symptoms, especially in patients aged 55 years or less.[2] In some patients, PVD may create an objective "floater scotoma" detectable by optical coherence tomography (OCT).[3] However, the real significance of PVD is that it may be a harbinger of retinal tears and detachment.

29.1.1 Clinical Features

PVD may be asymptomatic or may be associated with variable symptoms, typically new-onset floaters and/or photopsias. Characteristically, floaters move with eye movements and continue to show motion after eye movements have stopped. Patients sometimes have difficulty separating a truly floating dark spot from a central scotoma, which also moves with eye movements but remains in exactly the same position relative to the center of gaze.

Photopsias, or light flashes, may be caused by stimulation of the retina from a partial or complete detachment of the formed vitreous from the retina and are usually perceived as crescents of light in the peripheral visual field. Photopsias are most visible in the dark or in dim light conditions. In some cases, if vitreous hemorrhage accompanies the PVD, the presenting symptom may be blurred vision, which may vary in severity.

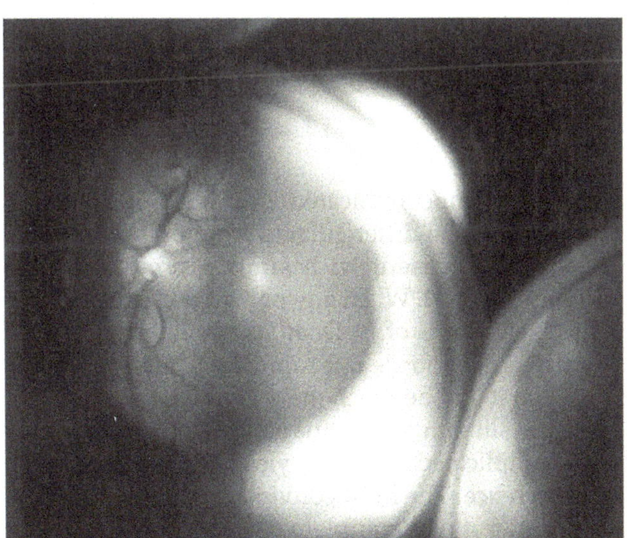

Fig. 29.1 Photograph of a Weiss ring in the midvitreous cavity. This annulus of tissue was previously adherent to the optic disc.

29.1.2 Diagnosis

Although a PVD is generally a benign occurrence, it must be differentiated from pathologic conditions that may present with similar symptoms and findings.

Differential diagnosis of Floaters and Photopsia

- Uncomplicated posterior vitreous detachment
- Vitreous hemorrhage
- Retinal tear or rhegmatogenous retinal detachment
- Retinal tear with bridging vessel
- Proliferative diabetic retinopathy
- Branch retinal vein occlusion with neovascularization
- Choroidal neovascularization with breakthrough bleeding into the vitreous
- Trauma
- Inflammatory conditions of retina/choroid/vitreous
- Multifocal choroiditis/panuveitis
- Sarcoidosis
- Pars planitis
- Toxoplasmosis
- Cytomegalovirus retinitis
- Idiopathic and other inflammatory conditions
- Intraocular lymphoma with vitreous infiltration
- Optic neuritis
- Migraine

Examination of the vitreous after an uncomplicated PVD may yield only subtle clues to its occurrence. The most convincing evidence of PVD is the finding of a complete or partial ring of tissue suspended in the vitreous cavity (Vogt or Weiss ring; ▸ Fig. 29.1), representing the fibrous remnants of the relatively tight attachment of the vitreous to the optic disc.[4] An optically empty zone posterior to biomicroscopically visible formed vitreous is frequently taken as evidence of PVD, although this often represents a pocket of liquified vitreous with a layer of cortical vitreous still adherent to the retina. The truly separated posterior hyaloid has a characteristic appearance, like that of wrinkled cellophane, anterior to an optically empty region.

The presence of anterior or posterior vitreous pigment clumps (also called "tobacco dust" or "Shafer's sign") in an eye that has not undergone surgery or other trauma is suggestive of a retinal tear. Vitreous white blood cells may indicate an inflammatory condition such as multifocal choroiditis/panuveitis, which often presents with both floaters and photopsias. Any inflammatory condition capable of producing vitreous inflammatory cells, or the presence of malignant cells in the case of intraocular lymphoma, can produce floaters.

The finding of blood in the vitreous cavity should prompt a search for sources of bleeding, particularly a retinal tear. An acute PVD with vitreous hemorrhage has an up to 70% incidence of retinal tears, compared with a 2 to 4% incidence in acute PVD without hemorrhage. Other sources of blood, with or without PVD, include retinal or optic disc neovascularization secondary to such etiologies as branch retinal vein occlusion or proliferative diabetic retinopathy, and choroidal neovascularization with breakthrough bleeding.

Special Considerations

- The presence of vitreous hemorrhage or pigment clumps after an acute PVD suggests the presence of an associated retinal tear.

29.1.3 Pathogenesis

The vitreous is an important structure during embryologic development, and undergoes three distinct stages of development.[5] Initially, the primary vitreous supplies vasculature to the developing eye. The primary vitreous reaches its most vascular stage near the ninth week of gestation, after which the vessels normally atrophy. The primary vitreous is then replaced by an avascular, clear secondary vitreous, leaving the primary vitreous occupying a central tubular structure extending from the optic disc to the posterior surface of the lens, Cloquet's canal. At the time of birth, the blood vessels have normally disappeared, although remnants of Cloquet's canal may persist near the posterior pole of the lens (Mittendorf dot) or on the optic disc (Bergmeister's papilla). Rarely, the primary vitreous fails to involute, and the resulting condition, persistent fetal vasculature (formerly called "persistent hyperplastic primary vitreous"), is associated with cataract, vitreous opacities, and a poor prognosis for vision.

Vitreous is comprised of 99% water. Contained in the water are collagen fibrils, cross-linking the entire volume of formed vitreous, and dissolved hyaluronic acid, forming a clear gel.[6] In the adult, the normally clear vitreous serves no apparent essential function, and changes in the vitreous can be responsible for a number of abnormal conditions.

In the normal young eye, the vitreous fills virtually the complete posterior cavity of the eye and is in contact with the entire retina. It is anchored most securely at the vitreous base, a zone of 3 to 4 mm that extends from the pars plana posteriorly across the ora serrata and into the anterior retina. Weaker zones of vitreous attachment include the optic disc, retinal vessels, and sites of abnormal vitreoretinal conditions, such as at the margins of lattice degeneration.

As a consequence of aging, the vitreous fibrils condense and shrink. Initially, large clear spaces or lacunae, which may be difficult to differentiate from vitreous detachment, may be visible at the slit lamp. With continued shrinkage of the vitreous body, the vitreous usually separates from the retina beginning at the macula. Once vitreous detachment has begun, it typically proceeds rapidly to a funnel-shaped configuration, with attachment anteriorly in a large annulus at the vitreous base; posteriorly, a small annulus is attached to the optic disc. Finally, the attachment at the disc releases and the posterior hyaloid becomes free-floating. Once the posterior hyaloid face has completely separated from the retina up to the vitreous base, no further spontaneous separation can occur (▶ Fig. 29.2).

29.1.4 Management and Course

The most important consideration in the management of a patient with PVD is to search for retinal tears. Once the symptoms of floaters and/or photopsias have begun, the patient should be examined at intervals until the separation has completed. A reexamination in 4 to 6 weeks after the symptoms have begun is generally appropriate, along with the admonition to return sooner if symptoms increase or change substantially.

Pearls

- Retinal tears occur most commonly around the time of a PVD. A thorough examination is generally recommended soon after the onset of flashes and floaters. If no tears are found, patients are advised to return in 4 to 6 weeks, and sooner if there is any change or increase in symptoms.

29.2 Retinal Tears

Following the introduction of the ophthalmoscope by Helmholtz in 1850, retinal tears were recognized in association with retinal detachment, but their role in the pathogenesis of retinal detachment was not understood. Von Graefe incorrectly believed that fluid traveled from the choroid into the subretinal space and that the tear relieved some of this excess pressure. Gonin realized that fluid from the vitreous cavity proceeded through the tear and showed that treatment of the tear could repair some retinal detachments.

Not all retinal tears lead to retinal detachment, and various clinical and autopsy studies have estimated a prevalence of retinal breaks at between 4 and 18% of adult eyes in the United States.[7,8,9,10]

29.2.1 Clinical Features

The term *retinal tear* is usually used to describe a full-thickness defect or break in the retina caused by traction exerted from the vitreous. A tear, as opposed to a round hole, contains a flap that gives the characteristic appearance of a horseshoe (▶ Fig. 29.3). In contrast, atrophic retinal holes are full-thickness retinal defects in which vitreous traction is not the primary pathogenetic mechanism. The term *hole* should not be used interchangeably with *tear* because their appearance, pathogenesis, and risk for associated retinal detachment are different (▶ Fig. 29.4).

Occasionally, the flap of a retinal tear will separate and create a free-floating operculum. In an operculated tear, vitreous traction on the retina is released. The resulting retinal defect is usually round, and the avulsed flap of retina (the operculum) can be seen floating in the vitreous cavity in the vicinity of the tear (▶ Fig. 29.5).

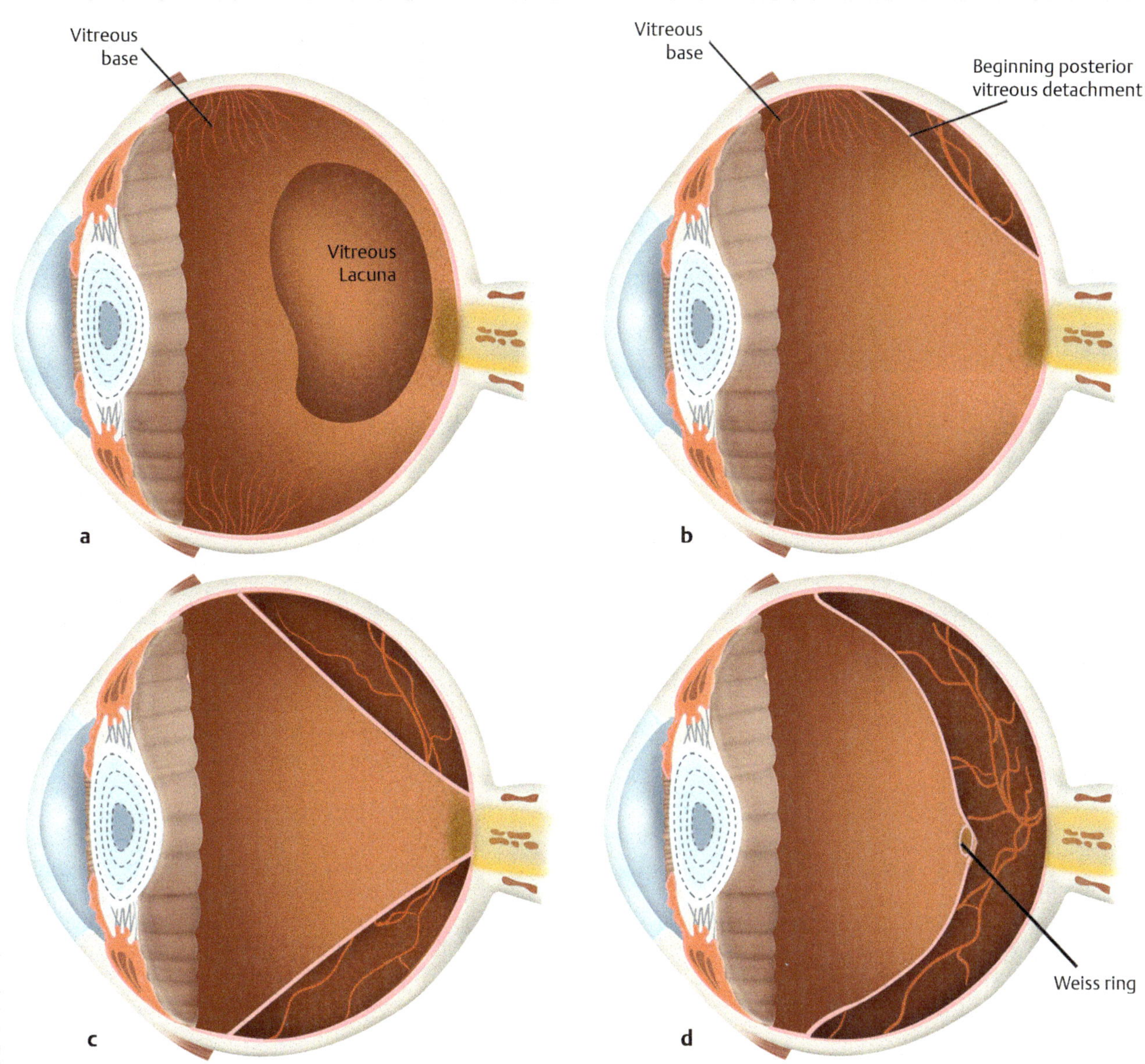

Fig. 29.2 (**a**) Cross-sectional schematic showing a vitreous lacuna that can simulate posterior vitreous detachment at the slit lamp. (**b**) Beginning posterior vitreous detachment. (**c**) Vitreous remaining attached at the vitreous base anteriorly and at the optic disc posteriorly. The remainder of the posterior hyaloid is no longer in contact with the retina. (**d**) Complete posterior vitreous detachment. The glial annulus of attachment to the optic disc (Weiss ring) is free-floating.

Lattice retinal degeneration may be associated with atrophic holes, retinal tears, or both.[11] Lattice is found in about 5 to 10% of the population and is bilateral in one-third of affected individuals. It can have a variable ophthalmoscopic appearance. Often, there is increased pigmentation in lattice lesions, and the overlying blood vessels may appear white, giving the appearance of latticework (▶ Fig. 29.6). Another variant of lattice is termed *"snail track" degeneration*, in which the appearance is white rather than hyperpigmented.[12] There may be a pocket of fluid in the overlying cortical vitreous and retinal thinning (▶ Fig. 29.7). Increased vitreoretinal adhesion at the edge of lattice may give rise to retinal tears at the posterior margin.

Lattice retinal degeneration typically occurs in curvilinear patches between the equator and ora serrata, near the posterior margin of the vitreous base. These patches are usually oriented circumferentially in one or more rows, although lattice may occur radially along retinal blood vessels. Atypical presentations of lattice degeneration may be seen in hereditary vitreoretinal degenerations (e.g., Wagner's syndrome, Stickler's syndrome) in which multiple patches of lattice, some of which are radial, occur in conjunction with a liquified or optically empty vitreous cavity. Retinal tears may occur at the margins of lattice degeneration. Byer[11] noted, however, that in eyes with lattice degeneration, many retinal tears that occur do so in previously normal-appearing retina.

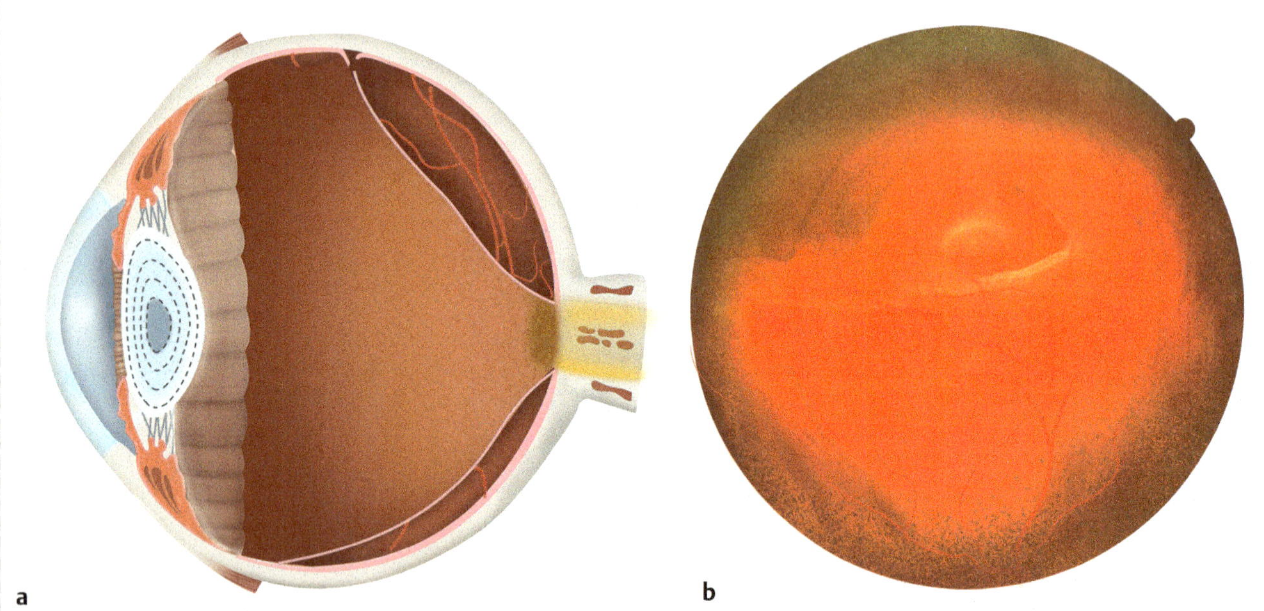

Fig. 29.3 (a) Retinal tear results from an abnormally tight localized vitreoretinal adhesion in the setting of a detaching posterior vitreous. The vitreous is always adherent to the anterior flap of retina and produces traction on the tear. (b) Typical horseshoe appearance of a retinal tear with an associated retinal detachment.

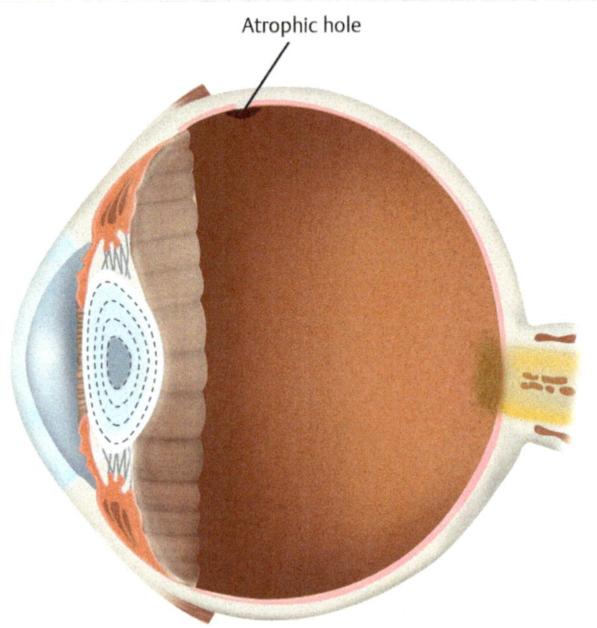

Fig. 29.4 An atrophic hole arises not from vitreous traction but from a thinning and ultimate dehiscence of the retina. These retinal holes by themselves have a low risk of progressing to retinal detachment.

Pearls

- In eyes with patches of lattice degeneration, retinal tears often occur at the edge of the lattice. However, it is also not unusual for retinal tears to occur in previously normal-appearing retina.

In contrast to lattice degeneration, cobblestone or pavingstone degeneration is a peripheral fundus finding that is not associated with retinal breaks and that should not be confused with lattice degeneration. Areas of cobblestone are sharply demarcated zones through which bare sclera or large choroidal vessels may be seen (▶ Fig. 29.8).

Retinal tears may range in size from only a fraction of a millimeter up to several clock hours. A giant retinal tear, by definition, extends 3 or more clock hours (=90 degrees).[13] The vitreous is adherent to the anterior retina in a giant retinal tear, just as it is in a horseshoe tear. The posterior edge of retina has no adherent vitreous, which allows it to detach and scroll up, exposing a large area of bare retinal pigment epithelium (RPE) (▶ Fig. 29.9). On casual viewing, the exposed RPE may have the appearance of a normal fundus, but closer scrutiny reveals the absence of retinal vessels.

A type of retinal break that may be confused with a giant retinal tear is a retinal dialysis. Unlike other retinal tears, which typically occur at the posterior margin of the vitreous base, a retinal dialysis (from the Greek for "separation") occurs at the ora serrata. Therefore, in a dialysis, the vitreous spans the break and is adherent to both the anterior and the posterior retinal edges (▶ Fig. 29.10). This very important difference from a giant tear prevents the posterior edge of the retina from folding over, and helps to give the dialysis a far better surgical prognosis.[14] As with the giant retinal tear, a dialysis can extend circumferentially over several clock hours. The most common location for a dialysis is in the inferotemporal quadrant, but it may also occur in the superonasal quadrant following blunt trauma.

29.2.2 Diagnosis

The detection of retinal breaks may be an arduous task, the success of which depends greatly on the skill and experience of the

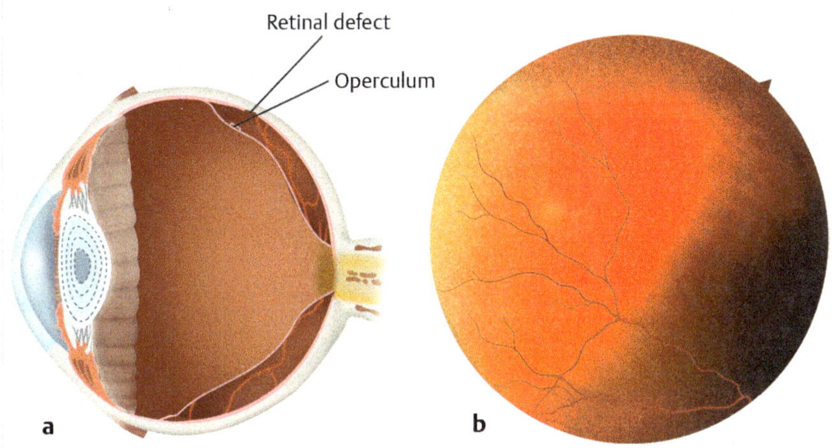

Fig. 29.5 (**a**) An operculated tear results if the flap of retina that is adherent to the vitreous separates from the surrounding retina. Such a tear usually does not have any residual vitreous traction acting on it. (**b**) Typical appearance of an operculated tear; note the small cuff of subretinal fluid.

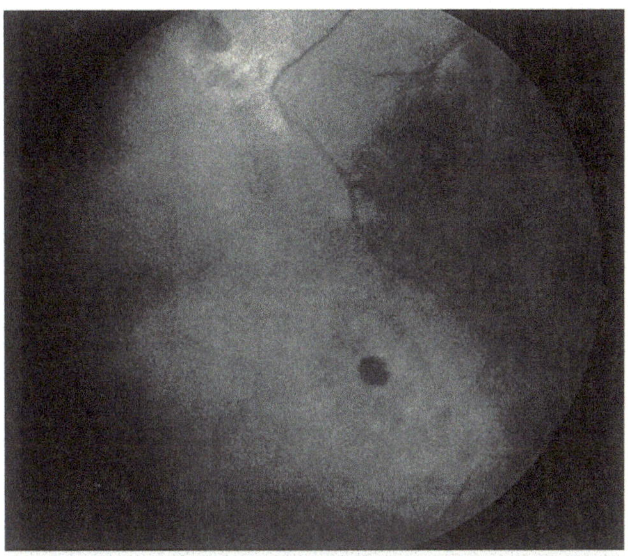

Fig. 29.6 Clinical appearance of lattice retinal degeneration. Atrophic holes are present within the patches of lattice.

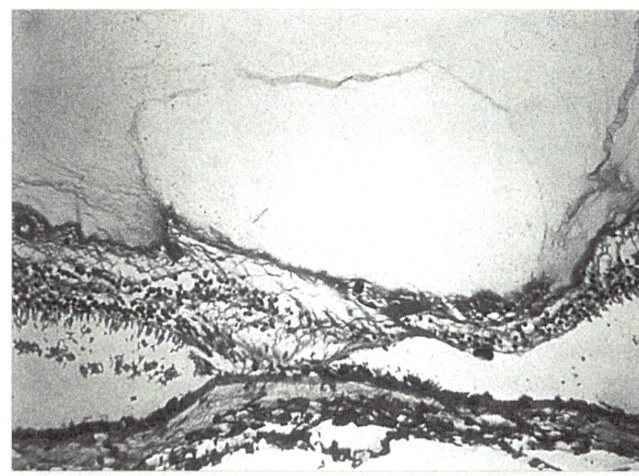

Fig. 29.7 Photomicrograph of lattice retinal degeneration. Note the overlying pocket of liquefied vitreous, prominent, adherent vitreous gel at the margin of the lesion, and thinning or atrophy of the inner retinal layers.

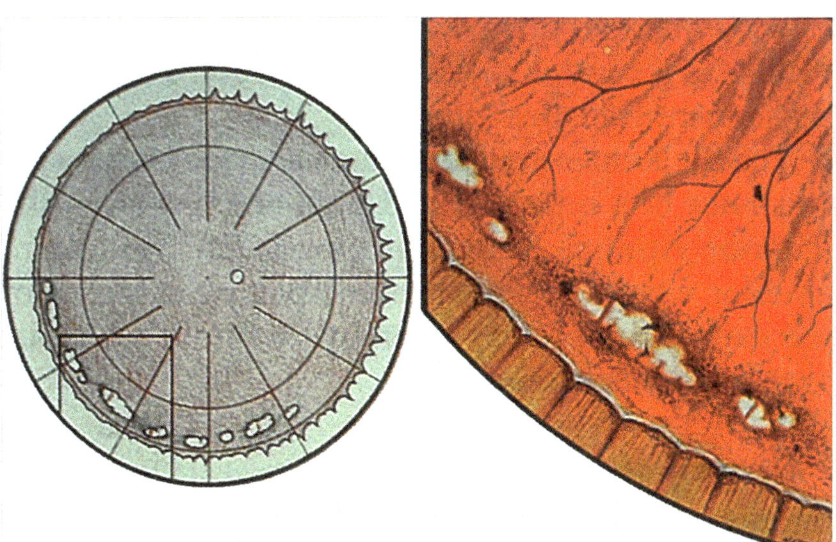

Fig. 29.8 Drawing depicting the typical location and appearance of cobblestone degeneration. The lesions have distinct borders, and on scleral depression there is no thinning of the overlying retina. (Reproduced with permission from Karlin DB, Cortain BJ. Peripheral chorioretinal lesions and axial length of the myopic eye. Am J Ophthalmol 1976;81:625–635.)

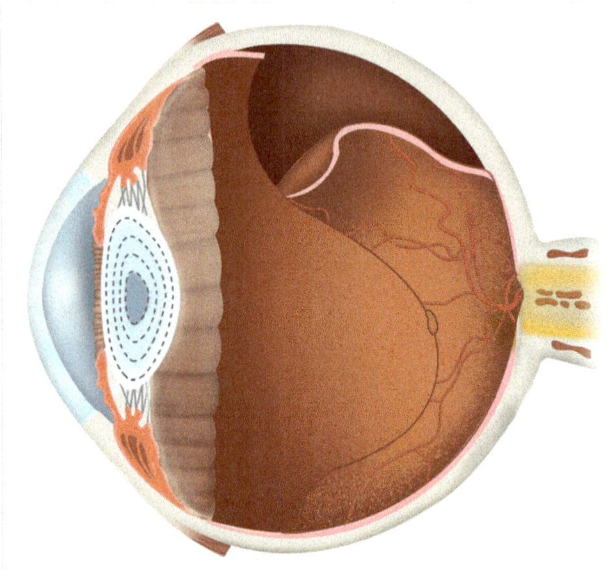

Fig. 29.9 Schematic cross-section of a giant retinal tear: The vitreous is not adherent to the posterior retinal edge, which allows the retina to detach and roll over in some cases.

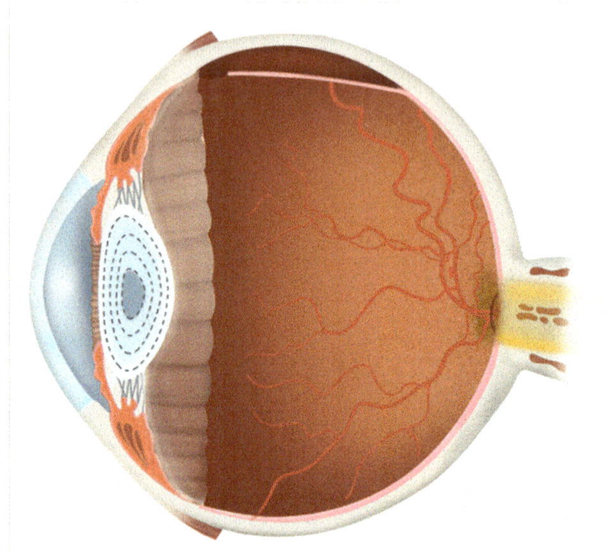

Fig. 29.10 A retinal dialysis differs from a giant retinal tear in that the vitreous spans the retinal defect and provides some stability to the posterior retinal edge. Dialyses usually do not arise directly as the result of posterior vitreous separation.

examiner, using slit-lamp biomicroscopy with hand-held condensing lenses, indirect ophthalmoscopy, or both. Scleral depression may be very helpful for viewing the retina in profile. Because retinal flap tears are three-dimensional, viewing the retina in profile with scleral depression may allow detection of breaks that are not visible when viewed frontally.

29.2.3 Pathogenesis

Retinal tears generally occur during a PVD, especially in eyes with abnormal vitreoretinal relationships, such as preexisting lattice degeneration.[15] However, retinal tears may occur in ophthalmoscopically normal retina, presumably due to excessively tight adhesion of the vitreous to the retina. If there is a wide zone of abnormal vitreoretinal adhesion, the tear may extend circumferentially into a giant retinal tear.

Blunt trauma can produce a number of different findings, depending on the amount of energy delivered to the eye by the blow, as well as on how that energy is distributed to various ocular structures. A finding unique to blunt trauma is avulsion of the vitreous base, which is recognized by a ribbon of pigmented material loosely draped across the peripheral retina, suspended within the vitreous cavity. Although trauma may precipitate horseshoe tears or giant retinal tears, there is usually nothing in their appearance that serves to distinguish traumatic from spontaneous breaks.[16]

29.2.4 Management and Course

Because retinal tears and holes are relatively common clinical and autopsy findings, and because retinal detachment as a consequence of such breaks is relatively uncommon, not all breaks require treatment. As with any therapeutic decision, the proper choice should be based on the known risks of the condition being treated, the risks of the treatment being considered, and to what extent that treatment favorably alters the natural history.

There is general agreement that an acutely symptomatic retinal horseshoe tear should be treated in an effort to reduce the risk for subsequent retinal detachment. Most retinal detachments occur within the first 6 weeks after the onset of symptoms associated with the retinal tear. By 3 months after the development of a tear, the likelihood of a retinal detachment arising from that tear is much less common.[9,17] These facts make the recognition of symptoms an important factor in the decision-making process.[18] A natural history study reported that treatment of the acutely symptomatic retinal tear is the first line of defense against retinal detachment.[19]

On the other hand, the proper response to the finding of a retinal break in an asymptomatic patient is less certain. In these situations, ancillary findings combined with clinical judgement must prevail. Few absolute guidelines exist for deciding which lesions may benefit from treatment. Some relative risk factors that might push the decision toward treatment are listed below.

Conditions Associated with Retinal Breaks That Increase the Risk for Retinal Detachment

- Vitreoretinal traction (elevated flap)
- Prior retinal detachment in fellow eye
- Aphakia/pseudophakia
- Impending cataract surgery
- High myopia
- Large size
- Superior location

In the fellow eye of a patient who has already experienced a retinal detachment, many clinicians consider treatment of lesions similar to the ones that led to the detachment in the first eye. These lesions could include flap tears or atrophic holes.

Controversial Points

- Most acutely symptomatic retinal tears are treated to reduce the risk of retinal detachment. The management of asymptomatic tears, however, is not as clear-cut and requires taking into consideration various features of both the involved and the fellow eyes.

The finding of an asymptomatic retinal tear in an otherwise normal, phakic eye may not require treatment. Pigment around a tear is evidence of chronicity and probable stability. The pigment does not itself provide additional adhesion, but it is a marker of the presence of the tear without change over time and is reassuring of its benign nature. The progression of asymptomatic tears to detachment is rare.

The American Academy of Ophthalmology's Preferred Practice Patterns recommends that acute symptomatic horseshoe tears be treated promptly, while traumatic retinal breaks are "usually treated" and other lesions are generally observed.[20]

When treatment is deemed appropriate, the immediate goal is to reduce the risk of a retinal detachment. A chorioretinal adhesion that prevents access of liquid vitreous into the subretinal space can be produced with either cryopexy or photocoagulation.

Cryopexy is a convenient treatment modality for treating retinal breaks anterior to the equator and can be applied in the setting of mild to moderate media opacity (vitreous hemorrhage, cataract) so long as the retinal break can be visualized. Treatment can be performed in the office examining chair or in a minor surgery area. Topical, subconjunctival or retrobulbar anesthesia may be employed, although if retrobulbar anesthesia can be avoided, the patient's cooperation in directing gaze is helpful. While treatment is being applied, the surgeon watches the white spot develop and releases the freezing pedal when the white freezing reaction reaches the retina. Treating posterior tears can be difficult with cryopexy, as the conjunctival fornix may limit the posterior positioning of the cryo probe.

If large tears are treated with cryopexy, treatment should be kept away from the center of the tear, where freezing risks liberating viable RPE cells into the vitreous cavity. Such cells may lead to epiretinal membrane formation or proliferative vitreoretinopathy (PVR).

Pearls

- When using cryopexy to treat large retinal tears, applications to the center of the tear should be avoided. Freezing this area may release viable retinal pigment epithelial cells into the vitreous cavity and promote epiretinal membrane formation or PVR.

Photocoagulation has some theoretical advantages compared with cryopexy in situations in which the optical media are clear. Laser may provoke less inflammatory response and breakdown of the blood–ocular barrier and, therefore, poses less risk for cellular proliferation and epiretinal membrane formation. Photocoagulation may be delivered by a slit lamp or indirect laser delivery system.

29.3 Acute and Chronic Retinal Detachments

Epidemiologic studies have estimated the incidence of rhegmatogenous retinal detachment in the general population to be about 1 case in every 10,000 persons per year.[21] Although retinal detachment is seen most often in middle-aged and older patients, retinal detachments can be found in all age groups, including infants.

Most retinal detachments are acutely symptomatic and prompt the patient to seek medical attention quickly. Some, however, are more indolent, and they may be present chronically and found only as an incidental finding on routine examination.

29.3.1 Clinical Features

Usually, the occurrence of rhegmatogenous retinal detachment is preceded by the symptoms of PVD a few days to weeks before. The location of floaters and photopsias, however, has very little localizing value.

Many patients will want to know, "Why did my retina detach?" Although specific reasons can rarely be given, understanding that there are identifiable risk factors may be helpful (see below). It is important to remember that some patients without any obvious risk factors will develop retinal detachment, and some patients with multiple risk factors will not.

29.3.2 Risk Factors for Retinal Detachment

- Family history of retinal detachment
- History of previous ocular surgery, especially for cataract (surgical complications, e.g., vitreous loss, further increase risk)
- Axial myopia
- History of ocular trauma
- Lattice degeneration
- Miotic therapy for glaucoma

29.3.3 Diagnosis

Rhegmatogenous retinal detachment is characterized by the clinical appearance of elevated retina in conjunction with one or more retinal breaks. Even if no retinal break can be found, it is important to remember that there is always at least one. In a recent retinal detachment, the detached portion of the retina becomes edematous almost immediately, and this edema is manifested by retinal whitening and a characteristic wrinkled appearance (▶ Fig. 29.11). Biomicroscopy of the freshly detached retina demonstrates that the wrinkling is confined to the outer retina only. In contrast, tracing the course of blood vessels, which lie on the inner retina, demonstrates smooth paths without any wrinkling. The outer retina, when swollen, is able to throw itself into folds, but the inner limiting membrane, being relatively inelastic, keeps the inner retina smooth.

In chronic retinal detachments, which are usually inferior in location, the edema ultimately disappears, and the detached retina becomes thin, atrophic, and relatively transparent. The transparency may make detection of the retinal breaks much more difficult than in a recent detachment and may cause confusion with degenerative retinoschisis (see below).

A number of other conditions may resemble retinal detachment and must be understood to ensure appropriate management. A partial list of causes for real and apparent retinal elevation is given below. Of the long list of differential diagnoses, the entities most often confused with retinal detachment are degenerative retinoschisis, choroidal melanoma, choroidal detachment, and exudative (serous) retinal detachment.

Differential Diagnosis of Rhegmatogenous Retinal Detachment

- **Exudative Retinal Detachment**
  - (See also Chapter 30)
  - Idopathic
  - Surgical or postsurgical
  - Inflammatory/autoimmune
  - Hematologic/vascular
  - Renal failure
  - Infectious
  - Neoplastic
  - Medications
- **Traction Retinal Detachment**
  - Proliferative diabetic retinopathy
  - Other proliferative retinopathies (sickle cell, sarcoid, etc.)
- **Choroidal Detachment**
  - Serous
  - Hemorrhagic
- **Retinoschisis**
  - Juvenile
  - Degenerative (senile)
- **Other Entities**
  - Pheripheral "white-without pressure"

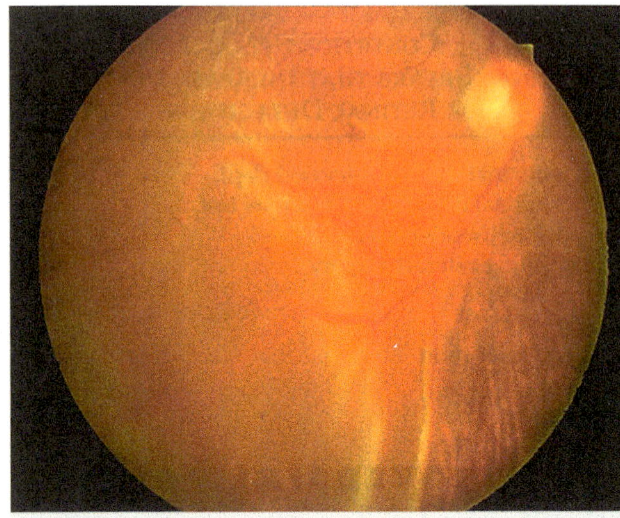

Fig. 29.11 Photograph of recent rhegmatogenous retinal detachment. The corrugated appearance of the outer retina is the result of edema or swelling. The inner retina has a smoother contour, as evidenced by the relatively smooth course of the retinal blood vessels.

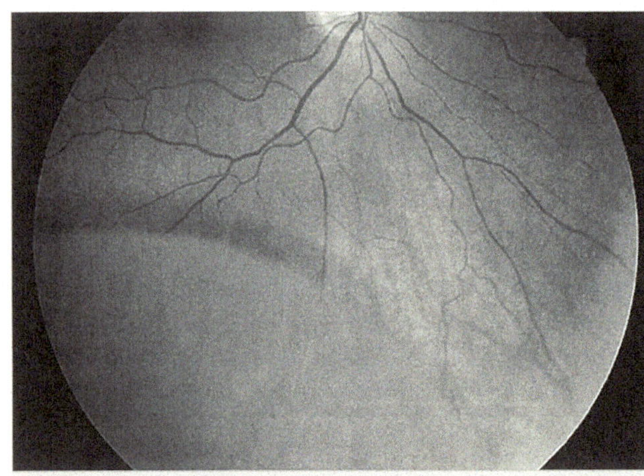

Fig. 29.12 Clinical photograph of degenerative retinoschisis. The inner retina is highly bullous and tense. Retinoschisis may be difficult to distinguish from chronic, full-thickness retinal detachment in some cases.

Degenerative retinoschisis is often difficult to distinguish from chronic retinal detachment (▶ Fig. 29.12). It is typically asymptomatic and found as an incidental finding on retinal examination. The inner retinal layer is very thin and transparent, and has a rather tense-appearing dome shape. The most frequent location of degenerative retinoschisis is the inferotemporal quadrant, and the condition is often bilateral, although it can be very asymmetric. Very tiny retinal breaks may occur in the inner retina, and these may be exceedingly difficult to detect against the transparent inner retinal layer. Outer layer defects, on the other hand, tend to be larger, round holes and may resemble Swiss cheese breaks. In most cases, the outer retinal layer remains in normal contact with the RPE and, therefore, pigmented demarcation lines are seen less commonly in association with retinoschisis than with rhegmatogenous retinal detachment.

Although the photoreceptors may show near-normal microanatomy in the outer layer of retinoschisis, they are functionally disconnected from the inner retina, and an absolute scotoma results. In relatively posterior cases, visual field testing may be useful, because retinoschisis produces an absolute scotoma, while rhegmatogenous retinal detachment produces only a relative scotoma. Perhaps more useful in relatively posterior cases, OCT can often distinguish intraretinal fluid, more consistent with retinoschisis, from subretinal fluid, more consistent with retinal detachment.

Although degenerative retinoschisis is generally a benign condition with little propensity to progress toward the macula, it can coexist with rhegmatogenous retinal detachment when both inner and outer layer breaks are present.[22]

Choroidal melanoma may be associated with nonrhegmatogenous (serous) retinal detachment. In most patients, the distinction between rhegmatogenous and nonrhegmatogenous retinal detachment can be made readily on clinical examination or with A- and B-scan echography. Choroidal melanoma classically presents as a dome-shaped or "collar button" elevation

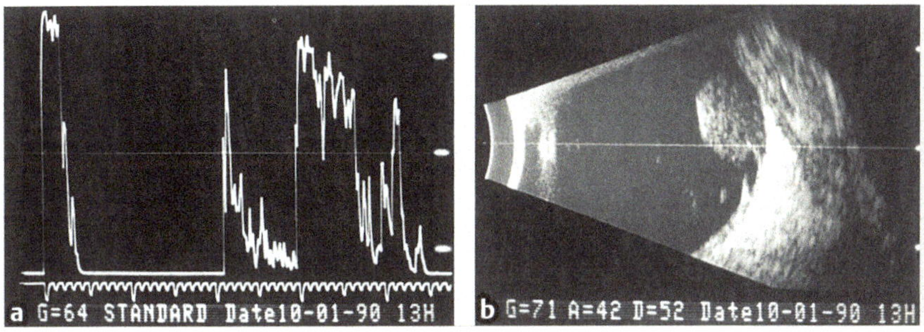

Fig. 29.13 (a) A-scan ultrasound through a choroidal malignant melanoma. The typical echographic pattern is a rapidly decaying internal echo and low internal reflectivity. (b) B-scan ultrasound typically shows a mushroom-shaped solid mass lesion.

behind the retina. Usually, the solid mass can be seen behind the retina, with a variable amount of subretinal fluid between the tumor and the retina. Occasionally, there is a more extensive associated exudative retinal detachment, which may progress to a complete detachment. The finding of any area of unusual coloration deep to the retina, either pigmented or nonpigmented, warrants an ultrasound evaluation if there is any question of a solid nature to the area. Choroidal melanomas produce characteristic ultrasound A-scan echoes demonstrating low internal reflectivity and a rapidly declining amplitude (▶ Fig. 29.13).

Choroidal detachment may be seen in the postoperative course of several types of ocular surgery, but most often it occurs following glaucoma filtering procedures, cataract surgery, or scleral buckling surgery for retinal detachment. Rather than the gray-white, wrinkled, and billowing appearance of detached retina, choroidal detachment is characterized as darker gray, smooth, and solid appearing, with little motion on saccadic movements (▶ Fig. 29.14). Another clue that an elevation is choroidal rather than retinal is the fact that whereas retinal detachments are limited anteriorly by the ora serrata, choroidal detachments do not respect this boundary and frequently extend anteriorly to the extent that they push the ora into view without scleral depression, and they may shift the iris forward, shallowing the anterior chamber. Still further typical findings in choroidal detachment include inability to visualize the scleral depressor during examination of an involved area, circumferential involvement for 360 degrees anteriorly, and relative hypotony. Ultrasound examination can be useful in differentiating serous choroidal detachment, in which no internal echoes are seen, from hemorrhagic choroidal detachment, in which red blood cells produce internal reflections.

An exudative (serous) retinal detachment from any cause is virtually always inferior in location and demonstrates "shifting fluid." The margins of exudative detachments are not well defined and will change with head position as the subretinal fluid gravitates to the most inferior portion of the eye. By contrast, in rhegmatogenous retinal detachment the fluid may shift slightly with changes in head position, but the boundaries of the detachment remain stable. Pigmented or red blood cells in the anterior vitreous are typically lacking in serous detachments, but white cells may be seen if the exudation is related to an inflammatory condition (see Chapter 25).

Pure traction retinal detachments usually are not a source of diagnostic confusion with rhegmatogenous detachments, but rhegmatogenous and tractional components may be present in the same detachment. The configuration of a purely tractional detachment is concave on its inner surface, as opposed to the convex configuration of a purely rhegmatogenous detachment

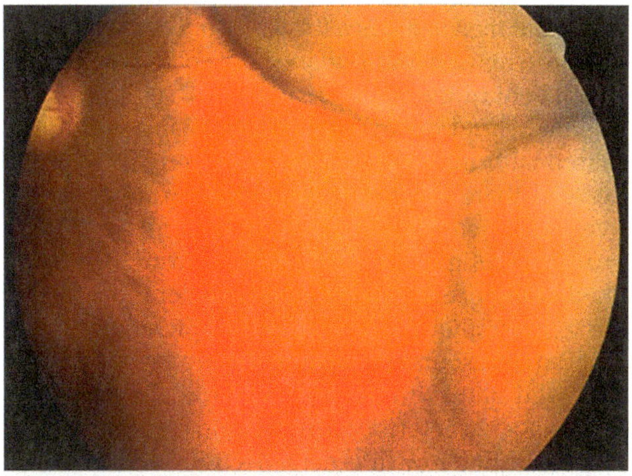

Fig. 29.14 Clinical photograph of choroidal detachment following ocular surgery. The elevation is solid appearing, has the normal color of choroid/retinal pigment epithelium, and may extend 360 degrees anteriorly.

(▶ Fig. 29.15). Traction detachments do not extend anteriorly to the ora serrata unless there is also a full-thickness retinal break, whereas clinical rhegmatogenous detachments nearly always reach the ora.

White without pressure can resemble retinal detachment in that peripheral geographic areas of retinal whitening can at first give the impression of being elevated. Scleral depression, however, will quickly demonstrate the absence of any subretinal fluid. White without pressure is observed most often in darkly pigmented individuals.

29.3.4 Pathogenesis

The retina is normally kept in apposition to the RPE by a balance of hydrostatic forces. The RPE is able to keep the subretinal potential space relatively fluid free through both osmotic and metabolically active fluid pumping mechanisms. For a rhegmatogenous retinal detachment to occur, by definition a full-thickness defect in the retina must be present, even if it cannot be detected on examination. In addition, two other factors are usually present: (1) traction on the retinal defect and (2) fluid currents or convection forces within the eye that result from normal eye movements. Atrophic round holes are a relatively uncommon cause of retinal detachment.

In a horseshoe retinal tear, all requirements for detachment exist inherently because of the vitreous pulling on the anterior flap of retinal tissue and normal eye movements producing the internal fluid currents. Even in the presence of all the requisite

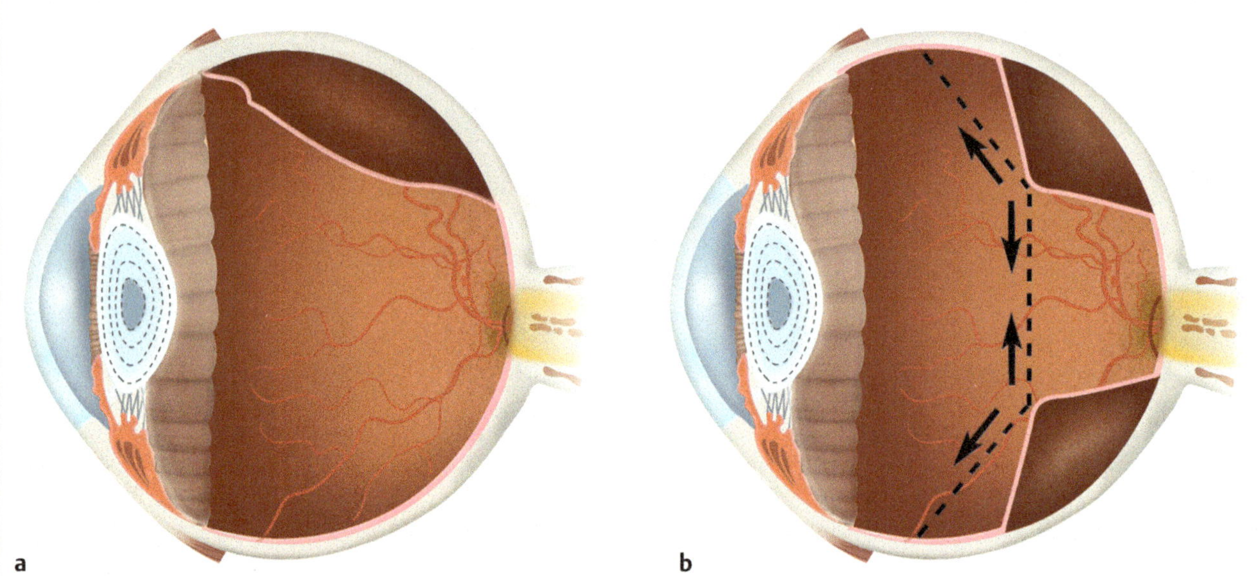

Fig. 29.15 (a) Schematic cross-section of a rhegmatogenous retinal detachment with convex contour, extending to the ora serrata. (b) Purely traction retinal detachment has a concave inner contour and does not extend to the ora serrata.

factors, some retinas do not detach if the hydrostatic tendency of the retina to remain attached is not overwhelmed by the forces that work to dissect it away.

Histopathologic changes of the detached retina occur primarily in the outer layers, which depend on the choroidal circulation for oxygen and nutrients. The photoreceptors show disorganized structure within days of retinal detachment. The inner and outer nuclear layers subsequently degenerate and become atrophic, and in very long-standing cases even the inner retinal ganglion cells are lost. With prompt surgical reattachment of the retina, the early degenerative changes are reversible, with substantial recovery of photoreceptor outer segments. Visual acuity improvement after successful repair of macula-off rhegmatogenous retinal detachment is highly variable and unpredictable.

29.3.5 Management and Course

The progression of a retinal detachment is affected by the location of the initiating retinal tear(s). Detachments beginning in the superior quadrants tend to progress relatively rapidly, spreading both inferiorly and posteriorly. Detachments arising from inferior quadrant tears progress more slowly. The knowledge of how detachments spread can be useful to locate retinal tears in detached retina (▶ Fig. 29.16).

Some detachments, particularly those resulting from inferior breaks, may progress very slowly or not at all for years. These chronic detachments often demonstrate pigmented demarcation lines, which represent "high water" marks where the detachment had remained stable for a period of time, before advancing further, producing another "high water" line more posteriorly. These concentric demarcation lines usually center around the causative retinal break.

Because the chronic detachment may produce visual field changes very slowly, it may not be recognized by the patient until it ultimately breaks through sufficiently posteriorly to be bothersome. A chronic detachment anterior to a fresh posterior detachment can give the appearance of a large area of absent retina because the atrophy of the chronically detached area contrasts with the more typical white and wrinkled fresh portion.

The various techniques for repair of rhegmatogenous retinal detachment are discussed in Chapter 40. The ultimate postoperative visual recovery of an eye with a retinal detachment depends strongly on whether or not the macula is involved. If the macula is still attached at the time of presentation, prompt surgery is generally recommended so that the macula is not allowed to detach. What exactly constitutes "prompt" repair of a rhegmatogenous retinal detachment depends on a variety of factors.[23] In one retrospective single-surgeon case series of 199 patients with macula-on retinal detachment, there were no statistically significant differences in single-operation success rate (SOSR) or postoperative best-corrected visual acuity at any time within the first 3 days after presentation, suggesting that at least some patients may be delayed for a short period of time.[24]

If surgery is delayed, eliminating internal fluid currents may be helpful in slowing progression toward the macula. Traditionally, some authorities have suggested the use of bed rest and bilateral patching, which may be beneficial but may not be feasible.

29.4 Proliferative Vitreoretinopathy

If retinal detachment surgery fails to achieve retinal reattachment, the most likely cause is one or more missed retinal breaks. However, if retinal detachment surgery initially succeeds, and subsequent recurrent retinal detachment develops, then the most likely cause is proliferative vitreoretinopathy (PVR). Typical reported incidences of PVR following retinal reattachment surgery are around 5% of cases in most series. Varying degrees of PVR can also be seen in detached retinas that have not had surgery, especially chronic cases.[25]

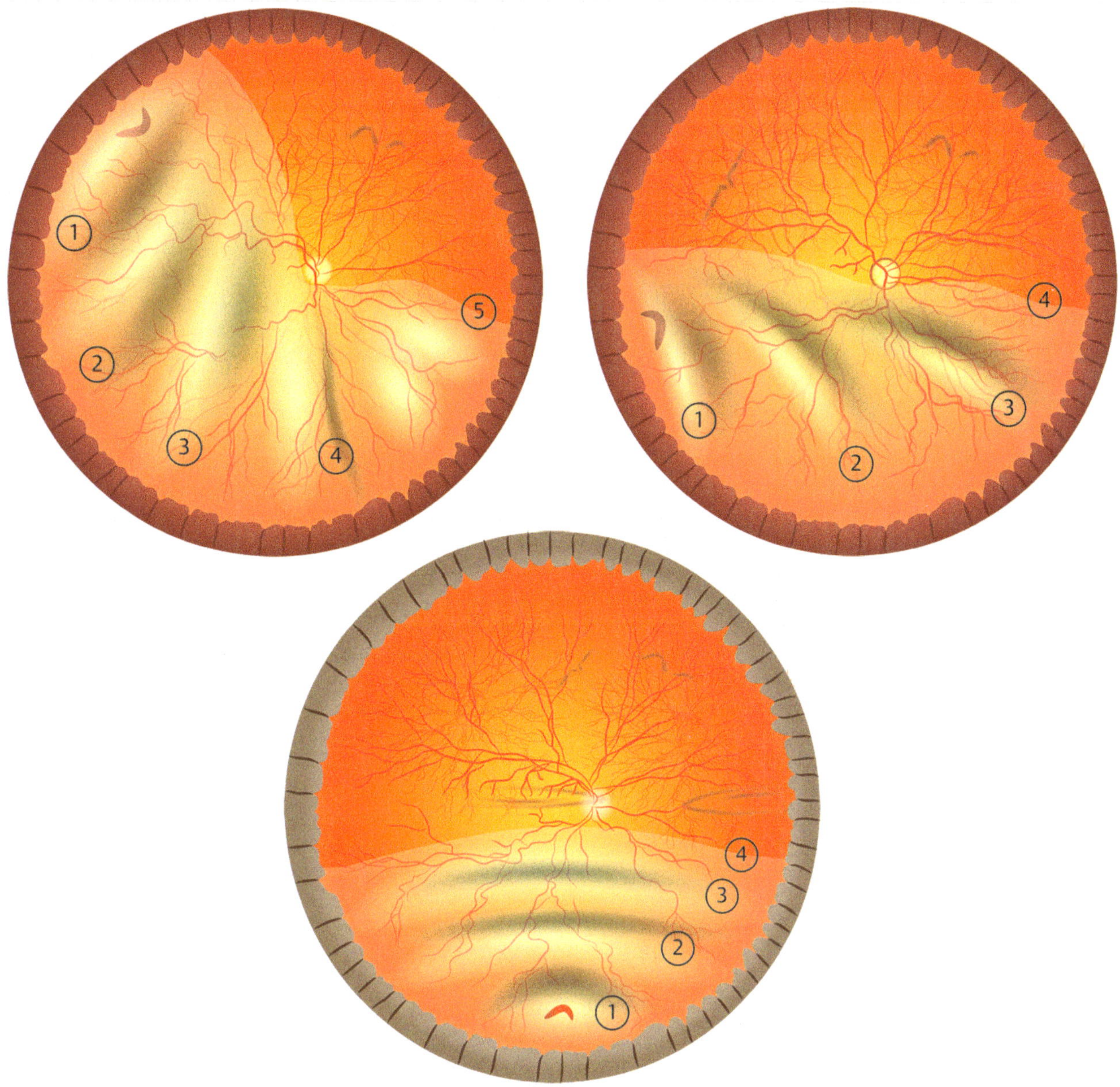

Fig. 29.16 If a single retinal tear is the cause of a retinal detachment, the progression of detachment is quite predictable, given the location of the tear. This fact can be useful in finding tears that are difficult to see clinically. In each of these three examples, the retinal tear progressed from a limited retinal detachment (1) to successively more extensive detachments (2-5)

Special Considerations

- PVR is an important cause of failure of retinal detachment surgery. The process can develop either before or after retinal detachment surgery.

Risk factors for development of PVR include intraocular inflammation, vitreous hemorrhage, large or giant retinal tears, and surgical complications (e.g., vitreous loss or retinal incarceration associated with external drainage of subretinal fluid).[25] Current terminology grades PVR according to severity and location, which have significant implications as to surgical prognosis.[26,27]

29.4.1 Clinical Features

The onset of recurrent retinal detachment associated with PVR usually produces symptoms quite different from those of the original detachment. Particularly if the detachment is primarily a tractional one, the patient rarely is aware of the "dark shadow" so prominent with primary detachment. Rather, the typical complaint is of "darkness" or simply generally decreased vision. If the proliferation causes reopening of the original retinal break or creation of a new break and a more rhegmatogenous type of detachment, the symptoms may be indistinguishable from those of primary rhegmatogenous retinal detachment.

29.4.2 Diagnosis

Advanced PVR usually manifests itself as fixed folds and stiffness in detached retina. Epiretinal or subretinal membranes may be visible, causing wrinkling that involves the retinal vessels and the internal limiting membrane, in contrast to the outer layer wrinkling of freshly detached retina described earlier. This inner distortion gives rise to characteristic fixed folding of the retina, or star folds. Star folds are most common in the inferior retinal quadrants, but extensive proliferation can occur over the entire retina (▶ Fig. 29.17).

Pearls

- The characteristic finding of significant PVR is fixed retinal star folds, most frequently inferiorly.

When proliferation occurs under detached retina, the appearance can be quite different and may take the form of subretinal strands or a reticular pattern of lacy fibers (▶ Fig. 29.18).

The original Retina Society classification scheme for PVR utilized grades from A to D to describe severity, and modifying numbers for grades C and D to subdivide the extent of proliferations in further detail (▶ Table 29.1).[26] This classification scheme is still used, although an updated classification was devised in 1991, which reflects a better understanding of the disease as well as implications for surgical management.[27] The updated scheme kept grades A and B, modified grade C, and eliminated grade D. ▶ Table 29.2 and ▶ Table 29.3 summarize the distinguishing features of this classification scheme.

29.4.3 Pathogenesis

PVR arises from the growth of a fibrocellular matrix or membranes on the inner retinal surface, in the subretinal space, or along the posterior hyaloid face (in nonvitrectomized eyes).[28] The cells that participate in this proliferative response may be derived from both glial and RPE cells. RPE cells are able to gain access into the vitreous cavity or preretinal space through any full-thickness retinal break. The availability of access is related to the size of the retinal defect, and access may be encouraged by liberating viable RPE cells with cryopexy or any form of chorioretinal treatment (e.g., laser or cryopexy) from their normal attachment to Bruch's membrane. Any intraocular inflammation may aggravate the situation further by causing breakdown of the blood–retinal barrier.

Ultimately, contraction of the fibrous membranes, which are tightly adherent to the retinal surface, causes a traction detachment of the retina or a combined traction–rhegmatogenous detachment by opening preexisting retinal breaks or producing new breaks (stretch holes). Less severe contraction may produce only local but sometimes severe wrinkling of the retina, as in macular pucker following retinal detachment surgery.

Less severe macular wrinkling may be seen in idiopathic epiretinal membrane formation without full-thickness retinal defects. Following PVD, a local break in the inner limiting membrane may permit cells to proliferate on the retinal surface with limited potential for contraction and retinal distortion (see Chapter 18).

29.4.4 Management and Course

The clinical course of PVR, once underway, is generally unfavorable, possibly progressing to total retinal detachment, hypotony, and phthisis bulbi. The rare occurrence of spontaneous peeling of proliferative membranes has, however, been reported.[29] The only satisfactory treatment for PVR at this time is through the use of vitreoretinal surgical techniques that involve peeling or sectioning of all contracted membranes to relieve tractional forces and closure of all retinal breaks, with either scleral buckling or internal tamponade (gas or silicone oil).[28,30] In the cases in which the retina is severely contracted, retinotomy or retinectomy may be needed to allow adequate mobilization for reattachment (see Chapter 40). Even with a satisfactory anatomic result, visual outcomes may be disappointing.

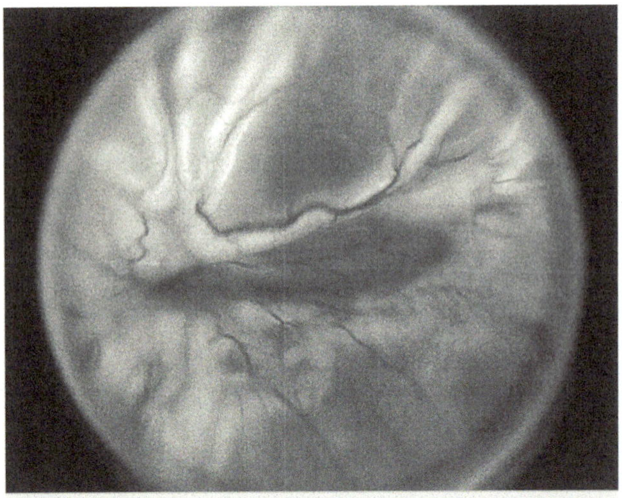

Fig. 29.17 Photograph of extensive star folds in proliferative vitreoretinopathy: The disc is obscured because of the tight funnel-shaped detachment.

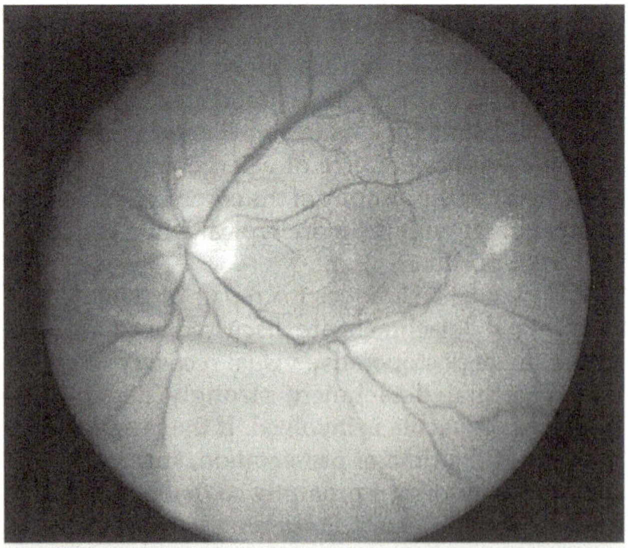

Fig. 29.18 Photograph of subretinal strands. Chronic inferior retinal detachment with a circumferential subretinal band along the inferotemporal arcade.

Table 29.1 Original Retina Society Classification of Proliferative Vitreoretinopathy (1983)

Grade	Name	Clinical signs	
A	Minimal	Vitreous haze, vitreous pigment clumps	
B	Moderate	Wrinkling of the inner retinal surface, rolled edge of retinal break, retinal stiffness, vessel tortuosity	
C	Marked	Full-thickness fixed retinal folds	
		C-1	One quadrant
		C-2	Two quadrants
		C-3	Three quadrants
D	Massive	Fixed retinal folds in four quadrants	
		D-1	Wide funnel shape
		D-2	Narrow funnel shape
		D-3	Closed funnel (optic nerve head not visible)

Table 29.2 Updated Classification of Proliferative Vitreoretinopathy (1991) (changes from original only)

Grade	Features
CP 1–12	Posterior to equator: focal, diffuse, or circumferential full-thickness folds[a]; subretinal strands[a]
CA 1–12	Anterior to equator: focal, diffuse, or circumferential full-thickness folds[a]; subretinal strands[a]; anterior displacement[a]; condensed vitreous with strands

[a]Expressed per number of clock hours involved.

Table 29.3 Grade C proliferative vitreoretinopathy described by contraction type (updated classification, 1991)

Type	Location in relation to equator	Features
Focal	Posterior	Star fold posterior to vitreous base
Diffuse	Posterior	Confluent star folds posterior to vitreous base optic disc may not be visible
Subretinal	Posterior/Anterior	Proliferations under the retina: annular strand near disc; linear strands; "moth-eaten"-appearing sheets
Circumferential	Anterior	Contraction along the posterior edge of vitreous base with central displacement of the retina: peripheral retina stretched; posterior retina in radial folds
Anterior displacement	Anterior	Vitreous base pulled anteriorly by proliferative tissue: peripheral retinal trough; stretched ciliary processes; iris retraction

When performing retinal reattachment surgery, PVR cannot be prevented, but its risks may be reduced by ensuring closure of all retinal breaks, minimizing chorioretinal treatment and subsequent dispersion of RPE cells, minimizing postoperative inflammation, avoiding intraoperative bleeding, and exercising care during drainage of subretinal fluid to prevent hemorrhage, retinal incarceration, or vitreous loss.

References

[1] Weber-Krause B, Eckardt C. Incidence of posterior vitreous detachment in the elderly [in German]. Ophthalmologe. 1997; 94(9):619–623

[2] Wagle AM, Lim WY, Yap TP, Neelam K, Au Eong KG. Utility values associated with vitreous floaters. Am J Ophthalmol. 2011; 152(1):60–65.e1

[3] Schwartz SG, Flynn HW, Jr, Fisher YL. "Floater scotoma" demonstrated on spectral-domain optical coherence tomography and caused by vitreous opacification. Ophthalmic Surg Lasers Imaging Retina. 2013; 44(4):415–418

[4] Foos RY. Anatomic and pathologic aspects of the vitreous body. Trans Am Acad Ophthalmol Otolaryngol. 1973; 77(2):OP171–OP183

[5] Fine BS, Yanoff M. Ocular Histology: A Text and Atlas. New York: Harper & Row; 1972:110

[6] Jaffe NS. The Vitreous in Clinical Ophthalmology. St. Louis, MO: CV Mosby; 1969

[7] Foos RY. Tears of the peripheral retina; pathogenesis, incidence and classification in autopsy eyes. Mod Probl Ophthalmol. 1975; 15:68–81

[8] Byer NE. Clinical study of retinal breaks. Trans Am Acad Ophthalmol Otolaryngol. 1967; 71(3):461–473

[9] Byer NE. The natural history of asymptomatic retinal breaks. Ophthalmology. 1982; 89(9):1033–1039

[10] Okun E. Gross and microscopic pathology in autopsy eyes. III. Retinal breaks without detachment. Am J Ophthalmol. 1961; 51:369–391

[11] Byer NE. Long-term natural history of lattice degeneration of the retina. Ophthalmology. 1989; 96(9):1396–1401, discussion 1401–1402

[12] Aaberg TM, Stevens TR. Snail track degeneration of the retina. Am J Ophthalmol. 1972; 73(3):370–376

[13] Kanski JJ. Giant retinal tears. Am J Ophthalmol. 1975; 79(5):846–852

[14] Smiddy WE, Green WR. Retinal dialysis: pathology and pathogenesis. Retina. 1982; 2(2):94–116
[15] Teng CC, Chi HH. Vitreous changes and the mechanism of retinal detachment. Am J Ophthalmol. 1957; 44(3):335–356
[16] Freeman HM, Cox MS, Schepens CL. Traumatic retinal detachments. Int Ophthalmol Clin. 1974; 14(4):151–170
[17] Yanoff M, Fine BS. Retina. In: Ocular Pathology: A Text and Atlas. 2nd ed. Philadelphia, PA: Harper & Row; 1982:473–585
[18] Combs JL, Welch RB. Retinal breaks without detachment: natural history, management and long term follow-up. Trans Am Ophthalmol Soc. 1982; 80:64–97
[19] Byer NE. Natural history of posterior vitreous detachment with early management as the premier line of defense against retinal detachment. Ophthalmology. 1994; 101(9):1503–1513, discussion 1513–1514
[20] Olsen TW, Adelman RA, Flaxel CJ, et al. Preferred Practice Pattern: Posterior Vitreous Detachment, Retinal Breaks, and Lattice Degeneration. San Francisco, CA: American Academy of Ophthalmology; 2014:10
[21] Michaelson IC, Stein R. A national study on the prevention of retinal detachment. Isr J Med Sci.. 1972; 8:1421-3
[22] Byer NE. Long-term natural history study of senile retinoschisis with implications for management. Ophthalmology. 1986; 93(9):1127–1137
[23] Wykoff CC, Flynn HW, Jr, Scott IU. What is the optimal timing for rhegmatogenous retinal detachment repair? JAMA Ophthalmol. 2013; 131(11):1399–1400
[24] Wykoff CC, Smiddy WE, Mathen T, Schwartz SG, Flynn HW, Jr, Shi W. Fovea-sparing retinal detachments: time to surgery and visual outcomes. Am J Ophthalmol. 2010; 150(2):205–210.e2
[25] Yoshizumi MO, Kreiger AE, Sharp DM. Risk factors associated with the development of massive periretinal proliferation. In: Ryan SJ, Dawson AK, Little HL, eds. Retinal Diseases. Orlando, FL: Grune & Stratton; 1984
[26] The Retina Society Terminology Committee. The classification of retinal detachment with proliferative vitreoretinopathy. Ophthalmology. 1983; 90 (2):121–125
[27] Machemer R, Aaberg TM, Freeman HM, Irvine AR, Lean JS, Michels RM. An updated classification of retinal detachment with proliferative vitreoretinopathy. Am J Ophthalmol. 1991; 112(2):159–165
[28] Ryan SJ. Traction retinal detachment. XLIX Edward Jackson Memorial Lecture. Am J Ophthalmol. 1993; 115(1):1–20
[29] de Juan E, Jr, Machemer R. Spontaneous reattachment of the retina despite proliferative vitreoretinopathy. Am J Ophthalmol. 1984; 97(4):428–433
[30] Schwartz SG, Flynn HW, Jr, Lee WH, Wang X. Tamponade in surgery for retinal detachment associated with proliferative vitreoretinopathy. Cochrane Database Syst Rev. 2014; 2:CD006126

30 Exudative and Tractional Retinal Detachments

Matthew D. Cooke, Robert A. Mittra, and Dennis P. Han

30.1 Introduction

Exudative retinal detachment refers to separation of the neurosensory retina from the underlying retinal pigment epithelium (RPE) due to abnormalities of the normal hydrostatic/osmotic pressure gradients or transport mechanisms that maintain the physical apposition of these two tissue layers or to excessive production of extracellular fluid. In contrast, *tractional retinal detachment* refers to separation of these tissue layers secondary to anatomically recognizable forces that physically pull on the retina. Importantly, neither type of retinal detachment is associated with retinal breaks. The common clinical features, pathogenesis, and differential diagnosis of exudative and tractional detachments are discussed later. Those entities not covered elsewhere in this book are presented in greater detail in this chapter.

30.2 Exudative Retinal Detachments

30.2.1 Clinical Features

Exudative or "serous" retinal detachments are characterized by separation of the neurosensory retina and RPE without the presence of a retinal break or vitreoretinal traction. They can be further differentiated from rhegmatogenous detachments by the lack of retinal folds or rugae on their surface (▶ Fig. 30.1). Exudative detachments can develop in all age groups when defects occur in the normal mechanisms for clearance of subretinal fluid or when these mechanisms are overwhelmed by excessive exudation. Such abnormalities are seen in a variety of disease states involving the RPE, Bruch's membrane, choroidal vasculature, or the retina. Exudative detachments display a dome or convex configuration, and their lateral extent can vary greatly, from a few disc diameters to the entire retina. The height of the detachment can likewise vary, and in some severe cases, the retina may be visible just posterior to the lens (▶ Fig. 30.2). In large exudative detachments, the subretinal fluid may shift to dependent areas of the fundus with changes in the patient's head position. Exudative detachments of the retina frequently coexist with detachments of the choroid.

Patients present with a history of decreased visual acuity, visual field defects, metamorphopsia, or floaters. Photopsia may be present as well, but when this history is elicited, patients should be examined carefully for the presence of a retinal break. The visual acuity depends on the chronicity and extent of the detachment as well as associated RPE and choroidal derangements. Visual acuity can vary from 20/20 in cases of central serous chorioretinopathy (CSC) to count fingers or worse in age-related macular degeneration with massive exudative detachment. The intraocular pressure can be decreased in the presence of ciliary body inflammation or detachment but is often normal. The anterior segment examination will frequently reveal clues to the diagnosis, such as conjunctival and episcleral injection in scleritis or anterior chamber cell and flare in Vogt–Koyanagi–Harada (VKH) syndrome. Fundus examination demonstrates single or multiple dome-shaped retinal elevations, with larger detachments exhibiting the phenomenon of shifting subretinal fluid.

Fluorescein angiography can be instrumental in diagnosis if the subretinal fluid is clear and the detachment is not too bullous. Fluorescein angiography may demonstrate small foci of hyperfluorescence in cases of CSC or characteristic patterns of lacy hyperfluorescence in choroidal neovascularization from a variety of causes. It can also help confirm various characteristic vascular changes of retinal diseases that can lead to exudative retinal detachments, such as leakage from macroaneurysms in

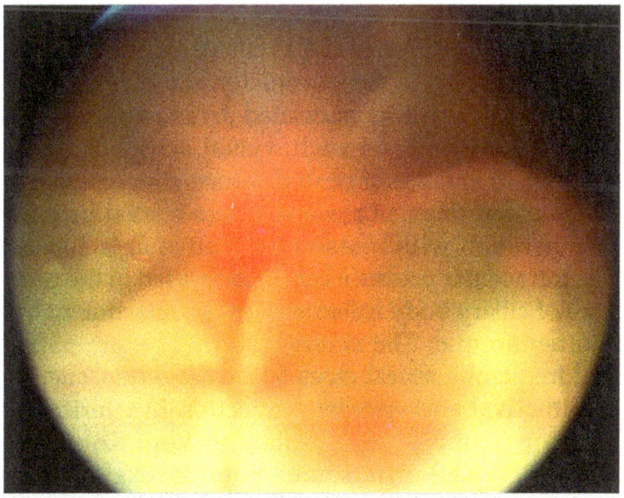

Fig. 30.1 Exudative retinal detachment. Fundus photograph taken with the patient in the upright position; the subretinal fluid has mainly settled inferiorly from the effects of gravity. Note also the smooth, dome-shaped appearance and the absence of any retinal rugae.

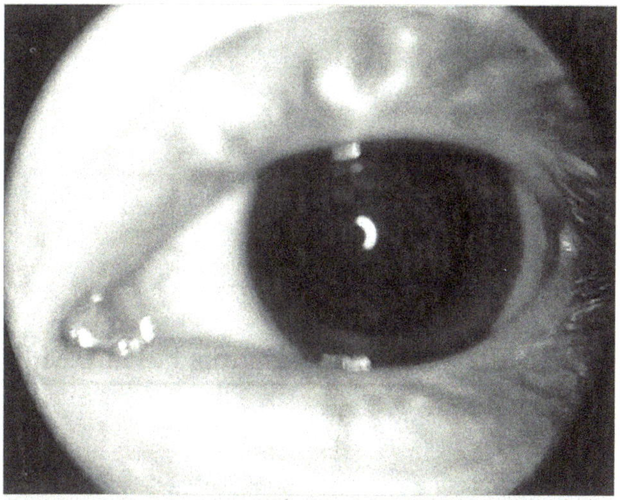

Fig. 30.2 Total exudative retinal detachment with loss of the red reflex and retina visible behind the lens in a patient with Coats' disease.

Coats' disease. In certain diseases, fluorescein angiography can be used to guide laser photocoagulation therapy. Indocyanine green (ICG) angiography may be useful in showing areas of increased choroidal vascular permeability in CSC or hyperfluorescent nodules with late hypofluorescence in polypoidal choroidal vasculopathy. Ocular coherence tomography (OCT) can show subretinal fluid and cysts in choroidal neovascularization and, with enhanced depth imaging (EDI), can be instrumental in making the diagnosis of CSC if the choroidal layer is thickened. Ultrasonography is helpful in eyes with both hazy and clear media. It may reveal the presence, location, and size of intraocular tumors; show scleral or choroidal thickening in inflammatory disorders; and display any coexisting choroidal detachment. Computed tomography (CT) or magnetic resonance imaging (MRI) can provide similar information in cases in which an ultrasound examination cannot be performed because of lack of patient cooperation (e.g., in a child) or because pressure from the ultrasound probe has potential for damage to the eye (e.g., in posttraumatic cases). Finally, CT or MRI can help with diagnosis of orbital and intracranial disorders (e.g., arteriovenous fistulas), which can occasionally manifest secondary exudative detachments.

30.2.2 Differential Diagnosis

This chapter will focus on entities capable of causing extensive exudative retinal detachments extending beyond the macula. The differential diagnosis of exudative retinal detachment is summarized below.

Conditions Causing Exudative Retinal Detachments

- Idiopathic
  - Central serous chorioretinopathy
  - Idiopathic uveal effusion/nanophthalmos
- Surgical or postsurgical
  - Wound leak/hypotony
  - Scleral buckle
  - Panretinal photocoagulation
- Inflammatory/autoimmune
  - Posterior Scleritis
  - Benign reactive lymphoid hyperplasia
  - Vogt–Koyanagi–Harada syndrome
  - Sympathetic ophthalmia
- Hematologic/vascular
  - Disseminated intravascular coagulation
  - Toxemia of pregnancy
  - Malignant hypertension
  - Goodpasture's syndrome
  - Thrombotic thrombocytopenic purpura
  - Collagen vascular disease (systemic lupus erythematosis)
  - Granulomatosis with polyangiitis (Wegener's granulomatosis)
  - Organ transplantation/hemodialysis
  - HELLP syndrome
  - Waldenström's macroglobulinemia
  - Renal failure
  - Choroidal neovascularization (any cause)
  - Coats' disease
  - Retinopathy of prematurity
  - Familial exudative vitreoretinopathy
  - Arteriovenous fistula/carotid obstruction
  - Retinal vein occlusion
- Infectious
  - Syphilis
  - Toxoplasmosis
  - Herpes zoster
  - *Pseudomonas*
- Neoplastic
  - Melanoma/nevus
  - Metastatic disease
  - Choroidal hemangioma
  - Lymphoma
  - Leukemia
  - Multiple myeloma
  - Bilateral diffuse uveal melanocytic proliferation
- Medications
  - Interferon-a
  - Ribavirin

Abbreviation: HELLP, hemolysis, elevated liver enzymes, low platelets.

30.2.3 Pathogenesis

The mechanisms responsible for maintaining a fluid-free subretinal space are numerous and complex. Intraocular hydrostatic pressure, osmotic pressure from choroidal extracellular protein, the interphotoreceptor matrix, and metabolic fluid transport by the RPE are all thought to play a role.[1] Tight junctions between RPE cells, which combine to form the outer blood–retinal barrier, provide high resistance to osmotic fluid flow across the retina. Without breakdown of this barrier, experiments have shown that RPE-mediated fluid transport is the predominant mechanism for deturgescence of the subretinal space.[1] With focal damage to this barrier, fluid is eliminated according to oncotic pressure gradients,[1,2] which promote fluid egress from the subretinal space due to high protein concentration of the choroid.

Spitznas[3] and Marmor[4] have hypothesized that a widespread deficit in RPE transport function is necessary to generate and maintain an exudative retinal detachment. In affected patients, the diseased RPE cells are barely able to prevent a detachment in their resting state, and when confronted with excess stress (e.g., ischemia), the system is overwhelmed and a detachment results. A small RPE defect (as often noted in patients with CSC) may be needed to provide a source of subretinal fluid entry. However, a serous detachment may be maintained only in the setting of diseased remaining RPE cells unable to prevent detachment yet still present to prevent fluid egress by oncotic pressure gradients that work in the absence of intact RPE.[5] In addition, inflammatory subretinal fluid may have increased protein content, reducing the oncotic pressure gradient between the subretinal space and the choroid.[2]

Widespread RPE damage may explain several etiologies of exudative retinal detachment, but some disease states, such as disseminated intravascular coagulation and hypertension, appear primarily to affect blood flow of the choroidal vasculature. Experimental serous retinal detachments have been created by using rose bengal as a photosensitizer to damage retinal and choroidal vessels selectively.[6] These detachments can be created with choroidal occlusion as well as lesser focal damage to endothelial cells of the choriocapillaris, resulting in increased permeability. Marmor and Yao argue that three conditions are needed for exudative detachment formation: a source of subretinal fluid entry (likely from the choriocapillaris); a blood–retinal barrier defect allowing fluid to reach the subretinal space; and impaired fluid transport or a high fluid entry rate that overwhelms normal transport mechanisms.[7]

30.2.4 Specific Entities

Idiopathic

Central Serous Chorioretinopathy

The typical patient with CSC is a man in his third to fifth decade of life with a unilateral visual disturbance and a localized exudative detachment of the neurosensory retina (and sometimes RPE) in the macula. Fluorescein angiography is instrumental in establishing the diagnosis. Characteristically, it shows a pinpoint focus of dye leakage at the level of the RPE under or near the detached retina. ICG angiography may be helpful in differentiating CSC from choroidal neovascularization and typically reveals midphase inner choroid staining that fades late in the study.[8] OCT images with EDI show a thickened choroid in the affected and the fellow eye in many cases. Most cases resolve spontaneously by 4 to 6 months, usually with good recovery of visual function, although over half of patients experience recurrent disease.[9] Cases that are chronic, recurrent, or bilateral may benefit from photodynamic therapy to facilitate subretinal fluid resorption and to improve visual outcomes.[10] Early photodynamic therapy may also be beneficial for acute CSC.[11] Laser photocoagulation directed to the area of leakage on fluorescein angiography may cause fluid resorption in refractory cases, although it may result in choroidal neovascularization and scotomas.[12,13] Potential roles for mineralocorticoid receptor antagonists have been explored.[14]

Pearls

- The fluorescein leakage spot in CSC may be located in the superior fundus, distant from the fluid in the macula. The fluorescein angiogram should, therefore, include views of the superior paramacular region and midperiphery to establish the diagnosis if no leakage site is seen in the macula.

Rarely, CSC may present with large, bullous, and sometimes bilateral exudative retinal detachments.[15,16] Misdiagnosis as VKH syndrome, uveal effusion, leukemia, or choroidal tumor can occur. Some cases have been presumed to be rhegmatogenous and have undergone unsuccessful and unnecessary surgery.[15] Many early cases were treated with systemic corticosteroids for serous macular detachments consistent with typical CSC, and widespread bullous detachments with whitish subretinal exudate subsequently developed. It is now known that corticosteroid use is contraindicated in CSC because of its association with more severe and recurrent disease.[17,18] Steroid use may increase the permeability of the choriocapillaris to larger proteins.

Because steroid use and surgery are contraindicated in any form of CSC, accurate diagnosis is essential. As noted earlier, the differential diagnosis of the "bullous" variant of CSC includes VKH syndrome, choroidal tumors, and uveal effusion syndrome (UES). VKH syndrome occurs in patients with dark skin pigmentation and usually is associated with systemic symptoms, such as headache, malaise, nausea, and vomiting, before onset of visual symptoms. Vitreous and anterior chamber cells are characteristically present. The presence of an inflamed optic nerve head, choroidal thickening, or cerebrospinal fluid pleocytosis favors the diagnosis of VKH syndrome. Furthermore, the serous detachments in VKH syndrome are not associated with RPE detachments, as is common with CSC. Choroidal tumors can usually be diagnosed by fundus appearance and ultrasound examination. UES displays ciliochoroidal edema and detachment on ultrasound and exhibits prominent shifting of subretinal fluid. For difficult cases, fluorescein angiography, ICG angiography, and ultrasonography should be performed to rule out other etiologies before the institution of any therapeutic measure.

Both endogenous and exogenous corticosteroids are associated with initiation, exacerbation, and prolongation of CSC.[19] CSC is also associated with increased stress, organ transplantation, pregnancy, steroid use, and hemodialysis, all known to increase cortisol levels.[20,21,22] Several studies have documented hyperpermeable choroidal circulation in the area of RPE detachment, and steroid use or elevated cortisol may increase this effect.[8,23] The mechanism by which corticosteroids contribute to CSC remains unclear, and intraocular steroid administration is only rarely associated with CSC development.[24] (See Chapter 16 for a more detailed discussion of the diagnosis and treatment of CSC.)

Uveal Effusion Syndrome/Nanophthalmos

The spontaneous development of peripheral choroidal and retinal detachments in middle-aged hyperopic patients is the hallmark of the UES.[25] UES is idiopathic and a diagnosis of exclusion, as similar findings may be caused by surgery, trauma, scleritis, or pars planitis.[26] Patients usually present with complaints of gradual loss of the superior visual field due to dependent shifting of subretinal fluid, although fluid may also be submacular, causing central vision loss. Episcleral vessel dilation and vitreous cells are frequently present, and the intraocular pressure is usually normal. Fundus examination reveals a combined exudative retinal and choroidal detachment with shifting subretinal fluid. A pattern of RPE hyperplasia with fluorescein angiographic transmission defects can be seen during or after resolution of long-standing detachments. Ultrasonography demonstrates peripheral detachments as well as choroidal thickening and decreased axial length in some patients. The syndrome is not inflammatory and does not respond to corticosteroid therapy. Analysis of subretinal fluid reveals markedly elevated protein levels, up to three times that of serum.[27] The augmented protein content produces the marked shifting of subretinal fluid seen in this condition.

Nanophthalmos is a rare bilateral disorder characterized by a small eye with a small cornea, shallow anterior chamber, high lens-to-eye ratio, thick sclera, and predisposition to uveal effusion.[26,28,29] Angle-closure glaucoma often occurs as a consequence of the crowded anterior segment. Historically, surgical manipulations for glaucoma and cataract were fraught with complications that included spontaneous retinochoroidal detachments.

In both UES and nanophthalmos, exudative detachment is caused by atypically thick sclera causing vortex vein compression, elevated choroidal venous pressure, and diminished outflow.[30] Sclera from UES patients displays abnormal deposition of glycosaminoglycans, which likely impedes fluid flow and increases scleral thickness. The finding of uveal effusion in Hunter's syndrome supports the idea that abnormal scleral glycosaminoglycan deposition is responsible for the clinical syndrome.

Special Considerations

- In both the UES and nanophthalmos, the pathogenesis of exudative detachment is related to atypically thick sclera with possible compression of the vortex veins resulting in diminished transscleral and choroidal venous outflow.

The uveal effusions can be treated effectively with both vortex vein decompression and scleral resection.[31] These operations decompress the engorged choroid and provide surface area for fluid transport. Scleral resection away from the vortex veins is less technically challenging and results in fewer complications. The use of topical mitomycin C along with creation of a scleral window has been described.[32] Modern techniques such as phacoemulsification have greatly reduced the risk of surgical complications from cataract extraction in these patients, although such procedures continue to be high risk.[33]

Postsurgical

Exudative retinal detachments and uveal effusions may occur following a wide variety of surgical procedures. Significant hypotony following an intraocular procedure can lead to serous choroidal detachment up to several months after surgery, often associated with an overlying exudative retinal detachment.[34,35] A postoperative exudative retinal detachment without choroidal detachment is unusual. The term *expulsive choroidal detachment* refers to massive serous or hemorrhagic choroidal detachments during intraocular surgery that cause loss or prolapse of intraocular contents, such as vitreous and uveal tissue.[36] This tends to occur in patients with increased choroidal venous pressure with Valsalva maneuvers (e.g., coughing) during the operation or in patients with risk factors such as glaucoma, myopia, advanced age, hypertension, and arteriosclerosis (see Chapter 35).

Exudative retinal and choroidal detachments can occur after any intraocular procedure but most commonly follow scleral buckling procedures. In such cases, they may be related to prolonged hypotony from subretinal fluid drainage, compression of vortex veins by the encircling band causing elevated choroidal venous pressure, damage to choroidal vasculature by cryotherapy or photocoagulation, or by creation of scleral slits to allow for passage of the scleral buckle in cases in which the buckle is not sewn in.[37] Aggressive panretinal photocoagulation can also lead to uveal effusion and exudative retinal detachment and may even cause anterior chamber shallowing or angle-closure glaucoma from anterior ciliary body rotation.[38] Both laser and cryotherapy cause thermal damage, leading to inflammation, choroidal vascular damage, and breakdown of the blood–retinal barrier.

Inflammatory

Posterior Scleritis

Pain and decreased visual acuity or visual field loss are the classic presenting symptoms of posterior scleritis. The level of pain is consistent with the amount of anterior scleritis and may be absent if this is minimal.[39,40] Ocular findings may include anterior chamber cells, optic disc edema, choroidal detachment with surrounding folds, and serous retinal detachment (▶ Fig. 30.3). The choroidal lesion may simulate a mass, and misdiagnosis of choroidal melanoma, metastatic carcinoma, choroidal hemangioma, or benign reactive lymphoid hyperplasia (BRLH) can occur.[41,42,43] Inaccurate diagnosis has unfortunately led to enucleation in a few cases.

Fluorescein angiography displays mottled early fluorescence, with multiple pinpoint spots of leakage at the level of the RPE in the middle phases and intense late staining of the exudative retinal detachment (Fig. 30.3). The ultrasonogram is the most helpful diagnostic test.[42,44] The B-scan reveals significant sclerochoroidal thickening with overlying retinal detachment (▶ Fig. 30.4). Retrobulbar edema is often seen as an echolucency behind the area of choroidal inflammation. Optic disc swelling and a distended optic nerve sheath may be noted. The A-scan demonstrates high reflectivity of any discrete mass-like formation that may be present. These combined findings are virtually pathognomonic for posterior scleritis.

Posterior scleritis is often associated with a systemic illness, such as rheumatoid arthritis, granulomatosis with angiitis (Wegener's granulomatosis), systemic vasculitis, systemic lymphoma, or multiple myeloma.[41,45] In other cases, infectious etiologies such as herpes zoster or toxoplasmosis may play a role. Many cases are idiopathic. Treatment for noninfectious disease typically begins with oral nonsteroidal anti-inflammatory drugs or oral corticosteroids. Other options include immunomodulatory therapy (e.g., methotrexate). Refractory cases may be treated with tumor necrosis factor antagonists (e.g., infliximab).[45]

Benign Reactive Lymphoid Hyperplasia (Inflammatory Pseudotumor)

Benign reactive lymphoid hyperplasia (BRLH) is a rare disorder characterized by a diffuse mononuclear uveal tract infiltration. The diagnosis is difficult to make and often made only after enucleation. The disease affects older adults, is typically unilateral, and may have anterior chamber cells.[46] Secondary angle closure from ciliary body infiltration and exudative retinal detachments often occur, causing decreased visual acuity. External signs are usually absent, although late proptosis may be noted. Salmon-pink conjunctival nodules may be present and accessible for biopsy.[47] Fundus examination reveals a

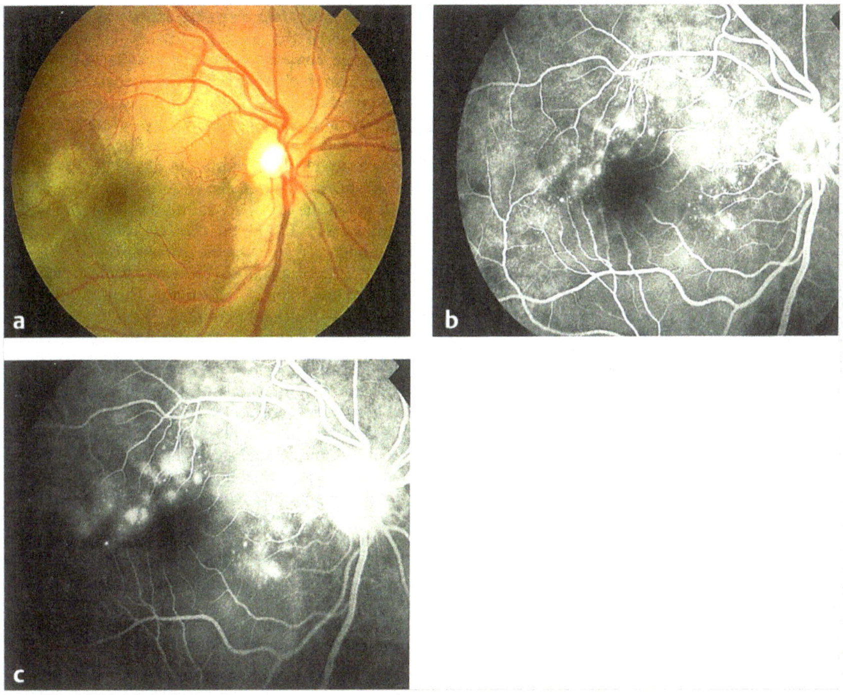

Fig. 30.3 Posterior scleritis. (**a**) A localized, serous (*exudative*) retinal detachment of the macula. The corresponding fluorescein angiogram shows (**b**) multiple dots of hyperfluorescence at the level of the retinal pigment epithelium and (**c**) late leakage of dye into the subretinal space.

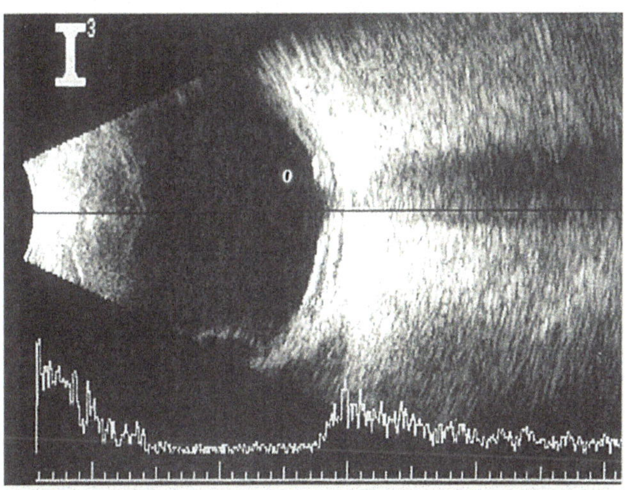

Fig. 30.4 Posterior scleritis. B-scan ultrasonography shows scleral thickening with an adjacent area of echolucency corresponding to edema in the posterior sub-Tenon's space.

diffuse, yellow-white choroidal mass with RPE pigment mottling. The infiltration may extend to the far periphery and ciliary body, resulting in ability to view the pars plana without scleral depression.

The differential diagnosis of this disease includes diffuse malignant melanoma, UES, metastatic carcinoma, posterior scleritis, systemic lymphoma, sarcoidosis, and infectious etiologies. Systemic lymphoma can often be differentiated from BRLH by extraocular manifestations of lymphoma before discovery of eye involvement. Although central nervous system large-cell lymphoma can rarely exhibit a serous retinal detachment, vitreous cellular aggregations and discrete, yellow-white subretinal and choroidal infiltrates readily distinguish this disorder. Differentiation of the other entities listed earlier, however, can be quite difficult clinically, and given the nonspecific fluorescein angiographic findings with BRLH, the clinician must rely mainly on echography to make the distinction.

Echographically, BRLH reveals a diffuse choroidal mass of low internal reflectivity. There is often evidence of extrascleral peripapillary nodule formation in advanced disease. In contrast, patients with posterior scleritis often have pain, and they typically display a highly reflective thickening of the sclera and choroid with an adjacent echolucent area of edema in Tenon's space on ultrasound.[48] Unlike patients with BRLH, patients with uveal effusion exhibit highly reflective, diffuse thickening of the choroid with extensive peripheral serous ciliochoroidal detachments. Metastatic disease typically presents with one solitary or several discrete lesions of the choroid bilaterally with medium to high internal reflectivity.

Diffuse melanoma remains the most difficult and important diagnosis to exclude when BRLH is suspected. Melanoma is usually more pigmented and does not respond rapidly to steroid therapy, as BRLH does. Both show low internal reflectivity and often display extraocular extension on ultrasound. These extrascleral nodules can distinguish the two echographically when present.[48] In BRLH, the nodules are adjacent to the optic nerve, with intact sclera visible between the choroidal tumor and nodule. Intact sclera is not seen with echography in diffuse melanoma with extraocular extension, as these tumors destroy the sclera during migration. Also, the nodules of BLRH often disappear with steroid therapy.

Pathologically, the infiltrates in BRLH appear similar to malignant lymphoma but can be reliably differentiated by immunohistochemical analysis.[49] In one series, many cases initially diagnosed as BRLH were actually low-grade B-cell lymphomas, although there were no deaths from systemic lymphoma in any misdiagnosed cases.[50] Biopsy with orbitotomy of extrascleral nodules, if present, may prevent unnecessary enucleation. If there is no evidence of systemic involvement, high-dose steroids may be initiated and usually cause disease regression. Some cases may require additional low-dose radiation for control.

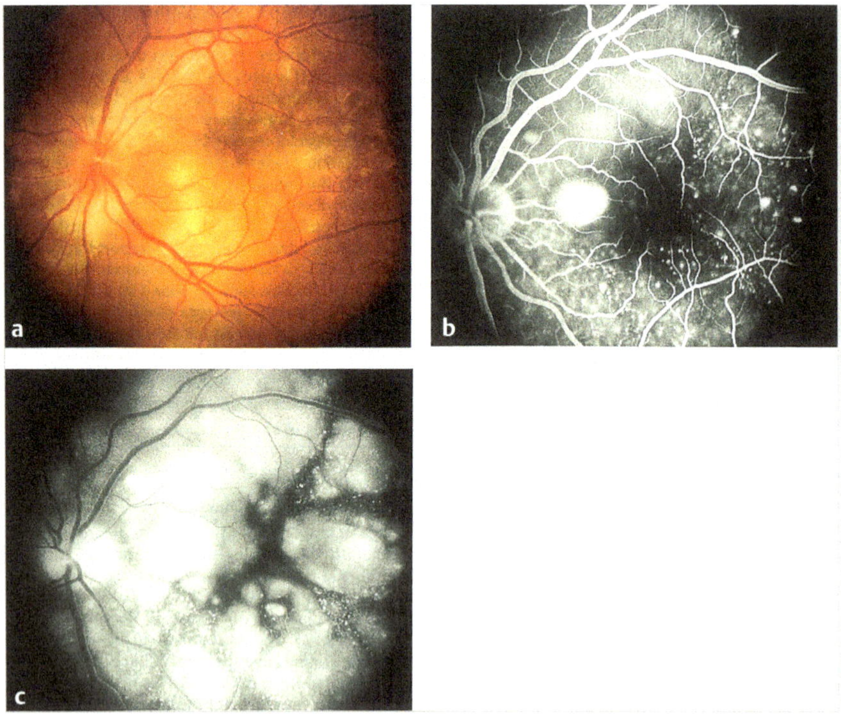

Fig. 30.5 (**a**) Vogt–Koyanagi–Harada syndrome with a localized exudative retinal detachment in the posterior pole. (**b**) The corresponding fluorescein angiogram shows multiple punctate hyperfluorescent dots in the early phase (**c**) with late leakage of dye into the subretinal fluid.

Pearls

- Diffuse melanoma is the most difficult and important diagnosis to differentiate from BRLH.

30.2.5 Vogt–Koyanagi–Harada Syndrome and Sympathetic Ophthalmia

VKH syndrome is a chronic, multisystem disorder seen in pigmented individuals characterized by bilateral exudative retinal detachments with panuveitis and RPE changes (▶ Fig. 30.5). Ocular signs may be preceded by flu-like symptoms, tinnitus, hearing loss, and lymphocytic pleocytosis of cerebrospinal fluid. Weeks to months after the ocular signs develop, patients can variably manifest poliosis, alopecia, and perilimbal and cutaneous vitiligo. Fluorescein angiography is helpful in differentiating this entity from other causes of bilateral exudative retinal detachment. Typically, multiple pinpoint leaks at the level of the RPE are seen early, with dye accumulation in the subretinal space and disc staining as the angiogram progresses. Metastatic carcinoma and leukemia may have a similar fluorescein angiographic appearance, but ultrasound examination reveals a low internal reflectivity in VKH.[51] With ultrasound, it is difficult to distinguish between scleral and choroidal thickening, leading to confusion of VKH syndrome with posterior scleritis. However, posterior scleritis is typically unilateral and often accompanied by pain, whereas VKH is bilateral.

Sympathetic ophthalmia is a related disorder with bilateral eye findings similar to VKH, but it occurs as a result of surgical or accidental ocular trauma in one eye, followed by findings in the other eye after a latent period. As in VKH, systemic skin and neurologic findings can be seen in sympathetic ophthalmia.[52]

VKH and sympathetic ophthalmia are typically treated with extended courses of high-dose oral or intravenous corticosteroids. Given significant disease recurrence off of corticosteroid therapy, treatment with immunomodulatory therapy, such as with cyclosporine, is necessary and may be used as first-line therapy with or without corticosteroids.[53] Other options include intravitreal corticosteroids and antitumor necrosis factor agents (e.g., infliximab).[54,55] In cases of sympathetic ophthalmia recalcitrant to corticosteroids and other immunomodulatory agents, high-dose, short-term, chlorambucil therapy has been associated with drug-free remission and preservation of visual function.[56]

Pearls

- VKH syndrome, sympathetic ophthalmia, and posterior scleritis can have very similar-appearing angiographic findings, with multiple pinpoint leaking spots at the level of the RPE and a hyperfluorescent optic nerve head. Associated ocular and systemic symptoms and signs, however, should readily allow for differentiation of the conditions.

Hematologic/Vascular

Several systemic diseases cause widespread coagulation (e.g., disseminated intravascular coagulation) or focal arteriolar narrowing and damage to vessel walls with secondary occlusion by platelet–fibrin thrombi (e.g., malignant hypertension). Ocular involvement in these conditions consists of occlusion of small arterioles and capillaries of the choroid with subsequent acute RPE necrosis. This frequently results in a secondary exudative retinal detachment.

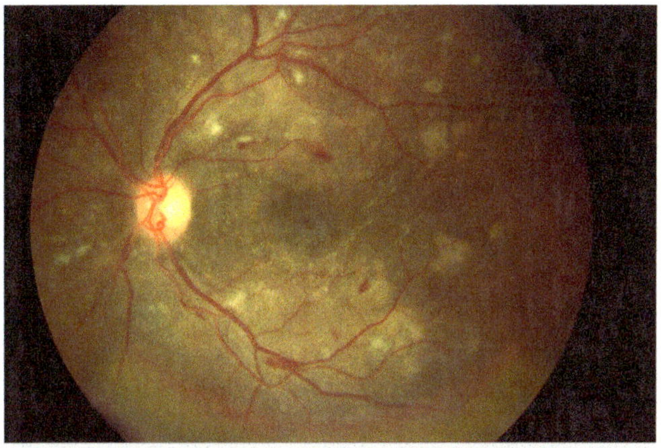

Fig. 30.6 Fundus photograph of a patient with malignant hypertension who had retinal vascular changes, intraretinal hemorrhages, multiple gray spots at the level of the retinal pigment epithelium, and an inferior exudative retinal detachment (not shown).

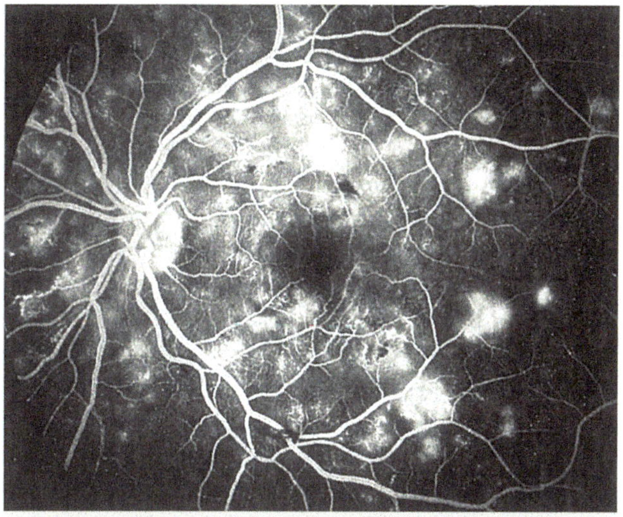

Fig. 30.7 Midphase fluorescein angiogram photograph of the eye shown in ▶ Fig. 30.6. Multiple areas of hyperfluorescence are evident that correspond to the deep gray spots seen clinically. These hyperfluorescent lesions represent areas of focal choroidal ischemia resulting from occlusion of the choroidal vasculature.

Disseminated Intravascular Coagulation

Disseminated intravascular coagulation is a complex disorder resulting in widespread thrombosis of small blood vessels, with ensuing depletion of clotting factors, platelets, and fibrinogen. The disorder always occurs secondarily, such as from sepsis, collagen vascular disease, or abruptio placentae. It primarily affects the kidneys, heart, and brain. Ocular involvement has been demonstrated with histopathologic and fluorescein angiographic evidence of derangement of the choroidal vasculature that may be associated with exudative retinal detachment.[57] Choroidal hypoperfusion, exudative detachments, and Elschnig's spots have also been seen in thrombotic thrombocytopenic purpura,[58,59] toxemia of pregnancy,[60,61] the HELLP syndrome (hemolysis, elevated liver enzymes, low platelets, and abdominal pain), and granulomatosis with polyangiitis (Wegener's granulomatosis).[62,63]

Malignant Hypertension

Malignant hypertension develops in 1% of patients with essential hypertension and can result in a variety of neurologic, cardiac, renal, and gastrointestinal complications. Large, bilateral exudative retinal detachments can be seen with malignant hypertension, but more frequently patients present with pronounced disc edema, intraretinal and preretinal hemorrhage, and a small inferior serous retinal detachment (▶ Fig. 30.6).[64] Fluorescein angiography often reveals areas of both retinal vascular and choroidal vascular leakage and nonperfusion (▶ Fig. 30.7). Choroidal vasculature can also be affected by linear deposition of immunoglobulins in vessel basement membranes. This has been shown histopathologically in cases of serous retinal detachment with both Goodpasture's syndrome and systemic lupus erythematosus.[65,66]

Renal Failure

Renal failure can result in exudative retinal detachment, either with or without coexistent hypertension and choroidal vascular occlusion.[67] The mechanism of detachment formation in cases without elevated blood pressure remains unknown. Treatment of the underlying renal disease causes resolution of the serous detachment, which has led some to cite electrolyte imbalance and fluid shifting as plausible etiologies. Exudative retinal detachments can occur after organ transplantation, possibly due to impaired postoperative renal function, although the high-dose steroids used may also precipitate CSC.[68]

Miscellaneous Vascular Etiologies

The exudative form of age-related macular degeneration is characterized by hemorrhagic or serous detachments of the neurosensory retina or RPE. These changes, caused by underlying choroidal neovascularization, are typically limited to the macula. Occasionally, a massive retinal detachment may develop, with or without associated lipid exudate or blood.[69] Other conditions producing choroidal neovascularization, such as ocular histoplasmosis syndrome or high myopia, may result in exudative macular detachments, but these are usually more limited in extent compared to those seen in age-related macular degeneration. Rarely, choroidal neovascularization may present in the peripheral fundus and cause exudative changes first in this area, a presentation that has been called *peripheral disciform degeneration*. Idiopathic polypoidal choroidal vasculopathy causes recurrent serosanguinous RPE and neurosensory retinal detachments due to abnormal choroidal vasculature. These detachments are typically limited to the macula, but large recurrent bullous detachments have been reported after photodynamic therapy.[70] Coats' disease, typically seen in young male patients, can produce immense exudative detachments from congenital telangiectatic retinal vessels that can be hard to differentiate from exophytic retinoblastoma.[71] Retinitis pigmentosa with a Coats' disease–type response can also occur. Although retinopathy of prematurity usually produces a tractional or rhegmatogenous detachment, cases of exudative detachment have been reported including late occurrences after laser photocoagulation or bevacizumab treatment.[72,73] Dural arteriovenous fistulas have been associated with spontaneous development of choroidal detachments that resolved after treatment.[74] Extensive exudative retinal detachments have been reported after central or hemicentral retinal vein occlusions.[75]

Infectious

Recurrent nonrhegmatogenous retinal detachment, uveal effusion, and choroidal thickening have been reported in a case of secondary syphilis in which treponemas were found in the subretinal fluid.[76] Serous detachments in cases of syphilis may resolve after initiation of antibiotic treatment.[77] Rarely, orbital cellulitis or infectious scleritis from toxoplasmosis, herpes zoster, or *Pseudomonas* infection can cause a secondary exudative retinal detachment.

Neoplastic

Choroidal nevus, melanoma, hemangioma, lymphoma, leukemia, and metastatic disease can all produce localized or diffuse exudative retinal detachments. In some cases, the diagnosis may be difficult, and fluorescein angiography, ultrasonography, and CT may differentiate these entities from others as discussed in detail earlier (and in Chapter 28).[78,79] Bilateral diffuse uveal melanocytic proliferation (BDUMP) is a rare paraneoplastic syndrome in patients with often occult systemic carcinoma. BDUMP is characterized by multiple round red patches at the RPE level with early associated hyperfluorescence seen with fluorescein angiography, multiple pigmented and nonpigmented uveal melanocytic tumors and diffuse uveal tract thickening, rapidly progressive cataracts, and exudative retinal detachments.[80]

Medications

Extensive exudative retinal detachments have been reported in patients with hepatitis C virus infection treated with interferon-a and ribavirin, along with other findings similar to VKH syndrome. The exudative detachments may improve with cessation of interferon-a and ribavirin and initiation of corticosteroid therapy.[81]

30.3 Tractional Retinal Detachment

30.3.1 Clinical Features

Patients with tractional retinal detachments present with decreased visual acuity and visual field loss. Floaters, metamorphopsia, and photopsia may also be present. Anterior segment, vitreous, and fundus appearance depend on the underlying etiology. Constant signs include a neurosensory retinal elevation with a concave surface and visible vitreoretinal membrane formation above or below the retina (▶ Fig. 30.8). These detachments, unlike rhegmatogenous detachments, rarely extend to the ora serrata and are not highly elevated. If the fundus is not visible because of media opacity (e.g., vitreous hemorrhage), ultrasound examination will easily differentiate this type of detachment by its concave or "table top" configuration and lack of undulating movement with kinetic ultrasonographic viewing (▶ Fig. 30.9).

Tractional retinal detachments occur in a variety of diseases that produce fibrous or fibrovascular membranes. The differential diagnosis is more limited than that of exudative detachment, and accurate diagnosis can usually be made with fundus examination alone. Traction membranes form after partial regression of neovascularization, as in diabetes or retinopathy of prematurity, after rhegmatogenous retinal detachment with metaplasia and RPE migration in proliferative vitreoretinopathy, or after trauma with fibrous ingrowth and contraction of membranes. Histopathologically, traction membranes consist of fibrin and glial and RPE elements. A complete differential diagnosis appears below. The presentation and management of specific entities are discussed in detail in other chapters of the book.

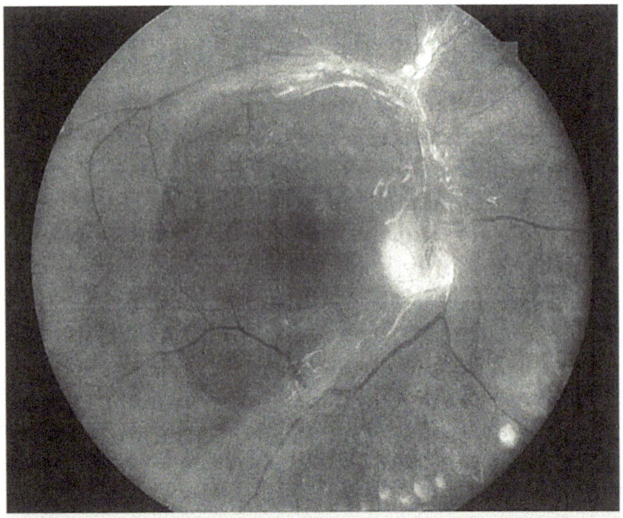

Fig. 30.8 Traction retinal detachments. Extensive fibrovascular proliferation with associated traction retinal detachments along the major arcades in an eye with mostly regressed proliferative diabetic retinopathy.

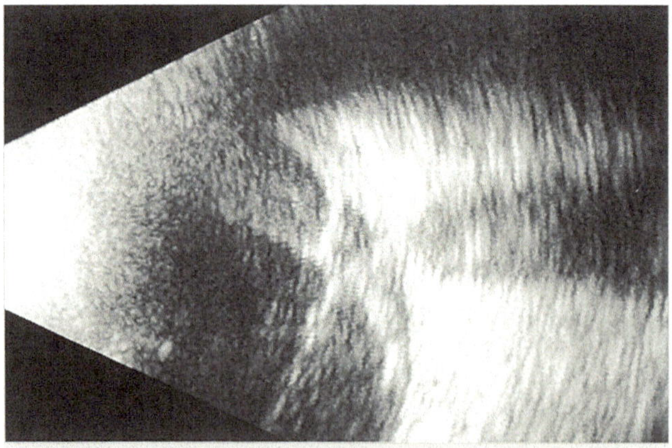

Fig. 30.9 B-scan ultrasonography of an eye with a diabetic retinopathy–related vitreous hemorrhage, partial posterior vitreous separation, and traction retinal detachment around the optic nerve head.

Conditions Causing Tractional Retinal Detachments

- **Neovascular**
  - Proliferative diabetic retinopathy
  - Retinopathy of prematurity
  - Familial exudative vitreoretinopathy
  - Sickle cell retinopathy
  - Sarcoidosis with peripheral neovascularization
  - Eales' disease
  - Branch and central retinal vein occlusion
  - Optic nerve hypoplasia or coloboma
  - Radiation retinopathy
- **Hereditary**
  - Norrie's disease
  - Incontinentia pigmenti
  - Autosomal dominant neovascular inflammatory vitreoretinopathy
  - von Hippel–Lindau syndrome
  - X-linked retinoschisis
- **Congenital**
  - Persistent fetal vasculature
- **Inflammatory**
  - *Toxocara canis* infection
  - Pars planitis
  - Proliferative vitreoretinopathy
- **Idiopathic**
  - Vitreomacular traction syndrome
- **Trauma/postsurgical**
  - Posttraumatic vitreous hemorrhage
  - Penetrating ocular injury
  - Proliferative vitreoretinopathy

30.3.2 Pathogenesis

The basic mechanism of tractional retinal detachments is relatively straightforward. The vitreoretinal attachments formed in these entities exert traction on the retina in a circumferential or anteroposterior direction. To result in neurosensory retinal detachment, the membranes must pull with more force than is generated by the mechanisms that normally keep the retina attached (e.g., RPE pump). Tractional detachments are usually addressed with vitrectomy surgery in which the adherent membranes are divided or stripped from the retina. Intravitreal anti-VEGF treatment just prior to vitrectomy may be beneficial to reduce vascular activity and risk of bleeding from fibrovascular membranes in proliferative diabetic retinopathy,[82] and may be considered for other proliferative retinopathies. However, it can also cause contraction of neovascular tissues and increase risk of tractional detachment.[83] Thus, in cases of severe and active neovascular proliferation, vitrectomy is often performed a few to several days after anti-VEGF treatment, enough time for vascular inactivation to occur, but before significant tissue contraction develops, to optimize its effect. Scleral buckling surgery or retinotomy/retinectomy may be necessary for peripheral tractional detachments that cannot be alleviated successfully with other vitreoretinal techniques.

30.3.3 Specific Entities

Neovascular

In patients with proliferative diabetic retinopathy, tractional retinal detachments with vitreoretinal adhesions develop at sites of active or regressing neovascularization. Because these occur primarily along major vascular arcades, tractional elevation of the macula is common. In children with retinopathy of prematurity or familial exudative vitreoretinopathy, peripheral neovascularization develops. In some cases, this disappears without incident, but vitreoretinal traction at the junction of vascularized and avascular retina may lead first to peripheral and then to total retinal detachment. These detachments often have complex shapes (e.g., funnel-shaped, closed anteriorly, open posteriorly) because the avascular retina present has a tremendous ability to stretch in response to the vitreous traction. Congenital optic nerve anomalies, such as optic nerve hypoplasia or coloboma, may be associated with peripheral neovascularization and tractional detachment due to incomplete retinal perfusion (▶ Fig. 30.10). Careful optic disc examination is thus critical in children with tractional retinal detachments. Conversely, assessment for peripheral retinal nonperfusion is important in children with optic nerve anomalies.[84] Sickle cell disease, sarcoid, Eales' disease, radiation retinopathy, and retinal vein occlusions all can be associated with tractional detachments due to peripheral neovascularization.

Hereditary

In patients with Norrie's disease and incontinentia pigmenti, tractional detachments can develop secondary to peripheral neovascularization. Those with autosomal dominant von Hippel–Lindau syndrome can develop vitreous traction to peripheral capillary hemangiomas, with localized tractional retinal detachments. Autosomal dominant neovascular inflammatory

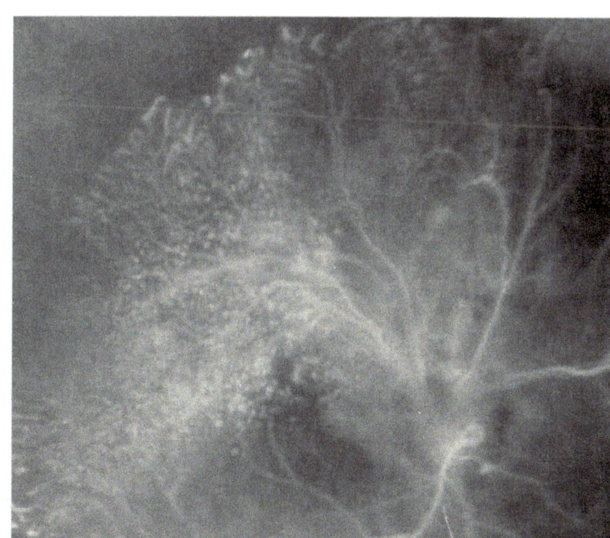

Fig. 30.10 Fluorescein angiogram illustrating peripheral retinal nonperfusion in a child with optic nerve hypoplasia. Shallow tractional retinal detachment was present in the superotemporal paramacular region (not shown).

vitreoretinopathy, a rare disease, can present with tractional detachment. Congenital X-linked retinoschisis is a rare disease in male patients with bilateral foveal schisis that may be complicated by tractional retinal detachment.

Congenital

Persistent fetal vasculature is a sporadic, unilateral disorder in which persistence of the fetal hyaloid system is associated with microphthalmia, cataract, and a fibrous stalk between the optic nerve and the lens. Occasionally, this stalk may contain a falciform fold of retina.

Inflammatory

Toxocara canis is a parasite that causes marked vitreous inflammation when it dies. This vitritis can organize into fibrous bands with strong retinal adhesions around the worm; these subsequently pull and detach the retina (▶ Fig. 30.11). Pars planitis, with its predominantly inferior peripheral vitritis, can cause tractional detachments by the same mechanism.

Idiopathic

Vitreomacular traction syndrome is a rare condition that results in retinal edema and lipid exudation in the macula. Occasionally, the vitreous can actually detach a portion of the macula if the traction generated is strong enough.

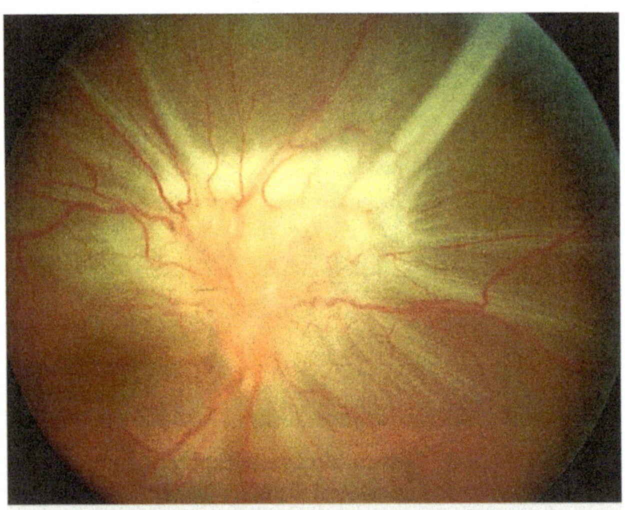

Fig. 30.11 Tractional retinal detachment associated with a focal *Toxocara canis* granuloma.

Trauma

An admixture of hemorrhage or disrupted lens material along a vitreous tract induced by penetrating injury is particularly likely to initiate a fibrovascular proliferative response with secondary retinal traction. Even severe blunt (nonpenetrating) globe injury can result in preretinal fibrous membranes and tractional retinal detachments (▶ Fig. 30.12). In general, with severely traumatized eyes, surgical intervention is preferred before this often exuberant proliferative vitreoretinopathy response develops to a significant degree (see Chapter 32).

30.4 Conclusion

In conclusion, the differential diagnosis for exudative or tractional retinal detachment is large. Differentiation of tractional, exudative, and rhegmatogenous retinal detachment is of utmost importance and is often achieved through the clinical examination alone. In cases of retinal detachment of uncertain cause, fundus fluorescein and ICG angiography, ultrasonography, and various laboratory studies may be critical for correct diagnosis and treatment. In cases of tractional retinal detachment, timely surgical intervention is paramount for good visual outcome. Appropriate actions by the physician may thus affect both the systemic and visual status of the patient.

References

[1] Negi A, Marmor MF. The resorption of subretinal fluid after diffuse damage to the retinal pigment epithelium. Invest Ophthalmol Vis Sci. 1983; 24 (11):1475–1479

[2] Negi A, Marmor MF. Experimental serous retinal detachment and focal pigment epithelial damage. Arch Ophthalmol. 1984; 102(3):445–449

[3] Spitznas M. Pathogenesis of central serous retinopathy: a new working hypothesis. Graefes Arch Clin Exp Ophthalmol. 1986; 224(4):321–324

[4] Marmor MF. New hypotheses on the pathogenesis and treatment of serous retinal detachment. Graefes Arch Clin Exp Ophthalmol. 1988; 226(6):548–552

[5] Marmor MF. Control of subretinal fluid: experimental and clinical studies. Eye (Lond). 1990; 4(Pt 2):340–344

[6] Wilson CA, Royster AJ, Tiedeman JS, Hatchell DL. Exudative retinal detachment after photodynamic injury. Arch Ophthalmol. 1991; 109(1):125–134

[7] Marmor MF, Yao XY. Conditions necessary for the formation of serous detachment. Experimental evidence from the cat. Arch Ophthalmol. 1994; 112 (6):830–838

[8] Spaide RF, Hall L, Haas A, et al. Indocyanine green videoangiography of older patients with central serous chorioretinopathy. Retina. 1996; 16(3):203–213

[9] Fok AC, Chan PP, Lam DS, Lai TY. Risk factors for recurrence of serous macular detachment in untreated patients with central serous chorioretinopathy. Ophthalmic Res. 2011; 46(3):160–163

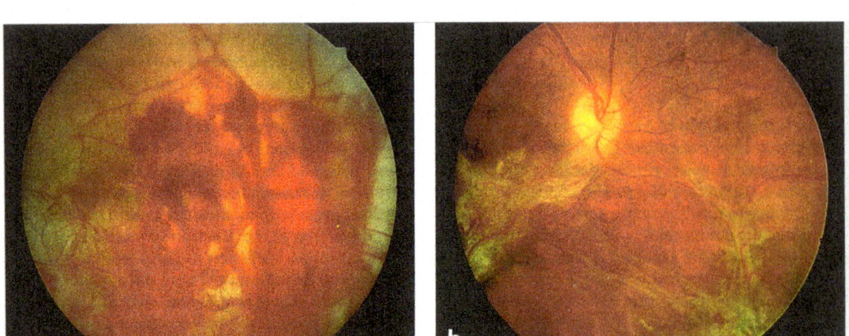

Fig. 30.12 (a) Blunt trauma with preretinal and subretinal hemorrhage. (b) The same eye several weeks later with clearing of the vitreous hemorrhage and extensive preretinal fibrous proliferation inferiorly and secondary localized traction retinal detachments. (Images provided courtesy of Carl D. Regillo, MD.)

[10] Chan WM, Lam DS, Lai TY, Tam BS, Liu DT, Chan CK. Choroidal vascular remodelling in central serous chorioretinopathy after indocyanine green guided photodynamic therapy with verteporfin: a novel treatment at the primary disease level. Br J Ophthalmol. 2003; 87(12):1453–1458

[11] Chan WM, Lai TY, Lai RY, Liu DT, Lam DS. Half-dose verteporfin photodynamic therapy for acute central serous chorioretinopathy: one-year results of a randomized controlled trial. Ophthalmology. 2008; 115(10):1756–1765

[12] Burumcek E, Mudun A, Karacorlu S, Arslan MO. Laser photocoagulation for persistent central serous retinopathy: results of long-term follow-up. Ophthalmology. 1997; 104(4):616–622

[13] Gilbert CM, Owens SL, Smith PD, Fine SL. Long-term follow-up of central serous chorioretinopathy. Br J Ophthalmol. 1984; 68(11):815–820

[14] Bousquet E, Beydoun T, Zhao M, Hassan L, Offret O, Behar-Cohen F. Mineralocorticoid receptor antagonism in the treatment of chronic central serous chorioretinopathy: a pilot study. Retina. 2013; 33(10):2096–2102

[15] Gass JDM. Bullous retinal detachment. An unusual manifestation of idiopathic central serous choroidopathy. Am J Ophthalmol. 1973; 75(5):810–821

[16] Otsuka S, Ohba N, Nakao K. A long-term follow-up study of severe variant of central serous chorioretinopathy. Retina. 2002; 22(1):25–32

[17] Gass JDM, Little H. Bilateral bullous exudative retinal detachment complicating idiopathic central serous chorioretinopathy during systemic corticosteroid therapy. Ophthalmology. 1995; 102(5):737–747

[18] Quillen DA, Gass DM, Brod RD, Gardner TW, Blankenship GW, Gottlieb JL. Central serous chorioretinopathy in women. Ophthalmology. 1996; 103 (1):72–79

[19] Bouzas EA, Karadimas P, Pournaras CJ. Central serous chorioretinopathy and glucocorticoids. Surv Ophthalmol. 2002; 47(5):431–448

[20] Gass JDM, Slamovits TL, Fuller DG, Gieser RG, Lean JS. Posterior chorioretinopathy and retinal detachment after organ transplantation. Arch Ophthalmol. 1992; 110(12):1717–1722

[21] Gass JDM. Central serous chorioretinopathy and white subretinal exudation during pregnancy. Arch Ophthalmol. 1991; 109(5):677–681

[22] Gass JDM. Bullous retinal detachment and multiple retinal pigment epithelial detachments in patients receiving hemodialysis. Graefes Arch Clin Exp Ophthalmol. 1992; 230(5):454–458

[23] Prünte C, Flammer J. Choroidal capillary and venous congestion in central serous chorioretinopathy. Am J Ophthalmol. 1996; 121(1):26–34

[24] Baumal CR, Martidis A, Truong SN. Central serous chorioretinopathy associated with periocular corticosteroid injection treatment for HLA-B27-associated iritis. Arch Ophthalmol. 2004; 122(6):926–928

[25] Gass JDM, Jallow S. Idiopathic serous detachment of the choroid, ciliary body, and retina (uveal effusion syndrome). Ophthalmology. 1982; 89(9):1018–1032

[26] Elagouz M, Stanescu-Segall D, Jackson TL. Uveal effusion syndrome. Surv Ophthalmol. 2010; 55(2):134–145

[27] Wilson RS, Hanna C, Morris MD. Idiopathic chorioretinal effusion: an analysis of extracellular fluids. Ann Ophthalmol. 1977; 9(5):647–653

[28] Singh OS, Simmons RJ, Brockhurst RJ, Trempe CL. Nanophthalmos: a perspective on identification and therapy. Ophthalmology. 1982; 89(9):1006–1012

[29] Ryan EA, Zwaan J, Chylack LT, Jr. Nanophthalmos with uveal effusion: clinical and embryologic considerations. Ophthalmology. 1982; 89(9):1013–1017

[30] Trelstad RL, Silbermann NN, Brockhurst RJ. Nanophthalmic sclera. Ultrastructural, histochemical, and biochemical observations. Arch Ophthalmol. 1982; 100(12):1935–1938

[31] Johnson MW, Gass JDM. Surgical management of the idiopathic uveal effusion syndrome. Ophthalmology. 1990; 97(6):778–785

[32] Suzuki Y, Nishina S, Azuma N. Scleral window surgery and topical mitomycin C for nanophthalmic uveal effusion complicated by renal failure: case report. Graefes Arch Clin Exp Ophthalmol. 2007; 245(5):755–757

[33] Steijns D, Bijlsma WR, Van der Lelij A. Cataract surgery in patients with nanophthalmos. Ophthalmology. 2013; 120(2):266–270

[34] Chu TG, Green RL. Suprachoroidal hemorrhage. Surv Ophthalmol. 1999; 43 (6):471–486

[35] Dawidek GMB, Kinsella FM, Pyott A, Hughes DS, Kyle PM, Lane CM. Delayed ciliochoroidal detachment following intraocular lens implantation. Br J Ophthalmol. 1991; 75(9):572–574

[36] Ruiz RS, Salmonsen PC. Expulsive choroidal effusion. A complication of intraocular surgery. Arch Ophthalmol. 1976; 94(1):69–70

[37] Ambati J, Arroyo JG. Postoperative complications of scleral buckling surgery. Int Ophthalmol Clin. 2000; 40(1):175–185

[38] Weiter JJ, Brockhurst RJ, Tolentino FI. Uveal effusion following pan-retinal photocoagulation. Ann Ophthalmol. 1979; 11(11):1723–1727

[39] Saikia P, Nashed A, Helbig H, Hillenkamp J. Bilateral posterior scleritis: an idiopathic painless presentation. Ocul Immunol Inflamm. 2010; 18(6):452–453

[40] McCluskey PJ, Watson PG, Lightman S, Haybittle J, Restori M, Branley M. Posterior scleritis: clinical features, systemic associations, and outcome in a large series of patients. Ophthalmology. 1999; 106(12):2380–2386

[41] Finger PT, Perry HD, Packer S, Erdey RA, Weisman GD, Sibony PA. Posterior scleritis as an intraocular tumour. Br J Ophthalmol. 1990; 74(2):121–122

[42] Brod RD, Saul RF. Nodular posterior scleritis. Arch Ophthalmol. 1990; 108 (8):1170–1171

[43] Yap EY, Robertson DM, Buettner H. Scleritis as an initial manifestation of choroidal malignant melanoma. Ophthalmology. 1992; 99(11):1693–1697

[44] Hunyor AP, Harper CA, O'Day J, McKelvie PA. Ocular-central nervous system lymphoma mimicking posterior scleritis with exudative retinal detachment. Ophthalmology. 2000; 107(10):1955–1959

[45] Wieringa WG, Wieringa JE, ten Dam-van Loon NH, Los LI. Visual outcome, treatment results, and prognostic factors in patients with scleritis. Ophthalmology. 2013; 120(2):379–386

[46] Desroches G, Abrams GW, Gass JDM. Reactive lymphoid hyperplasia of the uvea. A case with ultrasonographic and computed tomographic studies. Arch Ophthalmol. 1983; 101(5):725–728

[47] Grossniklaus HE, Martin DF, Avery R, et al. Uveal lymphoid infiltration. Report of four cases and clinicopathologic review. Ophthalmology. 1998; 105 (7):1265–1273

[48] Chang TS, Byrne SF, Gass JDM, Hughes JR, Johnson RN, Murray TG. Echographic findings in benign reactive lymphoid hyperplasia of the choroid. Arch Ophthalmol. 1996; 114(6):669–675

[49] Stacy RC, Jakobiec FA, Schoenfield L, Singh AD. Unifocal and multifocal reactive lymphoid hyperplasia vs follicular lymphoma of the ocular adnexa. Am J Ophthalmol. 2010; 150(3):412–426.e1

[50] Cockerham GC, Hidayat AA, Bijwaard KE, Sheng ZM. Re-evaluation of "reactive lymphoid hyperplasia of the uvea": an immunohistochemical and molecular analysis of 10 cases. Ophthalmology. 2000; 107(1):151–158

[51] Forster DJ, Cano MR, Green RL, Rao NA. Echographic features of the Vogt-Koyanagi-Harada syndrome. Arch Ophthalmol. 1990; 108(10):1421–1426

[52] Dreyer WB, Jr, Zegarra H, Zakov ZN, Gutman FA. Sympathetic ophthalmia. Am J Ophthalmol. 1981; 92(6):816–823

[53] Paredes I, Ahmed M, Foster CS. Immunomodulatory therapy for Vogt-Koyanagi-Harada patients as first-line therapy. Ocul Immunol Inflamm. 2006; 14 (2):87–90

[54] Chang GC, Young LH. Sympathetic ophthalmia. Semin Ophthalmol. 2011; 26 (4–5):316–320

[55] Greco A, Fusconi M, Gallo A, et al. Vogt-Koyanagi-Harada syndrome. Autoimmun Rev. 2013; 12(11):1033–1038

[56] Patel SS, Dodds EM, Echandi LV, et al. Long-term, drug-free remission of sympathetic ophthalmia with high-dose, short-term chlorambucil therapy. Ophthalmology. 2014; 121(2):596–602

[57] Hoines J, Buettner H. Ocular complications of disseminated intravascular coagulation (DIC) in abruptio placentae. Retina. 1989; 9(2):105–109

[58] Wyszynski RE, Frank KE, Grossniklaus HE. Bilateral retinal detachments in thrombotic thrombocytopenic purpura. Graefes Arch Clin Exp Ophthalmol. 1988; 226(6):501–504

[59] Hartley KL, Benz MS. Retinal pigment epithelial tear associated with a serous retinal detachment in a patient with thrombotic thrombocytopenic purpura and hypertension. Retina. 2004; 24(5):806–808

[60] Fastenberg DM, Fetkenhour CL, Choromokos E, Shoch DE. Choroidal vascular changes in toxemia of pregnancy. Am J Ophthalmol. 1980; 89(3):362–368

[61] Mabie WC, Ober RR. Fluorescein angiography in toxaemia of pregnancy. Br J Ophthalmol. 1980; 64(9):666–671

[62] Kinyoun JL, Kalina RE, Klein ML. Choroidal involvement in systemic necrotizing vasculitis. Arch Ophthalmol. 1987; 105(7):939–942

[63] Gundlach E, Junker B, Gross N, Hansen LL, Pielen A. Bilateral serous retinal detachment. Br J Ophthalmol. 2013; 97(7):939–940, 949

[64] MacCumber MW, Flower RW, Langham ME. Ischemic hypertensive choroidopathy. Fluorescein angiography, indocyanine green videoangiography, and measurement of pulsatile blood flow. Arch Ophthalmol. 1993; 111(5):704–705

[65] Jampol LM, Lahov M, Albert DM, Craft J. Ocular clinical findings and basement membrane changes in Goodpasture's syndrome. Am J Ophthalmol. 1975; 79 (3):452–463

[66] Diddie KR, Aronson AJ, Ernest JT. Chorioretinopathy in a case of systemic lupus erythematosus. Trans Am Ophthalmol Soc. 1977; 75:122–131

[67] Paris GL, Macoul KL. Reversible bullous retinal detachment in chronic renal disease. Am J Ophthalmol. 1969; 67(2):249–251

[68] Scorolli L, Giardina D, Morara M, Corazza D, Meduri RA. Bilateral serous retinal detachments following organ transplantation. Retina. 2003; 23 (6):785–791

[69] Blair CJ, Aaberg TM. Massive subretinal exudation associated with senile macular degeneration. Am J Ophthalmol. 1971; 71(3):639–648

[70] Prakash M, Han DP. Recurrent bullous retinal detachments from photodynamic therapy for idiopathic polypoidal choroidal vasculopathy. Am J Ophthalmol. 2006; 142(6):1079–1081

[71] Shields JA, Shields CL. Review: coats disease: the 2001 LuEsther T. Mertz lecture. Retina. 2002; 22(1):80–91

[72] Moshfeghi DM, Silva RA, Berrocal AM. Exudative retinal detachment following photocoagulation in older premature infants for retinopathy of prematurity: description and management. Retina. 2014; 34(1):83–86

[73] Ittiara S, Blair MP, Shapiro MJ, Lichtenstein SJ. Exudative retinopathy and detachment: a late reactivation of retinopathy of prematurity after intravitreal bevacizumab. J AAPOS. 2013; 17(3):323–325

[74] Harbison JW, Guerry D, Wiesinger H. Dural arteriovenous fistula and spontaneous choroidal detachment: new cause of an old disease. Br J Ophthalmol. 1978; 62(7):483–490

[75] Weinberg D, Jampol LM, Schatz H, Brady KD. Exudative retinal detachment following central and hemicentral retinal vein occlusions. Arch Ophthalmol. 1990; 108(2):271–275

[76] DeLuise VP, Clark SW, III, Smith JLS. Syphilitic retinal detachment and uveal effusion. Am J Ophthalmol. 1982; 94(6):757–761

[77] Fu EX, Geraets RL, Dodds EM, et al. Superficial retinal precipitates in patients with syphilitic retinitis. Retina. 2010; 30(7):1135–1143

[78] Kreiger AE, Meyer D, Smith TR, Riemer K. Metastatic carcinoma to the choroid with choroidal detachment. A case presenting as uveal effusion. Arch Ophthalmol. 1969; 82(2):209–213

[79] Muscat S, Parks S, Kemp E, Keating D. Secondary retinal changes associated with choroidal naevi and melanomas documented by optical coherence tomography. Br J Ophthalmol. 2004; 88(1):120–124

[80] Gass JDM, Gieser RG, Wilkinson CP, Beahm DE, Pautler SE. Bilateral diffuse uveal melanocytic proliferation in patients with occult carcinoma. Arch Ophthalmol. 1990; 108(4):527–533

[81] Modorati G, Matteo DF, Miserocchi E, Colucci A, Bandello F. Serous retinal detachments complicating interferon-a and ribavirin treatment in patients with hepatitis C. Case Rep Ophthalmol. 2011; 2(1):105–110

[82] Pokroy R, Desai UR, Du E, Li Y, Edwards P. Bevacizumab prior to vitrectomy for diabetic traction retinal detachment. Eye (Lond). 2011; 25(8):989–997

[83] Osaadon P, Fagan XJ, Lifshitz T, Levy J. A review of anti-VEGF agents for proliferative diabetic retinopathy. Eye (Lond). 2014; 28(5):510–520

[84] Shapiro MJ, Chow CC, Blair MP, Kiernan DF, Kaufman LM. Peripheral nonperfusion and tractional retinal detachment associated with congenital optic nerve anomalies. Ophthalmology. 2013; 120(3):607–615

31 Degenerative Retinoschisis

David C. Reed and Sunir J. Garg

31.1 Definitions and Histology

Degenerative (also called acquired or senile) retinoschisis is an acquired splitting of the retinal layers of unknown etiology. It has two subtypes, the typical form and the reticular form. In the typical form, the histological split is within the outer plexiform layer, and in the reticular form the split is within the nerve fiber layer (▸ Fig. 31.1).[1] A gradual accumulation of viscous fluid, rich in mucopolysaccharide, occurs within the schisis cavity. As the neural pathways of the retina become damaged due to the retinoschisis, patients develop an absolute scotoma in the affected area.

Retinal breaks can occur in the inner layer, the outer layer, or both, and do not necessarily cause a rhegmatogenous retinal detachment (RRD).[2] In fact, inner layer breaks by themselves cannot lead to a retinal detachment, since there is no path for fluid to enter the subretinal space.

Two types of retinal detachment are associated with retinoschisis:

1. *Schisis detachment*: This term describes a situation where there are outer layer holes without inner layer holes, and intraschisis fluid has migrated into the subretinal space.[2]
2. *Progressive RRD associated with retinoschisis*: This entity occurs when there are breaks in both the inner and outer layers, allowing liquefied vitreous to enter the subretinal space.

31.2 Clinical Features and Diagnosis

Degenerative retinoschisis can be seen in patients as young as 19 years, and the prevalence increases sharply after age 40 years.[3] It is associated with hyperopia, and occurs equally among males and females. Although it may appear in any quadrant, by far the most frequent location is the inferotemporal quadrant, followed by the superotemporal quadrant. Often, there are separate areas of involvement within the same eye that are not connected, because the disease is multicentric in origin. Bilateral involvement is present in more than 80% of cases.[2]

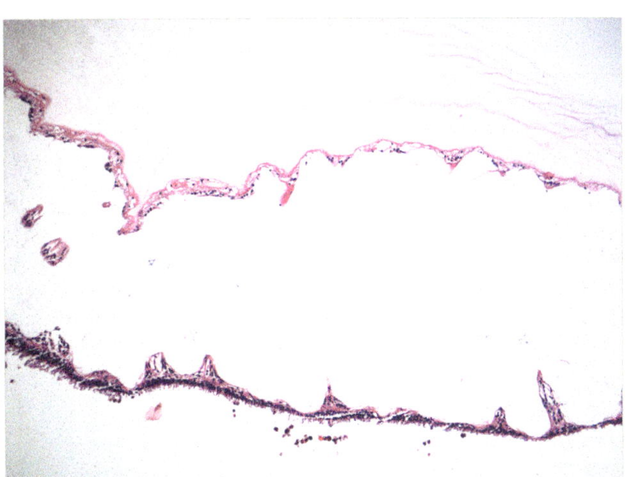

Fig. 31.1 Histological section of typical retinoschisis with splitting of the middle retinal layers. Note the normal cortical vitreous attached to the inner retinal surface. (Photo courtesy of Dr. Ralph Eagle.)

Retinoschisis with and without breaks is almost invariably asymptomatic, even when the extent of the retinoschisis is posterior to the equator.[2] Since the subretinal fluid of schisis detachments usually does not extend beyond the borders of the retinoschisis, schisis detachments are also usually asymptomatic. Cases of schisis detachment with posterior extension of subretinal fluid may be symptomatic, but this phenomenon is rare. In contrast, progressive RRD is usually symptomatic.

Retinoschisis typically is characterized by a smooth, uniform, inward convexity of the retina (▸ Fig. 31.2a,b). It is important to differentiate retinoschisis and peripheral subclinical retinal detachment secondary to small atrophic holes.

Retinoschisis is usually detected because of one of two findings: white lines in a vascular pattern in the inner layer, or the presence of tiny yellow-white flecks on the inner surface of the inner layer, colloquially called "snowflakes." These "snowflakes" are thought to be remnants of Müller cell footplates and neuronal connections between the inner and outer layers. The use of indirect ophthalmoscopy combined with scleral depression is essential in making the diagnosis of retinoschisis. By this method, it should be possible to demonstrate the presence of a fluid-filled layer between the outer and inner retinal layers. A characteristic feature of retinoschisis is that, upon scleral depression, the area of schisis tends to be displaced inward as a unitary enclosed structure. This helps to differentiate it from an RRD in which scleral depression tends to decrease, and flatten, the area of elevation, as some of the subretinal fluid may escape through retinal breaks into the vitreous space. In some patients, scleral depression produces the phenomenon of "white with pressure" arising from only the outer layer, and this is a confirmatory sign of the presence of retinoschisis. Optical coherence tomography can also be a useful means of distinguishing between retinoschisis and retinal detachment (▸ Fig. 31.3). Further, the outer layer in areas of retinoschisis will blanch with laser application, in contrast to areas of retinal detachment.[4] ▸ Table 31.1 compares the features of retinoschisis and retinal detachment.

Inner layer breaks are usually small, round, and difficult to detect (▸ Fig. 31.4). The prevalence of outer layer breaks in eyes with retinoschisis is between 11 and 24%.[2,5,6] Outer layer breaks tend to be much larger, more posterior, and often have rolled white edges (▸ Fig. 31.5).

Four clues pointing to a schisis detachment (▸ Fig. 31.6) include the following:

- The presence of an outer layer break.
- The appearance of the schisis is not uniform in height, texture, or transparency.
- There may be a curved yellowish line deep to the inner layer corresponding to the outer layer.
- There may be a pigmented demarcation line in chronic cases.

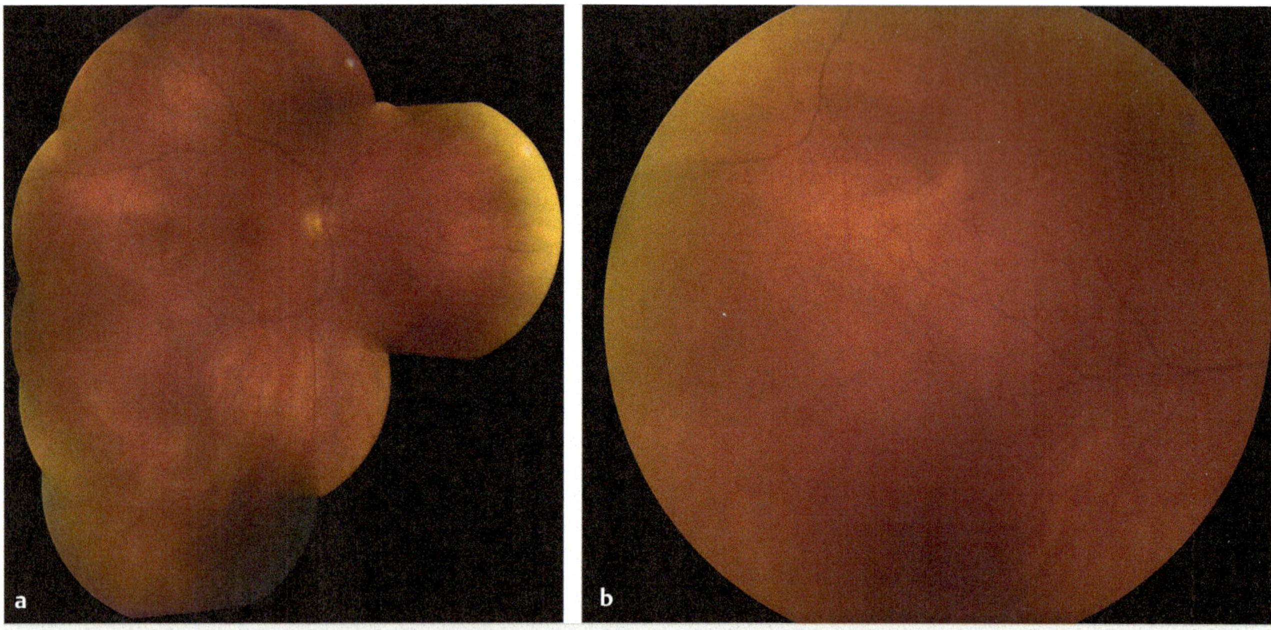

Fig. 31.2 (a) Smooth, dome-shaped bullous retinoschisis is seen inferotemporally. (b) Same eye as (a). Close-up of the transition between normal retina and schitic retina. Background diabetic retinopathy is noted coincidentally.

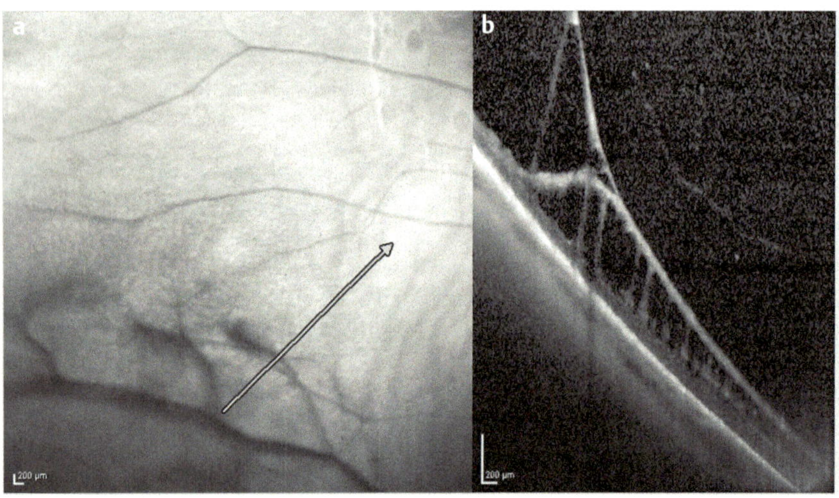

Fig. 31.3 (a) The arrow shows the orientation of the OCT slice. It starts in the area of retinoschisis and goes towards the normal retina. (b) Optical coherence tomography shows both bullous schisis of the nerve fiber layer (left hand side of image), schisis of the middle retinal layers (the middle of the image), and the nearly normal retina on the right hand side of the image.

Progressive RRD associated with retinoschisis is uncommon. Examination reveals opacified, corrugated retina typical of acute retinal detachment, but outer layer breaks are evident (▶ Fig. 31.7). Inner layer breaks may be difficult to detect.[7]

31.3 Prognosis

Prognosis of degenerative retinoschisis has been evaluated in a long-range natural history study of 218 eyes from a consecutive group of patients, followed without treatment over a period of 1 to 21 years (average, 9 years).[2] This revealed that the predominant tendency of degenerative retinoschisis over a period of years is either not to progress or to progress very slowly and almost imperceptibly. Posterior extension was found in 3% and lateral extension in 6% over the observation period. An increase in height was documented in 5%, but 5% decreased in height, with complete disappearance of lesions in 2% (five eyes). New retinal breaks were found in 6%. In 10% of eyes, new areas of retinoschisis appeared.

Extension of the retinoschisis to the macula is extremely rare,[8,9,10,11] and was not seen in the series mentioned earlier. In this regard, retinoschisis has another unusual and unexplained characteristic. In the relatively few cases in which the retinoschisis lesion does progress posteriorly, the extension usually stops approximately 3 disc diameters from the macula, with no further progression.

The most serious associated finding in the large natural history series was the development of schisis detachment in 6% (14 eyes). In the 13 cases that could be followed up, however, the schisis detachments remained localized, asymptomatic, and nonprogressive over an average observation period of 6 years, and none of these schisis detachments required treatment, even though in six eyes there were retinal breaks in both layers of the retinoschisis. The majority of outer layer breaks likely

Table 31.1 Comparison of retinoschisis and retinal detachment

Features	Retinoschisis	Retinal detachment
Typical patient age	Middle age to elderly	Middle age
Refractive association	Hyperopia	Myopia
Symptoms	Almost always absent	Acute: present
		Chronic: often absent
Scotoma	Absolute	Relative
"Tobacco dust" and vitreous hemorrhage	Absent	Common
Location	Inferotemporal, superotemporal	Acute: usually superior
		Chronic: usually inferior
Texture	Smooth	Acute: corrugated
		Chronic: smooth
Müller footplates	Common	Absent
Mobility	Relatively immobile	Acute: often very mobile
		Chronic: may be immobile
Movement with scleral depression	Moves as single unit	Height decreases
Color with scleral depression	"White with pressure" may be seen in outer layer	No "white with pressure"
Breaks	May be present	Present
Lattice in elevated retina	Unlikely	Suggestive
Retinal pigment epithelium	Normal (unless associated with retinal detachment, current or regressed)	Acute: normal
		Chronic: atrophy and demarcation lines may be present
Optical coherence tomography	Splitting of retinal layers	Subretinal fluid
Effect of laser application through retinal break[4]	Through inner layer break: uptake	Through full-thickness break: no uptake
Natural history	Progression rare and slow	Acute: progressive
		Chronic: may be nonprogressive or slowly progressive

lead to a schisis detachment. Symptomatic posterior extension of the subretinal fluid posterior to the area of schisis is rare.[12,13,14] When the fluid does progress posteriorly, it does so very slowly.[14] The relative stability of schisis detachment is likely due, at least in part, to the viscous nature of the intraschisis fluid, resulting in only some of the fluid traversing the outer layer break into the subretinal space.[15]

Breaks in both layers may occasionally lead to progressive RRD. The literature indicates, however, that the more likely course is for the retinoschisis to remain quiescent; in the large natural history study noted earlier, no cases of progressive RRD occurred. It has been calculated that only 1 in 2,000 cases of retinoschisis will develop into progressive RRD.[2]

Another question of considerable clinical importance is whether the prognosis of retinoschisis changes at the time of posterior vitreous detachment (PVD). This has been studied in 30 eyes with retinoschisis from a series of 350 consecutive eyes with acute PVD.[16] In four of these eyes, new tractional retinal tears occurred, but none were associated with areas of retinoschisis. Three of the eyes showed definite lowering in height of the retinoschisis following PVD. In the natural history study of retinoschisis, three eyes underwent cataract extraction (two intracapsular and one extracapsular) and no adverse effect on the retinoschisis was observed.[2] In the case of later cataract extraction or PVD, with preexisting retinoschisis, the lack of serious sequelae may be due to the fact that the essential pathology of retinoschisis is intraretinal rather than at the vitreoretinal interface and, therefore, does not produce abnormal vitreoretinal traction.

In the natural history study of 218 untreated eyes, the final vision was 20/25 or better in 196 eyes; in the 22 remaining eyes, the decreased vision was not believed to be related to retinoschisis.[2]

31.4 Management

In the past, many different methods of treatment for degenerative retinoschisis were recommended, including diathermy, cryotherapy, xenon arc photocoagulation, argon laser photocoagulation, various types of scleral surgery (resection, plication,

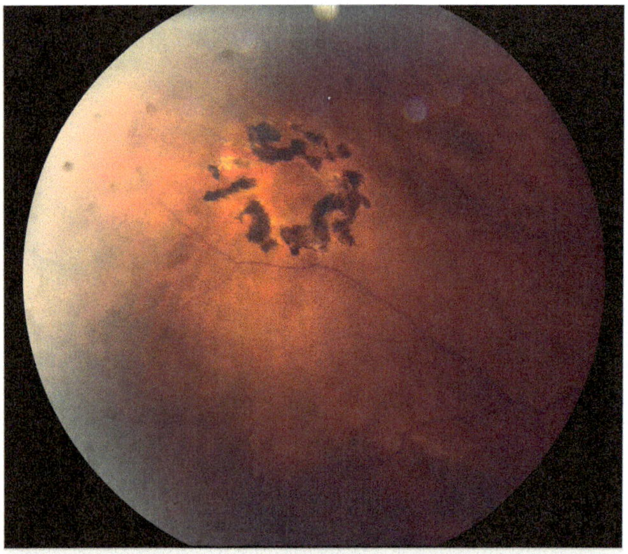

Fig. 31.4 A small round inner layer hole. Laser retinopexy had been attempted in order to surround the hole, but the telltale laser uptake within the break proves this is an inner layer hole of retinoschisis. (Photo courtesy of Dr. William Benson.)

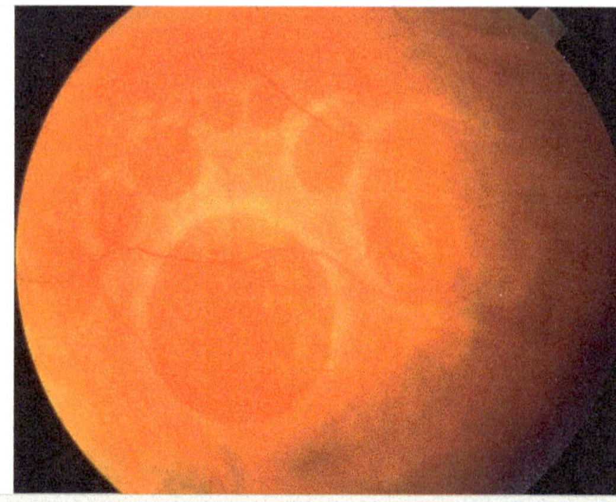

Fig. 31.5 Several large, round, posterior outer layer breaks. (Photo courtesy of Dr. William Tasman.)

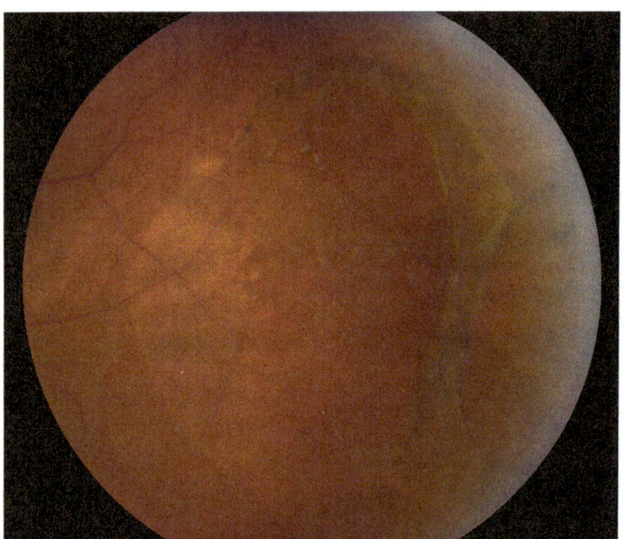

Fig. 31.6 An asymptomatic schisis detachment with a large posterior outer layer break and a crescent of subretinal fluid extending posterior to the schisis. Pigment clumping along the superior and anterior borders of the outer layer break denotes chronicity. "Snowflakes" are present in the inner layer "roof" of the outer layer break, corresponding to the remnants of Müller footplates and neuronal connections between the inner and outer layers.

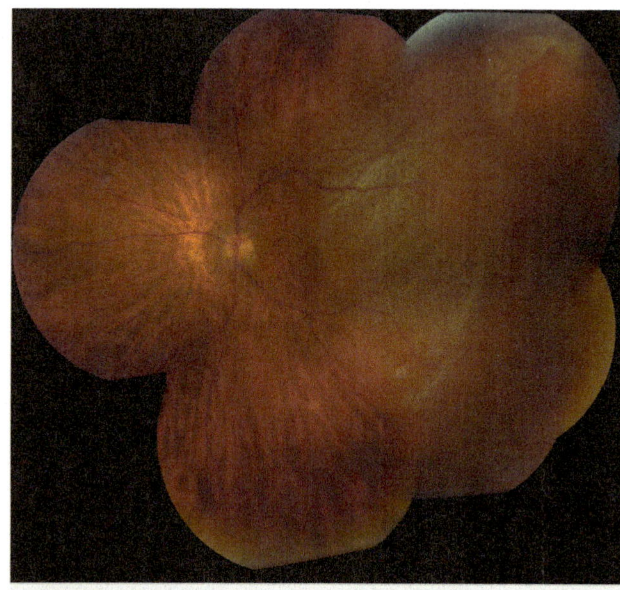

Fig. 31.7 A progressive rhegmatogenous retinal detachment associated with retinoschisis. Elevated, opacified, corrugated retina is seen, with subretinal fluid extending through the macula. A large superotemporal outer layer break is present, but no inner wall breaks are identified. (Photo courtesy of Dr. William Benson.)

or pockets), Silastic sponge exoplants, encircling buckles, and drainage of intraretinal fluid from the retinoschisis cavities (the latter procedure requiring newly created outer layer retinal breaks). These treatments have, however, been associated with significant postoperative complications, including retinal detachment, maculopathy, vitreous hemorrhage, new retinal breaks, and proliferative vitreoretinopathy. These types of treatment and complications recorded in the literature have been reviewed elsewhere.[2,17] It is important to note that no treatment has been proven to prevent the continued progression of degenerative retinoschisis. Many cases have been observed in which the process continued to advance beyond treatment demarcation lines or to arise de novo in previously uninvolved retinal areas. It is now known that the best management of almost all cases of retinoschisis is observation alone. The one indication for surgical treatment is symptomatic progressive RRD associated with retinoschisis (▸ Table 31.2).

The treatment of progressive RRD associated with retinoschisis follows the same surgical principles that are applicable to RRD, detailed elsewhere in this text. Principles specific to cases of progressive RRD associated with retinoschisis include the following:

Table 31.2 Summary of treatment guidelines for retinoschisis and related disorders

Stage of degenerative retinoschisis	Management
Without breaks	No treatment (except rarely)
With outer layer breaks	No treatment (except rarely)
With localized schisis detachment	No treatment (except rarely)
With symptomatic, posterior extension of schisis detachment (rare)	Prompt surgical repair
With progressive RRD	Prompt surgical repair

Abbreviation: RRD, rhegmatogenous retinal detachment.

Source: Adapted from Byer.[15]

- The surgical goal is to close the outer layer break, facilitating resolution of the subretinal fluid. Treatment of inner layer breaks is optional.[7]
- Collapsing the schisis cavity permanently may be attempted, but recurrence of the schisis cavity is common and its presence or absence is not usually related to visual outcome.[7] The scotoma caused by the retinoschisis is typically not symptomatic, and is not reversed with collapse of the schisis cavity.[18,19]
- Inner layer breaks are not caused by PVD. However, a PVD may cause full-thickness breaks away from the retinoschisis, leading to RRD. The lack of a PVD favors scleral buckling over pars plana vitrectomy, but both techniques can be used to repair the RRD.
- If the outer layer breaks are located anteriorly, scleral buckling may be advantageous over pars plana vitrectomy, whereas if the outer layer breaks are located posteriorly, pars plana vitrectomy may offer easier access to the breaks.[20]
- When performing pars plana vitrectomy in this context, it may be necessary to create an inner layer retinotomy over the outer layer break to drain the subretinal fluid, followed by endolaser to treat all breaks, with subsequent gas or oil tamponade.[7]

There now appears to be strong evidence that the wisest course in managing patients with degenerative retinoschisis is a deliberate policy of nontreatment, and that this carries less risk of serious complications and vision loss than does either surgical or so-called prophylactic treatment.[2] In the presence of an asymptomatic "schisis detachment" or of outer layer retinal breaks, patients should be rechecked approximately every 6 months. For other patients, reexamination every 2 to 3 years is sufficient. All patients should be informed of the presence of retinoschisis in their eyes, and asked to return promptly in case of any new visual symptoms.

It is important for ophthalmologists to recognize and understand this interesting disease, so that it can be differentiated from other important disease processes and so that unnecessary recommendations for treatment can be avoided.

Controversial Points

- Prophylactic treatment of posterior retinoschisis.
- Prophylactic treatment of outer layer breaks.
- Prophylactic treatment of schisis detachments.

The best natural history data available suggest that the vast majority of these findings will remain stable and do not require treatment.

Pearls

The Differentiation of Retinoschisis and Retinal Detachment

- With scleral depression, the entire schisis cavity will depress as one solitary, enclosed unit.
- With scleral depression, "white with pressure" of the outer layer confirms the presence of retinoschisis.
- The presence of lattice and/or retinal holes in either eye raises the suspicion for subclinical retinal detachment rather than retinoschisis.
- Tiny yellow-white flecks on the inner surface of the retina suggest retinoschisis.
- Sclerotic blood vessels suggest retinoschisis.
- Optical coherence tomography can help differentiate retinoschisis from RRD.

Special Considerations

- Treatment of retinoschisis should be reserved for cases of schisis detachment with symptomatic posterior extension of subretinal fluid and for progressive RRD. Both of these entities are rare.

31.5 Acknowledgments

We thank Dr. Byer, the author of this chapter in the first edition, for his foundational work on the natural history of retinoschisis. We also thank Dr. William Benson, for generously providing numerous images and critically reviewing the figures for accuracy of description, and Elaine Gonzales, RN, ophthalmic photographer, for her unflagging efforts to obtain publication-quality images for use in this chapter.

References

[1] Straatsma BR, Foss RY. Typical and reticular degenerative retinoschisis. Am J Ophthalmol. 1973; 75(4):551–575
[2] Byer NE. Long-term natural history study of senile retinoschisis with implications for management. Ophthalmology. 1986; 93(9):1127–1137
[3] Byer NE. Clinical study of senile retinoschisis. Arch Ophthalmol. 1968; 79 (1):36–44
[4] Lincoff H, Kreissig I, Stopa M. A modified laser test for the identification of retinoschisis. Am J Ophthalmol. 2003; 136(5):925–926
[5] Shea M, Schepens CL, von Pirquet SR. Retinoschisis: I. Senile type: a clinical report of one hundred seven cases. Arch Ophthalmol. 1960; 63:1–9

[6] Hirose T, Marcil G, Schepens CL, Freeman HM. Acquired retinoschisis: observations and treatment. In: Pruett RC, Regan DJ, eds. Retina Congress. New York, NY: Appleton-Century-Crofts; 1972:489–503

[7] Regillo CD, Custis PH. Surgical management of retinoschisis. Curr Opin Ophthalmol. 1997; 8(3):80–86

[8] Okun E, Cibis PA. The role of photocoagulation in the management of retinoschisis. Arch Ophthalmol. 1964; 72:309–314

[9] Brockhurst RJ. Discussion of: Dobbie JG. Cryotherapy in the management of senile retinoschisis. Trans Am Acad Ophthalmol Otolaryngol. 1969; 73:1060

[10] DiSclafani M, Wagner A, Humphrey W, Valone J, Jr. Pigmentary changes in acquired retinoschisis. Am J Ophthalmol. 1988; 105(3):291–293

[11] Gass JDM. Stereoscopic Atlas of Macular Diseases. 3rd ed. St. Louis, MO: Mosby; 1987:720–721

[12] Sulonen JM, Wells CG, Barricks ME, Verne AZ, Kalina RE, Hilton GF. Degenerative retinoschisis with giant outer layer breaks and retinal detachment. Am J Ophthalmol. 1985; 99(2):114–121

[13] Ambler JS, Gutman FA. Retinal detachment and retinoschisis. Ophthalmology. 1991; 98(1):1

[14] Watzke RC, Folk JC, Lauer AK. Foveal involvement by acquired retinoschisis: long-term visual outcomes. Retina. 2013; 33(3):606–612

[15] Byer NE. Perspectives on the management of the complications of senile retinoschisis. Eye (Lond). 2002; 16(4):359–364

[16] Byer N. Unpublished data

[17] Yu S, Gao Y, Liang X, Huang Y. Acquired retinoschisis resolved after 23Gage pars plana vitrectomy in posterior microphthalmos. BMC Ophthalmol. 2014; 14(1):65

[18] Lincoff H, Sarup V, Uram D, Kreissig I.. Progression and regression of retinoschisis in a single patient. Retinal Physician. 2010

[19] Byer NE. Spontaneous regression of senile retinoschisis. Arch Ophthalmol. 1972; 88(2):207–209

[20] Gotzaridis EV, Georgalas I, Petrou P, Assi AC, Sullivan P. Surgical treatment of retinal detachment associated with degenerative retinoschisis. Semin Ophthalmol. 2014; 29(3):136–141

32 Blunt and Penetrating Ocular Injuries

Liliya Shevchenko, Thomas M. Aaberg, Jr., and Paul Sternberg, Jr.

32.1 Introduction

Ocular trauma is one of the leading causes of visual impairment and monocular blindness in the United States.[1] Of the 2.5 million eye injuries that occur annually, 50,000 result in permanent partial or complete visual loss.[2] There are 55 million eye injuries reported worldwide each year, which result in limitation to daily activities. Of these injuries, 1.6 million are blinding.[3] According to the National Center for Health Statistics' Health Interview Survey conducted in 1977, approximately 1 million Americans were permanently visually impaired, and 75% of those patients were monocularly blind because of ocular trauma.[4,5] The personal, social, and economic impact of this problem is enormous. In recent years, there has been a significant shift of eye injuries from the workplace to the home setting.[2,4] However, current estimates of cost burden of eye injuries are still best extrapolated from those occurring in the workplace, due to the higher rate of injury reporting from work settings compared to home settings.[6,7,8] According to the National Safety Council, the cost of job-related eye injuries (which represents a third of all eye injuries) amounts to $300 million annually.[4] Based on several different reports, in the United States, the average annual rate of eye injury–related visits to an emergency department varied between 2.09 and 3.76 per 1,000 population during the last decade.[7,9,10] Injury is the leading cause for eye-related hospital admissions. The incidence rate of hospitalized cases for eye injuries (as a primary diagnosis) in the United States is 13.2 per 100,000 annually.[3,11] When all direct and indirect costs are included, Occupation Safety and Health Administration reports that, on average, the cost of an eye injury is $1,463.[12] Hospitalization costs secondary to penetrating ocular injuries alone are estimated to be $120 million annually. When personal expense, lost time from work, and social services are included, the financial burden of ocular trauma is immense, with estimates in excess of $1.3 billion annually.[13] Yet, 90% of these injuries are preventable.[4] For example, of more than 600 persons with work-related penetrating eye injuries reported to the National Eye Trauma System Registry between 1985 and 1991, only 6% were wearing safety glasses.[14] This highlights the potential role for the ophthalmologist as an educator and practitioner of preventive medicine.

The majority of ocular trauma occurs in three populations: children, young men, and the elderly. Nearly half (47.6%) of all eye injuries occur in young adults between 18 and 45 years of age.[4] From birth to age 75 years, men have a two to nine times higher risk of sustaining ocular trauma compared to women. Overall, 73% of eye injuries occur in males of all ages.[4,11] The incidence of annual hospitalization for patients with the principal diagnosis of ocular trauma as a function of age is bimodal, with one peak occurring between ages 15 and 35 years, and the other occurring after age 70 years.[11,13] BB gun use, immature motor skills, and curiosity are common factors that lead to eye injuries in children. Young men most commonly sustain injuries at home, workplace, or as a result of altercations, sports, or motor vehicle accidents. Ruptured surgical eye wounds in the elderly, who are prone to falling, account for 48% of ocular injuries in this population, according to one report.[2,7,13] Race is also an important risk factor for ocular trauma. Most studies report that nonwhite racial groups are most prone to ocular injuries. One study found that, in the United States, among individuals 25 to 65 years of age, African Americans and Hispanics have a 40 to 60% higher risk of eye injury compared to whites, while a more recent study found that American Indians and African Americans were most prone to ocular injuries.[7,15]

There are six general categories of trauma that can lead to vision loss:

1. Blunt trauma
2. Penetrating trauma
3. Perforating trauma
4. Intraocular foreign body (IOFB)
5. Chemical trauma
6. Thermal trauma

This chapter concentrates on the first four categories.

The Ocular Trauma Classification Group has devised a system to classify both closed- and open-globe injuries according to four variables[16]:

1. Type of injury (based on mechanism).
2. Grade of injury (defined by visual acuity upon presentation).
3. Pupil (based on presence or absence of relative afferent pupillary defect [APD]).
4. Zone of injury (defined by anteroposterior location).

To improve communication among physicians and to increase accuracy in clinical practice and research, a new, internationally standardized classification of ocular trauma terminology, which describes type of injury, has been developed (▶ Table 32.1).[17] The prognosis for visual recovery in each of these categories depends greatly on the ocular structures involved and the extent of the injury. In blunt trauma, damage depends on the tensile strength of the tissues involved. When these limits are exceeded, injury ranges from lid ecchymosis to fractures of the bony orbit or rupture of the globe. In penetrating ocular trauma, the extent of damage depends on the offending object, the site of entry, the depth of penetration, and the number of ocular structures disrupted. Similarly, in perforating trauma, injury depends on the same variables, with the addition of the location of the exit site. In ocular injuries resulting from penetration and retention of IOFBs, the extent of damage depends on the size and type of the foreign body, the velocity on impact, the site of impact, and the intraocular course.

Several studies looked into identifying factors that would be most predictive of visual recovery. Poor visual acuity and a relative APD on presentation have been consistently proven to be most predictive of both functional and anatomical outcome. One retrospective review of penetrating eye injuries demonstrated that eyes with a presenting visual acuity of 20/800 or better were 28 times more likely to achieve a final visual acuity of 20/800 or better compared to eyes presenting with a visual acuity of less than 20/800.[18] In another study, only 3% of eyes presenting with hand motions vision or better underwent enucleation, versus 39 to 89% of eyes presenting with light

Table 32.1 Standardized classification of ocular trauma terminology (Birmingham Eye Trauma Terminology)

Term	Definition
Eyewall	Sclera and cornea
Closed-globe injury	The eyewall does not have a full-thickness wound
Open-globe injury	The eyewall does have a full-thickness wound
Rupture	Full-thickness eyewall wound caused by a blunt object; the impact results in a momentary increase of the intraocular pressure and an inside-out injury mechanism
Laceration	Full-thickness wound of the eyewall, usually caused by a sharp object; the wound occurs at the impact site by an outside-in mechanism
Penetrating injury	Single laceration of the eyewall, usually caused by a sharp object
Intraocular foreign body injury	Retained foreign object(s) causing entrance laceration(s)
Perforating injury	Two full-thickness lacerations (entrance plus exit) of the eyewall, usually caused by a sharp object or missile

Table 32.2 Calculating the ocular trauma score: Variables and raw points

Variable	Raw points
Initial vision	
• NLP	60
• LP/HM	70
• 1/200 to 19/200	80
• 20/200 to 20/50	90
• >20/40	100
Rupture	-23
Endophthalmitis	-17
Perforating injury	-14
Retinal detachment	-11
Afferent pupillary defect	-10

HM, hand motion; LP, light perception; NLP, no light perception. Adapted from Kuhn F, Pieramici DJ. Ocular Trauma. Thieme. NY: 2002

Table 32.3 Calculating the ocular trauma score (OTS): Conversion of raw points into an OTS category, and calculating the likelihood of the final visual acuity in five categories

Sum of raw points	OTS	No light perception (%)	Light perception (%)	1/200 to 19/200 (%)	20/200 to 20/50 (%)	>20/40 (%)
0–44	1	74	15	7	3	1
45–65	2	27	26	18	15	15
66–80	3	2	11	15	31	41
81–91	4	1	2	3	22	73
92–100	5	0	1	1	5	94

Adapted from Kuhn F, Pieramici DJ. Ocular Trauma. Thieme. NY: 2002

perception or no light perception visual acuity, respectively.[19] With respect to the presence or absence of an APD, a multivariate analysis of 240 traumatized eyes found that 69% of eyes without an APD achieved a final visual acuity of 20/200 or better, compared to 34% of eyes with an APD.[20] A recent retrospective study of patients with open-globe injuries requiring vitrectomy showed that presence or absence of an APD was a significant predictive factor for visual outcome, while retinal detachment on initial presentation was predictive of anatomical outcome.[21]

The zones of eye injury were defined based on review of operative reports of open-globe repair and were grouped as such: zone I (cornea and limbus), zone II (anterior sclera within 5 mm of the limbus), and zone III (sclera 5 mm posterior from the limbus).[16,22]

The most recent advancement in predicting visual outcome in traumatized eyes comes from the development of an ocular trauma score (OTS) in 2002 by Kuhn et al. The authors analyzed 2,500 eye injuries and 100 variables. After statistical analysis, six variables were found to have prognostic significance in predicting long-term visual acuity in an injured eye. Each variable was assigned a raw point value and, based on the numerical sum of those points, an OTS on a scale from 1 to 5 was developed (▶ Table 32.2 and ▶ Table 32.3). Based on OTS, the physician can counsel the patient and family regarding triage, management, and expectations; decrease anxiety and some elements of uncertainty; and plan, evaluate, and reassess interventions in a standardized fashion.[23]

32.2 History and Examination

As with any medical emergency, the stability of the patient takes first priority. Because one-third to one-half of ocular injuries are associated with concomitant nonocular injuries,[24,25] a general neurologic and systemic examination, including assessment of vital signs, mental status, cardiac and pulmonary function (to rule out chest trauma), and the extremities (to rule out fractures), should be performed initially. For example, an elderly patient with previously normal mental status appeared in our emergency department confused after falling and sustaining blunt trauma to the eye and orbit. Although she had an open globe, her expanding subdural hematoma took medical precedence over any ocular damage. When it has been determined that other critical systems are stable and/or uninvolved, it is safe to proceed with the ophthalmic evaluation.

Pearls

- One-third to one-half of ocular injuries are accompanied by nonocular injuries. A comprehensive systemic evaluation is an important part of the initial work-up.

A detailed history of the injury is an essential part of the initial evaluation; it helps to guide management and clarify any medicolegal issues that may arise later. Important questions include the following:

- How did the injury occur (e.g., hammering metal on metal)?
- When did the injury occur?
- Where did the injury occur (e.g., work-related)?
- Was the patient wearing protective eyewear, glasses, or contact lenses?
- What emergency measures were taken (e.g., irrigation, tetanus, antibiotics)?
- Is there a possible IOFB?
- When was the patient's last meal (to time surgical intervention)?

Examination of both eyes should proceed with due caution. Excessive pressure on an open globe may result in extrusion of intraocular contents and further damage. The most critical components of the initial ocular examination are the visual acuity and pupillary examination for the reasons mentioned in the previous section. Careful external and slit-lamp examination can reveal orbital or facial bony abnormalities, subdermal air (crepitus), entry wounds, hyphema, lens rupture, prolapsed uvea or vitreous, and other anterior or posterior segment pathology. However, opening the lids of an uncooperative patient, such as a child or an inebriated patient, should be deferred until the patient is under anesthesia. The intraocular pressure should be measured in all cases unless there is an obvious anterior rupture site. If visualization of the lens, vitreous cavity, and retina is prevented by a miotic pupil, sterile dilating drops may be used to achieve mydriasis. The more information obtained during this initial examination, the better equipped the physician will be to make management decisions and plan any surgical intervention that may be needed.

32.3 Ancillary Tests

Ancillary tests, particularly various imaging modalities, are often used to help guide the timing or type of any necessary invasive procedure (▶ Table 32.4). The single most useful test in the initial evaluation of the ocular injury is *computed tomography* (CT). The physician ordering a CT scan should specify that the study include 1- to 1.5-mm axial and coronal cuts through the orbits and chiasm. If a small foreign body is suspected, overlapping slices may be requested.[26] CT can localize foreign bodies (▶ Fig. 32.1) and demonstrate scleral abnormalities and intraocular blood, and is the best imaging study for bones (▶ Fig. 32.2). However, bone-free projections are used to detect small radiolucent foreign bodies.[27] In an experimental study, investigators

Table 32.4 Comparison of imaging modalities

Imaging study	Metallic foreign body	Organic foreign body	Bone	Soft tissue	Foreign body localization
Computed tomography	+	+	++	+	±
Magnetic resonance imaging	-	+	-	++	+
Echography	+	±	±	+	+
Plain x-ray	+	±	+	-	-

+ and - signs indicate how well each one of the listed imaging modalities detects the listed materials/tissues.

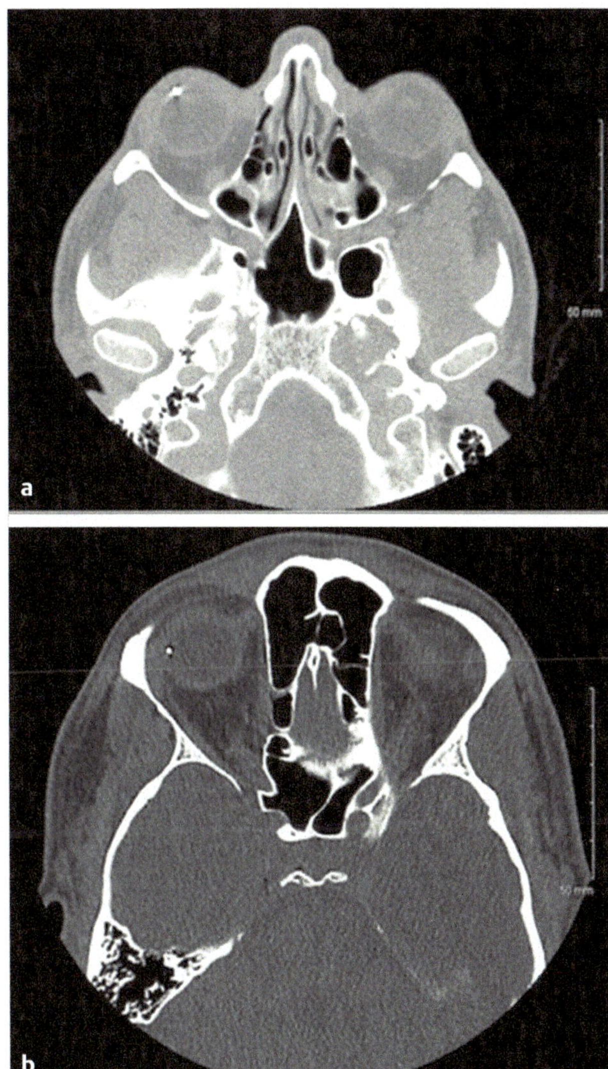

Fig. 32.1 (**a**) Computed tomography (CT) demonstrating metallic intraocular foreign body in the anterior chamber angle. (**b**) CT scan demonstrating metallic intraocular foreign body, which impacted the retina. Fortunately, minimal damage was done to surrounding tissues and the patient's visual acuity recovered to 20/25 after IOFB removal.

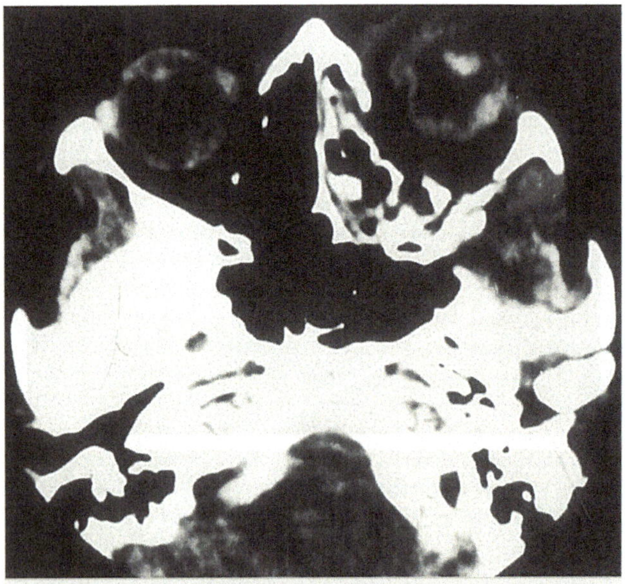

Fig. 32.2 Computed tomography (bone windows) demonstrating intraocular blood, an irregular scleral contour indicating a possible rupture site, and a tripod fracture.

implanted 21 metallic and nonmetallic foreign bodies in bovine eyes.[28] Except for polymethyl methacrylate intraocular lens (IOL), all objects (including glass, ceramic, metals, wood, stone, and porcelain) were visualized on CT. However, six of the objects (all metals) appeared 50 to 100% larger than their true size.

Pearls

- The single most useful ancillary test in the initial evaluation of ocular injury cases is CT.

CT has two main limitations. The first is that beam hardening (or scattering) artifact from metal may make exact localization or characterization of a metallic foreign body difficult. The second is that plastic and wood foreign bodies are low in Hounsfield units (similar to air) and, therefore, may not be apparent on CT.

32.3.1 B-scan Ultrasonography

B-scan ultrasonography is another useful imaging modality. It has resolution capabilities of up to 1 mm. Echographic examination is primarily useful in evaluating the lens and posterior segment when direct examination is precluded by media opacities (▸ Fig. 32.3). Ultrasonography is reliable in detecting vitreous incarceration, choroidal detachment, vitreous hemorrhage, vitreous separation, retinal tears and detachment, and areas of vitreoretinal adhesion. It is particularly useful in determining whether a small foreign body lies within or immediately outside the eye. A retrospective study of 46 eyes presenting with penetrating ocular injuries compared the preoperative echographic findings with the intraoperative findings. Echography proved 100% accurate in identifying retinal detachments, IOFBs, choroidal hemorrhages, and the presence of a posterior exit site, but posterior extensions of anterior lacerations were missed in 25%.[29] Echography can also detect the presence or absence of a lens, lens rupture or dislocation, and cyclitic membranes. Unfortunately, occult posterior scleral ruptures are often difficult to detect. Echographic clues such as incarcerated vitreous (▸ Fig. 32.4), retinal thickening or detachment, irregular scleral contours, decreased scleral reflectivity, and episcleral hemorrhage in the adjacent space may support a suspected diagnosis of scleral rupture. When the globe is open, echographic examination must be performed very gently and through closed lids, which can limit the resolution power. The usefulness of echography is also limited by shadowing caused by highly reflective surfaces such as air, reverberation artifacts created by some IOFBs, and the extent of the user's skill and familiarity with ocular pathology.[30]

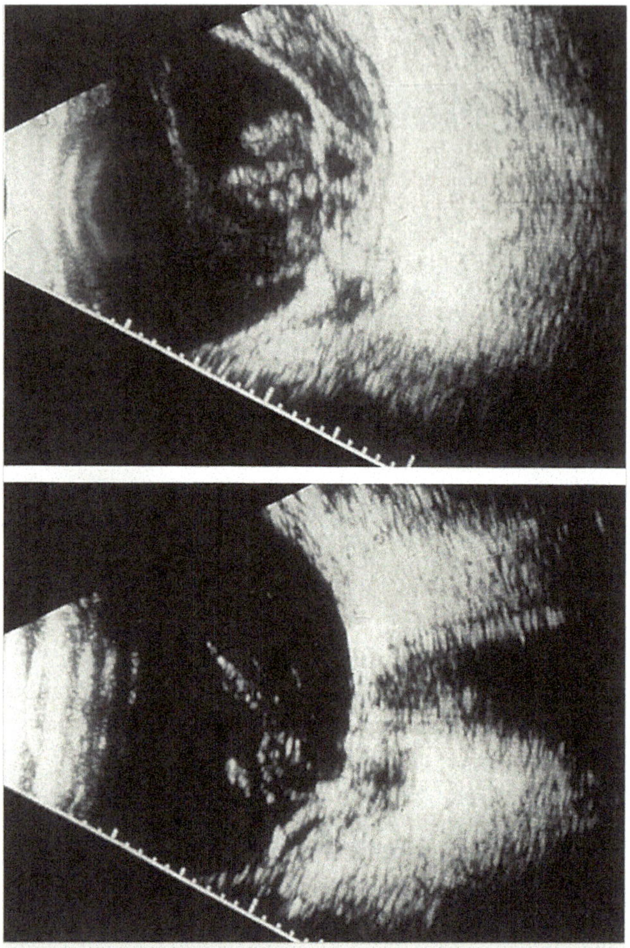

Fig. 32.3 B-scan ultrasonography of an eye with a perforating injury demonstrating vitreous strands to the wound, hemorrhagic choroidal detachment, retinal detachment, and a possible posterior exit site.

Controversial Points

- With an open globe, it is usually best to defer ultrasonographic examination until after the rupture site has been repaired. If an IOFB is suspected in this setting, CT should be used instead.

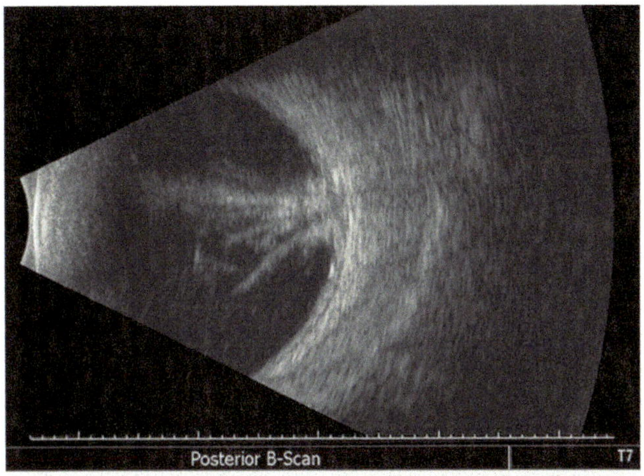

Fig. 32.4 B-scan ultrasonography of an eye demonstrating vitreous strands (highlighted by triamcinolone) to the wound. The cataract surgeon inadvertently injected triamcinolone acetonide into the vitreous cavity instead of sub-Tenon's space.

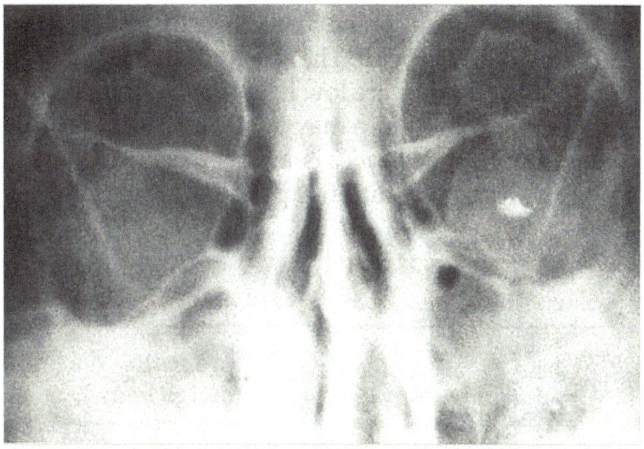

Fig. 32.5 Plain X-ray film demonstrating a metal foreign body in the left orbit. (In this view, it is not possible to know if the foreign body is intraocular or extraocular in location.)

32.3.2 Magnetic Resonance Imaging

Magnetic resonance imaging (MRI) has also been used in the evaluation of ocular trauma. Although the quality of MRI is excellent, it cannot image bone or metallic objects. Further, the magnetic fields and heat generated during MRI scanning preclude examination of patients with potential intraocular or intraorbital metallic foreign bodies. Investigators have shown that ferromagnetic foreign bodies implanted in animal eyes can move 7 to 8 mm in the suprachoroidal space and up to 10 mm in the vitreous space when subjected to the torsional forces of MRI.[28] In addition, retained intraocular ferromagnetic foreign bodies cause surrounding image distortion, making the globes themselves difficult to visualize. Image distortion can similarly occur from the paramagnetic effects in granite, solder, and mascara. The principle advantage of MRI over CT scan is that the former provides superior imaging of intraocular structures, accurately and safely detects vegetable, plastic, glass, and other radiolucent foreign bodies, and is safe during pregnancy.

32.3.3 Plain Roentgenograms

Plain roentgenograms are useful imaging studies to characterize the number and shape of metallic foreign bodies (▶ Fig. 32.5). Often, roentgenography is the first imaging study performed when the question of a foreign body exists. However, plain x-ray films may not detect nonmetallic objects or accurately determine whether objects are intraocular or intraorbital. Because of these limitations, many surgeons do not routinely use plain films and instead proceed directly to CT to expedite the initial evaluation.

32.3.4 Flash Visual Evoked Potential

Flash visual evoked potential (VEP) studies have been used as a prognostic examination. VEP is a measure of mass retinal response, providing information on central visual function. Patients with ocular trauma and normal VEP findings have been shown to have a mean visual acuity outcome of 20/100. In contrast, those with an absent response had a mean visual acuity of hand motions.[31] In the setting of a ruptured globe, this test would be performed after the eye has undergone the primary repair. Unfortunately, this test is not available in most eye centers.

32.3.5 Electroretinogram

Electroretinogram (ERG) can be used to gauge the visual potential of an injured eye in the setting of a nonverbal patient. It can also be used to assess retinal toxicity if a metallic intraocular or intraorbital foreign body is present.[27] In one study, the authors suggest that use of ERG and VEP within 2 weeks after primary severe eye injury repair may guide further intervention such as major reconstruction or enucleation to avoid sympathetic ophthalmia.[32]

32.4 Preoperative Management

For known or suspected ruptured globe cases, the primary surgical procedure should be performed as soon as possible. In preparation for surgery, the preoperative management includes the following:

- Nothing by mouth
- Rigid shield over the involved eye
- No narcotics or sedatives
- Antiemetics as needed
- Broad-spectrum intravenous antibiotics
- Updated tetanus immunity
- Notification of the operating team
- Laboratory tests
  - Serum electrolytes, blood urea nitrogen, and creatinine
  - Screening for human immunodeficiency virus, sickle cell, hepatitis, drugs, and alcohol
- Possible imaging (e.g., CT)

32.5 Blunt Trauma

In an urban setting, 60% of all eye injuries are caused by blunt trauma.[13] The etiologic object in blunt trauma does not

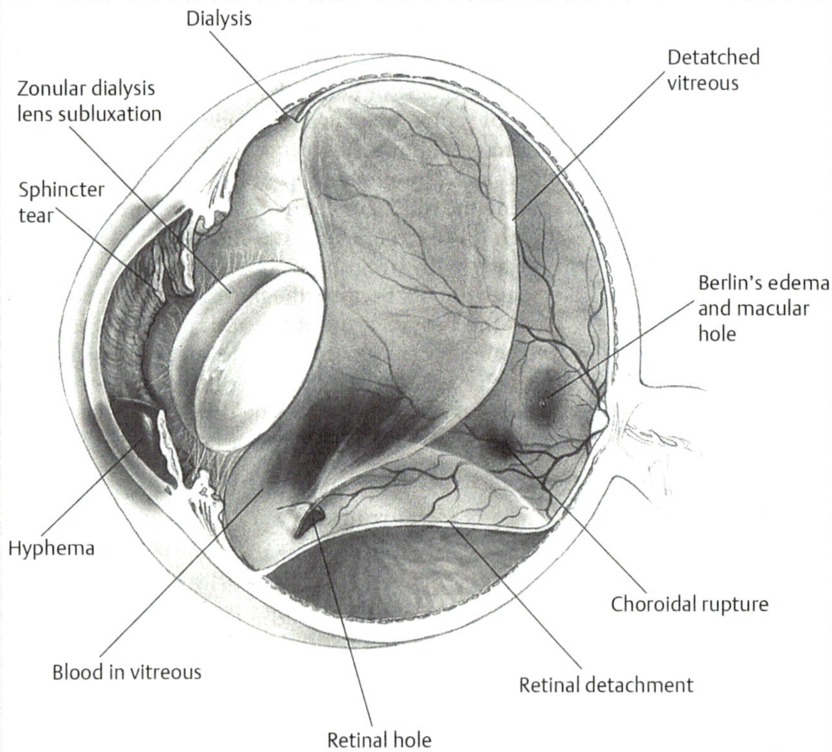

Fig. 32.6 Various intraocular injuries resulting from blunt trauma, including hyphema, iris sphincter tear, lens subluxation, posterior vitreous detachment, retinal dialysis, retinal tear and detachment, Berlin's edema, macular hole, and choroidal rupture with subretinal hemorrhage.

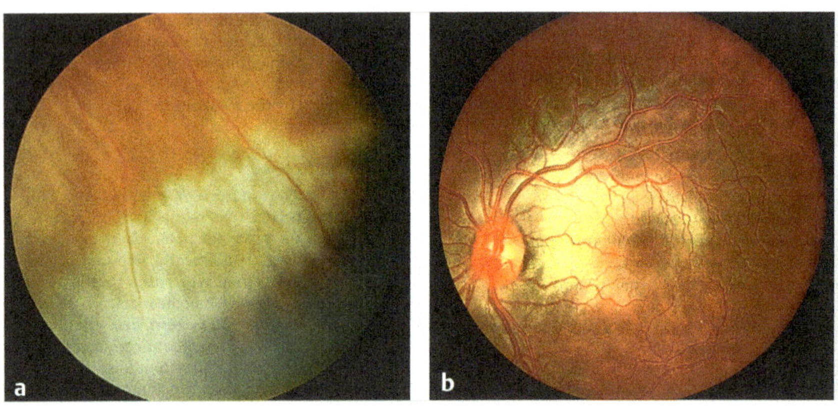

Fig. 32.7 Commotio retinae. **(a)** Retinal whitening in the periphery. **(b)** Retinal whitening in the macula (Berlin's edema).

penetrate the eye but may result in a variety of ocular injuries, including corneal abrasion, hyphema, iridodialysis, cyclodialysis, a dislocated or ruptured lens, vitreous hemorrhage, commotio retinae, sclopetaria, retinal tear or detachment, choroidal rupture, scleral rupture, and avulsion of the optic nerve (▶ Fig. 32.6). The damage incurred is a result of either direct tissue compression by the object or indirect tissue disruption by the resultant shock.

32.5.1 Commotio Retinae

Commotio retinae is a frequent complication of blunt trauma. It can occur in any retinal location but is most prominent in the posterior pole, where it is termed *Berlin's edema* (▶ Fig. 32.7). Clinically, commotio retinae appears as outer retinal whitening that is evident shortly after the injury. When the macula is involved, a cherry-red spot may be present, and visual acuity may be reduced to 20/200. Fluorescein angiography findings are usually normal, without leakage of fluorescein dye; however, breakdown of the outer blood–retinal barrier with leakage at the level of the retinal pigment epithelium (RPE) has been documented.[33] The retinal opacification was originally thought to be a form of retinal edema[34]; however, experimental and histopathologic studies have shown that it is the result of photoreceptor cell outer segment disruption and, perhaps, also some degree of damage to the RPE.[35,36,37] During the last decade, wide utilization of optical coherence tomography confirmed that the major site of retinal damage appears to be at the level of photoreceptor outer segments.[38,39] Typically, the retinal transparency and vision normalize within 4 days to 4 weeks of the injury as the photoreceptor outer segments regenerate. Although the prognosis for visual recovery is good, complete visual recovery occasionally does not occur, and this may be a result of underlying RPE damage or sometimes even secondary macular hole formation, the latter of which may be amenable to surgical repair.

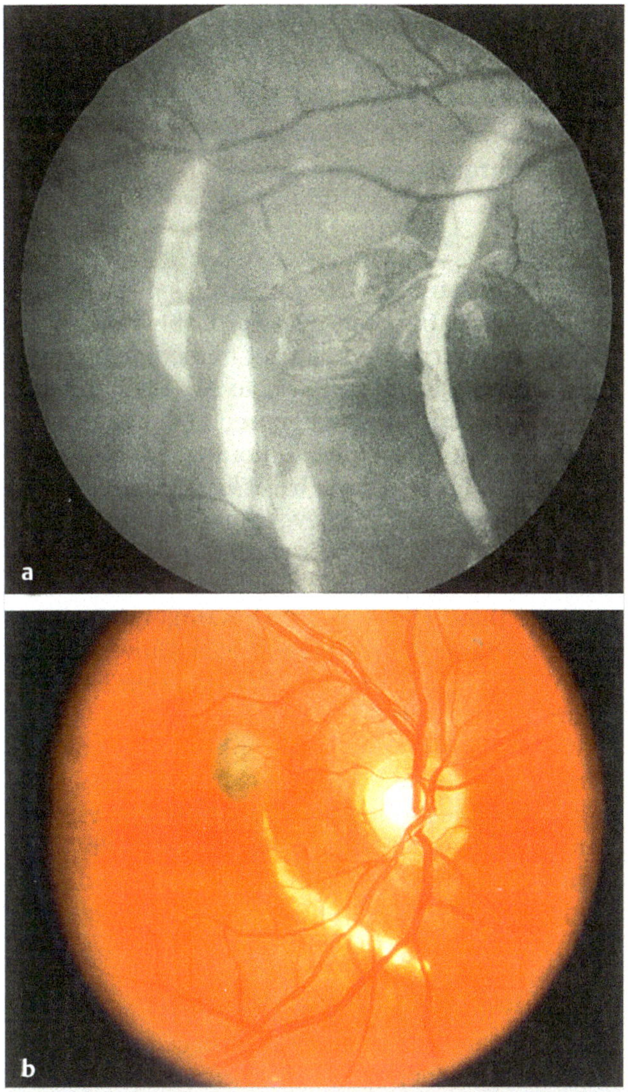

Fig. 32.8 Choroidal ruptures. (a) Multiple choroidal rupture sites in the macula with resolving subretinal hemorrhage. (b) Choroidal rupture site with secondary choroidal neovascularization (*subretinal gray-green membrane*) and associated subretinal fluid and hemorrhage.

32.5.2 Choroidal Rupture

When compression injury to the globe is sufficient, choroidal rupture(s) can result. Most often, the rupture is located posteriorly and is classically crescent-shaped and in an orientation concentric to the optic nerve head (▶ Fig. 32.8). Specifically, the injury represents rupture of the relatively inelastic Bruch's membrane and adjacent structures—that is, the overlying RPE and underlying choriocapillaris. Neurosensory retina, outer choroid, and sclera are intact. Of note, patients with angioid streaks are particularly vulnerable to choroidal rupture secondary to a brittle Bruch's membrane.[40] The curvilinear rupture site is yellow-white, but initially it may be obscured, at least in part, by subretinal and or sub-RPE hemorrhage. The associated blood at presentation is derived from the disrupted choriocapillaris. With time, the blood resorbs and varying degrees of surrounding RPE atrophy, RPE clumping, or subretinal fibrosis can be seen.[41]

Choroidal ruptures often occur in the macula and, in this location, usually result in some degree of decreased vision immediately (▶ Fig. 32.9). However, if the rupture is not directly under the fovea, either the vision is not affected or spontaneous visual improvement can occur once the adjacent thin layer of subretinal hemorrhage resorbs. Goldman et al reported successful pneumatic displacement of submacular hemorrhage associated with traumatic choroidal rupture with good visual recovery.[42] Late visual acuity loss can occur due to secondary choroidal neovascularization (CNV) at the edge of the rupture site (▶ Fig. 32.8). One study determined that proximity of the choroidal rupture site to the center of the fovea and its length serve as risk factors for development of CNV in traumatic choroidal ruptures.[43] Therefore, patients who initially have relatively good vision should be followed up regularly for the development of this complication, as early detection of CNV may allow for injections of anti–vascular endothelial growth factor medication or focal laser to help preserve vision (▶ Fig. 32.10).

32.5.3 Retinitis Sclopetaria

A concussive, nonpenetrating injury to the eyewall can sometimes cause disruption of both the retina and choroid,

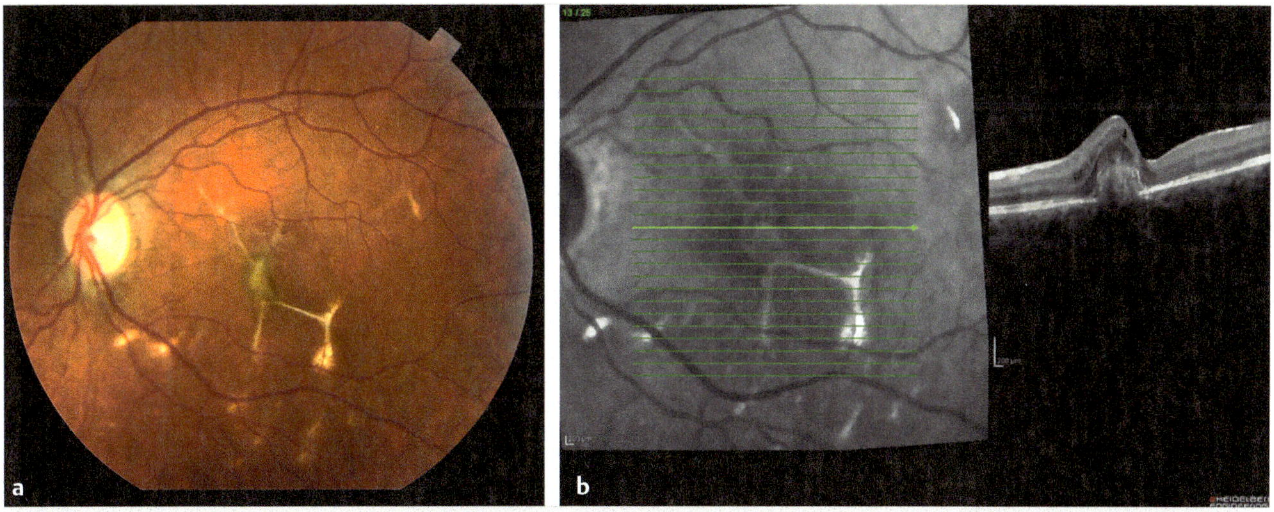

Fig. 32.9 (a) Color photograph demonstrating choroidal rupture after blunt eye injury. (b) Optical coherence tomography (OCT) demonstrating subretinal fibrosis and cystic changes in the overlying retina.

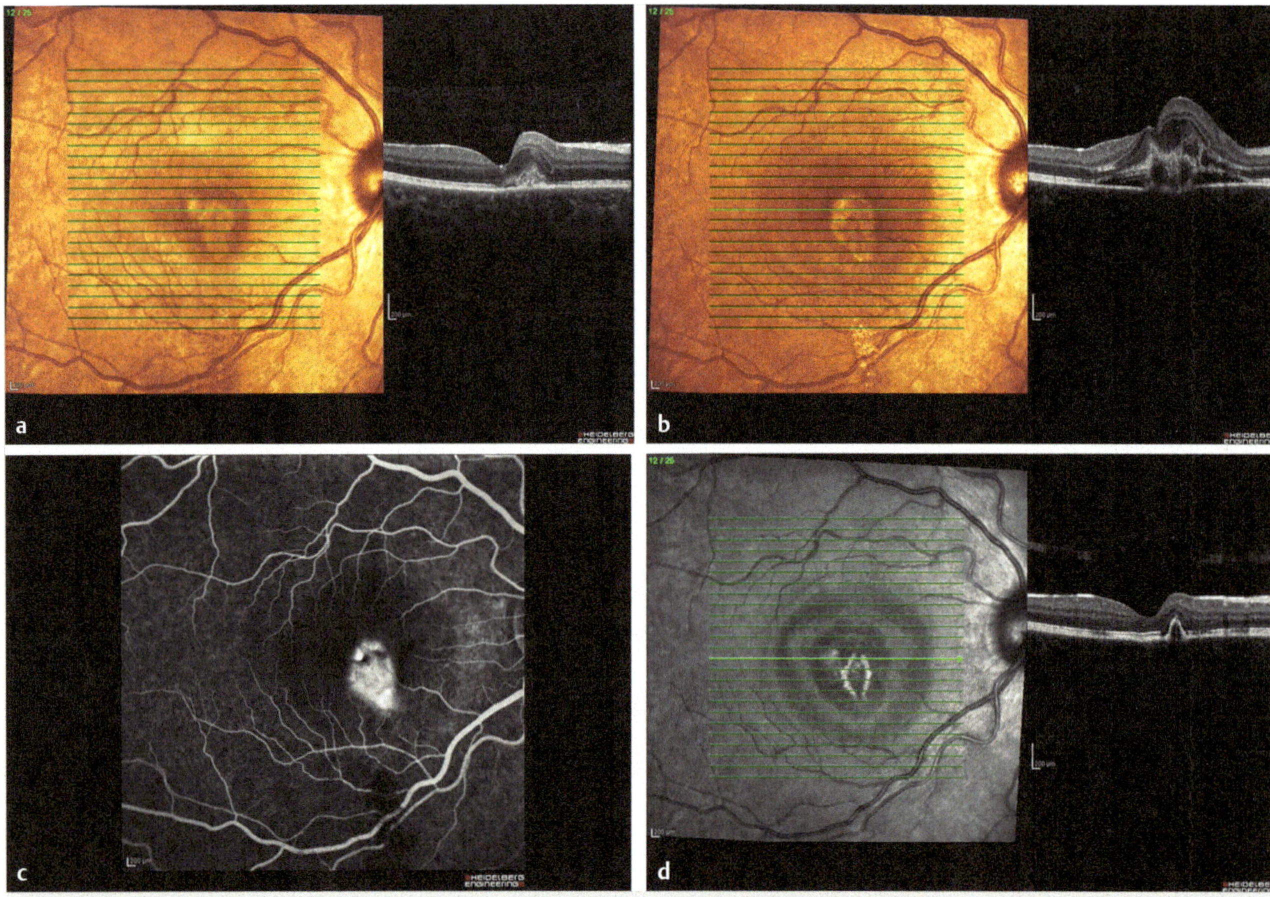

Fig. 32.10 Ocular coherence tomography demonstrating rapid onset of choroidal neovascularization (CNV) in a 20-year-old woman who suffered blunt ocular trauma. **(a)** Initial visual acuity was 20/40. **(b)** Within a month, her visual acuity declined to 20/400 as she developed CNV with submacular hemorrhage. **(c)** Fluorescein angiogram demonstrates dye leakage in the macular area. **(d)** After four injections of anti-VEGF medication, the fluid resolved and visual acuity improved to 20/25.

producing a clinical picture known as *retinitis sclopetaria* or *chorioretinitis sclopetaria*. This classically follows high-velocity missiles striking the orbit and traveling in close proximity to the eyeball, with the affected area usually located adjacent to the path of the missile (direct or coup injury) and in the posterior pole (indirect or contrecoup injury) caused by shock waves transmitted across the globe. On examination, those lesions frequently appear to coalesce.[44] Shock waves generated by the missile in the orbit are thought to be the primary mechanism of injury. Acutely, the ophthalmoscopic findings consist of large retinal breaks; surrounding areas of retinal opacification; subretinal, intraretinal, or vitreous hemorrhage; and areas of visible sclera. Initially, blood may dominate the clinical picture and obscure the retinal or choroidal disruption at first. As the blood resorbs, extensive chorioretinal scarring, typically with irregular, "clawlike" edges, becomes evident (▶ Fig. 32.11). Because the fibrosis often completely fuses the tissues around the retinal breaks, retinal detachment rarely occurs. Therefore, observation is all that is necessary in most cases. Should any retinal breaks appear not to be sealing down, however, laser or cryotherapy should be performed. If retinal detachment occurs, it is usually from another site.

32.5.4 Vitreous Hemorrhage

Among all patients presenting to an urban general eye clinic with vitreous hemorrhage, trauma was the underlying etiology in 18% of cases.[45] In patients younger than 40 years, trauma is the leading cause of vitreous hemorrhage.[45] Vitreous hemorrhage caused by blunt trauma results from damage to vessels of the ciliary body, retina, or choroid. The degree of hemorrhage varies but is usually visually significant, resulting in a visual acuity of 20/200 or worse in 74% of eyes.[45] Initially, the hemorrhages are often compartmentalized within a portion of the vitreous gel or in the subhyaloid space. Therefore, at the first examination, the location or configuration of the vitreous hemorrhage may provide clues to the origin. Particular attention should be paid to the peripheral fundus, with a search for retinal tears and detachments. The vitreous blood may eventually diffuse throughout the vitreous cavity, obscuring follow-up funduscopic examination. If a rupture site is evident or suspected, a depressed fundus examination should be deferred. If an adequate examination of the fundus cannot be performed, an echographic examination should be performed. Echography can accurately detect retinal detachments, posterior vitreous

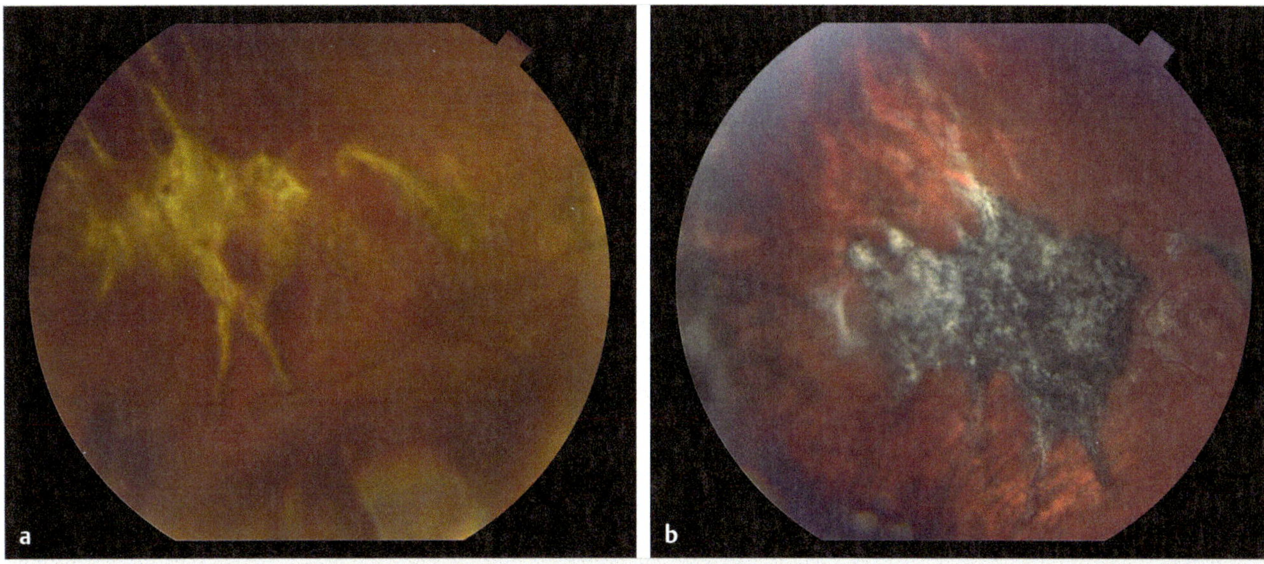

Fig. 32.11 Sclopetaria. (a) Subretinal hemorrhage and underlying "claw-like" chorioeretinal atrophy with fibrosis (b) Extensive chorioretinal scarring one year later after the hemorrhage resorbed.

detachments, and choroidal detachments. Retinal tears (without detachments) can also be seen, but small peripheral breaks may be missed; therefore, the lack of a retinal tear on ultrasonography does not rule out its presence. As mentioned earlier, occult scleral ruptures can be difficult to diagnose with ultrasound.

Special Considerations

- With a traumatized globe and significant media opacity, B-scan ultrasonography can detect retinal detachments and many retinal tears, but small peripheral retinal breaks and occult scleral ruptures can be missed.

The clinical information obtained from the examination and echography will direct management. In the absence of retinal tear or detachment, the patient should initially be observed with serial fundus and echographic examinations every 3 to 4 weeks. Bedrest with the patient's head elevated (30 degrees) at all times may facilitate clearing or settling of the vitreous blood. If a retinal tear is seen ophthalmoscopically, laser or cryotherapy should be performed to minimize the risk for subsequent retinal detachment. If a retinal tear is noted on ultrasound, it can be followed weekly with serial ultrasound examinations. During the follow-up period, the hemorrhage may clear and allow treatment. Some authors report success with ultrasound-guided cryopexy in patients with opaque media secondary to vitreous hemorrhage.[46,47] If a retinal detachment occurs, or if the hemorrhage is visually significant and does not clear within a few months, a standard three-port pars plana vitrectomy, with or without a scleral buckle, should be performed.

32.5.5 Retinal Tears and Detachments

Retinal tears and detachments can occur through direct and indirect mechanisms of injury.[48] Blunt trauma can cause anteroposterior compression of the globe and secondary equatorial expansion with traction at the vitreous base. This can lead to vitreous base avulsion, retinal tears at the posterior vitreous base, retinal tears at the pars plana (at the anterior vitreous base), and retinal dialyses. Direct impact to the eyewall itself (coup injury) can result in overlying focal retinal necrosis and ragged or irregular-appearing retinal tears at that site. Contrecoup injury from shock waves directed to a distant location, such as the posterior pole, can result in a traumatic macular hole. Of note is that head injury, without direct eye impact, is very unlikely to result in any type of retinal break or retinal detachment.

Retinal dialysis is the most common concussive retinal tear and is found in up to 84% of eyes with traumatic retinal detachments.[48,49,50,51,52] It is theorized that blunt trauma most often has its greatest impact on the eye in the inferotemporal quadrant, the location that is least protected by the orbital rim. This appears to account for the inferotemporal and superonasal predilection of traumatic retinal dialyses and other tears with coup and contrecoup mechanisms, respectively.[48,50,51,52] One prospective study found that 74% of traumatic dialyses occurred anterior to the ora serrata.[53] It is also important to distinguish retinal dialysis from giant retinal tear. In dialysis, the posterior edge does not roll on itself and become inverted because vitreous base is attached to posterior margin of the tear and posterior vitreous detachment is usually absent. Also, there is no radial posterior extension at the edge of dialysis, as is often present in giant tears.[53] Differentiating a dialysis from a giant retinal tear has a bearing on surgical approach and prognosis. A retinal dialysis may be accompanied by vitreous base avulsion (▶ Fig. 32.12). The presence of a vitreous base avulsion is thought to be pathognomonic for blunt ocular trauma.

Traumatic retinal tears are often multiple, found in the posterior vitreous base region, and located in the inferotemporal or superonasal quadrants. Although most traumatic tears probably occur at the time of the injury, they may not immediately lead to retinal detachment. Between 12 and 30% of "traumatic"

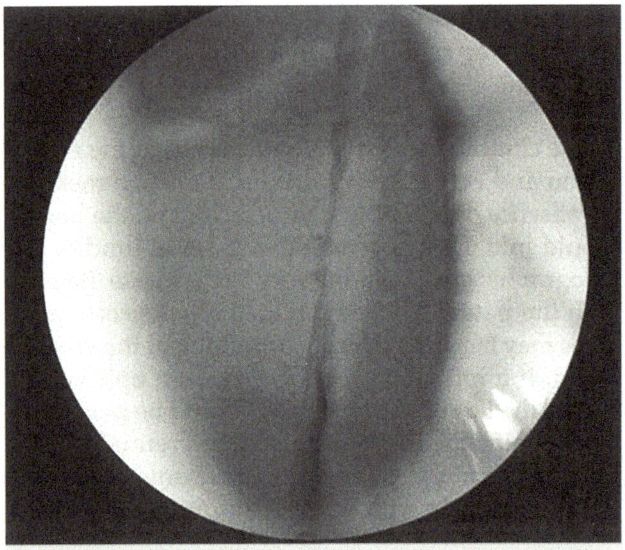

Fig. 32.12 Avulsed vitreous base with a linear band of pigment seen suspended just behind the lens in the pars plana region. (Image courtesy of William Tasman, MD.)

retinal detachments are diagnosed at the time of presentation, 30 to 40% within 1 month, and 80% within 2 years.[48,50,51] One study found that elapsed time from injury to detachment could be up to 40 years.[48] This is likely to be, at least in part, because most of the patients with eye trauma are young and, in such individuals, there is relatively little preexisting vitreous liquefaction. This also accounts for why many of these traumatic rhegmatogenous retinal detachments progress slowly and show signs of chronicity, such as multiple demarcation lines and intraretinal macrocysts.

Pearls

- Vitreous base avulsion is thought to be pathognomonic for blunt ocular trauma. It is typically located in the inferotemporal or superotemporal quadrants.

Most traumatic rhegmatogenous retinal detachments can be treated with conventional scleral buckling techniques alone unless significant vitreous hemorrhage or proliferative vitreoretinopathy (PVR) is present. Because traction may occur 180 degrees from the retinal break or impact site, we advocate using an encircling element.

32.5.6 Scleral Rupture

The National Eye Trauma System Registry from 1985 to 1991 found that posterior segment trauma occurred in 70% of assault-related eye injuries and 55% of the non–assault-related eye injuries.[14] The most serious posterior segment trauma is a scleral rupture. Of eyes that sustain severe blunt trauma, approximately 3.5% have a scleral rupture.[54] Because the thinnest portions of the sclera are at the limbus and under the insertions of the rectus muscles, scleral ruptures from blunt trauma most commonly occur in these locations.[55]

Diagnosing a scleral rupture in a patient with concurrent lid or orbital trauma can be difficult. Clinical findings with the greatest positive predictive value of a scleral rupture include severe periocular or intraocular hemorrhage with concurrent visual acuity of less than hand motions, intraocular pressure less than 5 mm Hg, anterior chamber depth asymmetry, and/or inability to visualize fundus details.[54,55,56] Although a low intraocular pressure may indicate a scleral rupture, normal or elevated intraocular pressure may also occur. Slit-lamp biomicroscopy may demonstrate vitreous streaming toward the rupture site. As discussed earlier, ancillary imaging studies may assist in the diagnosis of an occult rupture. If, however, the diagnosis is still in question, exploratory surgery must be performed.

Repair of scleral ruptures can be challenging. A 360-degree limbal peritomy should be performed with exploration of the entire globe. The examination should not be discontinued after one scleral rupture has been identified, as some eyes will have additional rupture sites. If the entirety or a portion of the wound is accessible, primary repair of each wound should be performed as it is found (suturing techniques are discussed in detail in the section on perforating injuries). If the wound extends very far posteriorly, complete closure may not be possible without undue pressure or deformation of the globe and possible extrusion of intraocular contents. In such cases, it is best to allow the most posterior portion of a large scleral laceration to close spontaneously by fibrosis. Eventual surgical closure of very posterior sites during subsequent procedures may or may not be needed.

Unfortunately, the probability of restoring good visual function in an eye with a large or posterior scleral rupture caused by blunt trauma is poor.[19,57] However, with better surgical instrumentation and a better understanding of the pathophysiology, more of these eyes are now able to maintain some degree of useful vision.

32.5.7 Optic Nerve Avulsion

The optic nerve is about 45 to 50 mm in length and its intraorbital section (20–30 mm) lies in a redundant S-shape fashion to allow unrestricted ocular rotation and some axial displacement. The optic nerve can be avulsed in three locations: optic disc, orbital apex, and optic chiasm.[58] Lang in 1901 reported the partial rupture of the lamina cribrosa and the optic nerve fibers at the papilla after blunt trauma.[59] Since that time, acute partial or complete optic nerve avulsion has been well documented. The possible mechanisms for optic nerve avulsion include the following:

- Extreme rotation and forward propulsion of the globe
- Displacement of the eye when an object intrudes between the globe and orbital wall
- Shearing trauma tearing the pia of the optic nerve
- Abrupt increase in the intraocular pressure, resulting in "expulsion" of the lamina and nerve
- Direct injury to the intraorbital optic nerve by a missile or knife

The diagnosis of partial or complete optic nerve avulsion is usually established during standard ophthalmologic examination. There is usually some degree of visual acuity loss and a relative

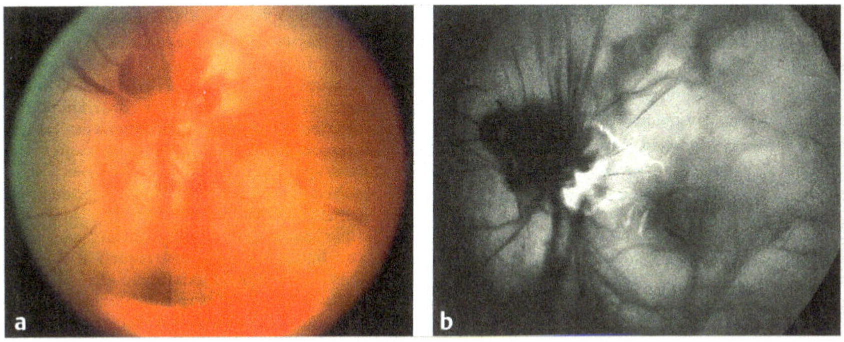

Fig. 32.13 Avulsed optic nerve. (**a**) Disruption of the tissue around the optic nerve head with vitreous gel and hemorrhage drawn into the area. (**b**) Corresponding fluorescein angiogram showing lack of retinal vascular filling and hyperfluorescence of the disc margin.

APD on the affected side. Ophthalmoscopically, there is a depression or excavation of the optic disc with a partial avulsion, and retraction of the entire nerve head within the sheath with a complete avulsion. Retinal vessels may either appear normal or end abruptly at the disc margin. Hemorrhage may be seen in the vitreous, prehyaloid, intraretinal, or subretinal spaces (▶ Fig. 32.13a). Fluorescein angiography shows a spectrum of retinal circulation patterns from normal to complete cessation of blood flow. Typically, there is hyperfluorescence of the affected disc margin in the late phases of the angiogram (▶ Fig. 32.13b). Histopathology reports demonstrate that the rupture occurs at the margin of the disc where Bruch's membrane terminates.[60]

The diagnosis of optic nerve avulsion is sometimes delayed because of a ring of vitreous hemorrhage that fans out from the disc, obscuring both disc and peripapillary details. Imaging techniques may be useful in making the diagnosis or ruling out other types of optic nerve dysfunction resulting from trauma, such as compression optic neuropathy. CT can accurately demonstrate complete nerve avulsion in some cases, but in others, it can be missed, probably because the nerve sheaths are usually intact. Nonetheless, CT may still be useful in ruling out other optic nerve problems related to the injury, as mentioned earlier. Although echography can also reveal an optic nerve avulsion directly by showing a defect in the anterior region of the optic nerve, only nonspecific findings, such as retrobulbar hemorrhage and increased optic nerve diameter, are evident in many cases. Therefore, echography is of limited value in this setting. In the realm of electrophysiology, the visual evoked cortical response is usually extinguished. ERG responses are highly variable, ranging from unrecordable to normal depending on associated damage to the retina. When the nerve is completely avulsed, glial proliferation can close the disc defect within 4 to 8 weeks of the injury, making the diagnosis sometimes more challenging if patients first present at this later stage. Electrophysiologic tests may help to support the diagnosis in such a scenario.

It is worth mentioning that optic nerve avulsion can occur at the anterior chiasm. Most of such cases are due to severe facial trauma, martial arts maneuvers, assault, and autoenucleation in psychiatric patients. A potentially devastating complication of such injury is that the visual field in the contralateral eye may be affected.[58]

There are no therapeutic options available that will alter the course of an avulsed optic nerve. Unless the avulsion is complete, in which case there will be no light perception, the final visual acuity is highly variable.

32.6 Penetrating Injuries

With current microsurgical techniques, the prognosis for achieving excellent visual acuity (20/60 or better) after a penetrating ocular injury is good. Predictors of excellent final visual acuity include a visual acuity of 20/200 or better at presentation, wound location anterior to the plane of insertion of the four rectus muscles (zone I or zone II), wound length of 10 mm or less, and a sharp mechanism of injury.[18,19]

Pearls

- In penetrating ocular injuries, predictors of excellent final visual acuity include a visual acuity of 20/200 or better at presentation, wound location anterior to the plane of insertion of the four rectus muscles, wound length of 10 mm or less, and a sharp mechanism of injury.

Certain basic surgical principles guide the repair of every open globe and are as follows:

- Restore the structural integrity of the globe.
- Reposit viable intraocular contents.
- Do not violate the visual axis, if possible.
- Avoid iatrogenic damage by minimizing intraocular manipulation during the primary repair.

These principles apply from the moment the patient arrives in the operating area and should guide the type of anesthesia, preparation techniques, and surgical procedures.

The type of anesthesia depends on factors such as patient age, level of anxiety, and health, and the extent and nature of the injury. In young, agitated, or anxious patients, general anesthesia is recommended. General anesthesia should also be used in patients with extensive lacerations, in patients with perforating injuries (even if only the anterior wound is being repaired), or in patients in which the extent of injury is unknown. Local peribulbar or retrobulbar anesthesia may be used safely in the repair of small corneal lacerations and in the removal of small IOFBs. We recommend giving a lid block when local anesthesia is elected, to minimize any potential pressure applied to the eye when patients squeeze their eyelids closed. The volume of anesthetic delivered should be kept to a minimum and delivered slowly to prevent excessive peribulbar pressure and consequent prolapse of intraocular contents.

The extent of the injury should be determined early on in the surgical repair. If a corneal laceration extends to the limbus, a conjunctival peritomy should be performed in that area, and the entire laceration should be explored. If a laceration extends under a rectus muscle that cannot be retracted easily, the muscle can be disinserted, isolated on a double-armed 5–0 or 6–0 Vicryl suture, and sutured back onto the insertion site after the laceration is closed. Particular attention should be given to possible vitreous or uveal prolapse or incarceration. In general, vitreous should be excised and uvea reposited, unless it is grossly necrotic. (This is discussed in greater detail later in this section.)

Following the basic principles of surgery, all wounds should be irrigated. We recommend irrigating the wound surface gently with balanced saline solution to debride the wound of possible foreign bodies, bacteria, and epithelial cells. If there is a clinical suspicion that the wound is contaminated or endophthalmitis is present, gently swab the wound, excise necrotic uvea, tap the aqueous humor, and send these specimens for culture and Gram's stain. The results of these cultures may help to guide future management of a possible infection.

"Simple" corneal lacerations without incarcerated uvea can be closed with interrupted 10–0 nylon suture. With the visual axis avoided if possible, sutures should be placed perpendicular to the laceration, with equal length and stromal depth on each side of the laceration (▶ Fig. 32.14). The ideal depth is about 80 to 90% of corneal thickness. Superficial passes may result in endothelial gaps and poor wound closure. Nonradial sutures may result in wound leaks and irregular corneal curvature. Long bites (1 mm from the wound edge) are preferable to shorter ones, as they are less prone to tear or "cheese wire" through damaged tissue and are easier to rotate, especially if the cornea is edematous. Manipulating the edges of the laceration with a forceps should be avoided, as macerating stromal tissue may prevent a watertight closure. If the arc of the 10–0 nylon cutting needle is utilized, a twisting motion can be used to pass the suture without need of another instrument for stabilization or counterpressure. If counterpressure is necessary, one can hold the limbus with a 0.12- or 0.3-mm forceps, or place forceps just distal to the exit site on the cornea. Closure of the wound can be achieved in a variety of ways, such as starting at one end and working to the other, or starting in the middle and continually bisecting the wound until it is closed. Most wounds are irregular, and the jagged edges provide landmarks for placement of cardinal sutures. Once the wound is stabilized, reinforcing sutures are then placed between the cardinal sutures. In such a fashion, the closure is most anatomic and minimizes irregular astigmatism. Because it is often difficult to predict how much tensile strength is necessary to close a wound adequately, it is often necessary to replace loose or tight sutures. Wounds can be closed more efficiently by using "slip knots" that can be adjusted as the wound is closed, which minimizes the time spent replacing sutures. Burying the knots of corneal sutures at the conclusion of the case improves wound healing and patient comfort.

Berdahl et al showed that dendritic polymer adhesive could be less traumatic than 10–0 nylon sutures in repair of full-thickness corneal lacerations up to 4.1 mm in length. Using an animal model, they showed that, at 28 days after repair, sutured corneas had much more inflammation, scarring, and anterior surface irregularity compared to glued corneas.[61] Prior to that, Velazquez et al, in their in vitro experiment on human eyes, showed that the corneas that were repaired with adhesive were able to withstand higher pressure in both stellate and linear lacerations compared to corneas that were repaired with suture, even though both methods were effective.[62]

Pearls

- Wounds can be closed efficiently by using "slip knots" that can be adjusted as the wound is closed.

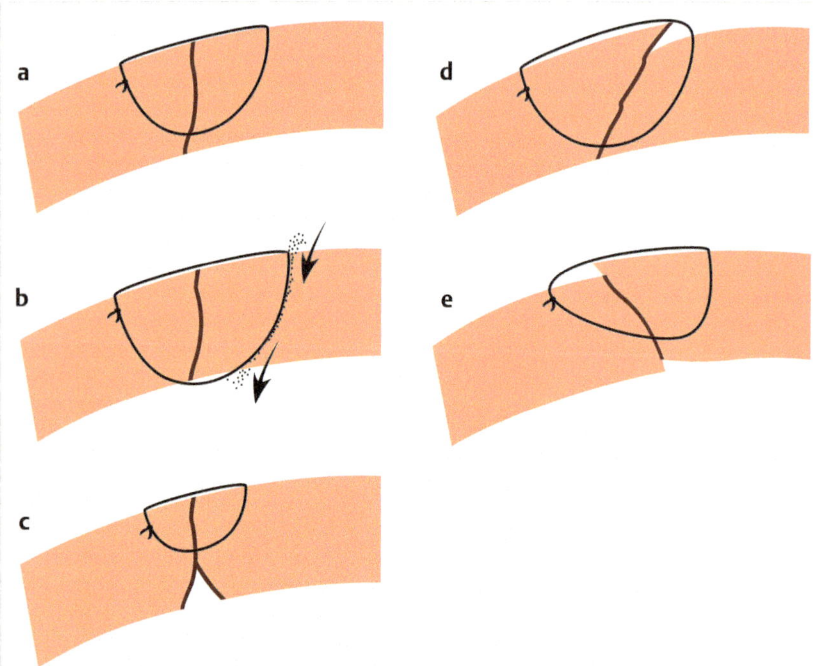

Fig. 32.14 (**a**) Proper suture placement for corneal lacerations. (**b**) Sutures that are too deep may serve as a tract for microbes to enter the eye. (**c**) Sutures that are too shallow can cause internal wound gape. Sutures of unequal (**d**) length or (**e**) depth can create wound override.

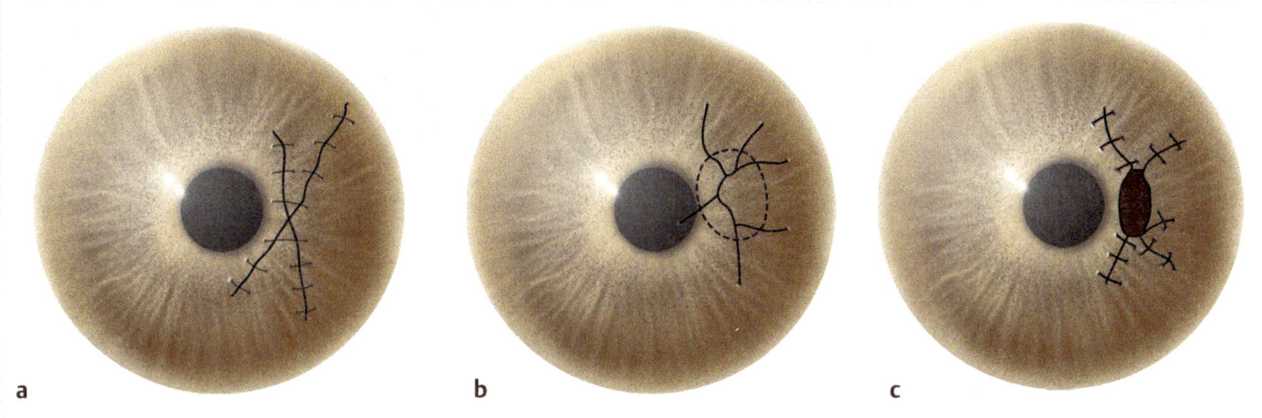

Fig. 32.15 Suturing to close stellate lacerations. Irregular surface appearance represents viscoelastic filling anterior chamber. Linear defect represent corneal laceration. (**a**) Interrupted, bridging sutures. (**b**) Purse-string suture. (**c**) Interrupted sutures and tissue glue.

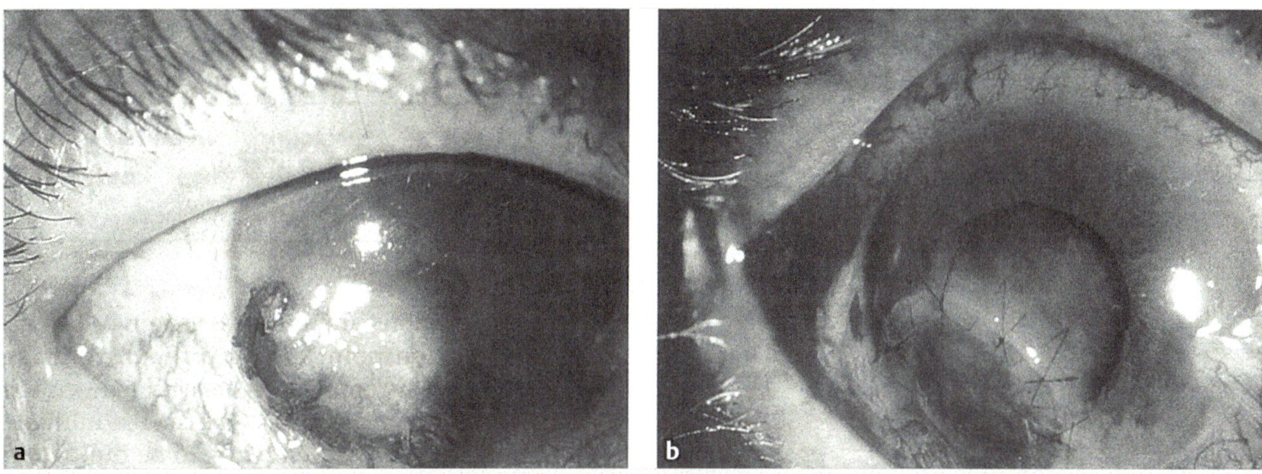

Fig. 32.16 Corneal patch graft for a large traumatic rupture of old corneal scar (**a**) before and (**b**) after surgical repair.

Stellate lacerations are more challenging to close, as the intersection point can be difficult to make watertight. A variety of methods have been described to seal such lacerations (▶ Fig. 32.15). One can use multiple crisscrossing sutures, but this method tends to be bulky and is often ineffective. Modified horizontal mattress sutures and purse-string sutures with the knot buried in the wound tend to produce the desired result. However, in some cases, the tissue at the intersection point is edematous, macerated, or missing, and a stable, watertight closure cannot be achieved. In cases with small leaks, cyanoacrylate tissue adhesive (Histocryl by Braun, or Bucrylate by Ethicon) can seal the leakage site. Because polymerization of the glue leaves a rough surface that can abrade the palpebral conjunctiva, a soft contact lens must be used after the glue has been applied. In cases with larger defects, a corneal or scleral patch graft may be necessary (▶ Fig. 32.16).

In corneal lacerations with incarcerated uveal tissue, it is best to try to control the intraocular contents before wound closure. When prolapsed uveal tissue appears very necrotic (usually when externalized more than 24 hours), it should be excised and sent to pathology for histopathologic examination and to microbiology for culture. Otherwise, as mentioned previously, uvea should be reposited. Before this is done, any epithelial membrane that has grown over the tissue should be either removed with a fine-tipped forceps or swept clean with a cotton-tipped applicator or dry cellulose sponge. A limbal paracentesis is then fashioned perpendicular to the orientation of the wound to provide the best lever arm for sweeping uvea from the wound. (For example, a paracentesis would be made at 12 o'clock position for a horizontally running laceration.) A blunt 27- or 30-gauge cannula attached to viscoelastic is inserted through the paracentesis and used to sweep the iris from the wound while delivering enough viscoelastic between the wound and iris to maintain a barrier to future iris prolapse (▶ Fig. 32.17). Too much viscoelastic will cause the wound to gap, making closure difficult and facilitating iris prolapse at another location. An alternative or supplement to this mechanical approach is to use miotics (e.g., acetylcholine and carbachol) to pull iris out of a peripheral laceration or mydriatics (e. g., neosynephrine and scopolamine) to help pull iris out of a central laceration.

With corneoscleral lacerations, landmarks such as the limbus or jagged corners should be approximated first using 9–0 nylon suture. The corneal component should be closed next with interrupted 10–0 nylon sutures, as described earlier. The scleral

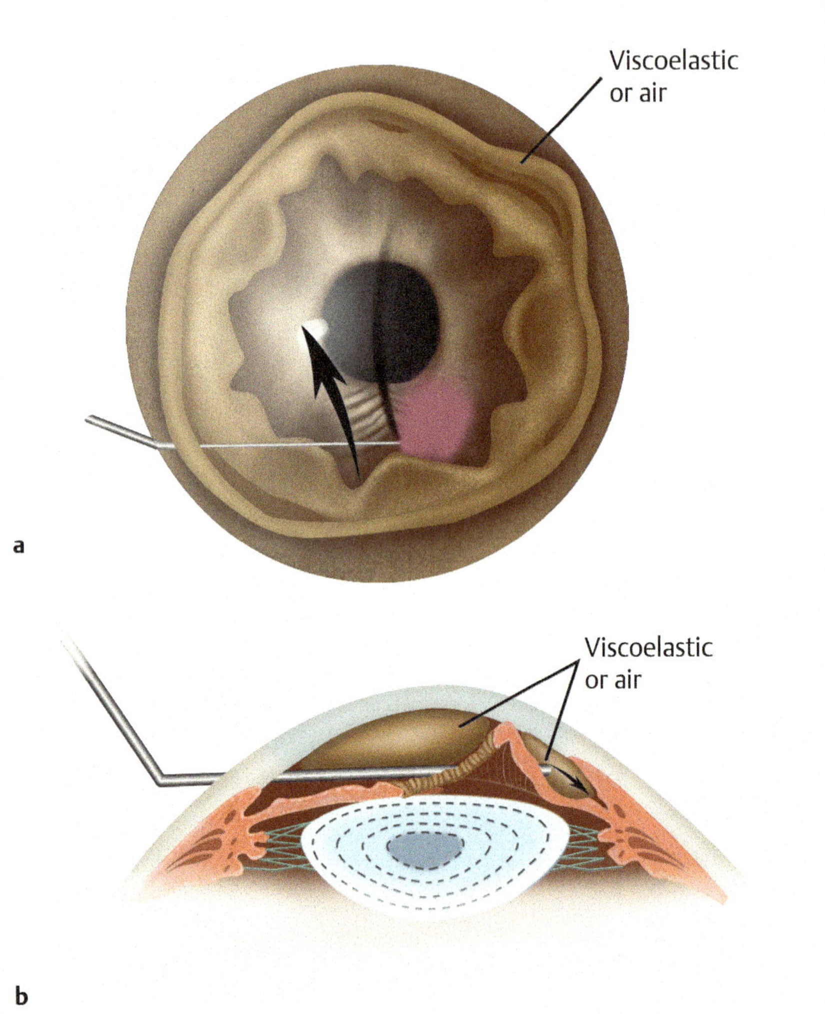

Fig. 32.17 Repositing iris by sweeping it from the wound and simultaneously injecting viscoelastic material to help seal the wound and maintain the anterior chamber.

component should be closed last with interrupted 8–0 nylon sutures, starting at the limbus and proceeding posteriorly. In some cases, the sclera can be closed nicely with a running shoestring technique, such as is used to close the incision made for a ganciclovir implant (▶ Fig. 32.18).

Pearls

- In some cases, a scleral laceration can be closed more efficiently with a running shoestring technique.

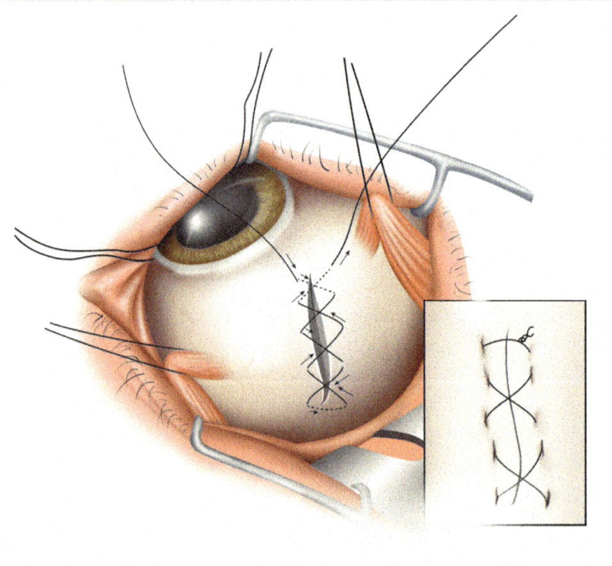

Fig. 32.18 Closing a scleral laceration with a running shoestring technique.

Corneoscleral lacerations are typically complicated by hyphema, lens disruption, uveal prolapse, vitreous prolapse, and sometimes even retinal prolapse. Again, the primary goal is to restore the integrity of the globe. Other considerations are secondary, such as lens removal or hyphema evacuation, and should be deferred to future surgical procedures when circumstances are more controlled. Incarcerated or prolapsed vitreous, uvea, or retina should be dealt with during the primary repair.

Vitreous should be excised from around the wound site, and this can be accomplished by using a dry cellulose sponge as a wick with scissors, the so-called Weck-Cel vitrectomy, or an automated vitreous cutting-aspirating instrument. When the vitrectomy instrument is used, care must be taken not to disrupt intraocular structures such as the lens, ciliary body, and retina. It is often best simply to clean around the wound without entering the site.

As noted earlier, all viable uveal tissue should be reposited. For uveal prolapse through the scleral component of the wound, it is often useful for the assistant to help reposit the uveal tissue with a blunt instrument such as a cyclodialysis spatula or the handle of a dry cellulose sponge while the surgeon places and ties the suture. We recommend passing the needle through each side of the wound completely and, utilizing slipknots, leaving the sutures loose. Once all the interrupted sutures are in place, the assistant holds the prolapsed uvea back with the blunt instrument as the surgeon cinches the sutures taut and closes the wound.

After the wound has been closed, intraocular pressure can be restored by injecting balanced saline solution via a 30-gauge needle passed through the pars plana. Before injection, the needle should be visualized in the vitreous space. If the visualization is prevented by media opacities, one should either slowly reform the eye via the anterior chamber (taking care not to break potentially weakened lens zonular complexes) or defer reforming the eye. Because the needle may be in the suprachoroidal or subretinal space, injecting blindly into the posterior segment is not recommended.

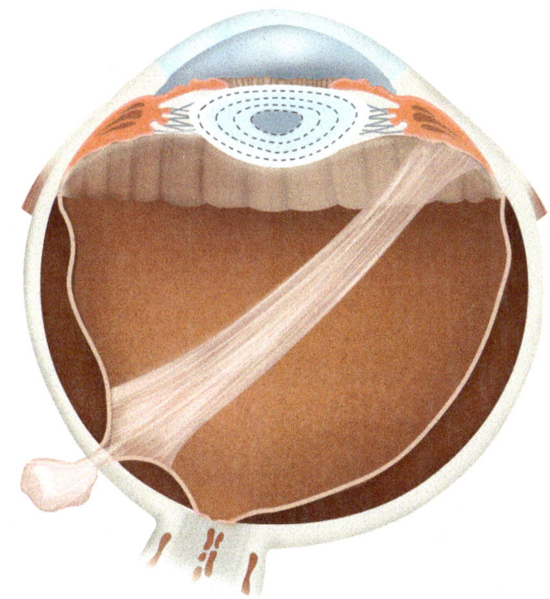

Fig. 32.19 Vitreous tract spanning the perforation sites; the vitreous tract can serve as a scaffold for fibrocellular proliferation and lead to complicated retinal detachments. (Modified from Tolentino FI. The vitreous in ocular trauma. Bull Soc Relge Ophthalmol 1987;223:179.)

Special Considerations

- During the primary repair of a ruptured globe, injecting blindly into the posterior segment for any reason is *not* recommended.

32.7 Perforating Injuries

In the treatment of perforating globe injuries, which by definition have an entry and an exit site, the same principles apply as for penetrating injuries. The prognosis for perforating injuries is poorer than for penetrating injuries[20,31,63] because immediate fibrocellular proliferation occurs along the scaffold of vitreous spanning the eye from the entry site to the exit site (▶ Fig. 32.19). This is a situation that is highly likely to evolve into a combined rhegmatogenous and traction retinal detachment.

The entry site should be repaired primarily with minimal intraocular irrigation, to avoid extruding intraocular contents through the posterior wound. Primary closure of the exit site is often difficult or impossible, and in most cases should be deferred. Experimental studies have shown that the posterior wound closes spontaneously within 7 days.[64] Therefore, a second procedure such as pars plana vitrectomy should be delayed for 7 to 10 days. These techniques are discussed in a later section.

32.8 Intraocular Foreign Bodies

Intraocular foreign bodies (IOFBs) are associated with 18 to 40% of penetrating ocular injuries and pose immediate and delayed threats to vision.[65,66] Acutely, foreign bodies cause mechanical damage and double the risk for posttraumatic endophthalmitis.[67] Delayed complications include PVR and retinal detachment, or toxicity from an oxidizing metallic foreign body (e.g., siderosis). Some compounds, such as plastic and glass, are well tolerated by the eye. In these cases, if there are no other complications, the eye can be observed after the entry wound is closed. However, in most cases the IOFB requires removal during or soon after the initial repair.

Historically, compared to nonferrous foreign bodies, ferrous foreign bodies were associated with a better prognosis because these could be removed with a magnet. However, with the advent of vitrectomy, the prognosis for visual recovery after penetrating trauma from any type of IOFB has improved dramatically. In a series reported in 1988, 79% of eyes with IOFBs achieved 5/200 visual acuity or better, with 60% achieving reading vision (20/40 or better).[68]

When choosing a surgical approach, it is helpful to know the composition of the IOFB, as well as its size and location. Often, the patient is able to tell you the composition of the IOFB. If not, family members can bring in the tool that the patient was using or a similar object (such as another BB or pellet), which can be tested for magnetic properties. However, because 80 to 90% of IOFBs are metallic and the vast majority are composed of iron, chances are good that the IOFB is magnetic.

As in penetrating and perforating injuries, the initial management steps should include a tetanus booster and broad-spectrum intravenous antibiotics. Other general principles in managing injuries with IOFB include the following:

- Restore the integrity of the globe first.
- Establish adequate visualization of the IOFB and important ocular structures before attempting IOFB removal.

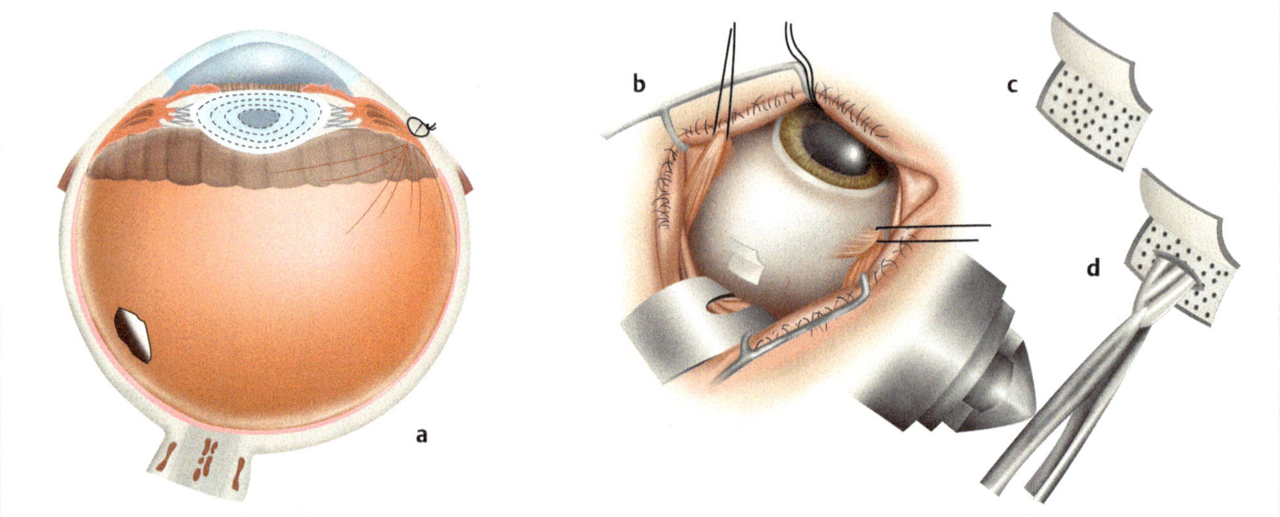

Fig. 32.20 Transscleral approach to intraretinal foreign body removal. (a) The location of the foreign body is determined by ophthalmoscopy. (b) A full-thickness scleral flap is then made over the foreign body. (c) The choroid is treated with diathermy and then incised. (d) The foreign body is removed with forceps and/or external magnet.

- Aim to minimize additional damage to the eye during removal:
  - Carefully plan the approach.
  - Make surgical wounds large enough to accommodate the extraction easily.
- Send the IOFB to microbiology for culture.

Foreign bodies in the anterior chamber or lens can usually be removed via a limbal wound. Many times an anterior chamber foreign body will fall into the inferior angle. Once the entry site is closed, reinflate the anterior chamber with viscoelastic via a paracentesis. Fashion a limbal wound large enough to accommodate the foreign body. Retrieve the object with either a forceps or magnet (if ferrous). The assistant can facilitate visualization with a gonioscopy lens. Irrigate the viscoelastic from the anterior chamber and close the surgical wound.

Intralenticular foreign bodies usually must be removed in concert with lens extraction. However, if the anterior capsule tear is small and the foreign body is composed of a nontoxic material, the capsular wound may fibrose, resulting in a localized, visually insignificant cataract that can be observed. If cataract formation has occurred, if the object is dirty, if the object is metallic, or if endophthalmitis is suspected, then both lens and foreign body extraction should be performed together.

Posteriorly located foreign bodies can be extracted in a variety of ways. Magnetic extraction has played an important historical role in the management of these cases and continues to be a useful alternative to vitrectomy. Some cases, such as a ferrous IOFB imbedded under the retina, are ideal for "trapdoor" magnetic extraction as opposed to pars plana vitrectomy (▶ Fig. 32.20). If visualization allows, the piece of metal is localized and the overlying sclera is marked. A full-thickness scleral "trapdoor" is fashioned, and the choroid is treated with diathermy. After the choroid is incised, the foreign body can be extracted with the magnet or forceps (touching the magnet to the forceps may further facilitate removal). The scleral flap is then closed with 8–0 nylon suture. If retina becomes incarcerated, a buckle should be placed. Because the choroid was treated with diathermy, cryotherapy is unnecessary.

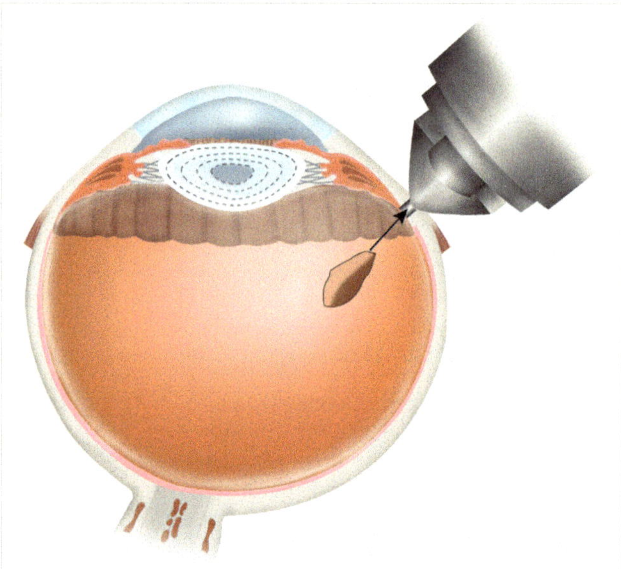

Fig. 32.21 Management of intravitreal foreign body with an external magnet held over a pars plana incision.

When an IOFB is removed from the vitreous with the external magnet, an area of the pars plana nearest to the IOFB and that is technically convenient should be used (▶ Fig. 32.21). The sclerotomy should be 4 mm posterior and parallel to the limbus in a phakic eye, and between 3 and 3.5 mm posterior and parallel to the limbus in an aphakic or pseudophakic eye. A radially oriented sclerotomy may extend posteriorly if a sharp IOFB is removed. The length of the sclerotomy should be large enough to accommodate the IOFB extraction. Preplacing a horizontal mattress suture will facilitate closure and decrease the chance for prolonged hypotony. While the external magnet is held over

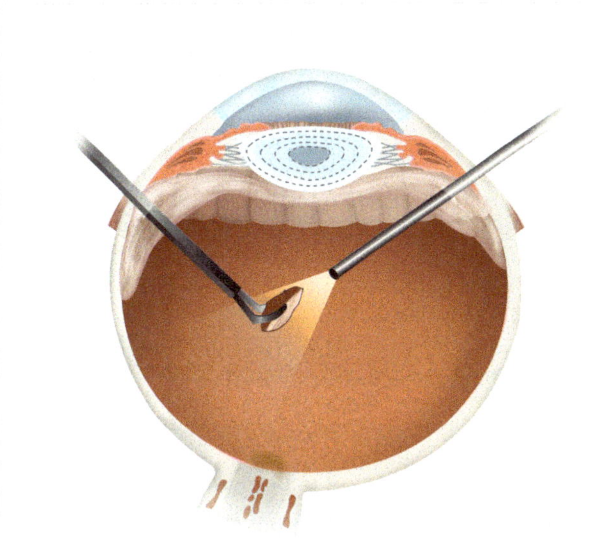

Fig. 32.22 Pars plana vitrectomy approach in managing an intraocular foreign body.

the sclerotomy, the IOFB can be observed with indirect ophthalmoscopy. Forceps may be necessary to remove the IOFB at the sclerotomy site. Magnetizing the forceps may help retrieve and stabilize the foreign body as you attempt to grasp it. Any prolapsed vitreous should be excised from the wound. Cryotherapy and scleral buckling in an eye without any other retinal pathology need not be performed.

Pearls

- Magnetizing the forceps may help retrieve and stabilize the foreign body as it is grasped.

Many surgeons prefer the control provided by pars plana vitrectomy (▶ Fig. 32.22). In eyes in which media opacities preclude an adequate view of the IOFB or status of the retina, vitrectomy is the best surgical approach. This can be combined with a pars plana lensectomy if there is a concomitant cataract. Pars plana vitrectomy will clear vitreous hemorrhage and release vitreous traction. Care should be taken to free the IOFB from the vitreous as completely as possible without allowing the object to roll around the eye. This can be accomplished by holding the IOFB with an illuminated forceps while performing the vitrectomy with the other hand. If the foreign body is engaged with the intraocular rare earth magnet, it should be transferred to a forceps before its removal, to prevent it becoming disengaged from the magnet, falling posteriorly, and damaging the macula.

Intraretinal foreign bodies are technically more challenging because retinal detachment can occur more easily than with an intravitreal foreign body. Once the visual axis is cleared of media opacities, the vitreous overlying the IOFB should be excised as completely and as safely as possible. At this point, the foreign body can be removed via either a transscleral or a transvitreal approach. When the transscleral approach is used, similar steps as described earlier should be followed. Again, if retina becomes incarcerated, a scleral buckle or radial element should be placed. When a transvitreal approach is used, the foreign body should be gently mobilized with the intraocular rare earth magnet, the intraocular forceps, or a pick. If the foreign body has been encapsulated, the capsule can be incised with a myringotomy blade and the foreign body then removed with the forceps or magnet.

In some eyes, a posterior vitreous detachment will already be present. However, because the majority of IOFBs occur in young men, it is likely that the posterior vitreous is still attached. It is important to create a posterior vitreous detachment in these eyes. If a posterior vitreous detachment is not obtained, postoperative vitreous contraction will likely result in retinal detachment or epiretinal membrane formation, as was seen in the early years of vitrectomy, when these complications developed in 90% of such eyes.[69] The posterior vitreous detachment can be created using high vacuum levels with either the vitrectomy instrument or a soft-tipped extrusion cannula, and carried out to the periphery with the vitrectomy cutter.

Eye injuries caused by BB pellets pose a special challenge to the vitreoretinal surgeon. These injuries have a grave prognosis; the vast majority of eyes either are enucleated or end up with nonambulatory vision.[70,71] Compared with other missiles, BB pellets are blunt and travel at relatively low velocity. If they penetrate the eye, they usually do not perforate the eye. Rather, they ricochet internally. Consequently, these missiles can cause significant intraocular damage. If the eye has maintained light perception, a vitrectomy should be attempted. Unfortunately, the size, spherical shape, and nonferrous composition of the BB make retrieval and removal difficult. Usually, the BB must be removed via the anterior chamber. After the wound is closed, a pars plana lensectomy/vitrectomy is performed. A limbal wound is fashioned. The BB is brought anteriorly, into the anterior chamber, and delivered through the limbal wound.

In some cases, the original corneal wound from the BB pellet is too large to close or precludes adequate visualization of the posterior segment. In these cases, the lensectomy and BB extraction may be best performed via an open-sky approach. A 360-degree conjunctival peritomy is performed. The four rectus muscles are isolated on 2–0 cotton suture, and a Flieringa ring is sutured to the sclera. The damaged cornea is trephined, removed, and placed in tissue culture medium. Lensectomy, vitrectomy, and BB extraction are then performed. If, thereafter, more intricate maneuvers and better visualization are necessary, a temporary keratoprosthesis can be used to complete the surgery.

32.9 Vitrectomy and Other Secondary (Delayed) Procedures

Secondary or delayed procedures for severe blunt trauma and penetrating or perforating injuries can be very complex because of myriad anterior and posterior segment conditions that can coexist, such as hyphema, cataract, suprachoroidal hemorrhage, vitreous hemorrhage, and retinal tears or detachments. The surgical repair requires a logical stepwise approach, beginning with a thorough preoperative assessment. Questions that are best answered preoperatively include the following:

- Will the corneal clarity allow adequate visualization of intraocular structures? If not, a keratoprosthesis or corneal graft will be needed.

- Will the surgery begin through a limbal incision or through a pars plana incision? Phakic or pseudophakic eyes will require a limbal incision to evacuate the anterior segment blood.
- Should the lens be removed, and if so, by what approach? The approach will be determined mainly by the status of the lens capsule or zonules and the presence of any associated pathology, such as cyclitic membranes and other posterior segment pathology.
- Are hemorrhagic choroidal detachments present? Hemorrhagic choroidal detachments should be drained before a vitrectomy is attempted. Preoperative B-scan ultrasonography not only will ascertain the presence or absence of choroidal detachments but also can provide information regarding the degree of clot organization or liquefaction through dynamic imaging (i.e., having the patient move the eye while the suprachoroidal space is imaged).
- What vitreoretinal abnormalities are present? Are retinal tears or detachments already forming? Is there incarceration of tissue into wound sites? Is PVR present? The surgeon needs to be prepared to perform complicated vitreoretinal maneuvers, such as membrane peeling or dissection and retinotomies. Surgical adjuncts such as perfluorocarbon liquid and silicone oil should be available if these problems are likely to be encountered.

The timing of any secondary procedures depends on the specific issue(s) to be addressed (▶ Fig. 32.23). Immediate intervention is needed for any suspected endophthalmitis. A delay of 7 to 10 days is usually best for managing choroidal detachments and most other posterior segment complications. Waiting several weeks or more for the eye to heal completely is ideal for penetrating keratoplasty or glaucoma procedures. A basic management scheme is outlined in ▶ Fig. 32.23.

The secondary repair of a severely traumatized eye with multiple problems should commence in a stepwise, anterior-to-posterior approach. However, often a scleral buckling procedure is required for a successful outcome. Some surgeons prefer to place an encircling band as the initial step in the procedure with final adjustments made at the conclusion of the case, whereas others prefer to place the buckle once visualization of the posterior segment is obtained. If the buckle is placed empirically, choose a wide element such as a 287 tire/240 band combination or, at the minimum, a 42 band. As with any scleral buckling procedure, the band should be placed under all four rectus muscles. However, in the case of a scleral laceration or rupture that could not be repaired primarily, particular attention should be paid to the fibrotic capsule overlying any portion of the scleral laceration. This capsule should not be incised. The buckle should be placed over the rupture to support as much of the area as possible. If the rupture is too posterior, the buckle should be positioned to support the vitreous base. Once the buckle is placed, bringing it to its final height should be deferred until the posterior segment is visualized and final adjustments can be made (i.e., adding radial elements and repositioning the buckle). Attention should then be directed to reconstructing the anterior segment.

If corneal opacities preclude adequate visualization of intraocular structures, a temporary keratoprosthesis will be needed. A penetrating keratoplasty should be avoided if at all possible, as postoperative inflammation significantly reduces the chance of long-term graft survival. If present, a hyphema is evacuated next. If the anterior chamber contains organized fibrin or blood clot, thrombolytic agents such as 10 to 15 µg of tissue plasminogen activator (tPA) can help facilitate its removal. For best results, at least 20 minutes is required for enzymatic clot lysis or fibrinolysis. Therefore, tPA should be injected into the anterior chamber either while the patient is in the holding room before surgery or as an initial step at the beginning of surgery before other procedures, such as scleral buckling, are begun. In aphakic eyes, the blood can be irrigated from the anterior chamber via a pars plana incision. A bent, 23- or 25-gauge butterfly needle connected to irrigating solution can be passed through a pars plana wound into the anterior chamber until adequately visualized, and the blood can be aspirated with the vitrectomy instrument by likewise passing it through a pars plana sclerotomy into the anterior chamber. In phakic eyes, anterior infusion can be delivered via a 21-, 23-, or 25-gauge butterfly cannula through a limbal wound or an anterior chamber maintainer. The blood can be aspirated or mechanically removed either with the vitrectomy unit or by delivering the clot through a limbal wound with the aid of an intraocular forceps (▶ Fig. 32.24). Because blood clots reach maximal consolidation by day 4 to 7, they are most amenable to removal in toto at that time.[70]

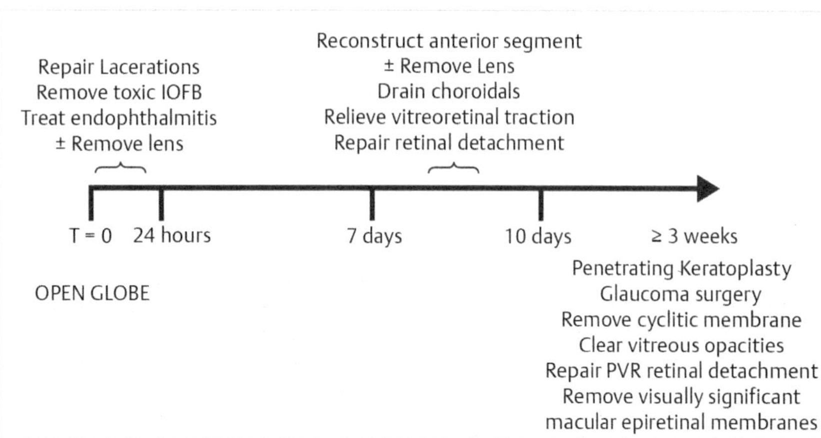

Fig. 32.23 General scheme for the timing of secondary (*delayed*) procedures.

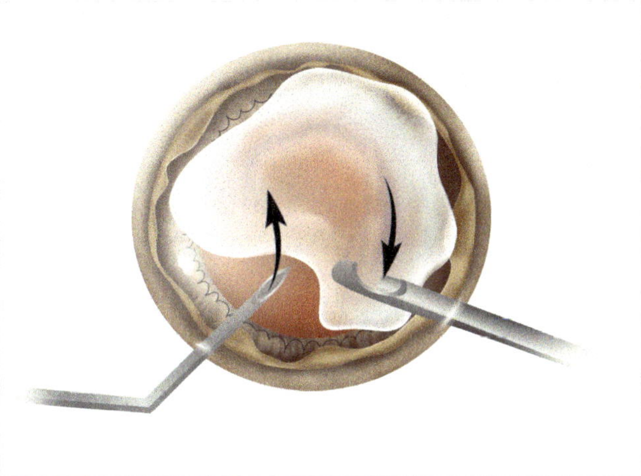

Fig. 32.24 Management of a hyphema in a phakic eye using a limbal approach: An angled 21-, 23-, or 25-gauge needle is used for infusion while the vitrectomy instrument is used to cut and aspirate the blood clot.

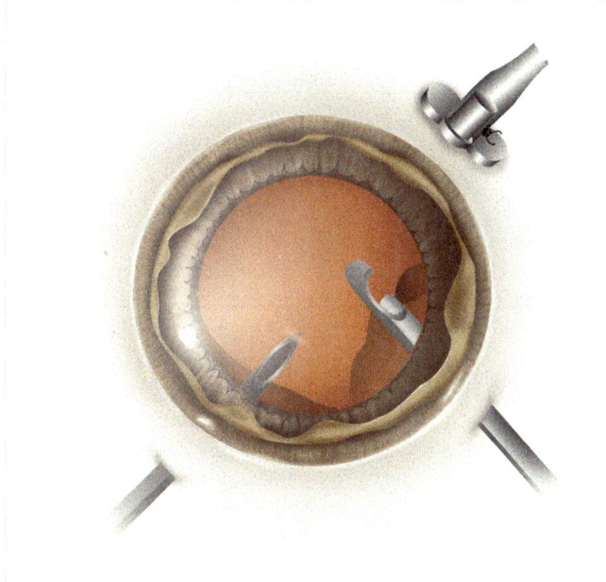

Fig. 32.25 Pars plana lensectomy. A vitrectomy or phacofragmatome instrument is used through one of the superior pars plana sclerotomies, and irrigation is supplied by a bent 20-, 23-, or 25-gauge bent butterfly needle (depending on the size of sclerotomy) placed directly into the lens through the other trocar cannula or sclerotomy.

Lensectomy is necessary in many cases to allow adequate visualization of the posterior segment. Furthermore, a unicameral eye enables safer and more complete anterior vitreous removal and membrane dissection, and facilitates postoperative care (e.g., fluid–air exchange, laser). Lens extraction can be performed in a variety of ways, depending on the preference of the surgeon, stability of the lens, and age of the patient. The softer lens in young patients can be aspirated with the automated cataract irrigation-aspiration instrument or a vitrectomy cutting-aspirating hand piece. The harder nuclei in older patients typically require phacoemulsification. Large wounds and extracapsular cataract extraction should be avoided in these cases. The lens can be removed via either the pars plana or limbus. We recommend the pars plana approach, as it minimizes the number of wounds and provides better stabilization of the lens. Sclerotomies should be placed 3 to 3.5 mm posterior to the limbus. With anterior infusion, liquefied choroidal blood can be drained from the sclerotomies; however, if uvea prolapses through the sclerotomy, the infusion should be stopped immediately. With use of a 20-, 23-, or 25-gauge bent butterfly needle (depending on the size of sclerotomies/trocar cannulas used) connected to irrigation through one sclerotomy and the phacofragmatome or vitrectomy cutter through the other sclerotomy, the lens and capsule can be removed (▸ Fig. 32.25). A complete excision is necessary to minimize any scaffold for subsequent PVR formation. If any lens fragments dislocate posteriorly, it is usually better to proceed with the vitrectomy before retrieving these fragments.

After the anterior media opacities are cleared, posterior vitrectomy is performed. It is critical that the posterior cortical vitreous be removed. In many severely traumatized eyes, a posterior vitreous detachment will have occurred spontaneously during the 7- to 10-day period. However, in some eyes, posterior vitreous attachment persists. In these eyes, a posterior vitreous detachment can usually be achieved with either automated or mechanical suction. It is critical to pay particular attention to vitreous traction on the edges of retinal tears, vitreous incarcerated in scleral wounds, vitreous attached to detached retina, and the vitreous base. If the anteroposterior and tangential traction to these areas cannot be alleviated adequately, they must be supported with a scleral buckle.

Once the vitrectomy is completed, the fundus must be examined thoroughly with a wide-angle viewing system or indirect ophthalmoscopy and scleral depression to look for retinal tears and detachments. All retinal tears should be treated with either endolaser or transscleral cryotherapy. Tears with persistent vitreous traction should be supported on an encircling buckle or radial element. If a retinal detachment is present, all traction to the causative break and detached retina must be relieved with membrane dissection and scleral buckling. Subretinal fluid is drained internally, either through the original peripheral retinal break or through a posterior drainage retinotomy. Internal tamponade of retinal breaks can be accomplished with the long-acting gases (e.g., perfluoropropane) or silicone oil.

Scleral lacerations and ruptures can be further complicated by incarceration of retina, which results in complicated retinal detachments. When retina is incarcerated anteriorly, it may be reattached with scleral buckling and vitrectomy. However, in some cases, particularly when retina is incarcerated posteriorly, retinotomy is necessary. This is performed most efficiently with an illuminated endodiathermy probe to provide hemostasis and either a vitrectomy instrument or vertical scissors to cut retina from the incarceration site. With these techniques, Han et al[71] achieved anatomic success in 73% of eyes; however, visual prognosis is still guarded, as only 40% of eyes in this series achieved ambulatory (5/200 or better) vision.

32.10 Prophylactic Scleral Buckling and Cryotherapy

A leading cause of poor visual outcome following eye trauma is delayed retinal detachment complicated by PVR. The Cleary–Ryan model of PVR utilizes a scleral laceration much like that seen in trauma patients. Retinal glial cells that have gained access to the inner retinal surface and vitreous cavity undergo metaplastic changes and acquire myoblastic features. Circumferential contraction of the vitreous base and anteroposterior traction of the fibroproliferative tissue, which may be incarcerated in the wound, commonly result in combined traction and rhegmatogenous detachments. Repair of such detachments is challenging, with a significant number of failures.

In the hope of countering the effects of PVR and preventing late retinal detachment, some clinicians have recommended prophylactic encircling scleral buckles in eyes in which the vitreous cavity has been penetrated. Published reports have demonstrated that the rate of delayed retinal detachment is reduced 43 to 70% in eyes prophylactically buckled in comparison with those not buckled.[20,31,72] It is presumed that the encircling scleral buckle reduces the tractional forces present within a traumatized eye, thereby decreasing the risk for delayed retinal detachments. Unfortunately, these studies likely have a selection bias, and a controlled clinical trial has not been performed to assess adequately the theoretic benefits of prophylactic scleral buckling. Most surgeons prefer to wait until the secondary repair to decide whether or not to use a scleral buckle rather than place it empirically at the initial repair of the ruptured globe. If used, the buckle should be relatively broad and positioned to support the entire vitreous base region.

Controversial Points

- Some clinicians recommend prophylactic scleral buckles in eyes in which the vitreous cavity has been penetrated.

Cryotherapy applied along the extent of the scleral laceration during the primary repair has been debated, but this practice has fallen out of favor. The theoretic benefit of cryotherapy is to increase the retinal adhesion surrounding the lacerated area, thereby decreasing the risk for retinal detachment. However, a possible risk of cryotherapy is extensive breakdown of the blood–retinal barrier and liberation and stimulation of RPE and glial cells, which will promote PVR and traction retinal detachment.[73] Furthermore, retinal breaks commonly occur 180 degrees away from the laceration site, because of the distant effects of vitreous incarceration. Further studies investigating cryotherapy need to be performed before a definitive answer can be given; however, we do not advocate such prophylactic treatment.

32.11 Lens Rupture and Primary Intraocular Lens Implantation

In cases in which the lens is disrupted and visualization is adequate, lens extraction at the initial repair can be performed after the laceration is closed (▶ Fig. 32.26). However, if the view is compromised by corneal opacities, hyphema, or anterior chamber fibrin, lens removal should be deferred. As will be discussed later, lens substrate is an excellent nidus for bacterial proliferation; if lens material is not removed, the risk for infectious postoperative endophthalmitis increases significantly. Because ocular trauma often occurs in the young, the lens can usually be removed by aspiration techniques alone. Primary placement of an IOL is usually well tolerated and does not appear to increase the risk for endophthalmitis or other postoperative complications. However, the IOL power selection may be inaccurate, and the surgeon may misjudge the intactness of the posterior capsule. In one series, 64% of patients who underwent lensectomy and IOL implantation at the time of primary repair of a penetrating ocular injury achieved 20/40 or better visual acuity.[74] Therefore, if capsular support allows, one can proceed with IOL placement. If too little capsule remains, an anterior chamber IOL or sutured posterior chamber IOL should be deferred as a second procedure. IOL implantation in children has become an accepted means of visual rehabilitation. In children ages 4 to 17 years, up to 87% of eyes with penetrating ocular injuries primarily managed with lens aspiration and IOL implantation achieved 20/40 or better visual acuity.[75] IOL implantation in infants, however, is still controversial and should probably be deferred until much later after the primary repair.

32.12 Prophylactic Antibiotics

Prophylactic subconjunctival, topical, and systemic antibiotics are used routinely in penetrating ocular trauma. Theoretically, prophylactic antibiotic use in the perioperative and postoperative period should help to decrease the risk for endophthalmitis. A prospective study of 30 ruptured globes identified prophylactic intravenous antibiotics as the only factor that significantly reduced the incidence of a culture-positive anterior chamber aspirate.[76] The fourth-generation fluoroquinolone, moxifloxacin, has a broad spectrum of coverage against most

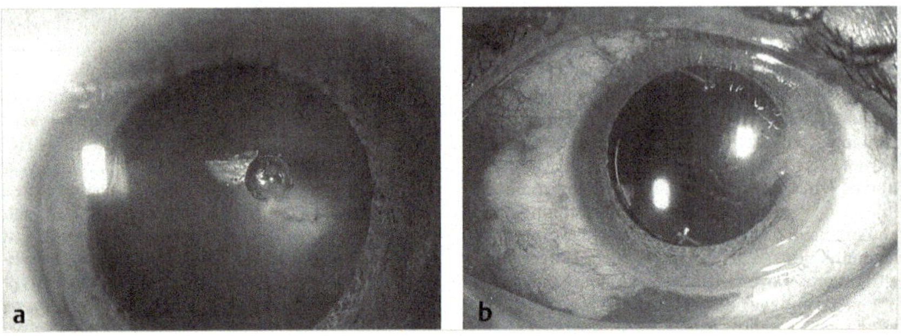

Fig. 32.26 (**a**) Corneal laceration with an intralenticular metallic foreign body and early cataract formation. (**b**) Postoperative photograph showing the repaired corneal laceration and a posterior chamber intraocular lens implant.

common organisms in endophthalmitis. It was shown to have a low minimal inhibitory concentration against 90% isolates and good vitreous penetration in noninflamed eyes when administered orally.[77] However, many other antibiotics do not adequately cross the blood–ocular barrier. Therefore, many systemically administered antibiotics will reach midvitreous concentrations that are not bactericidal or bacteriostatic and that are a fraction of what could be obtained with an intraocular injection of antibiotic. With this reasoning, some authors have proposed prophylactic use of intraocular antibiotics.[67,78,79] However, intraocular injections in a traumatized eye in which the anatomy may be disorganized and the needle may not be adequately visualized can lead to serious complications, such as retinal detachment, subretinal or suprachoroidal antibiotic delivery, or lens penetration. Retinal vascular infarction caused by aminoglycoside use has further dissuaded physicians from administering prophylactic intravitreal antibiotics.

We recommend using intraocular antibiotics in eyes for which the index of suspicion for endophthalmitis is high based on clinical signs or the setting of the injury. Specific preoperative and intraoperative signs and symptoms that should alert the physician to this possibility include severe pain, severe inflammation, hypopyon, vitreous opacification, or retinal vascular sheathing. In addition, injuries incurred in a rural setting should alert the physician to an increased risk for endophthalmitis.[80]

32.13 Endophthalmitis

The reported incidence of endophthalmitis following penetrating ocular trauma ranges from 2.5 to 14% and goes up to 15 and 30% if trauma occurred in a rural area or involved IOFB, respectively.[41,81,82] Many times, the initial diagnosis of posttraumatic endophthalmitis is obscured by the significant postoperative inflammation and pain that commonly afflict these eyes. The resultant delay, compounded by the virulent bacteria involved in such cases, makes the prognosis for recovery particularly grim.

In one retrospective investigation, potential risk factors for endophthalmitis after penetrating ocular trauma were subjected to univariate and multivariate analysis.[81] Only lens rupture was independently significant for the development of endophthalmitis, carrying a relative risk for infection of 15.8. Although the presence of an IOFB had a relative risk for infection of 1.9, it did not reach statistical significance. Scleral wounds, hyphema, uveal prolapse, retinal detachment, and suprachoroidal and vitreous hemorrhage were not associated with an increased risk for infection. The National Eye Trauma Study found a statistically significant increased incidence of endophthalmitis for eyes with a retained IOFB if surgical intervention took place more than 24 hours after the injury (13.4 vs. 3.5%; $p < 0.0001$).[14,24] Contrary to these findings, the report from Operation Iraqi Freedom found that urgent IOFB removal might not be necessary. In their study, 70 soldiers (79 eyes) underwent delayed IOFB removal (on average 21 days after trauma) and early systemic and topical antibiotic prophylaxis (levofloxacin and moxifloxacin) with no occurrence of endophthalmitis.[83]

Unlike the 60 to 75% of postoperative endophthalmitis cases caused by nonvirulent *Staphylococcus epidermidis*, posttraumatic endophthalmitis is frequently caused by virulent organisms. In addition, Jindal et al found that the microbiological spectrum of posttraumatic endophthalmitis over 14 years remained unchanged, with *Bacillus* being the most frequently encountered species.[84] *Bacillus cereus* is most commonly associated with soil-contaminated objects that have penetrated the eye, and although rarely seen in postoperative endophthalmitis, it accounts for 25 to 46% of posttraumatic endophthalmitis cases.[80] *B. cereus* endophthalmitis is characterized by rapid onset of severe pain and inflammation, hypopyon, chemosis, ring-shaped corneal infiltrate, and rapid progression to panophthalmitis.[85] Although there are reported cases of ambulatory-level visual acuity recovered after *B. cereus* endophthalmitis,[86] the multiple enzymes and exotoxins elaborated by this organism result in blindness or enucleation in the vast majority of eyes.[80] Gram-negative bacteria are responsible for another 5 to 20% of posttraumatic endophthalmitis cases.[87] Similarly, these cases also carry a poor prognosis, with a third of eyes ending up with no light perception or enucleation.[88] Polymicrobial infections may occur after open-globe injuries. Reported concomitant microorganisms in those cases include either *S. epidermidis* and *Streptococcus* species[89] or *Bacillus* with coagulase-negative *Staphylococcus*.[84] Fungal etiology, though uncommon, should be suspected in the setting of vegetable matter injury.

The basic surgical principles for managing an infected body cavity apply to the globe and include the following:

- Debridement of all necrotic tissue
- Drainage of abscesses
- Removal of foreign bodies
- Adjunctive antibiotic therapy

Cultures should include blood agar, chocolate agar, and thioglycolate broth incubated at 37 °C for bacteria, and Sabouraud's agar incubated at 25 °C for fungi. Gram's stains should also be obtained, as they may provide useful information for antibiotic selection.

The fundamental principles governing adjunctive antibiotics include the following:

- Administration of an antibiotic active against the etiologic organism
- Contact between the antibiotic and the organism
- Minimal toxic side effects

With these principles in mind, antibiotic delivery is administered via intravenous, oral, subconjunctival, intraocular, and topical routes. Although the Endophthalmitis Vitrectomy Study (EVS) did not show a benefit to using intravenous ceftazidime or aminoglycosides, it should be noted that the EVS included only eyes with acute-onset postoperative endophthalmitis following cataract extraction or secondary IOL implantation.[90] In posttraumatic endophthalmitis, systemic antibiotic use is still considered the standard of care. Intravenous vancomycin has good intraocular penetration and is effective against *Bacillus*, *Staphylococcus*, and *Streptococcus* species.[91] Intraocular antibiotics should be broad spectrum, and intraocular toxicity must be negligible. Vancomycin is active against gram-positive bacteria, is bactericidal, rarely promotes resistance, and is well tolerated by the eye in efficacious doses (1.0 mg). Ceftazidime is a beta-lactamase-stable, third-generation cephalosporin with excellent activity against most gram-negative bacteria, including *Neisseria*, *Haemophilus*, *Pseudomonas*, and *Acinetobacter*

Table 32.5 Antibiotic coverage

Route of administration	Gram-positive coverage	Gram-negative coverage
Intraocular[a]	Vancomycin 1.0 mg	Ceftazidime 2.25 mg or amikacin 400 µg
Subconjunctival[b]	Vancomycin 25 mg	Ceftazidime 100 mg or gentamicin 20 mg
Topical	Vancomycin 5%	Ceftazidime 5% or gentamicin 1.4%
Intravenous	Vancomycin 1 g every 12 h	Ceftazidime 1 g every 12 h, or gentamicin 1 to 2 mg/kg loading dose, then 1 mg/kg every 8 h[c]

[a]Delivered in 0.1 mL.

[b]Delivered in 0.5 mL.

[c]Peak and trough levels and renal status must be monitored.

species and most Enterobacteriaceae. Furthermore, it has activity against gram-positive bacteria, including penicillinase-producing *Staphylococcus aureus*. In one study, 40 cases of endophthalmitis were treated with intraocular ceftazidime (2.25 mg): 9 posttraumatic (22%), 4 endogenous (10%), and 27 postoperative (68%).[92] Of the 40 cases, 6 were caused by gram-negative bacteria. Sterilization was achieved in all cases, and macular toxicity was not observed in any case. Alternative intraocular antibiotics include clindamycin phosphate (450 µg) and amikacin (400 µg). See ▶ Table 32.5 for various antibiotic doses.

32.14 Enucleation and Sympathetic Ophthalmia

Because of the small risk for sympathetic ophthalmia, enucleation should be considered in a severely traumatized eye if there is thought to be no chance for any visual recovery. Primary enucleation is psychologically difficult for patients and should be used only when the eye has no light perception and is so disorganized that restoring the anatomic integrity of the globe is impossible. Delaying enucleation provides the physician the opportunity to assess postoperative visual acuity in a less acute setting, obtain consultation from other subspecialists (e.g., vitreoretinal surgery, oculoplastic surgery), and maximally stabilize both ocular and systemic problems. The patient benefits by having the time to acknowledge the loss of sight and disfigurement of the traumatized eye, and time to consult family and friends. In eyes that have maintained light perception or hand motions, a strategy used by some clinicians is to perform an exploratory vitrectomy, with the possibility of repair if the eye appears salvageable or enucleation if the eye is beyond repair.

There is a 0.19% incidence of sympathetic ophthalmia following penetrating ocular injuries, compared with 0.007 to 0.01% following intraocular surgery.[93,94] The risk for sympathetic ophthalmia can be minimized if the traumatized eye is enucleated within 10 to 14 days of the injury.[94] Typical clinical presentation of this potentially devastating uveitis is a bilateral granulomatous panuveitis characterized by ciliary injection, keratic precipitates, anterior chamber and vitreous cellular reaction, posterior iris synechiae, choroidal thickening, retinal vascular sheathing, and disc swelling. Dalen-Fuchs nodules develop in half or more of patients (▶ Fig. 32.27). Histologically, there is a lymphocytic and epithelioid cellular infiltration of the uveal tract, which often spares the choriocapillaris. The most important factor in maintaining or improving vision in the sympathizing eye is prompt aggressive medical treatment with anti-inflammatory drugs.

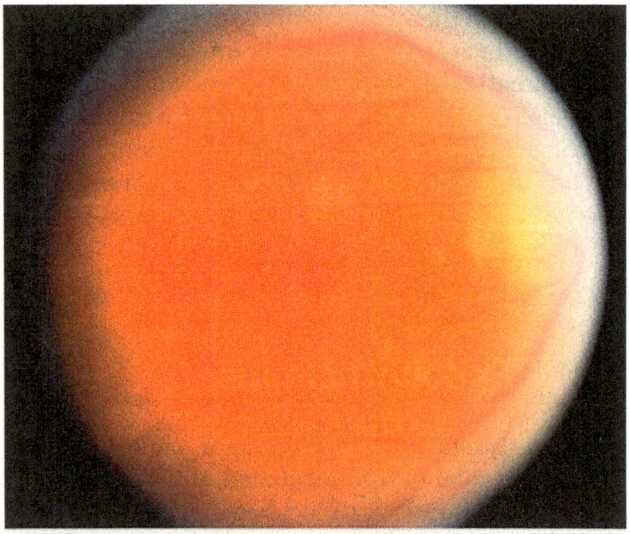

Fig. 32.27 Sympathetic ophthalmia with multiple subretinal yellow (*Dalen-Fuchs*) nodules evident in the posterior pole.

References

[1] Statistics on vision impairment: a resource manual. April 2002. Available online at: http://www.gesta.org/estudos/statistics0402.pdf. Accessed August 1, 2014

[2] Eye health statistics at a glance. April 2011. Available online at: http://development.aao.org/newsroom/upload/Eye-Health-Statistics-April-2011.pdf. Accessed August 1, 2014

[3] Négrel AD, Thylefors B. The global impact of eye injuries. Ophthalmic Epidemiol. 1998; 5(3):143–169

[4] US Eye Injury Registry. Available online at: http://www.useir.org. Accessed August 1, 2014

[5] National Society to Prevent Blindness. Eye Safety Is No Accident [Brochure]. Schaumburg, IL: The Society; 1990

[6] Kuhn F, Mester V, Berta A, Morris R. Epidemiology of serious ocular trauma: The United States Eye Injury Registry (USEIR) and the Hungarian Eye Injury Registry (HEIR). Ophthalmology. 1998; 95:332–343

[7] McGwin G, Jr, Owsley C. Incidence of emergency department-treated eye injury in the United States. Arch Ophthalmol. 2005; 123(5):662–666

[8] Kuhn F, ed. Ocular Traumatology. Berlin: Springer-Verlag; 2008

[9] CDC. QuickStats: average annual rate of eye-related emergency department visits for injuries and medical conditions, by age group—United States, 2007–2010. May 10, 2013. Available online at: http://www.cdc.gov/mmwr/preview/mmwrhtml/mm6218a9.htm/. Accessed August 1, 2014
[10] Healthcare Cost and Utilization Project. Agency for Healthcare Research and Quality. Emergency department visits related to eye injuries, 2008. Statistical Brief #112. May 2011. Available online at: http://www.hcup-us.ahrq.gov/reports/statbriefs/sb112.pdf. Accessed August 1, 2014
[11] Klopfer J, Tielsch JM, Vitale S, See LC, Canner JK. Ocular trauma in the United States. Eye injuries resulting in hospitalization, 1984 through 1987. Arch Ophthalmol. 1992; 110(6):838–842
[12] OSHA. Costs of accidents. Available online at: https://www.osha.gov/SLTC/etools/safetyhealth/mod1_costs.html/. Accessed August 1, 2014
[13] Zagelbaum BM, Tostanoski JR, Kerner DJ, Hersh PS. Urban eye trauma. A one-year prospective study. Ophthalmology. 1993; 100(6):851–856
[14] Dannenberg AL, Parver LM, Brechner RJ, Khoo L. Penetrating eye injuries in the workplace. The national eye trauma system registry. Arch Ophthalmol. 1992; 110:843–848
[15] Tielsch JM, Parver L, Shankar B. Time trends in the incidence of hospitalized ocular trauma. Arch Ophthalmol. 1989; 107(4):519–523
[16] Pieramici DJ, Sternberg P, Jr, Aaberg TM, Sr, et al. The Ocular Trauma Classification Group. A system for classifying mechanical injuries of the eye (globe). Am J Ophthalmol. 1997; 123(6):820–831
[17] Kuhn F, Morris R, Witherspoon CD, Heimann K, Jeffers JB, Treister G. A standardized classification of ocular trauma. Ophthalmology. 1996; 103(2):240–243
[18] Sternberg P, Jr, de Juan E, Jr, Michels RG, Auer C. Multivariate analysis of prognostic factors in penetrating ocular injuries. Am J Ophthalmol. 1984; 98 (4):467–472
[19] Esmaeli B, Elner SG, Schork MA, Elner VM. Visual outcome and ocular survival after penetrating trauma. A clinicopathologic study. Ophthalmology. 1995; 102(3):393–400
[20] Ahmadieh H, Soheilian M, Sajjadi H, Azarmina M, Abrishami M. Vitrectomy in ocular trauma. Factors influencing final visual outcome. Retina. 1993; 13 (2):107–113
[21] Pimolrat W, Choovuthayakorn J, Watanachai N, et al. Predictive factors of open globe injury in patients requiring vitrectomy. Injury. 2014; 45(1):212–216
[22] Burstein ES, Lazzaro DR. Traumatic ruptured globe eye injuries in a large urban center. Clin Ophthalmol. 2013; 7:485–488
[23] Kuhn F, Maisiak R, Mann L, Mester V, Morris R, Witherspoon CD. The ocular trauma score (OTS). Ophthalmol Clin North Am. 2002; 15(2):163–165, vi
[24] Dannenberg AL, Parver LM, Fowler CJ, The National Eye Trauma System Registry. Penetrating eye injuries related to assault. Arch Ophthalmol. 1992; 110 (6):849–852
[25] Hemady RK. Ocular injuries from violence treated at an inner-city hospital. J Trauma. 1994; 37(1):5–8
[26] Lakits A, Prokesch R, Scholda C, Bankier A. Orbital helical computed tomography in the diagnosis and management of eye trauma. Ophthalmology. 1999; 106(12):2330–2335
[27] Castellarin AA, Pieramici DJ. Open globe management. Compr Ophthalmol Update. 2007; 8(3):111–124
[28] Gunenc U, Maden A, Kaynak S, Pirnar T. Magnetic resonance imaging and computed tomography in the detection and localization of intraocular foreign bodies. Doc Ophthalmol. 1992; 81(4):369–378
[29] Rubsamen PE, Cousins SW, Winward KE, Byrne SF. Diagnostic ultrasound and pars plana vitrectomy in penetrating ocular trauma. Ophthalmology. 1994; 101(5):809–814
[30] Kramer M, Hart L, Miller JW. Ultrasonography in the management of penetrating ocular trauma. Int Ophthalmol Clin. 1995; 35(1):181–192
[31] Hutton WL, Fuller DG. Factors influencing final visual results in severely injured eyes. Am J Ophthalmol. 1984; 97(6):715–722
[32] Crews SJ, Thompson CR, Harding GF. The ERG and VEP in patients with severe eye injury. Doc Ophthalmol Proc Ser. 1978; 15:203–209
[33] Friberg TR. Traumatic retinal pigment epithelial edema. Am J Ophthalmol. 1979; 88(1):18–21
[34] Gregor Z, Ryan SJ. Blood-retinal barrier after blunt trauma to the eye. Graefes Arch Clin Exp Ophthalmol. 1982; 219(5):205–208
[35] Bunt-Milam AH, Black RA, Bensinger RE. Breakdown of the outer blood-retinal barrier in experimental commotio retinae. Exp Eye Res. 1986; 43(3):397–412
[36] Mansour AM, Green WR, Hogge C. Histopathology of commotio retinae. Retina. 1992; 12(1):24–28
[37] Sipperley JO, Quigley HA, Gass DM. Traumatic retinopathy in primates. The explanation of commotio retinae. Arch Ophthalmol. 1978; 96(12):2267–2273
[38] El Matri L, Chebil A, Kort F, Bouraoui R, Largueche L, Mghaieth F. Optical coherence tomographic findings in Berlin's edema. J Ophthalmic Vis Res. 2010; 5(2):127–129
[39] Ahn SJ, Woo SJ, Kim KE, Jo DH, Ahn J, Park KH. Optical coherence tomography morphologic grading of macular commotio retinae and its association with anatomic and visual outcomes. Am J Ophthalmol. 2013; 156(5):994–1001.e1
[40] Klien BA. Angloid streaks; a clinical and histopathologic study. Am J Ophthalmol. 1947; 30(8):955–968
[41] Aguilar JP, Green WR. Choroidal rupture. A histopathologic study of 47 cases. Retina. 1984; 4(4):269–275
[42] Goldman DR, Vora RA, Reichel E. Traumatic choroidal rupture with submacular hemorrhage treated with pneumatic displacement. Retina. 2014; 34 (6):1258–1260
[43] Secrétan M, Sickenberg M, Zografos L, Piguet B. Morphometric characteristics of traumatic choroidal ruptures associated with neovascularization. Retina. 1998; 18(1):62–66
[44] Dugel P, Win P, Ober R. Posterior segment manifestations of closed globe contusion injury. In: Ryan S, ed. Retina. Philadelphia, PA: Elsevier; 2006:2365–2377
[45] Dana MR, Werner MS, Viana MAG, Shapiro MJ. Spontaneous and traumatic vitreous hemorrhage. Ophthalmology. 1993; 100(9):1377–1383
[46] Schenek M, Rosenthal G, Klemperer I, Yagev R, Lifshitz T. Ultrasound guided cryotherapy for retinal tears in patients with opaque ocular media. Br J Ophthalmol. 1999; 83(5):628–629
[47] Kelley LM, Walker JP, Wing GL, Raskauskas PA, Schepens CL. Ultrasound-guided cryotherapy for retinal tears in patients with vitreous hemorrhage. Ophthalmic Surg Lasers. 1997; 28(7):565–569
[48] Cox MS, Schepens CL, Freeman HM. Retinal detachment due to ocular contusion. Arch Ophthalmol. 1966; 76(5):678–685
[49] Dumas JJ. Retinal detachment following contusion of the eye. Int Ophthalmol Clin. 1967; 7(1):19–38
[50] Johnston PB. Traumatic retinal detachment. Br J Ophthalmol. 1991; 75(1):18–21
[51] Ross WH. Traumatic retinal dialyses. Arch Ophthalmol. 1981; 99(8):1371–1374
[52] Zion VM, Burton TC. Retinal dialysis. Arch Ophthalmol. 1980; 98(11):1971–1974
[53] Hagler WS. Retinal dialysis: a statistical and genetic study to determine pathogenic factors. Trans Am Ophthalmol Soc. 1980; 78:686–733
[54] Kylstra JA, Lamkin JC, Runyan DK. Clinical predictors of scleral rupture after blunt ocular trauma. Am J Ophthalmol. 1993; 115(4):530–535
[55] Cherry PMH. Indirect traumatic rupture of the globe. Arch Ophthalmol. 1978; 96(2):252–256
[56] Russell SR, Olsen KR, Folk JC. Predictors of scleral rupture and the role of vitrectomy in severe blunt ocular trauma. Am J Ophthalmol. 1988; 105 (3):253–257
[57] Groessl S, Nanda SK, Mieler WF. Assault-related penetrating ocular injury. Am J Ophthalmol. 1993; 116(1):26–33
[58] Arkin MS, Rubin PAD, Bilyk JR, Buchbinder B. Anterior chiasmal optic nerve avulsion. AJNR Am J Neuroradiol. 1996; 17(9):1777–1781
[59] Lang W. Rupture of the lamina Cribrosa and Optic Nerve-Fibers at the Papilla. Tr. Ophth. Soc. U Kingdom. 1901:21–98
[60] Lister W. Some concussion changes met with in military practice. Br J Ophthalmol. 1924; 8(7):i1–i318
[61] Berdahl JP, Johnson CS, Proia AD, Grinstaff MW, Kim T. Comparison of sutures and dendritic polymer adhesives for corneal laceration repair in an in vivo chicken model. Arch Ophthalmol. 2009; 127(4):442–447
[62] Velazquez AJ, Carnahan MA, Kristinsson J, Stinnett S, Grinstaff MW, Kim T. New dendritic adhesives for sutureless ophthalmic surgical procedures: in vitro studies of corneal laceration repair. Arch Ophthalmol. 2004; 122 (6):867–870
[63] De Juan E, Jr, Sternberg P, Jr, Michels RG. Penetrating ocular injuries. Types of injuries and visual results. Ophthalmology. 1983; 90(11):1318–1322
[64] Topping TM, Abrams GW, Machemer R. Experimental double-perforating injury of the posterior segment in rabbit eyes: the natural history of intraocular proliferation. Arch Ophthalmol. 1979; 97(4):735–742
[65] Shock JP, Adams D. Long-term visual acuity results after penetrating and perforating ocular injuries. Am J Ophthalmol. 1985; 100(5):714–718
[66] Thompson JT, Parver LM, Enger CL, Mieler WF, Liggett PE, National Eye Trauma System. Infectious endophthalmitis after penetrating injuries with retained intraocular foreign bodies. Ophthalmology. 1993; 100(10):1468–1474

[67] Brinton GS, Topping TM, Hyndiuk RA, Aaberg TM, Sr, Reeser FH, Abrams GW. Posttraumatic endophthalmitis. Arch Ophthalmol. 1984; 102(4):547–550
[68] Williams DF, Mieler WF, Abrams GW, Lewis H. Results and prognostic factors in penetrating ocular injuries with retained intraocular foreign bodies. Ophthalmology. 1988; 95(7):911–916
[69] Slusher MM, Sarin LK, Federman JL. Management of intraretinal foreign bodies. Ophthalmology. 1982; 89(4):369–373
[70] Caprioli J, Sears ML. The histopathology of black ball hyphema: a report of two cases. Ophthalmic Surg. 1984; 15(6):491–495
[71] Han DP, Mieler F, Abrams GL, Williams GA. Vitrectomy for traumatic retinal incarceration. Arch Ophthalmol. 1988; 106:640–645
[72] Brinton GS, Aaberg TM, Reeser FH, Topping TM, Abrams GW. Surgical results in ocular trauma involving the posterior segment. Am J Ophthalmol. 1982; 93(3):271–278
[73] Mittra RA, Mieler WF. Controversies in the management of open-globe injuries involving the posterior segment. Surv Ophthalmol. 1999; 44(3):215–225
[74] Rubsamen PE, Irvin WD, McCuen BW, II, Smiddy WE, Bowman CB. Primary intraocular lens implantation in the setting of penetrating ocular trauma. Ophthalmology. 1995; 102(1):101–107
[75] Koenig SB, Ruttum MS, Lewandowski MF, Schultz RO. Pseudophakia for traumatic cataracts in children. Ophthalmology. 1993; 100(8):1218–1224
[76] Ariyasu RG, Kumar S, LaBree LD, Wagner DG, Smith RE. Microorganisms cultured from the anterior chamber of ruptured globes at the time of repair. Am J Ophthalmol. 1995; 119(2):181–188
[77] Hariprasad SM, Shah GK, Mieler WF, et al. Vitreous and aqueous penetration of orally administered moxifloxacin in humans. Arch Ophthalmol. 2006; 124 (2):178–182
[78] Peyman GA, Carroll CP, Raichand M. Prevention and management of traumatic endophthalmitis. Ophthalmology. 1980; 87(4):320–324
[79] Schemmer GB, Driebe WT, Jr. Posttraumatic Bacillus cereus endophthalmitis. Arch Ophthalmol. 1987; 105(3):342–344
[80] Boldt HC, Pulido JS, Blodi CF, Folk JC, Weingeist TA. Rural endophthalmitis. Ophthalmology. 1989; 96(12):1722–1726
[81] Thompson WS, Rubsamen PE, Flynn HW, Jr, Schiffman J, Cousins SW. Endophthalmitis after penetrating trauma. Risk factors and visual acuity outcomes. Ophthalmology. 1995; 102(11):1696–1701
[82] Reynolds DS, Flynn HW, Jr. Endophthalmitis after penetrating ocular trauma. Curr Opin Ophthalmol. 1997; 8(3):32–38
[83] Colyer MH, Weber ED, Weichel ED, et al. Delayed intraocular foreign body removal without endophthalmitis during Operations Iraqi Freedom and Enduring Freedom. Ophthalmology. 2007; 114(8):1439–1447
[84] Jindal A, Pathengay A, Mithal K, et al. Endophthalmitis after open globe injuries: changes in microbiological spectrum and isolate susceptibility patterns over 14 years. J Ophthalmic Inflamm Infect. 2014; 4(1):5
[85] Ahmed Y, Schimel AM, Pathengay A, Colyer MH, Flynn HW, Jr. Endophthalmitis following open-globe injuries. Eye (Lond). 2012; 26(2):212–217
[86] Foster RE, Martinez JA, Murray TG, Rubsamen PE, Flynn HW, Jr, Forster RK. Useful visual outcomes after treatment of Bacillus cereus endophthalmitis. Ophthalmology. 1996; 103(3):390–397
[87] Parrish CM, O'Day DM. Traumatic endophthalmitis. Int Ophthalmol Clin. 1987; 27(2):112–119
[88] Irvine WD, Flynn HW, Jr, Miller D, Pflugfelder SC. Endophthalmitis caused by gram-negative organisms. Arch Ophthalmol. 1992; 110(10):1450–1454
[89] Chhabra S, Kunimoto DY, Kazi L, et al. Endophthalmitis after open globe injury: microbiologic spectrum and susceptibilities of isolates. Am J Ophthalmol. 2006; 142(5):852–854
[90] Endophthalmitis Vitrectomy Study Group. Results of the Endophthalmitis Vitrectomy Study. A randomized trial of immediate vitrectomy and of intravenous antibiotics for the treatment of postoperative bacterial endophthalmitis. Arch Ophthalmol. 1995; 113(12):1479–1496
[91] Meredith TA, Aguilar HE, Shaarawy A, Kincaid M, Dick J, Niesman MR. Vancomycin levels in the vitreous cavity after intravenous administration. Am J Ophthalmol. 1995; 119(6):774–778
[92] Aaberg TM, Flynn HW, Murray TM. Intraocular ceftazidime as an alternative to the aminoglycosides in the treatment of endophthalmitis: two years' experience. Arch Ophthalmol. 1994; 112(1):18–19
[93] Gass JDM. Sympathetic ophthalmia following vitrectomy. Am J Ophthalmol. 1982; 93(5):552–558
[94] Liddy L, Stuart J. Sympathetic ophthalmia in Canada. Can J Ophthalmol. 1972; 7(2):157–159
[95] Albert DM, Diaz-Rohena R. A historical review of sympathetic ophthalmia and its epidemiology. Surv Ophthalmol. 1989; 34(1):1–14

33 Posterior Segment Manifestations of Systemic Trauma

Jason Hsu and Carl D. Regillo

33.1 Purtscher's Retinopathy

In 1910, Purtscher described a constellation of changes in the posterior pole of two patients with severe head trauma.[1] *Angiopathia retinae traumatica*, or *Purtscher's retinopathy*, as it is now known, consists of multiple patches of superficial retinal whitening and retinal hemorrhages around the optic nerve heads in both eyes. Similar fundus presentations have since been reported with a variety of traumatic and nontraumatic conditions.[2,3,4,5,6]

33.1.1 Clinical Features

Patients typically notice a marked, sudden loss of vision in one or both eyes. Ophthalmoscopic examination reveals multiple cotton-wool spots and intraretinal hemorrhages, all of which are clustered in the peripapillary region (▶ Fig. 33.1). Purtscher's flecken, characterized by larger areas of intraretinal whitening with a clear zone within 50 µm on either side of retinal arterioles, venules, and precapillary arterioles, are considered pathognomonic but occur in only about 50% of cases.[7] Some degree of asymmetry may be present. Rarely, a unilateral picture is observed.[8] The optic nerve heads usually appear normal early on, although disc swelling is sometimes noted. Retinal venous engorgement or tortuosity may also be present. The retinal periphery is usually uninvolved.

Optical coherence tomography may, in acute cases, show retinal edema and thickening. Fluorescein angiography demonstrates patchy capillary nonperfusion in the regions of retinal whitening, intraretinal leakage of dye from surrounding small retinal arterioles, and blocked fluorescence from intraretinal blood.[3,8] There may or may not be a delay in arteriovenous transit. Fluorescein angiography adds little to establishing the diagnosis and is not necessary in the work-up of patients with the condition.

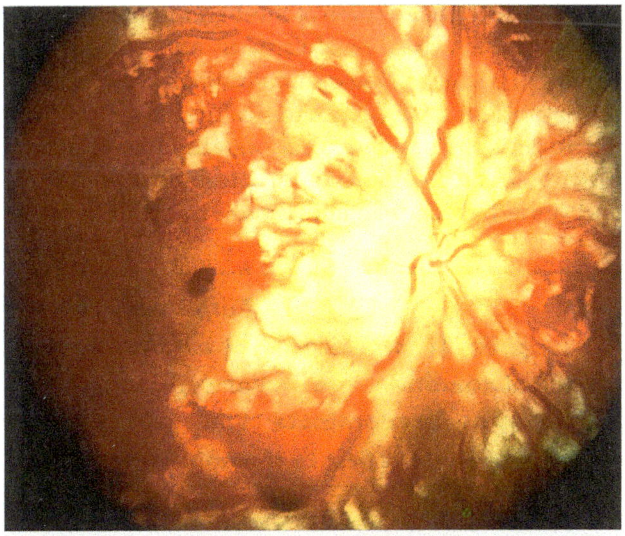

Fig. 33.1 Purtscher retinopathy: Peripapillary patches of retinal whitening (*cotton-wool spots*) and hemorrhage in the right eye of a patient who sustained massive head trauma.

33.1.2 Diagnosis

Purtscher's retinopathy has been associated with severe head trauma, significant chest compression injury, and extensive long-bone fractures.[2] In such cases, the associated trauma will be obvious and the diagnosis is readily made after fundus examination alone. No further testing is generally needed. However, when the fundus presentation occurs in conjunction with a systemic disease, the underlying cause may not be so easily recognizable. Medical conditions that have been described to produce a Purtscher-like retinopathy include acute pancreatitis, systemic lupus erythematosus, thrombotic thrombocytopenic purpura, chronic renal failure, and other, often autoimmune, systemic disease. With some of these conditions, the ocular symptoms may predominate over systemic symptoms and prompt the patient to present to the ophthalmologist first.[3] Finally, it is important to recognize that a fundus picture similar to that of Purtscher's retinopathy has also been described as a complication of retrobulbar anesthesia and steroid injection in and around the orbit.[9,10]

Conditions Associated with Purtscher's and Purtscher-like Retinopathy

- Purtscher's retinopathy
  - Trauma
    - Head injury
    - Chest compression
    - Long-bone fractures (fat embolism syndrome)
- Purtshcer's-like retinoplathy
  - Acute pancreatitis
  - Chronic renal failure
  - Autoimmune diseases
    - Systemic lupus erythematosus
    - Thrombotic thrombocytopenic purpura
    - Hemolysis, elevated liver enzymes, low platelets (HELLP) syndrome
    - Scleroderma
    - Dermatomyositis
    - Sjögren's syndrome
  - Amniotic fluid embolism
  - Retrobulbar anesthesia
  - Orbital steroid injection

Pearls

- When Purtscher's retinopathy is associated with a nontraumatic medical condition, the ocular symptoms may sometimes predominate and prompt the patient to present first to the ophthalmologist.

33.1.3 Pathogenesis and Histopathology

The pathogenesis of Purtscher's retinopathy is not well understood. There is, however, much clinical and experimental evidence to suggest that the underlying systemic condition results in the generation of various intravascular microparticles that occlude the small arterioles in the peripapillary retina and elsewhere.[2,3,6,11,12] Fibrin clots, platelet–leukocyte aggregates, fat emboli, air emboli, or other similarly sized particles have been implicated, depending on the nature of underlying systemic problem. Experimentally, injection of fibrin clots of about 0.15 to 1.0 mm in size into the ophthalmic artery of pigs results in a fundus picture identical to that of Purtscher's retinopathy.[12]

Histopathologic analyses show evidence for retinal capillary obliteration and inner retinal atrophy in areas corresponding clinically to retinal whitening. These findings are consistent with cotton-wool spots of a variety of etiologies.[13] Studies also confirm the clinical observation that pathology is confined mainly to the retina posterior to the equator. Recent indocyanine green angiography observations indicate that there may also be localized choroidal microvascular compromise in the posterior pole.[14] Nonspecific optic atrophy is present to various degrees both clinically and histopathologically. Histopathologic studies available to date have failed to reveal emboli or other intravascular particles, but data are limited to globes processed weeks or months after the acute event when such particles are likely to be no longer present.

33.1.4 Management and Course

Purtscher's retinopathy is essentially an acute ischemic event of the peripapillary retina and optic nerve for which there is no specific treatment. Visual acuity is decreased on the basis of infarction of either the foveal retina or the optic nerve. While corticosteroids have been used in the past, there is no evidence that they alter the visual prognosis. The retinal whitening and hemorrhages slowly disappear during weeks or months, but visual acuity often does not recover significantly. Optic atrophy and surrounding retinal pigment epithelial alterations are late findings. Therapy directed at the underlying systemic condition may help to reduce or eliminate ongoing embolic phenomena and the risk for additional retinal or optic nerve damage.

33.2 Terson's Syndrome

At the turn of the 20th century, the French ophthalmologist Albert Terson described the finding of vitreous hemorrhage associated with an acute subarachnoid hemorrhage.[15] The term *Terson's syndrome* is now used to refer to any intraocular hemorrhage present after either spontaneous or trauma-induced intracranial bleeding.

Some degree of intraocular hemorrhage is seen in approximately 20 to 40% of patients with various types of acute intracranial bleeds.[16,17,18] A smaller percentage of patients, around 3 to 5%, present with frank vitreous hemorrhage.[16,18,19] The intracranial hemorrhage is usually subarachnoid in location, and the most common reported cause is spontaneous rupture of an anterior communicating artery aneurysm.[17,18]

33.2.1 Clinical Features

At presentation, the most common ocular manifestation of Terson's syndrome is multiple retinal hemorrhages (▶ Fig. 33.2).[11,16] The hemorrhages are almost always bilateral and tend to be concentrated in the posterior pole. The amount of intraocular hemorrhage is often, but not consistently, proportional to the amount of intracranial hemorrhage.[17] Patients have varying degrees of decreased visual acuity, typically related to the extent of ocular hemorrhage. However, sparse hemorrhage that involves the fovea may sometimes cause a significant loss of acuity. Although the hemorrhages are occasionally subretinal, they are usually more superficial, being either just under the internal limiting membrane (ILM) or preretinal (subhyaloid) in location. There is some controversy as to which location is more common, as it can be difficult to distinguish between the two ophthalmoscopically. Significant vitreous hemorrhage also occurs and is thought to result from blood breaking through the ILM or posterior hyaloid face into the vitreous gel. This breakthrough bleeding can occur at any point in the clinical course and may be a cause for further worsening of visual acuity during follow-up.

Late-appearing sequelae include epiretinal membrane formation, macular holes, and, rarely, traction or rhegmatogenous retinal detachments.[20,21,22,23,24] Perimacular retinal folds, similar to what has been described in the shaken baby syndrome (SBS), have also been reported.[25] All these changes have the potential to limit visual recovery.

33.2.2 Diagnosis

Because the primary intracranial event typically dominates the clinical picture at presentation, the ophthalmologist is usually already aware that a significant intracranial hemorrhage has taken place. Therefore, the diagnosis is generally readily apparent at the initial ophthalmoscopic examination. Establishing the diagnosis of Terson's syndrome by documenting the

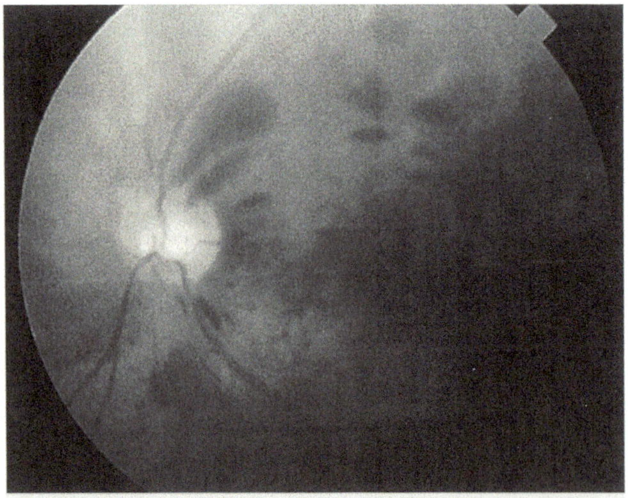

Fig. 33.2 Terson's retinopathy: Multiple superficial retinal hemorrhages of the posterior pole along with vitreous hemorrhage (*clouding the media*) in the left eye of a patient who had a spontaneous subarachnoid hemorrhage.

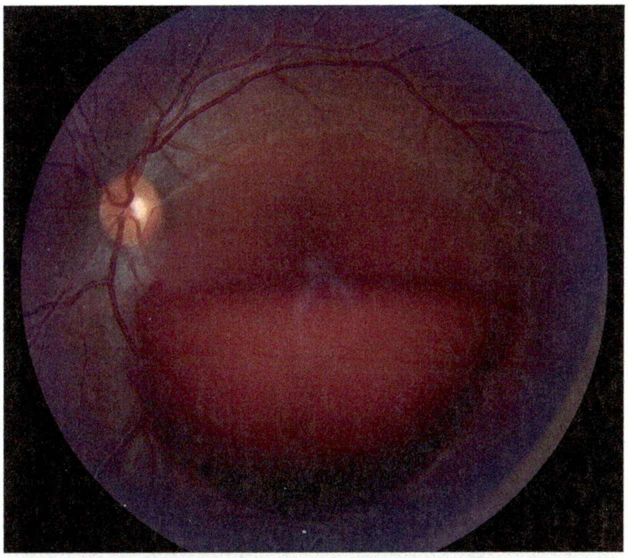

Fig. 33.3 Valsalva retinopathy: Large macular preretinal/subinternal limiting membrane hemorrhage.

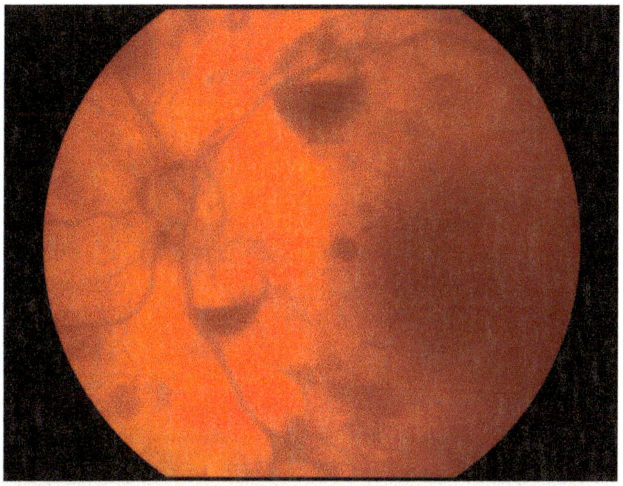

Fig. 33.4 Shaken baby syndrome: Multiple areas of subretinal, intraretinal, and preretinal hemorrhages in the posterior pole. (Image courtesy of Dr. Bruce Schnall.)

presence of intraocular hemorrhage may have systemic prognostic significance, as some series suggest that cases of intracranial hemorrhaging associated with intraocular bleeding have a higher mortality than those that do not have eye involvement.[16] In rare cases where patients present primarily to the ophthalmologist with fundus features suggestive of this diagnosis, emergency neuroimaging is essential.

A similar fundus appearance to that of Terson's syndrome can be seen after Valsalva maneuvers and with the SBS (▶ Fig. 33.3 and ▶ Fig. 33.4). In trauma cases, the findings of cotton-wool spots or retinal edema associated with the retinal hemorrhages are more consistent with Purtscher's retinopathy than with Terson's syndrome.

33.2.3 Pathogenesis and Histopathology

The mechanism of the intraocular hemorrhage has been the subject of debate for many years. Early on, it was thought that the subarachnoid hemorrhage tracked down within the optic nerve sheath and dissected directly into the eye.[11] This is an unlikely explanation for several reasons. First, there are no known communications between the subarachnoid space and the optic nerve. Second, the vitreous and retinal hemorrhages are not often contiguous with the optic nerve. Third, histopathologic studies indicate that, in many cases, the blood around the intraorbital optic nerve is actually subdural rather than subarachnoid and that the nerve sheath blood does not extend to the globe.[23,25,26]

Most investigators now believe that the intraocular hemorrhage is somehow related to the sudden rise in intracranial pressure that occurs at the time of the intracranial bleed.[17] It has been shown that the rapidity and magnitude of increase in intracranial pressure are directly correlated with the amount of ocular hemorrhage. The increased intracranial pressure either directly increases orbital venous pressure through its effects on the cavernous sinus or causes compression of both the ophthalmic vein and retinochoroidal anastomoses from a rapid effusion of cerebrospinal fluid or blood into the optic nerve sheath.[11,17] With either mechanism, there would be an acute obstruction to retinal outflow and this, in turn, is thought to result in rupture of epipapillary or retinal postcapillary venules.

Controversial Points

- Although the exact mechanism remains unclear, most investigators believe that the intraocular hemorrhage is related to the sudden rise in intracranial pressure that occurs at the time of the acute intracranial bleed.

33.2.4 Management and Course

In most cases of Terson's syndrome, the hemorrhage gradually clears and vision returns to normal.[11,16,17] Therefore, observation is usually all that is needed. Vision, however, may remain decreased from persistent vitreous hemorrhage or epiretinal membrane formation with surface wrinkling. Vitrectomy surgery is indicated in such cases to help restore or improve vision.[27] Early intervention should be considered in any case with significant bilateral involvement or in young children with either one or both eyes visually affected to prevent amblyopia. Surgery without delay will also be necessary should there be an associated retinal detachment. Even in cases without these significant complications, visual acuity loss may sometimes persist to some degree because of permanent pigmentary disruption or outer retinal damage from subretinal blood in the macula.

33.3 Shaken Baby Syndrome

The radiologist John Caffey is credited with first recognizing the association of some of the systemic and ocular manifestations of child abuse. In the 1940s, he described the findings of multiple long-bone fractures in abused infants who had subdural hematomas.[28] He later observed that many of the abused infants with brain damage lacked external signs of direct head trauma and had both intraocular and intracranial hemorrhage. In the 1970s, a whiplash type of mechanism was proposed to explain the injuries seen in such cases.[28,29]

It has since become apparent that the *shaken baby syndrome (SBS)*, as it is now called, is a common form of child abuse and, unfortunately, often results in significant morbidity and mortality. The syndrome is seen almost exclusively in children younger than 2 years, with most being under 12 months.[30,31] The age predilection is thought to be primarily a consequence of certain anatomic features that make the infant more likely to suffer from intracranial and intraocular bleeding as a result of shaking.[28,29] First, the head of an infant is proportionately larger and heavier relative to the body than in an older child or adult. Second, the head is not well stabilized by neck muscles at this age. Third, the average adult can generate relatively larger acceleration-deceleration forces in shaking an infant than in shaking a larger person. In addition to their anatomic susceptibility, infants may be more likely to be subjected to shaking abuse because of their inability to communicate verbally and their greater tendency to have prolonged episodes of crying.[30]

33.3.1 Clinical Features

In SBS, intraocular hemorrhage is the most common eye finding, occurring in approximately 85% of patients.[30,31,32,33] Subretinal, intraretinal, preretinal (subhyaloid), and vitreous hemorrhage have all been described. Of these types, intraretinal and preretinal hemorrhages predominate and are typically concentrated in the posterior pole region (▶ Fig. 33.4). Bilateral involvement is present in 58 to 100% of cases.[29,31] The extent or severity of the hemorrhages varies and may be directly correlated with the amount of acute neurologic injury.[34] The retinal hemorrhages usually resolve within several weeks or months after the abuse has stopped. Less commonly reported ocular findings at presentation include cotton-wool spots, macular edema, white-centered hemorrhages, retinoschisis, hemorrhagic posterior vitreous detachment, macular holes, retinal pigment epithelial tears, and papilledema.[11,28,31,35,36,37] Manifestations that are more chronic in nature include perimacular retinal folds, chorioretinal atrophy or scarring, optic atrophy, retinal neovascularization, and retinal detachment.[38,39,40]

The hallmark nonocular sign in SBS is intracranial hemorrhage. This is usually subdural in location and often involves both sides of the brain.[28,29,30,41] Subarachnoid or intracerebral blood is seen less commonly. Cerebral edema and elevated intracranial pressure are usually present to some degree. What results acutely is a spectrum of neurologic changes ranging from irritability and lethargy to seizures, coma, and death.[28] Bradycardia, apnea, and hypothermia can also be encountered. Computed tomography (CT) or magnetic resonance imaging (MRI) will be needed to confirm the underlying intracranial pathology. It is important to note that retinal hemorrhages may precede both clinical and radiologic recognition of subdural hematoma in SBS.[42] Therefore, repeated CT or MRI should be considered in cases in which SBS is strongly suspected. Cerebrospinal fluid and subdural aspirations may also be required to detect the presence of blood in the central nervous system.

Special Considerations

- Because retinal hemorrhages may occasionally precede both clinical and radiologic recognition of subdural hematoma in SBS, close follow-up with repeated neuroimaging should be considered when the diagnosis remains in question.

In some cases, subtle extracranial signs of shaking abuse may also be present and may help to establish the diagnosis of SBS, especially when a definitive history is not attainable. From shaking alone, bruises or fractures of the trunk or limbs can be seen. Cervical cord hematomas have also been described, and these are thought to be highly suggestive that a whiplash mechanism of injury has taken place.[41]

33.3.2 Diagnosis

SBS must be considered when intraocular hemorrhage is seen in an infant. As a history of abuse may be difficult to elicit with certainty, the clinician must maintain a high index of suspicion based on the clinical findings. However, intraocular hemorrhage alone is not specific for child abuse, as it can occur in a variety of other conditions at this age (see the following list).[28,31] Accidental injury to the head or a spontaneous subarachnoid hemorrhage can result in intraocular bleeding as described in the section on Terson's syndrome. Some studies, however, have suggested that intraocular hemorrhage may be uncommon in children with intracranial hemorrhage from nonabusive mechanisms, such as accidental or surgical trauma.[43] Cardiopulmonary resuscitation and vaginal delivery can also cause retinal hemorrhages. Furthermore, hemorrhages can be seen in conjunction with a number of different systemic conditions, such as arterial hypertension, blood dyscrasias, sepsis, meningitis, and vasculitis.

Differential Diagnosis of Retinal Hemorrhages in Infancy

- Shaken Baby Syndrome (SBS)
- Birth trauma (neonatal period only).
- Cardiopulmonary resuscitation.
- Spontaneous intracranial hemorrhage (e.g., Terson's syndrome).
- Direct head or chest trauma (accidental or nonaccidental).
- Blunt eye injury.
- Viral retinitis.
- Acute arterial hypertension.
- Systemic infections and meningitis.
- Hematologic disorders (e.g., malignancies, coagulopathies).
- Systemic (or retinal) vasculitis.

Optical coherence tomography may show focal vitreous separation in the macula, perimacular folds with vitreous attachment at the apices, epiretinal membrane, retinoschisis, lamellar or full-thickness macular hole, and even foveal detachment.[44,45,46] These findings appear to be consistent with shearing forces at the vitreoretinal interface due to shaking. Fluorescein angiography has demonstrated areas of peripheral nonperfusion in some cases.[47] However, the clinical implications of this finding are unclear given that some of these patients were observed and never developed neovascularization.

33.3.3 Pathogenesis and Histopathology

In the pathogenesis of SBS, the intracranial hemorrhage is thought to result primarily from tearing of the delicate bridging vessels between the cerebral cortices and venous sinuses as the brain forcefully shifts within the skull during shaking. Deceleration contusion injury to the cerebral cortices with bleeding and edema may also occur. The origin of the ocular hemorrhage remains somewhat debatable and is likely to be multifactorial. A Terson's syndrome–like mechanism may be at play should there be a rapid rise in intracranial pressure. The movement within the globe of the vitreous gel, which is strongly adherent to the ILM of the retina at this age, may cause enough traction to tear superficial retinal blood vessels. Increased venous pressure transmitted to the retina from chest compression during firm grasping or during choking may also contribute to the hemorrhaging, similar to Valsalva retinopathy.

Histopathologic analyses of the globes in SBS confirm what is seen clinically and demonstrate hemorrhage within all layers of the retina, between the retina and the retinal pigment epithelium, and in the vitreous.[32,33] Intraretinal edema, retinal folding, and retinal pigment epithelial alterations are other, not uncommon ocular findings. Intraorbital optic nerve sheath hemorrhage located in the corresponding subdural space is observed frequently and may be the cause of, or at least contribute to, optic disc edema or optic atrophy.[31,32,33] The blood in the nerve sheath is *not* usually contiguous with the intracranial blood.

33.3.4 Management and Course

Unfortunately, some degree of permanent visual loss is common in SBS.[30,31] Visual dysfunction can result from retinal, optic nerve, or cerebral cortex damage, and some combination of damage is often present.[28,31,38] Ocular signs indicative of at least a fair potential for adequate visual function are good pupillary reflexes, clear ocular media, retinal findings limited to intraretinal hemorrhages, and a normal optic nerve head.[28] In patients with vitreous hemorrhage dense enough to obscure the macula, vitrectomy surgery to clear the blood and prevent amblyopia should be considered if the bright flash electroretinographic response is preserved.[28] When surgical intervention is considered, it should be recognized that although the visual pathway may be relatively well preserved, the patient's overall function may still be very limited by other, severe neurologic damage.

Pearls

- When dense vitreous hemorrhage is present in SBS, early vitrectomy surgery to clear the blood and prevent amblyopia should be considered, but only if there is a preserved electroretinographic response.

33.4 Other Conditions

33.4.1 Fat Embolism Syndrome

Retinal changes are a well-described part of the *fat embolism syndrome* (FES). Within a few days after significant fracture of medullated bones, patients manifest a variety of systemic and ocular signs. Although only about 5% of patients presenting with long-bone fractures in general are found to have retinal findings, this figure can be as high as 60% when patients who meet the diagnostic criteria for FES are selected.[48]

The typical ophthalmoscopic findings in FES are bilateral cotton-wool spots and intraretinal hemorrhages.[11,48] In some cases, the fundus picture may resemble that of Purtscher's retinopathy, but in most, the white retinal infarcts and hemorrhages are usually smaller, less numerous, and scattered more peripherally.[2] Moreover, FES differs from Purtscher's retinopathy in that most patients acutely are asymptomatic or have only minor visual disturbance. Less common ocular signs include conjunctival petechiae, intravascular fat, and central retinal artery obstruction.[11,48]

The major systemic signs of FES consist of petechial rash, various central nervous system alterations, respiratory compromise, tachycardia, fever, anemia, and an elevated erythrocyte sedimentation rate. The syndrome is fatal in up to 20% of cases. The ophthalmologist is rarely involved during the acute phase of FES, as ocular symptoms are usually minimal, but may be called on to examine the eyes of patients suspected of having FES to help confirm the diagnosis. Furthermore, some patients have persistent paracentral scotomas.[48]

33.4.2 Whiplash Maculopathy

Whiplash injury in adults, such as from an automobile accident, can produce a somewhat unique ocular presentation called *whiplash maculopathy*.[42] The patient typically experiences bilateral, mild blurring of vision that is recognized immediately after a significant head and neck flexion-extension injury. Visual acuity is slightly decreased to about 20/30, and ocular examination shows only a faint, gray haze and a small depression of the foveal retina. A shallow posterior vitreous separation may also be seen. Fluorescein angiography findings are usually normal. Optical coherence tomography may demonstrate disruption of the ellipsoid zone (inner segment/outer segment hyperreflective line).[49]

The gray retinal discoloration fades and the vision returns to normal within several days. However, the small foveal depression, with or without a whitish border, can persist indefinitely. Mild commotio retinae of the central macula and sun gazing (solar retinopathy) can produce a similar fundus appearance.

33.4.3 Lightning Maculopathy

Being struck by lightning can produce both anterior and posterior segment manifestations.[50] The most common ocular change is cataract development, which occurs during the first 2 to 6 months after the injury. Mild, transient iritis and keratitis are other anterior segment signs that have been observed.

Infrequently, subtle retinal changes are also seen and consist mainly of punctate, deep retinal yellow deposits in the central macular area with or without minor pigmentary alterations.

The yellow deposits can resemble those seen at the base of a true macular hole even though a macular hole is not present or, if larger, they can mimic the changes seen in a pattern dystrophy. Surrounding reddish discoloration of the retina or cystic retinal edema can also be seen. Progression to a full-thickness macular hole has been reported but is probably rare. Recently, optical coherence tomography has demonstrated that the macular lesions simulating macular holes may actually represent foveal cysts.[51] With time, these cystic lesions tend to resolve spontaneously but may leave foveal atrophy. Usually, visual acuity is not significantly affected in lightning maculopathy, and patients typically have excellent visual outcomes after removal of the lightning-induced cataract.[50]

References

[1] Purtscher O. Angiopathia retinae traumatica. Lymphorrhagien des Augengrundes. Graefes Arch Clin Exp Ophthalmol. 1912; 82:347–371

[2] Gass JDM. 1987

[3] Power MH, Regillo MC, Custis PH. Thrombotic thrombocytopenic purpura associated with purtscher retinopathy. Arch Ophthalmol. 1997; 115(1):128–129

[4] Stoumbos VD, Klein ML, Goodman S. Purtscher's-like retinopathy in chronic renal failure. Ophthalmology. 1992; 99(12):1833–1839

[5] Jabs DA, Fine SL, Hochberg MC, Newman SA, Heiner GG, Stevens MB. Severe retinal vaso-occlusive disease in systemic lupus erythematous. Arch Ophthalmol. 1986; 104(4):558–563

[6] Roden D, Fitzpatrick G, O'Donoghue H, Phelan D. Purtscher's retinopathy and fat embolism. Br J Ophthalmol. 1989; 73(8):677–679

[7] Miguel AI, Henriques F, Azevedo LF, Loureiro AJ, Maberley DA. Systematic review of Purtscher's and Purtscher-like retinopathies. Eye (Lond). 2013; 27(1):1–13

[8] Burton TC. Unilateral Purtscher's retinopathy. Ophthalmology. 1980; 87(11):1096–1105

[9] Wilkinson WS, Morgan CM, Baruh E, Gitter KA. Retinal and choroidal vascular occlusion secondary to corticosteroid embolisation. Br J Ophthalmol. 1989; 73(1):32–34

[10] Lemagne JM, Michiels X, Van Causenbroeck S, Snyers B. Purtscher-like retinopathy after retrobulbar anesthesia. Ophthalmology. 1990; 97(7):859–861

[11] Williams DF, Mieler WF, Williams GA. Posterior segment manifestations of ocular trauma. Retina. 1990; 10 Suppl 1:S35–S44

[12] Behrens-Baumann W, Scheurer G, Schroer H. Pathogenesis of Purtscher's retinopathy. An experimental study. Graefes Arch Clin Exp Ophthalmol. 1992; 230(3):286–291

[13] Pratt MV, De Venecia G. Purtscher's retinopathy: a clinicohistopathological correlation. Surv Ophthalmol. 1970; 14(5):417–423

[14] Gomez-Ulla F, Fente B, Torreiro MG, Salorio MS, Gonzalez F. Choroidal vascular abnormality in Purtscher's retinopathy shown by indocyanine green angiography. Am J Ophthalmol. 1996; 122(2):261–263

[15] Terson A. De l'hémorrhagie dans le corps vitre au corps de l'hémorrhagie cérébrale. Clin Ophthalmol. 1900; 6:309–312

[16] Shaw HE, Jr, Landers MB, Sydnor CF. The significance of intraocular hemorrhages due to subarachnoid hemorrhage. Ann Ophthalmol. 1977; 9(11):1403–1405

[17] Garfinkle AM, Danys IR, Nicolle DA, Colohan AR, Brem S. Terson's syndrome: a reversible cause of blindness following subarachnoid hemorrhage. J Neurosurg. 1992; 76(5):766–771

[18] Fahmy JA. Fundal haemorrhages in ruptured intracranial aneurysms. I. Material, frequency and morphology. Acta Ophthalmol (Copenh). 1973; 51(3):289–298

[19] Toosi SH, Malton M. Terson's syndrome—significance of ocular findings. Ann Ophthalmol. 1987; 19(1):7–12

[20] Schultz PN, Sobol WM, Weingeist TA. Long-term visual outcome in Terson syndrome. Ophthalmology. 1991; 98(12):1814–1819

[21] García-Arumí J, Corcostegui B, Tallada N, Salvador F. Epiretinal membranes in Tersons syndrome. A clinicopathologic study. Retina. 1994; 14(4):351–355

[22] Velikay M, Datlinger P, Stolba U, Wedrich A, Binder S, Hausmann N. Retinal detachment with severe proliferative vitreoretinopathy in Terson syndrome. Ophthalmology. 1994; 101(1):35–37

[23] Weingeist TA, Goldman EJ, Folk JC, Packer AJ, Ossoinig KC. Terson's syndrome. Clinicopathologic correlations. Ophthalmology. 1986; 93(11):1435–1442

[24] Rubowitz A, Desai U. Nontraumatic macular holes associated with Terson syndrome. Retina. 2006; 26(2):230–232

[25] Keithahn MA, Bennett SR, Cameron D, Mieler WF. Retinal folds in Terson syndrome. Ophthalmology. 1993; 100(8):1187–1190

[26] Muller PJ, Deck JH. Intraocular and optic nerve sheath hemorrhage in cases of sudden intracranial hypertension. J Neurosurg. 1974; 41(2):160–166

[27] Clarkson JG, Flynn HW, Jr, Daily MJ. Vitrectomy in Terson's syndrome. Am J Ophthalmol. 1980; 90(4):549–552

[28] Greenwald MJ. The shaken baby syndrome. Semin Ophthalmol. 1990; 5:202–215

[29] Caffey J. The whiplash shaken infant syndrome: manual shaking by the extremities with whiplash-induced intracranial and intraocular bleedings, linked with residual permanent brain damage and mental retardation. Pediatrics. 1974; 54(4):396–403

[30] Spaide RF, Swengel RM, Scharre DW, Mein CE. Shaken baby syndrome. Am Fam Physician. 1990; 41(4):1145–1152

[31] Levin AV. Ocular manifestations of child abuse. Ophthalmol Clin North Am. 1990; 3:249–264

[32] Munger CE, Peiffer RL, Bouldin TW, Kylstra JA, Thompson RL. Ocular and associated neuropathologic observations in suspected whiplash shaken infant syndrome. A retrospective study of 12 cases. Am J Forensic Med Pathol. 1993; 14(3):193–200

[33] Riffenburgh RS, Sathyavagiswaran L. Ocular findings at autopsy of child abuse victims. Ophthalmology. 1991; 98(10):1519–1524

[34] Wilkinson WS, Han DP, Rappley MD, Owings CL. Retinal hemorrhage predicts neurologic injury in the shaken baby syndrome. Arch Ophthalmol. 1989; 107(10):1472–1474

[35] Brown SM, Bradley JC. Hemorrhagic posterior vitreous detachment without intraretinal hemorrhage in a shaken infant. Arch Ophthalmol. 2007; 125(9):1301

[36] Ou JI, Moshfeghi DM, Tawansy K, Sears JE. Macular hole in the shaken baby syndrome. Arch Ophthalmol. 2006; 124(6):913–915

[37] Ho LY, Goldenberg DT, Capone A, Jr. Retinal pigment epithelial tear in shaken baby syndrome. Arch Ophthalmol. 2009; 127(11):1547–1548

[38] Han DP, Wilkinson WS. Late ophthalmic manifestations of the shaken baby syndrome. J Pediatr Ophthalmol Strabismus. 1990; 27(6):299–303

[39] Massicotte SJ, Folberg R, Torczynski E, Gilliland MG, Luckenbach MW. Vitreoretinal traction and perimacular retinal folds in the eyes of deliberately traumatized children. Ophthalmology. 1991; 98(7):1124–1127

[40] Caputo G, de Haller R, Metge F, Dureau P. Ischemic retinopathy and neovascular proliferation secondary to shaken baby syndrome. Retina. 2008; 28(3) Suppl:S42–S46

[41] Hadley MN, Sonntag VK, Rekate HL, Murphy A. The infant whiplash-shake injury syndrome: a clinical and pathological study. Neurosurgery. 1989; 24(4):536–540

[42] Giangiacomo J, Khan JA, Levine C, Thompson VM. Sequential cranial computed tomography in infants with retinal hemorrhages. Ophthalmology. 1988; 95(3):295–299

[43] Schloff S, Mullaney PB, Armstrong DC, et al. Retinal findings in children with intracranial hemorrhage. Ophthalmology. 2002; 109(8):1472–1476

[44] Sturm V, Landau K, Menke MN. Optical coherence tomography findings in Shaken Baby syndrome. Am J Ophthalmol. 2008; 146(3):363–368

[45] Scott AW, Farsiu S, Enyedi LB, Wallace DK, Toth CA. Imaging the infant retina with a hand-held spectral-domain optical coherence tomography device. Am J Ophthalmol. 2009; 147(2):364–373.e2

[46] Muni RH, Kohly RP, Sohn EH, Lee TC. Hand-held spectral domain optical coherence tomography finding in shaken-baby syndrome. Retina. 2010; 30(4) Suppl:S45–S50

[47] Goldenberg DT, Wu D, Capone A, Jr, Drenser KA, Trese MT. Nonaccidental trauma and peripheral retinal nonperfusion. Ophthalmology. 2010; 117(3):561–566

[48] Chuang EL, Miller FS, III, Kalina RE. Retinal lesions following long bone fractures. Ophthalmology. 1985; 92(3):370–374

[49] McCannel CA. OCT III imaging of whiplash maculopathy. Eye (Lond). 2011; 25(4):531–532

[50] Lagrèze WD, Bömer TG, Aiello LP. Lightning-induced ocular injury. Arch Ophthalmol. 1995; 113(8):1076–1077

[51] Rivas-Aguiño PJ, Garcia RA, Arevalo JF. Bilateral macular cyst after lightning visualized with optical coherence tomography. Clin Experiment Ophthalmol. 2006; 34(9):893–894

34 Drug and Light Ocular Toxicity

Michael T. Andreoli, Robert A. Mittra, and William F. Mieler

Retinal toxicity may occur secondary to a variety of systemic medications. Fortunately, in many cases, the loss of visual function is mild, or is reversible with discontinuation of the inciting drug. Nevertheless, in some instances, permanent or progressive visual loss may occur. We present only those medications known to produce a well-described fundus abnormality. Others, which have not definitely been proven to cause retinal toxicity, are not included in this discussion.

Changes in fundus appearance and retinal function can also follow exposure to light waves. This can occur with visible (solar retinopathy, operating microscope toxicity, laser) as well as invisible (radiation retinopathy, welding arc retinopathy) light and radiation. These entities are presented along with suggestions for prevention.

34.1 Systemic and Topical Medication Toxicity

34.1.1 Disruption of the Retina and Retinal Pigment Epithelium

Phenothiazines

Thioridazine

Acute toxicity with thioridazine (Mellaril) is characterized by symptoms of blurred vision, dyschromatopsia (reddish or brownish discoloration of vision), and nyctalopia. In the earliest stages, the fundus appearance may be normal or display only mild granular pigment stippling posterior to the equator. An intermediate stage can then develop consisting of circumscribed nummular areas of retinal pigment epithelial (RPE) loss from the posterior pole to the midperiphery (▶ Fig. 34.1a).[1] Fluorescein angiography reveals disruption of the choriocapillaris in these zones (▶ Fig. 34.1b). In the late stages, more wide-spread areas of depigmentation alternating with hyperpigmented plaques, vascular attenuation, and optic atrophy are observed (▶ Fig. 34.2).

Retinal toxicity from thioridazine depends more on the total daily dose than on the cumulative amount received.[2] With higher daily doses, toxicity can develop rapidly, even within the first 2 weeks of therapy. Toxicity is rare at dosages of less than 800 mg/d, although a few cases have been reported with low doses given over several years.

In the initial stages, visual field testing may reveal mild constriction and paracentral or ring scotomas. The electroretinogram (ERG) is either normal or shows decreased oscillatory potentials. In the later stages, both the rod and cone functions of the ERG as well as the electrooculogram (EOG) are markedly abnormal. If the drug is stopped early, ERG testing improves within the first year.[3] Histologic studies demonstrate that atrophy and disorganization of photoreceptor outer segments occur before the loss of the RPE and choriocapillaris.

The early fundus changes associated with thioridazine often progress despite discontinuation of therapy following recognition of acute toxicity.[1] It is unclear whether this degeneration represents continued toxicity of the drug, or rather a nonspecific, delayed expansion of chorioretinal scarring to areas of subclinical, preexisting RPE damage.[3] Visual function, in contrast to fundus appearance, usually improves within the first year following a toxic reaction; this likely would not occur if thioridazine caused persistent toxicity. Nevertheless, in a few

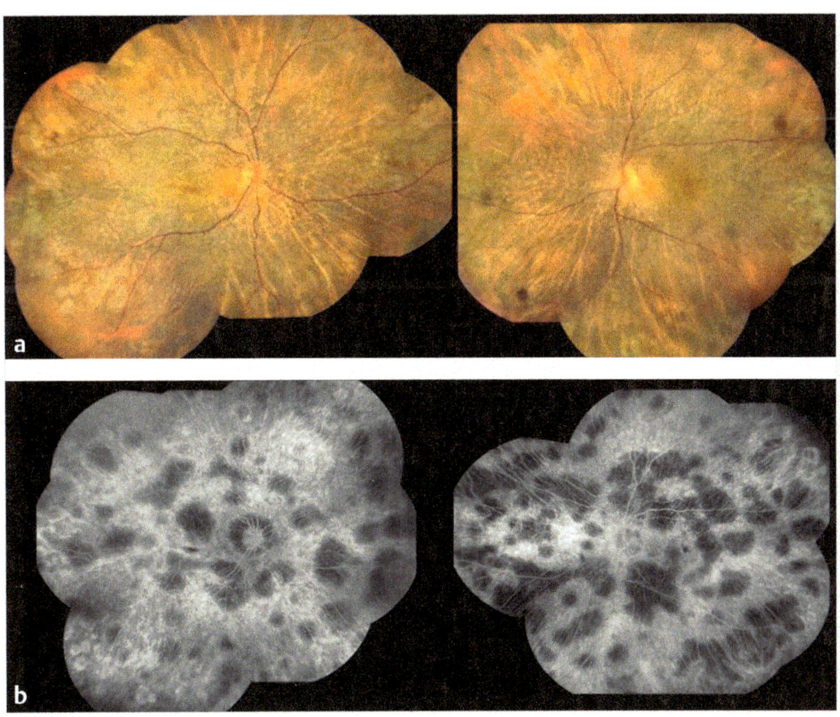

Fig. 34.1 (**a**) Fundus photograph and (**b**) fluorescein angiogram showing nummular pigment changes of intermediate thioridazine toxicity. (Image courtesy of Dr. David Sarraf.)

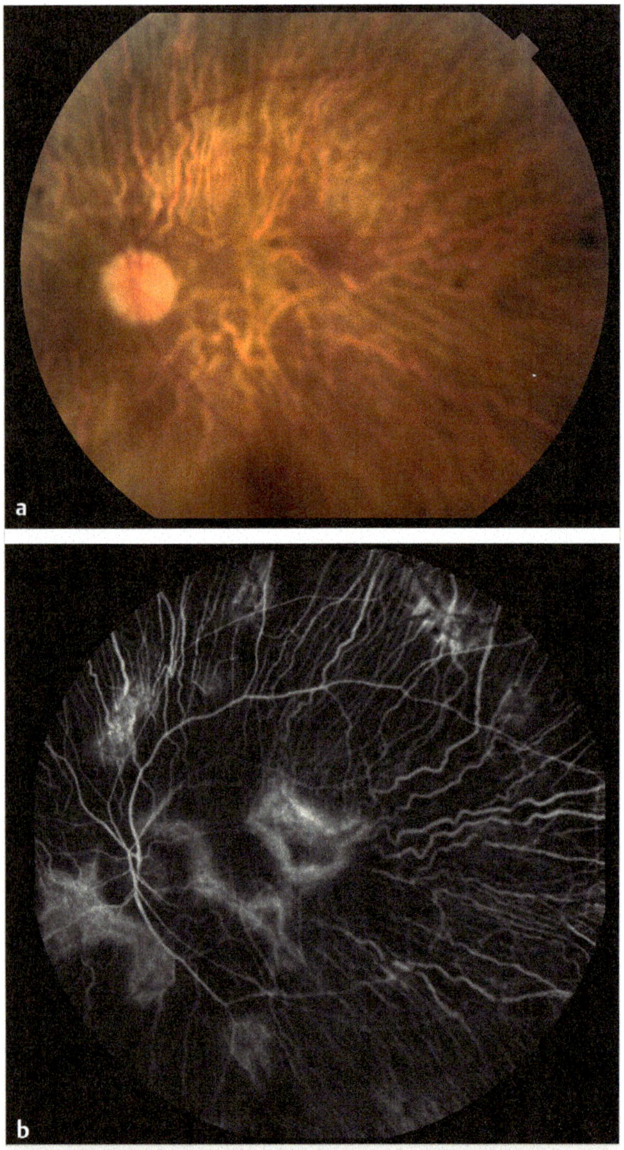

Fig. 34.2 (a) Fundus photograph and (b) fluorescein angiogram showing end-stage thioridazine toxicity with diffuse pigmentary and choriocapillaris atrophy, optic atrophy, and vascular attenuation. (Image courtesy of Dr. Daniel Kiernan.)

cases, there does appear to be a late, slow decline in functional ability as well as anatomic appearance. The precise mechanism of thioridazine-mediated toxicity is unknown, but mechanisms have been postulated involving dopamine receptor blockade or pathways leading to oxidative stress.[4,5] Many phenothiazines are known to bind to melanin granules of the RPE and uveal tissue, but not all commonly cause retinal toxicity. A compound, NP-207 (piperidyl chlorophenothiazine hydrochloride), has a very similar chemical composition to that of thioridazine, including the same piperidyl side chain. This drug was never marketed because of the pronounced pigmentary retinopathy that developed during clinical trials. This may account for the more retinotoxic effect of thioridazine in comparison with other phenothiazines, such as chlorpromazine, which do not have a piperidyl side chain. Experimental studies have shown an alteration of enzyme kinetics during phenothiazine administration and toxic inhibition of oxidative phosphorylation with subsequent abnormalities in rhodopsin synthesis. Further study is needed to determine whether these observed effects are involved in the pathogenesis of thioridazine toxicity.

The evaluation of patients on thioridazine should include a review of the daily and cumulative dose. Baseline fundus photography and possibly ERG testing may be helpful if future toxicity develops. Given the many antipsychotic medications available today, consideration of alternative agents may be discussed with the patient's psychiatrist. At the earliest sign of toxicity, thioridazine should be discontinued.

Chlorpromazine

Chlorpromazine (Thorazine) is a piperazine similar to thioridazine, but it lacks the piperidyl side chain, as mentioned earlier. The compound binds strongly to melanin and can cause pigmentation in the skin, conjunctiva, cornea, lens, and retina.[6] Other ocular effects include oculogyric crisis, miosis, and blurred vision secondary to paralysis of accommodation. Usual doses range from 40 to 75 mg/d, but doses up to 800 mg/d are not uncommon.

Retinal toxicity from chlorpromazine is rare. When massive doses are given, such as 2,400 mg/d for 12 months, they may cause pigmentary changes in the retina with attenuation of retinal vessels and optic nerve pallor. As with thioridazine, the development and extent of toxicity are more closely related to the daily dose than total amount of drug taken.

Chloroquine Derivatives

Chloroquine

Chloroquine (Aralen) was first used as an antimalarial drug in World War II. Currently, it is used for treatment of amebiasis, rheumatoid arthritis, and systemic lupus erythematosus. Retinal toxicity with degeneration of the RPE and neurosensory retina secondary to long-term daily use of chloroquine has been well described.[7] Most of the cases of retinopathy, however, developed when a higher than currently recommended dosage of 250 mg/d or 4 mg/kg per day was used. A daily dose exceeding 250 mg with a total dose of between 100 and 300 g is usually needed to produce toxicity.[8] One study showed a 19% incidence of chloroquine retinopathy (mean daily dose of 329 mg), which was increased in those older than 40 years and those with higher cumulative doses.[9] Conversely, with strict adherence to a low daily dose, the incidence of retinal abnormalities is minimal, even when total doses reach more than 1,000 g.

The earliest clinical sign of retinal toxicity may be a paracentral scotoma, which can precede the development of any ophthalmoscopic or ERG abnormality.[10] A high percentage of patients with chloroquine retinopathy also demonstrate color vision defects, predominantly blue-yellow deficiencies.[11] Subtle macular pigment stippling with a loss of the foveal light reflex usually appears on fundus examination before the development of a classic bull's-eye maculopathy, in which a ring of depigmentation surrounded by an area of hyperpigmentation is seen centered on the fovea (▶ Fig. 34.3). When the RPE abnormalities involve the center of the fovea, the visual acuity is affected. The peripheral retina can display pigment mottling, which may, in

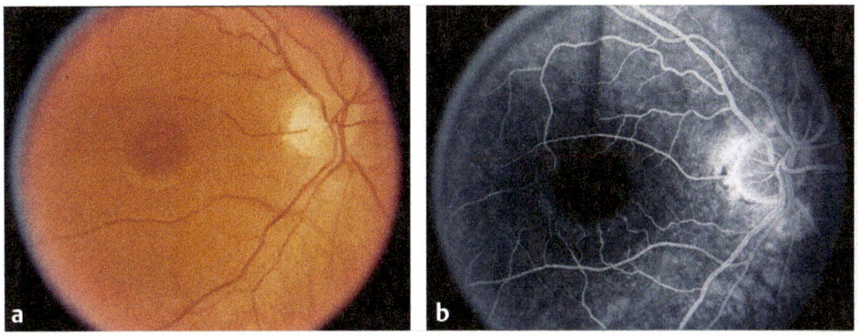

Fig. 34.3 (a) Fundus photograph and (b) fluorescein angiogram showing early chloroquine toxicity with perifoveal pigmentary changes.

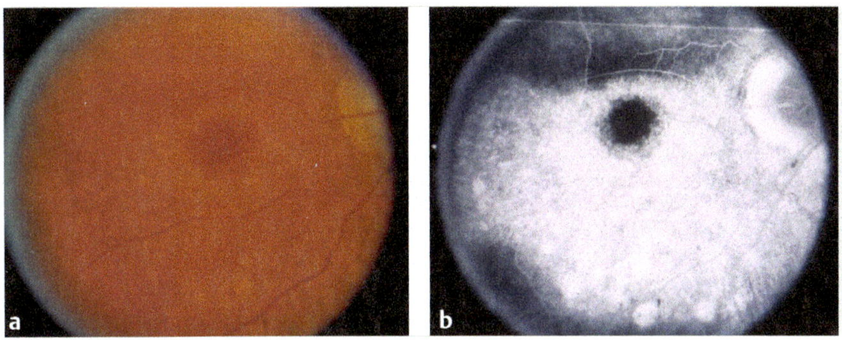

Fig. 34.4 (a) Fundus photograph and (b) fluorescein angiogram from the same patient as in Fig. 3 two years later, displaying marked progression with advanced bull's-eye pigmentary changes.

severe cases, develop the appearance of a primary tapetoretinal degeneration, with narrowed retinal vessels, optic disc pallor, and eventual blindness.

After the cessation of chloroquine treatment, early, subtle macular changes can revert to normal and advanced cases may progress (▶ Fig. 34.4a, b), but the large majority remain stable even with long-term follow-up.[12] Chloroquine is very slowly excreted from the body. It has been found in the plasma, red blood cells, and urine of patients up to 5 years after the last known ingestion. It is not surprising, therefore, that delayed onset of chloroquine retinopathy can be seen at an interval of up to 7 years or longer after discontinuation.

Fluorescein angiography can be helpful in the early demonstration of pigment abnormalities in the macula. There is minimal evidence of damage to the choriocapillaris on the fluorescein angiogram in the areas of pigment disturbance. The ERG and EOG may be abnormal early, although the EOG is sometimes supernormal initially. Multifocal ERG is capable of demonstrating evidence of toxicity before abnormalities develop on full-field ERG.[13] Histopathologic sections demonstrate loss of RPE pigmentation, with an accumulation of pigment-laden cells in the outer retinal layers and damage or reduction of photoreceptors. Electron microscopic studies reveal more widespread damage to the retina, with most of it occurring in the ganglion cell layer.

The mechanism of chloroquine-mediated retinal toxicity has not been fully elucidated. Like the phenothiazines, chloroquine is bound by melanin and concentrated in the RPE and uveal tissues. In vivo and in vitro rat models have revealed that chloroquine disrupts lysosomal function in retinal neurons and RPE.[14]

The American Academy of Ophthalmology (AAO) has issued toxicity screening recommendations for chloroquine and hydroxychloroquine (see "Hydroxychloroquine" section). If any abnormalities are detected, chloroquine therapy should be stopped.

Hydroxychloroquine

Hydroxychloroquine (Plaquenil) is also used for the treatment of rheumatoid arthritis and systemic lupus erythematosus. This medication can produce a retinopathy identical to that associated with chloroquine. With a daily dose of less than 6.5 mg/kg/d and lack of systemic renal disease, hydroxychloroquine is typically well tolerated. In many cases, cessation of therapy can result in stabilization of retinopathy; thus, regular surveillance is critical to detect early toxicity. The overall prevalence of hydroxychloroquine retinopathy is approximately 7.5%. Risk factors for the development of toxicity include daily dose per real body weight, daily dose per ideal body weight, duration of use, kidney disease, and concurrent tamoxifen treatment.[15]

Adjunctive testing now allows for earlier detection of hydroxychloroquine toxicity. Fundus autofluorescence (FAF) has become widely used imaging tool with a fairly high sensitivity for recognition of early toxicity. Mild retinopathy may show a pericentral ring of increased FAF, while more advanced stages may present as pericentral mottled loss of FAF with increased FAF in the adjacent retina. Late stages may demonstrate a complete loss of pericentral FAF.[16] Many regard multifocal ERG as the most definitive test of toxicity. An analysis of multifocal ERG findings in long-term hydroxychloroquine users revealed multiple patterns of abnormalities—paracentral loss, foveal loss, peripheral loss, and generalized loss (▶ Fig. 34.5).[17] The optical coherence tomographic (OCT) abnormalities associated with hydroxychloroquine toxicity include discontinuity of the inner segment/outer segment junction, thinning of the outer nuclear layer, and hyperscattering at the outer segment level (▶ Fig. 34.6).[18] However, perifoveal thinning of the inner plexiform and ganglion cell layers on OCT may precede structural changes to the photoreceptors.[19]

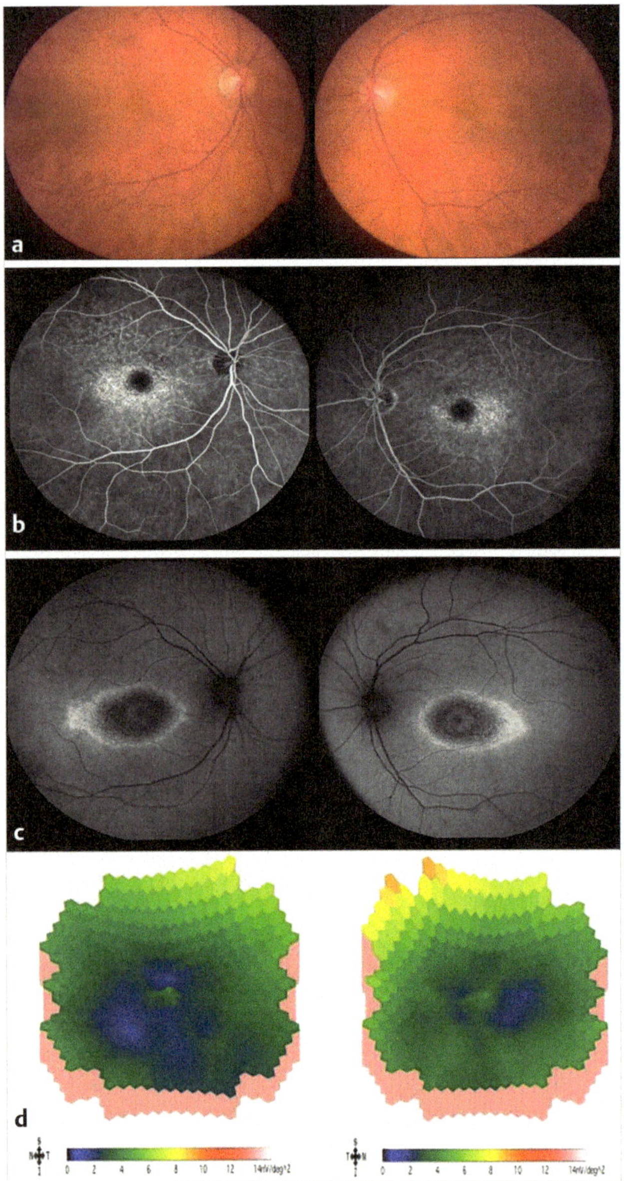

Fig. 34.5 Hydroxychloroquine toxicity: (**a**) Fundus photograph, (**b**) fluorescein angiogram, (**c**) fundus autofluorescence, and (**d**) multifocal electroretinogram demonstrating perifoveal pigmentary changes and diminished paracentral amplitudes in a patient taking hydroxychloroquine. (Image courtesy of Dr. David Sarraf.)

In early 2016, the American Academy of Ophthalmology (AAO) published revised and updated hydroxychloroquine screening guidelines. The update focused on a lowered recommended safe dosage to < 5.0 mg/kg per day of real body weight.

Additionally, it emphasized that some patients of Asian descent can demonstrate a pattern of perifoveal retinopathy, rather than central macular involvement. A final consideration is that one needs to be aware that co-existing renal disease and/or concurrent tamoxifen usage may increase or hasten development of hydroxychloroquine retinopathy. Otherwise, the recommended screening guidelines remain an annual examination, especially after 5 years of hydroxychloroquine usage, with SD-OCT, FAF, a Humphrey 10–2 Visual Field, and possible multifocal ERG.[20]

Quinine

Quinine was first used for the treatment of malaria in World War II, but currently it is prescribed for the management of nocturnal muscle cramps. The recommended daily dose is less than 2 g. Signs of systemic toxicity occur with doses greater than 4 g, and the fatal oral dose is 8 g. Ocular toxicity with quinine develops after an overdose, either by accidental ingestion or by attempted abortion or suicide. A syndrome known as *cinchonism* is rapidly produced and consists of nausea, vomiting, headache, tremor, and sometimes hypotension and loss of consciousness. When patients awake, they are often completely blind with dilated, unreactive pupils.[21] In the acute stages, fundus examination reveals mild venous dilation with minimal retinal edema and normal arterial caliber. The fluorescein angiogram displays minimal abnormalities. ERG testing shows an acute slowing down of the a-wave with increased depth, loss of oscillatory potentials, and a decreased b-wave. EOG and visual-evoked potential (VEP) testing are also abnormal.

During the next few days, visual acuity returns, but the patient is left with a small central island of vision. A progressive attenuation of the retinal arterioles with the development of optic disc pallor occurs during the next few weeks to months (▸ Fig. 34.7). The increased depth and slowing down of the a-wave revert to normal. The b-wave first normalizes, and then slowly decreases. The VEP remains abnormal, and dark adaptation reveals little or no rod function.[21] OCT demonstrates inner retinal atrophy.[22]

Early investigators believed the mechanism of quinine toxicity to be vascular in origin. This was based primarily on the fundus appearance several weeks after ingestion, which displays marked arteriolar attenuation and optic disc pallor. Recent experimental and clinical studies have demonstrated minimal involvement of the retinal vasculature in the early stages of quinine toxicity.[21] Furthermore, ERG and histologic studies show that the site of toxicity is likely the retinal ganglion, bipolar, and photoreceptor cells. The exact mechanism of quinine toxicity is unidentified, but some have suggested that it may act as an acetylcholine antagonist and disrupt cholinergic transmission in the retina.[23]

Clofazimine

Clofazimine is a red phenazine dye that has been used to treat dapsone-resistant leprosy, psoriasis, pyoderma gangrenosum, discoid lupus, and recently *Mycobacterium avium-intracellulare* complex infections in patients with AIDS. With treatment lasting several months, clofazimine crystals may accumulate in the cornea. Cases of bull's eye maculopathy with pigmentary retinopathy have been reported in patients with AIDS with doses of 200 to 300 mg/d (total dose of 40–48 g). Visual acuity was mildly affected, with reduced scotopic, photopic, and flicker ERG amplitudes. Cessation of treatment may result in the clearance of corneal deposits but does not appear to affect the retinopathy.

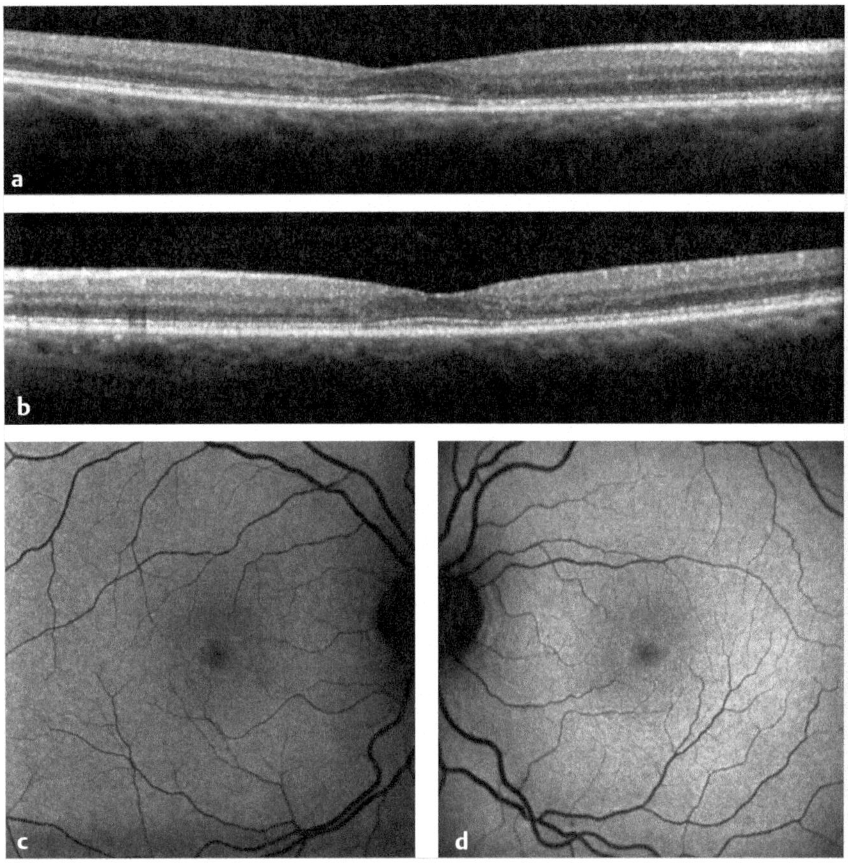

Fig. 34.6 Hydroxychloroquine toxicity: Optical coherence tomographic image of the (**a**) right and (**b**) left eye demonstrating perifoveal atrophy of the outer retinal layers and attenuation of the ellipsoid segment in a patient taking hydroxychloroquine for 9 years. Fundus autofluorescence of the (**c**) right and (**d**) left eye demonstrates a subtle bull's-eye pattern.

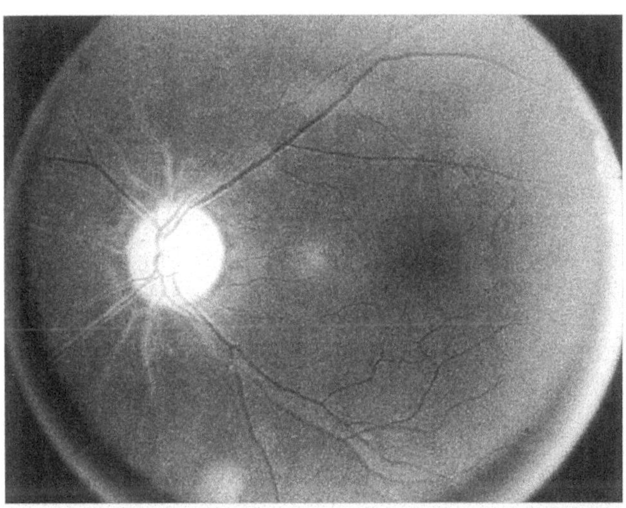

Fig. 34.7 Quinine toxicity: Fundus photograph displays the characteristic optic nerve head pallor with diffuse arteriolar attenuation.

Dideoxyinosine

A midperipheral pigmentary retinopathy (▶ Fig. 34.8) has been noted in children with AIDS receiving high-dose therapy with the antiviral 2',3'-dideoxyinosine. The cases were associated with ERG and EOG changes. Similar phenotypes have been observed in adults, with chorioretinal atrophy anterior to the vascular arcades with corresponding hypoautofluorescence or mottled hyperautofluorescence and hypoautofluorescence. OCT confirms severe chorioretinal atrophy in these regions.[24] The retinal toxicity typically stabilizes after discontinuation of the medication.

Deferoxamine

Intravenous and subcutaneous administration of deferoxamine (Desferal) has been used to treat patients who require repeated blood transfusions and in whom complications of iron overload subsequently develop. High-dose intravenous and subcutaneous therapy has produced visual loss, nyctalopia, peripheral and central field loss, reduced dark adaptation, ERG, and EOG responses.[25] Fundi can be normal initially, or there may be a faint graying of the macula.

Pigmentary changes in the macula and periphery develop within a few weeks. In some instances, toxicity may present as vitelliform macular lesions.[26] Accumulated material has been shown to deposit within the outer retina or in the Bruch's membrane–RPE complex on OCT.[27] Visual function returns with cessation of therapy. Deferoxamine forms chelates with many metals other than iron, and it is possible that the mechanism of toxicity may involve the removal of copper from the RPE.[25] Histopathologic changes occur primarily in the RPE and include loss of microvilli from the apical surface, patchy depigmentation, vacuolation of the cytoplasm, swelling and calcification of mitochondria, and disorganization of the plasma membrane.

Cisplatin and Carmustine

Cisplatin (Platinol) and carmustine (BCNU) are used for the treatment of malignant gliomas and metastatic breast cancer.

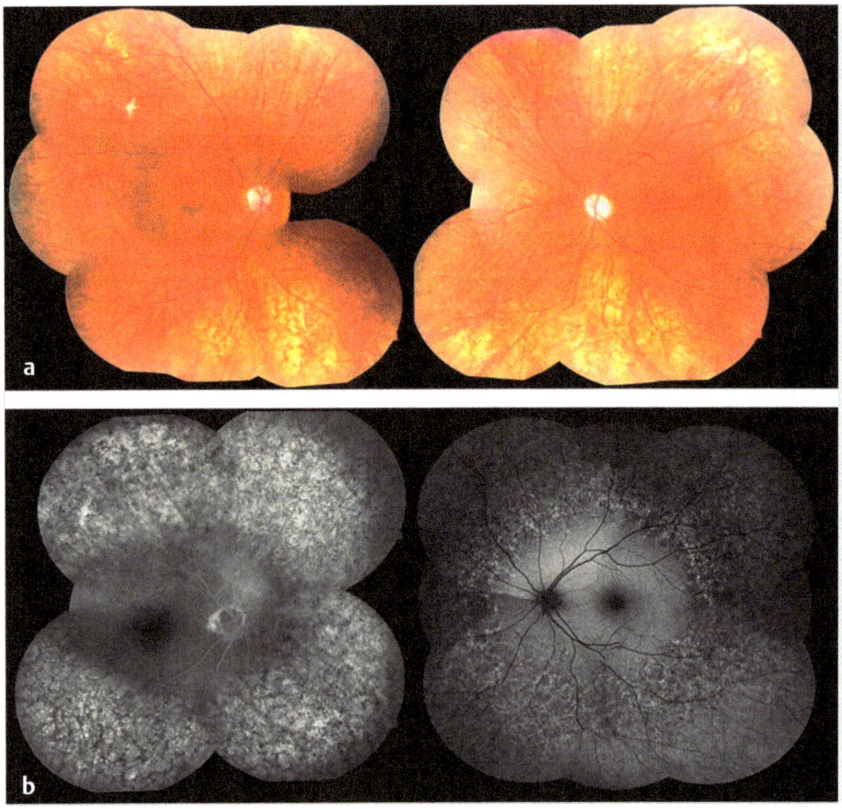

Fig. 34.8 Dideoxyinosine toxicity: (**a**) Fundus photograph displaying midperipheral pigmentary retinopathy. (**b**) Fluorescein angiogram of right eye and fundus autofluorescence of left eye demonstrating mottled hyperfluorescence and hyperautofluorescence in the midperiphery. (Image courtesy of Dr. David Sarraf.)

Retinal toxicity of three different types has been reported with these agents. A pigmentary retinopathy of the macula with markedly decreased visual acuity and abnormal ERG and EOG testing has been reported after administration of intra-arterial cisplatin and carmustine, and with cisplatin alone for malignant glioma.[28] In another study, intra-arterial cisplatin with intravenous carmustine caused macular pigmentary and decreased vision, but with a normal ERG.[29] These findings may be the result of platinum toxicity to the retina, as is seen with other metals, such as iron and copper. A retinopathy consisting of cotton-wool spots, intraretinal hemorrhages, and macular exudate and optic neuropathy with disc swelling have been reported after high-dose chemotherapy with cisplatin, cyclophosphamide, and carmustine and autologous bone marrow transplantation for metastatic breast cancer.[30] These changes were thought to be associated with a 1.2-fold higher cisplatin dose given to affected patients.

In approximately 65% of patients receiving intra-arterial carmustine alone or combined with cisplatin for malignant glioma, a vascular retinopathy or optic neuropathy develops that can include arterial occlusion, vasculitis, and papillitis.[28] These fundus changes are associated with profound visual loss that begins about 6 weeks after the start of therapy. Other ocular effects may include orbital pain, chemosis, secondary glaucoma, internal ophthalmoplegia, and cavernous sinus syndrome. Injection of the medication above the ophthalmic artery can still result in toxicity. Visual loss is usually progressive, and no treatment is known.

34.1.2 Vascular Damage

Cisplatin and Carmustine (BCNU)

Oral Contraceptives

Oral contraceptives have been implicated in some cases of central retinal vein occlusion, retinal and cilioretinal artery obstruction, and retinal edema. The synthetic estrogen and progesterone contained in contraceptive pills are thought to affect coagulation factors adversely and induce a hypercoagulable state leading to thromboembolic complications. Most of the studies reporting ocular complications are from the 1960s and 1970s, when the estrogen concentrations used in the contraceptive pills were much higher. Recent prospective studies have not shown an increased incidence of ocular pathology in patients taking oral contraceptives.[31]

Interferon

Interferons α2a and α2b were originally used as an antiviral agent, but it is currently used for Kaposi's sarcoma, hemangiomas of infancy, and chronic hepatitis C, in chemotherapy protocols, and experimentally for the treatment of choroidal neovascular membranes. Interferon therapy has been associated with the development of multiple cotton-wool spots and retinal hemorrhages (▶ Fig. 34.9).[32] Visual acuity is usually not affected. Changes are noted within the first 4 to 8 weeks of therapy and are seen more frequently in diabetic and hypertensive patients.

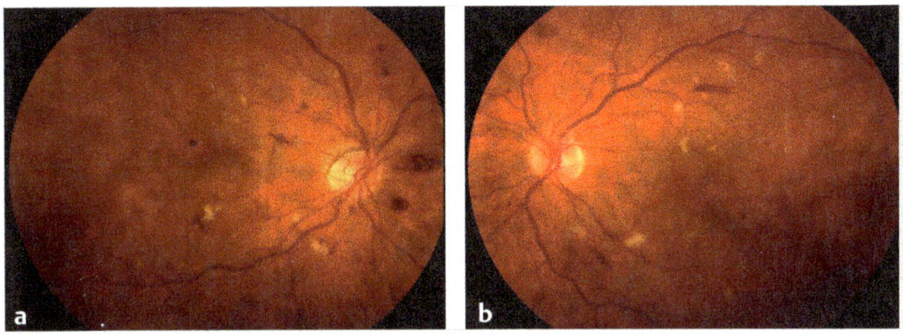

Fig. 34.9 Interferon toxicity. Fundus photograph demonstrating extensive cotton-wool spots and retinal hemorrhages. (Image courtesy of Dr. Joseph Maguire.)

Miscellaneous Agents

Ergot alkaloids in higher than recommended doses have been reported to cause retinal vasoconstriction, and over-the-counter phenylpropanolamine used in appetite suppressants and decongestants has been implicated in one case of central retinal vein occlusion.

34.1.3 Cystoid Macular Edema

Epinephrine

The use of topical epinephrine compounds for intraocular pressure control has been curtailed since the development of other, more efficacious glaucoma medicines. One of the side effects of topical epinephrine agents in aphakic eyes is macular edema that is indistinguishable clinically and angiographically from aphakic cystoid macular edema. In the largest controlled study, 28% of aphakic eyes treated with epinephrine and 13% of untreated aphakic eyes had macular edema, and the difference was found to be statistically significant.[33] Discontinuation of epinephrine therapy prompted resolution of cystoid edema in most cases. This medication should be avoided in the treatment of aphakic and pseudophakic eyes.

Nicotinic Acid (Niacin)

Nicotinic acid (niacin) in high doses can decrease serum lipid and cholesterol levels. Since the advent of more effective and better-tolerated 3-hydroxy-3methylglutaryl-coenzyme (HMG-CoA) reductase inhibitor agents, this medication is now seldom used. Fewer than 1% of patients taking nicotinic acid at doses greater than 1.5 g/d will complain of blurred central vision, sometimes associated with a paracentral scotoma or metamorphopsia. On fundus examination, the typical appearance of cystoid macular edema is present (▶ Fig. 34.10), but on fluorescein angiography, no retinal vascular leakage of dye is noted.[34] OCT has localized the cystoid spaces to the outer plexiform and inner nuclear layer.[35] With cessation of treatment, vision improves and the edema resolves. Given the rarity of this condition, only patients on high-dose niacin who have visual symptoms should be evaluated.

Latanoprost

Latanoprost (Xalatan) is a first-line prostaglandin analog used topically to lower intraocular pressure. New or recurrent cystoid macular edema has been observed in pseudophakic eyes.[36] The exact rate is not known, although a moderately-sized case series estimated the incidence of macular edema in latanoprost users to be 2%.[37] The incidence appears to be higher in aphakic and pseudophakia patients. The CME frequently resolves after 4 to 6 weeks of discontinuing the medicine.

Paclitaxel and Docetaxel

The chemotherapeutic agents, paclitaxel (Abraxane, Taxol) and docetaxel (Taxotere), belong to the taxane family of drugs which target the degradation of microtubules during cell division. These medications are used in the treatment of breast, lung, and prostate cancers. They have been implicated in the development of macular edema (▶ Fig. 34.11). Typically, fluorescein angiography does not exhibit associated leakage.[38,39] The macular edema may respond to carbonic anhydrase inhibitors or anti-VEGF therapy.

Fingolimod

Fingolimod (Gilenya) is an immunomodulatory agent targeting the sphingosine-1-phosphate receptor for the treatment of multiple sclerosis. This medication has been implicated in the development of cystoid macular edema, usually within 4 months of treatment initiation. The incidence of macular edema ranged from 0.3 to 1.2%, depending on the dosage. OCT localizes the cysts to the inner nuclear layer, and to a lesser extent, the outer nuclear layer. There may be associated perifoveal leakage on fluorescein angiography. Most cases resolve with discontinuation of the drug and administration of topical anti-inflammatory agents.[40]

34.1.4 Crystalline Retinopathy

Tamoxifen

Tamoxifen (Nolvadex) is an antiestrogen agent used in the treatment of breast carcinoma. Retinal toxicity consisting of decreased visual acuity and color vision with white intraretinal crystalline deposits, macular edema, and punctate retinal pigmentary changes can occur. The intraretinal deposits appear to reside in the inner retina and are most numerous in paramacular areas (▶ Fig. 34.12). Early reports were of patients who had received high doses (> 100 g total) of the drug. Recent studies have demonstrated that long-term low doses with a total of as little as 7.7 g can also result in ocular toxicity.[41] Even asymptomatic patients may exhibit intraretinal crystalline formation.[42] With discontinuation of the drug, visual function and edema improve, but the refractile deposits remain.

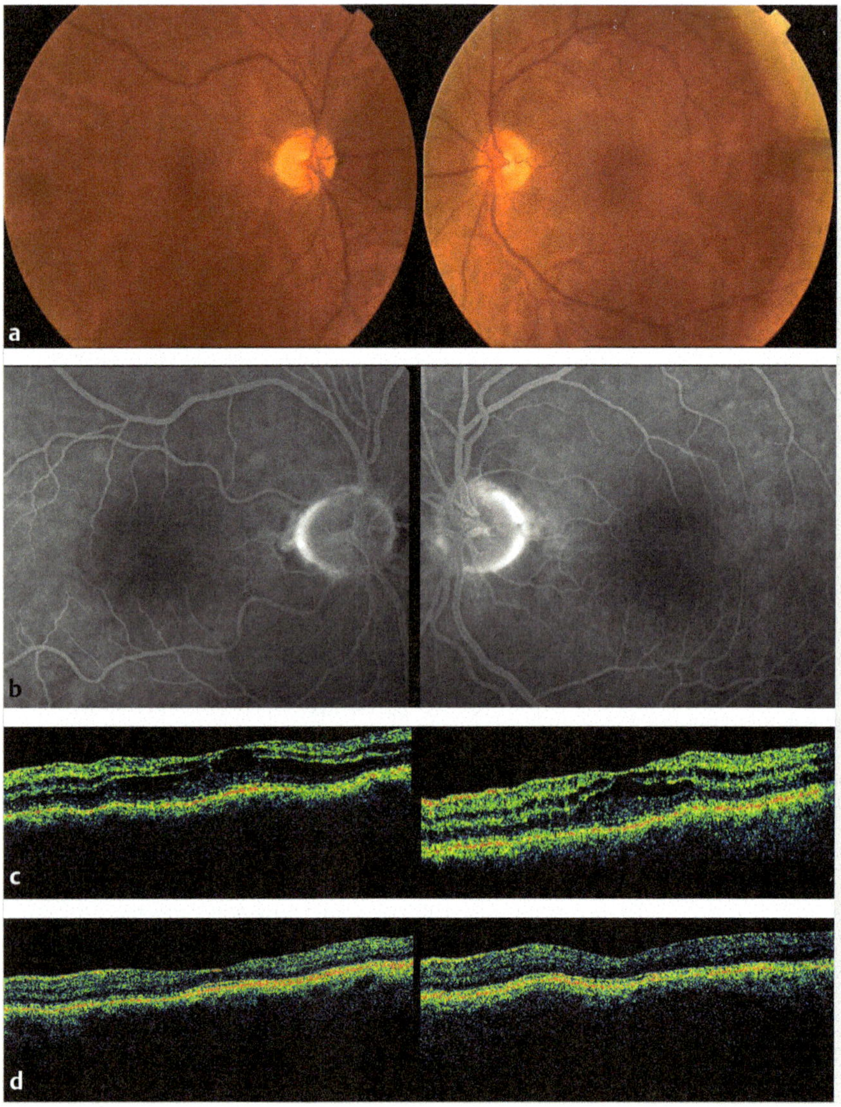

Fig. 34.10 Nicotinic acid maculopathy: (a) Fundus photograph displays a cystic appearance in the fovea. (b) There was no leakage on the fluorescein angiogram. (c) Optical coherence tomography demonstrates macular edema (d) with resolution 2 weeks after discontinuation of niacin. (Image courtesy of Dr. Lawrence Yannuzzi.)

Fluorescein angiography demonstrates late focal staining in the macula consistent with cystoid macular edema. Decreased photopic and scotopic a- and b-wave amplitudes are noted on ERG testing. Foveolar cystoid spaces on OCT have been demonstrated in some patients.[43] Light microscopy reveals lesions confined to the nerve fiber and inner plexiform layers that stain positively for glycosaminoglycans. Small (3–10 µm) intracellular and large (30–35 µm) extracellular lesions within axons are noted on electron microscopy.[44] The lesions appear to represent products of axonal degeneration similar to corpora amylacea. Decreased vision with bilateral optic disc swelling and retinal hemorrhages has been reported in a patient just 3 weeks after commencement of therapy with tamoxifen. These findings resolved completely after the drug was stopped. On current, low-dose therapy (20 mg/d), retinal lesions are rare and routine examination of asymptomatic patients is not indicated.[42] If a patient on tamoxifen is noted to have intraretinal crystals, fluorescein angiography to rule out juxtafoveal telangiectasis, which can have similar-appearing lesions, should be performed. With confirmed evidence of toxicity, the medication should be stopped.

Canthaxanthin

Canthaxanthin is a naturally occurring carotenoid. It is used as a food coloring, for skin pigmentation in the treatment of vitiligo, and for the treatment of photosensitivity disorders such as erythropoietic proto-porphyria, psoriasis, and photosensitive eczema. It has also been available over the counter and used in high doses as an oral tanning agent. Many reports have described a characteristic ring-shaped deposition of yellow-orange crystals in the superficial retina in persons taking high doses (usually a total dose > 19 g during 2 years) (▶ Fig. 34.13).[45,46] The crystals may be more prominent in eyes with other retinal diseases and with concurrent use of beta-carotene.[46]

Patients are usually asymptomatic. Fluorescein angiography is also usually normal. There have been scattered reports of both normal and abnormal ERG, EOG, dark adaptation, and static threshold perimetry. Even though crystals are clinically evident only in the macula, morphologically eyes display lipid-soluble crystals in the entire inner retina and ciliary body. They are, as would be expected, larger and more numerous surrounding the fovea. The crystals are located in spongy,

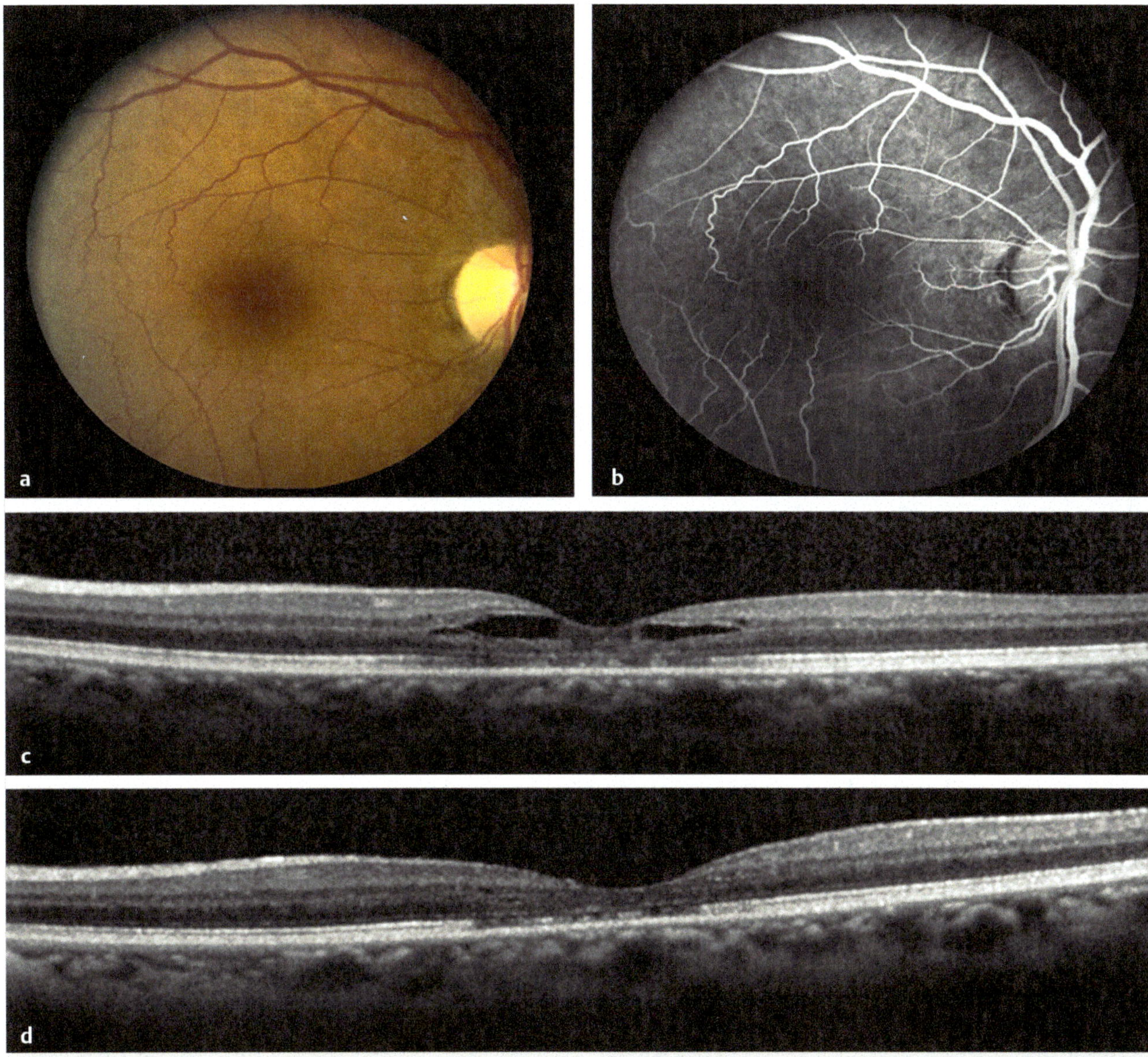

Fig. 34.11 Paclitaxel toxicity: (a) Fundus photograph showing macular edema without leakage on (b) fluorescein angiogram. (c) Optical coherence tomography of the left eye demonstrating macular edema (d) which improved after intravitreal injection of bevacizumab.

degenerated areas of the inner neuropil and are associated with atrophy of Müller's cells.

With discontinuation of treatment, deposits may slowly clear during many years. This slow reversal correlates with the detection of high plasma levels of canthaxanthin many months after discontinuation. Rarely, a fundus picture identical to that of canthaxanthin maculopathy can be seen in patients who have not taken extradietary canthaxanthin. High dietary intake along with preexisting retinal disease is thought to partially explain this phenomenon.

Methoxyflurane

Methoxyflurane (Penthrane) is an inhalational anesthetic that, when used for extended periods of time, especially in patients with renal insufficiency, causes irreversible renal failure secondary to deposition of calcium oxalate crystals in the kidney. These crystals are also deposited elsewhere throughout the body. Fundus examination of these patients reveals numerous yellow-white punctate lesions in the posterior pole or in a periarterial distribution.[47] Histologically, the deposits are located in both the RPE and inner retina.

Talc

While not a medicinal agent, talc particles in intravenous drug abusing patients, can result in a distinctive form of crystalline retinopathy.[48] Small, white crystals concentrated in the end arterioles of the posterior pole (▶ Fig. 34.14) may result from the intravenous injection of crushed oral medications such as methylphenidate hydrochloride (Ritalin) or methadone HCl, which contain talc as a filler material. Talc particles initially embolize to the pulmonary vasculature, and may enter the systemic circulation through collateral vessels that form with chronic abuse. An ischemic retinopathy may result, with associated capillary nonperfusion, microaneurysm formation, cotton-

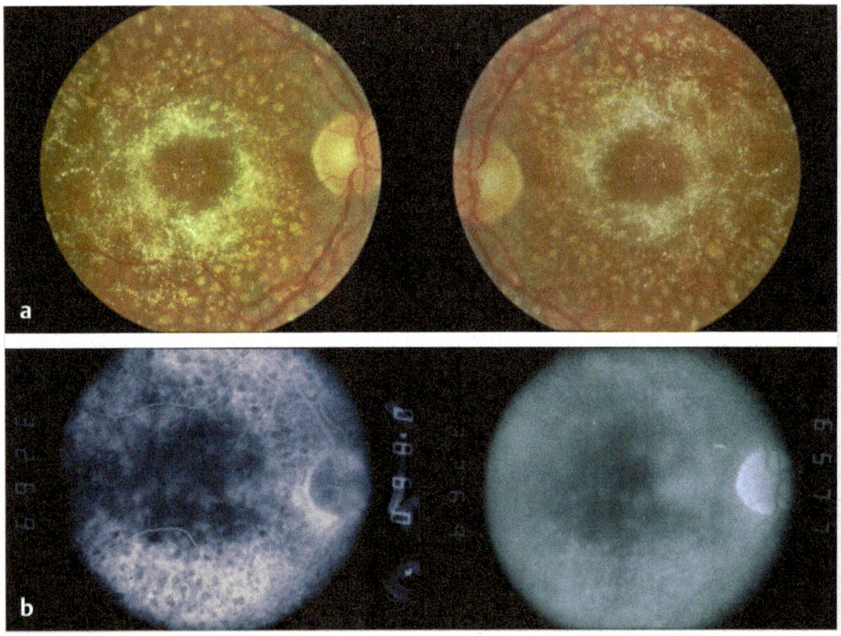

Fig. 34.12 Tamoxifen retinopathy: (**a**) fundus photographs OU displaying characteristic yellowwhite macular crystals, with (**b**) corresponding fluorescein angiogram revealing focal mid-frame and late frame staining

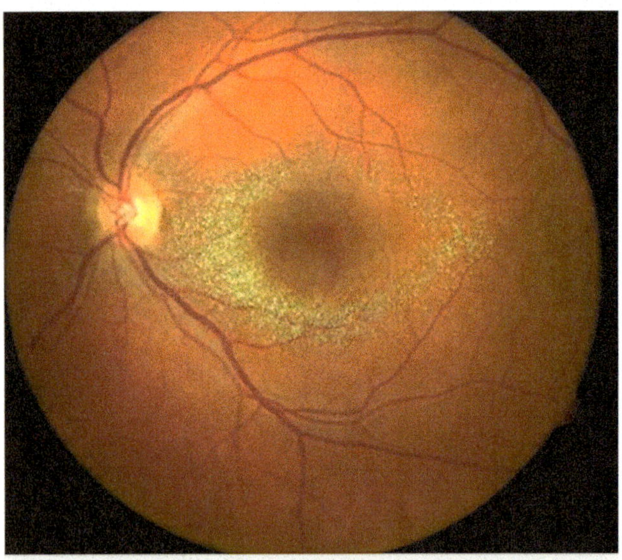

Fig. 34.13 Canthaxanthin retinopathy: Note the prominent, perifoveal punctate yellow deposits. Fluorescein angiography was essentially unremarkable.

wool spots, and venous loops.[49,50] Management of resulting neovascularization and vitreous hemorrhage may involve laser photocoagulation and pars plana vitrectomy as with proliferative diabetic retinopathy.

34.1.5 Retinal Folds

Sulfa Antibiotics, Acetazolamide, Ethoxyzolamide, Chlorthalidone, Hydrochlorothiazide, Topiramate, and Triamterene

Several medications, most with a structure similar to that of sulfanilamide, can cause a syndrome of transient acute myopia and anterior chamber shallowing. This phenomenon is thought to occur secondary to ciliary body swelling with subsequent forward rotation of the lens–iris diaphragm.[51] Retinal folds in the macula are seen in young patients with this syndrome (► Fig. 34.15), but fluorescein angiography does not reveal retinal leakage.[52] The folds presumably develop secondary to vitreous traction on the macula caused by the forward shift of the lens and iris.

34.1.6 Uveitis

Rifabutin

Rifabutin (Mycobutin) is a rifamycin antibiotic used for prophylaxis and treatment of disseminated *M. avium-complex* infection. A severe uveitic reaction may develop with bilateral involvement and hypopyon formation. This inflammatory response occurs more frequently when used in conjunction with clarithromycin, fluconazole, or itraconazole. Although the episodes more commonly represent an anterior uveitis, vitritis and retinal vasculitis have also been observed.[53,54] Treatment may consist of topical steroids or discontinuation of the medication.

Cidofovir

Cidofovir (Vistide) is a nucleotide analog used in the treatment of cytomegalovirus retinitis. Intravenous and intravitreal administration has been associated with anterior uveitis and hypotony.[55,56] The response may be due to a direct effect on the ciliary body.[57] This reaction may be treated with topical corticosteroids, cycloplegics, and oral probenecid.

34.2 Light Toxicity

Light can cause retinal toxicity through mechanical, photothermal, or photochemical effects, or through a combination of

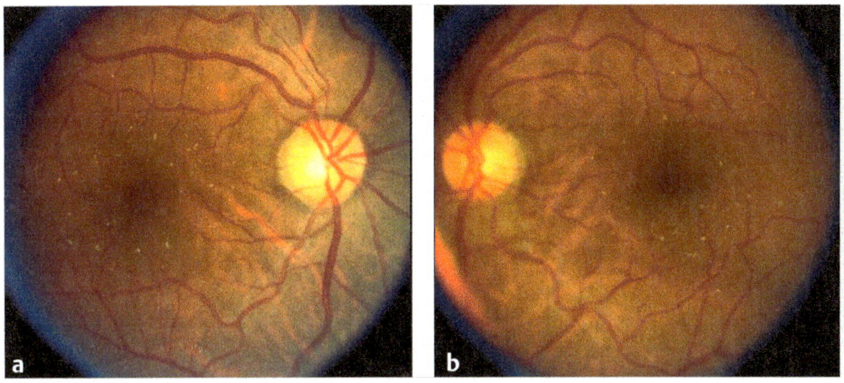

Fig. 34.14 Talc retinopathy: Fundus photograph demonstrating crystals present in end arterioles throughout posterior pole.

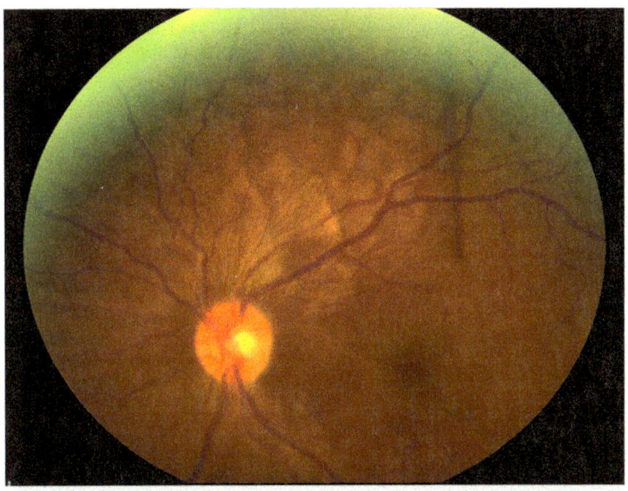

Fig. 34.15 Fundus photograph highlighting characteristic retinal striae in a patient using topiramate.

these factors. Mechanical damage occurs secondary to exposure to ultrashort Q-switched photodisruptor lasers, such as the neodymium:YAG (yttrium–aluminum–garnet), which cause ionization and disintegration of the target. Surrounding tissues are then mechanically disrupted by the shock and acoustic waves. Photocoagulative effects occur with longer exposure to focused laser beams (such as argon or krypton) or light, which heats the tissue to more than 10 to 20 °C above body temperature and causes thermal damage to retinal proteins. Photochemical damage results with exposure to visible or near-ultraviolet (UV) light, which causes retinal damage without an appreciable temperature elevation.

34.2.1 Solar Retinopathy

Solar retinopathy, which is also known as *eclipse burn* or *foveomacalar retinitis*, occurs in patients who have viewed an eclipse or gazed directly at the sun through a religious ritual, mental illness, influence of hallucinogenic drugs, malingering, or concocted therapeutic measure to strengthen the eye. Solar retinopathy has also been described in some patients who have been sunbathing or exercising outdoors with no direct sun-gazing behavior.[58] The typical patient is a young adult who is emmetropic. Shortly after gazing at the sun, the patient complains of decreased visual acuity, central scotoma, photophobia, and metamorphopsia. Vision is usually reduced bilaterally, but often more prominently in the dominant eye.

Acutely following exposure, the visual acuity is 20/30 to 20/100. This typically improves to 20/20 to 20/40 during the ensuing weeks to months. The fundus appearance varies according to the severity of injury. Those minimally afflicted will have normal fundi or a faint grayish thickening of the RPE in the foveal area. As the vision improves, these macular changes fade. With more extensive retinopathy, one or many small, yellow-white spots with surrounding gray patches develop in the center of the fovea (▶ Fig. 34.16). Within several days to 2 weeks, this lesion is replaced by a small (25- to 75-µm), reddish lamellar hole or depression in the foveal area. The depression is likely caused by loss of the retinal photoreceptors. In some patients with a particularly protracted exposure, larger lesions with pigment mottling of the RPE form during many weeks. Initially, the fluorescein angiogram is usually normal, but a few patients may exhibit a small focal area of staining in the macula (▶ Fig. 34.16b). In others, a transmission defect develops secondary to atrophic changes in the RPE.

The damage to the retina from sun gazing was originally thought to be a result of thermal injury, but Mainster has demonstrated that the temperature rise induced is insufficient for photocoagulation to occur.[59] Thus, photochemical or a combination of chemical and thermal effects results in solar retinopathy. Histologic tissue was obtained in a study in which patients with choroidal melanoma gazed at the sun for 1 hour a few days before an enucleation was scheduled.[60] Damage to pigment granules of the RPE was noted in all three cases. Similar effects on the apical melanosomes of the RPE after exposure to blue light have also been confirmed in laboratory studies.

Many factors may predispose patients to damage secondary to solar exposure, including young age, emmetropia, large pupillary size, increased body temperature, and clear ocular media. The cornea naturally absorbs light shorter than 300 nm, and the lens in older adults absorbs light in the 300- to 400-nm range. The lens develops this capability with a linear increase in absorption from age 20 to its peak at age 30. Thus, children, young adults, and aphakic individuals (or those with non–UV-absorbing intraocular lenses [IOLs]) are at the greatest risk for solar retinopathy. In experimental studies, the retina was found to be six times more sensitive to near-UV light (325–350 nm) than to blue light (441 nm). In addition, histologic lesions differed significantly from those produced with blue light and consisted of irreparable damage to the rod and cone photoreceptors.[61] Geophysical factors, such as the height of the ozone layer, have been

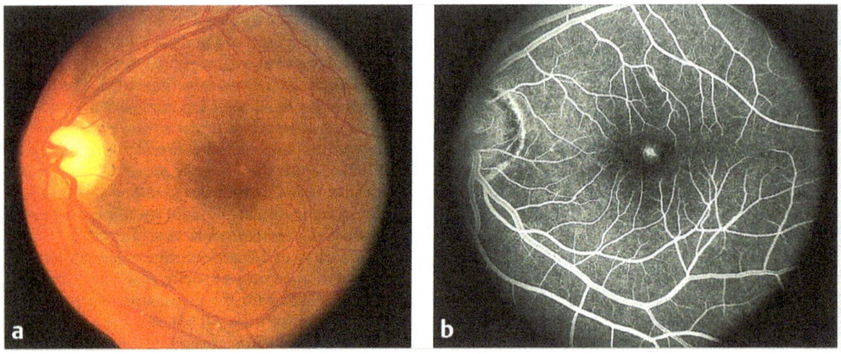

Fig. 34.16 (a) Fundus photograph and (b) fluorescein angiogram show the yellow foveal spot of solar retinopathy with a corresponding fluorescein angiographic window defect.

implicated in the pathogenesis of solar retinopathy in young individuals without direct sun-gazing activity.[58] Presumably, at times of low ozone protection, the increased UV transmission in conjunction with the young, clear lenses of these patients may result in retinal damage without direct sun gazing.

Diagnosis is usually straightforward, given the clinical history and characteristic fundus appearance. The fundus lesion should be differentiated from an aborted stage I macular hole or ocular trauma, which may also demonstrate a foveal depression. Increased public education, particularly before an eclipse, is likely to decrease the incidence of this condition. Also, young and aphakic/pseudophakic patients should be warned about the need to wear appropriate UV-filtering sunglasses in bright environmental situations, as when boating or snow skiing on a sunny day.

34.2.2 Welding Arc Retinopathy

Exposure to a welding arc without filtering goggles commonly results in a painful keratoconjunctivitis secondary to absorption of UV light by the cornea and lens. In addition, infrared (IR) radiation may cause a true exfoliation of the lens capsule, known as the "glassblower's cataract." Retinal damage secondary to exposure to welding arcs is rare; however, long, intensive exposure may result in facial burning, eyelid edema, and a central scotoma with foveal changes similar to those seen in solar maculopathy.[62] The clinical course and findings follow those of solar retinopathy, and available evidence suggests that photochemical injury of the retina results from exposure to visible blue and UV light.

34.2.3 Laser Exposure

Contact lenses used for fundus visualization during slit-lamp retinal photocoagulation procedures all have an antireflective coating to reduce the backscatter of harmful laser light. In addition, all modern slit-lamp photocoagulators and operating room endophotocoagulators have a filter that is switched into position with activation of the foot pedal to protect the surgeon. Assistants and other personnel near the operated eye, however, are subject to harmful reflections from the surface of the contact lens despite its antireflective coating. The reflected light may exceed occupational exposure limits if they are within 1 m of the contact lens.[63] Personnel in the operating room and laser suite should wear protective goggles appropriate for the wavelength of the laser used, and those in the laser suite should avoid the conical reflection zone behind the operator and slit-lamp contact lens.

Operators are not protected from the bright reflections associated with the aiming beam. Some have questioned whether the glare could cause ocular damage in surgeons and bystanders.[64] Experiments, however, alleged that aiming beam reflections were not hazardous.[63] Nevertheless, there have been several reports of decreased color contrast sensitivity among ophthalmologists who perform laser.[65] The defect correlated with the number of years of experience using lasers and number of patients treated. These ophthalmologists all used the argon blue-green laser, and retinal damage secondary to the blue portion of the aiming beam was postulated. Newer photocoagulators have an argon green-only aiming beam, and use of these has not resulted in toxicity to date.

Direct ocular exposure to hand-held recreational and commercial laser pointers has also been associated with retinal damage.[66] Clinically, disturbances may exhibit yellow deep retinal lesions. RPE disturbances may be present with accompanying window defects on fluorescein angiography. OCT may reveal disruption of the external limiting membrane and outer photoreceptors (▶ Fig. 34.17), as well as hyperreflective lesions extending from the external limiting membrane to the RPE.[67] Retinal architecture and visual defects may partially improve over time, though structural damage on occasion may be permanent, with indefinite visual impairment as well.

34.2.4 Operating Room Microscope Toxicity

Animal studies have shown that retinal toxicity can be created with exposure to light from a variety of ophthalmic instruments, including the slit lamp, indirect ophthalmoscope, operating microscope, and fiberoptic endoilluminator. The operating microscope is of particular concern, given that the retinal irradiance is three to four times higher than that of indirect ophthalmoscopes and 20 times that of overhead surgical lamps.[68] Human studies have not been able to produce retinal toxicity after 45 minutes of continuous macular exposure to the indirect ophthalmoscope (although the creation of corneal edema blocked light transmission to the retina), and no cases of slit-lamp–related toxicity have ever been reported. Beginning in 1983, however, numerous reports of operating microscope-induced maculopathy have appeared in association with many types of ocular surgery.[69,70]

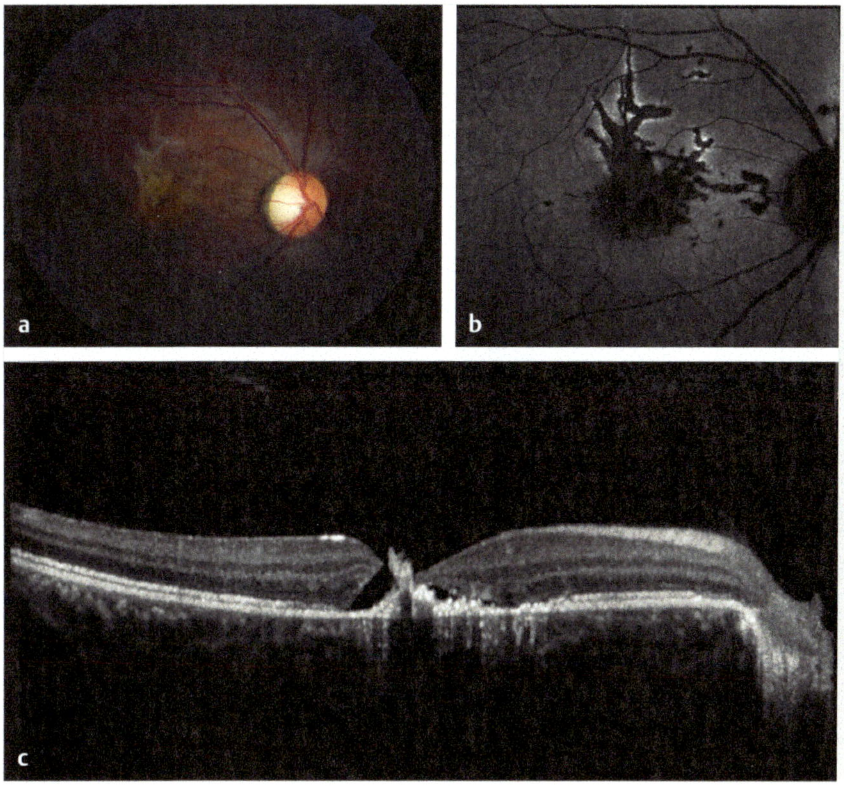

Fig. 34.17 (a) Fundus photograph, (b) fundus autofluorescence (FAF), and (c) SD-OCT images, demonstrating full-thickness retinal damage secondary to self-inflicted, repetitive, laser pointer exposure. Reprinted with permission from Freund KB, Sarraf D, Mieler WF, Yannuzzi L. The Retinal Atlas 2nd edition, Elsevier. NY: 2016

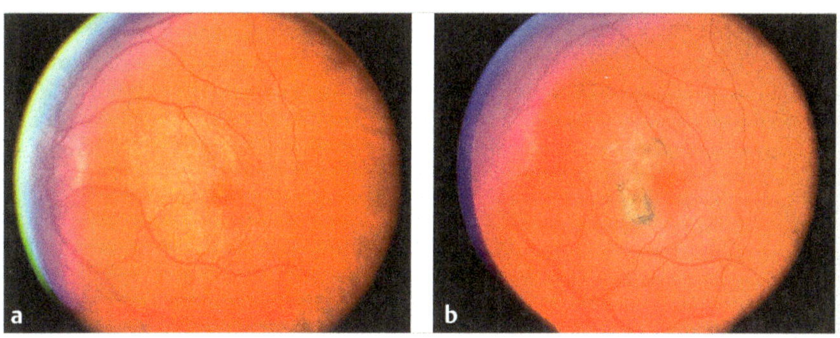

Fig. 34.18 Fundus photographs display the (a) acute and (b) chronic appearance of microscope light toxicity. Note the prominent retinal whitening acutely with the development of pigmentary changes chronically.

The retinal lesions secondary to operating microscope retinopathy are usually noted in the early postoperative period, and patients may complain of a paracentral scotoma. Visual impairment depends on the size and location of the defect. Fundus examination reveals an oval, yellow-white, deep retinal lesion located in the parafoveal area (▶ Fig. 34.18a). The inferior location is the most common because the customary use of a superior rectus bridle suture places the light image on this area of the retina.[70,71] In some cases, overlying serous fluid may be noted. The white retinal lesion fades during the first few weeks and is replaced by irregular pigment mottling, alternating with areas of pigment rarefaction (▶ Fig. 34.18b).

In a review of 135 consecutive cataract cases, the incidence of microscope toxicity was 7.4%.[70] The most critical risk factor for the generation of toxicity was the total operative time. All but one case exceeded 100 minutes in length. The greatest risk for retinal injury occurs after the IOL has been placed and a focused image is projected on the macula. Several authors have postulated that near-UV light is the cause of operating microscope retinopathy, and that the routine use of UV filters in microscopes and IOLs could diminish its incidence. Modern operating microscopes, however, do not produce an appreciable amount of light below 400 nm. Furthermore, classic lesions have been created in a patient with a blind eye (with clear phakic media) despite the use of an UV and IR filter.[72] Thus, lesions are most likely created after long exposures to visible blue light. Filtering this portion of the spectrum from 400 to 500 nm could theoretically eliminate toxicity, but it would change the color of the operating light to a faint yellow, which might affect surgical manipulations.

In an experimental model, retinal phototoxicity after light exposure was enhanced by increases in inspired oxygen during surgery.[73] Consequently, the use of higher levels of inspired oxygen than is absolutely necessary should be avoided. Retinal toxicity has also been reported with utilization of a fiberoptic endoilluminator during pars plana vitrectomy.[74] The risk appears to be highest with removal of epiretinal membranes. Lesions tend to spare the fovea, as do operating microscope defects, and this relative protection is thought to be mediated by macular xanthophyll. Animal studies have shown that an

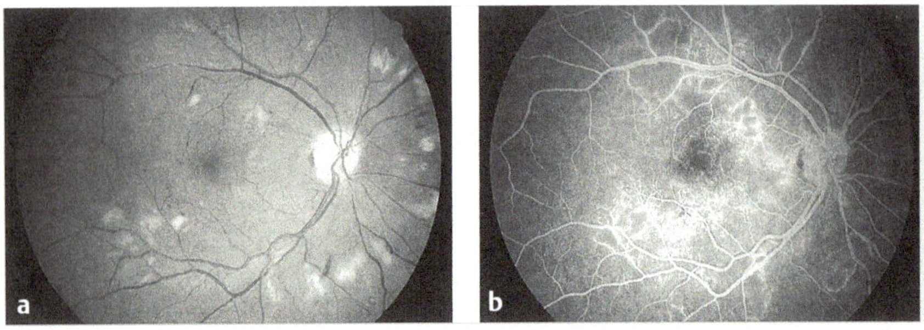

Fig. 34.19 (a) Fundus photograph and (b) fluorescein angiogram show the early stages of radiation retinopathy with cotton-wool spots, microaneurysms, and scattered capillary nonperfusion.

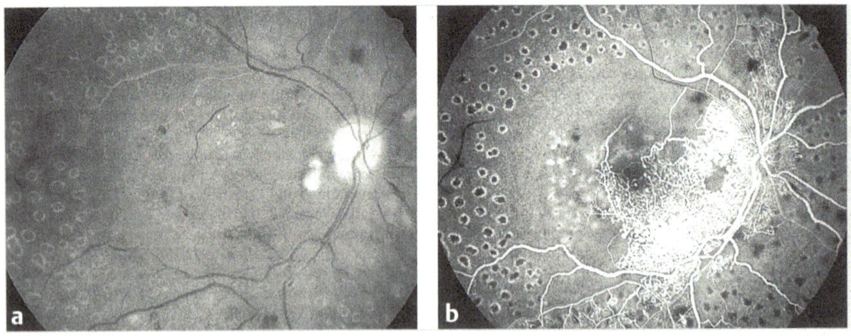

Fig. 34.20 (a) Fundus photograph and (b) fluorescein angiogram show the late stages of radiation retinopathy in the same patient as in ▶ Fig. 34.19. Widespread, nearly confluent retinal capillary dropout is now seen on the fluorescein angiogram. The patient has undergone panretinal photocoagulation for retinal neovascularization.

increase in temperature of the infusion fluid during vitrectomy markedly potentiates retinal toxicity to light; therefore, warmed infusion fluid should be avoided.

Several researchers have purported an association between near-UV radiation from the operating microscope and pseudophakic cystoid macular edema. However, a well-conducted prospective, randomized study failed to show an association. Based on current knowledge of the mechanism of development of cystoid macular edema, there does not appear to be good evidence to support this notion.[75]

34.3 Radiation Retinopathy

Radiation retinopathy was first described in 1933 by Stallard, who reported retinal changes after therapy for retinal capillary hemangiomas and retinoblastomas with radon seeds.[76] He noted hard exudates, RPE changes, and optic nerve head swelling and atrophy. Radiation retinopathy has more recently been described as a consequence of external beam, plaque, and charged particle radiotherapy.[77,78] Changes may occur secondary to treatment of ocular, orbital, and paranasal sinus tumors.[79]

The retinal microvasculature appears to be the most sensitive to the effects of radiation.[79] Fundus examination variably reveals hard exudates, intraretinal hemorrhages, microaneurysms, cotton-wool spots, telangiectases, arteriolar narrowing, and wide-spread capillary loss (▶ Fig. 34.19).[77] These changes are identical to those noted in diabetic retinopathy. Fluorescein angiography displays marked capillary dropout with increased permeability of the remaining vasculature. Acute radiation-induced optic neuropathy with disc swelling can also occur. With time, some cases may progress to retinal and optic nerve head neovascularization, vitreous hemorrhage, or anterior segment neovascularization. Visual loss from macular edema, macular ischemia, vitreous hemorrhage, choroidal neovascularization, neovascular glaucoma, or optic neuropathy may occur.

Human and animal histologic studies have confirmed the devastating effect of radiation on the inner retinal vasculature.[80] Early changes include loss of endothelial cells and pericytes of the deeper, smaller retinal vessels, followed by occlusion of larger vessels. With the advent of indocyanine green angiography, damage to the choroidal vasculature has also been demonstrated and appears to play a role in the visual loss associated with radiation retinopathy.[80] Patients usually present with findings of small-vessel disease, but occasionally large-vessel occlusions can occur before other signs of retinopathy.

Retinopathy can develop from 6 months to 8 years following radiation therapy; the average is 2 to 3 years. Long-term follow-up of radiated patients is essential for detection of this disorder.

The amount of radiation required to produce retinopathy has been widely debated. Both the total and the daily fractionated dose of external beam therapy appear to be important. Retinopathy is rare with a total dose of less than 3,000 rad but has been reported with as little as 1,500 rad. With a dose of 6,000 rad, retinopathy is seen in 50% of patients, and with 8,000 rad, it is seen in 85 to 90% of patients. Fraction sizes above 200 rad/d also seem to amplify the risk for retinopathy. Several important differences are noted with radioactive cobalt plaque therapy. The total dose needed to produce retinopathy is on average two to three times higher than that needed with external beam.[76] In addition, the mean latent time to development of retinopathy is shorter, and plaque therapy tends to produce more hard exudates and less neovascularization. Proton beam irradiation for choroidal melanoma results in retinopathy in 89% of patients, with the earliest and most common finding being macular edema.[78] A visual acuity of 20/200 or better was retained in 67% of these eyes with 3 years of follow-up.

With concurrent chemotherapy or diabetes mellitus, the radiation dose needed to produce retinopathy can be distinctly

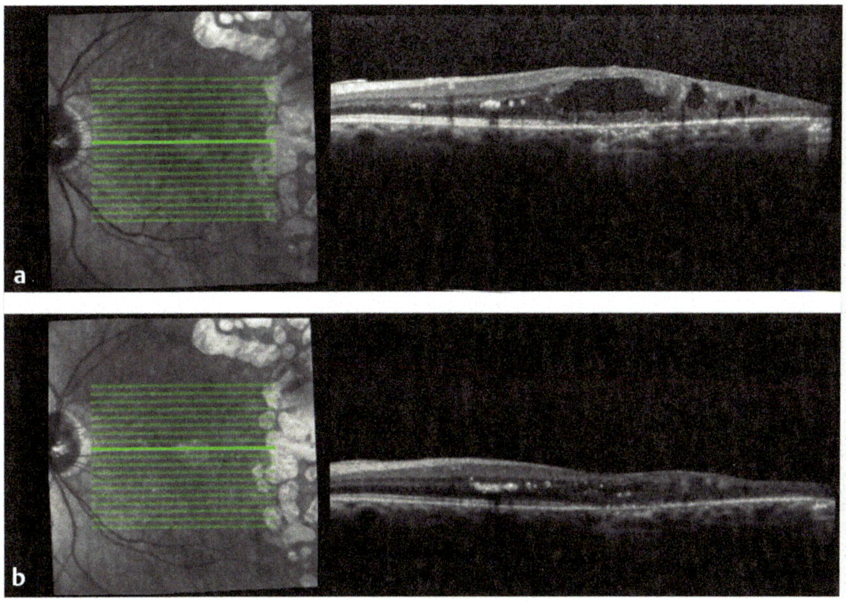

Fig. 34.21 (a) Before and (b) 1 month after intravitreal dexamethasone injection for macular edema which was previously refractory to intravitreal bevacizumab and triamcinolone in a patient with a history of proton beam therapy for uveal melanoma.

reduced. Very close follow-up is indicated in these patients, as a high incidence of eventual blindness has been reported.[77] A syndrome termed *bone marrow transplant retinopathy* has been described in which classic signs of radiation retinopathy develop after the patient has received only 1,200 rad of total body irradiation in conjunction with bone marrow transplant and high-dose cytarabine hydrochloride.[82] The authors hypothesize that high-dose chemotherapy sensitizes the retinal vasculature to radiation damage.

Therapy for macular edema associated with radiation retinopathy is evolving. Some have utilized photocoagulation modeled on treatment for diabetic macular edema.[83] This has resulted in partial resolution of the edema in most cases with modest improvement in visual acuity in 67% of eyes. Panretinal photocoagulation has likewise been successfully applied to patients with neovascular complications (▶ Fig. 34.20).[84] However, visual outcome with these treatments have remained poor. Recently, intravitreal steroids, including triamcinolone and dexamethasone, have emerged as a therapeutic option (▶ Fig. 34.21).[85,86] With the modern advances in intravitreal anti-VEGF therapy, these agents have become a first-line choice for many retinal specialists.[87] Vitrectomy techniques can be employed in those patients with nonclearing vitreous hemorrhage or tractional retinal detachment. Hyperbaric oxygen appears to exacerbate retinal damage from radiation when used concurrently, but it has been shown to have the potential to ameliorate radiation-induced optic neuropathy if given soon after visual loss.[88]

34.4 Conclusion

Exposure to a variety of systemic and topical medications may result in toxicity to the retina and RPE. Distinctive patterns of toxicity may occur, including loss or disruption of the RPE, development of vascular occlusive disease, cystoid macular and retinal edema, crystalline deposition, uveitis, and even retinal folds. Recognizing a medication as a potential cause of these findings is crucial to patient management. Early detection of the causative problem may lead to preservation of visual function.

Light toxicity can also occur from a variety of sources, including solar, arc welding, lasers, and even the operating microscope. It is imperative to recognize these various forms of light as being potentially destructive in select situations.

Finally, radiation from a variety of sources can cause extensive vascular damage, resulting in findings quite similar to diabetic retinopathy. Treatment often parallels what we do for diabetic retinopathy, yet the visual benefits are frequently quite limited.

References

[1] Meredith TA, Aaberg TM, Willerson WD. Progressive chorioretinopathy after receiving thioridazine. Arch Ophthalmol. 1978; 96(7):1172–1176

[2] Connell MM, Poley BJ, McFarlane JR. Chorioretinopathy associated with thioridazine therapy. Arch Ophthalmol. 1964; 71:816–821

[3] Marmor MF. Is thioridazine retinopathy progressive? Relationship of pigmentary changes to visual function. Br J Ophthalmol. 1990; 74(12):739–742

[4] Toler SM. Oxidative stress plays an important role in the pathogenesis of drug-induced retinopathy. Exp Biol Med (Maywood). 2004; 229(7):607–615

[5] Fornaro P, Calabria G, Corallo G, Picotti GB. Pathogenesis of degenerative retinopathies induced by thioridazine and other antipsychotics: a dopamine hypothesis. Doc Ophthalmol. 2002; 105(1):41–49

[6] Mathalone MB. Eye and skin changes in psychiatric patients treated with chlorpromazine. Br J Ophthalmol. 1967; 51(2):86–93

[7] Okun E, Gouras P, Bernstein H, Von Sallmann L. Chloroquine retinopathy; a report of eight cases with ERG and dark-adaptation findings. Arch Ophthalmol. 1963; 69:59–71

[8] Tobin DR, Krohel G, Rynes RI. Hydroxychloroquine. Seven-year experience. Arch Ophthalmol. 1982; 100(1):81–83

[9] Finbloom DS, Silver K, Newsome DA, Gunkel R. Comparison of hydroxychloroquine and chloroquine use and the development of retinal toxicity. J Rheumatol. 1985; 12(4):692–694

[10] Hart WM, Jr, Burde RM, Johnston GP, Drews RC. Static perimetry in chloroquine retinopathy. Perifoveal patterns of visual field depression. Arch Ophthalmol. 1984; 102(3):377–380

[11] Vu BL, Easterbrook M, Hovis JK. Detection of color vision defects in chloroquine retinopathy. Ophthalmology. 1999; 106(9):1799–1803, discussion 1804

[12] Brinkley JR, Jr, Dubois EL, Ryan SJ. Long-term course of chloroquine retinopathy after cessation of medication. Am J Ophthalmol. 1979; 88(1):1–11

[13] Kellner U, Kraus H, Foerster MH. Multifocal ERG in chloroquine retinopathy: regional variance of retinal dysfunction. Graefes Arch Clin Exp Ophthalmol. 2000; 238(1):94–97

[14] Mahon GJ, Anderson HR, Gardiner TA, McFarlane S, Archer DB, Stitt AW. Chloroquine causes lysosomal dysfunction in neural retina and RPE: implications for retinopathy. Curr Eye Res. 2004; 28(4):277–284

[15] Melles RB, Marmor MF. The risk of toxic retinopathy in patients on long-term hydroxychloroquine therapy. JAMA Ophthalmol. 2014; 132(12):1453–1460

[16] Kellner U, Renner AB, Tillack H. Fundus autofluorescence and mfERG for early detection of retinal alterations in patients using chloroquine/hydroxychloroquine. Invest Ophthalmol Vis Sci. 2006; 47(8):3531–3538

[17] Maturi RK, Yu M, Weleber RG. Multifocal electroretinographic evaluation of long-term hydroxychloroquine users. Arch Ophthalmol. 2004; 122(7):973–981

[18] Rodriguez-Padilla JA, Hedges TR, III, Monson B, et al. High-speed ultra-high-resolution optical coherence tomography findings in hydroxychloroquine retinopathy. Arch Ophthalmol. 2007; 125(6):775–780

[19] Pasadhika S, Fishman GA, Choi D, Shahidi M. Selective thinning of the perifoveal inner retina as an early sign of hydroxychloroquine retinal toxicity. Eye (Lond). 2010; 24(5):756–762, quiz 763

[20] Marmor MF, Kellner U, Lai TY, Melles RB, Mieler WF. Recommendations on Screening for Chloroquine and Hydroxychloroquine Retinopathy (2016 Revision). Ophthalmology. 2016; 123(6):1386-94.

[21] Brinton GS, Norton EW, Zahn JR, Knighton RW. Ocular quinine toxicity. Am J Ophthalmol. 1980; 90(3):403–410

[22] Christoforidis J, Ricketts R, Loizos T, Chang S. Optical coherence tomography findings of quinine poisoning. Clin Ophthalmol. 2011; 5:75–80

[23] Canning CR, Hague S. Ocular quinine toxicity. Br J Ophthalmol. 1988; 72 (1):23–26

[24] Gabrielian A, MacCumber MM, Kukuyev A, Mitsuyasu R, Holland GN, Sarraf D. Didanosine-associated retinal toxicity in adults infected with human immunodeficiency virus. JAMA Ophthalmol. 2013; 131(2):255–259

[25] Davies SC, Marcus RE, Hungerford JL, Miller MH, Arden GB, Huehns ER. Ocular toxicity of high-dose intravenous desferrioxamine. Lancet. 1983; 2 (8343):181–184

[26] Genead MA, Fishman GA, Anastasakis A, Lindeman M. Macular vitelliform lesion in desferrioxamine-related retinopathy. Doc Ophthalmol. 2010; 121 (2):161–166

[27] Viola F, Barteselli G, Dell'Arti L, et al. Multimodal imaging in deferoxamine retinopathy. Retina. 2014; 34(7):1428–1438

[28] Miller DF, Bay JW, Lederman RJ, Purvis JD, Rogers LR, Tomsak RL. Ocular and orbital toxicity following intracarotid injection of BCNU (carmustine) and cisplatinum for malignant gliomas. Ophthalmology. 1985; 92(3):402–406

[29] Kupersmith MJ, Seiple WH, Holopigian K, Noble K, Hiesiger E, Warren F. Maculopathy caused by intra-arterially administered cisplatin and intravenously administered carmustine. Am J Ophthalmol. 1992; 113(4):435–438

[30] Khawly JA, Rubin P, Petros W, Peters WP, Jaffe GJ. Retinopathy and optic neuropathy in bone marrow transplantation for breast cancer. Ophthalmology. 1996; 103(1):87–95

[31] Petursson GJ, Fraunfelder FT, Meyer SM. 6. Oral contraceptives. Ophthalmology. 1981; 88(4):368–371

[32] Guyer DR, Tiedeman J, Yannuzzi LA, et al. Interferon-associated retinopathy. Arch Ophthalmol. 1993; 111(3):350–356

[33] Thomas JV, Gragoudas ES, Blair NP, Lapus JV. Correlation of epinephrine use and macular edema in aphakic glaucomatous eyes. Arch Ophthalmol. 1978; 96(4):625–628

[34] Millay RH, Klein ML, Illingworth DR. Niacin maculopathy. Ophthalmology. 1988; 95(7):930–936

[35] Spirn MJ, Warren FA, Guyer DR, Klancnik JM, Spaide RF. Optical coherence tomography findings in nicotinic acid maculopathy. Am J Ophthalmol. 2003; 135(6):913–914

[36] Rowe JA, Hattenhauer MG, Herman DC. Adverse side effects associated with latanoprost. Am J Ophthalmol. 1997; 124(5):683–685

[37] Warwar RE, Bullock JD, Ballal D. Cystoid macular edema and anterior uveitis associated with latanoprost use. Experience and incidence in a retrospective review of 94 patients. Ophthalmology. 1998; 105(2):263–268

[38] Telander DG, Sarraf D. Cystoid macular edema with docetaxel chemotherapy and the fluid retention syndrome. Semin Ophthalmol. 2007; 22(3):151–153

[39] Joshi MM, Garretson BR. Paclitaxel maculopathy. Arch Ophthalmol. 2007; 125 (5):709–710

[40] Zarbin MA, Jampol LM, Jager RD, et al. Ophthalmic evaluations in clinical studies of fingolimod (FTY720) in multiple sclerosis. Ophthalmology. 2013; 120(7):1432–1439

[41] Griffiths MF. Tamoxifen retinopathy at low dosage. Am J Ophthalmol. 1987; 104(2):185–186

[42] Heier JS, Dragoo RA, Enzenauer RW, Waterhouse WJ. Screening for ocular toxicity in asymptomatic patients treated with tamoxifen. Am J Ophthalmol. 1994; 117(6):772–775

[43] Gualino V, Cohen SY, Delyfer MN, Sahel JA, Gaudric A. Optical coherence tomography findings in tamoxifen retinopathy. Am J Ophthalmol. 2005; 140 (4):757–758

[44] Kaiser-Kupfer MI, Kupfer C, Rodrigues MM. Tamoxifen retinopathy. A clinicopathologic report. Ophthalmology. 1981; 88(1):89–93

[45] Lonn LI. Canthaxanthin retinopathy. Arch Ophthalmol. 1987; 105(11):1590–1591

[46] Chang TS, Aylward W, Clarkson JG, Gass JD. Asymmetric canthaxanthin retinopathy. Am J Ophthalmol. 1995; 119(6):801–802

[47] Novak MA, Roth AS, Levine MR. Calcium oxalate retinopathy associated with methoxyflurane abuse. Retina. 1988; 8(4):230–236

[48] AtLee WE, Jr. Talc and cornstarch emboli in eyes of drug abusers. JAMA. 1972; 219(1):49–51

[49] Tse DT, Ober RR. Talc retinopathy. Am J Ophthalmol. 1980; 90(5):624–640

[50] Friberg TR, Gragoudas ES, Regan CD. Talc emboli and macular ischemia in intravenous drug abuse. Arch Ophthalmol. 1979; 97(6):1089–1091

[51] Ryan EH, Jr, Jampol LM. Drug-induced acute transient myopia with retinal folds. Retina. 1986; 6(4):220–223

[52] Sen HA, O'Halloran HS, Lee WB. Case reports and small case series: topiramate-induced acute myopia and retinal striae. Arch Ophthalmol. 2001; 119 (5):775–777

[53] Bhagat N, Read RW, Rao NA, Smith RE, Chong LP. Rifabutin-associated hypopyon uveitis in human immunodeficiency virus-negative immunocompetent individuals. Ophthalmology. 2001; 108(4):750–752

[54] Jacobs DS, Piliero PJ, Kuperwaser MG, et al. Acute uveitis associated with rifabutin use in patients with human immunodeficiency virus infection. Am J Ophthalmol. 1994; 118(6):716–722

[55] Davis JL, Taskintuna I, Freeman WR, Weinberg DV, Feuer WJ, Leonard RE. Iritis and hypotony after treatment with intravenous cidofovir for cytomegalovirus retinitis. Arch Ophthalmol. 1997; 115(6):733–737

[56] Friedberg DN. Hypotony and visual loss with intravenous cidofovir treatment of cytomegalovirus retinitis. Arch Ophthalmol. 1997; 115(6):801–802

[57] Banker AS, Arevalo JF, Munguia D, et al. Intraocular pressure and aqueous humor dynamics in patients with AIDS treated with intravitreal cidofovir (HPMPC) for cytomegalovirus retinitis. Am J Ophthalmol. 1997; 124(2):168–180

[58] Yannuzzi LA, Fisher YL, Krueger A, Slakter J. Solar retinopathy: a photobiological and geophysical analysis. Trans Am Ophthalmol Soc. 1987; 85:120–158

[59] Mainster MA. Spectral transmittance of intraocular lenses and retinal damage from intense light sources. Am J Ophthalmol. 1978; 85(2):167–170

[60] Tso MO, La Piana FG. The human fovea after sungazing. Trans Sect Ophthalmol Am Acad Ophthalmol Otolaryngol. 1975; 79(6):OP788–OP795

[61] Ham WT, Jr, Mueller HA, Ruffolo JJ, Jr, Guerry D, III, Guerry RK. Action spectrum for retinal injury from near-ultraviolet radiation in the aphakic monkey. Am J Ophthalmol. 1982; 93(3):299–306

[62] Uniat L, Olk RJ, Hanish SJ. Welding arc maculopathy. Am J Ophthalmol. 1986; 102(3):394–395

[63] Sliney DH, Mainster MA. Potential laser hazards to the clinician during photocoagulation. Am J Ophthalmol. 1987; 103(6):758–760

[64] Ward B. Mirror laser-treatment lenses: possible risks associated with lens design. Arch Ophthalmol. 1986; 104(11):1585–1586

[65] Arden GB, Berninger T, Hogg CR, Perry S. A survey of color discrimination in German ophthalmologists. Changes associated with the use of lasers and operating microscopes. Ophthalmology. 1991; 98(5):567–575

[66] Luttrull JK, Hallisey J. Laser pointer-induced macular injury. Am J Ophthalmol. 1999; 127(1):95–96

[67] Lee GD, Baumal CR, Lally D, Pitcher JD, Vander J, Duker JS. Retinal injury after inadvertent handheld laser exposure. Retina. 2014; 34(12):2388–2396

[68] Calkins JL, Hochheimer BF. Retinal light exposure from operation microscopes. Arch Ophthalmol. 1979; 97(12):2363–2367

[69] McDonald HR, Irvine AR. Light-induced maculopathy from the operating microscope in extracapsular cataract extraction and intraocular lens implantation. Ophthalmology. 1983; 90(8):945–951

[70] Khwarg SG, Linstone FA, Daniels SA, et al. Incidence, risk factors, and morphology in operating microscope light retinopathy. Am J Ophthalmol. 1987; 103(3, Pt 1):255–263

[71] Brod RD, Olsen KR, Ball SF, Packer AJ. The site of operating microscope light-induced injury on the human retina. Am J Ophthalmol. 1989; 107(4):390–397

[72] Robertson DM, McLaren JW. Photic retinopathy from the operating room microscope. Study with filters. Arch Ophthalmol. 1989; 107(3):373–375

[73] Jaffe GJ, Irvine AR, Wood IS, Severinghaus JW, Pino GR, Haugen C. Retinal phototoxicity from the operating microscope. The role of inspired oxygen. Ophthalmology. 1988; 95(8):1130–1141

[74] Michels M, Lewis H, Abrams GW, Han DP, Mieler WF, Neitz J. Macular phototoxicity caused by fiberoptic endoillumination during pars plana vitrectomy. Am J Ophthalmol. 1992; 114(3):287–296

[75] Jampol LM, Kraff MC, Sanders DR, Alexander K, Lieberman H. Near-UV radiation from the operating microscope and pseudophakic cystoid macular edema. Arch Ophthalmol. 1985; 103(1):28–30

[76] Stallard HB. Radiant energy as a pathogenic and a therapeutic agent in ophtahlmic disorder. Br J Ophthalmol. 1933; 6:1–126

[77] Brown GC, Shields JA, Sanborn G, Augsburger JJ, Savino PJ, Schatz NJ. Radiation retinopathy. Ophthalmology. 1982; 89(12):1494–1501

[78] Guyer DR, Mukai S, Egan KM, Seddon JM, Walsh SM, Gragoudas ES. Radiation maculopathy after proton beam irradiation for choroidal melanoma. Ophthalmology. 1992; 99(8):1278–1285

[79] Amoaku WM, Archer DB. Cephalic radiation and retinal vasculopathy. Eye (Lond). 1990; 4(Pt 1):195–203

[80] Irvine AR, Wood IS. Radiation retinopathy as an experimental model for ischemic proliferative retinopathy and rubeosis iridis. Am J Ophthalmol. 1987; 103(6):790–797

[81] Midena E, Segato T, Valenti M, Degli Angeli C, Bertoja E, Piermarocchi S. The effect of external eye irradiation on choroidal circulation. Ophthalmology. 1996; 103(10):1651–1660

[82] Lopez PF, Sternberg P, Jr, Dabbs CK, Vogler WR, Crocker I, Kalin NS. Bone marrow transplant retinopathy. Am J Ophthalmol. 1991; 112(6):635–646

[83] Kinyoun JL, Zamber RW, Lawrence BS, Barlow WE, Arnold AM. Photocoagulation treatment for clinically significant radiation macular oedema. Br J Ophthalmol. 1995; 79(2):144–149

[84] Kinyoun JL, Lawrence BS, Barlow WE. Proliferative radiation retinopathy. Arch Ophthalmol. 1996; 114(9):1097–1100

[85] Sutter FK, Gillies MC. Intravitreal triamcinolone for radiation-induced macular edema. Arch Ophthalmol. 2003; 121(10):1491–1493

[86] Shields CL, Demirci H, Dai V, et al. Intravitreal triamcinolone acetonide for radiation maculopathy after plaque radiotherapy for choroidal melanoma. Retina. 2005; 25(7):868–874

[87] Finger PT, Chin K. Anti-vascular endothelial growth factor bevacizumab (Avastin) for radiation retinopathy. Arch Ophthalmol. 2007; 125(6):751–756

[88] Borruat FX, Schatz NJ, Glaser JS, Feun LG, Matos L. Visual recovery from radiation-induced optic neuropathy. The role of hyperbaric oxygen therapy. J Clin Neuroophthalmol. 1993; 13(2):98–101

35 Posterior Segment Complications of Anterior Segment Surgery

Thalmon R. Campagnoli, William E. Smiddy, and Harry W. Flynn Jr.

35.1 Postoperative Endophthalmitis

Infectious endophthalmitis following ocular surgery is an uncommon clinical entity that often causes severe visual loss.[1] Pseudophakic endophthalmitis is the most frequently encountered postoperative endophthalmitis category in reported series, as would be expected because more than 1.8 million cataract operations were performed on Medicare beneficiaries alone in 2010.[2] Other types of intraocular surgery, such as secondary intraocular lens (IOL) implantation, corneal transplant, pars plana vitrectomy (PPV), and glaucoma filtering surgery, may also lead to endophthalmitis but are less frequent in clinical series.[3,4,5]

The overall incidence of postoperative endophthalmitis has decreased over a 10-year period from 0.05–0.37% to 0–0.11% (▶ Table 35.1).[6,7,8] The incidence of endophthalmitis after penetrating ocular trauma is much higher and ranges from 0 to 30% in reported trauma series.[9,10,11,12] A number of clinical factors are associated with a higher frequency of endophthalmitis after ocular surgery.[3,5,13,14,15,16,17]

Factors associated with higher acute-onset postoperative endophthalmitis incidence

Factors common to all surgical procedures

- Active blepharitis or conjunctivitis
- Contaminated eye drops
- Active systemic infection
- Cataract surgery
- Older age
- Vitreous loss
- Wound leak on POD1[a]
- Inferior incision
- Inferior bleb location
- Longer length of surgery
- Topical anesthesia
- Use of topical lidocaine gel before povidone
- Iodine
- Secondary IOL
- Repeated incisions in surgical limbus with potentially poor wound healing
- Lacrimal drainage system obstruction
- Contact lens wear
- Immune deficiency (e.g., diabetes mellitus, immunosuppressive medications)
- Filtering-bleb associated
- Bleb leakage
- Use of adjunctive antimetabolites
- Bleb manipulations
- History of bleb infection
- Corneal transplant
- Wound leakage
- Wound infection
- Infectious keratitis
- Topical corticosteroid use
- Suture manipulation or dehiscence

[a]Postoperative day 1.

35.1.1 Clinical Features and Diagnosis

The diagnosis of postoperative endophthalmitis is made by recognition of clinical features and microbiologic confirmation. The characteristic clinical feature of endophthalmitis after cataract surgery is marked intraocular inflammation (▶ Fig. 35.1), often with fibrin in the anterior chamber (AC) and hypopion.[1] Conjunctival congestion, corneal edema, and lid edema are common associated signs. Symptoms often include pain and marked loss of vision. The loss of vision is usually profound and out of proportion to the typical postoperative vision measured during the first days or weeks after intraocular surgery.

Pearls

- Pain is present in the majority of patients with postoperative endophthalmitis but may be minimal or absent, especially when the endophthalmitis is caused by less virulent organisms.
- The symptoms of acute-onset endophthalmitis historically occur during the first postoperative week; however, there is a tendency toward later occurrence (mean: 13 days postoperatively in one study) following clear cornea cataract surgery.[13,18]

When a clinical diagnosis of endophthalmitis is made, confirmation by microbiologic growth from intraocular specimens is attempted. Vitreous specimens are more likely to yield a

Table 35.1 Comparison of incidence of endophthalmitis over 25 years at the Bascom Palmer Eye Institute

	1984–1994[6]	1995–2001[7]	2002–2009[8]
Cataract surgery with or without IOL	0.08%	0.04%	0.03%
Secondary IOL implantation	0.37%	0.21%	0.06%
Pars plana vitrectomy	0.05%	0.03%	0.01%
Penetrating keratoplasty	0.18%	0.08%	0.11%
Glaucoma filtering surgery	0.12%	0.20%	0%

Abbreviation: IOL, intraocular lens.

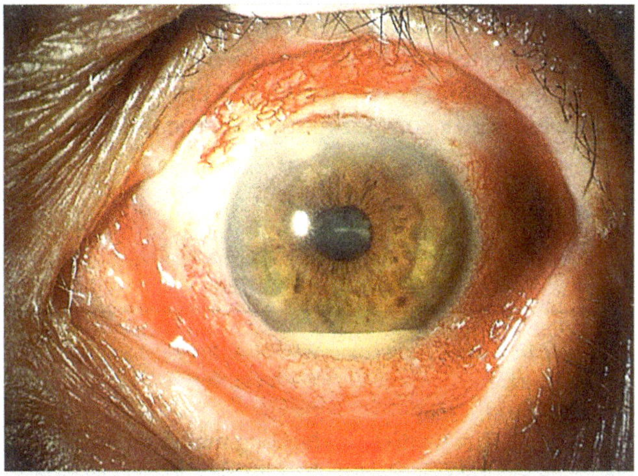

Fig. 35.1 Acute-onset endophthalmitis caused by *Staphylococcus aureus* presenting 3 days following cataract surgery with posterior chamber implant.

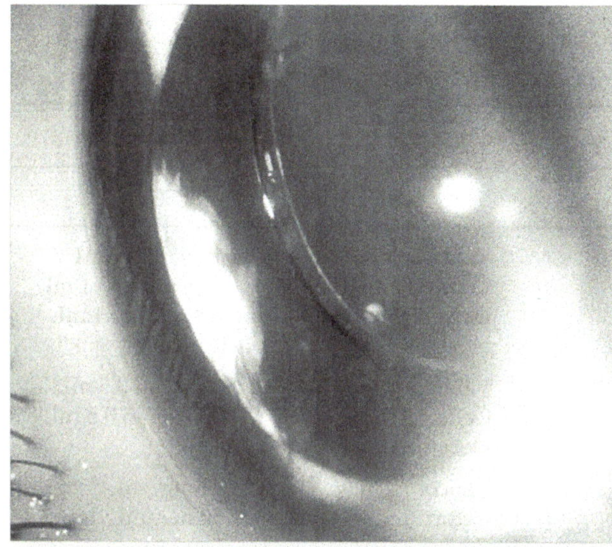

Fig. 35.2 Delayed-onset endophthalmitis caused by *Propionibacterium acnes* occurring 4 months after cataract surgery and showing a white intracapsular plaque with moderate intraocular inflammation.

positive culture result than are simultaneously obtained aqueous specimens.[19] An AC specimen is often obtained; a syringe with a 30-gauge needle is usually effective because aqueous is easily obtained, in contrast to vitreous. Two different techniques are utilized to procure vitreous specimens; either a needle tap or a vitrectomy (cutting–aspirating) instrument. In the needle tap technique, a 21- to 23-gauge needle is generally introduced through the pars plana and directed toward the midvitreous cavity. Neither a conjunctival incision nor a suture closure is necessary for the needle entry site. The vitrectomy cutter is used when the vitreous sample is obtained in an operating room setting, but some authors have described using a portable, in-office unit. The undiluted aspirate is collected through a syringe interposed proximally in the aspiration line. A small specimen (0.2–0.5 mL) is obtained and inoculated into culture media. If the diluted vitrectomy cassette is to be submitted, the specimen may be passed through a membrane filter system to concentrate the microorganisms on the filter paper. With sterile techniques, the filter paper sections are placed on appropriate culture media, into thioglycolate broth, and on slides for Gram stain.[20] There is a higher chance of achieving a positive culture using the vitrectomy cassette after PPV compared to a vitreous tap.[19,21]

The recommended culture media include blood agar, chocolate agar, Sabouraud's agar, Lowenstein-Jensen's agar, and anaerobic media[22] (▶ Table 35.2). If these are not available, the freshly collected vitreous specimen can be injected directly into blood culture bottles for analysis. Agar-based conventional media or blood culture bottles carry satisfactory sensitivity of microorganism detection with diluted or undiluted vitreous samples, but the culture yield increases when both techniques are combined.[19,20,21,23,24,25,26,27] The polymerase chain reaction (PCR) technique has emerged as a promising new development for microbiologic diagnosis in endophthalmitis due to its very high sensitivity even with very limited sample quantity and faster results than conventional culture methods.[28] The intrinsic low specificity carried by this technique might be surpassed with additional PCR-based tests (e.g., in situ hybridization).

Table 35.2 Recommended culture media

Blood agar	Most common bacteria and fungi
Chocolate agar	Fastidious organisms (*Neisseria gonorrhoeae, Haemophilus influenzae*)
Sabouraud's agar	Fungi
Thioglycolate media	Holding media for both bacteria and fungi
Anaerobic media	*Propionibacterium acnes* and other anaerobes

Pearls

- When the microbiology staff is not available to process the vitreous specimen in the standard way, blood culture bottles are particularly useful substitute for standard culture plates.

The source of the infecting organisms causing postoperative endophthalmitis is commonly the patient's flora from the lids, conjunctiva, and periocular tissues.[29] The American Academy of Ophthalmology "Cataract in the Adult Eye" Preferred Practice Patterns guidelines acknowledge this finding by reinforcing the necessity to follow stringent surgical site preparation before eye surgery—which includes application of 5% povidone iodine to the conjunctival cul-de-sac, periocular skin preparation with 10% povidone iodine, and careful sterile draping of the eyelid margins and eyelashes—to reduce resident flora.[30]

35.1.2 Management and Course: The Endophthalmitis Vitrectomy Study

The Endophthalmitis Vitrectomy Study (EVS) was a randomized prospective clinical trial evaluating treatment strategies for acute-onset endophthalmitis following cataract surgery or secondary IOL surgery.[31,32,33,34] Two management issues were investigated: immediate three-port PPV versus immediate tap/biopsy and the value of intravenous antibiotics (amikacin and ceftazidime) administered for a minimum of 5 days.

The EVS entry criteria are listed in the following text box. A double randomization scheme allowed four groups for analysis: immediate three-port PPV with intravenous antibiotics, immediate three-port PPV without intravenous antibiotics, immediate tap/biopsy with intravenous antibiotics, and immediate tap/biopsy without intravenous antibiotics.[31] All groups received intravitreal injections of vancomycin and amikacin along with subconjunctival injections of vancomycin, ceftazidime, and dexamethasone at the time of vitrectomy or vitreous tap. Ceftazidime has been widely substituted for intravitreal amikacin due to potential retinal toxicity and microbiologic sensitivity considerations.[21,35,36,37] Furthermore, all groups also received topical vancomycin, amikacin, and prednisolone acetate postoperatively. The value of subconjunctival injections has been questioned[38,39] and the authors no longer administer subconjunctival antibiotics and dexamethasone routinely.

EVS entry criteria

- Clinical diagnosis of endophthalmitis within 6 weeks of cataract surgery or secondary IOL implantation
- Hypopyon or clouding of AC or vitreous media sufficient to obscure clear visualization of second-order retinal arterioles
- Cornea and AC clear enough to visualize some part of iris
- Cornea clear enough to allow adequate visualization, possibly to perform PPV
- Visual acuity (VA) worse than 20/50 but at least light perception
- No serious coexisting diseases that might compromise visual outcomes

The microbiologic results of the EVS demonstrated bacterial growth in 69.3% of intraocular cultures.[31] The gram-positive, coagulase-negative micrococci (e.g., *Staphylococcus epidermidis*) comprised 70% of the EVS isolates. *Staphylococcus aureus* (9.9%), *Streptococcus* species (9.0%), *Enterococcus* species (2.2%), gram-negative organisms (5.9%), and miscellaneous gram-positive organisms (3.1%) occurred less often. All gram-positive organisms were sensitive to vancomycin, but two of the gram-negative organisms were resistant to both amikacin and ceftazidime.

The EVS treatment outcomes demonstrated no difference in final VA or media clarity outcomes whether or not systemic antibiotics were employed (see the following text box). Likewise, if the patient had hand motion or better vision on the initial examination, the EVS showed no difference in these outcomes between the immediate three-port PPV group versus the immediate tap/biopsy group. However, for patients with initial vision of light perception only (26% of patients in the EVS), much better outcomes occurred in the immediate three-port PPV group. On multivariate analysis, the presenting VA was the single most important factor in predicting EVS outcomes regardless of the treatment group.

EVS Results

- No difference in final VA or media clarity whether or not EVS systemic antibiotics were employed
- For patients with hand motion or better vision, no difference in outcomes between immediate three-port PPV versus tap/biopsy
- For patients with initial VA of light perception only, better visual results occurred in the immediate three-port PPV group (vs. tap/biopsy group)
  - Three times more likely to achieve > 20/40 (33 vs. 11%)
  - Two times more likely to achieve a 20/100 (56 vs. 30%)
  - Less likely to incur < 5/200 (20 vs. 47%)

The EVS VA outcomes can be stratified by microbiologic results.[18,33,34] The best EVS outcomes occurred in the groups with either no or equivocal growth, and in the coagulase-negative Micrococci group. EVS patients with gram-negative organisms had intermediate visual outcomes compared with the "other" gram-positive category (comprised mainly *S. aureus* and *Streptococcus* species), which had the poorest outcomes. In the EVS, all cataract surgeries were performed by extracapsular/scleral tunnel phacoemulsification technique. Lalwani et al[18] recently reported remarkably similar VA outcomes and microbiologic results in acute endophthalmitis after clear corneal cataract surgery—VA = 20/40 in 49% (vs. 53% in the EVS), = 20/100 in 71% (vs. 74% in the EVS), and 68% of coagulase-negative staphylococci cases (vs. 70% in the EVS).

Controversial Points

- The aminoglycosides have a narrow range of safety for intravitreal use during endophthalmitis treatment. Since vancomycin has been shown to cover almost 100% of gram-positive and ceftazidime has been shown to cover more than 90% of gram-negative organisms causing postoperative endophthalmitis,[22,36] the authors recommend intravitreal vancomycin and ceftazidime (instead of amikacin) for empirical coverage of organisms in the treatment of clinically diagnosed endophthalmitis.

The EVS evaluated amikacin and ceftazidime for intravenous use. Subsequently, other (possibly better) antibiotic choices (e.g., vancomycin) have become available, but there are no randomized data available to evaluate its use.[40,41,42] The EVS protocol included fortified topical antibiotics, and these are still generally used by clinicians treating endophthalmitis, but have not been evaluated separately from intravitreal antibiotics for efficacy. Orally administered antibiotics were not evaluated in the EVS. Owing to the lack of supporting evidence regarding the use of systemic antibiotics and the proven efficiency of intravitreal therapy guided by clinical response and culture results, the authors do not routinely use systemic antibiotics via any route in endophthalmitis treatment. Although systemic and even subconjunctival antibiotics are not uniformly used in the treatment of endophthalmitis, the drug dosages used in the EVS and the proper doses to use if the clinician chooses to use them are listed in ▶ Table 35.3.

Table 35.3 Endophthalmitis Vitrectomy Study medications compared with modified regimen for treatment of acute postoperative endophthalmitis

Site of Administration	EVS medications		EVS-modified regimen	
	Drug	Dose	Drug	Dose
Intravitreal	Vancomycin	1 mg in 0.1 mL	Vancomycin	1 mg in 0.1 mL
	Amikacin	0.4 mg in 0.1 mL	Ceftazidime	2.25 mg in 0.1 mL
	No intravitreal steroids		Dexamethasone	0.4 mg in 0.1 mL
Subconjunctival[a]	Vancomycin	25 mg in 0.5 mL	Vancomycin	25 mg in 0.5 mL
	Ceftazidime	100 mg in 0.5 mL	Ceftazidime	100 mg in 0.5 mL
	Dexamethasone	6 mg	Dexamethasone	12 mg
Topical[b]	Vancomycin	50 mg/mL drops	Vancomycin	50 mg/mL drops
	Amikacin	20 mg/mL drops	Ceftazidime	50 mg/mL drops
	Cycloplegics	various	Cycloplegics	various
	Prednisolone acetate drops	1%	Prednisolone acetate drops	1%
Systemic[c]	Ceftazidime	2 g IV q8h (1.5 g if weight less than 50 kg; modify for abnormal renal function)	Ceftazidime	1.0 g IV q12h
	Amikacin	7.5 mg/kg IV initially followed by 6 mg/kg IV q12h (modify for abnormal renal function)	Vancomycin	1.0 g IV q12h
	Prednisone	30 mg po bid (5–10 d)	No systemic steroids	N/A

Abbreviations: bid, twice a day; IV, intravenously; po, orally.

[a]The authors don't recommend subconjunctival antibiotic use anymore.

[b]Topical antibiotics are administered on an alternating regimen every hour if there is evidence for a wound leak or every 4 hours if the wound is secure. Other topical medicines are prescribed according to the level of inflammation.

[c]The authors don't recommend systemic antibiotic use anymore.

Pearls

- The frequency of resistance of coagulase-negative *Staphylococcus* species (the most common causative organisms of endophthalmitis) and *S. aureus* to methicillin/oxacillin[36,43] and third- and fourth-generation fluoroquinolones[13,18,22,35,43,44,45,46,47,48] has increased.

Systemic corticosteroids were used in all patients in the EVS. In the elderly postcataract surgery population, the use of systemic corticosteroids may often be contraindicated because of the high prevalence of diabetes mellitus and other medical conditions precluding the use of systemic corticosteroids. Intravitreal corticosteroids have generally supplanted systemic usage as an adjunct to intraocular antibiotics.[4] The authors recommend intravitreal dexamethasone as a part of the initial treatment in postoperative endophthalmitis (▶ Table 35.3).

Controversial Points

- There were 10 patients among the 420 patients in the EVS in whom acute-onset postoperative endophthalmitis developed, even though antibiotics were used in the irrigation solution during the cataract surgery. The European Society of Cataract and Refractive Surgery study group has advocated the use of prophylactic intracameral cefuroxime at the conclusion of cataract surgery[49] despite endophthalmitis rates comparable to subsequent publications not supporting this practice.[50,51] The use of irrigating solution antibiotics for routine cataract surgery or prophylactic intracameral antibiotics is generally discouraged due to toxicity concerns, risks of contamination when using compounding medication, and the potential to foster the emergence of multiresistant organisms.[52,53]

35.1.3 Other Postoperative Endophthalmitis Categories

Other postoperative categories include endophthalmitis associated with secondary IOL implantation, penetrating keratoplasty, or vitrectomy.[1,3] Because of coexisting ocular pathology, eyes with endophthalmitis after penetrating keratoplasty and PPV may have poorer visual prognoses compared to cases after secondary IOL implantation. Endophthalmitis may also occur following suture removal or manipulation,[16] or late-onset keratitis involving the wound.[54] The removal of 10–0 nylon sutures may facilitate entry of organisms in sufficient quantity through suture tracts to cause intraocular infection. The transition to sutureless cataract surgery has obviated this concern, but it bears consideration in contexts involving suture removal. Delayed-onset keratitis associated with a previous cataract wound may cause breakdown of the wound, allowing entry of organisms. These keratitis-associated cases are often caused by more virulent organisms and generally have a poor visual prognosis.[54]

Even though the EVS results apply only to cataract and secondary IOL surgery, some apply the EVS (or EVS-modified) antibiotic treatment regimen (▶ Table 35.3) to other etiologic categories of endophthalmitis, and use a vitreous tap and injection, unless the VA is light perception, in which case vitrectomy is more commonly pursued.

Delayed-Onset Endophthalmitis

Delayed-onset or chronic postoperative endophthalmitis occurs, by definition, more than 6 weeks after surgery, and is commonly associated with pseudophakia. These patients present with progressive intraocular inflammation and a chronic indolent course. The most frequently reported organisms include less virulent bacteria *Propionibacterium acnes*, *S. epidermidis*, and fungi.[55,56]

The clinical features of delayed-onset endophthalmitis observed on slit-lamp examination may help distinguish between these causative organisms. *P. acnes* cases are characterized by the presence of a large, white intracapsular plaque associated with chronic granulomatous inflammation that may seem to respond initially to topical corticosteroid treatment (▶ Fig. 35.2). These eyes may have large keratic precipitates on the corneal endothelium and beaded fibrin strands in the AC. In cases caused by *S. epidermidis*, chronic progressive vitritis is a typical feature, with no white intracapsular plaque.

Fungal endophthalmitis is a commonly overlooked cause of delayed-onset endophthalmitis and should be considered, especially when the clinical response to broad-spectrum antibiotics is poor. The AC may often be relatively quiet initially, but linear, white strands resembling a "string of pearls" may be present in the anterior vitreous, indicating the presence of Candida organisms (▶ Fig. 35.3). Because these organisms generally replicate more slowly, they may seem to respond to topical corticosteroid initially but frequently require vitrectomy combined with intravitreal therapy.[1] Characteristically, a more fulminant course eventually ensues. The efficacy of intravitreal antifungal agents has not been proven as has the efficacy of antibiotics for bacterial endophthalmitis, but intravitreal antifungal agents are generally recommended for suspected fungal endophthalmitis cases. Recommended doses for suspected yeast infections (e.g., Candida) include intravitreal amphotericin B 0.005 mg/0.1 mL or oral fluconazole 200 mg bid[57]; mold infections (e.g., *Aspergillus*) are generally resistant to these agents and sequential intravitreal voriconazole injections 0.05 to 0.1 mg/0.1 mL[58] are recommended.

PPV is commonly recommended for cases of delayed-onset endophthalmitis to establish the correct diagnosis by culture, as well as to remove offending organisms and localized foci of infectious material, such as the white intracapsular plaque, when present. Recurrent infection despite vitrectomy may require removal of the entire capsular bag and the IOL, and more prolonged antimicrobial treatment, including reinjection intravitreally.[59,60]

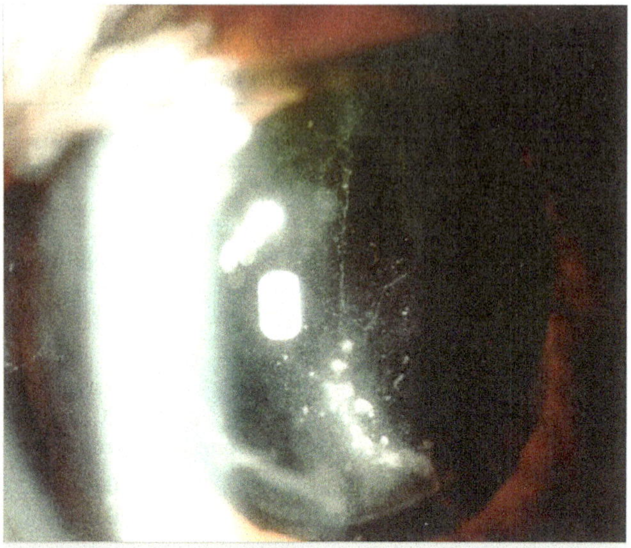

Fig. 35.3 Delayed-onset endophthalmitis caused by *Candida parapsilosis* occurring 6 weeks after cataract surgery and characterized by a "string of pearls" and white infiltrates in the anterior vitreous.

Endophthalmitis Associated with Filtering Blebs or Glaucoma Drainage Implants

Delayed-onset endophthalmitis can also be associated with conjunctival filtering blebs or glaucoma drainage implants (GDIs). A number of reports show incidence varying between 0.2 and 9.6% following glaucoma filtering surgery.[5,61,62,63,64] The offending organisms initially gain access to the bleb ("blebitis") and subsequently spread to involve the AC and adjacent intraocular structures. Blebitis may respond to periocular and topical therapy without the need for injection of intravitreal antibiotics, but close monitoring is recommended.[65]

The clinical features of conjunctival filtering bleb-associated endophthalmitis are similar to those of acute-onset postoperative endophthalmitis. These eyes may present with sudden onset of conjunctival congestion, intraocular inflammation, and pain months or years after previous glaucoma filtering surgery or cataract surgery with an unintentional bleb. The organisms in this category are often more virulent (*Streptococcus* or gram-negative organisms such as *Haemophilus*, *Pseudomonas*, or *Serratia* species) than the organisms present in other postoperative endophthalmitis categories.[5,17,61,64] Even with prompt treatment, the visual outcomes in this category are generally worse than for acute-onset pseudophakic cases.

Delayed-onset endophthalmitis associated with GDI is a rare event compared to conjunctival filtering bleb-associated endophthalmitis.[66,67,68] A major risk factor for its development is erosion of the conjunctiva overlying the tube. Manipulation of the tube may also be involved on its pathogenesis. Clinical features and causative organisms are similar to those associated with filtering bleb-associated endophthalmitis. The visual prognosis varies depending on the pathogen(s) involved and preexisting disease from glaucoma. Removal of the GDI at the time of management is controversial. Some cases are treated successfully only with vitreous tap and injection.[69] Prompt surgical conjunctival repair is advised if erosion is identified, and even placement of a patch graft over the tube at the time of the primary GDI procedure may be considered.

35.2 Suprachoroidal Hemorrhage

Suprachoroidal hemorrhage (SCH), also referred to as a hemorrhagic choroidal detachment, may occur during or after any form of intraocular surgery. Reported risk factors for SCH include glaucoma, aphakia, myopia, previous PPV, glaucoma surgery, dropped lens fragments (cataract surgery), phacoemulsification conversion, advanced age, arteriosclerotic cardiovascular disease, diabetes, hypertension, and intraoperative tachycardia.[70,71,72,73,74,75,76,77,78] Transient hypotony is a feature common to any intraocular surgery that may leave an eye susceptible to choroidal vascular congestion which, followed by rupture of long or short posterior ciliary arteries, may develop into a SCH. Rhegmatogenous retinal detachment (RRD), scleral buckling, dropped lens fragment, cryotherapy, external drainage of subretinal fluid, and use of aspirin or warfarin are associated with the occurrence of SCH during PPV.[79,80] Obstruction of vortex veins with scleral buckling may also predispose to the formation of choroidal effusions.

35.2.1 Clinical Features

The extent of a SCH may range from limited (and inconsequential) to massive (360-degree SCH), forcing the retinal surfaces into apposition in the midportion of the vitreous cavity ("kissing choroidals"); if there is an open wound, extrusion of intraocular contents may ensue ("expulsive choroidals"). Limited SCHs appear as dark gray-brown, dome-like elevations peripherally that have a solid appearance and are immobile. Chorioretinal folds may result from hypotony, and there may be some degree of overlying exudative retinal detachment which might be more visible at the margin of the SCH. Substantial intraocular pressure (IOP) elevation and eye pain are typically associated with the acute development of large SCHs. B-scan ultrasonography will show a relatively thick, dome-shaped elevation with little after movement and variable echogenicity within the suprachoroidal space.

35.2.2 Management and Course

For intraoperative SCH, all ocular incisions or wound leaks should be closed as quickly as possible. Most surgeons recommend removal of vitreous prolapse into the wound (if possible) and some recommend acute drainage of SCH if continued high IOP is present.[70,71,72,78,79,80] The only goal in pursuing primary intraoperative SCH drainage is to lower IOP sufficiently to avoid central retinal artery occlusion. Thus, intraoperative drainage of SCH should be considered only as a last resort, as the freshly clotted blood usually does not drain well, and lowering of the pressure often merely propagates more bleeding. The use of perfluorocarbon liquid or silicone oil tamponade has been advocated to provide long-term internal tamponade postoperatively.[78,81]

Drainage may be accomplished by making a full-thickness sclerotomy in any quadrant (preferably in the maximal choroidal elevation quadrant), approximately 4 to 8 mm posterior to the limbus. Generally, it is not necessary to make a drain posterior to the site corresponding to the ora serrata. The sclerotomy should be left open for continued postoperative drainage.

The timing of a secondary surgical intervention for either an intraoperative or postoperative massive SCH is somewhat controversial, but most surgeons recommend waiting 10 to 14 days to allow liquefaction of the SCH, which facilitates draining the hemorrhage. Some case reports demonstrated satisfactory benefit with injection of recombinant tissue plasminogen activator in the suprachoroidal space to induce earlier clot dissolution,[82,83] but this rarely seems necessary; further investigation is needed to support its use. Systemic and/or topical corticosteroids along with antiocular hypertensives and analgesics may be necessary during this observation period. Earlier surgical intervention, however, may be warranted for intractable pain or uncontrollable IOP elevation. There are no randomized prospective clinical trials addressing this timing issue because it is a rare problem with complex variables at play.

The surgical objective in treating patients with massive SCH is to drain as much hemorrhage as possible. If there is prolapsed vitreous gel or retinal detachment, vitrectomy is considered; a scleral buckle and/or intraocular gas tamponade are potential adjuncts if there is retinal detachment (▶ Fig. 35.4).[70,71,72,73] Perfluorocarbon liquids may be useful intraoperatively in managing a combined SCH and RRD.[78,81,84]

Risk factors for poor visual outcome include the presence of a RRD, more than two quadrants of SCH involvement, and extension to the posterior pole.[71,73,79]

35.3 Retinal Detachment following Cataract Surgery

Structural changes occur within the vitreous following cataract surgery that are likely initiated by biochemical changes which may lead to progressive syneresis, increased mobility of the vitreous gel, and eventual posterior vitreous detachment.[85] Hypotony might play a role in facilitating vitreous detachment. Acute posterior vitreous detachment is associated with retinal tears and subsequent retinal detachment in a small percentage of patients.[86,87] Although the incidence of RRD following cataract surgery is relatively low, it is an important cause of moderate to severe visual impairment consequent to cataract surgery. Patients undergoing cataract extraction should be aware of symptoms that could be indicative of a retinal tear or detachment, such as flashes, floaters, and a progressive loss of peripheral vision.

35.3.1 Clinical Features, Incidence, and Risk Factors

The reported incidence of retinal detachment following cataract surgery ranges from approximately 0.26 to 1.5%.[30,88,89,90,91] When patients are followed up for longer postoperative

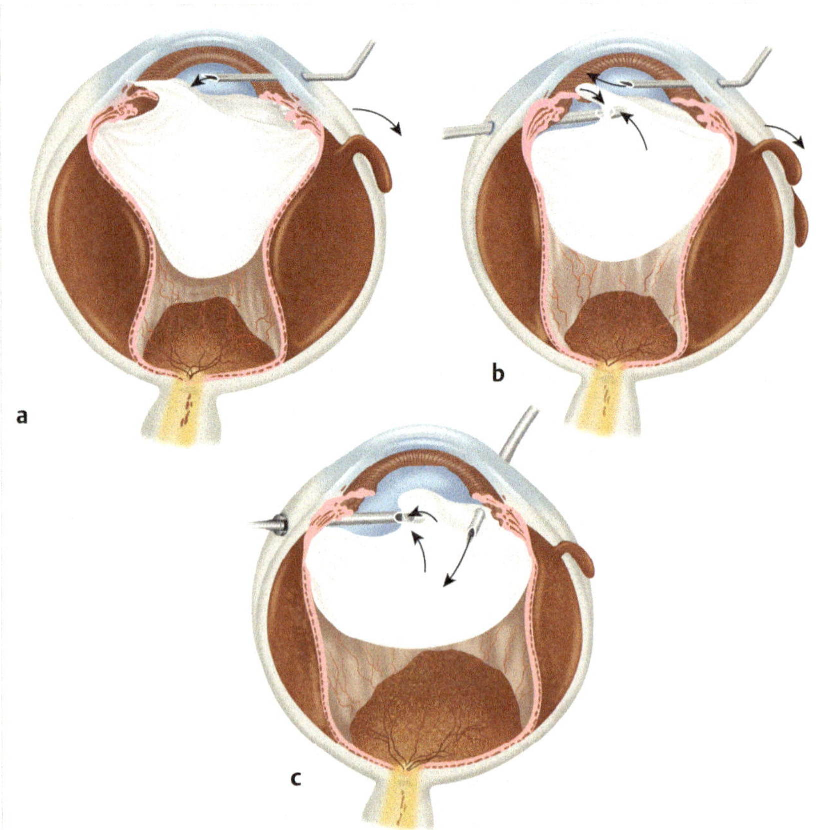

Fig. 35.4 Management of massive suprachoroidal hemorrhage: (**a**) Needle infusion into anterior chamber and scleral drainage of suprachoroidal hemorrhage. (**b**) Anterior vitrectomy and continued scleral drainage. (**c**) Posterior vitrectomy and continued scleral drainage.

intervals (8–20 years), the incidence has been reported to rise to 2.3%.[92,93] A 1991 retrospective study of 338,141 Medicare beneficiaries older than 65 years who underwent various forms of cataract surgery demonstrated incidences in retinal detachment of 1.6% after intracapsular surgery, 0.9% after extracapsular surgery, and 1.2% following phacoemulsification, during a 4-year follow-up period. The same study detected an increase to 5.0% when cataract surgery was accompanied by vitreous loss.[88] Recent studies have shown decreasing incidence of retinal detachment after phacoemulsification[90,93] and have corroborated evidence for vitreous loss during cataract surgery as a major factor for the development of retinal detachment after cataract surgery, increasing the risk at least four times.[94,95] A case–control study evaluating 63,298 cataract surgeries identified an increased risk for pseudophakic retinal detachment in patients with myopia (3 ×), RRD in the fellow eye (12 ×), zonule dehiscence (12 ×), and male gender (2 ×).[96] Other risk factors for retinal detachment after cataract surgery include loss of lens fragments into the vitreous cavity, lattice degeneration, younger age (< 60 years old) and white race.[86,87,88,89,90,91,92,93,94,95,96,97]

Another risk factor for retinal detachment that has been cited is the performance of YAG (yttrium–aluminum–garnet) laser capsulotomy.[89,93,96,98,99,100,101] The largest reported study involved Medicare patients who underwent extracapsular surgery in 1986 and 1987 and who were followed up for 1 to 2 years after YAG laser capsulotomy.[100] Overall, patients who underwent posterior capsulotomy were about two times more likely to have either retinal tears or retinal detachment during the follow-up interval. Later studies using a variety of methodologies showed variable but lower RD rates.[89,93,96,101]

Special Considerations

- The risk for retinal detachment after cataract surgery is between 0.26 and 1.5%. When cataract surgery is accompanied by vitreous loss, the incidence of retinal detachment or tear formation may increase more than four times.

35.3.2 Management and Course

The efficacy of prophylactic treatment of peripheral retinal disease before cataract surgery is controversial. While all symptomatic tears are generally treated, asymptomatic horseshoe retinal tears are commonly treated, and atrophic round holes or operculated holes are usually not treated. Likewise, lattice retinal degeneration, present in approximately 7% of the general population, is usually not treated before cataract surgery unless associated with a flap tear.[102]

Pneumatic retinopexy is not commonly performed in the early postoperative period following cataract surgery, especially when there is a limited view of the retinal periphery. Primary PPV with or without scleral buckling is more frequently used in these eyes. Sutures may be placed to reinforce the cataract surgery incision in selected patients. Potential complications from pseudophakic retinal detachment surgery include recurrent retinal detachment with proliferative vitreoretinopathy, choroidal detachment, and complications from drainage of subretinal fluid.[103]

35.4 Needle Penetration of the Globe

Cataract surgery today is usually performed under topical anesthesia using clear cornea incision and phacoemulsification. This technique obviates the concern of needle penetration of the globe during administration of traditional retrobulbar or peribulbar anesthesia. Because a retrobulbar or peribulbar block results in both deep anesthesia and akinesia, some anterior segment surgeons still prefer the various block techniques.

The Atkinson retrobulbar block employs an elevated and adducted eye position to place the needle tip into the muscle cone adjacent to the optic nerve. Because of the risk for needle entry into either the globe or the optic nerve, many ophthalmologists have adopted a peribulbar block, in which the eye is positioned straight ahead, the needle is directed more peripherally to the globe, and larger volumes of anesthetic are used to fill the orbit.[104] The delineation between peribulbar and retrobulbar is often indistinct. While some advocate a shorter needle than the traditional 1.5-inch, 25-gauge needle (which is not always inserted to the hub), this too is a somewhat artificial permutation because orbit sizes and other anatomic variations require a customized application of anesthetic for individual patients. Many also advocate a flat grind needle rather than the sharp end.

Factors predisposing to needle penetration of the globe include axial high myopia, posterior staphyloma, previous scleral buckling surgery, and poor patient cooperation with the injection.[105,106,107]

35.4.1 Clinical Features

Globe penetration during administration of the anesthesia should be suspected if any unusual resistance is felt by the surgeon during entry or if the IOP is noted to be either very low or very high after the block is given. The loss of the red reflex after the block is given could also indicate a needle penetration. Patients experience severe pain when needle entry of the globe occurs.

Pearls

- Factors that predispose to needle penetration of the globe during administration of a retrobulbar or peribulbar block include axial high myopia, posterior staphyloma, previous scleral buckling surgery, and poor patient cooperation with the injection.

When needle entry into the globe is suspected, the diagnosis can be confirmed by indirect ophthalmoscopy. One or two focal retinal penetration sites may be evident, and some degree of retinal disruption (retinal detachment) and subretinal or vitreous hemorrhage is typically present. Suprachoroidal detachments may also develop.

35.4.2 Management and Course

The early management of posterior segment needle entry wounds is controversial. Most authors recommend prompt laser treatment or retinocryopexy to peripheral visible retinal perforation sites, but blood or lens opacities may preclude a satisfactory view of the area. The patient can be followed up with serial echography examinations for the development of retinal detachment until the vitreous hemorrhage clears. If retinal detachment occurs, early intervention is recommended. The location of the retinal tears along with the type and extent of associated findings (e.g., hemorrhage, choroidal detachment) will determine the specific surgical approach utilized.

The visual prognosis usually depends on the presence or absence of retinal detachment and damage inflicted directly to the posterior pole by the needle. In one report, eyes that had retinal breaks without retinal detachment had a much better visual prognosis than eyes complicated by retinal detachment. In the former category, seven of nine cases without retinal detachment achieved 20/50 or better VA, whereas in the latter category, only 2 of 14 retinal detachment cases achieved 20/400 or better VA.[105]

35.5 Retained Lens Fragments

The complication of retained lens fragments after cataract surgery continues to occur. The most common clinical situation leading to retained lens fragments is posterior capsular rupture, with loss of lens fragments posteriorly into the vitreous cavity during the fragmentation phase of phacoemulsification. The displaced lens fragment may involve the entire nucleus or any fraction of it. The best estimate of the incidence of posteriorly displaced lens fragments is between 0.1 and 1.1%.[108,109,110] The phacoemulsification surgeon can minimize the risk for posterior migration of lens fragments by maintaining the integrity of the posterior capsule. If posterior capsule rupture occurs, the surgeon must proceed with extreme caution, retrieving displaced lens fragments, if necessary, using a larger incision and a lens loop or forceps to retrieve nuclear fragments before migration posteriorly. If the fragment falls posteriorly, further complication may occur with limbal-based retrieval attempts such as by probing posteriorly with a lens loop or other instruments, or by using high volumes of infusion fluid to create vortex currents to float the lens fragment anteriorly. Those maneuvers may be associated with giant retinal tears formation leading to poor prognosis, especially if vigorous attempts are made.[111] Performing, as indicated and possible, anterior vitrectomy, inserting the IOL, and closing the wound without vitreous incarceration are the most important steps the anterior segment surgeon can take to maximize ultimate outcome.

Special Considerations

- Attempts at retrieving a posteriorly dislocated nucleus from the limbus with high volumes of intraocular fluid or posterior aspiration with the phacoemulsification probe should be avoided, as these maneuvers are likely to increase the risk for retinal tears and detachments, complications that can compromise the visual prognosis.

35.5.1 Clinical Features

Posterior displacement of lens fragments is usually recognized intraoperatively by the cataract surgeon after posterior capsular rupture. Occasionally, retained lens fragments may cause a presentation with chronic intraocular inflammation and no visible fragments in the posterior pole. The degree of intraocular inflammation commonly correlates to the quantity of the retained lens material, the time interval since cataract surgery, individual inflammatory reactivity, and the extent of previous intraocular manipulations. Associated clinical signs, including corneal edema, glaucoma, uveitis, and vitreous opacities, are frequently mild, especially in the immediate postoperative interval, but these may worsen and lead to other complications, such as retinal detachment, causing profound visual loss.[112,113]

35.5.2 Management and Course

The size of the lens fragment and severity of intraocular inflammation usually form the basis for surgical intervention. Lens nucleus fragment leads to a worse visual prognosis[114] and, as a general rule, when larger than about 2 mm in diameter should probably be removed, as secondary inflammatory complications will virtually always ensue. Eyes with very small retained fragments have a better prognosis and can often be observed. However, if inflammation has not subsided by 1 to 2 weeks with aggressive topical nonsteroidal and steroidal medications, surgical intervention should be considered regardless of how small the retained fragment is, as occult fragments may be harbored behind the iris. As advances in cataract surgery have lowered the threshold for its indications, the visual goals and expectations have influenced the indications for intervention in management of complications such as retained lens fragments.

Many reports have addressed the timing for surgical intervention in eyes with retained lens fragments.[97,110,115,116,117,118,119,120,121,122,123,124,125,126,127,128] A few studies demonstrated superiority with same-day vitrectomy performance.[115,116,117,118,119] In contrast, other studies found no benefit in regard to VA outcomes or complications with same-day vitrectomy,[110,120,121,122] including no difference in the incidence of secondary glaucoma.[121,122] One major retrospective review[122] evaluated 569 eyes that underwent vitrectomy the same day, within 1 week, or more than 1 week after cataract surgery. The only benefit found on the same-day vitrectomy group was a diminished rate of corneal edema at last examination in comparison to 1-week and more than 1-week groups (9 vs. 12–19%, respectively). In this report, no differences were found in rates of cystoid macular edema, retinal detachment, elevated IOP, or SCH incidences between groups. Approximately 65% of patients achieved best-corrected VA 20/40 or better, while 5 to 15% were not able to reach more than 20/400 VA.

Chronic glaucoma may result with retained lens material. A report from 1992 showed chronic glaucoma to be more common when the subsequent vitrectomy was performed more than 3 weeks following surgery.[126] Recent reports, including a meta-analysis,[123] also found lower risk of developing glaucoma if early vitrectomy is performed.[116,128] Conversely, studies involving large pool of patients have not found outcome differences between earlier and later intervention,[97,110,119,120,121,122,124,127] although the retrospective nature of those studies brings potential selection bias due to the tendency of performing earlier vitrectomy in eyes with markedly elevated IOP. A study of 126 patients with posterior retained lens fragments after phacoemulsification but before vitrectomy demonstrated a 37% prevalence of IOP greater than 30 mm Hg.[97] The IOP normalized in all except 3% of patients after vitrectomy.

The patient's overall clinical situation influences timing, but usually surgery to remove retained lens material is optimized when performed about 1 week after the original cataract surgery. This window balances efforts to expedite visual rehabilitation, to break the cycle of progressive lens-induced inflammation, and to lessen risks for permanent, secondary lens-induced glaucoma. Logistically, these goals may also be accomplished when lens fragment removal can be performed during the original cataract operation. When this is not feasible, a delay of several days or even weeks is demonstrated to be equally effective, as the inflammation, corneal edema, and glaucoma will improve with topical treatment during the following several days.

Surgical Techniques

A variety of techniques have been described for use by the anterior segment surgeon at the time of displaced lens fragments. Although some cases may be satisfactorily managed through a limbal incision, PPV techniques probably offer superior results in most cases.[97,110,115,116,117,118,119,120,121,122,123,124,125,126,127,128,129,130,131]

There are three basic surgical techniques for lens fragment removal using a PPV approach: (1) ultrasonic fragmentation, (2) mechanical crushing of the nucleus between two instruments, and (3) limbal extraction of hard nuclear fragments. The availability of phacofragmentation units generally precludes the need for the latter two techniques, but they are options when fragmentation is unavailable or in cases with an extremely hard nuclear fragment.

There are three key elements in successful lens fragment removal technique: First, adequate initial vitrectomy avoids unintended vitreous traction during phacofragmentation (▶ Fig. 35.5). Second, reducing fragmentation power to only 5 to 10% of maximum allows more efficient nuclear extraction by continuous occlusion of the suction port, which minimizes the risk for mechanical retinal trauma from projectile fragments. This maneuver also minimizes the chance of fragments dropping back onto the retina, even though these fragments rarely strike the retina with sufficient force to damage it. Third, fragments should be cautiously aspirated from the retinal surface and moved to the midvitreous before ultrasonic fragmentation is activated to avoid suction or ultrasonic damage to the retina (▶ Fig. 35.6). Some authors have successfully used small-gauge vitrectomy to intervene in selected cases of retained lens fragments, benefiting from the option to convert one sclerotomy to a traditional 20-gauge when the use of fragmatome appears indispensable.[132,133,134,135,136,137]

Perfluorocarbon liquids are an option to float the nucleus anteriorly in order to facilitate removal,[138,139] but these are most useful when retinal detachment coexists.[140] Techniques for reattaching the retina when detachment is associated with retained lens fragments are similar to those for other complex retinal detachments.[119,141,142,143]

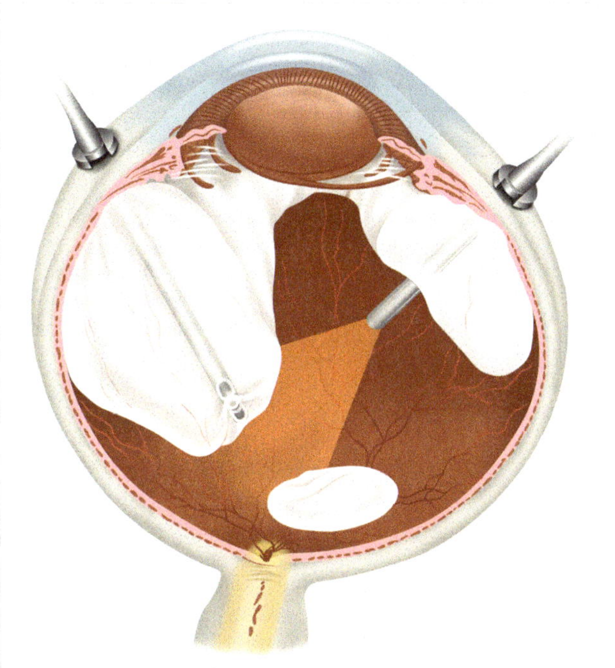

Fig. 35.5 Attention to complete central vitrectomy allows access to retained lens fragments.

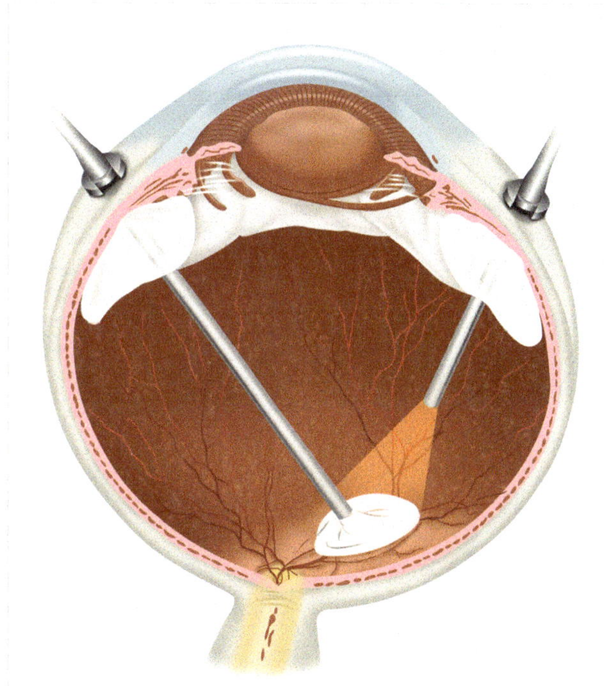

Fig. 35.6 Low ultrasonic fragmentation power allows more controlled removal of fragments.

Most anterior surgeons proceed to IOL insertion at the time of the original cataract surgery, despite the intraoperative complication of posteriorly displaced lens fragments, as most vitrectomy surgeons would recommend. However, sometimes the anterior segment surgeon defers to place the IOL initially, so the vitrectomy surgeon has to decide how to manage the aphakia. If there is sufficient capsular support, the vitrectomy surgeon may place the IOL in the sulcus in the posterior chamber (PC); if not, suture fixation techniques may be used[144,145,146,147,148,149,150] or the IOL may be placed in the AC. Various maneuvers have been used to facilitate transscleral suture placement, including the use of a mirror[151] or transillumination[152] to position the suture in the ciliary sulcus, but these are rarely necessary.

The important points in the management of posteriorly dislocated lens fragments for the cataract surgeon and vitreoretinal surgeon are summarized in the following text boxes, respectively.

Posterior Dislocation of Lens Fragments: Recommendations for the Cataract Surgeon

- Attempt lens fragment retrieval only if easily accessible (anteriorly located).
- Perform anterior vitrectomy to avoid postoperative vitreous adherence to the limbal wound.
- Insert IOL (PC or AC lens as safe and indicated).
- Perform standard wound closure and remove viscoelastic material.
- Administer frequent postoperative topical anti-inflammatory and IOP-lowering agents.
- Obtain prompt vitreoretinal consultation.

Posterior Dislocation of Lens Fragments: Recommendations for the Vitreoretinal Surgeon

- Initially observe patient on topical agents if inflammation is minimal or lens fragments are small.
- Perform surgical intervention if:
  - Inflammation or IOP is not well controlled.
  - Fragment size is estimated to be > 3 mm.
- Perform complete vitrectomy before attempting phacofragmentation.
- Use low ultrasonic fragmentation power (5–10%) for more efficient lens particle removal.
- Insert IOL as indicated.
- Carefully examine retinal periphery for retinal tears and detachments.

Outcomes after Vitrectomy

The visual results of managing cases of posteriorly dislocated or retained lens fragments are generally good (▶ Table 35.4). Postoperative VA of 20/40 or better has been reported in the majority of patients in many series. One of the earliest series reported only a 41% rate of 20/60 or better,[126] but subsequent series report 56 to 82% rates of 20/40 or better.[97,110,120,121,122,124,127,128,129,130,131] This apparent improvement may reflect changing patterns of cataract surgery technique, as a poorer prognosis tended to occur with displaced lens nuclei after expression extracapsular cataract extraction techniques are used compared to phacoemulsification, the almost universally employed technique today.

Table 35.4 Outcomes of vitrectomy for retained lens fragments

Study (date)	No. of patients	% with IOP > 30 mm Hg			Better VA with earlier PPV[a]
		% > 20/40	Before PPV	After PPV	
Hutton et al[129] (1978)	24	42	N/A	33	Yes
Fastenberg et al[130] (1991)	11	82	69	27	N/A
Gilliland et al[127] (1992)	56	50	52	25	No
Lambrou and Stew-ard[125] (1992)	8	88	N/A	N/A	N/A
Blodi et al[126] (1992)	32	41[b]	30	31	Yes
Kim et al[124] (1994)	62	68	46	13	No
Borne et al[110] (1996)	121	68	32	11	No
Kapusta et al[131] (1996)	25	71	60[c]	N/A	No
Vilar et al[97] (1997)	126	60	37	3	No
Scott et al[120] (2003)	343	56	25	2	No
Ho et al[128] (2009)	166	72	40[c]	2	No
Colyer et al[121] (2011)	172	67	10	5	No
Modi et al[122] (2013)	569	60	23	5	No

Abbreviations: IOP, intraocular pressure; PPV, pars plana vitrectomy; VA, visual acuity.

[a]Less than 3 weeks.

Postoperative complications related to vitrectomy surgery may be difficult to differentiate from those attributable to the complicated cataract surgery; these may include corneal edema, glaucoma, persistent intraocular inflammation, and new retinal detachment.[153] Retinal detachment coexisted with retained lens material in 5.8% of reported series, and retinal detachment has been reported after vitrectomy for removal of retained lens fragments in 6.9% of reported series (▶ Table 35.5). Thus, it is of critical importance to evaluate the retina intraoperatively in such patients.

35.6 Intraocular Lens Dislocation

Postoperative decentration of posterior chamber IOL (PCIOL) occurs in 0.2 to 3% of cases and usually does not require treatment.[154,155,156,157] A less common, but more significant, complication is IOL dislocation into the vitreous cavity. A common element in all cases is suboptimal posterior capsule support, usually resulting from posterior capsular rupture during cataract extraction. When dislocation occurs within the first few days or weeks after surgery, the cause may be less apparent and may be the result of poor IOL fixation—unknowing placement of the IOL through a posterior capsular defect onto the anterior hyaloid, or the result of subsequent IOL haptic rotation out of a zone of thin posterior capsule remnants. Late dislocation (more than 3 months after surgery) is less common and may be caused by traumatic[158] or spontaneous loss of zonular support, as in eyes with pseudoexfoliation syndrome,[159] high myopia,[160] vitreoretinal surgery,[161] retinitis pigmentosa,[162] and connective tissue disorders.[163]

35.6.1 Clinical Features

The presenting symptoms of patients with a dislocated IOLs range from minimally symptomatic lens decentration to complete luxation into the vitreous cavity. Decentration usually refers to mild malposition with the optic still covering more than half of the pupillary space. In many cases of decentration, one haptic is in the ciliary sulcus and the other is in the capsular bag. Progressive decentration may become apparent with progressive capsular constriction. Patients at this milder end of the spectrum usually present several weeks after cataract surgery with good VA and normal IOP and without inflammation. Visual symptoms usually are mild and may be related to glare from the edge of the optic.

PCIOLs completely dislocated into the vitreous cavity historically have been most commonly observed within the first week following surgery (26 of 32 cases in one series),[164] or less frequently during surgery. It seems now that they occur months after surgery, perhaps due to more pseudoexfoliation or trauma. The presenting VA with aphakic correction may be very good, but it tends to be decreased to a moderate degree despite best spectacle correction. Patients with a luxated or subluxated PCIOL may be symptomatic because of the variable position of the optic in the visual axis. In addition, a mobile PCIOL may also generate unique floater-like symptoms, or possibly lead to pupillary block glaucoma.

35.6.2 Management and Course

There are four general management options for dislocated IOL: observation, IOL removal, IOL exchange, and IOL

Table 35.5 Incidence of retinal detachment occurring before and after vitrectomy for removal of retained lens fragments

Series (date)	Initial coexisting RD	RD after vitrectomy	Combined
Hutton et al[129] (1978)	5/26 (19%)	5/26 (19%)	10/26 (38%)
Fastenberg et al[130] (1991)	3/13 (23%)	2/11 (18%)	5/11 (45%)
Blodi et al[126] (1992)	4/36 (11%)	3/32 (9%)	7/36 (19%)
Gilliland et al[127] (1992)	4/56 (7%)	4/56 (7%)	8/56 (14%)
Kim et al[124] (1994)	2/57 (3.5%)	2/57 (3.5%)	4/57 (7%)
Borne et al[110] (1996)	8/121 (6.6%)	11/121 (9.1%)	19/121 (16%)
Kapusta et al[131] (1996)	0/25 (10%)	0/25 (10%)	0/25 (10%)
Vilar et al[97] (1997)	11/126 (8.7%)	11/126 (8.7%)	22/126 (17.5%)
Scott et al[120] (2003)	25/343 (7.3%)	19/343 (5.5%)	44/343 (12.8%)
Ho et al[128] (2009)	3/166 (1.8%)	4/166 (2.4%)	7/166 (4.2%)
Colyer et al[121] (2011)	1/172 (0.6%)	6/172 (3.5%)	7/172 (4%)
Modi et al[122] (2013)	N/A	51/569 (9%)	51/569 (9%)
Total	66/1141 (5.8%)	118/1704 (6.9%)	74/1710 (10.8%)

Abbreviation: RD, retinal detachment.

repositioning.[164,165,166,167,168,169,170] The management plan and timing are formulated based on multiple clinical factors, such as the type of IOL, surgeon preferences, and any observed secondary complications.

Substantial intraocular inflammation, retinal detachment, or cystoid macular edema, especially when associated with vitreous to the cataract wound, constitute relative indications for surgery. Although a completely dislocated IOL may be well tolerated in many patients, the difficulties in visual rehabilitation necessitate surgical intervention in most. For significantly subluxated IOLs, surgery may be performed via a limbal or a pars plana approach. Patients with less subluxation can be managed through a limbal incision with minimal or no anterior vitrectomy if the posterior capsule is largely intact. However, if there is a substantial posterior capsular rent, vitrectomy using a pars plana approach may offer optimal control to achieve the goals of surgery and address unforeseeable intraoperative complications.

Observation

IOLs with mild decentration are usually satisfactorily managed by observation. Observation also may be considered for luxation if other, superseding medical or ocular problems prohibit further surgery, or if the patient simply elects not to pursue further surgery. Occasionally, management with topical miotics can be visually beneficial, especially for minor subluxations. In an earlier series of 15 patients with dislocated AC or iris plane IOL that were observed, a VA of 20/40 or better was reported in 60%, but retinal detachment occurred in two patients.[164]

Removal or Exchange

The IOL is usually exchanged when the IOL is damaged during surgical management (e.g., broken haptic), if available instrumentation to effect repositioning is lacking, or if IOL design features such as highly flexible haptics make the IOL unsuitable for sulcus fixation.

A circumstance in which IOL exchange may be considered is certain cases with a silicone plate haptic IOL. Silicone IOLs may be slippery and more difficult to grasp than acrylic or polymethylmethacrylate (PMMA) IOLs,[171] but can usually be engaged and elevated from the retinal surface with a vitreoretinal pick or a lighted pick. A serrated or diamond-dusted forceps may be necessary, but care should be exercised to avoid scratching the center of the optic if the IOL is to be repositioned, as some grasp site marks may persist. Although silicone and acrylic plate haptic IOLs are extremely floppy and may be difficult to manipulate, and the dimension of the IOL is designed for capsular fixation, they can usually be repositioned into the sulcus, on top of anterior capsular remnants satisfactorily.[172]

In patients for which repositioning a PCIOL proves problematic, an intraoperative decision can be made to remove and exchange it with an anterior chamber IOL (ACIOL) or scleral suture-fixated PCIOL. In anticipation of this possibility, it is advisable to obtain IOL power measurements preoperatively. Exchange for a suture-fixated PCIOL has been simplified by the availability of IOL designs that include holes (eyelets) in the haptics. However, explanting and reimplanting an IOL may risk more corneal trauma compared with repositioning techniques. Exchange for an ACIOL may be less traumatic to the corneal endothelium and may be easier and faster to accomplish. Newer ACIOL designs reportedly avoid complications caused by the mechanical effects of earlier ACIOL designs, such as peripheral anterior synechia and glaucoma. Reports have demonstrated good efficacy and safety profile with ACIOL implantation in comparison to PCIOL scleral fixation, but prospective, randomized clinical trial is required to exactly determine the superiority of a lens type and fixation site in regard to visual outcomes and complications.[173,174,175,176,177,178,179] In general, scleral suture fixation with a PCIOL may be preferred to ACIOL implantation. Foldable IOLs—the most commonly used IOL nowadays—are safely sutured in the sclera and, when necessary, are exchanged through smaller incisions, carrying benefits from both ACIOL implantation and PCIOL suture fixation.[179,180] An ancillary option is observation of the dislocated IOL, but visual rehabilitation with implantation of a second (usually AC) IOL.[181,182] This should be considered an option of last resort, however, as most surgeons would prefer not to exercise it. The authors have encountered cases in which the second IOL has presented symptoms sufficient to require removal. While techniques to accomplish this are more challenging, they are readily achievable with some caveats.[183]

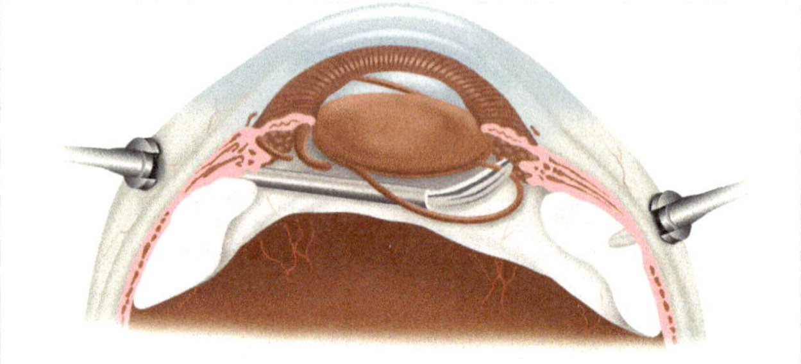

Fig. 35.7 Repositioning a posterior chamber intraocular lens into the ciliary sulcus, anterior to residual capsular remnants. Sometimes, it may be useful to bring one haptic anterior to the iris to facilitate accurate visualization of haptic placement over residual capsule.

Intraocular Lens Repositioning

IOL repositioning completes the initial surgical objectives of the cataract surgery and is the most commonly elected surgical approach. There are four basic approaches to IOL repositioning: (1) IOL repositioning without sutures using residual peripheral anterior or posterior capsule, (2) iris sutured fixation, (3) scleral suture fixation, and (4) scleral pocket.

IOL Repositioning without Sutures

Subluxated IOLs associated with an intact or mostly intact posterior capsule may be repositioned from an anterior approach if there is only moderate subluxation of the IOL. Usually, at least one haptic is posteriorly malpositioned—either protruding through an unseen zonular dehiscence, in an area without posterior capsular support, or posterior to the residual capsule. A pars plana approach is optimal for patients with large posterior capsule defects, for patients with IOL luxation into the vitreous cavity, and for patients with coexisting ocular complications, such as retinal detachment.

Recognizing and using adequate capsular support is as important for repositioning the PCIOL as it is for primary placement. Generally, the IOL remains well supported if at least 180 degrees of peripheral capsular material is intact (including the inferior meridians). More extensive support is necessary, however, when the inferior capsule is absent or if the margin of residual capsule where IOL haptics are to be placed is of questionable integrity. Repositioning by capsular fixation is the most common management technique in reported series[164,165,166,167,168,169,170] and is the authors' first choice when technically possible. Surgical success depends on accurate placement of the haptics into the ciliary sulcus, which requires visualization of the residual capsule.[184] Placement of iris retractors is useful in selected cases, although strategic local iris retraction with a hooked instrument usually allows confident visualization. A useful maneuver in a pars plana approach is to bring the IOL anteriorly and capture at least one haptic anterior to the iris. After the IOL is stabilized in the AC, the second haptic can be guided between the residual capsule and posterior iris surface, either by rotating the lens or by grasping the haptic with an intraocular forceps via the pars plana. Because of the widespread use of capsulorrhexis, the peripheral anterior capsule is usually intact and serves as an effective interface for sulcus fixation (▶ Fig. 35.7). Repositioning a PCIOL permanently into the AC also has been reported but is not recommended because of chronic chafing of the iris by the IOL and lens power considerations.[185]

Iris Suture Fixation

Iris fixation sutures were initially described for dislocated ACIOLs.[186] However, they have been modified for fixation of dislocated PC implants using a limbal or a pars plana approach.[187,188] This technique requires that a suture pass through cornea and iris, around the IOL haptic, and back out through the iris and cornea. Because accurate placement of the needle is difficult, it is challenging to optimize IOL centration. Also, concern regarding iris-mediated chronic inflammation and the technical difficulty encountered during suture placement has led to the development of other techniques. The use of iris-claw IOLs has been demonstrated to be a safe and effective option in selected cases.[173,175]

Scleral Suture Fixation

Scleral fixation sutures were first introduced for implantation of secondary IOLs and for primary IOL placement in the absence of satisfactory peripheral capsular support in a limbal or pars plana approach.[144,145,146,147,148,149,150] Early reports described pulling the haptic to or externally through a sclerotomy to sew a suture to a haptic before sewing to the deep part of the sclerotomy wound.[189,190,191] Subsequently, IOL repositioning by using transscleral fixation sutures, via a pars plana approach mimicking the techniques of secondary IOL fixation, was described. Numerous modifications have made the technique technically easier and safer and are reviewed later. Components common to all scleral suture fixation techniques include (1) retrieving the IOL, (2) introducing a suture loop through the ciliary sulcus region into the vitreous cavity, (3) passing the suture loop around the IOL haptic, (4) securing the suture to the sclera, and (5) covering or burying the scleral suture knot. A wide variety of techniques have been described to achieve these goals.

Most proposed techniques modify how the suture loop is introduced and attached to the IOL haptic. Such techniques have included imbricating the IOL haptic into the sutures used to close the sclerotomy,[192] externalizing the haptics to attach a suture,[193] using a needle guide to thread the suture around the haptic,[194] introducing a small needle intraocularly to capture the haptic,[195] suturing through IOL optic positioning holes,[196,197] backing a large needle into the eye to introduce a suture

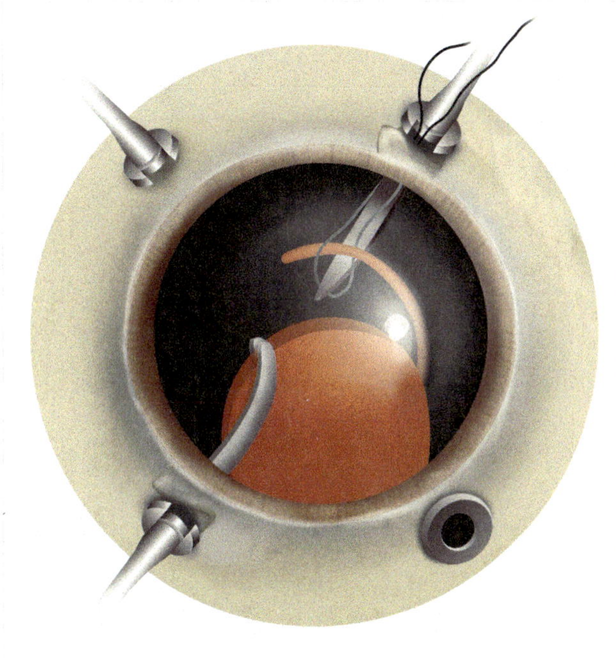

Fig. 35.8 Suture connected to one needle is threaded through a 27-gauge straight needle. The needle and suture are introduced into the vitreous cavity 1.0 mm posterior to the limbus through the bed of a partial-thickness scleral flap. Under direct visualization, the haptic is threaded through the loop along the shaft of the needle. A scleral plug is placed in the unused open sclerotomy.

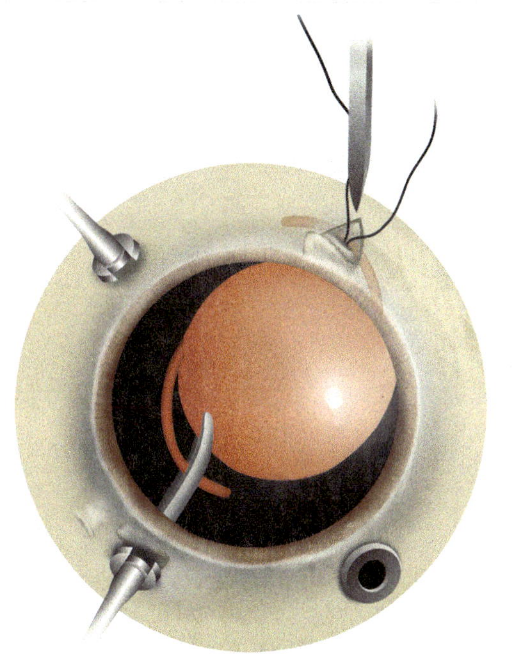

Fig. 35.9 The needle is withdrawn, and the suture is tied under the scleral flap in the usual fashion.

loop,[198] grasping a loop by intraocular forceps,[199,200] and introducing the suture from a third sclerotomy.[201] Other proposed variation techniques include achieving three- or four-point fixation to lessen lens torsion,[202] using specially designed, small-gauge forceps to aid in maneuvering the loop around the haptic,[203] and using perfluorocarbon liquids to place the implant in a convenient position for suturing.[204,205] Most posterior segment surgeons find the use of perfluorocarbon liquids unnecessary. A new technique utilizing Gore-Tex sutures with 4-point fixation IOL (Akreos AO, Bausch & Lomb) has become increasingly popular.

The current technique preferred by the authors is described and illustrated.[206,207] A standard three-port PPV is performed to remove the formed vitreous and mobilize the IOL. Partial-thickness, limbus-based scleral flaps are dissected, most conveniently in the 1 o'clock and 7 o'clock meridians to avoid the previous cataract wound and yet be accessible. A 5/8-inch, 25-gauge needle[207] is threaded with 9–0 polypropylene suture and introduced into the eye 1 mm posterior to the limbus in the bed of the partial-thickness scleral flap (▶ Fig. 35.8). Slack is created in the suture along the shaft of the needle by withdrawing it slightly. The IOL haptic is guided through this loop by using the intraocular forceps to grasp the optic. The haptic is captured in the loop as the needle is withdrawn (▶ Fig. 35.9). A partial-thickness scleral needle pass in the bed of the scleral flap allows fixation of the scleral suture. A similar procedure is repeated for the other haptic, unless capsular fixation is possible for the opposite haptic. Occasionally, it is necessary to guide the haptic through the loop by using intraocular forceps (▶ Fig. 35.10 and ▶ Fig. 35.11). The scleral flap is then closed with an absorbable suture and, if necessary, the vitrectomy is completed through the standard sclerotomies.

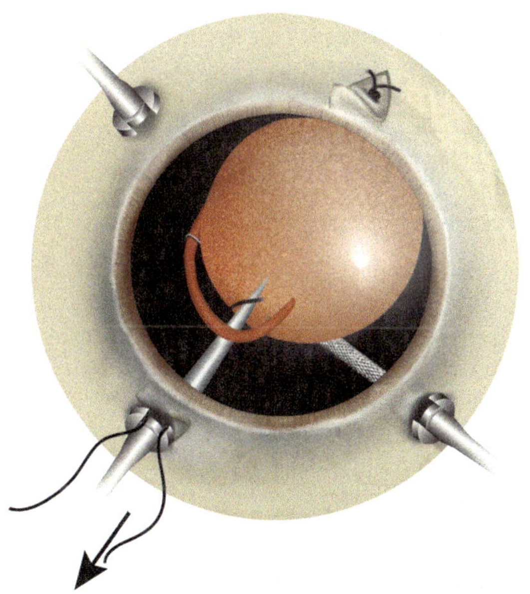

Fig. 35.10 A similar procedure is performed for the other haptic, unless the second haptic can be secured by capsular fixation.

Scleral suture fixation techniques for PCIOL placement have been reported to increase the risk for retinal detachment,[208,209,210,211,212] late postoperative endophthalmitis (with transscleral sutures serving as a conduit for bacteria to enter the globe),[213] and cystoid macular edema,[214,215] but these risks are relatively low, and may be less with newer techniques. ACIOL insertion in other settings has been reported to yield similar results as sutured PCIOL[149,216,217] and is a viable option in the absence of sufficient posterior capsular support. A randomized clinical trial performed a long-term comparison between posterior and AC IOL implantation in 438 eyes after extracapsular cataract extraction with vitreous loss, and found 20/40 or better vision in 91 and 79% in posterior and AC IOL implantation patients at 1 year, respectively.[218] Those results are congruent with another previous series that reported a higher rate of 20/40 or better final vision (80%) in eyes with PCIOL compared with eyes with ACIOL (62%),[124] but most other series have not reported a difference. If the cataract surgeon is reluctant to insert the IOL primarily, it can be inserted at the time of the subsequent vitrectomy.

Histopathologic and ultrasound biomicroscopic studies have shown that little or no fibrosis occurs around sutured PCIOL haptics,[219] but one study has shown cicatrization around the haptics.[220] Either way, it is vital to use a nondissolving suture material because it may provide the sole means of support at the ciliary sulcus.

IOL torsion and decentration can be avoided by accurate ciliary sulcus placement and by adequate excision of bulky capsular and cortical remnants. It may be necessary to exchange some IOLs that are too short from haptic to haptic for sulcus fixation. Anatomic studies have located the sulcus approximately 1 mm posterior to the limbus.[221] Consequently, suture placement more posteriorly may cause IOL optic torsion by forcing the circumferentially oriented haptic over radially oriented ciliary processes. Identification of the location of the ciliary sulcus can be facilitated by transillumination techniques.[152] The sutures must be placed diametrically apart for proper centration. Also, the IOL must be rotated minimally and cautiously to the center at the end of the case.

35.6.3 Scleral Sutureless Fixation

A recently described IOL sutureless fixation technique utilizes the construction of two lamellar scleral tunnels (scleral "pockets") in the setting of a standard three-port vitrectomy for the repositioning of a dislocated implant. With the use of a sharp 24-gauge needle, the 50% scleral thickness depth pockets are created 1.5 to 2 mm distant from the limbus in a parallel fashion, and exactly 180 degrees apart. Each IOL haptic is safely inserted in the correspondent pocket after being pulled out through the exit tract of the vitrectomy trocars. This technique has shown promising results, although it is only appropriate for a standard three-piece PCIOL.[222,223]

Outcomes of Surgery for Dislocated PCIOLs

The final VA probably depends not only on preoperative macular function but also on complications of the original cataract surgery, such as cystoid macular edema and retinal detachment. Still, previous series report a final VA of 20/40 or better in more than 90% of eyes (▶ Table 35.6). However, surgical series are difficult to compare accurately because of nonhomogeneity and the variety of management techniques.

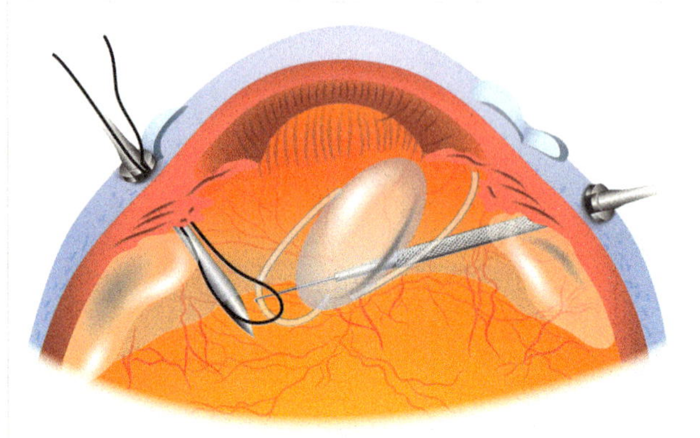

Fig. 35.11 Side view of Fig. 10 shows scleral fixation of first haptic and relationships in retrieving second haptic.

Table 35.6 Results of pars plana vitrectomy for dislocated intraocular lens

Study (date)	No. of patients	% = 20/40
Campo et al[194] (1989)	17	59
Flynn et al[167] (1990)	25	68
Smiddy and Flynn[164] (1991)	32	69
Chan[193] (1992)	12	92
Panton et al[168] (1993)	31	94
Smiddy et al[165] (1995)	46	50
Mello et al[166] (2000)	110	57
Sarrafizadeh et al[178] (2001)	31	53
Kim et al[180] (2008)	184	55

Postoperative Complications

An intraoperative or postoperative vitreous hemorrhage commonly occurs because sutures are placed through the vascular ciliary body, but these are almost always self-limited and of little clinical significance. Bacterial migration along the transscleral suture tract has been described as being the possible route of infection in cases of delayed-onset endophthalmitis.[167] The use of a partial-thickness scleral flap to cover the scleral suture knot should reduce the risk for this complication, but the suture knot can erode through the flap.

Other postoperative complications are difficult to separate from those that would be expected with complicated cataract surgery. Both cystoid macular edema and retinal detachment have been described after IOL repositioning surgery. Retinal detachment is reported to occur in about 2% of cases and may be less frequent than with retained lens fragments.[153] Some studies have reported that in approximately 10.8% of patients, retinal detachment will develop either at the time of or after the vitrectomy for the retained lens material, whereas within dislocated PC lens implants the prevalence seems much lower (▶ Table 35.7). Possible reasons for the disparity include less inflammation from IOL dislocation than from lens nuclear and cortical materials. Also, primary vitrectomy is often performed

Table 35.7 Incidence of retinal detachment occurring before and after vitrectomy for dislocated posterior chamber intraocular lens

Series (date)	Initial coexisting RD	RD after vitrectomy	Combined
Flynn et al[167] (1990)[a]	1/20 (5%)	0/20 (0%)	1/20 (5%)
Smiddy and Flynn[164] (1991)[a]	1/32 (3%)	1/32 (3%)	2/32 (6%)
Chan[193] (1992)	0/12 (0%)	0/12 (0%)	0/12 (0%)
Panton et al[168] (1993)	0/31 (0%)	0/31 (0%)	0/31 (0%)
Smiddy et al[165] (1995)[a]	0/59 (0%)	0/59 (0%)	0/59 (0%)
Mello et al[166] (2000)[a]	7/110 (6%)	7/110 (6%)	14/110 (13%)
Sarrafizadeh et al[178] (2001)	4/59 (7%)	6/59 (10%)	10/59 (17%)
Vote et al[210] (2006)	5/61 (8%)	5/61 (8%)	10/61 (16%)
Kim et al[180] (2008)	13/284 (5%)	11/284 (4%)	24/284 (8%)
Total	31/668 (4.6%)	30/668 (4.5%)	61/668 (9.1%)

Abbreviation: RD, retinal detachment.

[a]These three series are from the same institution and are listed here as consecutive series without overlap of cases.

from the limbus at the time the lens fragment is lost, whereas with the dislocated IOL, this is usually less aggressively performed. Surgical approach typically involves standard vitreoretinal surgical techniques, but perfluorocarbon liquids may be useful in selected cases to manipulate the IOL better while avoiding retinal trauma.

Recommendations for Management

For the anterior segment surgeon, avoiding PCIOL dislocation depends on accurate assessment of posterior capsule status intraoperatively. With the widespread use of phacoemulsification, capsular ruptures are generally central rather than peripheral, as was more commonly seen with expression extracapsular techniques. However, the anterior segment surgeon must take care to evaluate the integrity of the peripheral capsule carefully before implanting a PCIOL in the presence of a posterior capsular rupture. Generally, at least 6 clock hours of peripheral capsular support (including the inferior meridians) are necessary to maintain IOL positioning. Retracting the iris may be necessary to visualize the extent of peripheral capsular support directly before placing the PCIOL. Once it has been determined safe to proceed with IOL placement, it is vital that the haptics be placed precisely.

Recommendations to the anterior segment surgeon encountering PCIOL dislocation intraoperatively include performing anterior vitrectomy to avoid vitreous incarceration in the wound. Postoperatively, frequent topical corticosteroids and, as clinically indicated, IOP-reducing agents should be prescribed. For most cases, vitreoretinal referral for definitive management is advisable, but as described earlier, some cases are best observed or may be amenable to management with limbal incisions. Careful attention is necessary to evaluate for other complications, such as retinal detachment.

Recommendations to the vitreoretinal surgeon include careful assessment of existing capsular anatomy and coexisting complications to formulate a treatment plan in terms of timing and technique options. Generally, allowing a week or more for treatment and resolution of acute postoperative inflammation is advisable. The vitreoretinal surgeon should also be aware of IOL calculations from the cataract surgeon so that appropriate IOL power can be accurately selected if necessary. Newer techniques include the use of schleral pockets (Hoffman pockets and Gore-tex suture 4-point IOL fixation.[224,225]

References

[1] Scott IU, Flynn HW Jr. Endophthalmitis: categories, management and prevention. In: Tasman W, Jaeger EA, eds. Duane's Clinical Ophthalmology. Vol. 6, Ch. 64. Philadelphia, PA: Lippincott Williams & Wilkins; 2013

[2] Schein OD, Cassard SD, Tielsch JM, Gower EW. Cataract surgery among Medicare beneficiaries. Ophthalmic Epidemiol. 2012; 19(5):257–264

[3] Brod RD, Flynn HW Jr, Han DP, Miller D. Endophthalmitis: diagnosis, clinical findings and management. In: Spaeth GL, Danesh-Meyer HV, Goldberg I, Kampika, eds. Ophthalmic Surgery Principles and Practice. Philadelphia, PA: Elsevier; 2012:550–560

[4] Schwartz SG, Flynn HW Jr, Brod DR. Management of postoperative endophthalmitis. In: Narendran V, Kothari AR, eds. Principles and Practice of Vitreoretinal Surgery. Ch. 51. New Delhi, India: Jaypee Brothers Medical Publishers; 2014:481–489

[5] Leng T, Miller D, Flynn HW, Jr, Jacobs DJ, Gedde SJ. Delayed-onset bleb-associated endophthalmitis (1996–2008): causative organisms and visual acuity outcomes. Retina. 2011; 31(2):344–352

[6] Aaberg TM, Jr, Flynn HW, Jr, Newton J. Nosocomial endophthalmitis survey: a 10-year review of incidence and outcomes. Ophthalmology. 1998; 105:1004–1010

[7] Eifrig CW, Flynn HW, Jr, Scott IU, Newton J. Acute-onset postoperative endophthalmitis: review of incidence and visual outcomes (1995–2001). Ophthalmic Surg Lasers. 2002; 33(5):373–378

[8] Wykoff CC, Parrott MB, Flynn HW, Jr, Shi W, Miller D, Alfonso EC. Nosocomial acute-onset postoperative endophthalmitis at a university teaching hospital (2002–2009). Am J Ophthalmol. 2010; 150(3):392–398.e2

[9] Colyer MH, Weber ED, Weichel ED, et al. Delayed intraocular foreign body removal without endophthalmitis during Operations Iraqi Freedom and Enduring Freedom. Ophthalmology. 2007; 114(8):1439–1447

[10] Thompson WS, Rubsamen PE, Flynn HW, Jr, Schiffman J, Cousins SW. Endophthalmitis after penetrating trauma. Risk factors and visual acuity outcomes. Ophthalmology. 1995; 102(11):1696–1701

[11] Ahmed Y, Schimel AM, Pathengay A, Colyer MH, Flynn HW, Jr. Endophthalmitis following open-globe injuries. Eye (Lond). 2012; 26(2):212–217

[12] Boldt HC, Pulido JS, Blodi CF, Folk JC, Weingeist TA. Rural endophthalmitis. Ophthalmology. 1989; 96(12):1722–1726

[13] Miller JJ, Scott IU, Flynn HW, Jr, Smiddy WE, Newton J, Miller D. Acute-onset endophthalmitis after cataract surgery (2000–2004): incidence, clinical settings, and visual acuity outcomes after treatment. Am J Ophthalmol. 2005; 139(6):983–987

[14] Hatch WV, Cernat G, Wong D, Devenyi R, Bell CM. Risk factors for acute endophthalmitis after cataract surgery: a population-based study. Ophthalmology. 2009; 116(3):425–430

[15] Garcia-Arumi J, Fonollosa A, Sararols L, et al. Topical anesthesia: possible risk factor for endophthalmitis after cataract extraction. J Cataract Refract Surg. 2007; 33(6):989–992

[16] Henry CR, Flynn HW, Jr, Miller D, Schefler AC, Forster RK, Alfonso EC. Delayed-onset endophthalmitis associated with corneal suture infections. J Ophthalmic Inflamm Infect. 2013; 3(1):51

[17] Song A, Scott IU, Flynn HW, Jr, Budenz DL. Delayed-onset bleb-associated endophthalmitis: clinical features and visual acuity outcomes. Ophthalmology. 2002; 109(5):985–991

[18] Lalwani GA, Flynn HW, Jr, Scott IU, et al. Acute-onset endophthalmitis after clear corneal cataract surgery (1996–2005). Clinical features, causative organisms, and visual acuity outcomes. Ophthalmology. 2008; 115(3):473–476

[19] Donahue SP, Kowalski RP, Jewart BH, Friberg TR. Vitreous cultures in suspected endophthalmitis. Biopsy or vitrectomy? Ophthalmology. 1993; 100(4):452–455

[20] Rachitskaya AV, Flynn HW, Jr, Wong J, Kuriyan AE, Miller D. A 10-year study of membrane filter system versus blood culture bottles in culturing vitrectomy cassette vitreous in infectious endophthalmitis. Am J Ophthalmol. 2013; 156(2):349–354.e2

[21] Sharma S, Jalali S, Adiraju MV, Gopinathan U, Das T. Sensitivity and predictability of vitreous cytology, biopsy, and membrane filter culture in endophthalmitis. Retina. 1996; 16(6):525–529

[22] Schimel AM, Miller D, Flynn HW, Jr. Endophthalmitis isolates and antibiotic susceptibilities: a 10-year review of culture-proven cases. Am J Ophthalmol. 2013; 156(1):50–52.e1

[23] Kratz A, Levy J, Belfair N, Weinstein O, Klemperer I, Lifshitz T. Broth culture yield vs traditional approach in the work-up of endophthalmitis. Am J Ophthalmol. 2006; 141(6):1022–1026

[24] Yospaiboon Y, Saree S, Pasadhika S. Blood culture and conventional media for vitreous culture in infectious endophthalmitis. J Med Assoc Thai. 2005; 88(5):639–642

[25] Eser I, Kapran Z, Altan T, Eren H, Yilmaz OF. The use of blood culture bottles in endophthalmitis. Retina. 2007; 27(7):971–973

[26] Tan HS, Ghyczy-Carlborg EA, Spanjaard L, de Smet MD. The additional value of blood culture bottles in the diagnosis of endophthalmitis. Eye (Lond). 2011; 25(8):1069–1073

[27] Barza M, Pavan PR, Doft BH, et al. Evaluation of microbiological diagnostic techniques in postoperative endophthalmitis in the Endophthalmitis Vitrectomy Study. Arch Ophthalmol. 1997; 115(9):1142–1150

[28] Bharathi MJ, Murugan N, Rameshkumar G, et al. Comparative evaluation of uniplex, nested, semi-nested, multiplex and nested multiplex PCR methods in the identification of microbial etiology of clinically suspected infectious endophthalmitis. Curr Eye Res. 2013; 38(5):550–562

[29] Bannerman TL, Rhoden DL, McAllister SK, Miller JM, Wilson LA. The source of coagulase-negative staphylococci in the Endophthalmitis Vitrectomy Study. A comparison of eyelid and intraocular isolates using pulsed-field gel electrophoresis. Arch Ophthalmol. 1997; 115(3):357–361

[30] American Academy of Ophthalmology Cataract and Anterior Segment Panel. Preferred Practice Pattern® Guidelines. Cataract in the Adult Eye. San Francisco, CA: American Academy of Ophthalmology; 2011. Available at: http://www.aao.org/ppp. Accessed August 31, 2014

[31] Endophthalmitis Vitrectomy Study Group. Results of the Endophthalmitis Vitrectomy Study. A randomized trial of immediate vitrectomy and of intravenous antibiotics for the treatment of postoperative bacterial endophthalmitis. Arch Ophthalmol. 1995; 113(12):1479–1496

[32] Han DP, Wisniewski SR, Wilson LA, et al. Spectrum and susceptibilities of microbiologic isolates in the Endophthalmitis Vitrectomy Study. Am J Ophthalmol. 1996; 122(1):1–17

[33] The Endophthalmitis Vitrectomy Study Group. Microbiologic factors and visual outcome in the endophthalmitis vitrectomy study. Am J Ophthalmol. 1996; 122(6):830–846

[34] Johnson MW, Doft BH, Kelsey SF, et al. The Endophthalmitis Vitrectomy Study. Relationship between clinical presentation and microbiologic spectrum. Ophthalmology. 1997; 104(2):261–272

[35] Benz MS, Scott IU, Flynn HW, Jr, Unonius N, Miller D. Endophthalmitis isolates and antibiotic sensitivities: a 6-year review of culture-proven cases. Am J Ophthalmol. 2004; 137(1):38–42

[36] Gentile RC, Shukla S, Shah M, et al. Microbiological spectrum and antibiotic sensitivity in endophthalmitis: a 25-year review. Ophthalmology. 2014; 121(8):1634–1642

[37] Campochiaro PA, Lim JI, The Aminoglycoside Toxicity Study Group. Aminoglycoside toxicity in the treatment of endophthalmitis. Arch Ophthalmol. 1994; 112(1):48–53

[38] Iyer MN, Han DP, Yun HJ, et al. Subconjunctival antibiotics for acute postcataract extraction endophthalmitis—is it necessary? Am J Ophthalmol. 2004; 137(6):1120–1121

[39] Smiddy WE, Smiddy RJ, Ba'Arath B, et al. Subconjunctival antibiotics in the treatment of endophthalmitis managed without vitrectomy. Retina. 2005; 25(6):751–758

[40] Flynn HW, Jr, Meredith TA. Interpretation of EVS results. [Letter to Editor]. Arch Ophthalmol. 1996; 114:1027–1028

[41] Flynn HW, Jr, Scott IU. Legacy of the endophthalmitis vitrectomy study. Arch Ophthalmol. 2008; 126(4):559–561

[42] Meredith TA, Aguilar HE, Shaarawy A, Kincaid M, Dick J, Niesman MR. Vancomycin levels in the vitreous cavity after intravenous administration. Am J Ophthalmol. 1995; 119(6):774–778

[43] Major JC, Jr, Engelbert M, Flynn HW, Jr, Miller D, Smiddy WE, Davis JL. Staphylococcus aureus endophthalmitis: antibiotic susceptibilities, methicillin resistance, and clinical outcomes. Am J Ophthalmol. 2010; 149(2):278–283.e1

[44] Recchia FM, Busbee BG, Pearlman RB, Carvalho-Recchia CA, Ho AC. Changing trends in the microbiologic aspects of postcataract endophthalmitis. Arch Ophthalmol. 2005; 123(3):341–346

[45] Deramo VA, Lai JC, Fastenberg DM, Udell IJ. Acute endophthalmitis in eyes treated prophylactically with gatifloxacin and moxifloxacin. Am J Ophthalmol. 2006; 142(5):721–725

[46] Miller D, Flynn PM, Scott IU, Alfonso EC, Flynn HW, Jr. In vitro fluoroquinolone resistance in staphylococcal endophthalmitis isolates. Arch Ophthalmol. 2006; 124(4):479–483

[47] Harper T, Miller D, Flynn HW, Jr. In vitro efficacy and pharmacodynamic indices for antibiotics against coagulase-negative staphylococcus endophthalmitis isolates. Ophthalmology. 2007; 114(5):871–875

[48] Schimel AM, Miller D, Flynn HW, Jr. Evolving fluoroquinolone resistance among coagulase-negative Staphylococcus isolates causing endophthalmitis. Arch Ophthalmol. 2012; 130(12):1617–1618

[49] Endophthalmitis Study Group, European Society of Cataract & Refractive Surgeons. Prophylaxis of postoperative endophthalmitis following cataract surgery: results of the ESCRS multicenter study and identification of risk factors. J Cataract Refract Surg. 2007; 33(6):978–988

[50] Moshirfar M, Feiz V, Vitale AT, Wegelin JA, Basavanthappa S, Wolsey DH. Endophthalmitis rates after cataract surgery. Ophthalmology. 2007; 114:686–691

[51] Rudnisky CJ, Wan D, Weis E. Antibiotic choice for the prophylaxis of postcataract extraction endophthalmitis. Ophthalmology. 2014; 121(4):835–841

[52] Alfonso EC, Flynn HW, Jr. Controversies in endophthalmitis prevention. The risk for emerging resistance to vancomycin. Arch Ophthalmol. 1995; 113(11):1369–1370

[53] Schimel AM, Alfonso EC, Flynn HW, Jr. Endophthalmitis prophylaxis for cataract surgery: are intracameral antibiotics necessary? JAMA Ophthalmol. 2014; 132(11):1269–1270

[54] Henry CR, Flynn HW, Jr, Miller D, Forster RK, Alfonso EC. Infectious keratitis progressing to endophthalmitis: a 15-year study of microbiology, associated factors, and clinical outcomes. Ophthalmology. 2012; 119(12):2443–2449

[55] Al-Mezaine HS, Al-Assiri A, Al-Rajhi AA. Incidence, clinical features, causative organisms, and visual outcomes of delayed-onset pseudophakic endophthalmitis. Eur J Ophthalmol. 2009; 19(5):804–811

[56] Shirodkar AR, Pathengay A, Flynn HW, Jr, et al. Delayed- versus acute-onset endophthalmitis after cataract surgery. Am J Ophthalmol. 2012; 153(3):391–398.e2

[57] Essman TF, Flynn HW, Jr, Smiddy WE, et al. Treatment outcomes in a 10-year study of endogenous fungal endophthalmitis. Ophthalmic Surg Lasers. 1997; 28(3):185–194

[58] Kramer M, Kramer MR, Blau H, Bishara J, Axer-Siegel R, Weinberger D. Intravitreal voriconazole for the treatment of endogenous Aspergillus endophthalmitis. Ophthalmology. 2006; 113(7):1184–1186

[59] Winward KE, Pflugfelder SC, Flynn HW, Jr, Roussel TJ, Davis JL. Postoperative Propionibacterium endophthalmitis. Treatment strategies and long-term results. Ophthalmology. 1993; 100(4):447–451
[60] Fox GM, Joondeph BC, Flynn HW, Jr, Pflugfelder SC, Roussel TJ. Delayed-onset pseudophakic endophthalmitis. Am J Ophthalmol. 1991; 111(2):163–173
[61] Greenfield DS, Suñer IJ, Miller MP, Kangas TA, Palmberg PF, Flynn HW, Jr. Endophthalmitis after filtering surgery with mitomycin. Arch Ophthalmol. 1996; 114(8):943–949
[62] DeBry PW, Perkins TW, Heatley G, Kaufman P, Brumback LC. Incidence of late-onset bleb-related complications following trabeculectomy with mitomycin. Arch Ophthalmol. 2002; 120(3):297–300
[63] Sharan S, Trope GE, Chipman M, Buys YM. Late-onset bleb infections: prevalence and risk factors. Can J Ophthalmol. 2009; 44(3):279–283
[64] Jacobs DJ, Leng T, Flynn HW, Jr, Shi W, Miller D, Gedde SJ. Delayed-onset bleb-associated endophthalmitis: presentation and outcome by culture result. Clin Ophthalmol. 2011; 5:739–744
[65] Brown RH, Yang LH, Walker SD, Lynch MG, Martinez LA, Wilson LA. Treatment of bleb infection after glaucoma surgery. Arch Ophthalmol. 1994; 112 (1):57–61
[66] Al-Torbak AA, Al-Shahwan S, Al-Jadaan I, Al-Hommadi A, Edward DP. Endophthalmitis associated with the Ahmed glaucoma valve implant. Br J Ophthalmol. 2005; 89(4):454–458
[67] Gedde SJ, Scott IU, Tabandeh H, et al. Late endophthalmitis associated with glaucoma drainage implants. Ophthalmology. 2001; 108(7):1323–1327
[68] Wentzloff JN, Grosskreutz CL, Pasquale LR, Walton DS, Chen TC. Endophthalmitis after glaucoma drainage implant surgery. Int Ophthalmol Clin. 2007; 47(2):109–115
[69] Ahmed Y, Pathengay A, Flynn HW, Jr, Isom R. Delayed-onset endophthalmitis associated with Ex-PRESS mini glaucoma shunt®. Ophthalmic Surg Lasers Imaging. 2012; 43 Online:e62–e63
[70] Speaker MG, Guerriero PN, Met JA, Coad CT, Berger A, Marmor M. A case-control study of risk factors for intraoperative suprachoroidal expulsive hemorrhage. Ophthalmology. 1991; 98(2):202–209, discussion 210
[71] Reynolds MG, Haimovici R, Flynn HW, Jr, DiBernardo C, Byrne SF, Feuer W. Suprachoroidal hemorrhage. Clinical features and results of secondary surgical management. Ophthalmology. 1993; 100(4):460–465
[72] Lambrou FH, Jr, Meredith TA, Kaplan HJ. Secondary surgical management of expulsive choroidal hemorrhage. Arch Ophthalmol. 1987; 105(9):1195–1198
[73] Scott IU, Flynn HW, Jr, Schiffman J, Smiddy WE, Murray TG, Ehlies F. Visual acuity outcomes among patients with appositional suprachoroidal hemorrhage. Ophthalmology. 1997; 104(12):2039–2046
[74] Moshfeghi DM, Kim BY, Kaiser PK, Sears JE, Smith SD. Appositional suprachoroidal hemorrhage: a case-control study. Am J Ophthalmol. 2004; 138 (6):959–963
[75] Tuli SS, WuDunn D, Ciulla TA, Cantor LB. Delayed suprachoroidal hemorrhage after glaucoma filtration procedures. Ophthalmology. 2001; 108 (10):1808–1811
[76] Jeganathan VS, Ghosh S, Ruddle JB, Gupta V, Coote MA, Crowston JG. Risk factors for delayed suprachoroidal haemorrhage following glaucoma surgery. Br J Ophthalmol. 2008; 92(10):1393–1396
[77] Ling R, Kamalarajah S, Cole M, James C, Shaw S. Suprachoroidal haemorrhage complicating cataract surgery in the UK: a case control study of risk factors. Br J Ophthalmol. 2004; 88(4):474–477
[78] Tabandeh H, Flynn HW, Jr. Suprachoroidal hemorrhage during pars plana vitrectomy. Curr Opin Ophthalmol. 2001; 12(3):179–185
[79] Tabandeh H, Sullivan PM, Smahliuk P, Flynn HW, Jr, Schiffman J. Suprachoroidal hemorrhage during pars plana vitrectomy. Risk factors and outcomes. Ophthalmology. 1999; 106(2):236–242
[80] Chandra A, Xing W, Kadhim MR, Williamson TH. Suprachoroidal hemorrhage in pars plana vitrectomy: risk factors and outcomes over 10 years. Ophthalmology. 2014; 121(1):311–317
[81] Desai UR, Peyman GA, Chen CJ, et al. Use of perfluoroperhydrophenanthrene in the management of suprachoroidal hemorrhages. Ophthalmology. 1992; 99(10):1542–1547
[82] Kunjukunju N, Gonzales CR, Rodden WS. Recombinant tissue plasminogen activator in the treatment of suprachoroidal hemorrhage. Clin Ophthalmol. 2011; 5:155–157
[83] Murata T, Kikushima W, Imai A, Toriyama Y, Tokimitsu M, Kurokawa T. Tissue-type plasminogen activator-assisted drainage of suprachoroidal hemorrhage showing a kissing configuration. Jpn J Ophthalmol. 2011; 55(4):431–432
[84] Meier P, Wiedemann P. Massive suprachoroidal hemorrhage: secondary treatment and outcome. Graefes Arch Clin Exp Ophthalmol. 2000; 238 (1):28–32
[85] Brinton DA, Wilkinson CP. 2009
[86] Coppé AM, Lapucci G. Posterior vitreous detachment and retinal detachment following cataract extraction. Curr Opin Ophthalmol. 2008; 19(3):239–242
[87] Ripandelli G, Coppé AM, Parisi V, et al. Posterior vitreous detachment and retinal detachment after cataract surgery. Ophthalmology. 2007; 114 (4):692–697
[88] Javitt JC, Vitale S, Canner JK, Krakauer H, McBean AM, Sommer A. National outcomes of cataract extraction. I. Retinal detachment after inpatient surgery. Ophthalmology. 1991; 98(6):895–902
[89] Russell M, Gaskin B, Russell D, Polkinghorne PJ. Pseudophakic retinal detachment after phacoemulsification cataract surgery: ten-year retrospective review. J Cataract Refract Surg. 2006; 32(3):442–445
[90] Clark A, Morlet N, Ng JQ, Preen DB, Semmens JB. Risk for retinal detachment after phacoemulsification: a whole-population study of cataract surgery outcomes. Arch Ophthalmol. 2012; 130(7):882–888
[91] Boberg-Ans G, Villumsen J, Henning V. Retinal detachment after phacoemulsification cataract extraction. J Cataract Refract Surg. 2003; 29(7):1333–1338
[92] Sheu SJ, Ger LP, Ho WL. Late increased risk of retinal detachment after cataract extraction. Am J Ophthalmol. 2010; 149(1):113–119
[93] Erie JC, Raecker MA, Baratz KH, Schleck CD, Burke JP, Robertson DM. Risk of retinal detachment after cataract extraction, 1980–2004: a population-based study. Ophthalmology. 2006; 113(11):2026–2032
[94] Jakobsson G, Montan P, Zetterberg M, Stenevi U, Behndig A, Lundström M. Capsule complication during cataract surgery: retinal detachment after cataract surgery with capsule complication: Swedish Capsule Rupture Study Group report 4. J Cataract Refract Surg. 2009; 35(10):1699–1705
[95] Tuft SJ, Gore DM, Bunce C, Sullivan PM, Minassian DC. Outcomes of pseudophakic retinal detachment. Acta Ophthalmol (Copenh). 2012; 90(7):639–644
[96] Tuft SJ, Minassian D, Sullivan P. Risk factors for retinal detachment after cataract surgery: a case-control study. Ophthalmology. 2006; 113(4):650–656
[97] Vilar NF, Flynn HW, Jr, Smiddy WE, Murray TG, Davis JL, Rubsamen PE. Removal of retained lens fragments after phacoemulsification reverses secondary glaucoma and restores visual acuity. Ophthalmology. 1997; 104 (5):787–791, discussion 791–792
[98] Tielsch JM, Legro MW, Cassard SD, et al. Risk factors for retinal detachment after cataract surgery. A population-based case-control study. Ophthalmology. 1996; 103(10):1537–1545
[99] Ficker LA, Vickers S, Capon MRC, Mellerio J, Cooling RJ. Retinal detachment following Nd:YAG posterior capsulotomy. Eye (Lond). 1987; 1(Pt 1):86–89
[100] Javitt JC, Tielsh JN, Canner JK, et al. National outcome of cataract extraction, increased risk of retinal complications associated with Nd:YAG laser capsulotomy. Ophthalmology. 1992; 99:1486–1498
[101] Jahn CE, Richter J, Jahn AH, Kremer G, Kron M. Pseudophakic retinal detachment after uneventful phacoemulsification and subsequent neodymium: YAG capsulotomy for capsule opacification. J Cataract Refract Surg. 2003; 29 (5):925–929
[102] American Academy of Ophthalmology Retina Panel. Preferred Practice Pattern® Guidelines. Posterior Vitreous Detachment, Retinal Breaks, and Lattice Degeneration. San Francisco, CA: American Academy of Ophthalmology; 2013. Available at: http://www.aao.org/ppp. Accessed August 31, 2014
[103] Brinton DA, Wilkinson CP. Retinal Detachment. Principles and Practice [Monograph]. 3rd ed., Ch. 9. New York, NY: American Academy of Ophthalmology; 2009
[104] Grizzard WS. Ophthalmic anesthesia. In: Reineke R, ed. Ophthalmology Annual. New York, NY: Raven Press; 1989:265–294
[105] Hay A, Flynn HW, Jr, Hoffman JI, Rivera AH. Needle penetration of the globe during retrobulbar and peribulbar injections. Ophthalmology. 1991; 98 (7):1017–1024
[106] Duker JS, Belmont JB, Benson WE, et al. Inadvertent globe perforation during retrobulbar and peribulbar anesthesia. Patient characteristics, surgical management, and visual outcome. Ophthalmology. 1991; 98(4):519–526
[107] Morgan CM, Schatz H, Vine AK, et al. Ocular complications associated with retrobulbar injections. Ophthalmology. 1988; 95(5):660–665
[108] Leaming DV. Practice styles and preferences of ASCRS members—1994 survey. J Cataract Refract Surg. 1995; 21(4):378–385
[109] Pande M, Dabbs TR. Incidence of lens matter dislocation during phacoemulsification. J Cataract Refract Surg. 1996; 22(6):737–742

[110] Borne MJ, Tasman W, Regillo C, Malecha M, Sarin L. Outcomes of vitrectomy for retained lens fragments. Ophthalmology. 1996; 103(6):971–976

[111] Aaberg TM, Jr, Rubsamen PE, Flynn HW, Jr, Chang S, Mieler WF, Smiddy WE. Dropped nuclei and giant retinal tears as a complication of cataract surgery. Am J Ophthalmol. 1997; 124:222–226

[112] Irvine SR, Irvine AR. Lens-induced uveitis and glaucoma. Arch Ophthalmol. 1958; 60:829–840

[113] Epstein DL. Diagnosis and management of lens-induced glaucoma. Ophthalmology. 1982; 89(3):227–230

[114] Moisseiev E, Kinori M, Glovinsky Y, Loewenstein A, Moisseiev J, Barak A. Retained lens fragments: nucleus fragments are associated with worse prognosis than cortex or epinucleus fragments. Eur J Ophthalmol. 2011; 21 (6):741–747

[115] Vanner EA, Stewart MW, Liesegang TJ, Bendel RE, Bolling JP, Hasan SA. A retrospective cohort study of clinical outcomes for intravitreal crystalline retained lens fragments after age-related cataract surgery: a comparison of same-day versus delayed vitrectomy. Clin Ophthalmol. 2012; 6:1135–1148

[116] Chen CL, Wang TY, Cheng JH, Tai MC, Lu DW, Chen JT. Immediate pars plana vitrectomy improves outcome in retained intravitreal lens fragments after phacoemulsification. Ophthalmologica. 2008; 222(4):277–283

[117] Stefaniotou M, Aspiotis M, Pappa C, Eftaxias V, Psilas K. Timing of dislocated nuclear fragment management after cataract surgery. J Cataract Refract Surg. 2003; 29(10):1985–1988

[118] Romero-Aroca P, Fernández-Ballart J, Méndez-Marín I, Salvat-Serra M, Baget-Bernaldiz M, Buil-Calvo JA. Management of nucleus loss into the vitreous: long term follow up in 63 patients. Clin Ophthalmol. 2007; 1(4):505–512

[119] Moore JK, Scott IU, Flynn HW, Jr, et al. Retinal detachment in eyes undergoing pars plana vitrectomy for removal of retained lens fragments. Ophthalmology. 2003; 110(4):709–713, discussion 713–714

[120] Scott IU, Flynn HW, Jr, Smiddy WE, et al. Clinical features and outcomes of pars plana vitrectomy in patients with retained lens fragments. Ophthalmology. 2003; 110(8):1567–1572

[121] Colyer MH, Berinstein DM, Khan NJ, et al. Same-day versus delayed vitrectomy with lensectomy for the management of retained lens fragments. Retina. 2011; 31(8):1534–1540

[122] Modi YS, Epstein A, Smiddy WE, Murray TG, Feuer W, Flynn HW, Jr. Retained lens fragments after cataract surgery: outcomes of same-day versus later pars plana vitrectomy. Am J Ophthalmol. 2013; 156(3):454–9.e1

[123] Vanner EA, Stewart MW. Vitrectomy timing for retained lens fragments after surgery for age-related cataracts: a systematic review and meta-analysis. Am J Ophthalmol. 2011; 152(3):345–357.e3

[124] Kim JE, Flynn HW, Jr, Smiddy WE, et al. Retained lens fragments after phacoemulsification. Ophthalmology. 1994; 101(11):1827–1832

[125] Lambrou FH, Jr, Steward MW. Management of dislocated lens fragments after cataract surgery. Ophthalmology. 1992; 99:1260–1262

[126] Blodi BA, Flynn HW, Jr, Blodi CF, Folk JC, Daily MJ. Retained nuclei after cataract surgery. Ophthalmology. 1992; 99(1):41–44

[127] Gilliland GD, Hutton WL, Fuller DG. Retained intravitreal lens fragments after cataract surgery. Ophthalmology. 1992; 99(8):1263–1267, discussion 1268–1269

[128] Ho LY, Doft BH, Wang L, Bunker CH. Clinical predictors and outcomes of pars plana vitrectomy for retained lens material after cataract extraction. Am J Ophthalmol. 2009; 147(4):587–594.e1

[129] Hutton WL, Snyder WB, Vaiser A. Management of surgically dislocated intravitreal lens fragments by pars plana vitrectomy. Ophthalmology. 1978; 85 (2):176–189

[130] Fastenberg DM, Schwartz PL, Shakin JL, Golub BM. Management of dislocated nuclear fragments after phacoemulsification. Am J Ophthalmol. 1991; 112(5):535–539

[131] Kapusta MA, Chen JC, Lam WC. Outcomes of dropped nucleus during phacoemulsification. Ophthalmology. 1996; 103(8):1184–1187

[132] Cho M, Chan RP. 23-gauge pars plana vitrectomy for management of posteriorly dislocated crystalline lens. Clin Ophthalmol. 2011; 5:1737–1743

[133] Kongsap P. Combined 20-gauge and 23-gauge pars plana vitrectomy for the management of posteriorly dislocated lens: a case series. Clin Ophthalmol. 2010; 4:625–628

[134] Ho LY, Walsh MK, Hassan TS. 25-Gauge pars plana vitrectomy for retained lens fragments. Retina. 2010; 30(6):843–849

[135] Kiss S, Vavvas D. 25-Gauge transconjunctival sutureless pars plana vitrectomy for the removal of retained lens fragments and intraocular foreign bodies. Retina. 2008; 28(9):1346–1351

[136] Baker PS, Spirn MJ, Chiang A, et al. 23-Gauge transconjunctival pars plana vitrectomy for removal of retained lens fragments. Am J Ophthalmol. 2011; 152(4):624–627

[137] Bhandari R, Ernst BJ, Stafeeva K, Mandava N, Quiroz-Mercado H. 23-gauge vitrectomy for retained lens material. Ophthalmic Surg Lasers Imaging. 2012; 43(4):351–352

[138] Liu KR, Peyman GA, Chen MS, Chang KB. Use of high-density vitreous substitutes in the removal of posteriorly dislocated lenses or intraocular lenses. Ophthalmic Surg. 1991; 22(9):503–507

[139] Greve MD, Peyman GA, Mehta NJ, Millsap CM. Use of perfluoroperhydrophenanthrene in the management of posteriorly dislocated crystalline and intraocular lenses. Ophthalmic Surg. 1993; 24(9):593–597

[140] Lewis H, Blumenkranz MS, Chang S. Treatment of dislocated crystalline lens and retinal detachment with perfluorocarbon liquids. Retina. 1992; 12 (4):299–304

[141] Brod RD, Flynn HW, Jr, Clarkson JG, Blankenship GW. Management options for retinal detachment in the presence of a posteriorly dislocated intraocular lens. Retina. 1990; 10(1):50–56

[142] Smiddy WE, Flynn HW, Jr, Kim JE. Retinal detachment in patients with retained lens fragments or dislocated posterior chamber intraocular lenses. Ophthalmic Surg Lasers. 1996; 27(10):856–861

[143] Smiddy WE, Guererro JL, Pinto R, Feuer W. Retinal detachment rate after vitrectomy for retained lens material after phacoemulsification. Am J Ophthalmol. 2003; 135(2):183–187

[144] Lindquist TD, Agapitos PJ, Lindstrom RL, Lane SS, Spigelman AV. Transscleral fixation of posterior chamber intraocular lenses in the absence of capsular support. Ophthalmic Surg. 1989; 20(11):769–775

[145] Smiddy WE, Sawusch MR, O'Brien TP, Scott DR, Huang SS. Implantation of scleral-fixated posterior chamber intraocular lenses. J Cataract Refract Surg. 1990; 16(6):691–696

[146] Lewis JS. Sulcus fixation without flaps. Ophthalmology. 1993; 100(9):1346–1350

[147] McCluskey P, Harrisberg B. Long-term results using scleral-fixated posterior chamber intraocular lenses. J Cataract Refract Surg. 1994; 20(1):34–39

[148] Tomikawa S, Hara A. Simple approach to secondary posterior chamber intraocular lens implantation in patients without a complete posterior lens capsule support. Ophthalmic Surg. 1995; 26(2):160–163

[149] Lyle WA, Jin JC. Secondary intraocular lens implantation: anterior chamber vs posterior chamber lenses. Ophthalmic Surg. 1993; 24(6):375–381

[150] Regillo CD, Tidwell J. A small-incision technique for suturing a posterior chamber intraocular lens. Ophthalmic Surg Lasers. 1996; 27(6):473–475

[151] Tsai JC, Rowsey JJ, Fouraker BD, Stevens SX, Young DA, Polack PJ. Use of a mirror needle holder with transsclerally sutured posterior chamber intraocular lenses. Ophthalmic Surg Lasers. 1996; 27(8):720–724

[152] Horiguchi M, Hirose H, Koura T, Satou M. Identifying the ciliary sulcus for suturing a posterior chamber intraocular lens by transillumination. Arch Ophthalmol. 1993; 111(12):1693–1695

[153] Smiddy WE, Flynn HW, Jr. Managing retinal lens fragments and dislocated posterior chamber IOLs after cataract surgery. Focal Points.. 1996; 14(7):1–14

[154] Stark WJ, Worthen DM, Holladay JT, et al. The FDA report on intraocular lenses. Ophthalmology. 1983; 90(4):311–317

[155] Smith SG, Lindstrom RL. Malpositioned posterior chamber lenses: etiology, prevention, and management. J Am Intraocul Implant Soc. 1985; 11(6):584–591

[156] Mönestam EI. Incidence of dislocation of intraocular lenses and pseudophakodonesis 10 years after cataract surgery. Ophthalmology. 2009; 116 (12):2315–2320

[157] Clark A, Morlet N, Ng JQ, Preen DB, Semmens JB. Whole population trends in complications of cataract surgery over 22 years in Western Australia. Ophthalmology. 2011; 118(6):1055–1061

[158] Murphy GE. Traumatic dislocation of a shearing lens 31 months after implantation. Ophthalmic Surg. 1983; 14(1):53–54

[159] Naumann GO, Schlötzer-Schrehardt U, Küchle M. Pseudoexfoliation syndrome for the comprehensive ophthalmologist. Intraocular and systemic manifestations. Ophthalmology. 1998; 105(6):951–968

[160] Zech JC, Tanniére P, Denis P, Trepsat C. Posterior chamber intraocular lens dislocation with the bag. J Cataract Refract Surg. 1999; 25(8):1168–1169

[161] Yasuda A, Ohkoshi K, Orihara Y, Kusano Y, Sakuma A, Yamaguchi T. Spontaneous luxation of encapsulated intraocular lens onto the retina after a triple procedure of vitrectomy, phacoemulsification, and intraocular lens implantation. Am J Ophthalmol. 2000; 130(6):836–837

[162] Dikopf MS, Chow CC, Mieler WF, Tu EY. Cataract extraction outcomes and the prevalence of zonular insufficiency in retinitis pigmentosa. Am J Ophthalmol. 2013; 156(1):82–88.e2

[163] Cionni RJ. Surgical management of the congenitally subluxated crystalline lens using the modified capsular tension ring. In: Steinert RF, ed. Cataract Surgery: Technique, Complications, and Management. 2nd ed. Philadelphia, PA: Saunders; 2004:305–313

[164] Smiddy WE, Flynn HW, Jr. Management of dislocated posterior chamber intraocular lenses. Ophthalmology. 1991; 98(6):889–894

[165] Smiddy WE, Ibanez GV, Alfonso E, Flynn HW, Jr. Surgical management of dislocated intraocular lenses. J Cataract Refract Surg. 1995; 21(1):64–69

[166] Mello MO, Jr, Scott IU, Smiddy WE, Flynn HW, Jr, Feuer W. Surgical management and outcomes of dislocated intraocular lenses. Ophthalmology. 2000; 107(1):62–67

[167] Flynn HW, Jr, Buus D, Culbertson WW. Management of subluxated and posteriorly dislocated intraocular lenses using pars plana vitrectomy instrumentation. J Cataract Refract Surg. 1990; 16(1):51–56

[168] Panton RW, Sulewski ME, Parker JS, Panton PJ, Stark WJ. Surgical management of subluxed posterior-chamber intraocular lenses. Arch Ophthalmol. 1993; 111(7):919–926

[169] Smiddy WE, Flynn HW, Jr. Management options for posteriorly dislocated intraocular lenses. Ophthalmic Practice.. 1994; 12:72–77

[170] Gimbel HV, Sun R, Ferensowicz M, Anderson Penno E, Kamal A. Intraoperative management of posterior capsule tears in phacoemulsification and intraocular lens implantation. Ophthalmology. 2001; 108(12):2186–2189, discussion 2190–2192

[171] Smiddy WE. Management of dislocated foldable intraocular lenses. Retina. 2005; 25(5):576–580

[172] Schneiderman TE, Johnson MW, Smiddy WE, Flynn HW, Jr, Bennett SR, Central HL. Surgical management of dislocated plate haptic silicone posterior chamber intraocular lenses. Am J Ophthalmol. 1997; 123:629–635

[173] Güell JL, Verdaguer P, Elies D, et al. Secondary iris-claw anterior chamber lens implantation in patients with aphakia without capsular support. Br J Ophthalmol. 2014; 98(5):658–663

[174] Hazar L, Kara N, Bozkurt E, Ozgurhan EB, Demirok A. Intraocular lens implantation procedures in aphakic eyes with insufficient capsular support associated with previous cataract surgery. J Refract Surg. 2013; 29(10):685–691

[175] De Silva SR, Arun K, Anandan M, Glover N, Patel CK, Rosen P. Iris-claw intraocular lenses to correct aphakia in the absence of capsule support. J Cataract Refract Surg. 2011; 37(9):1667–1672

[176] Jin GJ, Crandall AS, Jones JJ. Changing indications for and improving outcomes of intraocular lens exchange. Am J Ophthalmol. 2005; 140(4):688–694

[177] Dadeya S, Kamlesh, Kumari Sodhi P. Secondary intraocular lens (IOL) implantation: anterior chamber versus scleral fixation long-term comparative evaluation. Eur J Ophthalmol. 2003; 13(7):627–633

[178] Sarrafizadeh R, Ruby AJ, Hassan TS, et al. A comparison of visual results and complications in eyes with posterior chamber intraocular lens dislocation treated with pars plana vitrectomy and lens repositioning or lens exchange. Ophthalmology. 2001; 108(1):82–89

[179] Wagoner MD, Cox TA, Ariyasu RG, Jacobs DS, Karp CL, American Academy of Ophthalmology. Intraocular lens implantation in the absence of capsular support: a report by the American Academy of Ophthalmology. Ophthalmology. 2003; 110(4):840–859

[180] Kim SS, Smiddy WE, Feuer W, Shi W. Management of dislocated intraocular lenses. Ophthalmology. 2008; 115(10):1699–1704

[181] Brockman EB, Franklin RM, Kaufman HE. Visual disability resulting from a dislocated intraocular lens. J Cataract Refract Surg. 1993; 19(2):312–313

[182] Sinskey RM. Posterior chamber implant removal with or without replacement. Cataract. 1983; 1:8–10

[183] Emanuelli A, Smiddy WE. Management of 2 intraocular lenses in the same eye. JAMA Ophthalmol. 2013; 131(1):86–87

[184] Eifrig DE. Two principles for repositioning intraocular lenses. Ophthalmic Surg. 1986; 17(8):486–489

[185] Allara RD, Weinstein GW. A new surgical technique for managing sunset syndrome. Ophthalmic Surg. 1987; 18(11):811–814

[186] McCannel MA. A retrievable suture idea for anterior uveal problems. Ophthalmic Surg. 1976; 7(2):98–103

[187] Sternberg P, Jr, Michels RG. Treatment of dislocated posterior chamber intraocular lenses. Arch Ophthalmol. 1986; 104(9):1391–1393

[188] Stutzman RD, Stark WJ. Surgical technique for suture fixation of an acrylic intraocular lens in the absence of capsule support. J Cataract Refract Surg. 2003; 29(9):1658–1662

[189] Lyons CJ, Steele AD. Report of a repositioned posteriorly dislocated intraocular lens via pars plicata sclerotomy. J Cataract Refract Surg. 1990; 16(4):509–511

[190] Moretsky SL. Suture fixation technique for subluxated posterior chamber IOL through stab wound incision. J Am Intraocul Implant Soc. 1984; 10 (4):477–480

[191] Insler MS, Mani H, Peyman GA. A new surgical technique for dislocated posterior chamber intraocular lenses. Ophthalmic Surg. 1988; 19(7):480–481

[192] Girard LJ, Nino N, Wesson M, Maghraby A. Scleral fixation of a subluxated posterior chamber intraocular lens. J Cataract Refract Surg. 1988; 14 (3):326–327

[193] Chan CK. An improved technique for management of dislocated posterior chamber implants. Ophthalmology. 1992; 99(1):51–57

[194] Campo RV, Chung KD, Oyakawa RT. Pars plana vitrectomy in the management of dislocated posterior chamber lenses. Am J Ophthalmol. 1989; 108 (5):529–534

[195] Smiddy WE. Dislocated posterior chamber intraocular lens. A new technique of management. Arch Ophthalmol. 1989; 107(11):1678–1680

[196] Koch DD. New optic hole configuration for iris fixation of posterior chamber lenses. Arch Ophthalmol. 1988; 106(2):163–164

[197] Nabors G, Varley MP, Charles S. Ciliary sulcus suturing of a posterior chamber intraocular lens. Ophthalmic Surg. 1990; 21(4):263–265

[198] Friedberg MA, Pilkerton AR. A new technique for repositioning and fixating a dislocated intraocular lens. Arch Ophthalmol. 1992; 110(3):413–415

[199] Maguire AM, Blumenkranz MS, Ward TG, Winkelman JZ. Scleral loop fixation for posteriorly dislocated intraocular lenses. Operative technique and long-term results. Arch Ophthalmol. 1991; 109(12):1754–1758

[200] Lawrence FC, II, Hubbard WA. "Lens lasso" repositioning of dislocated posterior chamber intraocular lenses. Retina. 1994; 14(1):47–50

[201] Bloom SM, Wyszynski RE, Brucker AJ. Scleral fixation suture for dislocated posterior chamber intraocular lens. Ophthalmic Surg. 1990; 21(12):851–854

[202] Anand R, Bowman RW. Simplified technique for suturing dislocated posterior chamber intraocular lens to the ciliary sulcus. Arch Ophthalmol. 1990; 108(9):1205–1206

[203] Chang S, Coll GE. Surgical techniques for repositioning a dislocated intraocular lens, repair of iridodialysis, and secondary intraocular lens implantation using innovative 25-gauge forceps. Am J Ophthalmol. 1995; 119(2):165–174

[204] Lewis H, Sanchez G. The use of perfluorocarbon liquids in the repositioning of posteriorly dislocated intraocular lenses. Ophthalmology. 1993; 100 (7):1055–1059

[205] Fanous MM, Friedman SM. Ciliary sulcus fixation of a dislocated posterior chamber intraocular lens using liquid perfluorophenanthrene. Ophthalmic Surg. 1992; 23(8):551–552

[206] Smiddy WE, Flynn HW, Jr. Needle-assisted scleral fixation suture technique for relocating posteriorly dislocated IOLs. Arch Ophthalmol. 1993; 111 (2):161–162

[207] Smiddy WE. Modification of scleral suture fixation technique for dislocated posterior chamber intraocular lens implants. Arch Ophthalmol. 1998; 116 (7):967

[208] Sheu SJ, Wu TD. Is a transsclerally sutured intraocular lens a poor prognostic factor for the management of rhegmatogenous retinal detachment? Ann Ophthalmol. 1996; 28:244–249

[209] Bourke RD, Gray PJ, Rosen PH, Cooling RJ. Retinal detachment complicating scleral-sutured posterior chamber intraocular lens surgery. Eye (Lond). 1996; 10(Pt 4):501–508

[210] Vote BJ, Tranos P, Bunce C, Charteris DG, Da Cruz L. Long-term outcome of combined pars plana vitrectomy and scleral fixated sutured posterior chamber intraocular lens implantation. Am J Ophthalmol. 2006; 141(2):308–312

[211] Bading G, Hillenkamp J, Sachs HG, Gabel VP, Framme C. Long-term safety and functional outcome of combined pars plana vitrectomy and scleral-fixated sutured posterior chamber lens implantation. Am J Ophthalmol. 2007; 144(3):371–377

[212] Kim SW, Kim MJ, Yang KS, Sohn JH, Huh K. Risk factors for pseudophakic retinal detachment after intraocular lens scleral fixation with or without pars plana vitrectomy. Retina. 2009; 29(10):1479–1485

[213] Epstein E. Suture problems. [Letter to Editor]. J Cataract Refract Surg. 1989; 15(1):116

[214] Uthoff D, Teichmann KD. Secondary implantation of scleral-fixated intraocular lenses. J Cataract Refract Surg. 1998; 24(7):945–950

[215] Busin M, Brauweiler P, Böker T, Spitznas M. Complications of sulcus-supported intraocular lenses with iris sutures, implanted during penetrating keratoplasty after intracapsular cataract extraction. Ophthalmology. 1990; 97(4):401–405, discussion 405–406

[216] Schein OD, Kenyon KR, Steinert RF, et al. A randomized trial of intraocular lens fixation techniques with penetrating keratoplasty. Ophthalmology. 1993; 100(10):1437–1443

[217] Pokroy R, Pollack A, Bukelman A. Retinal detachment in eyes with vitreous loss and an anterior chamber or a posterior chamber intraocular lens: comparison of the incidence. J Cataract Refract Surg. 2002; 28(11):1997–2000

[218] Collins JF, Gaster RN, Krol WF, Colling CL, Kirk GF, Smith TJ, Department of Veterans Affairs Cooperative Cataract Study. A comparison of anterior chamber and posterior chamber intraocular lenses after vitreous presentation during cataract surgery: the Department of Veterans Affairs Cooperative Cataract Study. Am J Ophthalmol. 2003; 136(1):1–9

[219] Pavlin CJ, Rootman D, Arshinoff S, Harasiewicz K, Foster FS. Determination of haptic position of transsclerally fixated posterior chamber intraocular lenses by ultrasound biomicroscopy. J Cataract Refract Surg. 1993; 19(5):573–577

[220] McDermott ML, Puklin JE. Pars plana cicatrization of sewn-in posterior chamber intraocular lens haptics. Ophthalmic Surg Lasers. 1997; 28(3):239–240

[221] Duffey RJ, Holland EJ, Agapitos PJ, Lindstrom RL. Anatomic study of transsclerally sutured intraocular lens implantation. Am J Ophthalmol. 1989; 108 (3):300–309

[222] Scharioth GB, Prasad S, Georgalas I, Tataru C, Pavlidis M. Intermediate results of sutureless intrascleral posterior chamber intraocular lens fixation. J Cataract Refract Surg. 2010; 36(2):254–259

[223] Kumar DA, Agarwal A, Jacob S, Prakash G, Agarwal A, Sivagnanam S. Repositioning of the dislocated intraocular lens with sutureless 20-gauge vitrectomy. Retina. 2010; 30(4):682–687

[224] Kan MA, Rahimy E, Gupta OP, Hsu J. Combined 270Gauge Pars Plana Vitrectomy and Scleral Fixation of an Akreos AO60 Intraocular Lens Using Gore-Tex Suture. Retina. 2016 Aug; 36(8):1602–4. doi: 10.1097/IAE.0000000000001147

[225] Budoff G, Miller CG, Halperin SJ, Jeng-Miller KW, Fine HF, Wheatly HM, Prenner JL. One-year outcomes of a novel technique for rescuing and scleral fixating a posterior dislocated intraocular lens-bag complex without conjunctival opening (Hoffman Pockets). Retina. 2016 Apr 25. [Epub ahead of print]

36 Congenital Fundus Abnormalities

Gary C. Brown

36.1 Vascular Anomalies of the Optic Disc

36.1.1 Prepapillary Vascular Loops

First described by Liebrich in 1871,[1] these vascular abnormalities were originally thought to be remnants of an incompletely regressed hyaloid system. Most evidence now suggests this is not the case, but rather that they occur because of aberrant development of the retinal vascular system.[2,3,4] Despite the fact that some of these anomalies appear dark and venous, approximately 95% of prepapillary loops are arterial.[3]

Clinically, the vessels present as loops that extend from the optic disc into the vitreous cavity and then back to the disc within Cloquet's canal (▶ Fig. 36.1). In contrast to a single hyaloid artery, each prepapillary loop has at least one ascending and one descending branch. Loops can assume a spiral or corkscrew shape (▶ Fig. 36.1), have a figure-of-eight appearance (▶ Fig. 36.2), or manifest with a simple hairpin-turn configuration.[3] Spontaneous movement or pulsations, coincident with the heartbeat, are seen in about one-half of the cases. Approximately 30% are encased by a white, glial-appearing sheath.

Arterial prepapillary loops average about 1.5 mm in height.[3] In contrast to a persistent hyaloid artery, arterial prepapillary loops achieve a maximum height of only about 5 mm and do not extend anteriorly to the posterior capsule of the lens. Bilaterality is present in 9 to 17% of cases,[4] and cilioretinal arteries have been noted in up to 75% of affected eyes. Consistent systematic associations have not been identified.

Histopathologically, a prepapillary arterial loop has been shown to contain intima but not an internal elastic lamina (▶ Fig. 36.3).[5] The loop was demonstrated to lie beneath a loose connective tissue sheath continuous with the internal limiting membrane of the retina.

Mann[2] has suggested that prepapillary arterial loops arise at about the 100-mm stage (3.5–4 mo) of gestation. At this time, mesenchymal cells- the precursors of retinal capillary endothelial cells- inadvertently grow anteriorly into the supporting

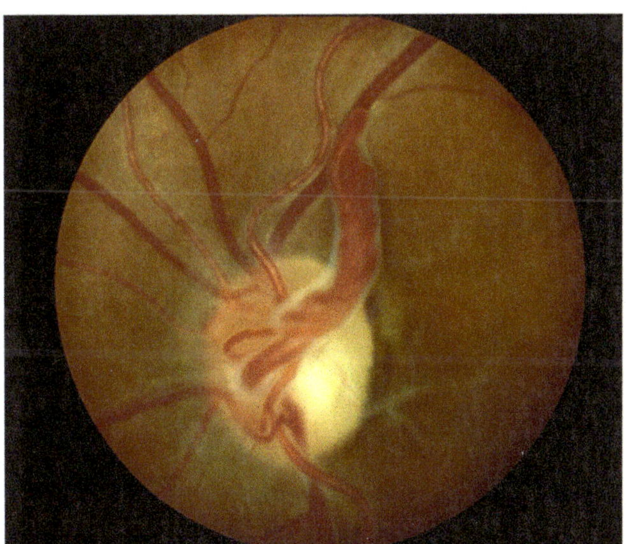

Fig. 36.1 Congenital prepapillary arterial loop with a corkscrew configuration in the left eye of a 33-year-old woman. The larger vessel in the center of the corkscrew is the central retinal artery, which divides into a superior papillary artery and inferior papillary artery within the loop. Note that the loop is sheathed. The cilioretinal artery at the 4 o'clock position on the optic nerve head is also sheathed for a different reason, severe eclampsia of pregnancy experienced at age 18 years.

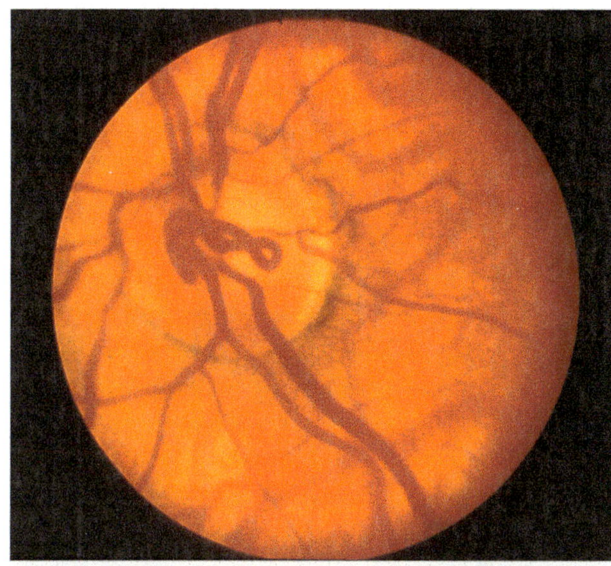

Fig. 36.2 Congenital prepapillary arterial loop with a figure-of-eight configuration. Despite the dark appearance of the vascular loop, it is arterial in origin. (Reproduced with permission from Brown and Tasman.[4])

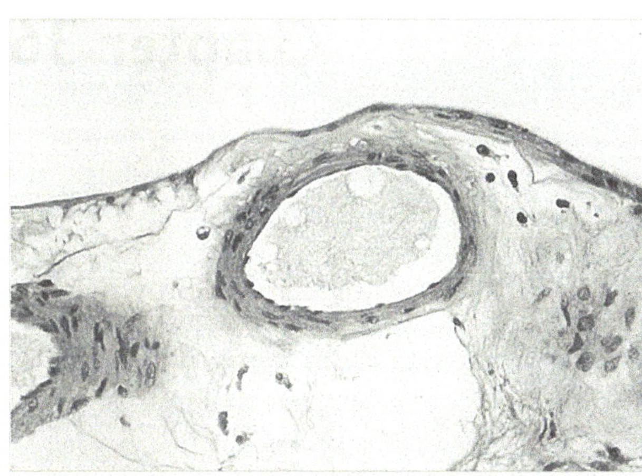

Fig. 36.3 Histopathology of prepapillary arterial loop. The vessel is located within amorphous connective tissue beneath the internal limiting membrane of Elschnig. (Hematoxylin and eosin, × 100.)

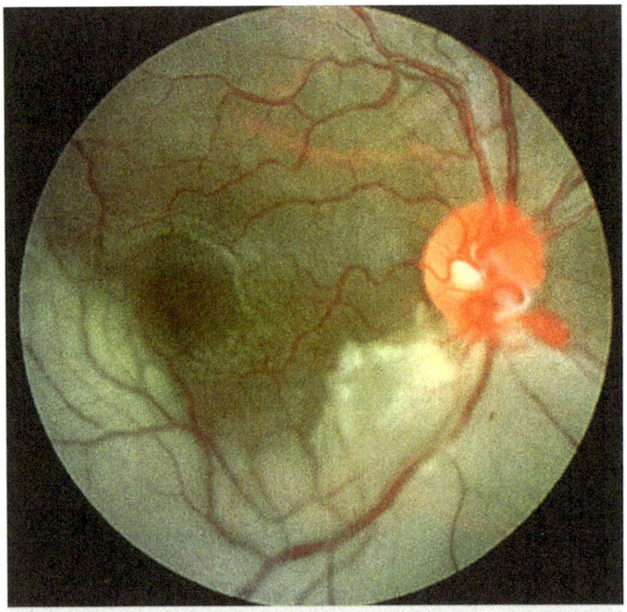

Fig. 36.4 Inferior branch retinal artery obstruction in the right eye of an 18-year-old youth with a prepapillary arterial loop. (Reproduced with permission of the Ophthalmic Publishing Company from Brown GC, Magargal L, Augsburger JJ, Shields JA. Preretinal arterial loops and retinal arterial occlusion. Am J Ophthalmol 1979; 87:646–651.)

tissue of Bergmeister's papilla overlying the optic nerve head. They then proceed back down onto the disc and on their course into the developing retina. Bergmeister's papilla subsequently regresses, leaving the vascular abnormality within Cloquet's canal.

The major complication associated with prepapillary arterial loops is retinal artery occlusion in the distribution of the area supplied by the loop (▶ Fig. 36.4).[4] Reported in approximately 10% of cases of prepapillary loops described in the literature, the occlusion has been hypothesized to occur secondary to turbulent flow, which predisposes to endothelial damage and thrombus formation. Vitreous hemorrhage and hyphema have also been noted.[3] It is likely that vitreous hemorrhage occurs in conjunction with the development of posterior vitreous detachment.

Pearls

- The major complication associated with prepapillary arterial loops is retinal artery occlusion, likely due to a clot in the loop. Rarely, vitreous hemorrhage and hyphema can also be seen.

Congenital prepapillary venous loops are usually single vessels that extend 0.5 mm or less into the vitreous cavity (▶ Fig. 36.5). Acquired prepapillary venous loops are often multiple (▶ Fig. 36.6), seen in adults, and found in conjunction with retinal venous occlusion or diseases associated with retinal venous occlusion, such as glaucoma, papilledema, or meningioma of the optic nerve or sphenoid wing.

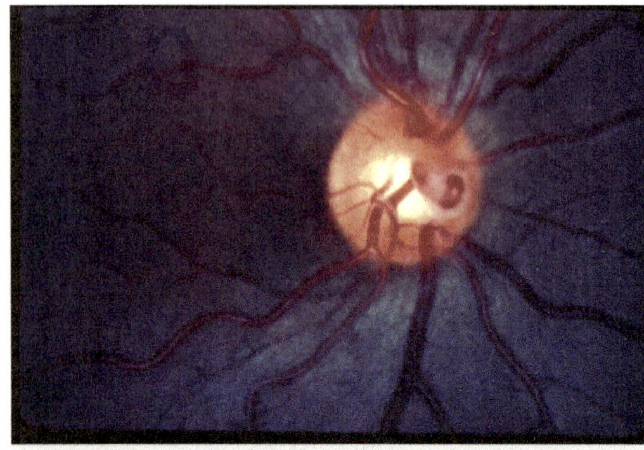

Fig. 36.5 Congenital prepapillary venous loop in the right eye. (Reproduced with permission from Brown and Tasman.[4])

36.1.2 Persistent Hyaloid Artery

A persistent hyaloid artery presents clinically as a single vessel that travels from the optic disc, through Cloquet's canal, and anteriorly to the posterior capsule of the lens.[4] The point of attachment to the posterior capsule, most often in a location inferonasal to the visual axis, is known as a *Mittendorf's dot* (▶ Fig. 36.7). Hyaloid artery remnants are seen in the eyes of premature infants in up to 95% of cases but are observed in only 3% of full-term infants.[6] The incidence in children and adults is less, but exact figures are lacking. Most commonly, a persistent hyaloid artery in a child is bloodless, but in rare instances it can contain blood and be associated with vitreous hemorrhage.[7] Ocular associations reported with persistent hyaloid artery include persistent hyperplastic primary vitreous (PHPV), coloboma of the optic disc, optic nerve hypoplasia, and posterior vitreous cysts.[4]

36.1.3 Persistent Bergmeister's Papilla

Although not a vascular abnormality in the strictest sense, Bergmeister's papilla develops around the posterior aspect of the fetal hyaloid artery. It has been described very elegantly by Mann.[8] Between the first and the second months of gestation, a group of neuroectodermal cells within the optic cup at the superior end of the embryonic fissure differentiate into a structure known as the *primitive epithelial papilla*. This primitive epithelial papilla becomes the optic nerve head when axons from retinal ganglion cells pass through it at 7 to 8 weeks of gestation. At the end of the fourth month of gestation, neuroectodermal glial cells on the surface of the optic disc multiply rapidly and form a sheath around the hyaloid artery that extends anteriorly for approximately one-third the length of the vessel (▶ Fig. 36.8). The sheath is maximally developed at about 5.5 months of gestation, following which atrophy occurs. The amount of regression determines, in part, the degree of physiologic cupping of the optic disc.

Incomplete regression of Bergmeister's papilla causes a persistent Bergmeister's papilla, also known as an *epipapillary veil*. Clinically, the entity appears as a tuft of glial tissue that is most

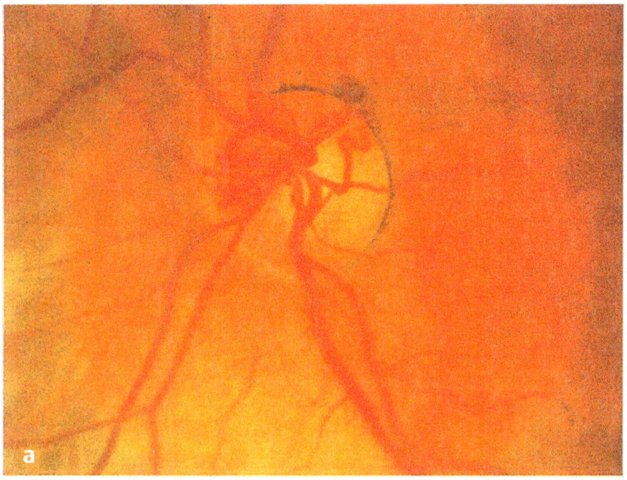

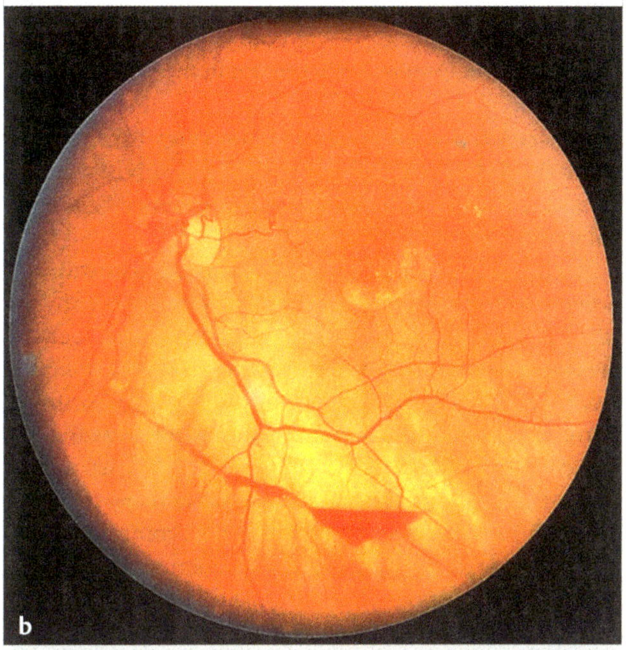

Fig. 36.6 (a) Multiple acquired prepapillary venous loops. (b) Larger field in same eye as in (a) discloses retinal vascular abnormalities in the superior macula, retinal pigment epithelial changes in the central macula, and preretinal blood resulting from a previous superotemporal retinal branch vein obstruction. (Reproduced with permission from Brown and Tasman.[4])

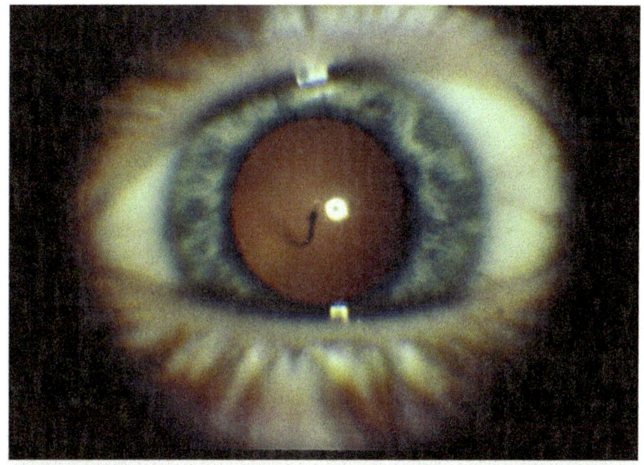

Fig. 36.7 Single loop of a persistent hyaloid artery extending anteriorly in the vitreous cavity to insert on the posterior capsule of the lens. The point of insertion is called a Mittendorf's dot.

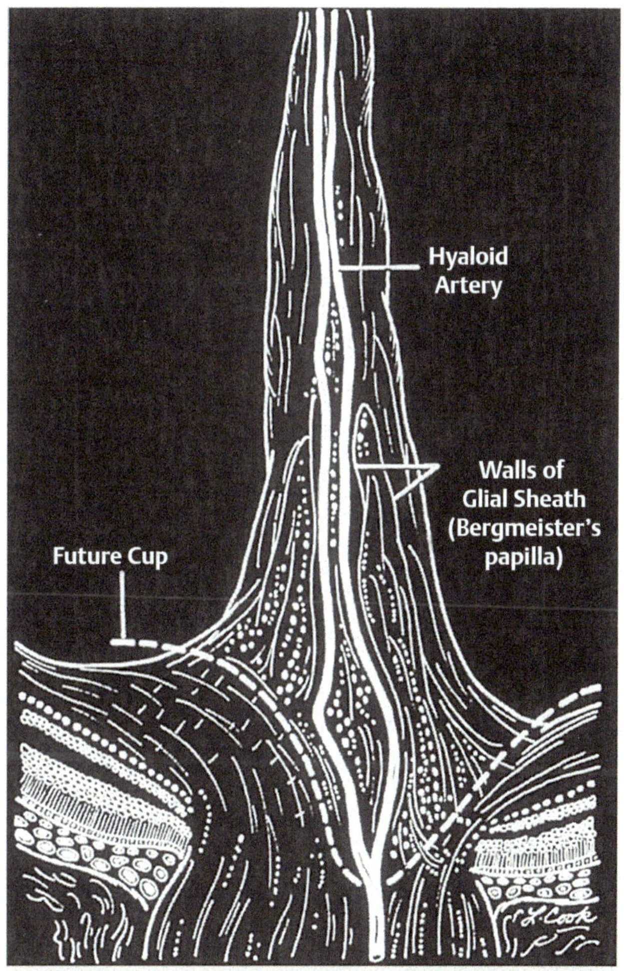

Fig. 36.8 Bergmeister's papilla at its maximum height during the fifth month of gestation. It extends approximately one-third of the way onto the vitreous cavity and usually regresses by birth. The degree of regression, in part, determines the amount of optic cupping. (Reproduced with permission from Brown and Tasman.[4])

commonly located on the nasal aspect of the nerve head (▶ Fig. 36.9). Absence of physiologic cupping can also be seen in affected eyes. The visual acuity is unaffected by the abnormality, and systemic associations are generally lacking.

36.1.4 Enlarged Vessels

Causes of enlarged vessels on the optic disc in children include arteriovenous malformations, retinal capillary hemangiomas (von Hippel's tumors), and retinoblastoma. Because the latter two conditions are most appropriately classified as tumors, they are not addressed in this section (see Chapter 27). Choroidal melanoma has also been associated with enlarged vessels on the optic disc,[9] but the tumor is rare in children.

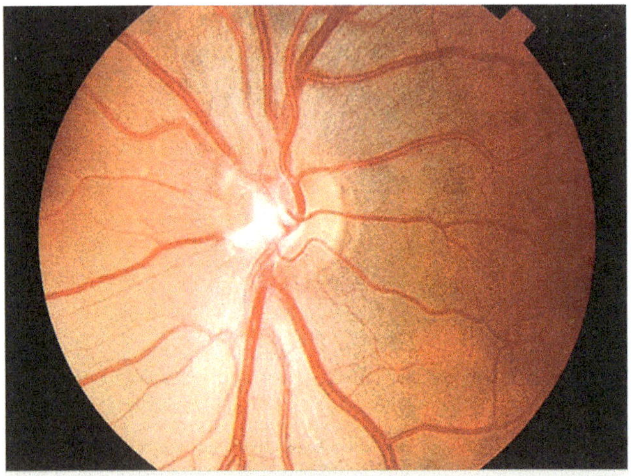

Fig. 36.9 White persistent Bergmeister's papilla in the nasal aspect of the optic disc in the left eye. Note that the optic disc has no cup. (Reproduced with permission from Brown and Tasman.[4])

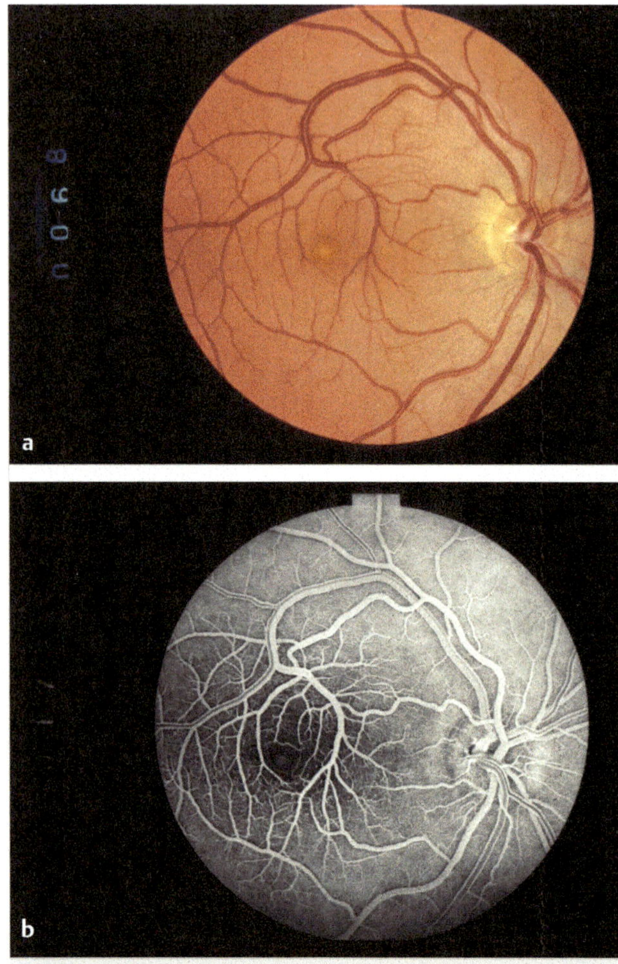

Fig. 36.10 (**a**) Congenital retinal macrovessel (grade I arteriovenous communication) in the right eye of a 31-year-old woman. The enlarged superotemporal vein drains retina both superior and inferior to the horizontal raphe. Visual acuity in the eye was 20/25 due to the presence of a central yellow macular cyst. Such cysts have been described in 28% of cases and tend to be transient. The cyst in this eye resolved a month later and the vision improved to 20/20. (**b**) Intravenous fluorescein angiogram corresponding to (a) at 17 seconds after injection. A round area of hyperfluorescence is present centrally corresponding to the macular cyst. Immediately superior to the hyperfluorescent cyst is a near-horizontal retinal vessel approximately 500 to 600 µm in length that is an arteriovenous communication between a retinal arteriole and retinal venule. Thus, a congenital retinal macrovessel is actually a grade I arteriovenous communication.

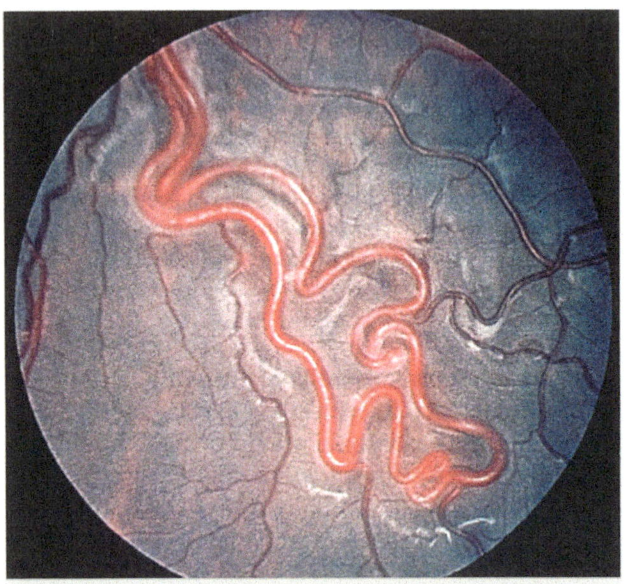

Fig. 36.11 Grade II arteriovenous communication in an 11-year-old boy. The visual acuity was 20/20 in the eye. (Reproduced with permission from Brown and Tasman.[4])

Arteriovenous malformations in the retina can be mild, moderate, or severe, and thus have been correspondingly classified by Archer et al[10] as grade I, II, and III abnormalities. They are predominantly unilateral. Grade I arteriovenous communications, the mildest variants, have also been noted as a subgroup of congenital macrovessels.[11] A congenital macrovessel is a single enlarged retinal vessel, usually a vein, that traverses both sides of the horizontal raphe (▶ Fig. 36.10). Most of these vessels are associated with arteriovenous communications, although some may be subtle. Cysts in the central fovea have been seen in association with congenital retinal macrovessels, but they may be transient and appear to affect the visual acuity only minimally.

Grades II and III arteriovenous communications have also been called *racemose angiomas* or *racemose hemangiomas*. The grade II variant is moderate and usually associated with normal vision (▶ Fig. 36.11), whereas in the grade III type the vision can be severely reduced due to replacement of optic nerve tissue by enlarged vessels (▶ Fig. 36.12).[12,13]

Both grades II and III arteriovenous communications can be associated with arteriovenous communications in the face, scalp, mandible, and central nervous system. The eponym *Wyburn-Mason's syndrome* has been applied to retinal arteriovenous communications associated with similar systemic abnormalities.[14] Rundles and Falls[15] found that among 34 cases of congenital retinal arteriovenous malformations reported through 1951,18 (53%) had associated central nervous system and/or dermatologic involvement.

Special Considerations

- Over 50% of congenital retinal arteriovenous malformations have the Wyburn-Mason's syndrome, retinal arteriovenous malformations in conjunction with malformations of the mandible, maxilla, cerebrum, brainstem, and/or spinal cord. Malformations in the cerebrum typically are deep and follow the optic tracts.

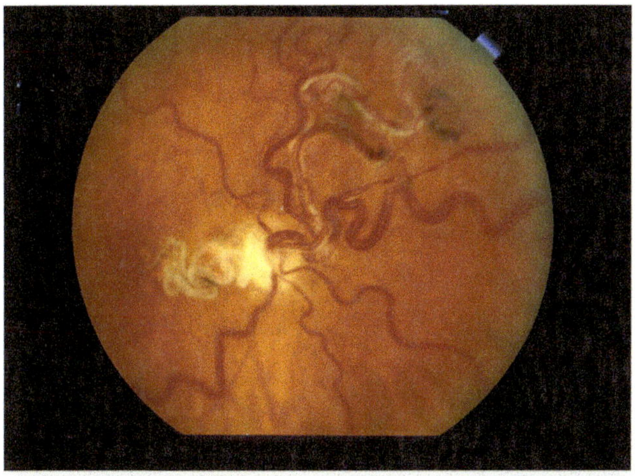

Fig. 36.12 Grade III arteriovenous communication. Visual acuity in the eye was no light perception, presumably due to replacement of the normal optic nerve tissue by the enlarged blood vessels. Note the retinal pigment epithelial hyperplasia surrounding the superonasal vessel. The vessels change shape over time. (Image courtesy of Dr. Jerry A. Shields.)

The lesions in the central nervous system are typically midline or unilateral on the same side as the ocular lesion, and tend to follow the optic tract. Because the optic tract is deep within the cerebrum, the arteriovenous anastomoses are rarely accessible surgically.

36.2 Colobomatous and Other Excavated Defects of the Optic Disc

36.2.1 Congenital Pit of the Optic Disc

Found in approximately 1 per 11,000 patients,[16] a congenital pit of the optic nerve head appears as a localized depression typically measuring from one to several diopters in depth. It can be yellow-white, gray, or black in color (▶ Fig. 36.13). The defect generally ranges in size from 0.25 to 0.40 disc diameters. More than 50% are located on the temporal side of the disc, and approximately one-third are located centrally (▶ Fig. 36.14).

Peripapillary retinal pigment epithelial disturbances are seen in 95% of eyes with optic pits that are not located centrally (▶ Fig. 36.13a,b).[17] In unilateral cases, the optic nerve head with the pit is larger than the normal fellow nerve head in 85% of patients. Most pits are single, but about 5% of affected eyes have more than one pit on the optic disc. Occasionally, the optic pits are located within the peripapillary region of the disc. Cilioretinal arteries are frequently associated with optic pits.

Approximately 40% of eyes with a congenital pit of the optic disc have an associated or previous serous retinal detachment of the sensory retina (▶ Fig. 36.15).[17,18,19] Retinal detachment is seen more commonly with larger, temporally located pits and usually involves the macula. Splitting of the retinal layers, or

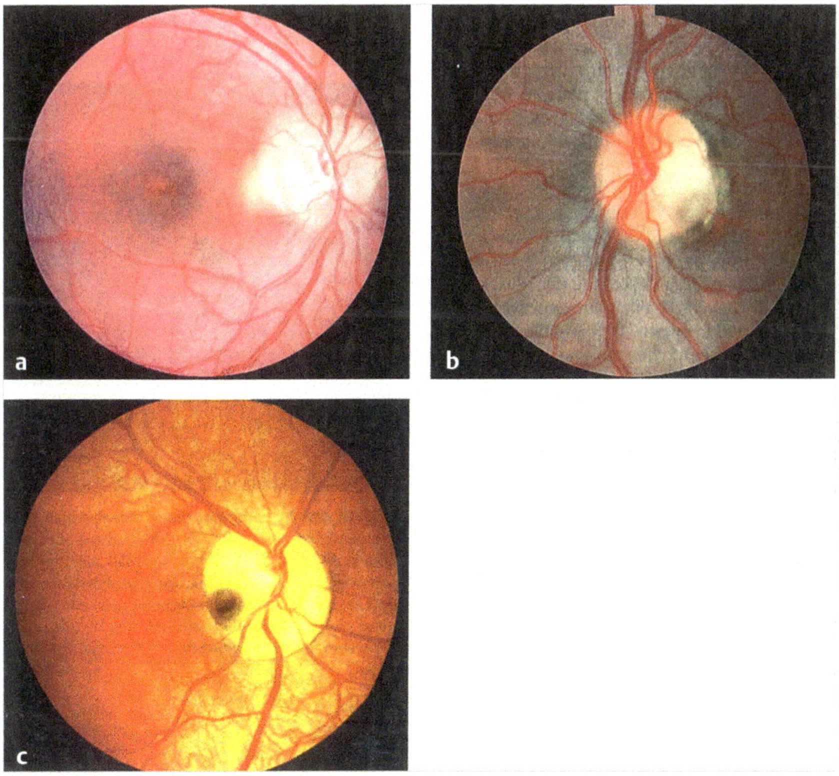

Fig. 36.13 (**a**) Yellow-white, (**b**) gray, and (**c**) black congenital pits of the optic nerve head. Peripapillary pigmentary changes in the vicinity of the optic pit are seen in (**a**) and (**b**).

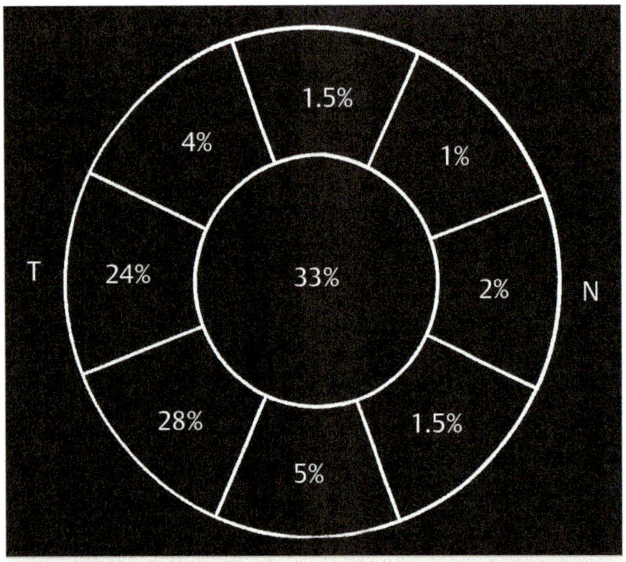

Fig. 36.14 Locations of congenital optic pits on the nerve head. N, nasal; T, temporal. (Reproduced with permission from Brown and Tasman.[4])

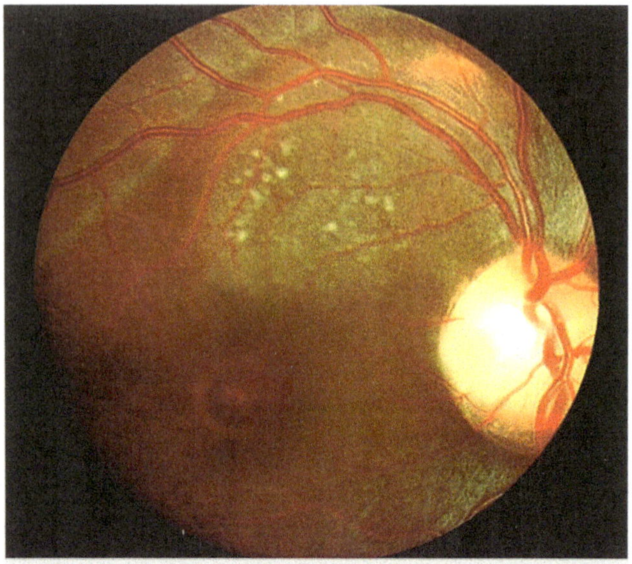

Fig. 36.15 Right eye of a patient with a temporal congenital optic pit and serous detachment of the sensory retina in the macular region. The vision was 20/800. An outer lamellar macular hole is present, with the internal limiting membrane remaining intact over it. Subretinal precipitates (probably deposits of retinal pigment epithelial cells imbibed by macrophages) are present on the outer surface of the superior retinal detachment. These precipitates resolve when the retinal detachment resolves.

macular retinoschisis, has also been described in eyes with congenital optic pits and retinal detachment.[20] Centrally located pits have not been associated with retinal detachment and/or retinoschisis. The subretinal fluid rarely extends beyond the posterior pole and, in most cases, can be seen extending to the optic disc in the vicinity of the optic pit. Cystic changes within the detached retina are found in two-thirds of cases, and a macular hole develops in about 25%. In contrast to most lamellar macular holes, in which absence of the inner retinal layers is observed, the macular holes noted in conjunction with optic pits tend to involve the outer retina, giving the appearance that the internal limiting membrane is intact.

The age of onset of the retinal detachment is variable, with a mean age of approximately 30 years.[17] We have observed retinal detachment developing in children as young as 6 years, as well as in patients in their 80 s.

Pearls

- Approximately 40% of eyes with a congenital pit of the optic nerve head have, or will have, an associated serous retinal detachment/retinoschisis.

Uncertainty exists as to the origin of the subretinal fluid seen in conjunction with congenital optic pits. Approximately 20% of collie dogs have either a congenital pit of the optic disc or optic nerve coloboma, and histopathologic evidence in the collie dog model suggests the subretinal fluid originates from the vitreous cavity.[18] Other possible origins of the subretinal fluid or retinoschisis fluid include cerebrospinal fluid from the subarachnoid space, leakage from choroidal vessels, and leakage from small vessels located at the base of the optic pit (▶ Fig. 36.16).[17]

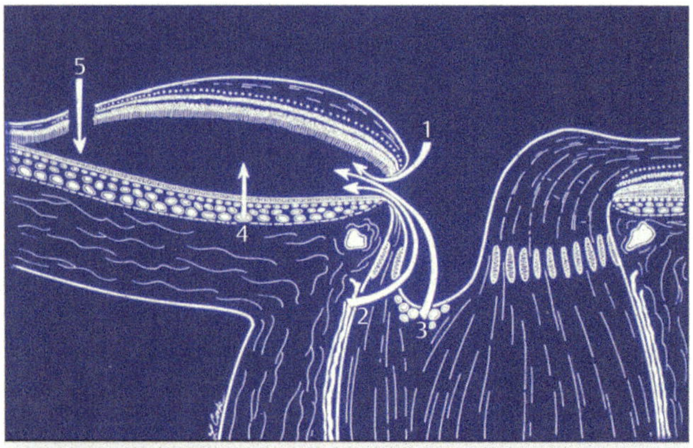

Fig. 36.16 Possible sources of the subretinal and intraretinal fluid associated with congenital optic pits. 1, from the vitreous cavity; 2, from the subarachnoid space; 3, from blood vessels located at the base of the pit; 4, from choroidal blood vessels; and 5, through a macular hole in instances in which such a hole is present. Histopathology of congenital optic pits with serous retinal detachment in collie dogs suggests the subretinal fluid comes from the vitreous cavity. (Reproduced with permission from Brown and Tasman.[4])

Evidence suggests that in the majority of instances, the presence of an associated retinal detachment in the posterior pole is visually disabling. Although the amount of subretinal fluid can wax and wane spontaneously, a Wills Eye Hospital report noted that, among 20 such untreated eyes followed for at least 1 year, the visual acuity was 20/100 or worse in 55%.[19] When the vision is decreased due to serous macular retinal detachment and/or retinoschisis, laser photocoagulation in the peripapillary region has been advocated to induce reattachment of the retina to the underlying retinal pigment epithelium and subsequent resorption of the subretinal fluid (▶ Fig. 36.17). The laser should

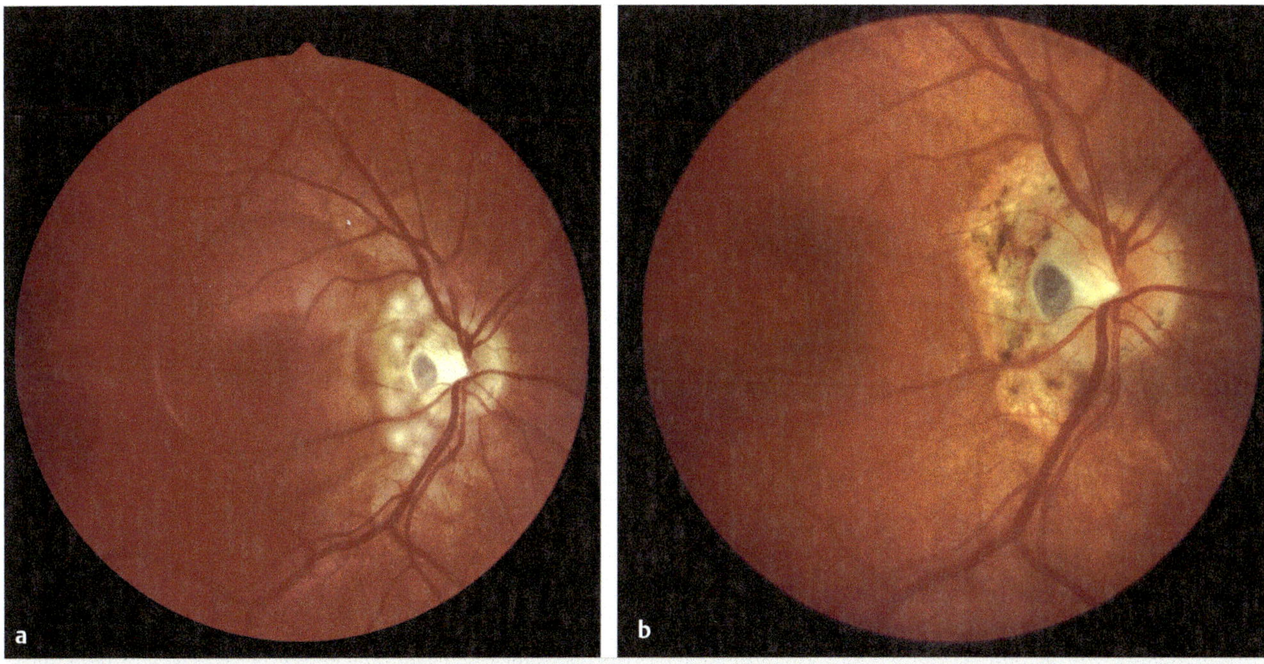

Fig. 36.17 (a) Peripapillary laser photocoagulation with 200-µm spot-size burns in the right eye of a 15-year-old girl with a congenital optic pit and serous retinal detachment. (b) Six weeks after laser photocoagulation. The subretinal fluid resolved and the vision improved from 20/200 before therapy to 20/25 at this time.

not involve the nerve fiber layer of the retina, but should extend into flattened retina both superiorly and inferiorly to the subretinal fluid/retinoschisis extending from the disc. This allows the retina to tack down to the retinal pigment epithelium from the edges. Laser therapy applied to an area greater than 120 degrees should be performed with caution and is compatible with 20/20 vision. Nonetheless, temporal peripapillary laser photocoagulation of 180 degrees or greater has been shown to cause counting fingers vision, likely due to loss of nerve fibers to the central fovea and/or damage to the ciliary vascular supply to the prelaminar optic nerve head (personal communication, Dr. Michael Klein, MD). Laser photocoagulation is successful in reattaching the retina in about 50% of cases, although it may have to be repeated at 2 to 4 months. The subretinal fluid may be present for a prolonged period of time without severely damaging the photoreceptors. We have noted vision to improve to 20/25 when a serous retinal detachment resolves at 9 months after the development of subretinal fluid. Rarely, subretinal choroidal neovascularization can develop at the edge of the laser photocoagulation.

With cases of severe vision loss that do not respond to laser photocoagulation, the possibility of repeat peripapillary laser photocoagulation in conjunction with either an injection of long-acting gas into the vitreous cavity or a pars plana vitrectomy and a gas/fluid exchange can be considered.[21,22] Overall, approximately 80% of eyes with a serous retinal detachment that does not resolve with laser therapy alone demonstrate resolution of the retinal detachment after laser therapy in conjunction with gas tamponade. Thus, approximately 90% of all serous retinal detachments associated with congenital optic pits can be flattened with interventions.

Pearls

- Peripapillary laser photocoagulation causes resolution of subretinal fluid in 50% of eyes with a congenital pit of the optic disc and an associated serous retinal detachment.

Fluorescein angiography typically reveals hypofluorescence of the pit, with progression to late hyperfluorescence. Associated visual field defects, excluding the larger blind spot present in 85% of cases with a larger optic disc in the eye with the pit, as well as serous retinal detachments, are present in approximately 62% of eyes.[19] These often mimic the field defects found with glaucoma. Included among the field defects are arcuate scotomas (▶ Fig. 36.18), altitudinal defects, paracentral scotomas, generalized and localized peripheral scotomas, sector defects extending from the disc, and nasal or temporal steps.

In general, systemic abnormalities have not been linked with congenital optic pits. Nevertheless, the association of a basal encephalocele with agenesis of the corpus callosum has been reported.[23] A hereditary pattern is not typically present, although an autosomal dominant inheritance pattern has been noted.[24] The defect is believed to arise, in most cases, from abnormal differentiation of the primitive epithelial papilla.[25]

36.2.2 Optic Nerve Coloboma

Occurring in approximately 1 per 12,000 patients,[19] an optic nerve coloboma has several identifying features (▶ Fig. 36.19 and ▶ Fig. 36.20). Included among these are (1) partial or total excavation of the optic disc, (2) enlargement of the peripapillary region and the posterior scleral foramen, (3) a glistening

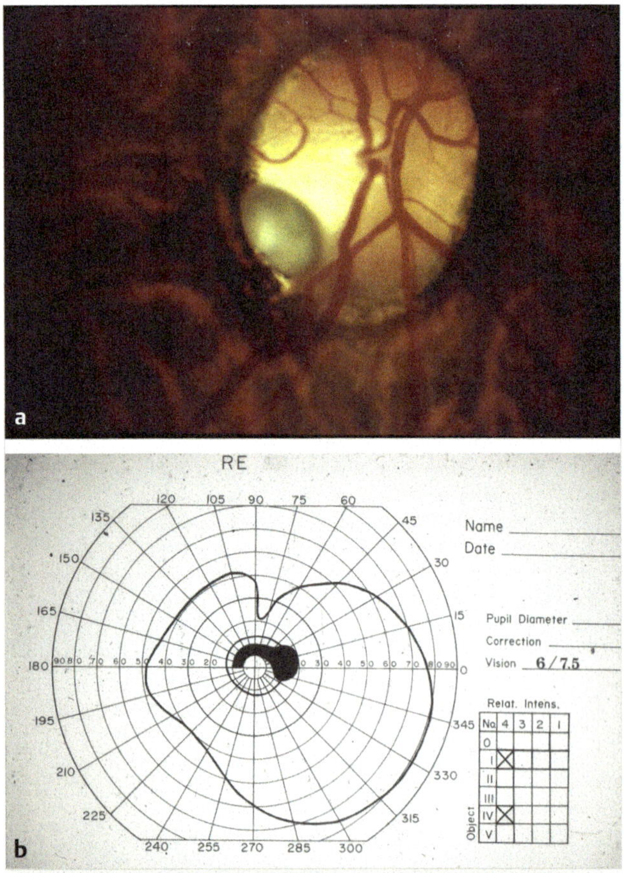

Fig. 36.18 (a) Inferotemporal congenital pit of the optic nerve head. (b) Visual field of the eye in (a) reveals a superior arcuate defect corresponding to the inferotemporal optic pit.

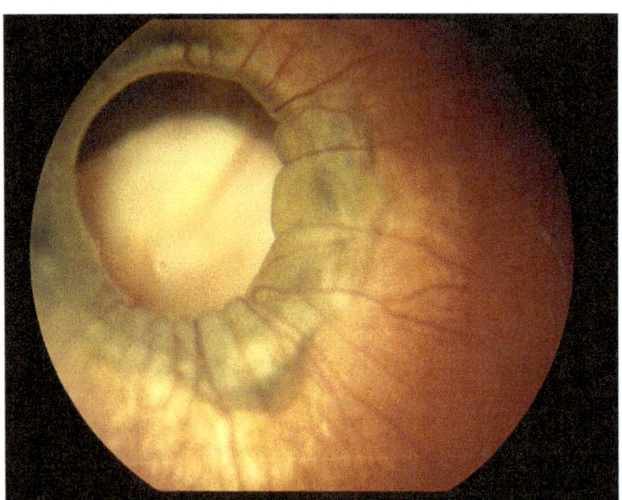

Fig. 36.20 Optic nerve coloboma with retinal vessels entering and exiting at the optic disc margins.

white surface, and (4) retinal blood vessels entering and exiting from the border of the defect. Depths are variable and may range up to 50 diopters (~17 mm).[26] Approximately 20% of collie dogs also have optic nerve colobomas or congenital pits of the optic nerve head, both of which look very similar to the respective defects in humans (▸ Fig. 36.21).

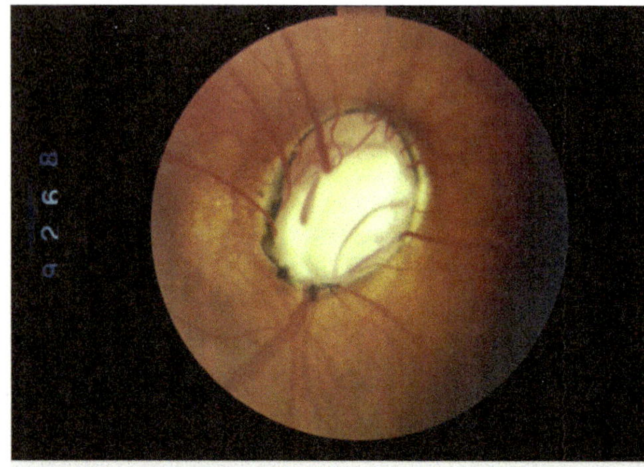

Fig. 36.19 Coloboma of the optic disc involving primarily the inferior optic disc. The retinal blood vessels enter and exit at the disc margins.

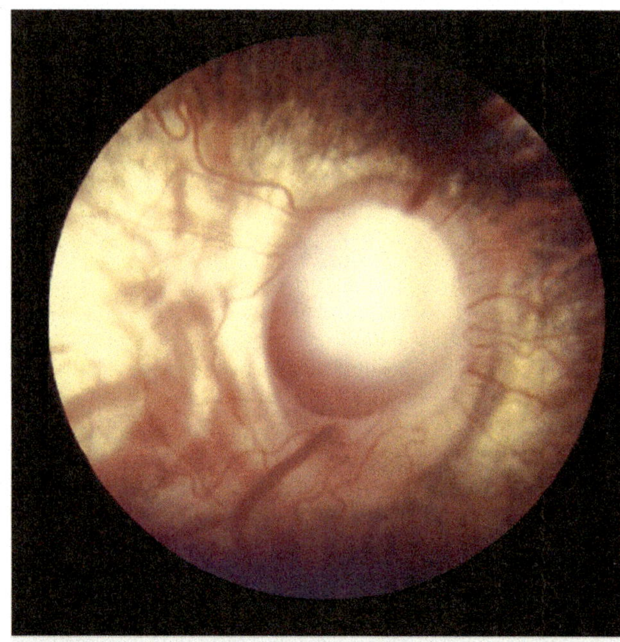

Fig. 36.21 Optic nerve coloboma in a collie dog. The appearance is similar to that of a human optic nerve coloboma.

The abnormality can be unilateral or bilateral. Visual acuity is variable and has been noted to range from normal to no light percepotion.[27] Concomitant retinochoroidal and/or iris colobomatous defects may also be present (▸ Fig. 36.22). An optic nerve coloboma is believed to occur secondary to incomplete closure of the embryonic fissure.[27] The embryonic fissure typically closes by approximately 5 to 6 weeks of gestation and begins to fuse centrally (▸ Fig. 36.23). Because of the initial central fusion, iris and posterior pole colobomas can be seen in conjunction with a normal midperipheral fundus.

Nonrhegmatogenous retinal detachment can be seen with optic nerve colobomas.[27] The detachment occurs most often in the second or third decade of life and typically extends outward from the optic disc.[24] Peripapillary laser photocoagulation in

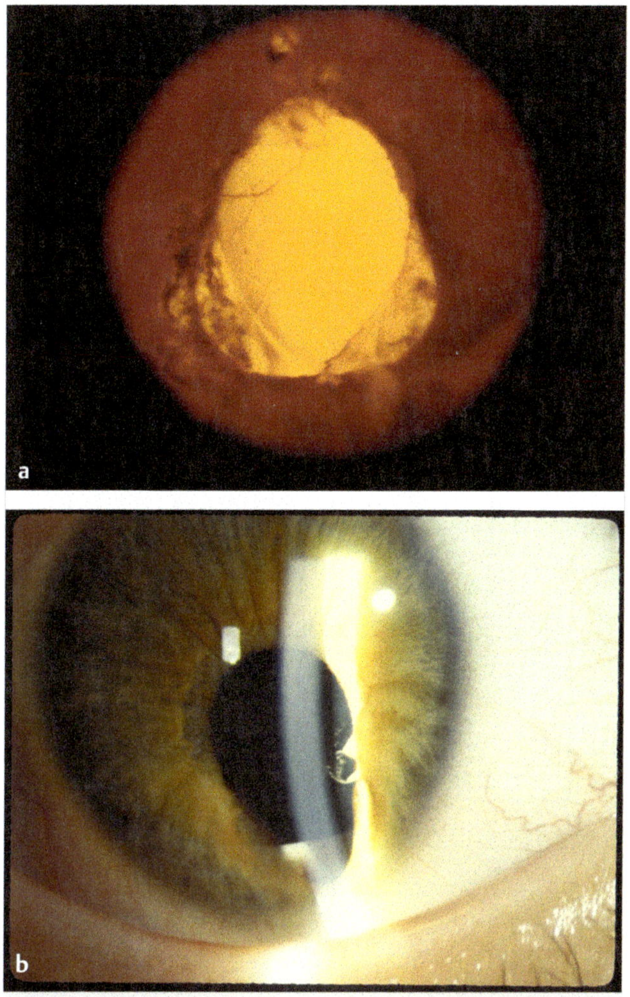

Fig. 36.22 (a) Equator-plus photograph demonstrating a retinochoroidal coloboma extending from the optic nerve head inferiorly. The optic nerve head is located within the superior coloboma. The peripheral inferior fundus is normal where the embryonic fissure partially closed. An iris coloboma was present anteriorly. This eye had a retinal detachment occurring secondary to a break in the intercalary membrane. During vitrectomy, laser photocoagulation was applied around the entire coloboma, treating the whole lesion as if it was the retinal break. The foveal region was not treated with laser photocoagulation. Laser spots are especially pronounced to the left of the coloboma. (b) Iris coloboma associated with the retinochoroidal coloboma shown in ▶ Fig. 36.24a.

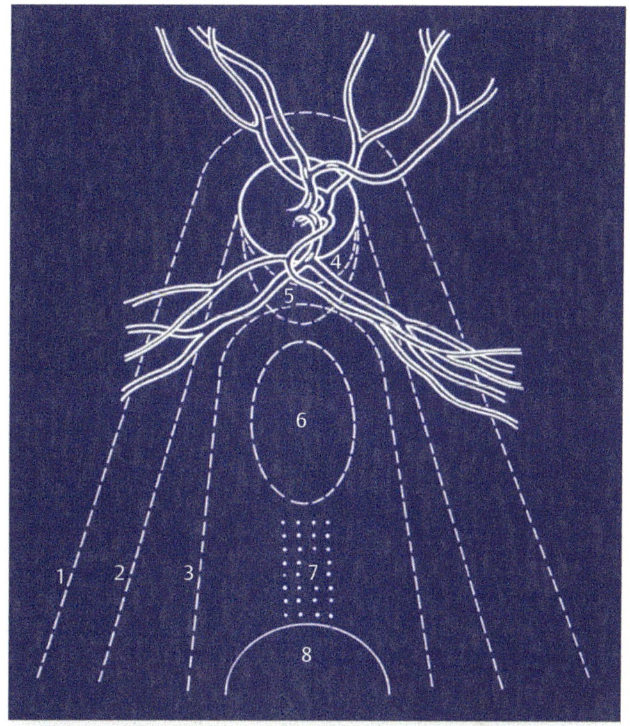

Fig. 36.23 Colobomas can affect the fundus along the line of closure of the embryonic fissure, as shown by the numbers. The fissure extends as far anteriorly as the pupillary frill of the iris and as far posteriorly as the optic nerve. Initial closure of the embryonic fissure, the whole of which is closed by 5 to 6 weeks of gestation, begins in the midperiphery (7 in the diagram) and extends anteriorly and posteriorly. (Reproduced with permission from Brown and Tasman.[4])

association with pars plana vitrectomy and gas/fluid exchange has been used successfully in our institution to flatten the retina (▶ Fig. 36.24).[21] The source of the subretinal fluid is uncertain, but most likely it is derived from the vitreous cavity or from cerebrospinal fluid via a connection between the coloboma and the subarachnoid space.

When there is an associated retinochoroidal coloboma, rhegmatogenous retinal detachments can also be encountered. These detachments typically result from one or more breaks in the intercalary membrane, the thin glial sheet over the retinochoroidal coloboma that is continuous with the sensory retina. Because there is no underlying pigmented retinal pigment epithelium to provide contrast, the breaks are often difficult to visualize. Breaks in the intercalary membrane may become visible during vitrectomy as the schlieren phenomenon can be seen when subretinal fluid is removed through an intercalary membrane break. Typically, treatment of such retinal detachments requires vitrectomy with internal drainage of subretinal fluid and a gas/fluid exchange. Laser photocoagulation is then applied along the entire border of the coloboma to isolate the colobomatous defect and associated intercalary break(s) from the surrounding retina. In essence, the entire coloboma is treated as the retinal break (▶ Fig. 36.22). An adequate laser-induced chorioretinal scar cannot be achieved directly around breaks in the intercalary membrane because of absence of a retinal pigment epithelium in this region.

Choroidal neovascularization can be seen at the edge of a retinochoroidal coloboma (▶ Fig. 36.25). Treatment can be initiated with intravitreal vascular endothelial growth factor inhibitors or laser photocoagulation, depending upon the location of the choroidal neovascularization and the discretion of the surgeon.

Numerous systemic abnormalities have been reported in conjunction with colobomatous defects in the eye.[19] Included among these are diseases of the cardiovascular, central nervous, dermatologic, gastrointestinal, genitourinary, nasopharyngeal, and musculoskeletal systems. Centrally located defects include basal encephalocele, cardiac wall defects, palatoschisis, and gastroschisis.[4] Of particular note is the CHARGE syndrome (coloboma, heart disease, atresia choanae, retarded growth, genital hypoplasia, ear anomalies and/or deafness).[28] Infants and young

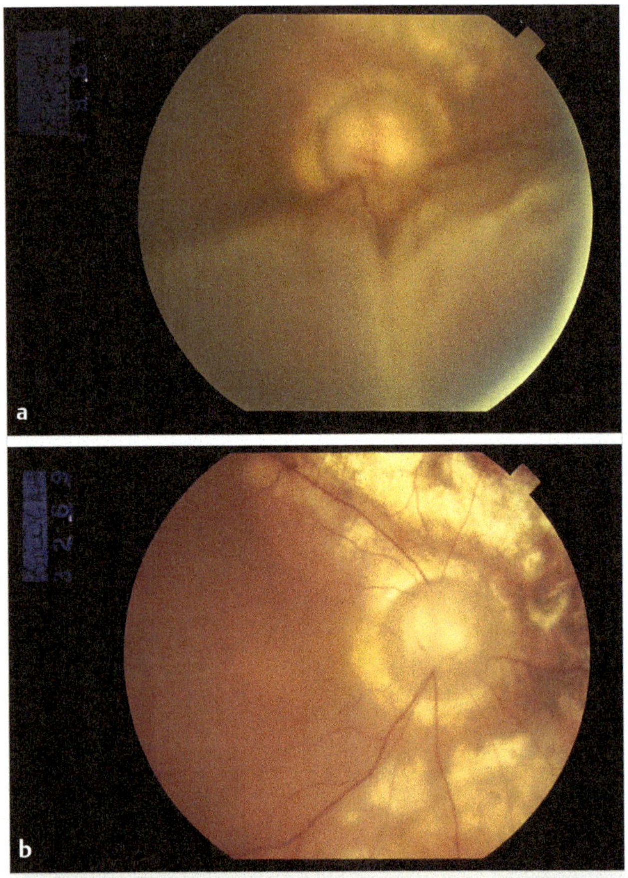

Fig. 36.24 (**a**) Optic nerve coloboma associated with a bullous inferior retinal detachment. (**b**) The retina was flattened after vitrectomy with peripapillary laser photocoagulation.

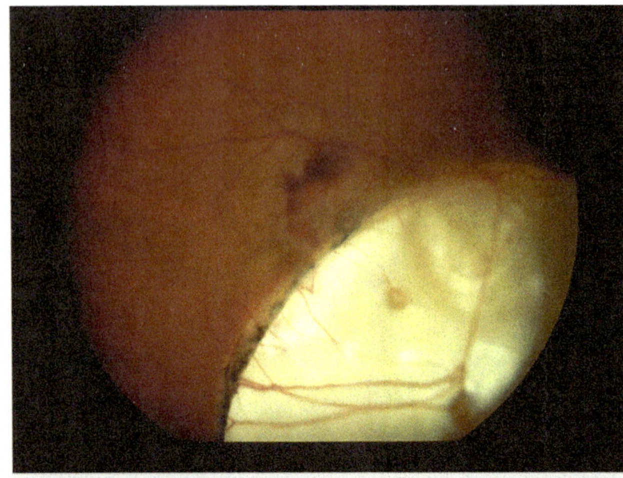

Fig. 36.25 Retinochoroidal coloboma associated with a choroidal neovascular membrane with blood at its border.

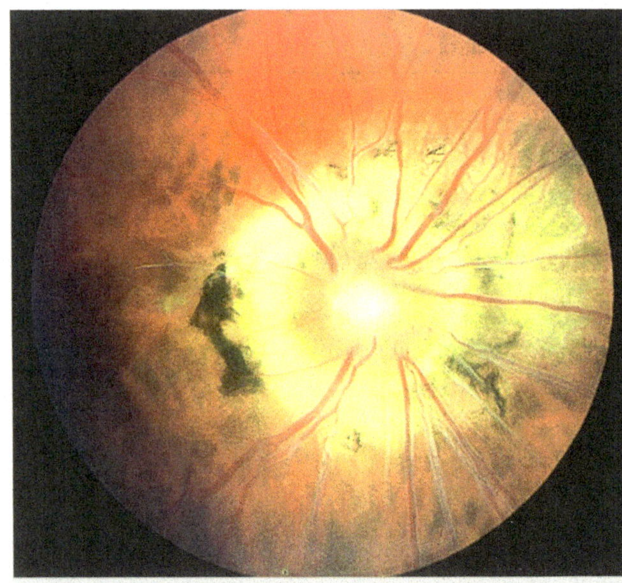

Fig. 36.26 Morning glory optic disc anomaly. The enlarged optic disc is excavated centrally and has a central tuft of fibroglial tissue, a peripapillary annulus of subretinal fibrovascular tissue, and straightened and sheathed retinal arteries.

children with colobomatous defects should undergo a general physical examination to rule out the possibility of coexistent systemic abnormalities.[4]

36.2.3 Morning Glory Disc Anomaly

In 1970, Kindler[29] reported the cases of 10 patients with a unilateral congenital optic nerve head anomaly that resembled the morning glory flower. Among the clinical features of the morning glory optic disc are (1) enlargement and excavation of the optic nerve head, (2) a central core of white fibroglial tissue, (3) a peripapillary annulus of variably pigmented subretinal tissue, and (4) retinal vessels that enter and exit from the borders of the defect. The retinal vessels, especially the arteries, are frequently straightened and sheathed (▶ Fig. 36.26). The entity has been seen in eyes with PHPV and Moyamoya disease.[30]

In approximately 30% of eyes, a nonrhegmatogenous retinal detachment develops.[29,31] It can involve only the posterior pole or extend to the fundus periphery. As is the case with optic nerve coloboma, the origin of the subretinal fluid is uncertain. Peripapillary laser photocoagulation in conjunction with vitrectomy and gas/fluid exchange can be of benefit in flattening the detached retina.[21] Nevertheless, in some instances it is very difficult to flatten the retina. As is the case with surgical repair of the retinal detachments associated with congenital pits of the optic nerve head and with optic nerve colobomas, the use of intravitreal silicone oil is controversial as it is not possible to be certain that there is no connection between the nerve head defect and the subarachnoid space.

The visual acuity in eyes with the morning glory disc anomaly and no retinal detachment can range from near-normal to hand motions.[19] Strabismus may be associated. In unilateral cases, the possibility of concomitant strabismic amblyopia should be considered, especially as the visual loss in affected eyes with bilateral cases does not seem to be as severe as the vision loss in unilaterally affected eyes.[32]

Basal encephalocele has been noted in conjunction with the morning glory disc anomaly.[33] Other congenital optic disc abnormalities that have been reported with basal encephalocele (▶ Fig. 36.27) include congenital optic pit, optic nerve coloboma, and megalopapilla.[19]

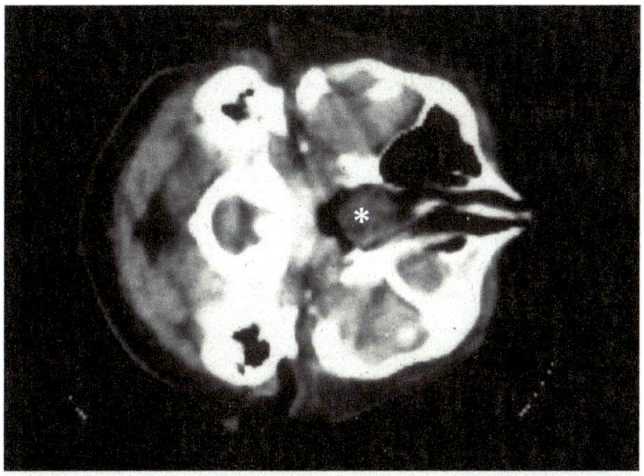

Fig. 36.27 Computed tomography scan of the base of the skull reveals a basal encephalocele with neural tissue (white star) extending inferiorly where the skull base is absent. The patient had a coloboma of the optic nerve.

Pearls

- Amblyopic therapy should be considered in unilateral cases of the morning glory disc anomaly associated with decreased vision.

36.2.4 Peripapillary Staphyloma

A rare congenital anomaly, the peripapillary staphyloma is an excavated defect caused by outpouching of the sclera surrounding the optic disc (▶ Fig. 36.28). The optic nerve head within the staphyloma typically appears normal. Atrophic changes in the choroid and retinal pigment epithelium are usually seen within the walls of the defect. Although the depth of the optic disc ranges from 1 to 20 diopters,[19] the macula may be emmetropic. The visual acuity may be normal in mild cases, but severe visual loss is generally seen with more pronounced defects.[19] Smooth muscle in the walls of larger staphylomas has been reported to cause spontaneous contractions.[34] Neither light nor accommodation appears to affect the contractions.

Pearls

- The optic nerve head associated with posterior staphyloma is frequently normal in appearance at the base of the staphyloma.

36.2.5 Tilted Disc Syndrome

The tilted disc syndrome has a number of alternative names, including *nasal fundus ectasia syndrome*, *Fuchs' coloboma*, *inverse myopia*, *inversion of the optic disc*, and *dysversion of the optic disc*. The entity may actually be a variant of a colobomatous defect.

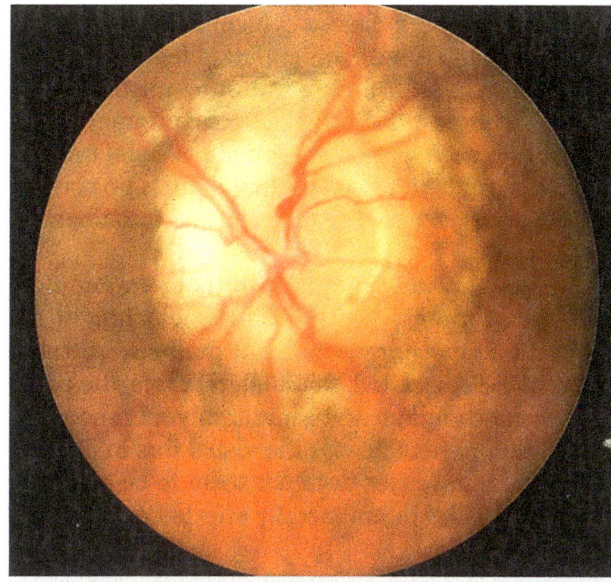

Fig. 36.28 Normal-appearing optic disc recessed at the base of a peripapillary staphyloma, a localized ectasia of the sclera, choroid, and retina surrounding the optic nerve.

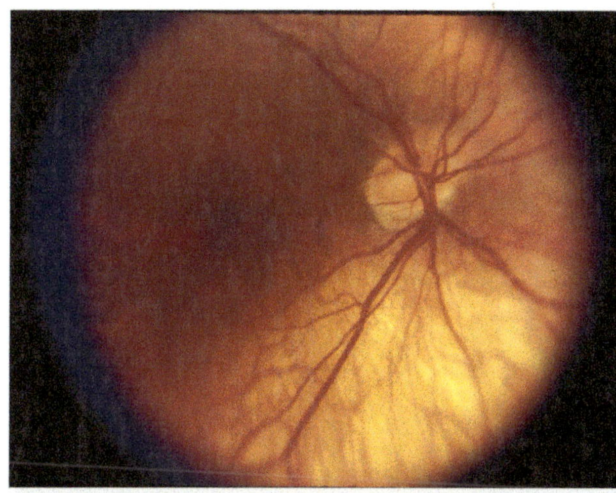

Fig. 36.29 Tilted disc syndrome. The optic nerve head is tilted inferiorly, there is slight haziness of the mildly elevated, superior disc margin, a classic Fuchs' coloboma is present inferiorly, and the inferior fundus is lightened when there is mild ectasia. There is mild situs inversus, signified by the inferotemporal vein traveling more nasally than usual before it heads temporally. This condition is often associated with vision of 20/25 to 20/50, although patients do not complain of vision loss since their vision has always been at this level.

Present in approximately 1 to 2% of the population, the tilted disc syndrome (▶ Fig. 36.29) has the clinical features listed in Table 36.1.[35,36] In the region of the inferior Fuchs' coloboma, both the retinal pigment epithelium and choroid are absent (▶ Fig. 36.30). The superior margin of the optic disc is often elevated due to the tilting effect, at times mimicking the appearance of papilledema. Bilaterality is seen in 75% of cases, and most eyes with the inferior lightened and ectatic fundus have associated superotemporal field defects (▶ Fig. 36.31). The field defects typically correspond to the inferior ectatic fundus and

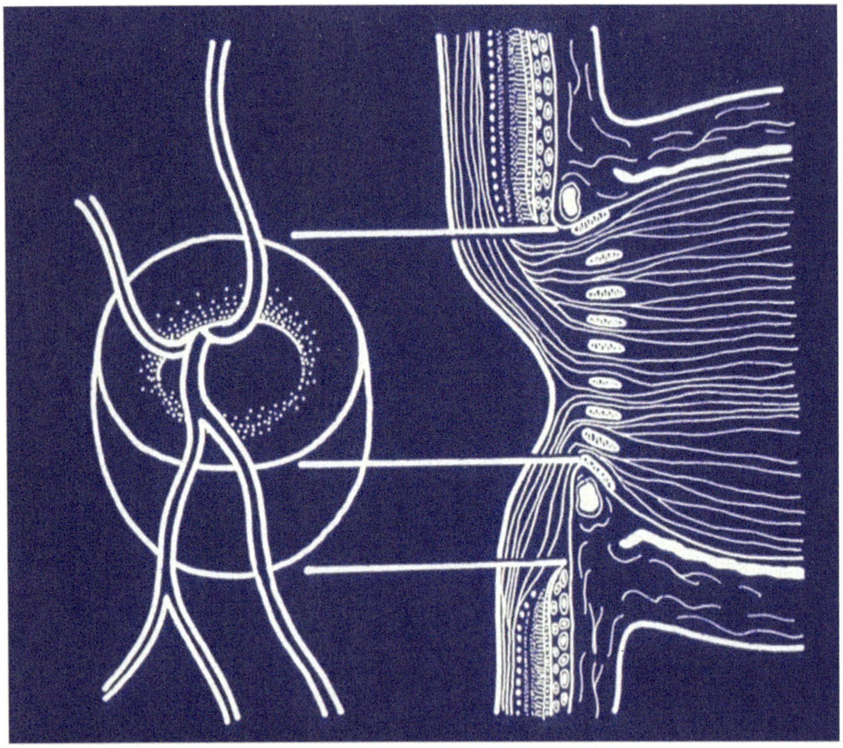

Fig. 36.30 Tilted disc syndrome. The retinal pigment epithelium and choroid are absent in the region of the inferior Fuchs' coloboma. The superior optic disc is slightly elevated.

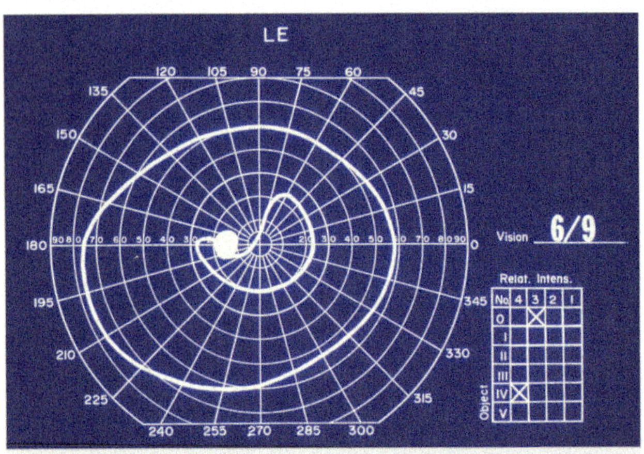

Fig. 36.31 Visual field from an eye with the tilted disc syndrome. The superotemporal field defect on the inner isopter crosses the midline, unlike the field defect with a pituitary tumor which typically respects the midline. The field defect corresponds to the lightened, ectatic inferior fundus.

can be absolute or relative. Minus lenses may eliminate the visual field defects in those cases in which they are relative.

Not all of the features are necessary to make the diagnosis (▶ Table 36.1). For example, inferonasal tilting of the optic disc is present in only 65% of cases (▶ Fig. 36.32). Bilateral optic disc elevation, decreased vision, and the superotemporal visual field defects in people with the tilted disc syndrome have led to the misdiagnosis of a pituitary tumor prior to the era of computed tomography scan and magnetic resonance imaging. Unlike the visual field abnormalities associated with perichiasmal lesions, which respect the vertical midline, those seen with the tilted disc syndrome often cross the vertical midline (▶ Fig. 36.31).[35,36]

Table 36.1 Tilted disc syndrome

Feature	Percentage of cases
Inferonasal disc tilting	65%
Inferonasal or inferior crescent	88%
Situs inversus of the retinal vessels	80%
Myopia (> 1 diopter)	85–90%
Astigmatism (> 1 diopter)	71%
Hypopigmented, inferior fundus ectasia	72–90%

In 75% of eyes with the tilted disc syndrome, the visual acuity is reduced to the 20/25 to 20/50 range. Despite the decreased acuities, these patients do not generally complain of vision loss as their vision has been at this level for their lifetimes. Thus, if a person with the tilted disc syndrome does complain of vision loss, or has vision less than 20/50, it should not be attributed to this entity. It is uncertain why the vision is decreased, but the possibility that obliquely oriented macular cones account for the loss has been proposed.[35] The Stiles–Crawford effect demonstrates that cones receiving light head-on, rather than at an angle, are the most sensitive. Choroidal neovascularization can occasionally be seen in association with the tilted disc syndrome (▶ Fig. 36.33).

Pearls

- The tilted disc syndrome is associated with vision in the 20/25 to 20/50 range in 75% of eyes.

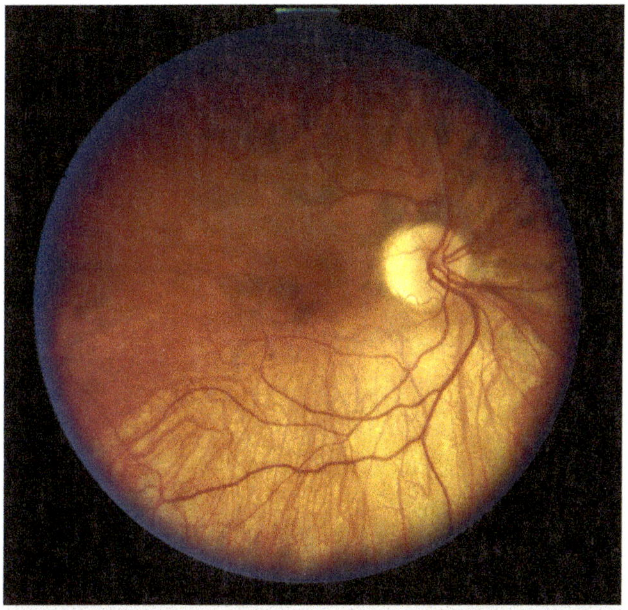

Fig. 36.32 Tilted disc syndrome. Prominent situs inversus of the retinal vessels is present and the inferior fundus is lightened and ectatic. There is temporal disc tilting in this myopic eye. Despite the absence of inferonasal tilting and a Fuchs' coloboma, this eye demonstrates a variant of the tilted disc syndrome.

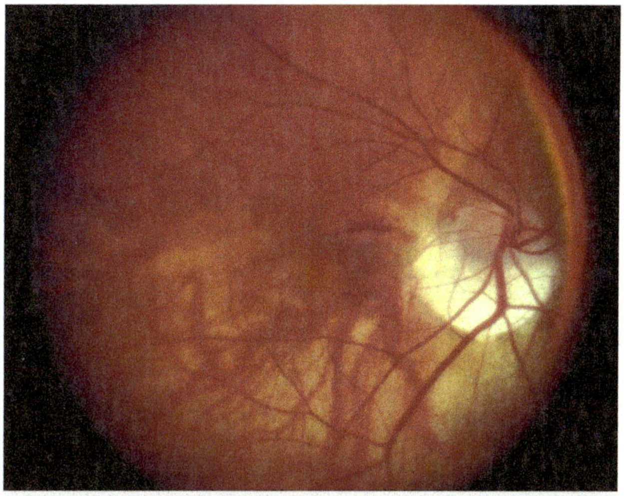

Fig. 36.33 The tilted disc syndrome with inferior tilting of the optic disc, a hazy superonasal disc border, situs inversus, a Fuchs' coloboma, and a lightened, ectatic inferior fundus. Subretinal blood occurring secondary to choroidal neovascularization is present at the juncture of the normal fundus with the ectatic inferior fundus.

36.3 Size Abnormalities of the Optic Disc

36.3.1 Optic Nerve Hypoplasia

Optic nerve hypoplasia can vary from almost imperceptible hypoplasia to severe involvement of the optic disc.[37,38,39,40] The typical funduscopic appearance is that of a small disc in which the retinal blood vessels enter and exit centrally (▶ Fig. 36.34), rather than in the more nasal location on the normal optic disc. The vessels are normal in caliber but may seem enlarged due to the small size of the disc.

Pearls

- Retinal blood vessels typically enter and exit centrally on the optic disc in cases of optic nerve hypoplasia.

A "double-ring sign" is typically present (▶ Fig. 36.34). The outer ring has been shown histopathologically to correlate with the juncture of the normal sclera and lamina cribrosa, the latter the specialized sclera within the posterior scleral foramen through which approximately 1,000 optic nerve fascicles pass. Each fascicle has approximately 1,250 retinal ganglion cell axons that terminate in the lateral geniculate nucleus. The inner ring is formed by the border of the remaining optic nerve tissue with the sensory retina and retinal pigment epithelium that extend abnormally posteriorly over the surface of the optic disc.

Optic nerve hypoplasia is believed to occur secondary to failure of development of the ganglion cell layer of the retina,[37,38] although retrograde degeneration associated with congenital lesions of the cerebral hemispheres has also been reported.[39] An autosomal dominant hereditary pattern has been rarely noted.[40] Pharmacologic insults that have been associated prenatally in mothers of children with optic nerve hypoplasia include the use of phenytoin,[41] quinine,[42] lysergic acid diethylamide, diuretics, and corticosteroids.[43] The entity has been noted in conjunction with congenital cytomegalovirus, as well as maternal syphilis and rubella.[43,44] Diabetes mellitus in the mother has also been associated in a number of cases.[43,45]

Unilateral and bilateral cases appear to occur with almost equal frequency. The visual acuity is variable and can range from normal to no light perception. Visual field abnormalities can be seen, including altitudinal defects, localized and generalized constriction, centrocecal scotomas, bitemporal hemianopsias, and binasal hemaniopsias.[19] Concomitant nystagmus and strabismus may be present, particularly in more severe cases. As with the morning glory disc anomaly, patients with unilateral optic nerve hypoplasia and milder vision loss may also respond to amblyopia therapy.

Optic nerve hypoplasia, both unilateral and bilateral, has been associated with a number of systemic abnormalities. Approximately 13% of affected patients have pituitary dysfunction associated with hypothalamic abnormalities, including anterior pituitary defects with growth hormone insufficiency, posterior pituitary dysfunction with diabetes insipidus, and panhypopituitarism.[46] Partial or complete absence of the septum pellucidum has been seen in 27% of patients with optic nerve hypoplasia.[46] Agenesis of the septum pellucidum in association with optic nerve hypoplasia is known as de Morsier's syndrome.[47] Hypoglycemia, neonatal seizures, cerebral dysgenesis, and cerebral palsy have been noted in conjunction with de Morsier's syndrome.[46]

Pearls

- Approximately 13% of patients with optic nerve hypoplasia have endocrine abnormalities associated with dysfunction of the hypothalamic–pituitary axis.

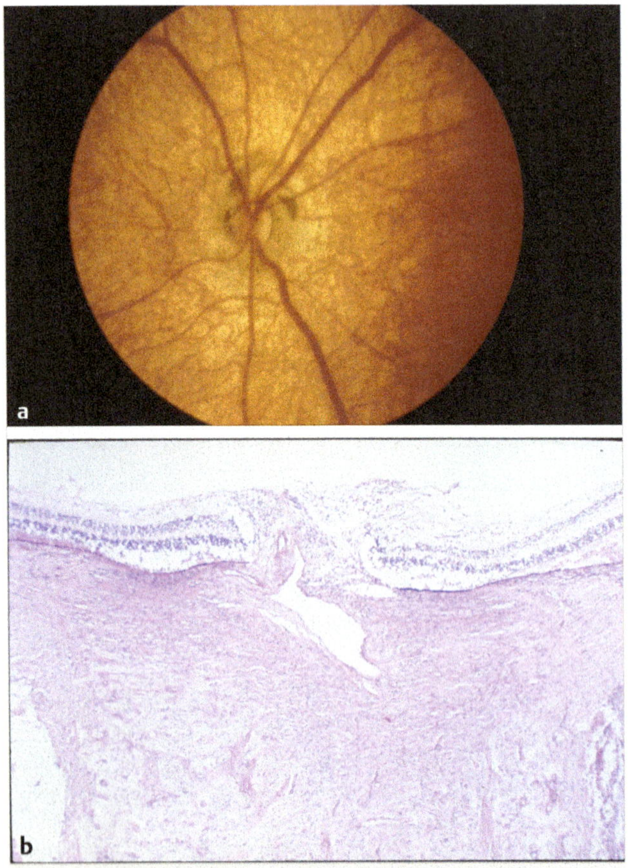

Fig. 36.34 (a) Hypoplastic optic disc of an infant who died from pneumoperitonitis. The optic disc is very small and is surrounded by a ring of yellow-white tissue filling in the region of the normal-sized optic nerve head. Note that the retinal blood vessels enter and exit centrally on the optic nerve head, whereas they are typically located more nasally in a normal optic nerve. Centrally located blood vessels on an optic disc should always at least arouse suspicion of the possibility of coexistent optic nerve hypoplasia. (b) Histopathology of the optic nerve head shown in (a). Optic nerve tissue is present centrally, the borders of which comprise the inner ring of the "double-ring" sign seen with optic nerve hypoplasia. Note that the sensory retina and the retinal pigment epithelium extend further posteriorly than normal to meet the remaining optic nerve tissue. The outer ring of the "double-ring sign" is formed by the juncture of the lamina cribrosa with the nonlaminar sclera. The outer ring corresponds to the size of a normal optic nerve. (Hematoxylin and eosin, x30.)

36.3.2 Optic Nerve Aplasia

With optic nerve hypoplasia, the retinal blood vessels and optic nerve are present. In contrast, with true optic nerve aplasia, both the optic disc and the retinal blood vessels are absent (▸ Fig. 36.35), as are also the retinal ganglion cells.[48] Fortunately, the entity is usually unilateral. Some earlier reported cases of optic nerve aplasia were probably variants of optic nerve hypoplasia instead, especially since some reported optic nerve tissue was present.

The visual acuity with optic nerve aplasia is no light perception. Fluorescein angiography discloses only choroidal filling. Electroretinography is subnormal, but a-waves and b-waves can be present.[48] Concurrent microphthalmos and retinochoroidal coloboma have been reported.[48]

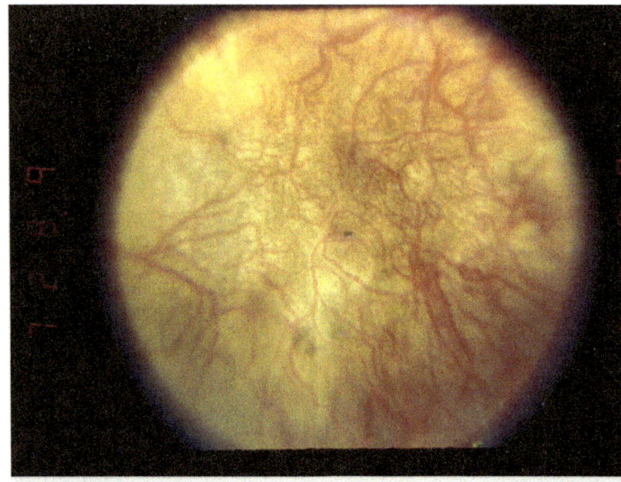

Fig. 36.35 Optic nerve aplasia. The optic nerve head and retinal blood vessels are absent. The vision was no light perception. (Image courtesy of Leonard Nelson, MD.)

Optic nerve aplasia can occur as an isolated finding, but it has been associated with cyclopia, partial agenesis of the central nervous system, and a Hallermann–Streiff-like syndrome.[48] It has also been linked to hypopituitarism.[49] Rare familial occurrence and genetic associations have been reported.[50]

36.3.3 Megalopapilla

Abnormalities associated with an enlarged optic include (1) coloboma of the optic disc, (2) congenital pit of the optic disc, (3) the morning glory disc anomaly, (4) high myopia, and (5) megalopapilla.[4] Clinically, megalopapilla manifests as an enlarged, but otherwise usually normal-appearing, optic disc (▸ Fig. 36.36). A mild peripapillary retinal pigment epithelial disturbance is frequently observed, but other intraocular abnormalities have not been consistently associated.

First described by Franceschetti and Bock in 1950,[51] megalopapilla is generally not associated with decreased visual acuity, although mild to moderate loss has been noted.[52] By strict definition, the entity includes optic discs with averaged horizontal and vertical diameters that measure 2.1 mm or greater (3 standard deviations from the norm of 1.62 mm^4). The embryologic derivation is uncertain, but it is thought to arise from abnormal development of the primitive epithelial papilla.[53]

An enlarged blind spot is present on visual field examination, and partial superotemporal quadrantanopsia has also been noted.[54] Systemic abnormalities described in conjunction with megalopapilla include basal encephalocele, palatoschisis, and mandibulofacial dysostosis.[52,53,54,55]

36.4 Other Congenital Fundus Abnormalities

36.4.1 Myelinated Nerve Fibers

Myelinated nerve fibers in the retina occur in the nerve fiber layer and manifest clinically as white or yellow-white superficial abnormalities with feathery margins (▸ Fig. 36.37). Because of their very superficial location, they often obscure the already

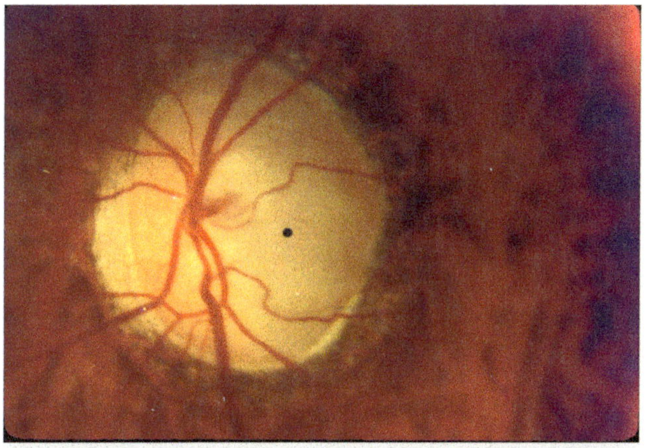

Fig. 36.36 Megalopapilla in the left eye. The distance between the temporal margin of the optic disc and the central fovea is approximately one disc diameter. The retinal vessels are normal in caliber, but appear small because of the enlarged size of the optic disc. By definition, an optic disc with a diameter of 2.1 mm or greater is a megalopapilla.

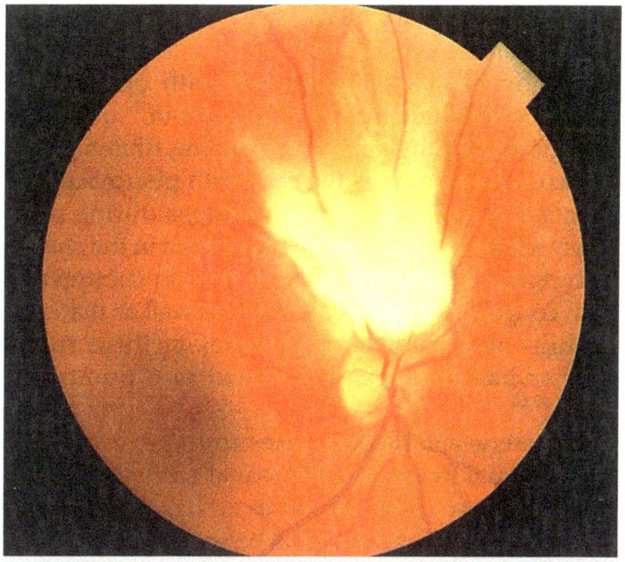

Fig. 36.37 Myelinated nerve fibers extending superiorly from the optic disc. The superficial nerve fibers obscure the retinal blood vessels.

superficial large retinal blood vessels. Myelinated nerve fibers are typically located adjacent to the optic disc, but also may occur as isolated anomalies in the peripheral retina. Since oligodendroglia, not normally present in the retina, are seen in conjunction with myelinated nerve fibers, it is surmised that abnormal rests of oligodendroglia are deposited in the peripheral retina in the instance of peripheral fundus myelination.

Myelination, or medullation, first occurs centrally and then spreads peripherally. By approximately 7.5 months of gestation, myelination has reached the optic chiasm. By term, it reaches the lamina cribrosa. Myelinated nerve fibers in the retina are believed to be congenital in most cases, but rarely can be acquired in childhood or adulthood.[56,57] Conversely, they can disappear after events such as optic neuritis and retinal arterial occlusion.[58]

Visual field defects can be encountered with myelinated nerve fibers in the distribution of the myelination. The field defects are typically relative, rather than absolute. While myelinated nerve fibers do not generally decrease the visual acuity, their presence in the central macula in severe cases may be associated with subnormal vision.

Myelinated nerve fibers can be seen in association with telangiectatic retinal vascular abnormalities and have also been associated with multiple basal cell nevi (Gorlin's) syndrome.[59] The association of myelinated retinal nerve fibers with amblyopia and myopia has also been described.[60]

36.4.2 Persistent Hyperplastic Primary Vitreous

Persistent hyperplastic primary vitreous (PHPV) is typically a unilateral ocular disease characterized by overgrowth of the fetal hyaloid vascular system in the vitreous cavity.[61] The term *persistent fetal vasculature* has also been proposed to describe the entity.[62]

In most cases, a fibrovascular membrane supplied by a persistent hyaloid artery is adherent to the posterior lens capsule. It can lead to cyclitic membrane and phthisis. It can also, however, invade the lens capsule, leading to sudden intumescence of the lens and acute glaucoma as the enlarged lens pushes the iris anteriorly and closes the anterior chamber angle.

The condition is more common in males and is usually associated with micophthalmia.[61] Leukocoria is a common presenting sign; in some instances, the ciliary processes that are dragged centrally by the retrolenticular membrane can be seen through a dilated pupil (▶ Fig. 36.38). The retina can be detached posteriorly, and in some cases the optic disc has the appearance seen with the morning glory disc anomaly.[63]

Ultrasonography and computed tomography can be helpful for making the diagnosis.[64,65] Ultrasonography often demonstrates a shortened eye, and both studies reveal an absence of calcium such as would be seen with retinoblastoma. Radiodense retrolental soft tissue can often be demonstrated along Cloquet's canal.

The visual prognosis in eyes with PHPV is generally poor. Among 25 patients managed nonsurgically at Iowa,[66] 23 had a visual outcome of 5/200 or worse. Two with mild cases had visual acuities of 20/100 and 20/30.

Because of the poor visual prognosis and the possibility of severe acute glaucoma, surgical intervention had been recommended for pronounced cases at any early age, usually within 3 months after birth.[67,68,69] This can be performed via an anterior segment approach or via pars plana vitrectomy. Both the lens and the retrolenticular fibrovascular membrane are removed. When a pars plana approach is employed, the incisions should be made no further back than 1.5 to 2.0 mm posterior to the limbus. Because of the thick, well-formed vitreous gel and small eyes, serious intraoperative complications, such as giant retinal tear, can occur.[69]

The surgical results vary, but are typically poor due to the small size of the eyes. Nevertheless, surgery can prevent severe glaucoma and phthisis. The results are improved when there is no posterior segment involvement. Pollard[68] found that 17% achieved 20/100 vision or better after surgery. Scott et al[67] noted slightly better results, but they also included some patients with solely congenital cataract.

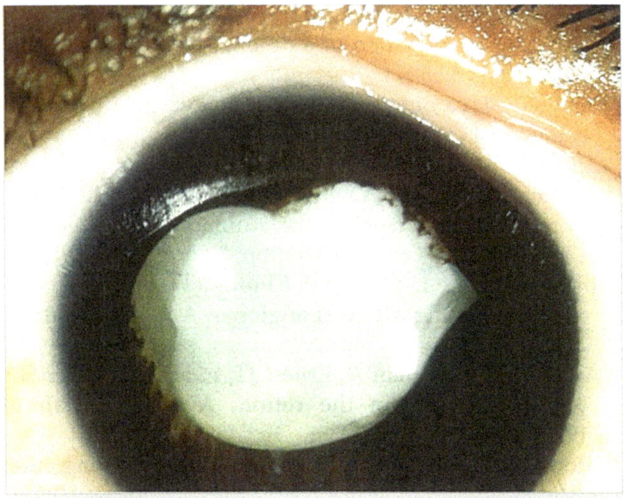

Fig. 36.38 Persistent hyperplastic primary vitreous (PHPV). The ciliary processes have been pulled centrally by the retrolental fibrovascular membrane. The lens is clear.

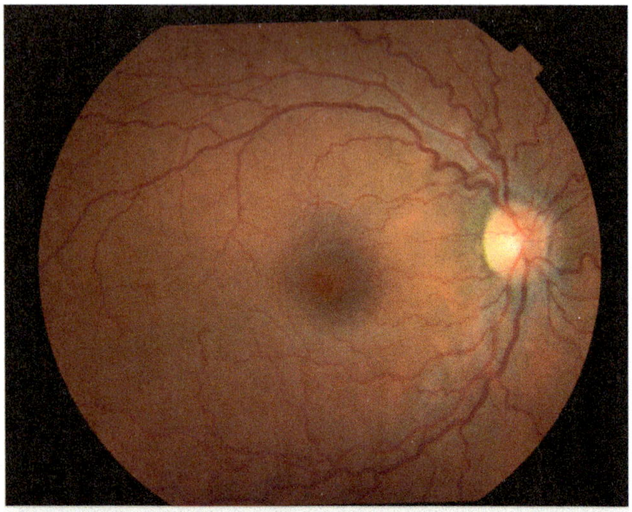

Fig. 36.39 Congenital tortuosity, primarily of the second-order (after the first branching) and third-order (after the second branching), of retinal arterioles and venules in the right eye of a 23-year-old woman in good systemic health.

36.4.3 Congenital Tortuosity of the Retinal Blood Vessels

Acquired causes of tortuosity of the retinal arteries include sickling hemoglobinopathies, retinal hemangioblastomas (von Hippel's tumors), and retinopathy of prematurity in the acute postnatal phases. Acquired causes of venous tortuosity include retinal vein occlusion and hyperviscosity syndromes.

Congenital tortuosity can occur within the retinal arterial system, in which case associated retinal hemorrhages are sometimes observed.[70] Occasionally, an autosomal dominant inheritance pattern can be seen.[70] The second-order and third-order vessels appear to be affected most commonly. In most instances of congenital tortuosity of the retinal arteries and/or veins, both the arteries (arterioles) and veins (venules) are tortuous to some degree (▶ Fig. 36.39).

References

[1] Liebrich R. Demonstration of diseases of the eye. Persistent hyaloid artery and vein. Trans Pathol Soc Lond. 1871; 22:221–224

[2] Mann I. Developmental Abnormalities of the Eye. 2nd ed. Philadelphia, PA: JB Lippincott; 1957:133–136

[3] Degenhart W, Brown GC, Augsburger JJ, Magargal L. Prepapillary vascular loops. Ophthalmology. 1981; 88(11):1126–1131

[4] Brown GC, Tasman WS. Congenital Anomalies of the Optic Disc. New York, NY: Grune & Stratton; 1983:31–93

[5] Shakin EP, Shields JA, Augsburger JJ, Brown GC. Clinicopathologic correlation of a prepapillary vascular loop. Retina. 1988; 8(1):55–58

[6] Jones HE. Hyaloid remnants in the eyes of premature babies. Br J Ophthalmol. 1963; 47:39–44

[7] Delaney WV, Jr. Prepapillary hemorrhage and persistent hyaloid artery. Am J Ophthalmol. 1980; 90(3):419–421

[8] Mann IC. Development of the Human Eye. 3rd ed. New York, NY: Grune & Stratton; 1969:27–28, 228–231

[9] Shields JA, Joffe L, Guibor P. Choroidal melanoma clinically simulating a retinal angioma. Am J Ophthalmol. 1978; 85(1):67–71

[10] Archer DB, Deutman A, Ernest JT, Krill AE. Arteriovenous communications of the retina. Am J Ophthalmol. 1973; 75(2):224–241

[11] Brown GC, Donoso LA, Magargal LE, Goldberg RE, Sarin LK. Congenital retinal macrovessels. Arch Ophthalmol. 1982; 100(9):1430–1436

[12] Cameron ME, Greer CH. Congenital arterio-venous aneurysm of the retina. A post mortem report. Br J Ophthalmol. 1968; 52:768–772

[13] Augsburger JJ, Goldberg RE, Shields JA, Mulberger RD, Magargal LE. Changing appearance of retinal arteriovenous malformation. Albrecht Von Graefes Arch Klin Exp Ophthalmol. 1980; 215(1):65–70

[14] Wynburn-Mason R. Arteriovenous aneurysm of midbrain and retina, optic nerve, chiasm, and brain. Brain. 1943; 66:165–203

[15] Rundles WZ, Falls HF. Congenital arteriovenous (race-mose) aneurysm of the retina; report of 3 cases. AMA Arch Ophthalmol. 1951; 46(4):408–418

[16] Kranenburg EW. Crater-like holes in the optic disc and central serous retinopathy. Arch Ophthalmol. 1960; 64:912–924

[17] Brown GC, Shields JA, Goldberg RE. Congenital pits of the optic nerve head. II. Clinical studies in humans. Ophthalmology. 1980; 87(1):51–65

[18] Brown GC, Shields JA, Patty BE, Goldberg RE. Congenital pits of the optic nerve head. I. Experimental studies in collie dogs. Arch Ophthalmol. 1979; 97 (7):1341–1344

[19] Brown GC, Tasman WS. Congenital Anomalies of the Optic Disc. New York, NY: Grune & Stratton; 1983:95–215

[20] Lincoff H, Lopez R, Kreissig I, Yannuzzi L, Cox M, Burton T. Retinoschisis associated with optic nerve pits. Arch Ophthalmol. 1988; 106(1):61–67

[21] Brown GC, Brown MM. Repair of retinal detachment associated with congenital excavated defects of the optic disc. Ophthalmic Surg. 1995; 26(1):11–15

[22] Cox MS, Witherspoon CD, Morris RE, Flynn HW. Evolving techniques in the treatment of macular detachment caused by optic nerve pits. Ophthalmology. 1988; 95(7):889–896

[23] Vannouhuys JM, Bruyn GW. Nasopharyngeal transsphenoidal encephalocele, craterlike hole in the optic disc and agenesis of the corpus callosum, pneumoencephalographic visualization in a case. Psychiatr Neurol Neurochir. 1964; 67:243–258

[24] Babel J, Farpour H. The genetic origin of colobomatous fossae of the optic nerve [in French]. J Genet Hum. 1967; 16(1):187–198

[25] Vossias A. Beitrag zur Lehne von den Angebroenen Conis. Klin Monatsbl Augenheilkd. 1885; 23:137–157

[26] Lyle DJ. Colomboma of the optic nerve. Am J Ophthalmol. 1932; 15:347–349

[27] Savell J, Cook JR. Optic nerve colobomas of autosomal-dominant heredity. Arch Ophthalmol. 1976; 94(3):395–400

[28] Pagon RA, Graham JM, Jr, Zonana J, Yong SL. Coloboma, congenital heart disease, and choanal atresia with multiple anomalies: CHARGE association. J Pediatr. 1981; 99(2):223–227

[29] Kindler P. Morning glory syndrome: unusual congenital optic disk anomaly. Am J Ophthalmol. 1970; 69(3):376–384

[30] Brodsky MC, Parsa CF. The moyamoya optic disc. JAMA Ophthalmol. 2015; 133(2):164

[31] Steinkuller PG. The morning glory disk anomaly: case report and literature review. J Pediatr Ophthalmol Strabismus. 1980; 17(2):81–87

[32] Beyer WB, Quencer RM, Osher RH. Morning glory syndrome. A functional analysis including fluorescein angiography, ultrasonography, and computerized tomography. Ophthalmology. 1982; 89(12):1362–1367

[33] Pollock JA, Newton TH, Hoyt WF. Transsphenoidal and transethmoidal encephaloceles. A review of clinical and roentgen features in 8 cases. Radiology. 1968; 90(3):442–453

[34] Wise JB, MacLean AL, Gass JDM. Contractile peripapillary staphyloma. Arch Ophthalmol. 1966; 75(5):626–630

[35] Riise D. The nasal fundus ectasia. Acta Ophthalmol Suppl. 1975(126):3–108

[36] Riise D. Visual field defects in optic disc malformation with ectasia of the fundus. Acta Ophthalmol (Copenh). 1966; 44(6):906–918

[37] Mosier MA, Lieberman MF, Green WR, Knox DL. Hypoplasia of the optic nerve. Arch Ophthalmol. 1978; 96(8):1437–1442

[38] Jerome B, Forster HW, Jr. Congenital hypoplasia, partial aplasia, of the optic nerve. Arch Ophthal. 1948; 39(5):669–672

[39] Ellenberger C, Jr, Runyan TE. Holoprosencephaly with hypoplasia of the optic nerves, dwarfism, and agenesis of the septum pellucidum. Am J Ophthalmol. 1970; 70(6):960–967

[40] Hackenbruch Y, Meerhoff E, Besio R, Cardoso H. Familial bilateral optic nerve hypoplasia. Am J Ophthalmol. 1975; 79(2):314–320

[41] Hoyt CS, Billson FA. Maternal anticonvulsants and optic nerve hypoplasia. Br J Ophthalmol. 1978; 62(1):3–6

[42] McKinna AJ. Quinine induced hypoplasia of the optic nerve. Can J Ophthalmol. 1966; 1(4):261–266

[43] Hotchkiss ML, Green WR. Optic nerve aplasia and hypoplasia. J Pediatr Ophthalmol Strabismus. 1979; 16(4):225–240

[44] Hittner HM, Desmond MM, Montgomery JR. Optic nerve manifestations of human congenital cytomegalovirus infection. Am J Ophthalmol. 1976; 81 (5):661–665

[45] Petersen RA, Walton DS. Optic nerve hypoplasia with good visual acuity and visual field defects: a study of children of diabetic mothers. Arch Ophthalmol. 1977; 95(2):254–258

[46] Acers TE. Optic nerve hypoplasia: septo-optic-pituitary dysplasia syndrome. Trans Am Ophthalmol Soc. 1981; 79:425–457

[47] DeMosier G. Agenesie du septum Lucidum avec malformation du tractus optique. La dysplasie septo-optique. Schweiz Arch Neurol Neurochir Psychiatr. 1956; 77:267–292

[48] Little LE, Whitmore PV, Wells TW, Jr. Aplasia of the optic nerve. J Pediatr Ophthalmol. 1976; 13(2):84–88

[49] Brodsky MC, Atreides SPA, Fowlkes JL, Sundin OH. Optic nerve aplasia in an infant with congenital hypopituitarism and posterior pituitary ectopia. Arch Ophthalmol. 2004; 122(1):125–126

[50] Meire F, Delpierre I, Brachet C, et al. Nonsyndromic bilateral and unilateral optic nerve aplasia: first familial occurrence and potential implication of CYP26A1 and CYP26C1 genes. Mol Vis. 2011; 17:2072–2079

[51] Franceschetti A, Bock RH. Megalopapilla; a new congenital anomaly. Am J Ophthalmol. 1950; 33(2):227–235, illust

[52] Strieff B. Uber Megalopapillae. Klin Monatsbl Augenheilkd. 1961; 139:824–827

[53] Badke G. Uber die Grossenanomalien der Papilla nervi optici, unter besonderer, Beruksichtig ung der schwarzen Megaloppapille. Klin Monatsbl Augenheilkd. 1959; 135:502–510

[54] Merin S, Harwood-Nash DC, Crawford JS. Axial tomography of optic nerve in diagnosis of children's eye and optic nerve defects. Am J Ophthalmol. 1971; 72:1122–1129

[55] Malbran JL, Roveda JM. Magalopapilla. Arq Oftal B Aires. 1951; 26:331–335

[56] Kushner BJ. Optic nerve decompression. Presumed postoperative development of medullated nerve fibers. Arch Ophthalmol. 1979; 97(8):1459–1461

[57] Baarsma GS. Acquired medullated nerve fibres. Br J Ophthalmol. 1980; 64:651

[58] Sharpe JA, Sanders MD. Atrophy of myelinated nerve fibres in the retina in optic neuritis. Br J Ophthalmol. 1975; 59(4):229–232

[59] De Jong PT, Bistervels B, Cosgrove J, de Grip G, Leys A, Goffin M. Medullated nerve fibers. A sign of multiple basal cell nevi (Gorlin's) syndrome. Arch Ophthalmol. 1985; 103(12):1833–1836

[60] Tarabishy AB, Alexandrou TJ, Traboulsi EI. Syndrome of myelinated retinal nerve fibers, myopia, and amblyopia: a review. Surv Ophthalmol. 2007; 52 (6):588–596

[61] Haddad R, Font RL, Reeser F. Persistent hyperplastic primary vitreous. A clinicopathologic study of 62 cases and review of the literature. Surv Ophthalmol. 1978; 23(2):123–134

[62] Goldberg MF. Persistent fetal vasculature (PFV): an integrated interpretation of signs and symptoms associated with persistent hyperplastic primary vitreous (PHPV). LIV Edward Jackson Memorial Lecture. Am J Ophthalmol. 1997; 124(5):587–626

[63] Brown GC, Gonder J, Levin A. Persistence of the primary vitreous in association with the morning glory disc anomaly. J Pediatr Ophthalmol Strabismus. 1984; 21(1):5–7

[64] Goldberg MF, Mafee M. Computed tomography for diagnosis of persistent hyperplastic primary vitreous (PHPV). Ophthalmology. 1983; 90(5):442–451

[65] Kaste SC, Jenkins JJ, III, Meyer D, Fontanesi J, Pratt CB. Persistent hyperplastic primary vitreous of the eye: imaging findings with pathologic correlation. AJR Am J Roentgenol. 1994; 162(2):437–440

[66] Karr DJ, Scott WE. Visual acuity results following treatment of persistent hyperplastic primary vitreous. Arch Ophthalmol. 1986; 104(5):662–667

[67] Scott WE, Drummond GT, Keech RV, Karr DJ. Management and visual acuity results of monocular congenital cataracts and persistent hyperplastic primary vitreous. Aust N Z J Ophthalmol. 1989; 17(2):143–152

[68] Pollard ZF. Results of treatment of persistent hyperplastic primary vitreous. Ophthalmic Surg. 1991; 22(1):48–52

[69] Federman JL, Shields JA, Altman B, Koller H. The surgical and nonsurgical management of persistent hyperplastic primary vitreous. Ophthalmology. 1982; 89(1):20–24

[70] Sutter FKP, Helbig H. Familial retinal arteriolar tortuosity: a review. Surv Ophthalmol. 2003; 48(3):245–255

37 Intravitreal Injections

Ingrid U. Scott and Harry W. Flynn Jr.

37.1 Introduction

Intravitreal injection was reported by Ohm in 1911 as a technique to introduce air for retinal tamponade and repair of retinal detachment.[1] Intravitreal administration of pharmacotherapies dates back to the mid-1940s with the use of penicillin to treat endophthalmitis.[2,3] Since that time, use of the intravitreal injection technique has steadily increased, with its usage for the treatment of retinal detachment,[4,5] endophthalmitis,[6,7] and cytomegalovirus (CMV) retinitis.[8,9] The introduction of anti-vascular endothelial growth factor (anti-VEGF) agents resulted in a dramatic increase in intravitreal injections.[10] An analysis of the United States Medicare claims database revealed that fewer than 5,000 intravitreal injections were performed in 2001, and 812,413 intravitreal injections were performed in 2007.[10] Currently, intravitreal injection is one of the most commonly performed medical procedures in the United States with well over 1 million injections performed annually.[11]

Pearls

- Although the intravitreal injection procedure dates back to 1911, the recent development of pharmacotherapies for various posterior segment diseases has led to a rapid increase in the use of this technique.

37.2 Risk of Endophthalmitis Associated with the Intravitreal Injection Procedure

With the widespread use of the intravitreal injection technique, there has been increased concern regarding the risk of endophthalmitis following intravitreal injection. The risk of endophthalmitis in eyes with CMV retinitis treated with intravitreal injection has been estimated to be 1.3% per eye and 0.1% per injection.[12] The risk of endophthalmitis following intravitreal triamcinolone acetonide injection has been estimated to be approximately 0.8% for noninfectious endophthalmitis[12,13,14] and 0.6 to 0.16% for infectious endophthalmitis.[12,15] Because most patients treated with anti-VEGF agents receive a series of injections over months or years, it is important to distinguish between per-injection rates of endophthalmitis versus per-patient (or cumulative) rates of endophthalmitis over the course of treatment. While reported per-injection rates of endophthalmitis are generally very low in series of patients treated with anti-VEGF agents, per-patient rates may be close to 1% over a 2-year course of therapy. Recent series from Florida (20 cases of endophthalmitis out of 121,285 intravitreal injections, or a rate of 0.016%),[16] Denmark (2 cases out of 7,584 injections, or a rate of 0.026%),[17] Australia (2 cases out of 9.162 injections, 0.022%),[18] and Massachusetts (3 cases out of 10,208 injections, 0.029%)[19] indicate an endophthalmitis rate of 1 per 3,000 intravitreal anti-VEGF injections or less. A population-based study in the United Kingdom estimated the per-injection rate of endophthalmitis following intravitreal anti-VEGF injection to be 0.025%.[20] A review of the United States Medicare claims database revealed a per-injection rate of 0.09% for endophthalmitis associated with intravitreal anti-VEGF injections administered to patients with age-related macular degeneration (AMD).[21] In the Comparison of Age-related Macular Degeneration Treatments Trials (CATT), a prospective, multicenter, randomized clinical trial comparing intravitreal ranibizumab (Lucentis, Genentech) and intravitreal bevacizumab (Avastin, Genentech) in 1,107 patients with neovascular AMD, the per-patient rate of endophthalmitis over 2 years was 0.7% with intravitreal ranibizumab and 1.2% with intravitreal bevacizumab ($p = 0.38$).[22] A recent meta-analysis of 43 studies reported that endophthalmitis occurred after 197 of 350,535 intravitreal anti-VEGF injections, for an endophthalmitis rate of 0.056%.[23]

37.3 Endophthalmitis after Intravitreal Injection: Spectrum of Causative Organisms Compared to Postsurgical Cases of Endophthalmitis

While the majority of postsurgical cases of endophthalmitis are believed to be related to the patient's baseline ocular surface flora, many cases of endophthalmitis associated with the intravitreal injection procedure may be related to droplet transmission from the patient or from the health care providers involved with the intravitreal injection. Several studies provide evidence that the patient's ocular surface flora may be the most common source of bacteria causing postoperative endophthalmitis, with the most common causative organisms being coagulase-negative *Staphylococcus* species.[24,25,26,27] *Streptococcus* species, which comprise at least 41% of culturable adult salivary flora,[28,29] are believed to contaminate operative fields by aerosolization or droplet spread.[30,31,32,33,34] Several studies have reported that *Streptococcus* species are significantly more likely to be the causative organism of endophthalmitis after intravitreal injection than of endophthalmitis after intraocular surgery. McCannel[35] summarized 54 cases of endophthalmitis following 105,532 intravitreal injections of anti-VEGF agents, and found that, of the culture-positive cases, *Staphylococcus* (*n* = 17; 65%) and *Streptococcus* (*n* = 8; 31%) were the most common causative organisms. In contrast, in series of postsurgical endophthalmitis cases, the proportion of culture-positive cases that were *Streptococcus* species ranged from 0 to 9%.[35] Similarly, Gregori et al[16] reported a series of 20 patients with endophthalmitis after 121,285 intravitreal injections of anti-VEGF agents; of the 9 (45%) culture-positive cases, 5 (56%) were *Streptococcus* species, 3 (33%) were coagulase-negative *Staphylococcus*, and 1 (11%) was nonanthracis Bacillus. Fileta et al[23] reported a meta-analysis which included 197 cases of endophthalmitis out of 350,535 intravitreal anti-VEGF injections; the most common organisms isolated were coagulase-negative *Staphylococcus* (38%) and *Streptococcus* (29%). An analysis of conjunctival flora in patients undergoing intravitreal injections identified *Streptococcus* species in only 3 of 71 (4.2%) cultured isolates, supporting the hypothesis that such organisms come from respiratory droplets instead of the patient's conjunctival flora.[36]

Special Considerations

- Several studies have reported that *Streptococcus* species are significantly more likely to be the causative organism of endophthalmitis after intravitreal injection than of endophthalmitis after intraocular surgery. Thus, an important source for some cases of endophthalmitis after intravitreal injection may be respiratory droplets from the patient or the health care providers involved with the intravitreal injection procedure.

37.4 Injection Procedure Guidelines

Strategies that may be important in reducing the risk of complications associated with intravitreal injection include attention to issues before, during, and after the injection. Guidelines developed as a result of round-table deliberations conducted after a review of published and unpublished studies and case series are summarized, and an appropriate sequence of events for the administration of intravitreal injection is provided in the following.[37]

Special Considerations

- Injection procedure guidelines include consideration of preexisting conditions, such as active external infection and eyelid abnormalities, povidone-iodine, lid speculum, gloves, anesthesia, injection site location, needle selection, intraocular pressure (IOP) and vision monitoring postinjection, patient counselling postinjection regarding signs and symptoms of complications, and follow-up.

Guideline Areas with General Agreement among Committee Members

- Povidone-iodine (5–10%) should be the last agent applied to the intended injection site before injection. If a gel anesthetic is used, povidone-iodine should be applied both before and after application of gel, as retained gel may prevent povidone-iodine from contacting the conjunctival surface of the injection site.
- Pre- peri-, or postinjection topical antibiotics are unnecessary.
- There is no evidence to support the routine use of a sterile drape.
- Avoid contamination of the needle and injection site by the eyelashes or the eyelid margins.
- Avoid extensive massage of the eyelids either pre- or postinjection (to avoid meibomian gland expression).
- Use adequate anesthetic for a given patient (topical drops, gel, and/or subconjunctival injection).
- Use of sterile or nonsterile gloves as consistent with modern office practice, combined with strong agreement regarding the need for handwashing before and after patient contact.
- Either surgical masks should be used or both the patient and providers should minimize speaking during the injection preparation and procedure to limit aerosolized droplets containing oral contaminants from the patient and/or provider.
- Monitor IOP both pre- and postinjection.
- Routine anterior chamber paracentesis is not recommended.

Source: Adapted from Avery et al.[37]

Guideline Areas with No Clear Consensus among Committee Members

- Need for povidone-iodine application to the eyelids, including the eyelashes and eyelid margins. All agreed that when povidone-iodine is applied to the eyelashes and eyelid margins, eyelid scrubbing or eyelid pressure adequate to express material from the meibomian gland should be avoided.
- Use of a speculum (some prevent contact between the needle/injection site and the eyelashes and eyelids with manual lid retraction).
- Need for pupillary dilation and postinjection dilated examination of the posterior segment (although some viewed the return of formed vision as sufficient, others routinely dilate the pupil and examine the posterior segment after injection).
- Use of povidone-iodine flush (most preferred drops only and saw no benefit to allowing the povidone-iodine to dry before injection).

(Adapted from Avery et al.[37])

Intravitreal Injection Procedure: An Appropriate Sequence of Events

1. Both the patient and providers should minimize speaking during the injection preparation and procedure.
2. Take a procedural time-out to verify patient, agent, and laterality.
3. Apply liquid anesthetic drops to the ocular surface.
4. Apply povidone-iodine to the eyelashes and eyelid margins (optional, most use 10%).
5. Retract the eyelids away from the intended injection site for the duration of the procedure
6. Apply povidone-iodine (most use 5%) to the conjunctival surface including the intended injection site, at least 30 seconds before injection.
7. If additional anesthetic is applied, reapply povidone-iodine to the intended injection site immediately before injection (most use 5%).
8. Insert the needle perpendicular to the sclera, 3.5 to 4.0 mm posterior to the limbus (3.0–3.5 mm in pseudophakic or aphakic eyes) between the vertical and horizontal rectus muscles.

Active external infection, including significant blepharitis, should be treated prior to injection. In addition, eyelid abnormalities such as ectropion are reported risk factors for endophthalmitis and should be considered. Ocular surface bacteria represent an important source of bacteria causing postoperative endophthalmitis[24,25,26,27] and post–intravitreal injection endophthalmitis.[23,35] Thus, one strategy to reduce the risk of endophthalmitis is to reduce or eliminate the bacteria on the patient's ocular surface and eyelids. While this may be achieved in various ways (povidone-iodine, topical antibiotics, eyelid hygiene, and sterile isolation of the surgical site), povidone-iodine is the only agent that has been demonstrated to reduce the risk of postoperative endophthalmitis in a prospective study of cataract surgery.[38] It is unknown whether the application of povidone-iodine in the form of drops versus a flush impacts on the ability of this agent to prevent endophthalmitis. Lid scrubs have been reported to be associated with a significant increase in bacterial flora; thus, excessive eyelid manipulation should be avoided (although the efficacy of lid scrubs in combination with povidone-iodine has not been reported). Since true contact allergy to povidone-iodine is rare, and anaphylaxis after ophthalmic application of povidone-iodine has not been reported, a reported history of contact allergy to povidone-iodine can be verified with a skin patch test. Conjunctival exposure to 5% povidone-iodine for a period of 30 seconds achieves a significant reduction in the bacterial colony-forming units and appears to be an adequate contact time before intravitreal injection.[39]

Topical antibiotics have been demonstrated to reduce ocular surface bacteria significantly, but have not been proven to reduce the risk of endophthalmitis.[40,41,42,43] Despite the evidence that topical antibiotics reduce the conjunctival bacterial load,[42,44,45] several studies have demonstrated that the addition of preinjection or postinjection topical antibiotics to povidone-iodine antisepsis does not decrease the rates of endophthalmitis compared with the use of povidone-iodine alone.[46,47,48] A similar conclusion was reached in a prospective study in which bacterial growth from conjunctival swabs was analyzed; preoperative application of moxifloxacin 0.5% offered no reduction in bacterial cultures beyond that of povidone-iodine alone.[49] Furthermore, use of topical antibiotics has been associated with increased bacterial resistance rates of ocular surface flora in patients undergoing intravitreal injections.[50,51,52] For example, one prospective study found that over a 1-year period, coagulase-negative *Staphylococcus* resistance to gatifloxacin and moxifloxacin roughly doubled, from rates of 39 and 34%, respectively, prior to treatment with intravitreal injections, to 67 and 70%, respectively, following treatment with intravitreal injections.[50,51] These eyes were initially treatment naïve, and all received four monthly intravitreal injections, followed by intravitreal injections as needed on an individual basis. After each injection, patients were administered one drop of their assigned fluoroquinolone to the injected eye and were instructed to instill one drop of their assigned fluoroquinolone to the injected eye four times per day for 4 days. Over the same 1-year study period, untreated fellow eyes of the same patients did not develop an increase in fluoroquinolone-resistant coagulase-negative *Staphylococcus* strains. Thus, due to emerging antimicrobial resistance and lack of evidence supporting a reduction in endophthalmitis rates, topical antibiotic use for prophylaxis of endophthalmitis following intravitreal injection is not the current standard of care.

Controversial Points

- Topical antibiotic use for prophylaxis of endophthalmitis following intravitreal injection is not the current standard of care due to concerns regarding emerging antimicrobial resistance and lack of evidence supporting a reduction in endophthalmitis rates.

Because of the evidence that the underlying causative mechanism for some cases of endophthalmitis after intravitreal injection might be related to respiratory droplet transmission from the patient or the health care providers involved with the intravitreal injection procedure, it is recommended that the patient and health care providers either wear surgical masks or minimize speaking during the injection preparation and procedure.[37,53] During the injection procedure, the use of a sterile lid speculum has been recommended to avoid needle contact with lids and lashes. However, the most recent "guidelines" paper listed the use of a lid speculum as having "no consensus" among the panel members because many members no longer used a speculum.[37] The use of a sterile drape is also optional but gloves, part of universal precautions, are appropriate. Sterile topical anesthetic is administered as the first step in the procedure. Ophthalmologists may consider subconjunctival anesthesia, but this requires additional instrumentation and manipulation which may be associated with increased surface flora. If subconjunctival anesthesia is used, keep in mind that the needle used for intravitreal injection passes through the subconjunctival space filled with anesthetic and that surface bacteria may have been introduced beneath the conjunctiva. Although lidocaine gel has been used with increased frequency for anterior segment surgery cases in recent years, and has been reported as providing satisfactory patient comfort during intravitreal injection procedures while causing less chemosis and hemorrhage than subconjunctival anesthesia,[54] another study identified lidocaine gel as a potential risk factor for endophthalmitis following cataract surgery.[55] Lidocaine gel may serve as a barrier, reducing the ability of povidone-iodine to contact the ocular surface and reduce the risk of endophthalmitis. Even if povidone-iodine is administered prior to lidocaine gel (in an attempt to bypass the potential barrier effect), it should be recognized that the commercially available lidocaine gel is not prepared as a sterile formulation and, therefore, the injection needle may become contaminated as it passes through the lidocaine gel and before it enters the intravitreal cavity. Thus, if a gel anesthetic is used, povidone-iodine should be applied both before and after the gel. Care should be taken to avoid pressure to the eyelids, eyelid margins, and the adnexa due to the potential for release of resident bacteria. According to one study,[56] 13% of the ophthalmic drugs obtained from multiple-use medication bottles tested positive for bacteria and 21% of the bottle tips were culture-positive.

Pearls

- It is recommended that the patient and health care providers involved in the intravitreal injection either wear surgical masks or minimize speaking during the injection preparation and procedure.

Intravitreal injections should be given between the horizontal and vertical rectus muscles at the pars plana, 3.5 to 4.0 mm posterior to the limbus in phakic eyes and 3.0 to 3.5 mm posterior to the limbus in pseudophakic or aphakic eyes. Although the inferotemporal quadrant is generally the preferred site of injection due to such factors as ease of exposure (no need to pass the needle over the bridge of the nose or the brow), quadrant selection should be dictated by patient-specific considerations and injection physician preference. Although oblique and tunneled needle insertions have been described as attempts to minimize drug reflux after injection, a perpendicular injection approach is convenient and preferred in most settings.[37]

Needle gauge is selected based on the drug being injected. A 30-gauge or smaller needle is generally preferred for nonviscous drugs. Larger gauge needles may be considered for suspensions and for more viscous solutions. Needle length should be 5/8 inch (18 mm) or shorter but long enough to permit complete penetration of the pars plana.[37]

37.5 Guidelines for Postinjection Management and Follow-Up

The intraocular pressure (IOP) is monitored postinjection, and therapy for persistently elevated IOP should be provided as indicated. The injecting physician confirms the presence of formed vision before the patient leaves the office and 24-hour emergency contact information should be provided to the patient. Patients and/or caregivers should be educated to avoid eye rubbing and to recognize and report the signs and symptoms of endophthalmitis, retinal detachment, or intraocular hemorrhage. Because of the relatively low risk of endophthalmitis associated with intravitreal injection, no study has compared different strategies for follow-up. As clinicians' comfort level with this procedure has increased, most clinicians no longer evaluate patients 1 day following intravitreal injection. However, patients should be instructed to contact the ophthalmologist immediately with signs and symptoms of complications (e.g., decreased vision, increased ocular redness, or discomfort compared to immediately after the injection).

37.6 Noninfectious Endophthalmitis

Both infectious and noninfectious endophthalmitis have been reported following intravitreal injections. Noninfectious endophthalmitis may represent dispersion of drug crystals (such as has been reported in association with triamcinolone acetonide)[57] in the anterior chamber (which may form a pseudohypopyon) and vitreous cavity or an acute inflammatory reaction to a component in the drug formulation. The incidence of noninfectious endophthalmitis following intravitreal triamcinolone acetonide injection has been reported to range from 0.2 to 1.6%.[58,59,60,61] Typical clinical features of noninfectious endophthalmitis include absence of, or mild, pain and eyelid edema, no increased conjunctival injection compared with that present immediately after injection, absence of fibrin and true hypopyon, and absent or mild vitreous opacities. Such patients should be monitored carefully to rule out progressive inflammation due to early endophthalmitis. In addition, patients should be instructed to contact the ophthalmologist immediately if they note any change in their ocular symptoms, such as pain, decreased vision, or increased ocular redness compared to that present immediately after the injection procedure. ▶ Table 37.1 summarize clinical features which may help to distinguish infectious from noninfectious inflammation after intravitreal injections.

Special Considerations

- Both infectious and noninfectious endophthalmitis have been reported following intravitreal injections. Clinical features may help to differentiate between infectious and noninfectious inflammation, but close monitoring is recommended for both conditions.

37.7 Conclusion

Intravitreal injection has become a commonly employed technique in the management of a variety of posterior segment diseases and is an important part of the retina specialist's armamentarium. In order to optimize the outcomes associated with intravitreal injection, careful attention should be paid to reducing the risk of complications. Ultimately, the outcomes of treatment depend not only on the safety and efficacy of the pharmacotherapy being delivered, but also on the safety and potential adverse events associated with the procedure itself.

Table 37.1 Distinguishing infectious from noninfections inflammation after intravitreal injections

	Infectious	Noninfectious
More common features		
Pain	Moderate to severe pain	Usually mild pain
Vision loss	Severe	Mid to moderate
Fibrin	Typically present	Rare
Hypopyon	Very common	Rare
Vitreous opacity	Usually prominent	Usually mild
Conjunctival vascular congestion	Very common	Often absent
Less common features		
Retinal infiltrates	Occasionally present	Absent
Intraretinal hemorrhages	Common	Rare
Whitening of retinal vessels	May be present	Absent
Clinical course	Rapidly progressive	Slow improvement

References

[1] Ohm J. Über die behandlung der netzhautablösung durch operative entleerung der subretinalen flössigkeit und einspritzung von luft in den glaskörper. Albrecht Von Graefes Arch Ophthalmol. 1911; 79:442–450
[2] Schneider J, Frankel SS. Treatment of late postoperative intraocular infections with intraocular injection of penicillin. Arch Ophthal. 1947; 37(3):304–307
[3] Rycroft BW. Penicillin and the control of deep intra-ocular infection. Br J Ophthalmol. 1945; 29(2):57–87
[4] Rosengren B. 300 cases operated upon for retinal detachment; method and results. Acta Ophthalmol (Copenh). 1952; 30(1):117–122
[5] Cibis PA, Becker B, Okun E, Canaan S. The use of liquid silicone in retinal detachment surgery. Arch Ophthalmol. 1962; 68:590–599
[6] Forster RK, Zachary IG, Cottingham AJ, Jr, Norton EWD. Further observations on the diagnosis cause, and treatment of endophthalmitis. Am J Ophthalmol. 1976; 81(1):52–56
[7] Peyman GA, Vastine DW, Raichand M. Experimental aspects and their clinical application. Ophthalmology. 1978; 85(4):374–385
[8] Henry K, Cantrill H, Fletcher C, Chinnock BJ, Balfour HH, Jr. Use of intravitreal ganciclovir (dihydroxy propoxymethyl guanine) for cytomegalovirus retinitis in a patient with AIDS. Am J Ophthalmol. 1987; 103(1):17–23
[9] Vitravene injection (fomivirsen sodium intravitreal injectable). Approval letter, pages 1–4. Vol. 2004. U.S. Food and Drug Administration Web site. Available at: www.fda.gov/cder/foi/nda/98/20961_Vitravene_Approv.pdf. Accessed April 29, 2004
[10] Ramulu PY, Do DV, Corcoran KJ, Corcoran SL, Robin AL. Use of retinal procedures in medicare beneficiaries from 1997 to 2007. Arch Ophthalmol. 2010; 128(10):1335–1340
[11] Peyman GA, Lad EM, Moshfeghi DM. Intravitreal injection of therapeutic agents. Retina. 2009; 29(7):875–912
[12] Cekiç O, Chang S, Tseng JJ, et al. Intravitreal triamcinolone injection for treatment of macular edema secondary to branch retinal vein occlusion. Retina. 2005; 25(7):851–855
[13] Antcliff RJ, Spalton DJ, Stanford MR, Graham EM, ffytche TJ, Marshall J. Intravitreal triamcinolone for uveitic cystoid macular edema: an optical coherence tomography study. Ophthalmology. 2001; 108(4):765–772
[14] Young S, Larkin G, Branley M, Lightman S. Safety and efficacy of intravitreal triamcinolone for cystoid macular oedema in uveitis. Clin Experiment Ophthalmol. 2001; 29(1):2–6
[15] Martidis A, Duker JS, Puliafito CA. Intravitreal triamcinolone for refractory cystoid macular edema secondary to birdshot retinochoroidopathy. Arch Ophthalmol. 2001; 119(9):1380–1383
[16] Gregori NZ, Flynn HW, Jr, Schwartz SG, et al. Current infectious endophthalmitis rates after intravitreal injections of anti-vascular endothelial growth factor agents and outcomes of treatment. Ophthalmic Surg Lasers Imaging Retina. 2015; 46(6):643–648
[17] Rasmussen A, Bloch SB, Fuchs J, et al. A 4-year longitudinal study of 555 patients treated with ranibizumab for neovascular age-related macular degeneration. Ophthalmology. 2013; 120(12):2630–2636
[18] Gillies MC, Walton R, Simpson JM, et al. Fight Retinal Blindness! Project Investigators. Prospective audit of exudative age-related macular degeneration: 12-month outcomes in treatment-naive eyes. Invest Ophthalmol Vis Sci. 2013; 54(8):5754–5760
[19] Englander M, Chen TC, Paschalis EI, Miller JW, Kim IK. Intravitreal injections at the Massachusetts Eye and Ear Infirmary: analysis of treatment indications and postinjection endophthalmitis rates. Br J Ophthalmol. 2013; 97(4):460–465
[20] Lyall DA, Tey A, Foot B, et al. Post-intravitreal anti-VEGF endophthalmitis in the United Kingdom: incidence, features, risk factors, and outcomes. Eye (Lond). 2012; 26(12):1517–1526
[21] Day S, Acquah K, Mruthyunjaya P, Grossman DS, Lee PP, Sloan FA. Ocular complications after anti-vascular endothelial growth factor therapy in Medicare patients with age-related macular degeneration. Am J Ophthalmol. 2011; 152 (2):266–272
[22] Martin DF, Maguire MG, Fine SL, et al. Comparison of Age-related Macular Degeneration Treatments Trials (CATT) Research Group. Ranibizumab and bevacizumab for treatment of neovascular age-related macular degeneration: two-year results. Ophthalmology. 2012; 119(7):1388–1398
[23] Fileta JB, Scott IU, Flynn HW, Jr. Meta-analysis of infectious endophthalmitis after intravitreal injection of anti-vascular endothelial growth factor agents. Ophthalmic Surg Lasers Imaging Retina. 2014; 45(2):143–149
[24] Speaker MG, Milch FA, Shah MK, Eisner W, Kreiswirth BN. Role of external bacterial flora in the pathogenesis of acute postoperative endophthalmitis. Ophthalmology. 1991; 98(5):639–649, discussion 650
[25] Bannerman TL, Rhoden DL, McAllister SK, Miller JM, Wilson LA. The source of coagulase-negative staphylococci in the Endophthalmitis Vitrectomy Study. A comparison of eyelid and intraocular isolates using pulsed-field gel electrophoresis. Arch Ophthalmol. 1997; 115(3):357–361
[26] Han DP, Wisniewski SR, Wilson LA, et al. Spectrum and susceptibilities of microbiologic isolates in the Endophthalmitis Vitrectomy Study. Am J Ophthalmol. 1996; 122(1):1–17
[27] Leong JK, Shah R, McCluskey PJ, Benn RA, Taylor RF. Bacterial contamination of the anterior chamber during phacoemulsification cataract surgery. J Cataract Refract Surg. 2002; 28(5):826–833
[28] Gordon DF, Jong BB. Indigenous flora from human saliva. Appl Microbiol. 1968; 16(2):428–429
[29] McCarthy C, Snyder ML, Parker RB. The indigenous oral flora of man. I. The newborn to the 1-year-old infant. Arch Oral Biol. 1965; 10:61–70
[30] Veringa E, van Belkum A, Schellekens H. Iatrogenic meningitis by Streptococcus salivarius following lumbar puncture. J Hosp Infect. 1995; 29(4):316–318
[31] Sherertz RJ, Reagan DR, Hampton KD, et al. A cloud adult: the Staphylococcus aureus-virus interaction revisited. Ann Intern Med. 1996; 124(6):539–547
[32] O'Kelly SW, Marsh D. Face masks and spinal anaesthesia. Br J Anaesth. 1993; 70(2):239
[33] McLure HA, Talboys CA, Yentis SM, Azadian BS. Surgical face masks and downward dispersal of bacteria. Anaesthesia. 1998; 53(7):624–626
[34] Trautmann M, Lepper PM, Schmitz FJ. Three cases of bacterial meningitis after spinal and epidural anesthesia. Eur J Clin Microbiol Infect Dis. 2002; 21 (1):43–45
[35] McCannel CA. Meta-analysis of endophthalmitis after intravitreal injection of anti-vascular endothelial growth factor agents: causative organisms and possible prevention strategies. Retina. 2011; 31(4):654–661
[36] Moss JM, Sanislo SR, Ta CN. Antibiotic susceptibility patterns of ocular bacterial flora in patients undergoing intravitreal injections. Ophthalmology. 2010; 117(11):2141–2145
[37] Avery RL, Bakri SJ, Blumenkranz MS, et al. Intravitreal injection technique and monitoring: updated guidelines of an expert panel. Retina. 2014; 34 (Suppl)(11):S1–S18
[38] Speaker MG, Menikoff JA. Prophylaxis of endophthalmitis with topical povidone-iodine. Ophthalmology. 1991; 98(12):1769–1775

[39] Friedman DA, Mason JO, III, Emond T, McGwin G, Jr. Povidone-iodine contact time and lid speculum use during intravitreal injection. Retina. 2013; 33 (5):975–981

[40] Isenberg SJ, Apt L, Yoshimori R, Khwarg S. Chemical preparation of the eye in ophthalmic surgery. IV. Comparison of povidone-iodine on the conjunctiva with a prophylactic antibiotic. Arch Ophthalmol. 1985; 103(9):1340–1342

[41] Grimes SR, Mein CE, Trevino S. Preoperative antibiotic and povidone-iodine preparation of the eye. Ann Ophthalmol. 1991; 23(7):263–266

[42] Ta CN, Egbert PR, Singh K, Shriver EM, Blumenkranz MS, Miño De Kaspar H. Prospective randomized comparison of 3-day versus 1-hour preoperative ofloxacin prophylaxis for cataract surgery. Ophthalmology. 2002; 109 (11):2036–2040, discussion 2040–2041

[43] Osher RH, Amdahl LD, Cheetham JK. Antimicrobial efficacy and aqueous humor concentration of preoperative and postoperative topical trimethoprim/polymyxin B sulfate versus tobramycin. J Cataract Refract Surg. 1994; 20(1):3–8

[44] Vasavada AR, Gajjar D, Raj SM, Vasavada V, Vasavada V. Comparison of 2 moxifloxacin regimens for preoperative prophylaxis: prospective randomized triple-masked trial. Part 2: residual conjunctival flora. J Cataract Refract Surg. 2008; 34(8):1383–1388

[45] Moss JM, Nguyen D, Liu YI, et al. Comparison of one-day versus one-hour application of topical gatifloxacin in eliminating conjunctival bacterial flora. Ophthalmology. 2008; 115(11):2013–2016

[46] Bhatt SS, Stepien KE, Joshi K. Prophylactic antibiotic use after intravitreal injection: effect on endophthalmitis rate. Retina. 2011; 31(10):2032–2036

[47] Moss JM, Sanislo SR, Ta CN. A prospective randomized evaluation of topical gatifloxacin on conjunctival flora in patients undergoing intravitreal injections. Ophthalmology. 2009; 116(8):1498–1501

[48] Cheung CS, Wong AW, Lui A, Kertes PJ, Devenyi RG, Lam WC. Incidence of endophthalmitis and use of antibiotic prophylaxis after intravitreal injections. Ophthalmology. 2012; 119(8):1609–1614

[49] Halachmi-Eyal O, Lang Y, Keness Y, Miron D. Preoperative topical moxifloxacin 0.5% and povidone-iodine 5.0% versus povidone-iodine 5.0% alone to reduce bacterial colonization in the conjunctival sac. J Cataract Refract Surg. 2009; 35(12):2109–2114

[50] Kim SJ, Toma HS. Ophthalmic antibiotics and antimicrobial resistance a randomized, controlled study of patients undergoing intravitreal injections. Ophthalmology. 2011; 118(7):1358–1363

[51] Kim SJ, Toma HS. Antimicrobial resistance and ophthalmic antibiotics: 1-year results of a longitudinal controlled study of patients undergoing intravitreal injections. Arch Ophthalmol. 2011; 129(9):1180–1188

[52] Milder E, Vander J, Shah C, Garg S. Changes in antibiotic resistance patterns of conjunctival flora due to repeated use of topical antibiotics after intravitreal injection. Ophthalmology. 2012; 119(7):1420–1424

[53] Schimel AM, Scott IU, Flynn HW, Jr. Endophthalmitis after intravitreal injections: should the use of face masks be the standard of care? Arch Ophthalmol. 2011; 129(12):1607–1609

[54] Kozak I, Cheng L, Freeman WR. Lidocaine gel anesthesia for intravitreal drug administration. Retina. 2005; 25(8):994–998

[55] Miller JJ, Scott IU, Flynn HW, Jr, Smiddy WE, Newton J, Miller D. Acute-onset endophthalmitis after cataract surgery (2000–2004): incidence, clinical settings, and visual acuity outcomes after treatment. Am J Ophthalmol. 2005; 139(6):983–987

[56] Høvding G, Sjursen H. Bacterial contamination of drops and dropper tips of in-use multidose eye drop bottles. Acta Ophthalmol (Copenh). 1982; 60 (2):213–222

[57] Moshfeghi AA, Scott IU, Flynn HW, Jr, Puliafito CA. Pseudohypopyon after intravitreal triamcinolone acetonide injection for cystoid macular edema. Am J Ophthalmol. 2004; 138(3):489–492

[58] Sutter FK, Gillies MC. Pseudo-endophthalmitis after intravitreal injection of triamcinolone. Br J Ophthalmol. 2003; 87(8):972–974

[59] Roth DB, Chieh J, Spirn MJ, Green SN, Yarian DL, Chaudhry NA. Noninfectious endophthalmitis associated with intravitreal triamcinolone injection. Arch Ophthalmol. 2003; 121(9):1279–1282

[60] Nelson ML, Tennant MT, Sivalingam A, Regillo CD, Belmont JB, Martidis A. Infectious and presumed noninfectious endophthalmitis after intravitreal triamcinolone acetonide injection. Retina. 2003; 23(5):686–691

[61] Jonas JB, Kreissig I, Degenring RF. Endophthalmitis after intravitreal injection of triamcinolone acetonide. Arch Ophthalmol. 2003; 121(11):1663–1664

38 Posterior Segment Drug Delivery

Sumit Sharma and Glenn J. Jaffe

38.1 Introduction

Posterior segment pathology can be treated with medications delivered by a variety of routes; however, the anatomy of the eye creates multiple barriers to prevent delivery of therapeutic doses of medications to the posterior segment. The blood–ocular barrier is maintained by the tight junctions of the retinal vascular endothelium, the retinal pigment epithelium (RPE), and the nonpigmented ciliary epithelium.[1] Drugs can be delivered to the posterior segment by topical drops, long-acting, slow-release conjunctival inserts, periocular injections, intravitreal injections, surgically implanted intravitreal sustained release implants, or injected intravitreal sustained release implants. In addition, various experimental techniques, based on advances in biomaterials and nanotechnology, have been developed to deliver drugs to the posterior segment. Systemic delivery is usually via oral, intramuscular, or intravenous routes. This chapter discusses the various local methods for posterior segment drug delivery excluding the intravitreal injection procedure, which is discussed in Chapter 37.

38.2 Periocular Injections

Drugs are absorbed following periocular injections by one of two ways: slow drainage from the injection site into the tear film and through the cornea or permeation across the sclera and choroid into the RPE, retina, and vitreous.[2] The amount of drug entering the eye after periocular injection is related to the ability of the drug molecule to penetrate the sclera, choroid, and RPE. Lipid-soluble molecules, such as prednisolone acetate, can be expected to penetrate the eye better than water-soluble compounds, such as tobramycin. The sclera permits the diffusion of molecules up to 70 kDa in size, while the cornea does not allow diffusion of molecules > 1kDa in size.[2] Periocular injections are a relatively inefficient delivery route; only 2 to 4% of the administered dose actually penetrates the eye.[3] However, they are an effective means of drug delivery to the posterior segment compared with systemic administration, with which a negligible percentage of drug reaches the eye.[2] In particular, lipophilic drugs, which may cause systemic toxicity, are delivered efficiently by the periocular route while limiting systemic toxicity.

Pearls

- Although the overall ocular bioavailability of drugs delivered by the periocular route is relatively low, it is still often significantly higher than when the drug is administered systemically, particularly with lipophilic compounds such as prednisolone acetate.

Periocular corticosteroid injections are given relatively commonly. Most often, they are used to treat noninfectious inflammation of the posterior segment and cystoid macular edema. The injections can be given as frequently as weekly for short periods of time, but are generally spaced much further apart. To maximize delivery to the posterior segment, injections are typically placed as posteriorly as possible in the sub-Tenon's space. Many techniques for periocular injections have been described. Either an inferotemporal or superotemporal approach can be used; however, it is felt that the superotemporal approach allows for more posterior placement of drug.[4] The superotemporal approach is associated with blepharoptosis and orbital fluocinolone acetonide prolapse. Both approaches may cause skin hypopigmentation, especially in darkly pigmented individuals, although this problem occurs more commonly with the inferotemporal approach.[5,6,7]

Pearls

- For sub-Tenon's injections, both inferior and superior approaches can be used. The latter approach, however, usually enables the injected medicine to be placed more posteriorly.

Posterior sub-Tenon's injection (PSTI) of triamcinolone has been used with excellent results to treat noninfectious anterior, intermediate, posterior, and panuveitis.[8,9,10,11,12] Multiple studies have shown that while PSTI of triamcinolone controls inflammation, the percentage of patients remaining inflammation-free decreases by 3 months; however, repeat injections can be given to achieve long-term control. Steroid-related side effects including elevated intraocular pressure (IOP) and cataract progression may limit the use of repeated injections.

Special Considerations

- The intraocular bioavailability of certain drugs administered by the periocular route may be reduced in inflamed eyes compared with noninflamed eyes.

A few initial studies that investigated PSTI of triamcinolone to treat diabetic macular edema (DME) showed promising results with improvement in visual acuity[13,14,15,16] and reduced side effects compared to intravitreal triamcinolone acetonide injection (IVTA).[17,18] The Diabetic Retinopathy Clinical Research Network (DRCR.net) performed a phase II, randomized, prospective, pilot study (Protocol E) to determine the safety and efficacy of PSTI of triamcinolone either alone or in combination with focal laser to treat mild DME. In this study, PSTI of triamcinolone was not beneficial, and was associated with adverse effects from the injections including elevated IOP and blepharoptosis.[19] This study included only patients with good visual acuity, so PSTI of triamcinolone may still be a useful adjunct for patients with diffuse DME and poor visual acuity when performed prior to grid focal laser, as has been suggested by other studies.[20,21]

The duration of effect has been found to be longer following IVTA compared to PSTI.[22,23] PSTI of triamcinolone is associated with increased IOP but the degree of IOP increase is lower than with IVTA.[24,25] Other side effects reported after PSTI of triamcinolone include reactivation of infectious retinitis,[26] cutaneous hypopigmentation,[5] retinal and choroidal vascular occlusion,[27] infectious crystalline keratopathy,[28] herpetic keratitis,[29] orbital abscess,[30,31,32] encapsulated cyst,[33] and infectious scleritis.[34]

Special Considerations

Potential adverse effects of periocular injections are as follows:

- Perforation of the globe
- Corticosteroid-induced glaucoma (prolonged with suspensions)
- Proptosis
- Fibrosis of extraocular muscles
- Allergic reaction (to the drug or vehicle)

38.3 Nonbiodegradable Implants

Nonbiodegradable sustained release implants are based on one of two designs: matrix or reservoir systems. Reservoir systems consist of a central drug core surrounded by layers of nonbiodegradable materials that are either semipermeable or impermeable.[35,36] By finely tweaking the design of the semipermeable and impermeable layers, the implant drug release rate can be controlled.[35,36] The release rate of reservoir implants is based on the surface area over which the drug is released, the thickness of the semipermeable coatings, the shape of the implant, and the ease with which the drug diffuses through the semipermeable coating. The release profile follows zero-order kinetics and is characterized by a minimal initial burst of drug release followed by constant drug release over time. In contrast, in matrix systems the drug is dispersed homogeneously within the matrix material. Drug release relies on the slow diffusion of the drug through the polymatrix material. Nonbiodegradable implants contain small amounts of drug but can produce therapeutic drug concentrations in the eye.

Drug delivery from nonbiodegradable implants generally depends on simple diffusion of the drug from the implant to the aqueous or vitreous. The vitreous is in contact with the retina, and indirectly with the choroid and sclera, the posterior chamber, and the posterior lens capsule. Drug molecules released from the implant diffuse throughout the vitreous and then move into the surrounding tissues. The vitreous concentration of any drug is dependent on the implant release rate, the volume of the posterior segment, intravitreal metabolism, and the drug elimination rate through the surrounding tissues. The ocular distribution volume is determined by the size of the eye, the amount of protein in the eye, and the lipophilicity of the surrounding tissues. Furthermore, despite its high water content, drug molecules are not distributed uniformly through the vitreous because the local concentration gradient is influenced by different elimination rates through each boundary tissue.[37]

Depending on drug solubility, the implant configuration, and polymeric coatings, nonbiodegradable drug delivery implants can be designed to release drug over extended time periods. Because of this long release duration, nonbiodegradable sustained release implants are particularly suitable for treating chronic conditions such as glaucoma, cytomegalovirus retinitis, age-related macular degeneration (AMD), diabetes, and uveitis.[35,38,39,40,41]

Two different sustained release fluocinolone acetonide implants have been approved for the treatment of ocular diseases: a nonbioerodable, extended release, implantable fluocinolone acetonide device (Retisert, Bausch and Lomb) which must be surgically implanted in the operating room (▸ Fig. 38.1) and a much smaller, nonbioerodable, injectable fluocinolone acetonide insert (Iluvien, Alimera) which can be injected in the outpatient clinic. The fluocinolone acetonide implant is currently approved in the United States for the

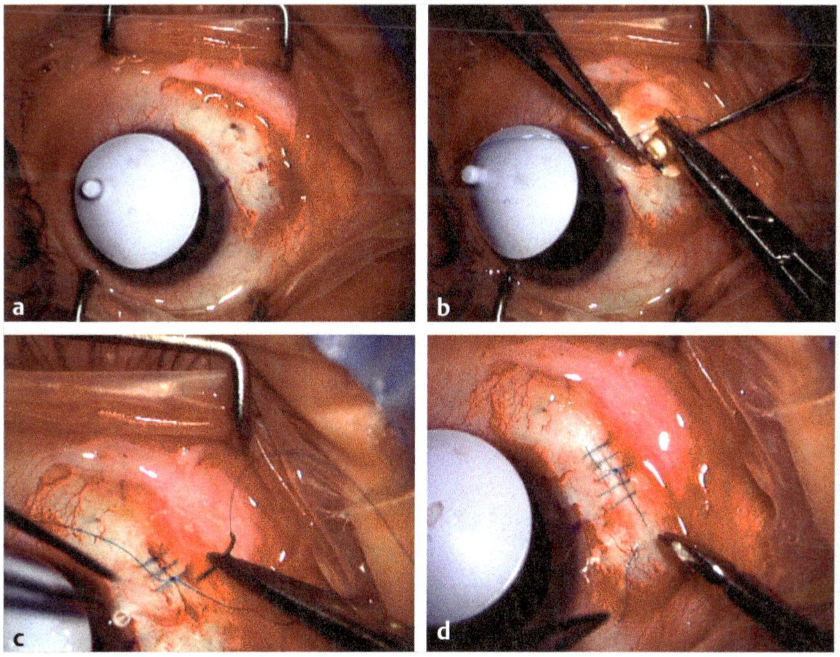

Fig. 38.1 Intravitreal implant surgical technique. **(a)** A 3.5-mm circumferential, full-thickness incision is made with a microvitreoretinal blade 3.75 mm posterior to the limbus. (Care is taken to incise the pars plana epithelium over the length of the incision.) **(b)** The implant is grasped with nontoothed forceps or needle holder and placed in the eye. (Previously, a double-armed 8–0 nylon suture was placed through the implant anchoring strut.) **(c)** The implant is secured to the sclera with full-thickness bites from the double-armed 8–0 polypropylene suture. The wound is then closed with interrupted 9–0 polypropylene sutures tied over the tails of the anchoring sutures. **(d)** The 8–0 suture is then trimmed short, at the edge of the furthest 9–0 suture, so that it rests flat on the sclera. The conjunctiva is then closed over the implant; Tenon's capsule may be closed as a separate layer to ensure the implant is well covered and the sutures do not erode through the conjunctiva.

treatment of noninfectious posterior uveitis.[42] The fluocinolone acetonide insert is approved for the treatment of DME in the United States and in certain countries in Europe.[43]

The surgically placed fluocinolone acetonide implant releases 0.59 µg/day of fluocinolone acetonide over 3 years.[42] This system provides constant drug release and thereby avoids the peak and trough effect of steroid solutions injected into the vitreous or by bioerodable implants. The fluocinolone acetonide implant has been used to treat severe uveitis refractory to conventional systemic immunosuppression and periocular steroid injections. A multicenter, randomized, dose-masked clinical trial was conducted to determine the safety and efficacy of a sustained release fluocinolone acetonide intravitreal implant in patients with posterior segment uveitis.[44] The fluocinolone acetonide implant reduced the aggregate recurrence rate for the implanted eyes from 51.4% in the 34 weeks preceding implantation to 6.1% postimplantation ($p < 0.0001$) in the study eyes, while there was a significant increase in the nonimplanted eye recurrence rate. Adjunctive therapy use was also significantly decreased postimplantation. The multicenter uveitis steroid treatment (MUST) trial randomized patients with intermediate, posterior, or panuveitis to the fluocinolone acetonide implant or corticosteroids plus systemic immunosuppression to evaluate the change in best-corrected visual acuity as the main outcome measure. While there was not a statistically significant difference in the improvement of visual acuity between the two groups, there was a trend towards better visual acuity in the fluocinolone acetonide implant group.[45] The implant group was found to have greater improvement in vision-related quality of life, lower rates of residual active uveitis, and lower rates of prescription requiring systemic infections. The most common serious adverse events observed by 2 years after placement of the fluocinolone acetonide implant were cataract progression requiring cataract extraction (80%), elevation of IOP by more than 10 mm Hg from baseline (65%), and filtering procedures (26%).[45,46] In this difficult-to-treat patient population, the fluocinolone acetonide implant controlled inflammation and was associated with visual acuity improvement in a significant proportion of the eyes studied; however, because of the fluocinolone implant's effect on IOP and lens clarity, these patients must be closely monitored in the postoperative period.

Pearls

- When replacing a previously placed bioerodable implant, the implant can separate from the strut which is sutured to the sclera. Care must be taken to ensure that both are removed from the eye. Using a posterior segment infusion can help "float" the implant out of the eye.

The fluocinolone acetonide implant has also been investigated to treat DME. A 4-year, randomized, prospective study of the fluocinolone acetonide implant versus additional laser in cases of persistent DME, despite focal laser 12 weeks prior to study entry, met the primary end point of a greater than 15 letter visual acuity gain at 6 months. The study also met the secondary end points of reduced central macular thickness and diabetic retinopathy severity score.[47] However, side effects were common, most notably cataract that required extraction in 91% of phakic patients, elevated IOP greater than 30 in 61.4% of eyes, and elevated IOP that required surgery in 33.8%. Because the implant requires placement in the operating room and causes a high incidence of IOP elevation requiring surgical intervention, there has been limited use of this implant in routine clinical practice to treat DME.

The injectable fluocinolone acetonide insert releases 0.2 or 0.5 µg/day of fluocinolone acetonide over 3 years[48] and is injected with a modified needle system. The ocular drug delivery rate for both doses peaks at 1 week and remains at that level for 2 months prior to declining to a steady state level for at least 12 months.[48] In two randomized, prospective, sham injection–controlled trials evaluating the efficacy and safety of the injectable 0.2- and 0.5-µg fluocinolone acetonide inserts, both doses met the primary study end point; 28% of eyes achieved a greater than 15 letter gain in visual acuity compared to 16% in the sham group.[49] At 2 years, the mean improvement in visual acuity was 4.4 and 5.4 letters for the 0.2 and 0.5 µg doses, respectively, compared to 1.7 letters for sham. The rate of incisional glaucoma surgery was 3.7 and 7.6% for the 0.2 and 0.5 µg doses, respectively. The results at 3 years were similar.[43] Nearly all phakic eyes required surgery by 3 years. In a subgroup analysis, the low-dose (0.2 µg) insert was found to be more effective for patients with DME of greater than 3 years' duration compared to those with DME of less than 3 years' duration.[50] This finding is significant as it represents a treatment option for patients with DME that is recalcitrant to other treatment options.

38.4 Biodegradable Implants

Biodegradable implants are useful as they do not need to be explanted and have increased flexibility in their shape. These implants are typically composed of polymers such as polylactic acid, polyglycolic acid, and polylactic-co-glycolic acid (PLGA) that allow dissolution of the implant and release of the biologically active drug over time. These materials are biocompatible, are widely used as suture materials, surgical scaffolds, bone screws, and vascular grafts, and have been repurposed to surround biologically active molecules and function as biodegradable implants. The rate of drug release from biodegradable implants depends on the total surface area of the implant, the percentage of loaded drug, the water solubility of the drug, and the speed of polymer degradation.[51] There are typically three phases of drug release from these materials: an initial burst from the implant surface, a diffusion phase as the implant is degraded, and a final burst when the implant disintegrates.

The dexamethasone implant (Ozurdex, Allergan, Inc) is a dexamethasone-containing intravitreal implant coated in PLGA and is approved by Food and Drug Administration (FDA) to treat DME, cystoid macular edema resulting from branch or central retinal vein occlusion, and noninfectious uveitis. The implant contains 0.7 mg of dexamethasone and is injected through the sclera into the eye in clinic with a preloaded single-use injector. It releases steroid into the vitreous cavity for approximately 6 months with peak concentrations in the first 2 months.[52] In a study that used optical coherence tomography–based monitoring of central macular thickness to determine the ideal retreatment interval after injection of the dexamethasone implant, there was a rapid and dramatic effect on macular edema for about 8 weeks and a modest effect up to week 32; the ideal retreatment point was felt to be week 20.[53]

A 26-week multicenter, randomized, prospective clinical trial evaluated the safety and efficacy of two different doses of the dexamethasone implant (0.7 and 0.35 mg) in noninfectious intermediate or posterior uveitis. In this trial, the number of eyes with no vitreous inflammation at 8 weeks was 47, 36, and 12% for the 0.7 mg, 0.35 mg, and sham treatment groups, respectively.[54] The percentage of eyes with IOP greater than 25 was 7.1, 8.7, and 4.2% for the 0.7 mg, 0.35 mg, and sham treatment groups, respectively.[54] Two large, randomized, prospective clinical trials evaluated the safety and efficacy of the dexamethasone implant when compared to sham, to treat DME. The percentage of eyes that met the primary end point of greater than 15 letter improvement in vision was 22.2, 18.4, and 12.0% for the 0.7 mg, 0.35 mg, and sham treatment groups, respectively.[55] A mean of approximately four treatments were needed during the 3 years of the trial. The mean reduction in central macular thickness was similar (~110 µm) in the two dexamethasone implant groups and was significantly less in the sham treatment group (~40 µm). Over three times as many eyes developed cataracts after the dexamethasone implant compared to sham. An IOP increase of > 10 mm Hg from baseline was observed in 27.7 and 24.8% eyes treated with the 0.7 and 0.35 mg doses, respectively. This elevated IOP was controlled with medications or monitoring in most cases; trabeculectomy was performed in two eyes treated with the 0.7 mg dose and one eye treated with the 0.35 mg dose. Similar results were found in a study that evaluated the dexamethasone implant to treat eyes with either branch or central retinal vein occlusion.[56] The results from these trials led the FDA to approve the 0.7 mg dexamethasone implant for use in DME, noninfectious uveitis, and cystoid macular edema due to branch or central retinal vein occlusion. It has been suggested that sustained low-dose release of corticosteroid into the vitreous may be more efficacious compared to higher bolus doses seen after IVTA injection.[57] Despite the larger gauge and use of a tunneled incision, dexamethasone implant injection was not found to be more painful than anti-VEGF injection.[58]

Aphakic and pseudophakic eyes are at risk of anterior migration of the dexamethasone implant, and vitrectomized eyes are at much higher risk of this complication than nonvitrectomized eyes.[59,60,61,62] Anterior migration of the implant is associated with corneal decompensation, pain, elevated IOP, and misidentification as a hypopyon. Fortunately, the implant can often be surgically repositioned into the vitreous cavity, but in selected cases, surgery may be required to remove the displaced implant. The dexamethasone implant has also been trapped anterior to the anterior hyaloid face, and between the posterior capsule and a silicon oil bubble. In both of these cases, the implant relocated spontaneously to the inferior vitreous cavity without any other complications.[63,64] Fragmentation of the implant has occurred during injection or shortly thereafter; fortunately, this event does not change the rate or duration of ocular drug delivery.[65,66,67,68] Inadvertent injection of the dexamethasone implant into the crystalline lens can be managed safely and successfully by standard cataract extraction with phacoemulsification.[69,70]

Special Considerations

- Vitrectomy and lensectomy both greatly decrease the half-life of intraocular drugs, regardless of their primary route of elimination from the eye. Ocular inflammation, however, can either increase or decrease the rate of elimination, depending on the specific drug and transport mechanism at hand.

38.4.1 Encapsulated Cell Technology

The encapsulated cell technology (ECT) system is a surgically placed polymeric implant containing a viable, immortalized, genetically modified human RPE cell line designed to overproduce a therapeutic protein. There are several advantages to the use of ECT: it offers the potential for any gene encoding a therapeutic protein to be engineered into a cell, the therapeutic protein is freshly synthesized and released in vivo, the availability of the protein in the eye can be continuous and long term, and the output of an ECT implant can be controlled to achieve the ideal dose for treatment. Thus, ECT may offer an effective means of sustained long-term delivery of proteins and polypeptides to the vitreous, retina, and choroid.

ECT has been used in the NT-501 implant (Renexus, Neurotech Pharmaceuticals, Inc.), which secretes ciliary neurotrophic factor (CNTF).[71,72] The NT-501 implant (▶ Fig. 38.2) is 1 mm in diameter and 6 mm long, and consists of a semipermeable polymer outer membrane with a titanium anchor at one end to facilitate suturing to the sclera and contains an internal polyethylene scaffold that supports human cells. It is surrounded by a capsule that allows nutrients and therapeutic molecules to diffuse freely across the membrane while preventing immune cell entry.[71,73] The implant is surgically implanted through a 2.0-mm sclerotomy through the pars plana and anchored with a single suture. The wound is closed with additional sutures. NT-501 is being investigated for the potential treatment of all stages of retinitis pigmentosa (RP) and geographic atrophy (GA) in nonneovascular AMD.[74] In a 2-year clinical trial, two versions of the implant, each secreting different amounts of CNTF, produced CNTF consistently over the 2-year period and had clinically viable cells throughout the 2 years of the study. Antibodies to the encapsulated cells and anti-CNTF antibodies were not detected in any of the patients.[74] While this study demonstrated long-term stability of the ECT implant for production of CNTF, further studies evaluating the efficacy of CNTF in the treatment of RP and AMD-associated GA are ongoing. Phase II, dose escalation studies of an anti-VEGF producing ECT implant, NT-503, have been completed in subjects with neovascular AMD. In these studies, the implant, which produces a soluble VEGF receptor protein similar to VEGF-trap for at least 2 years, was associated with sustained visual acuity gains and reduced central foveal thickness.[75] Additional modifications to the design of the device have augmented the total dose of drug produced by the implant.[75]

38.4.2 Implantable Sustained Release Drug Reservoirs

Implantable drug pumps have promise in the treatment of ocular disease but face multiple challenges: They require

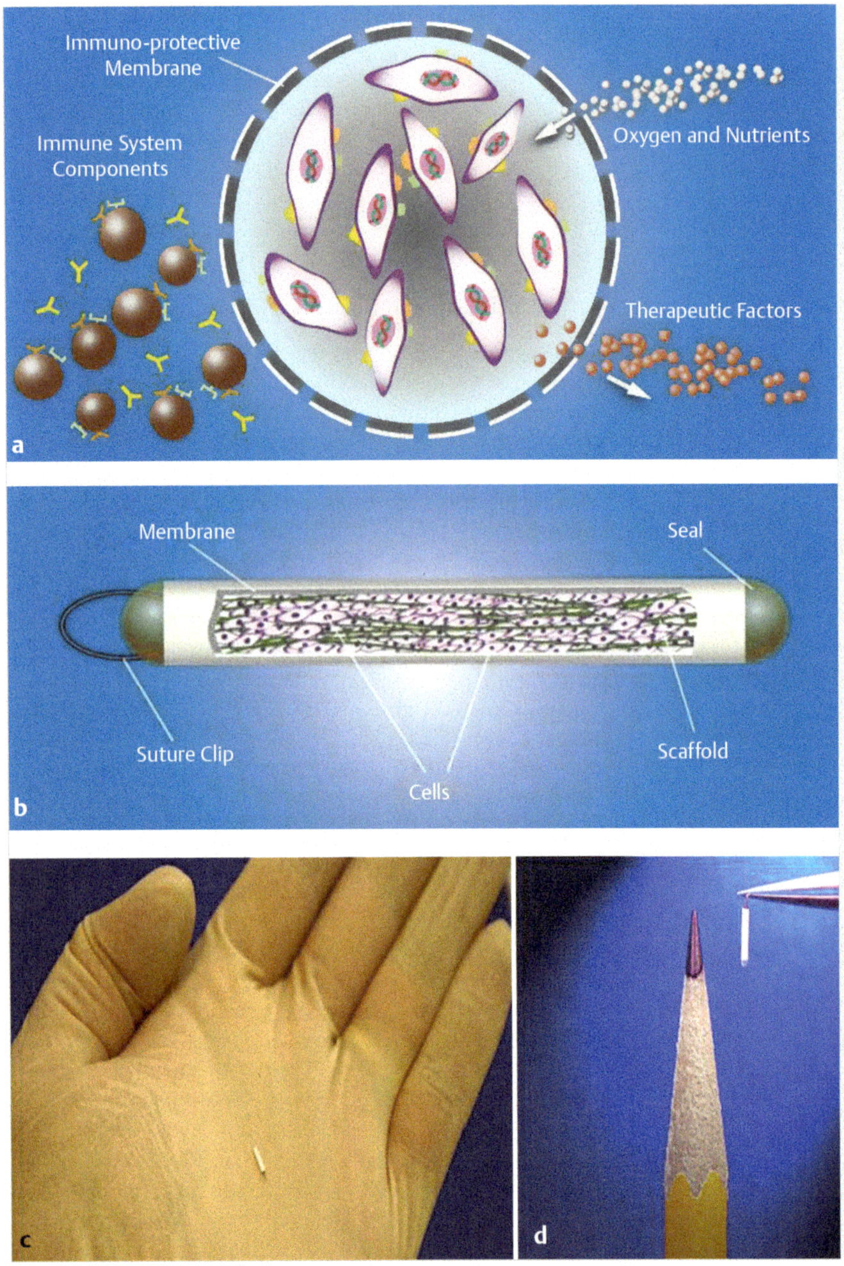

Fig. 38.2 Encapsulated cell technology implant. (**a**) semipermeable polymer outer membrane with (**b**) a titanium anchor at one end facilitates suturing to the sclera and contains an internal polyethylene scaffold that supports human cells. It is surrounded by a capsule that allows nutrients and therapeutic molecules to diffuse freely across the membrane while preventing immune cell entry. (**c,d**) The implant compared to a pencil tip.

miniaturization to allow for successful implantation around the eye, must contain drugs that are very potent with microdosing, and need to be programmable and refillable in a minimally invasive manner. Microelectromechanical system technology has been used in the Posterior MicroPump Drug Delivery System (PMP; Replenish, Inc). This system has been implanted in humans and delivers drug microdoses into the vitreous cavity.[76] The PMP (▶ Fig. 38.3) consists of five components: electronics in a hermetically sealed package that power the device and control drug delivery, a drug reservoir capable of storing 60 µL of drug, a one-way check valve, a refill port that can be accessed transconjunctivally with a 31-gauge needle, and an intraocular cannula through which drug is released.[77] The PMP is implanted in a manner similar to that used to implant a glaucoma drainage device and can be performed under peribulbar anesthesia. The port of the device is inserted into the vitreous cavity through the pars plana and the remainder of the implant rests subconjunctivally. A telemetry system wirelessly connects to the PMP to receive pump functionality information and to control drug delivery rate. The first human safety studies of the PMP found the implant was viable for 90 days, capable of delivering microdoses into the vitreous cavity, and demonstrated a trend toward efficacy, although the study was not powered to detect efficacy.[76] A 1-year feasibility study in dogs showed that the implant was well tolerated over this time period and paves the way for further studies in humans.[78]

Genentech has secured the exclusive worldwide rights for the proprietary, nonbiodegradable, refillable port delivery system (PDS-1.0) developed by ForSight VISION4 (ForSight Labs, LLC) to be used for sustained delivery of ranibizumab (Genentech).[79] This system Artist's rendering is surgically implanted under the conjunctiva with standard surgical techniques through a 3.2-mm scleral incision through the pars plana (▶ Fig. 38.4). No scleral sutures are needed. The implant is preloaded with a

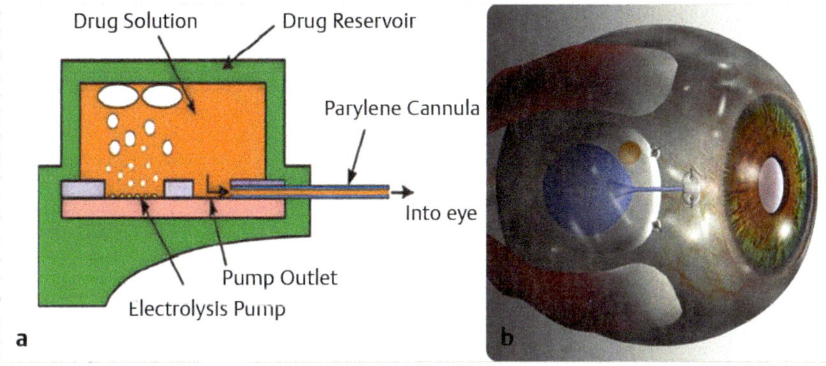

Fig. 38.3 (a) Schematic of Replenish MicroPump showing the drug reservoir filled with drug solution being drawn into the electrolysis pump and inserted into the eye through the parylene cannula. (b) Artist's rendering of the micropump resting on the sclera with the cannula inserted into the eye.

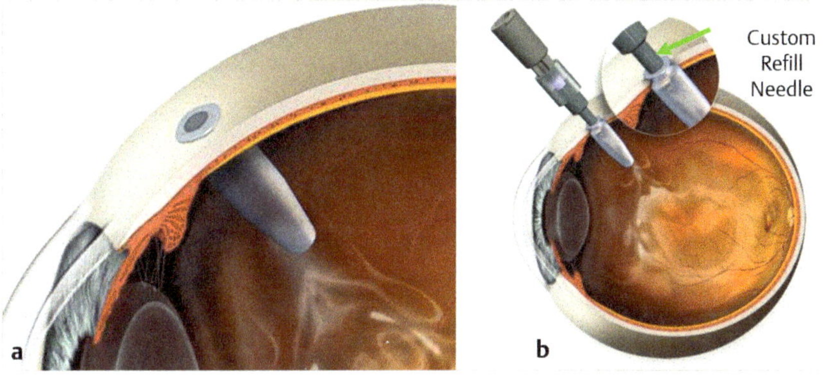

Fig. 38.4 (a) Port Delivery System implant resting in the sclera without sutures. (b) Artist's rendering of custom refill needle being used to refill the implant.

concentrated ranibizumab formulation and is refilled every 4 to 6 months in a minimally invasive office procedure and delivers a constant dose of drug in between refills. A preliminary, phase I, safety and efficacy trial was recently completed and phase II studies are underway.[80]

References

[1] Sasaki H, Yamamura K, Mukai T, et al. Enhancement of ocular drug penetration. Crit Rev Ther Drug Carrier Syst. 1999; 16(1):85–146

[2] Raghava S, Hammond M, Kompella UB. Periocular routes for retinal drug delivery. Expert Opin Drug Deliv. 2004; 1(1):99–114

[3] Kovacs K, Wagley S, Quirk MT, et al. Pharmacokinetic study of vitreous and serum concentrations of triamcinolone acetonide after posterior sub-tenon's injection. Am J Ophthalmol. 2012; 153(5):939–948

[4] Nussenblatt RB, Whitcup SM. Philosophy, goals and approaches to medical therapy. In Nussenblatt RB, Whitcup SM, eds. Uveitis: fundamentals and clinical practice. 3rd ed. Philadelphia, PA: Mosby;2004:95–136

[5] Gallardo MJ, Johnson DA. Cutaneous hypopigmentation following a posterior sub-tenon triamcinolone injection. Am J Ophthalmol. 2004; 137(4):779–780

[6] Dal Canto AJ, Downs-Kelly E, Perry JD. Ptosis and orbital fat prolapse after posterior sub-Tenon's capsule triamcinolone injection. Ophthalmology. 2005; 112:1092–1097

[7] Ferrante P, Ramsey A, Bunce C, Lightman S. Clinical trial to compare efficacy and side-effects of injection of posterior sub-Tenon triamcinolone versus orbital floor methylprednisolone in the management of posterior uveitis. Clin Experiment Ophthalmol. 2004; 32(6):563–568

[8] Sen HN, Vitale S, Gangaputra SS, et al. Periocular corticosteroid injections in uveitis: effects and complications. Ophthalmology. 2014; 121(11):2275–2286

[9] Salek SS, Leder HA, Butler NJ, Gan TJ, Dunn JP, Thorne JE. Periocular triamcinolone acetonide injections for control of intraocular inflammation associated with uveitis. Ocul Immunol Inflamm. 2013; 21(4):257–263

[10] Leder HA, Jabs DA, Galor A, Dunn JP, Thorne JE. Periocular triamcinolone acetonide injections for cystoid macular edema complicating noninfectious uveitis. Am J Ophthalmol. 2011; 152(3):441–448.e2

[11] Sajnani D. Posterior sub-Tenon's triamcinolone injections in the treatment of uveitis. Eye (Lond). 1999; 13(Pt 5):703–704

[12] Tanner V, Kanski JJ, Frith PA. Posterior sub-Tenon's triamcinolone injections in the treatment of uveitis. Eye (Lond). 1998; 12(Pt 4):679–685

[13] Verma LK, Vivek MB, Kumar A, Tewari HK, Venkatesh P. A prospective controlled trial to evaluate the adjunctive role of posterior subtenon triamcinolone in the treatment of diffuse diabetic macular edema. J Ocul Pharmacol Ther. 2004; 20(4):277–284

[14] Bakri SJ, Kaiser PK. Posterior subtenon triamcinolone acetonide for refractory diabetic macular edema. Am J Ophthalmol. 2005; 139(2):290–294

[15] Entezari M, Ahmadieh H, Dehghan MH, Ramezani A, Bassirnia N, Anissian A. Posterior sub-tenon triamcinolone for refractory diabetic macular edema: a randomized clinical trial. Eur J Ophthalmol. 2005; 15(6):746–750

[16] Javadzadeh A. The effect of posterior subtenon methylprednisolone acetate in the refractory diabetic macular edema: a prospective nonrandomized interventional case series. BMC Ophthalmol. 2006; 6:15

[17] Choi YJ, Oh IK, Oh JR, Huh K. Intravitreal versus posterior subtenon injection of triamcinolone acetonide for diabetic macular edema. Korean J Ophthalmol. 2006; 20(4):205–209

[18] Ozdek S, Bahçeci UA, Gürelik G, Hasanreisoglu B. Posterior subtenon and intravitreal triamcinolone acetonide for diabetic macular edema. J Diabetes Complications. 2006; 20(4):246–251

[19] Chew E, Strauber S, Beck R, et al. Diabetic Retinopathy Clinical Research Network. Randomized trial of peribulbar triamcinolone acetonide with and without focal photocoagulation for mild diabetic macular edema: a pilot study. Ophthalmology. 2007; 114(6):1190–1196

[20] Shimura M, Nakazawa T, Yasuda K, Shiono T, Nishida K. Pretreatment of posterior subtenon injection of triamcinolone acetonide has beneficial effects for grid pattern photocoagulation against diffuse diabetic macular oedema. Br J Ophthalmol. 2007; 91(4):449–454

[21] Chung EJ, Freeman WR, Azen SP, Lee H, Koh HJ. Comparison of combination posterior sub-tenon triamcinolone and modified grid laser treatment with intravitreal triamcinolone treatment in patients with diffuse diabetic macular edema. Yonsei Med J. 2008; 49(6):955–964

[22] Yalcinbayir O, Gelisken O, Kaderli B, Avci R. Intravitreal versus sub-tenon posterior triamcinolone injection in bilateral diffuse diabetic macular edema. Ophthalmologica. 2011; 225(4):222–227

[23] Nan K, Sun S, Li Y, et al. Characterisation of systemic and ocular drug level of triamcinolone acetonide following a single sub-Tenon injection. Br J Ophthalmol. 2010; 94(5):654–658
[24] Iwao K, Inatani M, Kawaji T, et al. Frequency and risk factors for intraocular pressure elevation after posterior sub-Tenon capsule triamcinolone acetonide injection. J Glaucoma. 2007; 16:251–256
[25] Hirano Y, Ito T, Nozaki M, et al. Intraocular pressure elevation following triamcinolone acetonide administration as related to administration routes. Jpn J Ophthalmol. 2009; 53(5):519–522
[26] Yamamoto Y, Kato Y, Tabuchi H, Fukushima A. Case of cytomegalovirus retinitis aggravated by sub-Tenon injection of triamcinolone acetonide with subsequent metastatic liver cancer. Clin Ophthalmol. 2013; 7:411–415
[27] Moshfeghi DM, Lowder CY, Roth DB, Kaiser PK. Retinal and choroidal vascular occlusion after posterior sub-tenon triamcinolone injection. Am J Ophthalmol. 2002; 134(1):132–134
[28] Hollander DA, Clay EL, Sidikaro Y. Infectious crystalline keratopathy associated with intravitreal and posterior sub-Tenon triamcinolone acetonide injections. Br J Ophthalmol. 2006; 90(5):656
[29] Hashizume K, Nabeshima T, Fujiwara T, Machida S, Kurosaka D. A case of herpetic epithelial keratitis after triamcinolone acetonide subtenon injection. Cornea. 2009; 28(4):463–464
[30] Azarbod P, Mohammed Q, Akram I, Moorman C. Localised abscess following an injection of subtenon triamcinolone acitonide. Eye (Lond). 2007; 21 (5):672–674
[31] Engelman CJ, Palmer JD, Egbert P. Orbital abscess following subtenon triamcinolone injection. Arch Ophthalmol. 2004; 122(4):654–655
[32] Kusaka S, Ikuno Y, Ohguro N, Hori Y, Tano Y. Orbital infection following posterior subtenon triamcinolone injection. Acta Ophthalmol Scand. 2007; 85 (6):692–693
[33] Chan CK, Mohamed S, Tang EW, Shanmugam MP, Chan NR, Lam DS. Encapsulated triamcinolone cyst after subtenon injection. Clin Experiment Ophthalmol. 2006; 34(4):360–362
[34] Gharaee H, Khalife M, Poor SS, Abrishami M. Infectious scleritis after subtenon triamcinolone acetonide injection. Ocul Immunol Inflamm. 2011; 19 (4):284–285
[35] Ashton P, Blandford DL, Pearson PA, Jaffe GJ, Martin DF, Nussenblatt RB. Review: implants. J Ocul Pharmacol. 1994; 10(4):691–701
[36] Jaffe GJ, Yang CH, Guo H, Denny JP, Lima C, Ashton P. Safety and pharmacokinetics of an intraocular fluocinolone acetonide sustained delivery device. Invest Ophthalmol Vis Sci. 2000; 41(11):3569–3575
[37] Tojo K, Isowaki A. Pharmacokinetic model for in vivo/in vitro correlation of intravitreal drug delivery. Adv Drug Deliv Rev. 2001; 52(1):17–24
[38] Musch DC, Martin DF, Gordon JF, Davis MD, Kuppermann BD, The Ganciclovir Implant Study Group. Treatment of cytomegalovirus retinitis with a sustained-release ganciclovir implant. N Engl J Med. 1997; 337(2):83–90
[39] Jaffe GJ, Yang CS, Wang XC, Cousins SW, Gallemore RP, Ashton P. Intravitreal sustained-release cyclosporine in the treatment of experimental uveitis. Ophthalmology. 1998; 105(1):46–56
[40] Jaffe GJ, Ben-Nun J, Guo H, Dunn JP, Ashton P. Fluocinolone acetonide sustained drug delivery device to treat severe uveitis. Ophthalmology. 2000; 107 (11):2024–2033
[41] Gooch N, Molokhia SA, Condie R, et al. Ocular drug delivery for glaucoma management. Pharmaceutics. 2012; 4(1):197–211
[42] Callanan DG, Jaffe GJ, Martin DF, Pearson PA, Comstock TL. Treatment of posterior uveitis with a fluocinolone acetonide implant: three-year clinical trial results. Arch Ophthalmol. 2008; 126(9):1191–1201
[43] Campochiaro PA, Brown DM, Pearson A, et al. FAME Study Group. Sustained delivery fluocinolone acetonide vitreous inserts provide benefit for at least 3 years in patients with diabetic macular edema. Ophthalmology. 2012; 119 (10):2125–2132
[44] Jaffe GJ, Martin D, Callanan D, Pearson PA, Levy B, Comstock T, Fluocinolone Acetonide Uveitis Study Group. Fluocinolone acetonide implant (Retisert) for noninfectious posterior uveitis: thirty-four-week results of a multicenter randomized clinical study. Ophthalmology. 2006; 113(6):1020–1027
[45] Kempen JH, Altaweel MM, Holbrook JT, et al. Multicenter Uveitis Steroid Treatment (MUST) Trial Research Group. Randomized comparison of systemic anti-inflammatory therapy versus fluocinolone acetonide implant for intermediate, posterior, and panuveitis: the multicenter uveitis steroid treatment trial. Ophthalmology. 2011; 118(10):1916–1926
[46] Friedman DS, Holbrook JT, Ansari H, et al. MUST Research Group. Risk of elevated intraocular pressure and glaucoma in patients with uveitis: results of the multicenter uveitis steroid treatment trial. Ophthalmology. 2013; 120 (8):1571–1579
[47] Pearson PA, Comstock TL, Ip M, et al. Fluocinolone acetonide intravitreal implant for diabetic macular edema: a 3-year multicenter, randomized, controlled clinical trial. Ophthalmology. 2011; 118(8):1580–1587
[48] Campochiaro PA, Hafiz G, Shah SM, et al. Famous Study Group. Sustained ocular delivery of fluocinolone acetonide by an intravitreal insert. Ophthalmology. 2010; 117(7):1393–9.e3
[49] Campochiaro PA, Brown DM, Pearson A, et al. FAME Study Group. Long-term benefit of sustained-delivery fluocinolone acetonide vitreous inserts for diabetic macular edema. Ophthalmology. 2011; 118(4):626–635.e2
[50] Cunha-Vaz J, Ashton P, Iezzi R, et al. FAME Study Group. Sustained delivery fluocinolone acetonide vitreous implants: long-term benefit in patients with chronic diabetic macular edema. Ophthalmology. 2014; 121(10):1892–1903
[51] Shive MS, Anderson JM. Biodegradation and biocompatibility of PLA and PLGA microspheres. Adv Drug Deliv Rev. 1997; 28(1):5–24
[52] Chang-Lin JE, Attar M, Acheampong AA, et al. Pharmacokinetics and pharmacodynamics of a sustained-release dexamethasone intravitreal implant. Invest Ophthalmol Vis Sci. 2011; 52(1):80–86
[53] Mathew R, Pearce E, Muniraju R, Abdel-Hay A, Sivaprasad S. Monthly OCT monitoring of Ozurdex for macular oedema related to retinal vascular diseases: re-treatment strategy (OCTOME Report 1). Eye (Lond). 2014; 28 (3):318–326
[54] Lowder C, Belfort R, Jr, Lightman S, et al. Ozurdex HURON Study Group. Dexamethasone intravitreal implant for noninfectious intermediate or posterior uveitis. Arch Ophthalmol. 2011; 129(5):545–553
[55] Boyer DS, Yoon YH, Belfort R, Jr, et al. Ozurdex MEAD Study Group. Three-year, randomized, sham-controlled trial of dexamethasone intravitreal implant in patients with diabetic macular edema. Ophthalmology. 2014; 121 (10):1904–1914
[56] Haller JA, Bandello F, Belfort R, Jr, et al. OZURDEX GENEVA Study Group. Randomized, sham-controlled trial of dexamethasone intravitreal implant in patients with macular edema due to retinal vein occlusion. Ophthalmology. 2010; 117(6):1134–1146.e3
[57] Yilmaz T, Cordero-Coma M, Lavaque AJ, Gallagher MJ, Padula WV. Triamcinolone and intraocular sustained-release delivery systems in diabetic retinopathy. Curr Pharm Biotechnol. 2011; 12(3):337–346
[58] Moisseiev E, Regenbogen M, Rabinovitch T, Barak A, Loewenstein A, Goldstein M. Evaluation of pain during intravitreal Ozurdex injections vs. intravitreal bevacizumab injections. Eye (Lond). 2014; 28(8):980–985
[59] Khurana RN, Appa SN, McCannel CA, et al. Dexamethasone implant anterior chamber migration: risk factors, complications, and management strategies. Ophthalmology. 2014; 121:67–71
[60] Kishore SA, Schaal S. Management of anterior chamber dislocation of dexamethasone implant. Ocul Immunol Inflamm. 2013; 21(1):90–91
[61] Collet B. Management of ozurdex in the anterior chamber. JAMA Ophthalmol. 2013; 131(12):1651–1652
[62] Vela JI, Crespí J, Andreu D. Repositioning of dexamethasone intravitreal implant (Ozurdex) migrated into the anterior chamber. Int Ophthalmol. 2012; 32(6):583–584
[63] Wai Ch'ng S, Padroni S, Banerjee S. Anterior vitreous displacement of the intravitreal dexamethasone implant (Ozurdex). Eye (Lond). 2014; 28(2):238–239
[64] Banerjee PJ, Petrou P, Zvobgo TM, Charteris DG. Spontaneous relocation of a trapped retrolenticular slow-release dexamethasone implant (Ozurdex) in a silicone oil-filled eye of a pseudophakic patient. Eye (Lond). 2014; 28 (8):1036–1037
[65] Agrawal R, Fernandez-Sanz G, Bala S, Addison PK. Desegmentation of Ozurdex implant in vitreous cavity: report of two cases. Br J Ophthalmol. 2014; 98 (7):961–963
[66] Rishi P, Mathur G, Rishi E. Fractured Ozurdex™ implant in the vitreous cavity. Indian J Ophthalmol. 2012; 60(4):337–338
[67] Roy R, Hegde S. Split Ozurdex implant: a caution. Can J Ophthalmol. 2013; 48 (1):e15–e16
[68] Donmez O, Parlak M, Yaman A, Saatci AO. Splitting of a dexamethasone implant (Ozurdex) following the Injection. Case Rep Ophthalmol Med. 2013; 2013:247949
[69] Berarducci A, Sian IS, Ling R. Inadvertent dexamethasone implant injection into the lens body management. Eur J Ophthalmol. 2014; 24(4):620–622
[70] Coca-Robinot J, Casco-Silva B, Armadá-Maresca F, García-Martínez J. Accidental injections of dexamethasone intravitreal implant (Ozurdex) into the crystalline lens. Eur J Ophthalmol. 2014; 24(4):633–636
[71] Emerich DF, Thanos CG. NT-501: an ophthalmic implant of polymer-encapsulated ciliary factor-producing cells. Curr Opin Mol Ther. 2008; 10:506–515

[72] Dunn KC, Aotaki-Keen AE, Putkey FR, Hjelmeland LM. ARPE-19, a human retinal pigment epithelial cell line with differentiated properties. Exp Eye Res. 1996; 62(2):155–169

[73] Sieving PA, Caruso RC, Tao W, et al. Ciliary neurotrophic factor (CNTF) for human retinal degeneration: phase I trial of CNTF delivered by encapsulated cell intraocular implants. Proc Natl Acad Sci U S A. 2006; 103:3896–3901

[74] Kauper K, McGovern C, Sherman S, et al. Two-year intraocular delivery of ciliary neurotrophic factor by encapsulated cell technology implants in patients with chronic retinal degenerative diseases. Invest Ophthalmol Vis Sci. 2012; 53:7484–7491

[75] Neurotech Pharmaceuticals. Treating the symptoms of wet AMD. NT-503. 2015

[76] Humayun M, Santos A, Altamirano JC, et al. Implantable MicroPump for drug delivery in patients with diabetic macular edema. Transl Vis Sci Technol. 2014; 3(6):5

[77] Saati S, Lo R, Li PY, Meng E, Varma R, Humayun MS. Mini drug pump for ophthalmic use. Curr Eye Res. 2010; 35(3):192–201

[78] Gutiérrez-Hernández JC, Caffey S, Abdallah W, et al. One-year feasibility study of replenish MicroPump for intravitreal drug delivery: a pilot study. Transl Vis Sci Technol. 2014; 3(4):8

[79] Genentech. Genentech announces first milestone payment to device-maker ForSight VISION4, Inc. in development of sustained delivery lucentis. 2012

[80] ClinicalTrials.gov. Preliminary safety and efficacy of the PDS-1.0 in patients with neovascular age related macular degeneration (AMD). 2015

39 Laser for Vitreoretinal Diseases

Yannis M. Paulus and Mark S. Blumenkranz

Retinal laser therapy was developed more than 50 years ago and has had a profound and lasting impact on the treatment of numerous vitreoretinal and choroidal disorders. Since the introduction of the ruby laser in 1960,[1] the safety and efficacy of retinal lasers have been investigated in several large clinical trials. Significant advances have been achieved in laser technology and the molecular understanding of laser–tissue interactions to minimize collateral tissue damage while retaining the therapeutic effects of laser therapy. This chapter gives a brief history of retinal lasers, discusses the science behind lasers and laser–tissue interactions, reviews delivery systems and current clinical applications and trials evaluating lasers, and discusses promising recent innovations in retinal laser therapy. The important clinical role of lasers is highlighted in proliferative diabetic retinopathy (PDR), diabetic macular edema (DME), central retinal vein occlusions (CRVOs), branch retinal vein occlusions (BRVOs), central serous chorioretinopathy (CSCR), choroidal neovascularization (CNV), retinal tumors, polypoidal choroidal vasculopathy, retinal tears, and numerous additional retinal conditions.

39.1 History

In 1900, Max Planck published the relationship between energy and the frequency of radiation. In 1917, Albert Einstein proposed the concept of stimulated emission; that is, electrons could be stimulated to emit light of a particular wavelength, creating the theoretical framework for the development of the laser.[2] The first device to utilize these concepts was not developed until 1954, when American physicists Charles H. Townes, Herbert J. Zeiger, and James P. Gordon produced the first MASER (microwave amplification by stimulated emission of radiation) at Columbia University. In March 1960, Townes and Arthur L. Schawlow at Bell Labs were granted a patent for a similar device using optical light: a LASER (light amplification by stimulated emission of radiation). In May 1960, Theodore H. Maiman, a physicist at Hughes Research Laboratories in California, constructed the first laser using synthetic ruby and photographic flashlamps as a pump source and, thus, the laser was born. By 1961, several companies were producing commercial lasers.[3]

Although lasers were not developed until 1960,[1] retinal photocoagulation dates back to Socrates, who observed solar retinitis or solar eclipse burns of the retina. Czerny, in 1867,[4] and Deutschmann, in 1882,[5] demonstrated burns in rabbit retinas by focusing sunlight through dilated pupils. However, utilizing the sun proved to be suboptimal for medical applications due to its motion, dependence on weather, and large angular size (0.52 degrees). In 1944, Eccles and Flynn[6] provided some insight into the relationship between the time of exposure and the heat intensity required to produce a solar burn in rabbit retinas. In 1955, Byrnes et al[7] demonstrated that rabbit retinas exposed to nuclear explosions had burns similar to those in retinas exposed to sunlight. The following year, Guerry et al[8] and Ham et al[9] carried out quantitative measurements of exposure time and intensity of retinal burns produced with a carbon arc lamp.

In 1945, after noting retinal damage associated with gazing at a solar eclipse, Dr. Gerhard Rudolph Edmund Meyer-Schwickerath[10] surmised that focused radiant energy could be used to create an intentional, therapeutic chorioretinal lesion. He demonstrated that sunlight could be used for this purpose. However, the inability to regulate the power led him to the carbon arc and eventually the xenon arc.[11] By 1956, the xenon arc had gained widespread acceptance, proving to be a convenient source of intense, polychromatic white light emitting all wavelengths from 400 to 1600 nm and producing a full-thickness chorioretinal burn without selective tissue targeting.

The xenon arc has since been supplanted by the more selective laser. The laser emits a discrete wavelength and has a high degree of collimation, permitting a focused, smaller spot size. Clinical investigation with Maiman's ruby laser was carried out in 1963 by Kapany et al[12] and Zweng et al.[13] Difficulty in producing a full-thickness retinal burn and the risk of subretinal hemorrhage with a pulsed laser were attributed to the 2-ms pulse duration and the emitted red wavelength; this stimulated the development of the continuous-wave (CW) gas ion lasers for use in ophthalmology.

The argon blue-green laser was introduced by Dr. Francis A. L'Esperance in 1968,[14] and it rapidly gained wide acceptance by the mid-1970s for its several advances over the ruby laser. This was followed by the krypton laser in 1972[15] and the indirect laser ophthalmoscope in 1981.[16] The tunable organic dye laser was introduced to ophthalmology in 1981, initially as a source of photodynamic therapy (PDT) and then for photocoagulation therapy. The dye laser enabled variation of output wavelength to target specific ocular tissues.

The semiconductor laser diode was developed in 1962, but clinical applications were limited by low power outputs. Advances in technology led to the development of the gallium aluminum arsenide laser diode, which can emit CW, monochromatic, coherent laser light in excess of 1 W. Emission from this laser is in the near-infrared range with wavelengths between 780 and 840 nm. In 1987, Puliafito et al[17] first performed retinal photocoagulation lesions using a diode laser endophotocoagulation delivery system. McHugh et al[18] in 1989 described the use of clinical transpupillary retinal photocoagulation with the diode for treating a variety of retinal vascular diseases. Diode lasers are now available in many delivery modes: transpupillary slit-lamp biomicroscope and indirect ophthalmoscope, transscleral, and endoprobe.

39.2 Laser Principles

LASER (light amplification by stimulated emission of radiation) is achieved by pumping energy into an active medium to stimulate atoms from a lower, more stable state to a higher energy level through the absorption of a discrete quantum of energy. From this excited state, they return to the lower steady state with the emission of energy. With ordinary light sources, the excited atoms emit light independently and in a variety of wavelengths, which is referred to as spontaneous emission. In a

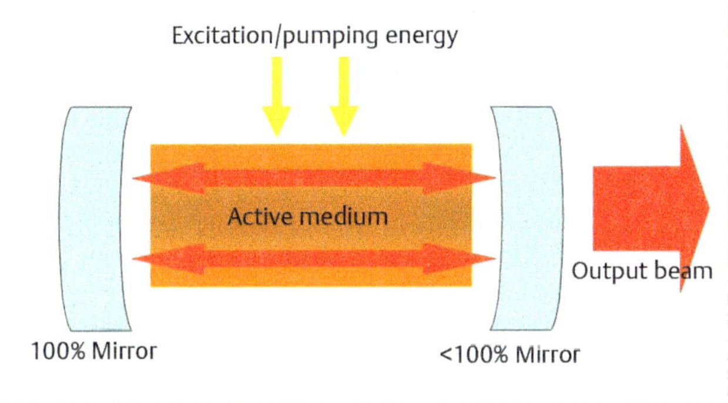

Fig. 39.1 Schematic of a basic laser cavity demonstrating the excitation/pumping energy source, active medium, and optical cavity with one partially transparent mirror allowing a laser output beam.

laser, stimulated transition releases photons which are in phase and at the same frequency as that of the stimulating light.

Lasers comprise three basic elements: an active medium, a resonant cavity, and an excitation or pumping mechanism. The basic laser cavity is set up by placing an active medium into a resonant cavity with coaxial mirrors at opposite ends (▶ Fig. 39.1). One of the mirrors allows partial transmission of laser light as output. A pumping source introduces energy into the active medium to excite the atoms to a higher energy level and to achieve population inversion. Population inversion refers to the situation in which more atoms reside in a higher energy level than at the lower energy level. Spontaneously emitted radiation occurs in all directions, rarely striking the mirrors. Only stimulated emission strikes the mirror. All stimulated emission is of the same wavelength and in the same direction. In this way, amplified, coherent, collimated light energy is released as laser energy. Laser systems differ in the active laser medium and the way this medium is pumped.

Several qualities of lasers make them a unique source of stimulated emission. These include monochromaticity, spatial coherence, collimation, and ability to produce short pulses. *Monochromaticity* refers to the ability to emit a very narrow band of wavelengths. *Spatial coherence* refers to the ability to be focused to a very small spot size. *Collimation* refers to the lack of divergence of the light waves. These properties allow laser energy to be directed at specific target tissue in a carefully controlled manner.

39.2.1 Laser Output Modes

Lasers can be classified according to the variation of their power output with time. Laser output can be operated in either a continuous wave (CW) or a pulsed mode. A CW laser is one in which the power output undergoes little or no fluctuation with time. There is a steady flow of coherent energy, such as in the helium ion, argon gas, or carbon dioxide lasers. A pulsed mode laser has an output beam power that fluctuates with time, such as an Nd:YAG laser. Pulse duration can range from microseconds (10^{-6}) to nanoseconds (10^{-9}), picoseconds (10^{-12}), or femtoseconds (10^{-15}). Concentrating energy in short pulse durations results in high peak power. A laser whose output is normally continuous can also be turned on and off to create pulses of light.

There are a variety of ways to produce a short laser pulse. One way is to take a CW laser and mechanically open and close a shutter. It is difficult to produce pulses shorter than 1 µs with mechanical shutters. One disadvantage of this technique is that much of the energy is wasted when the shutter is closed.

A more efficient method to produce short pulses is by pulsing the laser medium itself, for instance, with a flashlamp. Many current solid-state lasers operate in this mode. The shortest flashlamp pulse available is of the order of 1 µs.

Q-switching and mode locking are two methods that allow for compression of the laser output in time to achieve high peak power. The Q-switch is an intracavity shutter that requires an active medium allowing atoms to remain in a high-energy state for a relatively long time to create high peak power. At the appropriate time, the Q-switch shutter is opened, exposing the mirror. Oscillation and stimulated emission follow quickly with the emission of a single, brief, high-power pulse. Q refers to the quality factor of the laser cavity, which is defined as the energy stored in the cavity divided by the energy lost per cycle. Rapid extraction of high power is accomplished as the Q-switch changes the quality factor of the cavity (Q) from high to low. Q-switching can be accomplished electro-optically, acousto-optically, or even mechanically. This is compatible with either a CW or a pulse mode.

Mode locking is a technique whereby ultrashort pulses with picosecond to femtosecond pulse durations can be produced. Normally, a laser oscillates at several frequencies. By synchronizing these modes with a shutter near one of the cavity mirrors, a process called *mode locking*, even shorter, more powerful pulses can be obtained. Maximum outputs of most ophthalmic models are 10 to 30 mJ and 4.5 mJ for Q-switched and mode-locked lasers, respectively.

39.2.2 Laser Media

Lasers are characterized by their *active medium*. Depending on the physical state of this substance, lasers are described as solid, liquid, gas, or semiconductor. Moreover, because the spectrum of wavelengths emitted by each element is unique, lasers are named for the excitable medium from which they are generated.

Solid-State Lasers

Solid-state lasers include the ruby, Nd:YAG, and erbium:YAG lasers. The active element in the ruby laser is the chromium ion incorporated into the crystalline sapphire. In the Nd:YAG laser, the yttrium-aluminum-garnet crystal is doped with neodymium ions.

Gas Ion Lasers

Gas ion lasers include the argon, krypton, He-Neon, and carbon dioxide lasers. Ion lasers have an ionized gas as their active medium. Carbon dioxide, in combination with nitrogen and helium, is the active medium in carbon dioxide lasers. Gas discharge lasers do not require a pumping lamp. Instead, a long narrow tube with mirrors at each end contains the gas. The exact wavelength is determined by the coating on the mirrors, which is a good reflector for only one particular wavelength.

Disadvantages of gas ion lasers include the need for a special high-voltage power supply and plumbing for water cooling. In addition, they are large, expensive, and not portable.

Liquid Lasers

The operation of tunable dye lasers is based on transitions of organic dye molecules dissolved in solutions. These transitions are broad, and when a series of dye solutions is used, wavelengths from near ultraviolet to near infrared are available. For a given dye, monochromatic output can be obtained by using an intracavity tuning element, usually an etalon, prism, or grating. New solid-state tunable lasers are increasingly popular and are replacing certain tunable dye lasers.

Semiconductor Lasers

Diode lasers are made from semiconductor crystals of gallium arsenide or indium phosphide. The wavelength of the emitted light is a property of the semiconductor crystal. Gallium arsenide doped with aluminum is the most common semiconductor laser crystal in current use and can emit wavelengths between 780 and 850 nm. Other wavelengths can be produced by doping with other materials, but the low power output of these lasers limits their clinical applications. Diode lasers can be used in many delivery modes: transpupillary slit-lamp biomicroscope and laser indirect ophthalmoscope (LIO), transscleral, and endoprobe.

Technical advantages of the diode laser include its compact size and portability. The laser can be powered from an ordinary wall electric current. Additionally, because of their high electric efficiency, little heat is generated and no special plumbing or water cooling system is required. Due to advances in semiconductor technology, diode lasers are relatively inexpensive.

Disadvantages of the diode laser include a nonstandard delivery system with a greater beam divergence cone angle than that of standard argon and krypton lasers. This can make focusing a uniform round laser spot on the retina more difficult. Moreover, infrared laser reflection of up to 10% of the incident beam can occur off the front surface of current laser treatment lenses. This increases the potential danger to unprotected assistants in the treatment room. Standard lenses have antireflective coatings effective in the visible spectrum from 400 to 700 nm. Newer lenses have additional antireflective coatings effective in the near-infrared range.

39.2.3 Laser–Tissue Interactions

The interaction of laser light with a particular target depends on properties of both the laser and the target. The most important laser parameters include wavelength, pulse duration, spot size, and power. The wavelength is a function of the laser cavity's active medium. According to the principle of wave–particle duality, radiation is propagated in the form of waves and photons. Thus, radiation of a given wavelength is associated with photons of a given energy such that $E = hc/?$, where h = Planck's constant, c = speed of light, and $?$ = wavelength. The frequency and energy increase as the wavelength decreases.

The effects of lasers can be considered in several main categories depending on the parameters of laser wavelength, irradiance, and duration of exposure: photochemical, photothermal, photocoagulation, photodisruption, photovaporization, and photoablation. Photochemical refers to nonthermal light-induced chemical reactions, for example, phototransduction in the retina or photosynthesis in plants. Photothermal refers to light absorption in tissue leading to heating. Photocoagulation, a thermal effect, is the most common therapeutic application for retinal lasers. The main disadvantage of lasers that rely on the mechanism of photocoagulation is their dependence on the absorption of radiation by pigment such as melanin or hemoglobin for absorption of radiation.

Photocoagulation occurs when photon absorption or mechanical vibrations produce a critical temperature rise sufficient to denature biomolecules, resulting in thermally induced structural changes within target tissues. The rise in temperature is proportional to the absorption of light in target tissues. That is determined by the ability of molecules to absorb photons of a given wavelength. The increase in retinal temperature is associated with disruption of hydrogen and van der Waals forces stabilizing molecular configuration. These changes, manifested as a loss of biologic activity or structural integrity, result in cell necrosis, hemostasis, and coagulation. The degree and extent of destruction within a tissue are also related to the laser power, laser absorption, laser spot size, and pulse duration.

Photodisruption and photoablation have joined photocoagulation as established medical laser procedures.[19] Unlike photocoagulation, they do not depend on pigment absorption of radiation. Photodisruption is a process in which high-peak-power, ionizing laser pulses are used to disrupt tissue. Energy is concentrated in time and space to create optical breakdown or ionization of the target medium, with the formation of plasma. Photoablation uses high-energy ultraviolet photons to break molecular bonds directly at the irradiated surface into smaller volatile fragments without heating the remaining substrate, resulting in the removal of tissue.

39.2.4 Tissue Variables

The efficiency of converting light energy to heat energy in a particular tissue depends on how effectively light is absorbed at that site. Several ocular factors determine the effect of the laser on the target tissue. The laser must first be transmitted through the ocular media to reach the target tissue. The ocular media include the cornea, anterior chamber, lens, and vitreous. The cornea may have a stromal scar, the anterior chamber may have a hyphema, the lens may be cataractous, and the vitreous may be hazy secondary to inflammation or the presence of blood. Fluid within or beneath the retina behaves similarly to vitreous haze.

The first law of photochemistry (the Grotthus–Draper law) states that photons must be absorbed by a target for a chemical reaction to be initiated.[20] A chromophore is a molecule that absorbs a photon of a particular energy. Depending on the photon's energy, a chromophore can undergo bond breakage, ionization, or various types of molecular excitation. In the visible spectrum (400–800 nm), the primary chromophores involved in retinal photocoagulation include: hemoglobin in the red blood cells, macular xanthophyll, melanin in the retinal pigment epithelium (RPE) and pigmented choroid, rhodopsin and cone photopigments in photoreceptors, and lipofuscin in the

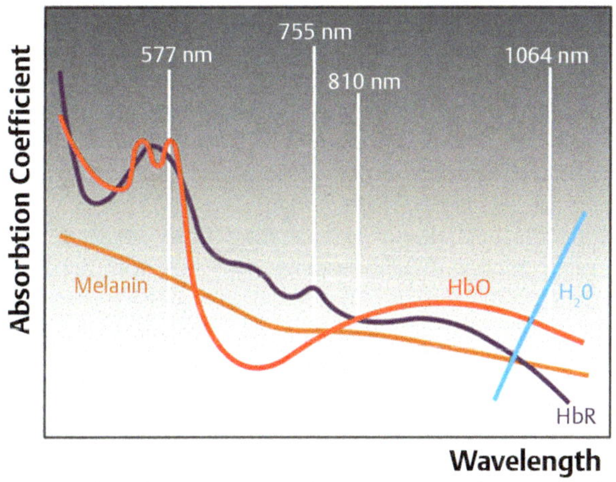

Fig. 39.2 Relative absorption coefficient versus wavelength for melanin, oxygenated and reduced (deoxygenated) hemoglobin, and water. (1) Hemoglobin has excellent blue, green, and yellow light absorption but much poorer red light absorption; (2) light absorption maxima for oxyhemoglobin are located at 542 nm (green) and 577 nm (yellow); (3) reduced (venous) hemoglobin has better krypton red light absorption than does oxygenated hemoglobin. (Image courtesy of Laser and Health Academy.)

RPE. The amount and distribution of these pigments in the region of irradiation determine the level of photocoagulation.

Hemoglobin is located in the blood vessels of the inner retina and choroid, as well as in the extravascular tissues. The absorption spectrum of hemoglobin varies with its oxygen saturation. Oxyhemoglobin absorbs maximally at 542 nm (green) and 577 nm (yellow), whereas reduced deoxyhemoglobin absorbs maximally at 555 nm (yellow). Blue, green, and yellow are absorbed well, in contrast to red and infrared, which are absorbed poorly (▶ Fig. 39.2).

Xanthophyll, located within the inner and outer plexiform layers of the macula and in some cataracts, absorbs well below 500 nm. Blue light is absorbed well, green light poorly, and yellow and red light minimally. The use of blue light results in absorption by the inner retina, in addition to the RPE and choroid. Therefore, utilizing blue light for macular photocoagulation can result in damage to the neurosensory retina.

Melanin, the best absorber of all the pigments, is located in the RPE and the pigmented choroid. The shorter the wavelength, the greater the melanin absorption. It has a maximal absorption of 400 to 700 nm. The greater the fundus pigmentation, the greater the absorption of light and the more intense the burn for a given amount of power. Thus, in treating a lightly pigmented fundus with laser, one may require a higher power setting.

39.3 Delivery Systems

Three main retinal delivery systems are in clinical use today: the slit-lamp biomicroscope with or without a contact lens, the LIO with a condensing lens, and the endophotocoagulation probe inserted through a pars plana incision. Selection of the appropriate delivery system for treatment will depend on the location to be treated, the setting in which the system is to be used (e.g., clinic vs. operating room), patient comfort, and physician preference.

39.3.1 Slit-Lamp Biomicroscope

The slit-lamp biomicroscope is the most commonly employed delivery system today. The essential components of a functional system are a laser source, an attachment system that connects the laser source to the slit lamp, and a slit-lamp microscope to direct the laser beam to the target tissue.

Photocoagulators are differentiated based on their wavelength, active medium, attachment system, pulse duration, power, and spot size selection system. Photocoagulators are available with a variety of wavelengths. The attachment system may be a fiberoptic cable or an articulated mirror arm. The fiberoptic cable offers greater flexibility, whereas the mirror arm offers maintained beam structure with smaller spot sizes. Spot size selectors are of two varieties, parfocal and defocal. In the parfocal system, the spot size is not changed by altering the focal plane of the treatment beam. Instead, changing the magnification varies the spot size. With the defocal system, the spot size is increased by anterior displacement of the focal plane of the treatment beam. Most photocoagulators today have a mixed spot size selector system, with the parfocal system used in the 50 to 200 µm range and the defocal system in the range greater than 200 µm.

The slit-lamp delivery system can be used with or without a contact lens. The majority of posterior segment applications require a contact lens that serves as a coupling device for laser application. A variety of contact lenses are in use today that differ in magnification, spot size, and field of view. These are important parameters in determining the appropriate lens for a particular area of treatment. The conventional Goldmann three-mirror lens has been used for both anterior and posterior segment applications since biomicroscopic laser photocoagulation began.[21] Its limited field of view at any given instant led to the development of newer lenses to optimize treatment of specific posterior segment structures.

Lenses in use are classified as positive (concave) or negative (convex). The various Mainster lenses and the Rodenstock panfunduscopic lens are positive lenses that create a real, inverted image. The Goldmann and Krieger lenses are negative lenses that create a virtual, erect image. Inverted-image lenses provide a considerably greater field of view than erect-image lenses, permitting treatment of large areas of the retina while maintaining visualization of the optic disc and macula to ensure proper orientation.

Mainster et al[22] compared the magnification, spot size, and field of view of four commonly used lenses: Goldmann three-mirror, Krieger, Rodenstock panfunduscopic, and Mainster standard retinal laser lenses. The Goldmann and Mainster standard lenses have similar magnification, whereas the Rodenstock panfunduscopic and Krieger lenses have 24 and 29% less magnification, respectively. The Mainster standard, Krieger, and Rodenstock panfunduscopic lenses have a working field of view greater than that of the Goldmann lens by 58, 8, and 84%, respectively. The working field of view is the maximum field obtained with a 15-degree tilt of the lens to either side of the optical axis. The field of view of each lens varies with the refractive status of the eye (increased in myopic eyes and decreased in hyperopic eyes). The actual size of the retinal burn varies from the spot size setting of the biomicroscope depending on the specific contact lens used. For the Goldmann, Mainster standard, Krieger, and Rodenstock panfunduscopic lenses, the actual retinal spot size is 8, 5, 53, and 41% greater, respectively, than the aerial spot size setting.[22]

The Mainster high-magnification laser lens provides 1.25 × magnification and is useful for the treatment of macular lesions. It provides a 75-degree field of view with a 43-degree stereoscopic field of view. The retinal spot size is 20% less than the actual spot size setting. The Mainster wide-field lens provides a 125-degree view with 0.68 × magnification and is useful for panretinal photocoagulation (PRP). The retinal spot size is 47% greater than the spot size setting.

39.3.2 Laser Indirect Ophthalmoscope

Since its introduction in 1981, the LIO has become an integral part of most vitreoretinal practices.[16] Its wide field of view and versatility offer many advantages over the traditional slit-lamp delivery system. It is available to deliver argon, krypton, and diode irradiation. It expanded the scope of laser photocoagulation by allowing PRP for patients unable to position at a slit lamp. It facilitates the ease of photocoagulation in eyes with intraocular gas or air. It provides an alternative to cryotherapy for the treatment of peripheral retinal breaks. Studies have indicated that photocoagulation with the indirect ophthalmoscope is as effective as cryotherapy for the treatment of retinopathy of prematurity.[23] The energy efficiency of the diode laser allows greater portability, making it the ideal treatment of choice in neonatal intensive care units.

Disadvantages of the LIO include instability of the optical delivery system and a five- to sevenfold decrease in magnification compared with the slit-lamp delivery system, resulting in variations in burn size and intensity.[24] Additionally, Friberg[25] demonstrated that the precision of burn placement to the intended target is accurate only to ±200 µm. When using the LIO with scleral depression, less power is necessary to create a retinal burn. The variability in burn size, intensity, and placement minimizes the utility of this procedure for macular photocoagulation, but it is ideally suited for treating the peripheral retina.

The retinal spot size depends on the distance of the ophthalmic surgeon from the patient, the power of the condensing lens, and the patient's refractive status. The retinal spot size increases as the power of the condensing lens increases and as the plus power of refraction of the eye increases. Vitreous substitutes also affect spot size; the presence of air and gas results in decreased spot size, whereas silicone and perfluorocarbon cause an increase in spot size. Scleral depression, by decreasing the posterior nodal point of the eye, results in a decreased spot size.

39.3.3 Endophotocoagulation

Endophotocoagulation is a technique whereby energy is delivered to the retina via a fiberoptic cable inserted through a pars plana sclerotomy. Early endolaser systems using xenon required placement of the probe in close proximity to the retina, and they could not be positioned through intraocular gas because this resulted in thermal damage to the probe.[26] Because of these limitations, the xenon system has been largely abandoned.

The introduction of the argon laser for endophotocoagulation was an important event in the evolution of vitreous surgery.[27] Laser, with its inherent lack of beam divergence, has increased the safety of endophotocoagulation by permitting treatment at a safe distance from the retina. In addition, it has allowed treatment through a gas-filled eye.

During the past several years, considerable advances have been made in endoprobe technology, especially with the diode laser, with an increase in range of functions of each individual endoprobe. Endoprobes incorporating laser capability with aspiration and infusion function are now available and eliminate the need for repeated forays into the eye with separate instruments.[28] In addition, endoprobes combining diode laser capability with illuminating fiberoptics permit a clear view of structures that may have been obscured through the operating microscope.[29]

Endophotocoagulation has made numerous vital vitreoretinal surgical maneuvers possible, including internal drainage of subretinal fluid, retinectomy, and retinotomy. The intraocular laser delivery system has increased both the scope and safety of vitreous surgery.

39.4 Techniques and Settings

39.4.1 Settings

Three interrelated factors control the amount of energy that arrives at the tissue: laser power, spot size, and pulse duration. The wavelength determines the tissue to which energy is delivered.

Wavelength

For retinal therapy, the laser must be able to penetrate the ocular media (cornea, aqueous, lens, and vitreous) to interact with the target tissue in the posterior segment. There is 75 to 90% transmission of electromagnetic radiation in the visible range (wavelength of 400 to 1,064 nm) through the ocular media. Most lasers for photocoagulation emit radiation in the visible portion of the electromagnetic spectrum, with the exception of the diode and long-pulsed Nd:YAG lasers that emit in the infrared portion. By utilizing a wavelength of light that is selectively absorbed by the target tissue, sufficient heat is generated to selectively coagulate the target tissue. To maximize the desired therapeutic effect while minimizing surrounding tissue effects, one can select a laser with a wavelength of emission that matches the absorption characteristics of the target tissue (▶ Table 39.1).

Argon Green

The argon laser was initially a blue-green laser emitting 60 to 70% blue light. The blue-green laser had several disadvantages, principally associated with the blue wavelength: increased scatter and absorption by cataractous lenses, uptake by macular xanthophyll to cause undesired inner retinal damage, and potential for photochemical toxicity. For these reasons, the argon green laser has largely replaced the blue-green laser for the treatment of retinal vascular abnormalities and macular

Table 39.1 Principal wavelengths of common retinal lasers

Laser	Wavelength (nm)
Argon	
Blue-green	488
Green	514
Krypton	
Yellow	568
Red	647
Tunable dye	570–630
Frequency doubled Nd:YAG	532
Diode	805 (780–850)
Nd:YAG	1,064

photocoagulation. Green light is well absorbed by melanin and hemoglobin and poorly by xanthophyll, thereby producing a cone-shaped lesion sparing the inner retina.[30] It is good for direct vessel coagulation, resulting in shrinkage around vessel walls, and hemoglobin heating, resulting in formation of thrombi. Argon green is a commonly employed laser for PRP.

Krypton Red

Krypton red is well absorbed by melanin but poorly absorbed by hemoglobin. Additionally, it is minimally absorbed by xanthophyll and, thus, may be useful in the treatment of subretinal neovascularization adjacent to the fovea. Krypton red light has the advantage of better penetration than argon green through hazy media and mild vitreous or shallow subretinal hemorrhages. Because of its longer wavelength, krypton red penetrates more deeply than argon green and, as a result, applications may be more painful.

The main difference between argon green and krypton red laser light in retinal photocoagulation is that argon green light is well absorbed by hemoglobin, whereas krypton red light is minimally absorbed. Thus, argon green light may produce primary damage to CNV, whereas the thermal effects of krypton red light probably result from light absorption and heating in pigmented tissues surrounding the new vessels and not from direct absorption of light by hemoglobin. Adequate melanin is required in the vicinity of the CNV to produce thermal coagulation of the abnormal vessels. Moreover, a hemorrhage resulting from krypton red laser treatment may be difficult to stop because of poor absorption by hemoglobin.

Dye Yellow

Tunable dye lasers have output that can be tuned over a wide range of wavelengths. The advantages of dye yellow laser include minimal scatter, low xanthophyll absorption, and little potential for photochemical damage. Moreover, it is maximally absorbed by oxyhemoglobin, with the highest oxyhemoglobin-to-melanin absorption ratio and a high oxyhemoglobin-to-deoxyhemoglobin absorption ratio.[31] Dye yellow appears useful for destroying vascular structures while minimizing damage to adjacent pigmented tissue, and therefore many surgeons prefer it for the treatment of retinal vascular and subretinal neovascular lesions.

Diode (Infrared)

Diode lasers emit in the near-infrared range, demonstrating clinical similarity to the krypton red laser. The laser energy is able to penetrate through cataracts and has better penetration through vitreous hemorrhage than the argon laser. Additionally, the diode laser demonstrates excellent penetration through serous fluid and retinal edema. The 800-nm diode laser requires more power and longer exposures to achieve photocoagulation. Moreover, there is less absorption in the RPE and choriocapillaris, resulting in penetration of energy to the deeper choroid.

Power

The output of photocoagulation lasers is expressed in units of power (watts), whereas the outputs for photodisruption and ablation lasers are expressed in units of energy (joules). The power (watts) is equal to the energy (joules) divided by the time period (seconds). The shorter the time over which a given amount of power is delivered, the lower the safety window and the greater the risk for tissue rupture and hemorrhage. Although up to 1 W may be necessary for photocoagulation depending on the laser and ocular media, several hundred milliwatts is generally sufficient for most purposes.

Spot Size

Irradiance, the power per unit area measured in watts per square meter, increases as the spot size decreases. Smaller spot sizes are more affected by dissipation of heat to surrounding tissue and, hence, higher irradiance is needed to achieve the same central effect as with larger spots.

A spot size of 50 µm can be used to target individual vessels or in the presence of media opacity, whereas spot sizes of 50 to 100 µm are generally used for photocoagulation of the macula and peripheral retina, respectively. Small spot sizes have decreased safety windows and can result in inadvertent choroidal rupture and hemorrhage.

Contact lenses used for delivery of laser energy to the posterior segment can also affect spot size significantly. It is important to understand the effect on spot size of the variety of commercially available contact lens systems. Selecting the appropriate lens and spot size setting is necessary to achieve the desired effect while minimizing complications. For example, the Goldmann and Mainster standard lenses have spot size settings that correlate closely with the actual size of the retinal burn produced. However, the Rodenstock, Krieger, and Mainster wide-field lenses produce retinal lesions that are larger than the spot size setting by about 40 to 50%. The disparity should be kept in mind and laser settings adjusted when these lenses are used.

Pulse Duration

For a given power, decreasing the pulse duration can alter the tissue reaction. Short pulse durations may result in photodisruption, whereas longer pulse durations may lead to photocoagulation. The amount of light energy is proportional to the duration of the burn. If the duration is increased, the power should be reduced. Photocoagulation is classically performed at pulse durations of 100 to 200 ms, but recent studies have shown that shorter pulse durations of 10 to 100 ms can result in clinically efficacious burns with an increased speed of treatment. Pulse duration can be increased to about 500 ms in cases of ocular media opacity.

39.4.2 Techniques

Before Laser Surgery

Patients should have a complete work-up, including medical history. The ocular examination should include best-corrected visual acuity (BCVA), slit-lamp biomicroscopy, and indirect ophthalmoscopy. Ancillary imaging testing such as fluorescein angiography, color fundus photography, optical coherence tomography (OCT), and indocyanine green angiography can be performed depending on the underlying diagnosis. When all the data have been collected and the diagnosis has been made, the physician should consider possible treatment alternatives, keeping in mind the natural history of the condition. If the condition is amenable to laser, the physician should weigh the potential benefits and risks of laser therapy.

The physician should discuss with the patient and family the patient's condition and the risks and benefits of laser therapy in comparison with the natural history of the condition. Once the patient has been informed and has elected to undergo laser treatment, the patient should read and sign an informed consent form that describes the treatment objectives, risks, benefits, and alternatives.

Depending on the laser procedure, imaging studies can be projected to help direct treatment. Before laser treatment, the involved eye is typically dilated with 2.5% phenylephrine and 1% tropicamide. In patients with poor pupillary dilation, 10% phenylephrine can be used.

Treatment

The laser is turned on and allowed to warm up. The spot size, wavelength, and pulse duration are selected, and the power is set below the expected appropriate power level. The patient is then taken to the slit lamp, where the eye is anesthetized with a drop of proparacaine or tetracaine ophthalmic. Once the eye is anesthetized, care is taken to adjust the slit lamp so that the patient is comfortable, with the chin on the chin rest and forehead against the bar. Often, a head strap is used to remind patients to keep their head still and up against the bar during the procedure.

Once the patient is in the appropriate position, the intensity of the light beam and aiming beam are adjusted so that they are visualized clearly and excessive glare is avoided. Next, the foot pedal is adjusted so that it is in a comfortable range, and a test fire in the standby position is performed to prepare the patient for the sound made by the laser. A contact lens is then placed on the eye, and the fundus is examined through the contact lens, with the physician noting the landmarks and area of pathology. For macular laser procedures, the fundus is compared with the angiogram and foveal landmarks are localized carefully so that they can be recognized easily during treatment. When the physician is ready to initiate therapy, the control panel is switched to the on position and treatment is begun. Frequent reorientation with fundus landmarks is a good idea to ensure the proper retinal areas are treated.

Peripheral Scatter Laser Treatment Principles

Panretinal photocoagulation (PRP) is performed with the slit-lamp biomicroscope and contact lens or the LIO with a condensing lens. Several retinal vascular conditions may be treated with peripheral scatter laser, including most commonly diabetic retinopathy, retinal vein occlusions, sickle-cell retinopathy, hyperviscosity syndromes, retinal embolization, radiation retinopathy, ocular ischemic syndrome, retinopathy of prematurity, familial exudative vitreoretinopathy (FEVR), retinal vasculitis, uveitis, Eales' disease, sarcoidosis, chronic retinal detachment, carotid-cavernous fistula, Coats' disease, retinal artery macroaneurysms, and incontinentia pigmenti. The rationale for PRP is that it reduces the stimulus for neovascularization through destruction of hypoxic retina, especially the metabolically active photoreceptors, and may improve oxygen perfusion to the remaining viable retina.[32]

PRP is typically performed with a semiconductor, argon green, or krypton red laser. An initial complete treatment consists of applying 1,000 to 2,000 medium-intensity burns in the peripheral retina for 360 degrees. Burns are spaced one-half to one spot width apart and are distributed from just outside the disc and temporal vascular arcades to the periphery. To minimize complications, laser spots should not be applied directly to major retinal vessels, posterior ciliary arteries and nerves, intraretinal hemorrhages, or large neovascular fronds.

Classically, PRP was given in two or more sessions to reduce patient pain and postlaser exacerbation of macular edema. However, the Diabetic Retinopathy Clinical Research Network (DRCR.net) conducted a nonrandomized, prospective, multicenter clinical trial comparing PRP in one session and four sessions and found no clinical difference. While the central macular thickness (CMT) was slightly higher and vision slightly worse at 3 days and 4 weeks postlaser in the one-session group, the primary end point of 34 weeks showed a reversal, with the four-session group having a CMT 8 µm thicker and visual acuity two letters worse than the one-session group.[33] If PRP treatment is split into multiple sessions, burns should first be placed in the inferior retina to avoid delay in treatment should a vitreous hemorrhage occur before the next treatment session.

Laser parameters for the slit-lamp biomicroscope include a 200- to 500-µm-diameter spot size and a 10- to 200-ms pulse duration. A power setting of about 200 mW is used to start and titrated up in 20- to 50-mW increments until a burn of the desired intensity is achieved (▶ Fig. 39.3). The power used will vary depending on the media clarity, presence of retinal edema, and degree of fundus pigmentation. Laser therapy is typically titrated to a visible clinical effect (graying or whitening of the retina), which corresponds to necrosis of the photoreceptors and, at higher settings, to the inner retina.

When the LIO is used for PRP or any other retinal laser work, care should be taken to line up the laser beam from the indirect

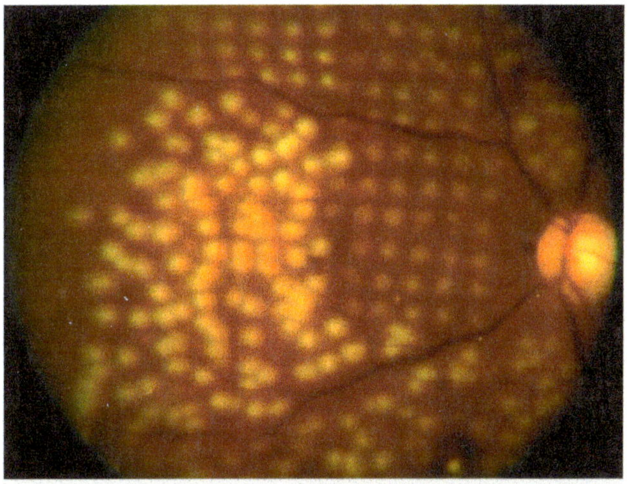

Fig. 39.3 Fundus photograph comparing conventional laser (lower left laser spots in the image) with patterned scanning laser (upper right laser spots in the image; PASCAL, Topcon) demonstrating more uniformly spaced, smaller, and less intense laser spots with PASCAL.

source with the condensing lens to the retinal target. A 20-diopter condensing lens should be used to minimize the spot size in hyperopic eyes or eyes with vitreous substitutes, such as silicone oil. A 28-diopter lens can be used to magnify the spot size in eyes with high myopia and in gas-filled eyes.

Macular Laser Treatment Principles

In general, macular laser work is either localized, ablative treatment for discrete lesions, such CNV, or light "focal" or "grid" therapy for intraretinal edema associated with conditions such as diabetic retinopathy or branch vein occlusions. The mechanism by which focal or grid laser photocoagulation reduces macular edema is unclear. Possible explanations include: a laser-induced reduction in retinal blood flow; replacement of compromised RPE cells with new, healthy cells; increase in the inner retinal oxygen supply; and reinforcement of the outer or inner blood–retinal barriers by stimulation of the proliferation of endothelial cells in capillaries and venules overlying the laser spot.[34]

There are several requirements for wavelength selection in macular photocoagulation, including: effective transmission through the ocular media; low absorption by macular xanthophyll; and penetration through subretinal fluid, retinal edema, or thin layers of intraretinal and subretinal hemorrhages. The techniques and laser parameters for various conditions are described in the section on indications later in this chapter.

After Laser Surgery

Once treatment is complete, the laser is turned to the standby position and the contact lens and head strap are removed. The eye can be rinsed. The laser parameters, including wavelength, power, pulse duration, spot size, and number of treatment spots, are documented in the patient's chart. Instructions including postoperative expectations and cautions are discussed, and the patient is scheduled for a postoperative appointment.

39.5 Complications

Laser photocoagulation, as with any surgical procedure, may be associated with complications. Proper patient selection, patient education, and laser parameters can minimize the most serious complications of excessive energy or misdirected light.

Misdirected light can result in burns of the cornea, iris, and lens in addition to inadvertent burns of the fovea. Anterior segment burns can occur during the use of contact lenses with mirrors to treat the peripheral retina. In addition, they can occur when the LIO is used; thus, when the LIO is used and laser burns become more sporadic, photocoagulation should be stopped and the cornea and lens should be inspected for burns.[35] Anterior segment burns with the LIO result from poor focus. Burns of the iris may result in iritis, accommodative difficulties, or posterior synechiae.[36] Focal lens opacifications occur most frequently in eyes with a senescent crystalline lens after the absorption of light by lens pigments. This can be avoided by using longer wavelengths, such as krypton red.

Although highly effective clinically at halting angiogenesis, laser photocoagulation can lead to unwanted side effects, including significant discomfort during application,[37] permanent retinal scarring, laser spot enlargement postoperatively, rupture of Bruch's membrane and development of CNV, scotoma, exudative retinal detachment, optic neuritis, RPE tears, subretinal fibrosis, visual field loss, dyschromatopsia, nyctalopia, and decreased peripheral vision.[38,39] Systematic clinicopathological analysis of laser-induced retinal lesions over time has demonstrated that exposures of 100 ms and longer typically produce retinal lesions that affect not only RPE and photoreceptors, but also the inner nuclear layer, ganglion cell layer, and nerve fiber layer (NFL). Arcuate nerve fiber and visual field defects can result from laser lesions that affect the inner retina. PRP can also exacerbate DME. Permanent retinal scarring has multiple detrimental effects: (1) it distorts the normal retinal architecture and replaces it with gliotic/fibrotic matrix; (2) it disrupts normal retinal connectivity; (3) it is associated with an infiltrative/inflammatory process involving cell loss; (4) lack of photoreceptors and/or other retinal cells in the scarred areas directly reduces the visual field sensitivity; (5) loss of one class of retinal cells may, by trans-synaptic degeneration and by incitement of inflammation, result in loss of other retinal neurons.[40,41]

Inadvertent foveal burns can occur if the eye moves during photocoagulation and the ophthalmic surgeon is not aware that treatment is occurring within the macula, or if the fovea cannot be identified. When using a contact lens with mirrors, the surgeon should frequently check the location of the macula by looking through the center of the contact lens before treating peripheral retina through the selected mirror. Difficulty in determining the center of the fovea that is not resolved with fluorescein angiography may be a contraindication to macular treatment.

Heavy PRP can result in elevated intraocular pressure, choroidal effusion, cystoid macular edema (CME), nyctalopia, and visual field loss. A transient increase of intraocular pressure can also occur. The majority of pressure rises are of an open-angle variety, the etiology of which is not known. Less commonly, heavy treatment can result in choroidal effusion with angle closure and subsequent elevation of intraocular pressure, which may persist for several days.[42] Dividing treatment into several sessions may reduce the risk of this complication.

Direct treatment of retinal blood vessels or retinal neovascularization may result in hemorrhage. Hemorrhages can occur as an early or late complication of laser photocoagulation. Bleeding into the retina and vitreous can occur during treatment with intense power and small spot size; this may stop spontaneously or with direct laser therapy or digital pressure. Immediate or delayed hemorrhage can occur with photocoagulation of CNV. Immediate bleeding can occur at the area of photocoagulation or from a remote site, whereas delayed bleeding typically occurs from inadequately treated CNV. Intense, confluent treatment of CNV, including a rim of surrounding retina, should decrease the frequency of this complication.

The treatment of CNV can lead to unique complications, including RPE tears and macular holes. Rips of the RPE have been described, particularly with the krypton laser.[43] These occur most frequently in the presence of a pigment epithelial detachments, and Gass[44] hypothesized that when spontaneous tears occur in pigment epithelial detachments, the detachments are associated with occult CNV. Macular holes have also been described following laser photocoagulation of CNV.[45] It is thought that contraction of the photocoagulation scars results in tangential forces to the fovea, resulting in a macular hole.

Delayed complications of photocoagulation include secondary CNV, subretinal fibrosis, and macular pucker. These complications generally occur in areas where small spot size combined with intense burns has resulted in ruptures in Bruch's membrane. Contraction of an epiretinal membrane with visual distortion can occur after photocoagulation of retinal vascular conditions, especially those associated with inner retinal hemorrhages. This may be a consequence of damage to the inner limiting membrane.

Complications of laser affect not only the patient but also the ophthalmic surgeon. There is now conclusive evidence that subtle but definite alterations in color vision can result from chronic exposure to argon blue light.[46] Therefore, ophthalmic surgeons should minimize their exposure to argon blue light and all laser light by installing appropriate safety filters, blocking blue laser light, or using a different laser wavelength.

39.6 Indications

It is useful to consider some clinical applications for laser photocoagulation and the mechanism by which laser achieves its clinical effect. Only the most common conditions and techniques are discussed here. The number of laser-treatable diseases is far greater than the number of unique laser modalities. Since many diseases have common pathologic components, the examples of clinical applications provided in this chapter can serve as paradigms for such entities.

39.6.1 Diabetic Macular Edema

Diabetic mellitus is growing at epidemic proportions worldwide. Diabetic retinopathy is the leading cause of blindness in persons between the ages of 20 and 64 years, affects 40 to 45% of the 29.1 million Americans with diabetes, and accounts for 12% of all new cases of blindness each year in the United States.[47] The prevalence and degree of retinopathy increase with the duration of diabetes mellitus.

The most common cause of decreased vision in diabetics is macular edema. DME is diagnosed with slit-lamp biomicroscopy and OCT. It is further subdivided into focal and diffuse forms. Focal macular edema is characterized by discrete areas of retinal thickening associated with specific points of leakage on fluorescein angiography. Diffuse macular edema is characterized by widespread thickening and diffuse leakage of fluorescein dye that reflects extensive breakdown of the blood–retinal barrier.

Although anti–vascular endothelial growth factor (anti-VEGF) therapy has become a mainstay of primary treatment for DME, and is discussed elsewhere in this book, laser continues to play an important role in modern practice. For many years prior to the availability of anti-VEGF agents, laser was the only effective therapy available for DME. The Early Treatment Diabetic Retinopathy Study (ETDRS) was a multicenter, randomized, controlled clinical trial enrolling between 1980 and 1985 a total of 3,711 patients with mild-to-severe nonproliferative diabetic retinopathy (NPDR) or PDR without high-risk features followed at least every 4 months. Eyes were categorized by the extent of retinopathy and the presence of macular edema and were randomized to receive immediate or deferred focal laser. Focal photocoagulation consisted of direct focal treatment of microaneurysms more than 500 µm from the foveal center but treatment up to 300 µm from the foveal center was allowed if vision was 20/40 or worse. Grid photocoagulation was applied to areas of diffuse leakage and capillary nonperfusion on fluorescein angiography. Focal laser settings were 50 to 100 µm spot size, 50 to 100 ms pulse duration, and power titrated to whiten the microaneurysm. Grid laser settings were 50 to 200 µm spot size, 50 to 100 ms pulse duration, and power titrated to achieve mild burn intensities. The primary outcome was defined as "moderate vision loss" (a loss of =15 letters, or 3 lines, of ETDRS vision). The ETDRS demonstrated that laser photocoagulation could reduce moderate vision loss by 50% in eyes with clinically significant macular edema (CSME). Eyes with macular edema that did not meet criteria for CSME did not show a benefit with focal laser, whereas those with CSME with central foveal involvement had a reduction in moderate vision loss from 33% in controls to 13% with focal laser. Patients with CSME without central foveal involvement had a reduction in moderate vision loss from 16% in controls to 6% with focal laser.[48] The ETDRS definition of CSME was based on the presence of any one of the following three characteristics[49]:

1. Retinal thickening within 500 µm of the foveal center.
2. Hard exudate within 500 µm of the foveal center with associated retinal thickening.
3. Retinal thickening larger than one disc area in size within one disc diameter of the foveal center.

Olk[50] defined diffuse DME as two or more disc areas of retinal thickening involving the foveal avascular zone, and this is a form of CSME.

Laser treatment or other pharmacotherapy, such as anti-VEGF or steroids, is indicated for eyes with CSME.[48] The treatment approach of laser photocoagulation depends on whether there is focal or diffuse leakage. *Focal laser photocoagulation* implies the treatment of areas of focal leakage, with direct therapy to leaking microaneurysms. The early phase of the fluorescein angiogram can guide and ensure adequate treatment. *Grid laser photocoagulation* is performed in eyes with diffuse retinal thickening (DRT) and involves the application of uniformly spaced spots in the areas of diffuse leakage and nonfoveal capillary nonperfusion on the fluorescein angiogram. A combination of focal and grid laser is referred to as a *modified grid laser* and involves direct treatment to areas of focal leakage combined with grid treatment to areas of diffuse leakage.[50]

Since the landmark ETDRS study, clinicians have sought to continue the therapeutic benefit of focal laser with less intense laser lesions. The DRCR.net developed "modified ETDRS" (mETDRS) guidelines in which all microaneurysms are treated between 500 and 3,000 µm from the foveal center with 50 µm, 50 to 100 ms lesions with power titrated to produce a grey-white burn. Grid laser is applied to all areas with edema from 500 to 3,000 µm in all directions and up to 3.5 mm temporally from the foveal center with laser spots that are 50 µm, 50 to 100 ms pulse duration separated by 2 burn diameters with power titrated to barely visible laser spots. Mild macular grid (MMG) laser burns are lighter that mETDRS burns and are given throughout the macula in both thickened and unthickened retina. MMG is applied 500 to 3,000 µm in all directions and up to 3.5 mm temporally from the foveal center with laser spots that are 50 µm, 50 to 100 ms pulse duration, barely visible with 200 to 300 burns evenly distributed approximately 2 to 3 burn widths apart. Comparison of the mETDRS with MMG in 263 patients found that, at 1 year, the mETDRS grid photocoagulation was associated with a reduced central macular thickness (CMT) of 88 µm, whereas MMG was associated with a CMT reduction of 49 µm. The mean visual acuity of the mETDRS group was stable, whereas the MMG group lost 2 letters of vision at 1 year. Thus, mETDRS remains the standard of care.[51]

Response to laser therapy has also been shown to depend on subclassification of the condition. OCT can be used to subclassify DME into four categories: diffuse retinal thickening (DRT), cystoid macular edema (CME), serous retinal detachment (SRD), and vitreomacular interface abnormalities (VMIA). In a study of 70 eyes in 45 patients who underwent focal laser photocoagulation with different subcategories of DME, patients with DRT were found to achieve a greater reduction in retinal thickness and greater improvement in visual acuity than patients with CME or VMIA.[52] Patients with SRD had significant reduction in retinal thickness without improvement in visual acuity.[52]

For treatment, several contact lenses including the Area Centralis (Volk Optical Inc), Mainster high-magnification lens, or the Yannuzzi lens can be used. In the ETDRS, initial focal treatment with the argon laser involved direct treatment of leaking microaneurysms between 500 µm and two disc diameters of the center of the macula. Typical settings include a spot size of 50 to 100 µm and a pulse duration of 0.05 to 0.1 second. Traditionally, the power was adjusted to produce whitening of the microaneurysms, but a less intense burn probably suffices. For grid treatment, laser should be applied 2 to 3 burn widths apart in areas of retinal thickening by ophthalmoscopy and OCT and leakage on fluorescein angiography from 500 to 3,000 µm from the foveal center superiorly, inferiorly, and nasally and from 500 to 3,500 µm from the foveal center temporally. The usual laser parameters consist of a spot size of 100 µm and an exposure time of 0.1 second.[53,54] The power should be adjusted to obtain a light burn. Argon green, krypton red, or diode laser may be used.

39.6.2 Proliferative Diabetic Retinopathy

Another indication for laser photocoagulation is PDR and, in distinction to DME, laser remains the first-line therapy for patients with PDR. Early attempts at laser therapy of PDR relied on direct and intense targeting of neovascular elements, but this could exacerbate the problem. It is now accepted that PRP should be performed with several thousand laser burns placed in the peripheral retina. The Diabetic Retinopathy Study (DRS), begun in 1971, was a prospective, multicenter, randomized, controlled clinical trial sponsored by the National Eye Institute. It included more than 1,700 patients at 15 centers, and was designed to evaluate the timing of PRP in eyes with advanced NPDR and PDR. One eye of each patient was randomly assigned to immediate laser treatment with either a xenon arc or argon laser and the second eye served as a control without treatment. Patients were included if they had a BCVA of 20/100 or better in both eyes and the presence of PDR in one eye or severe NPDR in both eyes. The primary outcome measurement was severe vision loss, defined as a BCVA less than 5/200 at two consecutive visits 4 months apart.[55] The DRS noted the 2-year risk of developing severe vision loss increased dramatically in patients with at least three of the following high-risk characteristics: (1) presence of vitreous or preretinal hemorrhage, (2) presence of neovascularization, (3) location of neovascularization on or near the optic disc (NVD), and (4) severity of neovascularization.[56] In eyes with high-risk characteristics, PRP decreased the incidence of severe vision loss at 2 years from 26% of controls to 11% of treated eyes. This increased to 44% of control eyes and 20% of treated eyes at 4 years.[57]

The DRS found that xenon arc was associated with a higher rate of complications and thus recommended argon laser photocoagulation. In the xenon arc cohort, 19% of patients lost 1 or more lines of vision and 11% of patients lost 2 or more lines, compared to 11 and 3%, respectively, in the argon group. A quarter of patients in the xenon arc group had peripheral field constriction compared to less than 5% of patients in the argon group.

The British Xenon Arc Coagulation Study, performed at a similar time, was also a multicenter, randomized controlled trial where one eye of each patient was randomly assigned to immediate laser treatment with xenon arc and the second eye served as a control without treatment in 99 patients. The mean visual acuity decreased by less than 1 line in treated eyes but more than 2 lines in controls. This decrease was most significant in patients who initial vision was 20/20 to 20/30. There was no difference in patients with BCVA of 20/120 or worse. Treatment was thus recommended in patients particularly with better visual acuity.[58]

Based on the DRS, the efficacy of treatment in patients with NPDR or PDR without high-risk characteristics was unclear. The role of aspirin 650 mg daily was evaluated along with early PRP or deferral of treatment until development of high-risk characteristics. Early PRP was given either in full scatter (similar to the DRS argon with 1,200 to 1,600 spots, 500 µm burn diameter, and 100 ms pulse duration to the equator delivered in two sittings) or in mild scatter (400 to 650 spots more widely spaced in one sitting) along with two macular treatments which are described in the previous section. Neovascularization elsewhere was treated directly as in the DRS. The primary outcome was severe vision loss, defined the same as in the DRS with BCVA less than 5/200 at two consecutive visits 4 months apart, or necessitating vitrectomy. The ETDRS reported a 5-year rate of severe vision loss of 2.6% in the treatment group and 3.7% in the control group. However, both groups had a low rate of severe vision loss, and side effects of PRP were noted in the treated group. Thus, the study recommended careful follow-up without PRP for mild or moderate NPDR.[59] The ETDRS found no difference in progression to high-risk PDR or vision loss between the placebo and aspirin groups but did find a 17% decrease in cardiovascular morbidity and mortality in the aspirin group compared to the placebo group.[60]

In eyes with CSME and high-risk PDR, it is generally best to deliver focal treatment before or at the same time as the PRP. For example, one can perform focal treatment for macular edema and PRP of the nasal or inferior quadrants in the first sitting and then complete the PRP during the subsequent weeks. This will help minimize the risk of the PRP exacerbating the macular edema.

39.6.3 Central Retinal Vein Occlusion

A central retinal vein occlusion (CRVO) is caused by an obstruction of retinal venous outflow at the lamina cribrosa. A CRVO presents clinically with intraretinal hemorrhages in all four quadrants and dilation and tortuosity of the retinal veins. Nerve fiber layer (NFL) infarcts, optic disc swelling, and retinal edema may also be present. Macular pathologic changes are the most common cause of decreased vision in acute CRVO and consist of macular edema, intraretinal hemorrhages, and capillary nonperfusion. Other causes include vitreous hemorrhage and arteriolar occlusion. The visual prognosis is highly variable, ranging from normal vision to no light perception. Decreased vision long term is caused by capillary nonperfusion, retinal atrophy, chronic macular edema, retinal arteriole occlusion, macular hole formation, vitreous hemorrhage, retinal detachment, retinal or disc neovascularization, iris neovascularization, and neovascular glaucoma.[61,62]

Clinical examination and fluorescein angiography can further classify CRVO into "ischemic" and "nonischemic" types, which have significant prognostic and management implications. A nonischemic CRVO is one with minimal or no retinal capillary nonperfusion on fluorescein angiography and is associated with a better visual prognosis. An ischemic CRVO is one with more widespread retinal capillary nonperfusion and is more likely to result in severe visual loss and neovascular complications.[63]

The Central Vein Occlusion Study (CVOS), sponsored by the National Eye Institute, was a multicenter, randomized, controlled clinical trial designed to evaluate the natural history of CRVO, the effect of grid laser photocoagulation for macular edema, and the efficacy of PRP in preventing or promoting regression of anterior segment neovascularization.[64] In contrast to the Branch Vein Occlusion Study (BVOS), the CVOS did not find grid laser photocoagulation to be of visual benefit in patients with macular edema associated with the retinal vein occlusion.[65] In the CVOS, grid laser reduced angiographic leakage but did not significantly improve the visual acuity at any point during follow-up.

All patients with CRVO should be observed closely with careful slit-lamp biomicroscopic examination of the anterior segment (including gonioscopy) and funduscopic examination, especially during the first 3 to 6 months. Patients who have acute CRVO with poor initial vision, moderate to severe venous tortuosity, numerous intraretinal hemorrhages, and 30 or more disc areas of capillary nonperfusion have a 45 to 80% risk for the development of anterior segment neovascularization during the first 3 to 6 months after CRVO.[66,67] The CVOS found that although prophylactic PRP decreased the risk of iris or angle neovascularization in such eyes, prompt regression of neovascularization was more likely to occur in eyes that did not receive prior laser therapy.[68] Therefore, in most cases, it was preferable to observe and administer PRP at the first signs of iris or angle neovascularization rather than to deliver laser prophylactically in all acute ischemic CRVO cases. The creation of a laser-induced chorioretinal venous anastomosis in eyes with nonischemic CRVO and progressive visual loss has been explored.[69]

39.6.4 Branch Retinal Vein Occlusion

Branch retinal vein occlusion (BRVO) occurs most commonly at an arteriovenous crossing point. Ophthalmoscopic findings of an acute BRVO include intraretinal hemorrhages, retinal edema, and NFL infarcts in a sector of retina drained by the involved vein.

Acutely, the vision may be reduced secondary to macular edema, intraretinal hemorrhages, or capillary nonperfusion. Later, retinal hemorrhages resolve and capillary collaterals may form to permit resolution of edema with possible improvement of vision, or there may be progressive closure of capillaries. As with CRVO, macular abnormalities are the most common cause of permanent visual loss and include capillary nonperfusion, retinal atrophy, chronic macular edema, epiretinal membrane, and subretinal fibrosis. Other causes of visual loss include vitreous hemorrhage and tractional or rhegmatogenous retinal detachment.

Photocoagulation is considered for two situations in patients with BRVO: chronic macular edema in eyes with an intact foveal vasculature, and neovascularization of the optic disc, retina, or iris. In eyes with macular edema of greater than 3 months' duration and visual acuity of 20/40 to 20/200, the BVOS demonstrated that macular grid laser photocoagulation significantly improves the visual outcome.[70] Treated eyes were more likely to gain two lines of vision (65%) in comparison with untreated eyes (37%). Furthermore, treated eyes were more likely to have 20/40 or better vision at 3 years' follow-up than were untreated eyes (60 vs. 34%, respectively). Overall, mean visual acuity in the treated group was in the 20/40 to 20/50 range, and in the untreated group it was 20/70.

Once a decision is made to treat, a fluorescein angiogram less than 1 month old should be available to guide treatment. As in eyes with diffuse DME, treatment consists of applying a light grid pattern of laser spots to the area of macular thickening and leakage on the fluorescein angiogram using a 100- to 200-µm spot size. No spots should be placed within 500 µm of the foveal center during the initial treatment. Eyes are then reevaluated, and repeat treatment can be considered in areas of persistent leakage if the visual acuity remains decreased.

Eyes with BRVO and large areas of associated retinal capillary nonperfusion are at relatively greater risk for posterior segment (disc and retinal) neovascularization. The BVOS concluded that ischemia alone is not an indication for sector PRP. Instead, the study recommended that PRP be initiated at the first signs of neovascularization. Such treatment reduces the risk for vitreous hemorrhage by 50%.[71]

Scatter photocoagulation should be applied to achieve medium-intensity burns spaced one burn width apart and covering the entire involved segment. A semiconductor or argon green laser with settings similar to PRP can be used.

39.6.5 Other Proliferative Conditions

A variety of retinal vascular and inflammatory disorders may potentially benefit from scatter laser photocoagulation. These include vascular occlusions, sickling hemoglobinopathies, hyperviscosity syndromes, retinal embolization, radiation retinopathy, ocular ischemic syndrome, retinopathy of prematurity, FEVR, retinal vasculitis, uveitis, Eales' disease, sarcoidosis, chronic retinal detachment, carotid-cavernous fistula, retinal artery macroaneurysms, Coats' disease, and incontinentia pigmenti, to mention a few.

39.6.6 Macular Degeneration

Age-related macular degeneration (AMD) is the leading cause of irreversible blindness in the developed world, causing 14 million people to be blind worldwide and affecting more than 1.5 million people in the United States.[72] Many patients with significant vision loss from AMD have CNV. Blurry vision and distortion, most evident at close range, are the most common symptoms in affected patients. If CNV is suspected based on signs and symptoms, a fluorescein angiogram, OCT, and possibly indocyanine green angiogram should be obtained. Therapy with anti-VEGF agents should generally be considered as the first choice for patients with exudative AMD due to the favorable visual acuity outcomes and safety profile of those agents in large randomized clinical trials as well as the development of significant scotomata with thermal ablative laser therapy in regions near or beneath the center of the fovea following laser and the high rates of CNV recurrence following laser. Laser treatment can be considered for angiographically determined, well-delineated extrafoveal CNV along with occult, or poorly delineated CNV in a minority of cases or special circumstances such as the unavailability of, or medical contraindication to, anti-VEGF therapy. Photodynamic laser therapy (described later) may also be considered for primary or adjunctive therapy in similar cases or for those with suboptimal responses to anti-VEGF therapy.[73]

The Macular Photocoagulation Study (MPS), sponsored by the National Eye Institute, was a multicenter, prospective, randomized clinical trial designed to evaluate the role of laser photocoagulation in patients with well-defined CNV associated with AMD or ocular histoplasmosis and in patient with idiopathic CNV. Well-defined CNV was classified into three types based on its location relative to the center of the fovea on fluorescein angiogram.

1. Extrafoveal: 200 to 2,500 µm from the foveal center
2. Juxtafoveal: 1 to 199 µm from the foveal center
3. Subfoveal: directly beneath the foveal center

The initial MPS trial evaluated the role of argon blue-green laser for the treatment of well-defined, extrafoveal CNV, and demonstrated that at 18 months' follow-up, laser photocoagulation reduced the risk of severe visual loss from 69% in untreated eyes to 25% in treated eyes.[74] This benefit remained significant, but not as great, at 5 years: 64% of untreated eyes versus 46% of treated eyes. At 5 years' follow-up, 54% of the laser-treated eyes had a recurrence.[75]

The MPS also evaluated the role of krypton red laser for the treatment of juxtafoveal CNV. At 3 years, the risk for severe visual loss was reduced from 58% in untreated eyes to 49% in treated eyes.[76] The major cause of visual loss in both groups was persistent or recurrent CNV. At the time of these studies, the benefit of treating recurrences in the foveal center was not known. The benefit of photocoagulation in both of these substudies may have been better had recurrences been treated.

The MPS conducted two additional studies in eyes with subfoveal CNV. The first, the subfoveal study, evaluated the effect of krypton and argon green laser in previously untreated CNV.[77] The second, the subfoveal recurrence study, was performed because of the high rate of recurrent and persistent CNV in the previous studies.[78] The MPS reported that the treatment of subfoveal neovascular membranes was better than observation alone in both studies, but only if the neovascular complex was relatively small.[77,78]

Before treatment, patients should be informed that laser treatment will create an absolute scotoma in the area of treatment. If the CNV is subfoveal, an immediate reduction in vision will likely occur, and patients should understand that the goal of treatment is not to improve vision, but to prevent severe visual loss.

The MPS treatment protocol recommends projection of a fluorescein angiogram less than 72 hours old to permit orientation to retinal vascular and CNV landmarks. Initially, a test burn should be placed at the nonfoveal edge of extrafoveal or juxtafoveal CNV or the inferior edge of subfoveal CNV using a 200-µm spot size and a 0.2- to 0.5-second duration to determine the appropriate power setting. Next, the perimeter of the membrane is outlined with overlapping burns. Finally, the membrane is treated with confluent, heavy white burns.[78,79] Because of availability, the argon blue-green laser was the wavelength used initially by the MPS.[74] This laser fell out of favor because the blue light was absorbed by xanthophyll, resulting in thermal damage to the inner retina.[80] The juxtafoveal arm of the MPS employed krypton red because of the theoretical advantage of penetration through xanthophyll and hemorrhage with uptake in the RPE and inner choroid.[76] The subfoveal trials found no difference between the argon green and krypton red wavelengths.[77]

In occult CNV, indocyanine green angiography can be used as an adjunct to fluorescein angiography to improve visualization of the neovascular complex and guide laser photocoagulation in selected cases.[73,81,82] Selectivity may also be increased using exogenous dyes and different types of laser light. However, the advent of anti-VEGF therapy has greatly reduced the clinical utilization of laser in patients with AMD.

39.6.7 Retinal Tear

Several studies have demonstrated a 5 to 7% incidence of retinal breaks in the general population.[83,84] Any retinal break can result in a retinal detachment if liquefied vitreous passes through the break into the potential space between the neurosensory retina and the RPE. The majority of retinal breaks, however, are asymptomatic, small, atrophic holes located in the far periphery and rarely lead to retinal detachment. Treatment of asymptomatic individuals with small, atrophic holes is typically not indicated. On the other hand, retinal horseshoe tears are breaks with persistent vitreous traction and are much more likely to lead to rhegmatogenous retinal detachment. Such breaks should be treated to prevent retinal detachment, especially if the tear is acute and symptomatic. For the broad spectrum of retinal breaks between these two extremes, the decision of whether or not to treat is made after multiple variables are considered.

Prophylactic treatment of retinal breaks can be accomplished with laser retinopexy or transscleral cryotherapy. The advantages of photocoagulation over cryotherapy include more localized treatment, avoiding the liberation of RPE cells that has been shown to occur during cryopexy, and less scarring.[85] Photocoagulation without scleral buckling surgery or internal tamponade can be used to treat retinal breaks with small localized retinal detachments measuring approximately two disc diameters in size. Larger amounts of fluid typically require reattachment of the retina first, such as with a gas injection, and then application of the laser afterward. Treatment can be accomplished by using the LIO or the slit-lamp biomicroscope with the Goldmann three-mirror or Mainster wide-field contact lens. Laser therapy with either slit-lamp delivery systems or the LIO has largely supplanted cryopexy for the treatment of peripheral retinal pathology.

The technique consists of surrounding the edges of the tear by at least three rows of confluent laser burns with edges touching each other. If subretinal fluid is present, treatment should extend beyond the fluid to reach attached retina. The aim of treatment is to produce inflammation around the retinal tear to produce a chorioretinal scar. Care must be taken to ensure adequate photocoagulation along the anterior margin of the break because continuing vitreous traction can pull the flap through a laser scar, resulting in a retinal detachment.

39.7 Types of Retinal Laser Therapy

39.7.1 Dye-Enhanced Laser Photocoagulation

Dye-enhanced laser photocoagulation relies on the administration of an exogenous dye that concentrates in the target tissue. The laser effect can be localized by utilizing a wavelength of emission that is absorbed by the dye. This permits more selective treatment of the target tissue while minimizing damage to adjacent tissues. Dye-enhanced photocoagulation is relatively rare in modern clinical practice with the availability of photodynamic techniques now.

Fluorescein dye has been used to enhance argon blue-green laser therapy of retinal angiomas. Indocyanine green, a water-soluble tricarbocyanine intravenous dye,[73,81,82] has a peak wavelength of absorption of 805 nm, which is similar to the wavelength of emission of the diode laser. Thus, intravenous indocyanine green administration before diode laser treatment allows for more selective photocoagulation of CNV with less energy.[86,87]

39.7.2 Photodynamic Therapy

Laser application can also be modulated and targeted through the intravenous administration of photosensitizers such as verteporfin, called photodynamic therapy (PDT). PDT targets abnormal vessels while minimizing damage to the surrounding retinal tissues through utilizing low-intensity light to activate photosensitized tissues without an increase in temperature and associated photothermal collateral damage. A photosensitive agent is injected intravenously and activated with irradiation of the target tissue at the absorption maximum of the dye. Longer wavelengths are typically chosen because of their greater depth of penetration. A photochemical interaction between the photosensitizing agent and light results in the production of reactive oxygen, including singlet oxygen ($^1O_2$)[88] and superoxide radicals that interact with various cellular constituents. This interaction results in direct cellular injury, including vascular endothelial cell injury and vessel thrombosis, while preserving the surrounding retina, RPE, and choroid.[89] Selective tissue targeting occurs as the photochemical agent preferentially concentrates in the tissue of choice.[90] This technique permits nonthermal and selective occlusion of abnormal vessels while minimizing damage to surrounding retinal tissues.

Several photosensitizers have been developed for PDT, the majority of which are based on the molecular structure of porphyrin. PDT has been utilized to treat intraocular retinoblastoma and melanoma.[91,92,93] Therapy with various photosensitizers has induced closure of experimental iris and CNV in animals. SnET2, a second-generation photosensitizer, has been proven effective for the photodynamic occlusion of normal choriocapillaris and choroidal vessels in pigmented rabbits.[91,92,93,94,95,96,97,98] Multicenter, randomized clinical trials (TAP and VIP) have established PDT with verteporfin as an effective therapy to reduce visual acuity loss in patients with CNV associated with AMD, although in head-to-head trials against ranibizumab, the latter was shown to be more effective in reducing vision loss and increasing vision improvement either singly or in combination for patients with classic and occult CNV.[99,100] Side effects of PDT with verteporfin include photosensitivity reactions, dye extravasation, transient visual disturbances, and infusion-related back pain.

Another important clinical application of PDT is CSCR. Full-dose and half-dose and low-fluence PDT have been associated with more rapid anatomic resolution of subretinal fluid compared to observation in numerous clinical studies.[101,102,103,104,105] Some studies also report an improvement in visual acuity.[106]

PDT is also employed for polypoidal choroidal vasculopathy, a variant of AMD with branching choroidal vessels with terminal, polyp-like aneurysmal lesions associated with serous and hemorrhagic detachments of the RPE noted frequently in Asians, particularly Japanese.[107] In the EVEREST study, a multicenter, randomized, double-masked, indocyanine green angiography–guided trial, PDT combined with ranibizumab was superior to ranibizumab monotherapy in achieving complete polyp regression (77.8 vs. 28.6%; $p < 0.01$) with improved visual acuity (mean gain of 10.9 letters vs. 9.2 letters, respectively).[108] Additional studies with up to 3-year follow-up have found PDT for polypoidal effective with a long-lasting effect.[109,110]

While PDT remains in use for CSCR and polypoidal choroidal vasculopathy, PDT has decreased in popularity for AMD in recent years due to the efficacy of anti-VEGF agents in halting and reversing vision loss due to CNV. The EVEREST trial, however, suggests there may be a role for PDT as adjunctive treatment to anti-VEGF or other pharmacologic therapy in various vitreoretinal diseases. Treatment selectivity may be achieved using laser-activated gold nanoparticles to selectively target tissue, which has been demonstrated in animal models for oncologic applications but has not been applied in retinal lasers to date.[111]

39.7.3 Improving Selectivity of Millisecond Pulse Duration Laser

Investigations have been performed using shorter millisecond pulse duration lasers (with pulse durations ranging from 1 to 100 ms) compared to conventional laser.[112] Shorter millisecond pulse durations resulted in decreased lesion size for an equivalent clinical appearance of a lesion and improved lesion localization but were associated with a reduced safety window with respect to rupture of Bruch's membrane (▶ Fig. 39.4).[112] A pulse duration of 20 ms was reported to adequately balance safety with speed (▶ Fig. 39.5).[112] Further modifications have been proposed, including spatial and temporal modulation of laser beams,[113] pattern scanning retinal photocoagulation,[114] and reduced lesion intensity.[115,116] Two clinical pattern scanning laser photocoagulation systems are available: the PASCAL (Topcon Corp) and the Visulas 532s VITE (Carl Zeiss Meditec). Another advance has been image-guided, planned laser application (▶ Fig. 39.6).

These delivery systems allow for the creation of well-aligned arrays of retinal lesions in a shorter time. A clinical grading system was devised to describe laser burns: barely visible, mild, moderate, intense, very intense, and rupture.[112] A barely visible lesion was one that just crossed the limit of clinical detection and produced no retinal whitening, whereas a mild lesion was described as one that produced some blanching but no whitening. A moderate lesion was one that produced some retinal whitening but did not have a ring of edema, while an intense lesion had an area of central whitening and a halo of translucent edema. A very intense lesion had a very pronounced area of opaque central retinal whitening and a larger ring of edema. A rupture was assumed when a vapor bubble or discontinuity in retinal architecture was visualized with or without bleeding. Investigations of retinal photocoagulation have found that 10- to 20-ms exposures can produce retinal lesions of all clinical grades if power is increased accordingly.[112] In addition, shorter pulse durations result in improved lesion localization, as compared to conventional 100-ms exposures (▶ Fig. 39.7). Patterned scanning laser typically utilizes settings of 532 nm wavelength, 200 µm, 20 ms, and powers from 300 to 750 mW.

Several small pilot clinical studies have been performed comparing photocoagulation performed with 10 to 20 ms pulses to conventional 100-ms exposures. In a study by Sanghvi et al, 10 to 20 ms pulse duration photocoagulation was performed in 75 eyes of 60 patients and was reported to be safe and effective.[117] In a study by Al-Hussainy et al, 20 patients were treated with a conventional laser (100 ms, 180 mW) and short pulse duration (20 ms, 500 mW), each lesion type in half of every treated retina. Following laser treatment, patients were asked to rate the pain of each of the two treatments from 0 (no pain) to 10 (worst pain ever experienced). Conventional PRP resulted in a pain score of 5.11, whereas short pulse duration had a mean pain score of 1.4.[118] Additional studies have also confirmed that shorter duration laser burns cause less perceived pain than conventional laser lesions.[119] A study by Muqit and colleagues evaluated the evolution of the lesions produced by 10- and 20-ms

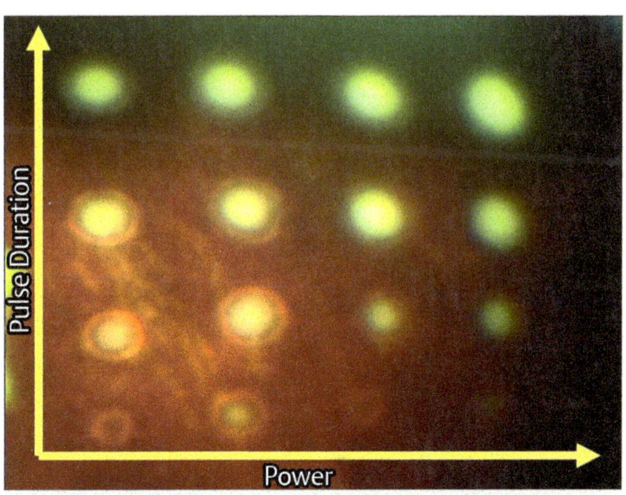

Fig. 39.4 Fundus photograph of the rabbit retina with laser burns produced at various pulse durations (10–100 ms) and powers (50–250 mW). The burns appear increasingly intense and larger with increases in either pulse duration or power.

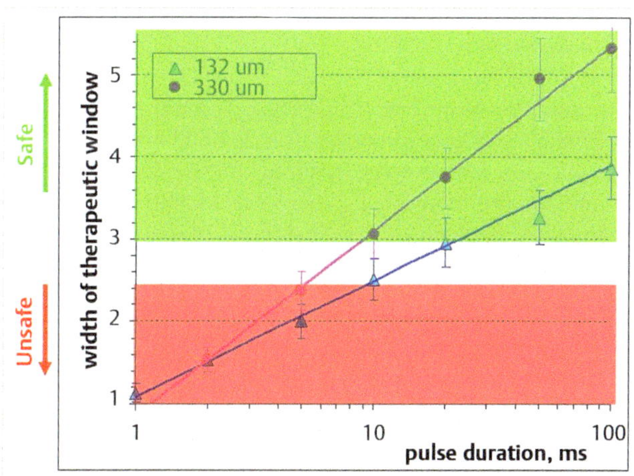

Fig. 39.5 Semi-logarithmic plot of the therapeutic window (the ratio of the threshold of rupture to that of a light burn) as a function of pulse duration for retinal laser spot sizes of 132 and 330 µm, demonstrating that 20-ms pulse durations result in a safe therapeutic window.

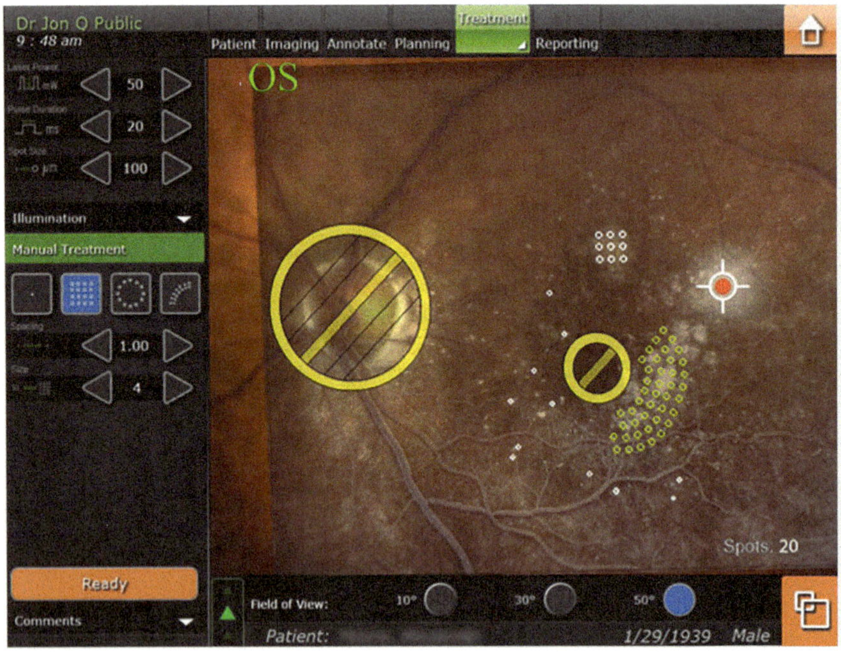

Fig. 39.6 The Navilas laser platform demonstrating preplanning of laser spots. (Image courtesy of OD-OS Retina Navigation Co.)

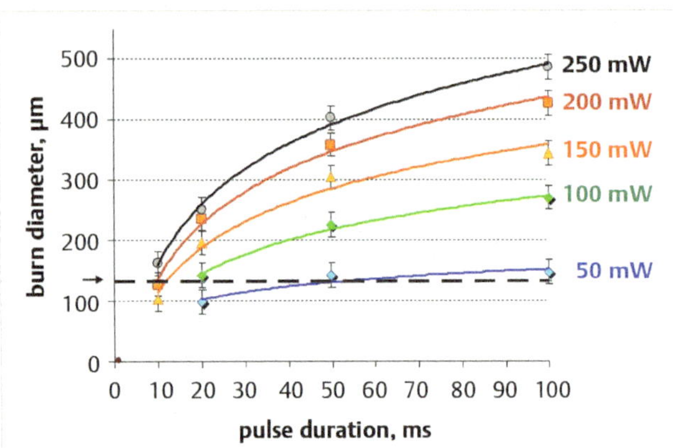

Fig. 39.7 Retinal burn diameter plotted as a function of laser pulse durations ranging from 10 to 100 ms with a retinal laser spot size 132 μm for varying laser powers. The dashed line represents a laser spot size of 132 μm at the retinal plane.

pulse duration using ophthalmoscopy, spectral-domain OCT, and fundus autofluorescence in 17 eyes of 11 patients. Short pulse duration lesions were localized to the outer retina and RPE and showed more predictable lesion characteristics at 18 months posttreatment.[120] A retrospective study comparing 41 eyes with newly diagnosed high-risk PDR treated with argon green laser before 2007 to 41 eyes treated with PASCAL after 2007 found that 73% of PASCAL-treated patients experienced persistence or recurrence of any persistent or recurrent neovascularization within 6 months of treatment compared to 34% treated with conventional laser ($p < 0.0008$).[121] Twenty percent of PASCAL-treated eyes had persistence of neovascularization, 73% had neovascularization of the disc (NVD) or neovascularization elsewhere (NVE), 10% had neovascularization of the iris (NVI), 5% had neovascular glaucoma (NVG), and 37% had vitreous hemorrhage. However, in this study a similar number of laser spots was applied in each of the two groups (1,438 spots in PASCAL vs. 1,386 spots in conventional) which, given the decreased retinal lesion size with each PASCAL burn, means that a smaller area of the retina was treated in the PASCAL eyes. Up to 6,924 PASCAL burns could be required to cause regression of severe PDR.[122,123]

Modifications have also been described using OCT to guide selective focal laser treatment. OCT-guided focal laser was associated with 2.5 letters of improved vision ($p = 0.04$) and a 45.56 μm reduction in central subfield thickness ($p < 0.001$) compared to conventional mETDRS focal laser at 1 year.[124] Further modifications have been described using laser dosimetry to empirically titrate to barely visible burns. The power is reduced from this level and has been shown to result in invisible burns funduscopically but visible on fluorescein angiography and OCT at 50 to 75% of barely visible level and invisible burns at 30 to 50% of barely visible level using a software termed *Endpoint Management*.[125] A small clinical study of 16 patients with chronic CSCR of more than 4 months' duration treated with 30% of barely visible pulse energy reported a gain of 12 letters of vision by 2 months ($p < 0.001$) with a decrease in CMT from 350 to 282 μm ($p = 0.004$).[126] Subvisible laser burns have been shown to result in upregulation of inflammatory markers after laser application[127] and improved response to oxidative stress.[128]

Recent evidence suggests that reduced intensity and pulse duration retinal lesions might not be permanent, and that the outer retina can fill the damaged areas in animal models, including rats, rabbits, and snakes (▶ Fig. 39.8).[129,130,131] This has been shown to result in restoration of both retina structure and function in these laser spots with intact retinal ganglion cells in the laser region through retinal remodeling.[132] This restoration of morphology has also been shown in humans with OCT following less intense laser burns.[133,134]

39.7.4 Transpupillary Thermotherapy

Another approach to retinal treatment is transpupillary thermotherapy (TTT). In a more intense, destructive modality, TTT

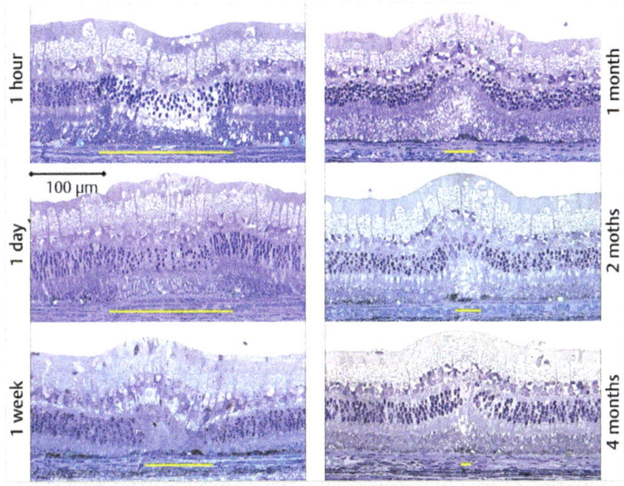

Fig. 39.8 Toluidine blue histopathology of 7-ms pulse duration "barely visible" laser burns from 1 hour to 4 months following laser application demonstrating photoreceptors filling in the damaged area after initial photoreceptor loss in rabbits. A retinal beam diameter of 330 µm and power of 175 mW were used. The yellow bar indicates the extent of damage at the RPE-photoreceptor junction. By 4 months, there is a continuous photoreceptor layer. (Reproduced with permission from Paulus et al[129]; Copyright 2008 by the Association for Research in Vision and Ophthalmology.)

is used for the treatment of less than 5 mm thick retinal and choroidal tumors, including choroidal melanoma, metastases, and retinoblastoma, since 1995 and CNV associated with AMD since 1999.[135,136,137,138] TTT involves long exposures (approximately 60 seconds) of a large spot (1.2–3 mm) at low irradiance (~10 W/cm^2), using a near-infrared laser. Numerous small clinical trials have demonstrated the efficacy of sublethal phototherapy of the retina in several eye conditions. A retrospective review of 77 patients with occult CNV demonstrated that TTT was associated with visual stabilization (47%) or improvement (22%) in the majority of patients.[139] Other retrospective reviews have similarly shown a closure of approximately 75% of classic and occult CNV membranes in patients after TTT.[140]

39.7.5 Micropulse Laser

In contrast to the long exposure durations and large spots used in TTT, shorter bursts of near-infrared radiation (810 nm) with small spot sizes (100–200 µm) have also been applied for nondamaging retinal phototherapy, termed subvisible diode micropulse (SDM) laser therapy. In this technique, treatment of retinal vascular disease is performed with the express goal of avoiding cellular destruction. Mathematical models of SDM have demonstrated that the hyperthermia in this approach does not exceed the threshold of cell toxicity and has a high degree of selectivity. Low-intensity/high-density SDM allows for complete and confluent (high-density) coverage of the entire diseased retina, such as the areas of macular thickening constituting DME or ischemic retina in PDR. Subthreshold micropulse laser delivers a series of short pulses to allow thermal dissipation between each pulse.[141] Subthreshold laser has been shown in pathologic and histochemical analyses to reduce the changes to the surrounding choroidal and retinal cells.[142]

The micropulse 810 nm diode, low-intensity/high-density subvisible photocoagulator has also been shown to be clinically effective in the treatment of DME and PDR in small clinical series. SDM has been shown to be as effective as mETDRS focal laser in the treatment of clinically significant DME in some small studies. SDM resulted in improved clinical examination and retinal thickness measurement with OCT without producing visible retinal damage.[143] Beneficial effects in the treatment of retinal neovascularization from PDR have also been reported[144] along with DME[145] and CSCR.[146] These studies, however, are limited by their sample size and the duration of patient follow-up.

39.7.6 Selective Retinal Therapy with Microsecond Pulse Duration Laser

One method to provide retinal phototherapy without severe permanent damage is selective treatment of the RPE by decreasing the laser pulse duration, termed selective retinal therapy (SRT). It has been demonstrated that microsecond (µs) pulse durations that are absorbed by melanin can selectively destroy RPE without damaging the retina (▶ Fig. 39.9).[147] Due to minimal thermal heat diffusion, microsecond and nanosecond laser pulses can produce explosive vaporization of melanosomes, resulting in selective damage to the RPE while sparing the photoreceptors and the inner retina. Subsequent RPE proliferation and migration restores RPE continuity. SRT has also been shown to cause a release of inflammatory markers, including matrix metalloproteinases 2 and 9, which may play a role in its treatment efficacy.[148] Multifocal ERG and histology following SRT have demonstrated no significant retinal change 30 days after SRT laser application.[149]

The first RPE-selective retinal laser treatment was achieved using 5-µs argon laser pulses at 514 nm and a repetition rate of 500 Hz.[150] Currently, several microsecond-pulsed laser systems are available.[151,152,153] Recently, an alternative SRT approach has been developed based on a rapidly scanning CW laser, such that RPE cells are exposed to a scanning laser light to achieve dwell times of a few microseconds.[154,155] This technique has been further refined using an automatic, energy ramping, noncontact, reflectometric dosimetry technique.[156]

Several small clinical studies have demonstrated the efficacy of SRT in diabetic retinopathy, DME, CSCR, and subfoveal fluid after a rhegmatogenous retinal detachment.[157,158] A randomized prospective study of 30 patients with chronic CSCR of at least 3 months' duration with 14 eyes randomized to SRT and 16 eyes as controls found a statistically significant improvement in mean visual acuity, with 12.7 letters gained in the laser group versus 6.3 letters gained in the control group ($p = 0.04$). SRT also resulted in less subretinal fluid with a decrease of 203 µm in retinal thickness with laser versus 41 µm in control patients at 3 months ($p = 0.005$).[159,160] A prospective uncontrolled study of 39 patients with DME found an improvement of 2.4 letters of vision 6 months after laser application ($p = 0.02$). Eighty-four percent of eyes had either stable or improved vision, and there were no adverse events associated with SRT.[161]

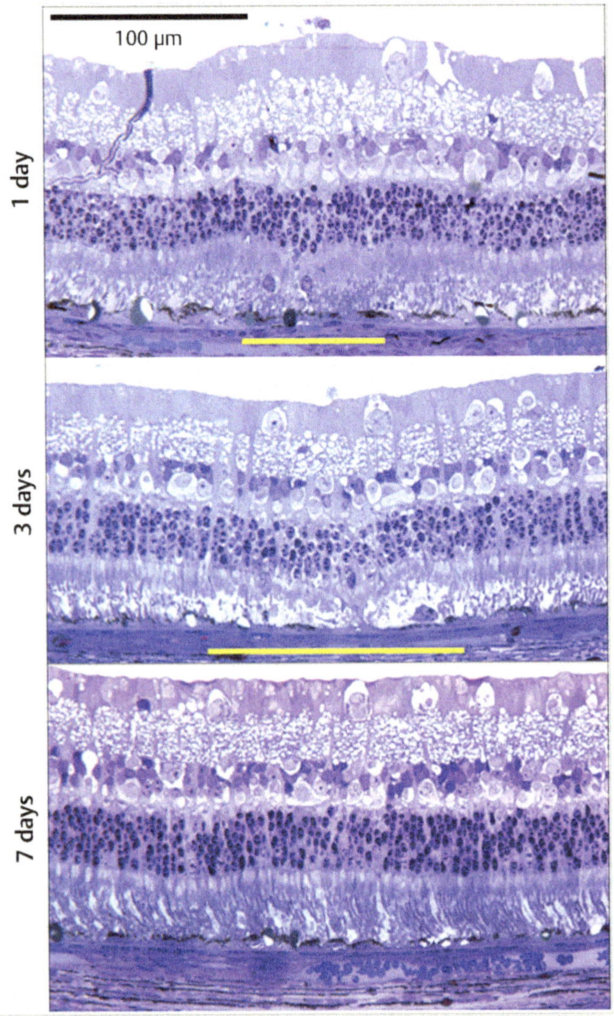

Fig. 39.9 Selective retinal therapy histology in rabbits. RPE-selective treatment in clinically invisible lesion at 1 day, 3 days, and 7 days after treatment. Beam diameter 66 μm, dwell time 15 μs, power 1100 mW. At 1 day, there is RPE cell collapse and outer segment hyperpigmentation and increased density. At 3 days, damage to the outer segments expands to a width twice that of the laser beam with edema. By 1 week, the damage has largely resolved.

39.8 Future

We stand on the cusp of a transformation in our care of patients through the use of personalized, targeted therapy, and novel laser treatments promise to play an important role in numerous retinal conditions. Advances in laser technology have created new treatments, including scanners, micropulse laser, and SRT, that minimize collateral tissue damage and could allow for safe treatment of the macula. Studies have indicated that laser power approximately half that of barely visible burns produces cellular changes while minimizing tissue injury.[162] Further studies are needed to elucidate the mechanisms of cellular response leading to clinical efficacy of laser therapy. To prove the clinical utility of these new modalities, larger randomized control clinical trials with longer follow-up are required to ensure that these treatment modalities meet or exceed the current clinical standard of care.

In addition to laser monotherapy trials as were performed in the past, further clinical trials are also needed of laser treatment in combination with pharmacologic therapy. Concomitant laser and anti-VEGF or steroid therapy has been shown to improve polyp regression in polypoidal choroidal vasculopathy, and further trials are needed with DME and BRVO.

New techniques are being developed to further automate and standardize laser application to increase the specificity and safety of laser therapy. These include optoacoustic monitoring of retinal temperature in real time to achieve real-time automatic dosimetry for more reproducible, homogenous photocoagulation lesions. In addition, retinal navigated laser photocoagulation using eye tracking and registered diagnostic imaging with scanning slit ophthalmoscope (NAVILAS) allows one to register fluorescein angiographic and other imaging data to better guide photocoagulation delivery.

In addition, lasers could be used in the future for photodisruption, a process in which explosive vaporization is used for tissue dissection. Similar to laser technology used in refractive surgery for creation of cornea flaps, high-intensity laser beams have also been described for dissection of preretinal fibrovascular tissue with diabetes.[163] While this has, to date, had limited applicability due to difficulty in axial differentiation between the retina and preretinal membrane and strong optical aberrations, further developments in the technology may overcome this hurdle.

39.9 Conclusion

Lasers are an indispensable component in the management of diseases of the vitreous and retina. Laser therapy has revolutionized the treatment of many ocular conditions, including diabetic retinopathy, retinal vein occlusions, sickle-cell retinopathy, CSCR, retinal tumors, polypoidal choroidal vasculopathy, retinal ischemic diseases, CNV, retinal tears, and AMD. Improved understanding of laser–tissue interactions has permitted increased targeting of select tissue while minimizing damage to the surrounding tissue. Selective therapeutic approaches permit desirable biochemical, cellular, and tissue effects while excluding unwanted damage, and will improve our understanding of the function and pathology of posterior segment structures. Continuous innovations in laser technology and progress in the understanding of retinal pathology make us believe that improvements in the treatment of retinal diseases using laser therapy are likely to continue for many years to come.

References

[1] Maiman TH. Stimulated optical radiation in ruby. Nature. 1960; 187:493–494

[2] Einstein A. Zur quantentheorie der Strahlung. Physiol Zool. 1917; 18:121–128

[3] Rose M. A history of the laser: A trip through the light fantastic. Photon Spectra. 2010; 44(5):58–69

[4] Czerny V. Ueber Blendung der netzhaut durch Sonnenlicht. Klin Monatsbl Augenheilkd. 1867; 5:393–395

[5] Deutschmann R. Ueber die blendung der netzhaut durch directes Sonnenlicht. Albrecht Von Graefes Arch Klin Exp Ophthalmol. 1882; 28:241–254

[6] Eccles JC, Flynn AJ. Experimental photoretinitis. Med J Aust. 1944; 1:339–342

[7] Byrnes VA, Brown DV, Rose HW, Cibis PA. Retinal burns: new hazard of the atomic bomb. J Am Med Assoc. 1955; 157(1):21–22

[8] Guerry D, III, Ham WT, Jr, Ruffin RS, et al. The transmission of light; through the ocular media of the rabbit eye. Am J Ophthalmol. 1956; 42(6):907–910

[9] Ham WT, Jr, Wiesinger H, Guerry D, III, et al. Experimental production of flash burns in the rabbit retina. Am J Ophthalmol. 1957; 43(5):711–718

[10] Meyer-Schwickerath G. Indications and limitations of light coagulation of the retina. Trans Am Acad Ophthalmol Otolaryngol. 1959; 63:725–738

[11] Meyer-Schwickerath G. Light coagulation; a method for treatment and prevention of the retinal detachment [in German]. Albrecht Von Graefes Arch Ophthalmol. 1954; 156(1):2–34

[12] Kapany NS, Peppers NA, Zweng HC, Flocks M. Retinal photocoagulation by lasers. Nature. 1963; 199:146–149

[13] Zweng HC, Flocks M, Kapany NS, Silbertrust N, Peppers NA. Experimental laser photocoagulation. Am J Ophthalmol. 1964; 58:353–362

[14] L'Esperance FA, Jr. An opthalmic argon laser photocoagulation system: design, construction, and laboratory investigations. Trans Am Ophthalmol Soc. 1968; 66:827–904

[15] L'Esperance FA, Jr. Clinical photocoagulation with the krypton laser. Arch Ophthalmol. 1972; 87(6):693–700

[16] Mizuno K. Binocular indirect argon laser photocoagulator. Br J Ophthalmol. 1981; 65(6):425–428

[17] Puliafito CA, Deutsch TF, Boll J, To K. Semiconductor laser endophotocoagulation of the retina. Arch Ophthalmol. 1987; 105(3):424–427

[18] McHugh JD, Marshall J, Ffytche TJ, Hamilton AM, Raven A, Keeler CR. Initial clinical experience using a diode laser in the treatment of retinal vascular disease. Eye (Lond). 1989; 3(Pt 5):516–527

[19] Krasnov MM. Laser puncture of the anterior chamber angle in glaucoma (a preliminary report) [in Russian]. Vestn Oftalmol. 1972; 3:27–31

[20] Longsworth JW. Photophysics. In: Regan JD, Parrish JA, eds. The Science of Photomedicine. New York, NY: Plenum;1982:43

[21] Fankhauser F, Lotmar W. Photocoagulation through the Goldmann contact glass. Arch Ophthalmol. 1967; 77(3):320–330

[22] Mainster MA, Crossman JL, Erickson PJ, Heacock GL. Retinal laser lenses: magnification, spot size, and field of view. Br J Ophthalmol. 1990; 74 (3):177–179

[23] McNamara JA, Tasman W, Brown GC, Federman JL. Laser photocoagulation for stage 3 + retinopathy of prematurity. Ophthalmology. 1991; 98(5):576–580

[24] Benner JD, Huang M, Morse LS, Hjelmeland LM, Landers MB, III. Comparison of photocoagulation with the argon, krypton, and diode laser indirect ophthalmoscopes in rabbit eyes. Ophthalmology. 1992; 99(10):1554–1563

[25] Friberg TR. Clinical experience with a binocular indirect ophthalmoscope laser delivery system. Retina. 1987; 7(1):28–31

[26] Charles S. Endophotocoagulation. Ophthalmol Times. 1979; 4:68–69

[27] Fleischman JA, Swartz M, Dixon JA. Argon laser endophotocoagulation. An intraoperative trans-pars plana technique. Arch Ophthalmol. 1981; 99 (9):1610–1612

[28] Peyman GA, Lee KJ. Multifunction endolaser probe. Am J Ophthalmol. 1992; 114(1):103–104

[29] Uram M. Ophthalmic laser microendoscope endophotocoagulation. Ophthalmology. 1992; 99(12):1829–1832

[30] Trempe CL, Mainster MA, Pomerantzeff O, et al. Macular photocoagulation. Optimal wavelength selection. Ophthalmology. 1982; 89(7):721–728

[31] Mainster MA. Wavelength selection in macular photocoagulation. Tissue optics, thermal effects, and laser systems. Ophthalmology. 1986; 93(7):952–958

[32] Wolbarsht ML, Landers MB, III. The rationale of photocoagulation therapy for proliferative diabetic retinopathy: a review and a model. Ophthalmic Surg. 1980; 11(4):235–245

[33] Brucker AJ, Qin H, Antoszyk AN, et al. Diabetic Retinopathy Clinical Research Network. Observational study of the development of diabetic macular edema following panretinal (scatter) photocoagulation given in 1 or 4 sittings. Arch Ophthalmol. 2009; 127(2):132–140

[34] Okisaka S, Kuwabara T, Aiello LM. The effects of laser photocoagulation in the retinal capillaries. Am J Ophthalmol. 1975; 80(4):591–601

[35] Irvine WD, Smiddy WE, Nicholson DH. Corneal and iris burns with the laser indirect ophthalmoscope. Am J Ophthalmol. 1990; 110(3):311–313

[36] Lobes LA, Jr, Bourgon P. Pupillary abnormalities induced by argon laser photocoagulation. Ophthalmology. 1985; 92(2):234–236

[37] Fong DS, Girach A, Boney A. Visual side effects of successful scatter laser photocoagulation surgery for proliferative diabetic retinopathy: a literature review. Retina. 2007; 27(7):816–824

[38] Shimura M, Yasuda K, Nakazawa T, Tamai M. Visual dysfunction after panretinal photocoagulation in patients with severe diabetic retinopathy and good vision. Am J Ophthalmol. 2005; 140(1):8–15

[39] Higgins KE, Meyers SM, Jaffe MJ, Roy MS, de Monasterio FM. Temporary loss of foveal contrast sensitivity associated with panretinal photocoagulation. Arch Ophthalmol. 1986; 104(7):997–1003

[40] Stone JL, Barlow WE, Humayun MS, de Juan E, Jr, Milam AH. Morphometric analysis of macular photoreceptors and ganglion cells in retinas with retinitis pigmentosa. Arch Ophthalmol. 1992; 110(11):1634–1639

[41] Birnbach CD, Järveläinen M, Possin DE, Milam AH. Histopathology and immunocytochemistry of the neurosensory retina in fundus flavimaculatus. Ophthalmology. 1994; 101(7):1211–1219

[42] Blondeau P, Pavan PR, Phelps CD. Acute pressure elevation following panretinal photocoagulation. Arch Ophthalmol. 1981; 99(7):1239–1241

[43] Gass JD. Retinal pigment epithelial rip during krypton red laser photocoagulation. Am J Ophthalmol. 1984; 98(6):700–706

[44] Gass JD. Serous retinal pigment epithelial detachment with a notch. A sign of occult choroidal neovascularization. Retina. 1984; 4(4):205–220

[45] Lim JI, Schachat AP, Conway B. Macular hole formation following laser photocoagulation of choroidal neovascular membranes in a patient with presumed ocular histoplasmosis. Arch Ophthalmol. 1991; 109(11):1500–1501

[46] Arden GB, Berninger T, Hogg CR, Perry S. A survey of color discrimination in German ophthalmologists. Changes associated with the use of lasers and operating microscopes. Ophthalmology. 1991; 98(5):567–575

[47] National Institute of Diabetes and Digestive and Kidney Diseases. National Diabetes Statistics fact sheet: general information and national estimates on diabetes in the United States, 2005. Bethesda, MD: U.S. Department of Health and Human Services, National Institute of Health; 2005

[48] Early Treatment Diabetic Retinopathy Study Research Group. Early photocoagulation for diabetic retinopathy. ETDRS report number 9. Ophthalmology. 1991; 98 5 Suppl:766–85

[49] Early Treatment Diabetic Retinopathy Study Research Group. Photocoagulation for diabetic macular edema. Early Treatment Diabetic Retinopathy Study report number 1. Early Treatment Diabetic Retinopathy Study research group. Arch Ophthalmol. 1985; 103(12):1796–1806

[50] Olk RJ. Modified grid argon (blue-green) laser photocoagulation for diffuse diabetic macular edema. Ophthalmology. 1986; 93(7):938–950

[51] Writing Committee for the, Diabetic Retinopathy Clinical Research Network Fong DS, Strauber SF, Aiello LP, et al. Comparison of the modified Early Treatment Diabetic Retinopathy Study and mild macular grid laser photocoagulation strategies for diabetic macular edema. Arch Ophthalmol. 2007; 125 (4):469–480

[52] Kim NR, Kim YJ, Chin HS, Moon YS. Optical coherence tomographic patterns in diabetic macular oedema: prediction of visual outcome after focal laser photocoagulation. Br J Ophthalmol. 2009; 93(7):901–905

[53] Early Treatment Diabetic Retinopathy Study Research Group. Treatment techniques and clinical guidelines for photocoagulation of diabetic macular edema. Early Treatment Diabetic Retinopathy Study Report Number 2. Ophthalmology. 1987; 94(7):761–774

[54] The Early Treatment Diabetic Retinopathy Study Research Group. Techniques for scatter and local photocoagulation treatment of diabetic retinopathy: Early Treatment Diabetic Retinopathy Study Report no. 3. Int Ophthalmol Clin. 1987; 27(4):254–264

[55] Diabetic Retinopathy Study. Reports Number 6 Design, methods, and baseline results. Report Number 7. A modification of the Airlie House classification of diabetic retinopathy. Prepared by the Diabetic Retinopathy. Invest Ophthalmol Vis Sci. 1981; 21 (1 Pt 2):1–226

[56] The Diabetic Retinopathy Study Research Group. Four risk factors for severe visual loss in diabetic retinopathy. The third report from the Diabetic Retinopathy Study. Arch Ophthalmol. 1979; 97(4):654–655

[57] The Diabetic Retinopathy Study Research Group. Photocoagulation treatment of proliferative diabetic retinopathy. Clinical application of Diabetic Retinopathy Study (DRS) findings, DRS Report Number 8. Ophthalmology. 1981; 88(7):583–600

[58] British Multicentre Study Group. Photocoagulation for diabetic maculopathy. A randomized controlled clinical trial using the xenon arc. Diabetes. 1983; 32(11):1010–1016

[59] Early Treatment Diabetic Retinopathy Study Research Group. Early photocoagulation for diabetic retinopathy. ETDRS report number 9. Ophthalmology. 1991; 98(5) Suppl:766–785

[60] ETDRS Investigators. Aspirin effects on mortality and morbidity in patients with diabetes mellitus. Early Treatment Diabetic Retinopathy Study report 14. JAMA. 1992; 268(10):1292–1300

[61] Brown GC. Central retinal vein obstruction with lipid exudate. Arch Ophthalmol. 1989; 107(7):1001–1005
[62] Weinberg D, Jampol LM, Schatz H, Brady KD. Exudative retinal detachment following central and hemicentral retinal vein occlusions. Arch Ophthalmol. 1990; 108(2):271–275
[63] Hayreh SS. Classification of central retinal vein occlusion. Ophthalmology. 1983; 90(5):458–474
[64] Baseline and early natural history report. The Central Vein Occlusion Study. Arch Ophthalmol. 1993; 111(8):1087–1095
[65] Evaluation of grid pattern photocoagulation for macular edema in central vein occlusion. The Central Vein Occlusion Study Group M report. Ophthalmology. 1995; 102(10):1425–1433
[66] Natural history and clinical management of central retinal vein occlusion. The Central Vein Occlusion Study Group. Arch Ophthalmol. 1997; 115 (4):486–491
[67] Quinlan PM, Elman MJ, Bhatt AK, Mardesich P, Enger C. The natural course of central retinal vein occlusion. Am J Ophthalmol. 1990; 110(2):118–123
[68] A randomized clinical trial of early panretinal photocoagulation for ischemic central vein occlusion. The Central Vein Occlusion Study Group N report. Ophthalmology. 1995; 102(10):1434–1444
[69] McAllister IL, Constabl, e IJ. Laser-induced chorioretinal venous anastomosis for treatment of nonischemic central retinal vein occlusion. Arch Ophthalmol. 1995; 113(4):456–462
[70] The Branch Vein Occlusion Study Group. Argon laser photocoagulation for macular edema in branch vein occlusion. Am J Ophthalmol. 1984; 98 (3):271–282
[71] Branch Vein Occlusion Study Group. Argon laser scatter photocoagulation for prevention of neovascularization and vitreous hemorrhage in branch vein occlusion. A randomized clinical trial. Arch Ophthalmol. 1986; 104 (1):34–41
[72] Friedman DS, O'Colmain BJ, Muñoz B, et al. Eye Diseases Prevalence Research Group. Prevalence of age-related macular degeneration in the United States. Arch Ophthalmol. 2004; 122(4):564–572
[73] Regillo CD, Benson WE, Maguire JI, Annesley WH, Jr. Indocyanine green angiography and occult choroidal neovascularization. Ophthalmology. 1994; 101(2):280–288
[74] Macular Photocoagulation Study Group. Argon laser photocoagulation for senile macular degeneration. Results of a randomized clinical trial. Arch Ophthalmol. 1982; 100(6):912–918
[75] Macular Photocoagulation Study Group. Argon laser photocoagulation for neovascular maculopathy. Five-year results from randomized clinical trials. Arch Ophthalmol. 1991; 109(8):1109–1114
[76] Macular Photocoagulation Study Group. Persistent and recurrent neovascularization after krypton laser photocoagulation for neovascular lesions of age-related macular degeneration. Arch Ophthalmol. 1990; 108(6):825–831
[77] Macular Photocoagulation Study Group. Laser photocoagulation of subfoveal neovascular lesions in age-related macular degeneration. Results of a randomized clinical trial. Arch Ophthalmol. 1991; 109(9):1220–1231
[78] Macular Photocoagulation Study Group. Subfoveal neovascular lesions in age-related macular degeneration. Guidelines for evaluation and treatment in the macular photocoagulation study. Arch Ophthalmol. 1991; 109 (9):1242–1257
[79] Macular Photocoagulation Study Group. Krypton laser photocoagulation for neovascular lesions of age-related macular degeneration. Results of a randomized clinical trial. Arch Ophthalmol. 1990; 108(6):816–824
[80] Smiddy WE, Fine SL, Quigley HA, Hohman RM, Addicks EA. Comparison of krypton and argon laser photocoagulation. Results of stimulated clinical treatment of primate retina. Arch Ophthalmol. 1984; 102(7):1086–1092
[81] Guyer DR, Puliafito CA, Monés JM, Friedman E, Chang W, Verdooner SR. Digital indocyanine-green angiography in chorioretinal disorders. Ophthalmology. 1992; 99(2):287–291
[82] Yannuzzi LA, Slakter JS, Sorenson JA, Guyer DR, Orlock DA. Digital indocyanine green videoangiography and choroidal neovascularization. Retina. 1992; 12(3):191–223
[83] Foos RY. Retinal holes. Am J Ophthalmol. 1978; 86(3):354–358
[84] Byer NE. Clinical study of retinal breaks. Trans Am Acad Ophthalmol Otolaryngol. 1967; 71(3):461–473
[85] Campochiaro PA, Kaden IH, Vidaurri-Leal J, Glaser BM. Cryotherapy enhances intravitreal dispersion of viable retinal pigment epithelial cells. Arch Ophthalmol. 1985; 103(3):434–436
[86] Guyer DR, Duker JS, Puliafito CA. Indocyanine green angiography and dye-enhanced diode laser photocoagulation. Semin Ophthalmol. 1992; 7 (3):172–176
[87] Reichel E, Puliafito CA, Duker JS, Guyer DR. Indocyanine green dye-enhanced diode laser photocoagulation of poorly defined subfoveal choroidal neovascularization. Ophthalmic Surg. 1994; 25(3):195–201
[88] Gibson SL, Havens JJ, Nguyen ML, Hilf R. Delta-aminolaevulinic acid-induced photodynamic therapy inhibits protoporphyrin IX biosynthesis and reduces subsequent treatment efficacy in vitro. Br J Cancer. 1999; 80(7):998–1004
[89] Ben-Hur E, Orenstein A. The endothelium and red blood cells as potential targets in PDT-induced vascular stasis. Int J Radiat Biol. 1991; 60(1-2):293–301
[90] Henderson BW, Dougherty TJ. How does photodynamic therapy work? Photochem Photobiol. 1992; 55(1):145–157
[91] Murphree AL, Cote M, Gomer CJ. The evolution of photodynamic therapy techniques in the treatment of intraocular tumors. Photochem Photobiol. 1987; 46(5):919–923
[92] Tse DT, Dutton JJ, Weingeist TA, Hermsen VM, Kersten RC. Hematoporphyrin photoradiation therapy for intraocular and orbital malignant melanoma. Arch Ophthalmol. 1984; 102(6):833–838
[93] Favilla I, Barry WR, Gosbell A, Ellims P, Burgess F. Phototherapy of posterior uveal melanomas. Br J Ophthalmol. 1991; 75(12):718–721
[94] Miller JW, Stinson WG, Gregory WA, el-Koumy HA, Puliafito CA. Phthalocyanine photodynamic therapy of experimental iris neovascularization. Ophthalmology. 1991; 98(11):1711–1719
[95] Kliman GH, Puliafito CA, Grossman GA, Gregory WA. Retinal and choroidal vessel closure using phthalocyanine photodynamic therapy. Lasers Surg Med. 1994; 15(1):11–18
[96] Kliman GH, Puliafito CA, Stern D, Borirakchanyavat S, Gregory WA. Phthalocyanine photodynamic therapy: new strategy for closure of choroidal neovascularization. Lasers Surg Med. 1994; 15(1):2–10
[97] Baumal CR, Puliafito CA, Pieroth L, et al. Photodynamic therapy of experimental choroidal neovascularization with tin ethyl etiopurpurin. Invest Ophthalmol Vis Sci. 1996; 37:S:122
[98] Peyman GA, Moshfeghi DM, Moshfeghi A, et al. Photodynamic therapy for choriocapillaris using tin ethyl etiopurpurin (SnET2). Ophthalmic Surg Lasers. 1997; 28(5):409–417
[99] TAP Study Group. Photodynamic therapy of subfoveal choroidal neovascularization in age-related macular degeneration with verteporfin: one-year results of 2 randomized clinical trials—TAP report. Treatment of age-related macular degeneration with photodynamic therapy (TAP) Study Group. Arch Ophthalmol. 1999; 117:1329–1345
[100] Verteporfin in Photodynamic Therapy Study Group. Photodynamic therapy of subfoveal choroidal neovascularization in pathologic myopia with verteporfin. 1-year results of a randomized clinical trial—VIP report no. 1. Ophthalmology. 2001; 108(5):841–852
[101] Tseng CC, Chen SN. Long-term efficacy of half-dose photodynamic therapy on chronic central serous chorioretinopathy. Br J Ophthalmol. 2015; 99 (8):1070–1077
[102] Zhao M, Zhang F, Chen Y, et al. A 50% vs 30% dose of verteporfin (photodynamic therapy) for acute central serous chorioretinopathy: one-year results of a randomized clinical trial. JAMA Ophthalmol. 2015; 133(3):333–340
[103] Fujita K, Imamura Y, Shinoda K, et al. One-year outcomes with half-dose verteporfin photodynamic therapy for chronic central serous chorioretinopathy. Ophthalmology. 2015; 122(3):555–561
[104] Ma J, Meng N, Xu X, Zhou F, Qu Y. System review and meta-analysis on photodynamic therapy in central serous chorioretinopathy. Acta Ophthalmol (Copenh). 2014; 92(8):e594–e601
[105] Reibaldi M, Cardascia N, Longo A, et al. Standard-fluence versus low-fluence photodynamic therapy in chronic central serous chorioretinopathy: a nonrandomized clinical trial. Am J Ophthalmol. 2010; 149(2):307–315.e2
[106] Lim JI, Glassman AR, Aiello LP, Chakravarthy U, Flaxel CJ, Spaide RF, Macula Society CSC Collaborative Study Group, Research and Education Committee and Website Committee. Collaborative retrospective macula society study of photodynamic therapy for chronic central serous chorioretinopathy. Ophthalmology. 2014; 121(5):1073–1078
[107] Yannuzzi LA, Sorenson J, Spaide RF, Lipson B. Idiopathic polypoidal choroidal vasculopathy (IPCV). Retina. 1990; 10(1):1–8
[108] Koh A, Lee WK, Chen LJ, et al. EVEREST study: efficacy and safety of verteporfin photodynamic therapy in combination with ranibizumab or alone versus ranibizumab monotherapy in patients with symptomatic macular polypoidal choroidal vasculopathy. Retina. 2012; 32(8):1453–1464
[109] Gomi F, Oshima Y, Mori R, et al. Initial versus delayed photodynamic therapy in combination with ranibizumab for treatment of polypoidal choroidal vasculopathy: The Fujisan Study. Retina. 2015; 35(8):1569–1576

[110] Wong CW, Cheung CM, Mathur R, et al. Three-year results of polypoidal choroidal vasculopathy treated with photodynamic therapy: Retrospective study and systematic review. Retina. 2015; 35(8):1577–1593

[111] Zharov VP, Galitovskaya EN, Johnson C, Kelly T. Synergistic enhancement of selective nanophotothermolysis with gold nanoclusters: potential for cancer therapy. Lasers Surg Med. 2005; 37(3):219–226

[112] Jain A, Blumenkranz MS, Paulus Y, et al. Effect of pulse duration on size and character of the lesion in retinal photocoagulation. Arch Ophthalmol. 2008; 126(1):78–85

[113] Sramek C, Paulus Y, Nomoto H, Huie P, Brown J, Palanker D. Dynamics of retinal photocoagulation and rupture. J Biomed Opt. 2009; 14(3):034007

[114] Blumenkranz MS, Yellachich D, Andersen DE, et al. Semiautomated patterned scanning laser for retinal photocoagulation. Retina. 2006; 26(3):370–376

[115] Bandello F, Polito A, Del Borrello M, Zemella N, Isola M. "Light" versus "classic" laser treatment for clinically significant diabetic macular oedema. Br J Ophthalmol. 2005; 89(7):864–870

[116] Bandello F, Brancato R, Menchini U, et al. Light panretinal photocoagulation (LPRP) versus classic panretinal photocoagulation (CPRP) in proliferative diabetic retinopathy. Semin Ophthalmol. 2001; 16(1):12–18

[117] Sanghvi C, McLauchlan R, Delgado C, et al. Initial experience with the Pascal photocoagulator: a pilot study of 75 procedures. Br J Ophthalmol. 2008; 92 (8):1061–1064

[118] Al-Hussainy S, Dodson PM, Gibson JM. Pain response and follow-up of patients undergoing panretinal laser photocoagulation with reduced exposure times. Eye (Lond). 2008; 22(1):96–99

[119] Rüfer F, Flöhr CM, Poerksen E, Roider J. Retinal laser coagulation with the pattern scanning laser—report of first clinical experience [in German]. Klin Monatsbl Augenheilkd. 2008; 225(11):968–972

[120] Muqit MM, Gray JC, Marcellino GR, et al. Fundus autofluorescence and Fourier-domain optical coherence tomography imaging of 10 and 20 millisecond Pascal retinal photocoagulation treatment. Br J Ophthalmol. 2009; 93 (4):518–525

[121] Chappelow AV, Tan K, Waheed NK, Kaiser PK. Panretinal photocoagulation for proliferative diabetic retinopathy: pattern scan laser versus argon laser. Am J Ophthalmol. 2012; 153(1):137–42.e2

[122] Muqit MM, Marcellino GR, Henson DB, Young LB, Turner GS, Stanga PE. Pascal panretinal laser ablation and regression analysis in proliferative diabetic retinopathy: Manchester Pascal Study Report 4. Eye (Lond). 2011; 25 (11):1447–1456

[123] Palanker D, Lavinsky D, Blumenkranz MS, Marcellino G. The impact of pulse duration and burn grade on size of retinal photocoagulation lesion: implications for pattern density. Retina. 2011; 31(8):1664–1669

[124] Shin JY, Byeon SH, Kwon OW. Optical coherence tomography-guided selective focal laser photocoagulation: a novel laser protocol for diabetic macular edema. Graefes Arch Clin Exp Ophthalmol. 2015; 253(4):527–535

[125] Lavinsky D, Sramek C, Wang J, et al. Subvisible retinal laser therapy: titration algorithm and tissue response. Retina. 2014; 34(1):87–97

[126] Lavinsky D, Palanker D. Nondamaging photothermal therapy for the retina: initial clinical experience with chronic central serous retinopathy. Retina. 2015; 35(2):213–222

[127] Sramek C, Mackanos M, Spitler R, et al. Non-damaging retinal phototherapy: dynamic range of heat shock protein expression. Invest Ophthalmol Vis Sci. 2011; 52(3):1780–1787

[128] Iwami H, Pruessner J, Shiraki K, Brinkmann R, Miura Y. Protective effect of a laser-induced sub-lethal temperature rise on RPE cells from oxidative stress. Exp Eye Res. 2014; 124:37–47

[129] Paulus YM, Jain A, Gariano RF, et al. Healing of retinal photocoagulation lesions. Invest Ophthalmol Vis Sci. 2008; 49(12):5540–5545

[130] Busch EM, Gorgels TG, Van Norren D. Filling-in after focal loss of photoreceptors in rat retina. Exp Eye Res. 1999; 68(4):485–492

[131] Zwick H, Edsall P, Stuck BE, et al. Laser induced photoreceptor damage and recovery in the high numerical aperture eye of the garter snake. Vision Res. 2008; 48(3):486–493

[132] Sher A, Jones BW, Huie P, et al. Restoration of retinal structure and function after selective photocoagulation. J Neurosci. 2013; 33(16):6800–6808

[133] Lavinsky D, Cardillo JA, Mandel Y, et al. Restoration of retinal morphology and residual scarring after photocoagulation. Acta Ophthalmol (Copenh). 2013; 91(4):e315–e323

[134] Koinzer S, Saeger M, Hesse C, et al. Correlation with OCT and histology of photocoagulation lesions in patients and rabbits. Acta Ophthalmol (Copenh). 2013; 91(8):e603–e611

[135] Parrozzani R, Boccassini B, De Belvis V, Radin PP, Midena E. Long-term outcome of transpupillary thermotherapy as primary treatment of selected choroidal melanoma. Acta Ophthalmol (Copenh). 2009; 87(7):789–792

[136] Aaberg TM, Jr, Bergstrom CS, Hickner ZJ, Lynn MJ. Long-term results of primary transpupillary thermal therapy for the treatment of choroidal malignant melanoma. Br J Ophthalmol. 2008; 92(6):741–746

[137] Oosterhuis JA, Journée-de Korver HG, Kakebeeke-Kemme HM, Bleeker JC. Transpupillary thermotherapy in choroidal melanomas. Arch Ophthalmol. 1995; 113(3):315–321

[138] Reichel E, Berrocal AM, Ip M, et al. Transpupillary thermotherapy of occult subfoveal choroidal neovascularization in patients with age-related macular degeneration. Ophthalmology. 1999; 106(10):1908–1914

[139] Ahuja RM, Benner JD, Schwartz JC, Butler JW, Steidl SM. Efficacy of transpupillary thermotherapy (TTT) in the treatment of occult subfoveal choroidal neovascularization in age-related macular degeneration. Semin Ophthalmol. 2001; 16(2):81–85

[140] Newsom RS, McAlister JC, Saeed M, McHugh JD. Transpupillary thermotherapy (TTT) for the treatment of choroidal neovascularisation. Br J Ophthalmol. 2001; 85(2):173–178

[141] Sivaprasad S, Elagouz M, McHugh D, Shona O, Dorin G. Micropulsed diode laser therapy: evolution and clinical applications. Surv Ophthalmol. 2010; 55(6):516–530

[142] Fedoruk NA, Fedorov AA, Bol'shunov AV. Morphological and histochemical effects of subthreshold laser therapy on the chorioretinal complex [in Russian]. Vestn Oftalmol. 2013; 129(5):73–81

[143] Luttrull JK, Musch DC, Mainster MA. Subthreshold diode micropulse photocoagulation for the treatment of clinically significant diabetic macular oedema. Br J Ophthalmol. 2005; 89(1):74–80

[144] Luttrull JK, Musch DC, Spink CA. Subthreshold diode micropulse panretinal photocoagulation for proliferative diabetic retinopathy. Eye (Lond). 2008; 22 (5):607–612

[145] Luttrull JK, Spink CJ. Serial optical coherence tomography of subthreshold diode laser micropulse photocoagulation for diabetic macular edema. Ophthalmic Surg Lasers Imaging. 2006; 37(5):370–377

[146] Malik KJ, Sampat KM, Mansouri A, Steiner JN, Glaser BM. Low-intensity/high-density subthreshold microPulse diode laser for chronic central serous chorioretinopathy. Retina. 2015; 35(3):532–536

[147] Roider J. Laser treatment of retinal diseases by subthreshold laser effects. Semin Ophthalmol. 1999; 14(1):19–26

[148] Brinkmann R, Roider J, Birngruber R. Selective retina therapy (SRT): a review on methods, techniques, preclinical and first clinical results. Bull Soc Belge Ophtalmol. 2006; 302(302):51–69

[149] Treumer F, Klettner A, Baltz J, et al. Vectorial release of matrix metalloproteinases (MMPs) from porcine RPE-choroid explants following selective retina therapy (SRT): towards slowing the macular ageing process. Exp Eye Res. 2012; 97(1):63–72

[150] Kim HD, Han JW, Ohn YH, Brinkmann R, Park TK. Functional evaluation using multifocal electroretinogram after selective retina therapy with a microsecond-pulsed laser. Invest Ophthalmol Vis Sci. 2015; 56(1):122–131

[151] Roider J, Michaud NA, Flotte TJ, Birngruber R. Response of the retinal pigment epithelium to selective photocoagulation. Arch Ophthalmol. 1992; 110 (12):1786–1792

[152] Framme C, Schuele G, Roider J, Kracht D, Birngruber R, Brinkmann R. Threshold determinations for selective retinal pigment epithelium damage with repetitive pulsed microsecond laser systems in rabbits. Ophthalmic Surg Lasers. 2002; 33(5):400–409

[153] Roider J, Brinkmann R, Wirbelauer C, Laqua H, Birngruber R. Retinal sparing by selective retinal pigment epithelial photocoagulation. Arch Ophthalmol. 1999; 117(8):1028–1034

[154] Framme C, Alt C, Schnell S, Sherwood M, Brinkmann R, Lin CP. Selective targeting of the retinal pigment epithelium in rabbit eyes with a scanning laser beam. Invest Ophthalmol Vis Sci. 2007; 48(4):1782–1792

[155] Paulus YM, Jain A, Nomoto H, et al. Selective retinal therapy with microsecond exposures using a continuous line scanning laser. Retina. 2011; 31 (2):380–388

[156] Park YG, Seifert E, Roh YJ, Theisen-Kunde D, Kang S, Brinkmann R. Tissue response of selective retina therapy by means of a feedback-controlled energy ramping mode. Clin Experiment Ophthalmol. 2014; 42(9):846–855

[157] Roider J, Brinkmann R, Wirbelauer C, Laqua H, Birngruber R. Subthreshold (retinal pigment epithelium) photocoagulation in macular diseases: a pilot study. Br J Ophthalmol. 2000; 84(1):40–47

[158] Elsner H, Pörksen E, Klatt C, et al. Selective retina therapy in patients with central serous chorioretinopathy. Graefes Arch Clin Exp Ophthalmol. 2006; 244(12):1638–1645

[159] Koinzer S, Elsner H, Klatt C, et al. Selective retina therapy (SRT) of chronic subfoveal fluid after surgery of rhegmatogenous retinal detachment: three case reports. Graefes Arch Clin Exp Ophthalmol. 2008; 246(10):1373–1378

[160] Klatt C, Saeger M, Oppermann T, et al. Selective retina therapy for acute central serous chorioretinopathy. Br J Ophthalmol. 2011; 95(1):83–88

[161] Roider J, Liew SH, Klatt C, et al. Selective retina therapy (SRT) for clinically significant diabetic macular edema. Graefes Arch Clin Exp Ophthalmol. 2010; 248(9):1263–1272

[162] Ohkoshi K, Yamaguchi T. Subthreshold micropulse diode laser photocoagulation for diabetic macular edema in Japanese patients. Am J Ophthalmol. 2010; 149(1):133–139

[163] Cohen BZ, Wald KJ, Toyama K. Neodymium:YLF picosecond laser segmentation for retinal traction associated with proliferative diabetic retinopathy. Am J Ophthalmol. 1997; 123(4):515–523

40 Vitreous Surgery

Thanos D. Papakostas, Dean Eliott, and Ingrid U. Scott

40.1 Introduction

Robert Machemer is considered the father of modern vitreous surgery as he developed the instrumentation and was the first to perform pars plana vitrectomy (PPV). He also paved the way for our understanding of the role of the vitreous and the etiology of abnormal cellular proliferation in many vitreoretinal disorders.

Initially, vitrectomy was reserved only for select cases such as nonclearing vitreous hemorrhage and complicated retinal detachment. With increased surgeon experience and improved technology and instrumentation, the indications for vitrectomy expanded, and today it is the most commonly performed surgical procedure by retinal specialists. Advances in technology have made vitrectomy surgery safer and more effective, and after the introduction of microincisional vitrectomy surgery in the 2000s, vitrectomy has become an even more efficient procedure with less morbidity. There are myriad indications for vitrectomy which are summarized in ▶ Table 40.1.

The purpose of this chapter is to describe the essential principles of vitrectomy and highlight the outcomes of common disorders managed with vitrectomy.

40.2 Preoperative Considerations

The patient who will undergo vitrectomy needs to have a thorough preoperative ophthalmic examination and a general medical evaluation by an internist or a member of the anesthesia team. The surgeon should discuss with the patient the goals of the surgery and the potential risks, benefits, and alternatives. The patient must show understanding of the information provided. The patient needs to be able to lie flat (or nearly flat) for the duration of the vitrectomy and patients with claustrophobia, moderate to severe anxiety, or dementia may benefit from having vitrectomy performed under general anesthesia.

Preoperative examination should include detailed slit-lamp biomicroscopy. The clarity of the cornea is noted. In cases of significant corneal opacity, a temporary keratoprosthesis with subsequent penetrating keratoplasty can be considered. Alternatively, an endoscopic approach can be followed. The anterior chamber is examined and its depth is noted. A potentially occludable angle may necessitate the creation of a prophylactic peripheral iridotomy. Gonioscopy is important in diabetic patients undergoing vitrectomy as well as in patients with uveitis. Dilation of the pupil is important for any vitreoretinal procedure. The lens status and clarity of the crystalline lens in phakic patients should always be noted. In pseudophakic patients, the type of implant, its position in the capsular bag or sulcus, and the integrity of the posterior capsule should be known by the surgeon before proceeding to the operating room. For example, silicone oil placement in an eye with a silicone intraocular lens (IOL) and an open posterior capsule may result in accumulation of silicone oil droplets on the posterior surface of the lens.

A thorough posterior segment examination is of paramount importance before any vitreoretinal procedure. The anterior vitreous is inspected with the slit lamp and any cells are noted. Then, a 90-diopter or a 78-diopter lens is used for the examination of the posterior pole. The 90-diopter lens provides a wider field of view, while the 78-diopter lens provides higher magnification. The presence or absence of a posterior vitreous detachment (PVD) is noted, and the optic nerve, macula, and retinal vessels are examined carefully. Identification of presence or absence of PVD is one of the most important preoperative considerations, as it may impact the surgical approach. The peripheral retina is examined with binocular indirect ophthalmoscopy with and without scleral depression. The lenses typically used are the 28-diopter or the 20-diopter lens. The 28-diopter lens offers a wider field of view than the 20-diopter lens and the 20-diopter lens offers higher magnification. The authors prefer the 28-diopter lens, especially in eyes with a preexisting gas bubble.

Digital imaging aids the surgeon in preoperative decision making. An important imaging modality is optical coherence tomography (OCT), which shows the relation of the posterior hyaloid to the retina, presence or absence of epiretinal membrane (ERM), foveal contour, and retinal thickness. Cystoid macular edema and subtle subretinal fluid can be detected with OCT. Other imaging modalities that may be helpful are digital fundus photographs of the macula and the more recently introduced panoramic wide-field views of the retina (▶ Fig. 40.1). Fluorescein angiography may be performed before diabetic vitrectomy to assess retinal perfusion and neovascularization.

When media opacities preclude visualization of the posterior segment, B-scan ultrasonography should be performed in both static and dynamic fashion. The presence or absence of PVD should be assessed. Any retinal breaks, traction, or detachment should be noted. In patients with prior traumatic open-globe injuries, care should be taken during the ultrasonographic examination to identify any area of retinal incarceration. Computed tomography is the standard of care in the identification of intraocular foreign body (IOFB).

Most vitreoretinal procedures can be performed under local anesthesia with monitored anesthesia care. In patients who are unable to cooperate, in pediatric patients, and in patients with open-globe trauma, general anesthesia is recommended. General anesthesia may also be considered in cases with long expected surgical durations or in cases requiring a scleral buckle.

40.3 Surgical Techniques

40.3.1 Visualization

Vitreoretinal surgery is always performed with an operating microscope. Historically, the lenses used for vitrectomy were planoconcave or biconcave lenses, which allow a limited field of view (20–35 degrees).[1] Prism lenses were also used to increase

Table 40.1 Indications for vitrectomy

Diabetic retinopathy	Choroidal neovascularization
• Nonclearing or repeated vitreous hemorrhage	Massive subretinal hemorrhage
• Traction retinal detachment	Macular translocation
• Combined traction and rhegmatogenous retinal detachment	Transplantation of retinal photoreceptors or retinal pigment epithelium
• Progressive fibrovascular proliferation	*Pediatric retinal disorders*
• Macular distortion by fibrovascular proliferation	• Retinopathy of prematurity
• Macular edema resulting from a taut posterior hyaloid	• Persistent hyperplastic primary vitreous
Retinal detachment	• Familial exudative vitreoretinopathy
• Retinal detachment with proliferative vitreoretinopathy	• Giant retinal tears/dialysis
• Giant retinal tears	• Juvenile retinoschisis
• Retinal detachment secondary to posterior retinal breaks	• Juvenile rheumatoid arthritis
	• Retinal detachment secondary to choroidal coloboma
• Selected primary retinal detachments	• Retinal detachment in "morning glory" syndrome or optic nerve colobomas
Complications of anterior segment surgery	*Tumors*
• Dislocated lens fragments	• Internal resection of choroidal melanoma
• Dislocated intraocular lens	• Complications of retinal angiomatosis
• Aphakic or pseudophakic cystoid macular edema	• Combined hamartoma of the retina and retinal pigment epithelium
• Endophthalmitis	• Intraocular lymphoma
• Malignant glaucoma	• Diagnostic vitrectomy
• Choroidal hemorrhage	• Retinal biopsy
• Epithelial downgrowth	*Uveitis*
• Anesthetic needle perforation	• Viral retinitis—cytomegalovirus, acute retinal necrosis
Trauma	• Intraocular infections—bacterial, viral, fungal, parasitic
• Hyphema evacuation	• Ophthalmomyiasis
• Traumatic cataract or dislocated lens	• Inflammatory conditions—sarcoidosis, Behçet's disease, uveal effusion
• Posterior penetrating injuries with vitreous hemorrhage and/or retinal detachment	• Pars planitis
• Reactive intraocular foreign body	• Whipple's disease
• Subretinal membranes or hemorrhage	• Familial amyloidosis
• Traumatic macular holes	• Hypotony
Macular surgery	
• Macular pucker	
• Macular hole	
• Vitreomacular traction syndrome	
• Serous retinal detachment secondary to optic pit	

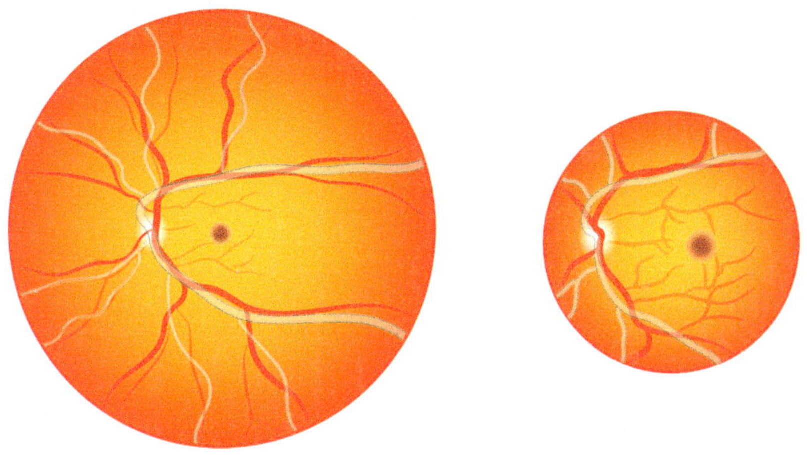

Fig. 40.1 The panoramic system allows adequate stereoscopic assessment of the retina with a wider field of view.

the field of view to 60 degrees.[2] The retinal periphery was difficult to visualize with these viewing systems, making the surgery technically cumbersome. Wide-angle viewing systems were developed that revolutionized vitreoretinal surgery as surgeons gained access to the peripheral vitreous and retina where substantial vitreoretinal pathology is often present. These systems are based on the principles of binocular indirect ophthalmoscopy and require an image inverter mounted on the operating microscope. Two types of wide-angle viewing systems for vitrectomy surgery exist: contact and noncontact systems. Contact systems (Volk Reinverting Operating Lens System, Volk; AVI Panoramic Wide-Angle Viewing System, AVI) provide 10 degrees greater field of view than noncontact systems and eliminate corneal aberrations. However, surgeons are dependent on a skilled assistant. The most popular noncontact systems are the Binocular Indirect Ophthalmomicroscope (BIOM) by Oculus and the Resight 700 system incorporated in the Lumera operating microscope by Zeiss. Noncontact systems require greater ocular rotation for viewing the periphery than contact systems. Surgeons switching from contact systems to noncontact systems are faced with a steep learning curve. The field of view with the BIOM depends primarily on the distance between the noncontact lens surface of the operating microscope and the corneal surface. As the noncontact lens approaches the cornea, the observed field becomes wider. Also, focusing the operating microscope sharpens the image. Focusing the BIOM can be complicated for beginners due to difficulty in maintaining a suitable distance between the indirect lens and the corneal surface and in maintaining the optimal distance between the height of the operating microscope and the corneal surface. However, once the surgeon becomes accustomed to the BIOM system, most vitreoretinal procedures can be performed safely and efficiently. More recently, another noncontact system, the Resight 700, was introduced by Zeiss and is becoming increasingly popular. It has a unique focusing system that allows the reduction lens set to be moved automatically inside the operating microscope. That allows the surgeon to obtain a high-resolution wide-angle view of the retina. Most surgeons perform macular surgery with a plano contact lens which provides high magnification and good lateral and axial resolution and other vitreoretinal procedures with the BIOM or Resight system Image.

40.3.2 Illumination

The current method of endoillumination, using a fiberoptic probe inserted into the vitreous cavity, was first introduced in the 1970s for 20-gauge vitrectomy.[3] In the 20-gauge era, illumination was made possible with a halogen bulb. However, when using a small-gauge fiberoptic probe with a conventional halogen light source, only 50% or less of the brightness found with the 20-gauge system is obtained. To compensate, xenon and mercury vapor bulbs were introduced. These systems provide superior illumination even with 25- or 27-gauge systems. Concerns regarding phototoxicity have been raised with these powerful illuminating systems, especially when the endoilluminator is close to the retina for a prolonged period of time.[4] More recently, wide-angle illumination probes were introduced[5] that provide a field of view close to 100 degrees compared to the standard 50 or 80 degree field of view that focal probes produce. A chandelier illumination system, which permits the surgeon to perform bimanual maneuvers, may also be used. The retina can tolerate this type of endoillumination for a prolonged period of time without evidence of toxicity compared to the conventional endoilluminator (▶ Fig. 40.2).

40.3.3 Chromovitrectomy

The term "chromovitrectomy" refers to the use of vital dyes during vitreoretinal surgery to assist with the identification of preretinal tissues and membranes.[6] It was first introduced by Kadonosono in 2000 when he used indocyanine green (ICG) to stain the internal limiting membrane (ILM) in macular hole surgery.[7] ICG binds to ILM, thus facilitating ILM visualization and aiding in its removal. It has also been proposed for visualization of ERM. There are concerns, however, as some investigators have reported suspected toxicity.[8] Other vital dyes used for ILM peeling are trypan blue and brilliant blue. Triamcinolone acetonide is superior in staining the vitreous and the posterior hyaloid but is not as good as ICG, trypan blue, or brilliant blue for ILM staining. Triamcinolone acetonide is used commonly by many surgeons to visualize the vitreous and ensure removal of the entire posterior vitreous cortex during surgery.

Controversial Points

- Intraoperative dyes such as ICG or brilliant blue can assist in visualization of the ILM. There is a concern regarding their potential toxic effects to the retina.

40.3.4 Cannula-Trocar Systems

Historically, 20-gauge surgery was performed for all pars plana vitrectomies; however, during the last decade, there has been a shift to transconjunctival MIVS with cannulated sclerotomies. In 2002, Fujii et al[9] introduced the 25-gauge transconjunctival sutureless vitrectomy system. The 25-gauge vitrectomy creates a smaller, self-sealing incision 0.55 mm in diameter, approximately half the size of the 1.15-mm incision created during 20-gauge vitrectomy. Initially, there were limitations with the 25-gauge instruments given their high flexibility and increased fragility. Eckardt introduced the 23-gauge system in 2005[10] with an incision size of 0.72 mm in diameter (▶ Fig. 40.3), and in 2010, Oshima et al introduced the 27-gauge system[11] with an incision size of 0.4 mm. The initial limitations with the early vitrectomy probes were later overcome as new stiffer probes were designed. Advantages of modern MIVS include less conjunctival disruption and faster surface recovery with less postoperative discomfort, quick entry and exit from the eye, lower incidence of entry site–associated retinal breaks, lower flow rates and possibly less retinal traction, smaller cutter port size and closer proximity to the probe tip with more precise end cutting ability, and valved cannulas that eliminate sclerotomy leakage. Currently, the majority of vitreoretinal procedures are performed with 23- or 25-gauge transconjunctival cannula-trocar–based systems; 20-gauge systems are typically reserved for some trauma cases or in cases with an IOFB. Three sclerotomies are created for vitrectomy through the pars plana, 3.5 to 4.0 mm posterior to the limbus in phakic eyes and 3.0 to 3.5 mm posterior to the limbus in pseudophakic or aphakic eyes (▶ Fig. 40.4). One sclerotomy is placed inferotemporally and provides continuous infusion of a saline solution. Two additional sclerotomies are placed (superonasally and superotemporally) and provide access for the endoilluminator and the vitreous cutter. Many surgeons prefer to displace the conjunctiva before the trocar insertion. Conjunctival displacement is essential for the transconjunctival sutureless technique, to provide containment of a vitreous wick as well as to prevent access of the tear film to the sclerotomies, thereby potentially reducing the endophthalmitis risk. In addition, the majority of surgeons prefer to enter the globe in a two-plane approach. The initial insertion is approximately 30 degrees relative to the sclera and the second trajectory is perpendicular to the sclera. This results in the creation of more stable and watertight wounds. After cannula placement, it is very important to confirm with direct visualization that the infusion cannula tip is in the vitreous cavity before the infusion is turned on, thus avoiding the possibility of infusing into the suprachoroidal space.

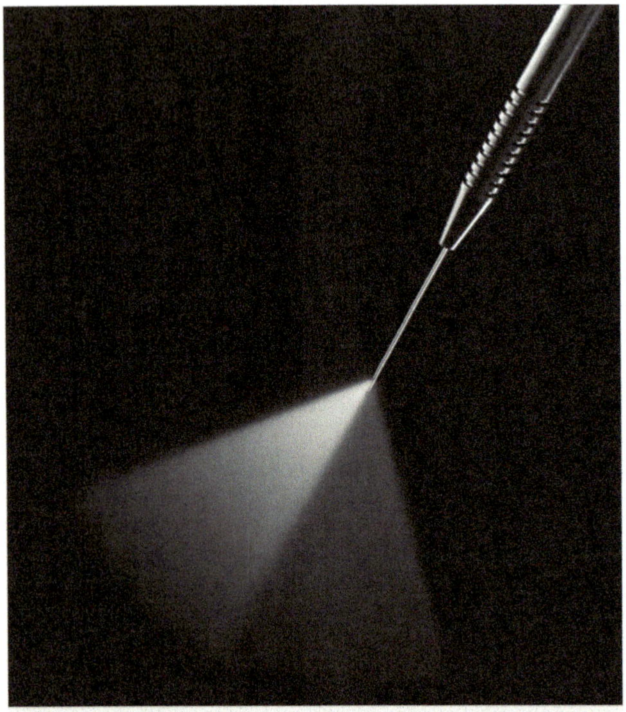

Fig. 40.2 23-gauge xenon endoilluminator. (Image courtesy of Alcon, Alcon Laboratories.)

40.3.5 Vitrectomy Systems

Machemer introduced the vitreous infusion suction cutter in 1970.[12] The original instrumentation was 17 gauge with an external diameter of 1.5 mm. Douvas developed the rotoextractor in the early 1970s,[13] and subsequently, O'Malley and Heintz

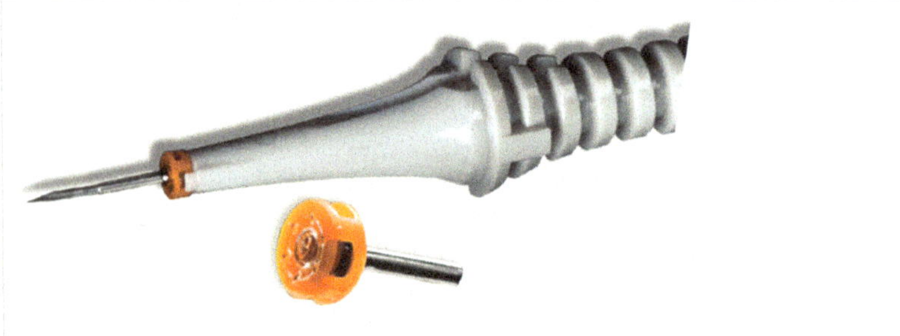

Fig. 40.3 23-gauge valved cannula and trocar. (Image courtesy of Alcon, Alcon Laboratories.)

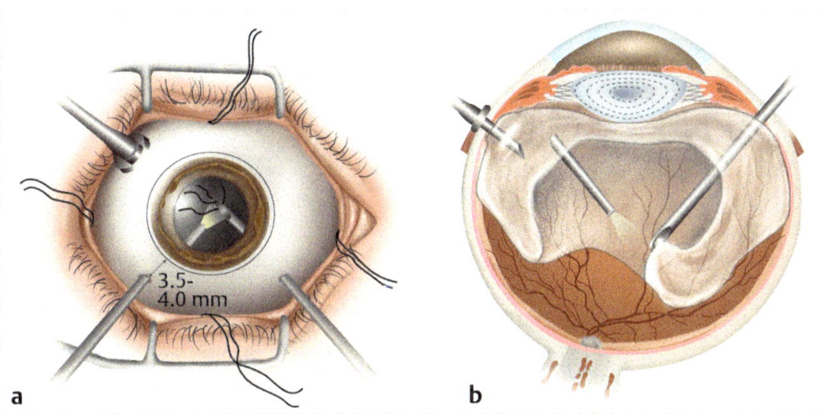

Fig. 40.4 Standard three-port pars plana vitrectomy. (**a**) Top and (**b**) cross-sectional views. The infusion cannula is secured inferotemporally. The two superior sclerotomies support the endoillumination probe and the vitrectomy handpiece

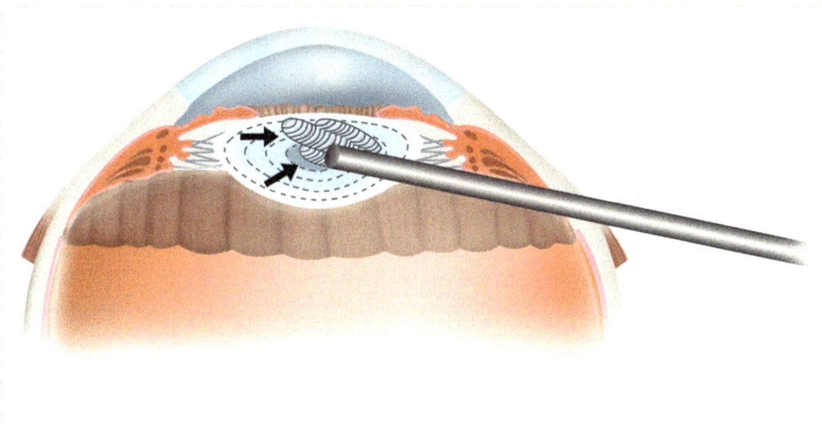

Fig. 40.5 Pars plana lensectomy is performed with an ultrasonic fragmenter or the vitrectomy cutter that is passed into the lens at its equator.

introduced the Berkley Bioengineering Ocutome 800, a 20-gauge vitrectomy probe with a 0.9-mm external diameter and 0.47-mm internal diameter.[14] This was the first lightweight pneumatic probe with surgeon foot pedal–controlled on-off aspiration. Over the ensuing years, several additional vitrectomy probes were developed, and in the mid-1990s, Alcon developed the first integrated vitrectomy system, the Accurus. This included an advanced graphical user interface with soft keys, vented gas-forced infusion, integrated fragmatome, silicone oil injector, and a halogen light source. The Accurus could provide cutting speeds of up to 2,500 cuts per minute. A similar system, the Millenium Microsurgical System, was developed by Bausch & Lomb. For almost 30 years, 20-gauge vitrectomy surgery was the standard until MIVS was introduced in the early 2000s. The Accurus was later substituted with the Constellation vitrectomy system, which provided cutting speeds of up to 7,500 cuts per minute. Similarly, the Millennium was substituted with the Stellaris PC. Higher cutting speeds are considered preferable because there is less retinal traction as the vitreous is cut. In addition to increasing safety by decreasing retinal traction and mobility, increased cut rates may also increase efficiency by enhancing flow through the cutter. An integral component contributing to the dynamics of vitreous flow into the cutter is the duty cycle. Duty cycle is defined as the proportion of time the port stays open during the entire length of the open-close cycle. Modern vitrectomy machines such as the Constellation vitrectomy system allow the surgeon to control the duty cycle.

Pearls

- Higher vitrectomy cutting speeds result in less traction on the retina and make maneuvers closer to the retina safer.
- Compared to 20-gauge vitrectomy, 23- and 25-gauge vitrectomy are associated with shorter operative times, faster recovery, and less postoperative inflammation.

40.3.6 Lensectomy

Pars plana lensectomy is performed (▸ Fig. 40.5) when there is a cataract precluding adequate visualization of the fundus or when the crystalline lens is subluxated or dislocated. In some cases, the capsular bag can be retained for simultaneous or possible future IOL implantation; however, removal of the lens and the entire capsule is recommended in cases of significant trauma and/or anterior proliferative vitreoretinopathy (PVR). If the crystalline lens and/or the capsule are retained in eyes with advanced anterior PVR, the capsule may serve as a scaffold for the proliferation of membranes, possibly resulting in recurrent retinal detachment and hypotony. In the pre-MIVS era, a 20-gauge fragmatome (sleeveless straight ultrasonic probe) was used for removal of the lens nucleus and cortex. However, with the advent of MIVS, many surgeons utilize the 23-gauge cutter to remove the lens. If the lens nucleus is exceptionally hard, it can be removed with the fragmatome, which requires enlargement of the 23-gauge wound. When using the fragmatome, the surgeon should be careful not to engage any vitreous in the tip of the probe as it will result in vitreous traction. Almost all cases of lensectomy are performed with a pars plana infusion. If there is a white cataract with no visualization posteriorly, an anterior chamber maintainer can be placed until there is sufficient view to visualize the pars plana infusion cannula tip so that the infusion fluid can be turned on safely. If an IOL is placed, a silicone IOL should be avoided in cases that may require future silicone oil tamponade.

40.3.7 Vitrectomy

Briefly, vitrectomy consists of first removing the vitreous around the sclerotomies, followed by removal of the core vitreous, induction of a PVD if it is not already present, peripheral vitreous shaving, and removal of any ERM. All steps of the vitrectomy should be performed under direct visualization. The vitreous cutter is placed through the superotemporal sclerotomy to perform the initial portion of the vitrectomy as access through the superotemporal sclerotomy provides a greater range of motion for the vitreous cutter. In phakic eyes, the nasal vitreous can be accessed by placing the cutter through the superonasal sclerotomy, thus minimizing the risk of traumatizing the crystalline lens. It is important to remove the vitreous near the sclerotomies before proceeding to the subsequent steps as it minimizes the chances of iatrogenic retinal breaks close to the sclerotomies.

40.3.8 Epiretinal Membrane Dissection

The first steps are to remove the vitreous around the sclerotomies, perform a core vitrectomy, and then induce a PVD if it is not already present. Most cases of idiopathic ERM are associated with a PVD, but if a PVD is not present, then a soft silicone tip or the vitreous cutter is used to create a PVD by using high aspiration adjacent to the optic nerve. Once the posterior hyaloid is engaged, it can be elevated and stripped to the periphery by gently moving the silicone tip or the cutter anteriorly. In some eyes with a strongly adherent posterior hyaloid, a pick or microvitreoretinal (MVR) blade can be used to initiate this process.

Machemer performed ERM peeling shortly after he developed vitrectomy.[15] He used a 23-gauge bent needle to engage and lift the ERM. Subsequently, O'Malley introduced the pick, a rounded-tip instrument, and Steve Charles developed end-grasping forceps (▶ Fig. 40.6). Most surgeons nowadays prefer to use forceps to peel the ERM, while some prefer to do this after the ERM has been stained with one of the dyes discussed previously. If an ERM edge cannot be identified, then a pick, an MVR blade, or a diamond-dusted scraper introduced by Tano can be used to develop an edge. Some surgeons have suggested peeling the ILM in all cases of ERM removal in order to minimize the risk of ERM recurrence; however, this remains controversial.

In cases of proliferative diabetic retinopathy with traction retinal detachment (TRD), different techniques are utilized in order to relieve traction on the macula. In these cases, the surgical goal is to relieve anterior-posterior and tangential traction of the posterior hyaloid and ERM. The techniques commonly used are segmentation, delamination, and en-bloc dissection. Segmentation involves the vertical cutting of ERM between epicenters (individual neovascular connections from the retina to the membrane) into small segments (▶ Fig. 40.7). Delamination (▶ Fig. 40.8) involves removal of fibrovascular tissue from the retina using horizontal scissors to sever the individual neovascular connections from the retinal surface. Segmentation or delamination can be performed with either specially designed vertical (▶ Fig. 40.9) or horizontal scissors, curved scissors, or even with the vitreous cutter probe. In en-bloc delamination, a small window in the partially detached posterior hyaloid is made so that a horizontal scissors can be introduced into the retrohyaloid space. Gentle traction from the vitreous immobilizes the fibrovascular membrane, and exposes areas of adhesion between the membrane and the retina, which facilitates membrane excision. The endoilluminator or illuminated forceps can be used to facilitate the dissection. When the membranes have been completely separated from the retina, the remaining posterior hyaloid complex can be removed with the vitreous cutter. Current MIVS cutters have the port close to the tip, which makes segmentation and delamination safer. Alternatively, one may use scissors to segment and forceps to dissect. Viscoelastic devices can be also used to create a plane for dissection and protect the retinal surface. In cases of strongly adherent membranes, bimanual techniques are often used with a lighted pick and forceps or a chandelier, scissors, and forceps.

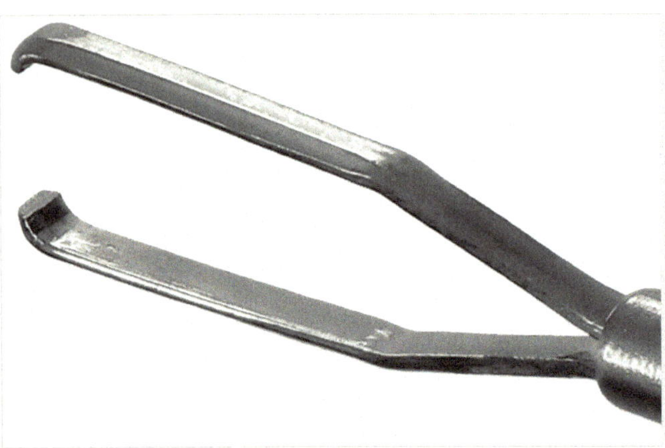

Fig. 40.6 End-grasping forceps for epiretinal and internal limiting membrane removal. (Image courtesy of Alcon, Alcon Laboratories.)

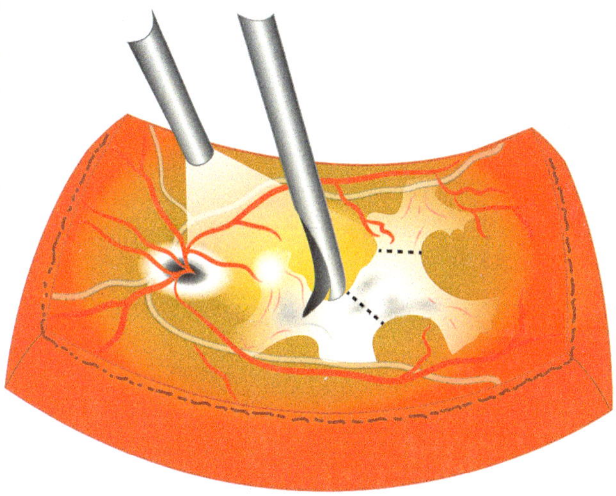

Fig. 40.7 Segmentation: Vertical sectioning of epiretinal fibrovascular tissue relieves tangential traction over the retina but leaves islands of fibrovascular tissue.

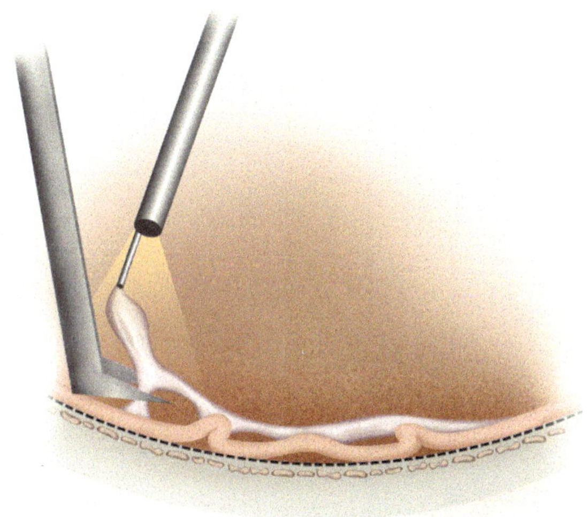

Fig. 40.8 Delamination: Using a bimanual technique, fibrovascular membranes are gently lifted with the fiberoptic tissue manipulator, while adhesions of the membranes to the retina are cut with horizontal scissors.

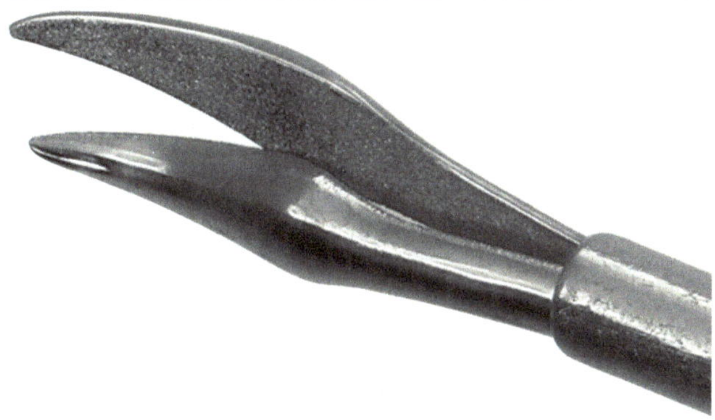

Fig. 40.9 Curved vertical scissors that are used for segmentation and delamination of adherent epiretinal membranes. (Image courtesy of Alcon, Alcon Laboratories.)

Pearls

- Complete separation of the posterior hyaloid is critical, especially in eyes with macular hole or diabetic tractional detachment.

40.3.9 Retinotomy–Retinectomy

Retinotomy and retinectomy were first described by Machemer in cases of PVR and trauma.[16] The term retinotomy refers to creating a hole in the retina, whereas retinectomy indicates excision of a portion of retina. There are two types of retinotomies: access and drainage. These are usually created in a healthy area of retina in order to enter the subretinal space. An access retinotomy can be performed for removal of subretinal tissues such as choroidal neovascular membrane and/or blood, or subretinal substances such as retained subretinal perfluorocarbon liquid (PFCL) or silicone oil, and subretinal foreign body. A drainage retinotomy is performed to remove subretinal fluid during retinal detachment surgery. Drainage retinotomies are usually performed superiorly so that they are in better contact with the gas or silicone oil tamponade. If possible, retinotomies should be performed along the distal course of nerve fibers to minimize nerve fiber bundle defects.[17]

Retinectomy is performed when there is an area of retinal traction with significant epiretinal or subretinal proliferation that does not lend itself to adequate removal (unrelieved traction) or when there is retinal contraction/foreshortening such that retinal attachment cannot be achieved without retinectomy. The most common indication is PVR. Another indication is when there is retina incarcerated in a scleral wound following trauma. Retinectomies are performed in the area of pathologic retina and usually extend to healthy retina for a clock hour on either side and are commonly performed in the peripheral retina. We prefer to apply diathermy at the edge of the intended retinectomy to minimize bleeding. When the retinectomy is oriented circumferentially, the edges should reach the ora by a right angle, if possible, and circumferential retinectomies are generally more stable than radial retinectomies. The vitreous cutter is usually used to perform the retinectomy, but vertical

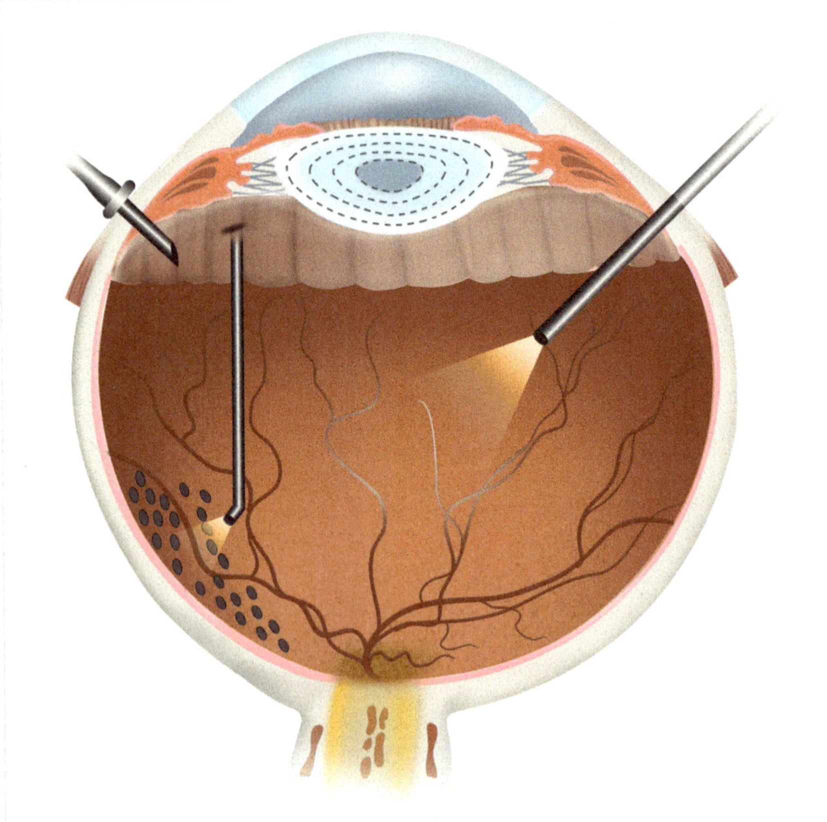

Fig. 40.10 Laser is applied internally with a fiberoptic probe. Curved probes allow more effective treatment of the retinal periphery than straight probes

scissors can be used to cut areas where there is very low lying retinal detachment to avoid damage to the underlying retinal pigment epithelium and choroid. In cases of PVR requiring circumferential retinectomy, it is recommended to remove the anterior retina all the way to the ora as residual nonperfused retina can promote fibrous proliferation and neovascularization.

40.3.10 Endophotocoagulation

Endophotocoagulation is applied around all retinal breaks and at the edges of the retinotomy/retinectomy, except when a retinotomy is within the macula. Typically, three rows of laser are applied and the burns should be gray in appearance. Intense laser burns should be generally avoided as new breaks can form at the edges of the laser spots. In cases of rhegmatogenous retinal detachment with extensive peripheral vitreoretinal pathology, 360-degree endophotocoagulation is advocated by some surgeons. There are a wide variety of laser probes available including illuminated and curved laser probes. Curved laser probes are extremely useful in phakic patients for the treatment of retinal pathology in the far periphery. Illuminated laser probes permit the surgeon to perform simultaneous scleral depression of the areas of interest. In most cases of diabetic vitrectomy, we apply 360-degree panretinal laser photocoagulation all the way to the ora serrata (▶ Fig. 40.10).

40.3.11 Perfluorocarbon Liquid

Chang introduced PFCL in vitreous surgery in 1987.[18] PFCLs have several physical properties that have made them popular in vitreoretinal surgery (▶ Fig. 40.11). The high density and specific gravity of PFCLs allow flattening of the retina and unrolling of retinal folds. They also help the surgeon avoid a posterior retinotomy to drain the subretinal fluid. They are optically clear and, therefore, allow for surgical manipulations under them. In addition, immiscibility with water resists incursion by saline and blood and allows a clear operating field despite intraoperative hemorrhage. Also, immiscibility with silicone oil allows PFCL–silicone oil exchange, which is helpful when treating giant retinal tears (GRTs) by reducing the risk of retinal slippage. There is no interference between PFCLs and laser wavelengths, thus allowing endolaser under PFCL. Furthermore, the low viscosity of PFCLs allows easy injection and aspiration.

PFCLs are invaluable in PVR and GRT surgery. The use of PFCLs has revolutionized the treatment of GRTs, as the surgeon can unroll the GRT with the patient in the supine position.

40.4 Surgical Complications

There are many possible complications that can occur with vitreous surgery. Modern techniques and instrumentation have significantly reduced the rate of complications; however, they are still relevant. Herein, we discuss the most important complications that can occur during or after vitrectomy.

40.4.1 Intraoperative Complications

If the cannula/trocar is inserted too anteriorly, bleeding can occur if the trocar penetrates the ciliary body. In addition, if the cannula/trocar has contact with the crystalline lens, a cataract

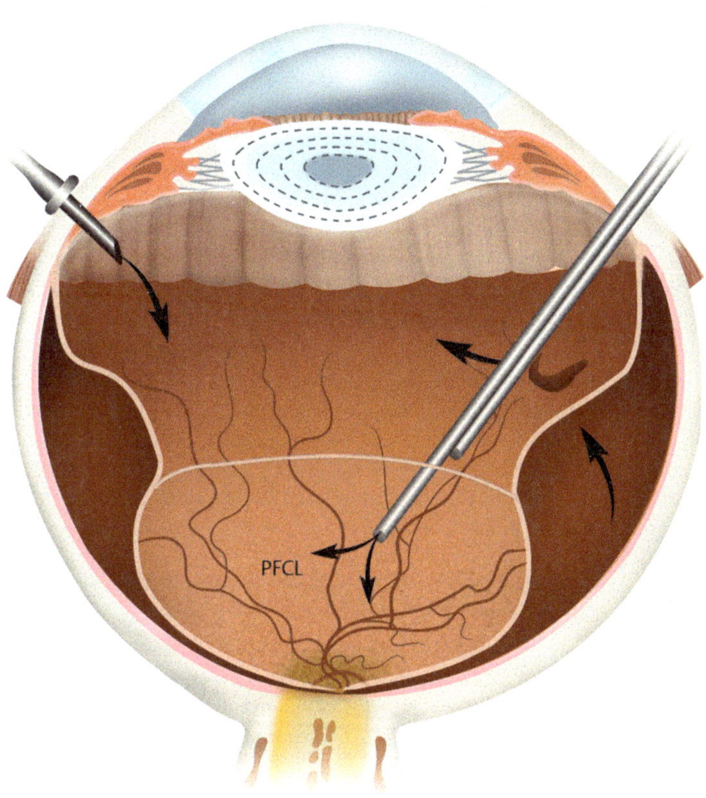

Fig. 40.11 The injection of perfluorocarbon liquid intraoperatively reattaches the retina in a posterior-to-anterior direction. The subretinal fluid is displaced through an existing peripheral retinal break as the fluid is instilled

may form, making visualization during the vitrectomy challenging. If the cannula/trocar is inserted too far posteriorly, a retinal break with or without retinal detachment may occur. Cannula placement should be 3.0 to 3.5 mm posterior to the limbus in aphakic and pseudophakic eyes and 3.5 to 4.0 mm in phakic eyes. Another possible complication during the first steps of surgery is suprachoroidal infusion of infusion fluid. This occurs when the tip of the infusion cannula is placed in the suprachoroidal space instead of the vitreous cavity. This can be avoided by direct visualization of the infusion cannula tip before the infusion fluid is turned on, and it is an important part of every vitrectomy procedure. This complication can also occur during vitrectomy if the cannula tip inadvertently slips into the suprachoroidal space. When this happens, the infusion line should be turned off immediately and removed from the displaced cannula and inserted into another cannula and turned on after direct visualization. Peripheral iatrogenic breaks may occur during vitrectomy. They typically occur in close proximity to the sclerotomy sites when there is incomplete vitreous removal and traction occurs during repeated insertion/removal of instruments. Further, they can occur in the peripheral retina during PVD induction as the posterior hyaloid is detaching from the retina near the vitreous base. More posterior breaks usually happen with ERM removal, such as in cases with PVR and in diabetic TRD. It is very important to recognize breaks during surgery and to apply endophotocoagulation and internal tamponade. The peripheral retina should be examined carefully under scleral depression at the end of the vitrectomy and before the eye is filled with gas in order to identify iatrogenic breaks.

Care should be taken during surgery to avoid contact of any instrument with the crystalline lens. Lens touch can markedly diminish visualization and a lensectomy may become necessary. Vascular occlusions may occur during vitrectomy, especially when operating under a high intraocular pressure (IOP) for a prolonged period of time. The patency of the central retinal artery and the perfusion status of the nerve should be monitored throughout the surgery. Another potentially devastating complication is suprachoroidal hemorrhage. This risk can be minimized by avoiding intraoperative hypotony, tachycardia, or Valsalva maneuvers (e.g., bucking on the tube during general anesthesia), as well as extensive cryopexy or endolaser.

40.4.2 Postoperative Complications

If a sclerotomy is leaking at the conclusion of surgery, hypotony and choroidal effusion may be observed in the immediate postoperative period. Furthermore, choroidal hemorrhage may occur. It is strongly recommended to suture a sclerotomy that is not self-sealing at the end of surgery. Elevation of IOP can occur after vitrectomy surgery, and there are multiple potential mechanisms. Anterior chamber inflammation and/or blood, as well as gas or oil, complications are the most likely causes. Gas can cause early IOP spikes in aphakic eyes by means of a pupillary block mechanism, and this can be prevented by proper postoperative face-down positioning. When silicone oil is used in aphakic eyes, pupillary block is avoided by making an inferior peripheral iridotomy and recommending strict face-down positioning.

Cataract formation or progression is the most common complication after vitrectomy. More than half of patients (60–98%) will develop clinically significant nuclear sclerosis in the first 2 years after vitrectomy.[19,20,21,22] Several authors have implicated increased oxygen tension after vitrectomy in the mechanism of cataract formation.[23]

Endophthalmitis is a potentially devastating complication after vitrectomy. The rate of endophthalmitis after 20-gauge vitrectomy was reported to be 0.15% in a study published in 1984.[24] Other subsequent studies reported rates between 0.03 and 0.05%.[25,26,27] As MIVS gained popularity in the mid-2000s, authors raised concerns about the increased rate of endophthalmitis with 25-gauge transconjunctival sutureless vitrectomy. Kunimoto and Kaiser[28] reported a 12-fold and Scott et al[29] reported a 28-fold higher rate of postoperative endophthalmitis when they evaluated the outcomes of 25-gauge versus 20-gauge vitrectomy. However, after significant modifications were made to the MIVS procedure, Scott et al and other investigative groups found no significant difference in endophthalmitis rates between 20-gauge and small incision vitrectomy.[30,31,32,33]

40.5 Outcomes of Vitrectomy

40.5.1 Proliferative Vitreoretinopathy

PVR accounts for roughly three-quarters of all primary surgical failures in retinal detachment surgery.[34] Risk factors for PVR include multiple previous surgeries, aphakia, choroidal detachment, trauma, young age, and retinal detachments involving greater than two quadrants of the eye.[34] There are various classification systems for the severity of PVR. The Retina Society Terminology Committee classified PVR as minimal, moderate, marked, and massive (A–D).[35] A different classification system was proposed by the Silicone Oil Study Group differentiating between anterior and posterior forms of PVR,[36] and Machemer further revised this system to offer more information regarding the extent of the PVR, its location, and its severity.[37] PVR is incompletely understood, and many growth factors have been implicated in its pathogenesis (vascular endothelial growth factor [VEGF], platelet-derived growth factor, transforming growth factor- ß, fibroblast growth factor, tumor necrosis factor-a, tumor necrosis factor-ß).[38]

Advancements in vitreoretinal surgery have allowed surgeons to use 23- and 25-gauge instrumentation in the management of retinal detachments with PVR. Inferior retinectomy and scleral buckle are important adjuncts to vitrectomy for retinal detachment with PVR. PVR is gravity dependent and is, therefore, most prevalent in the inferior clock hours. If an inferior retinectomy is needed, we prefer to perform an inferior retinectomy from 3 to 9 o'clock position as the vulnerable edges for reproliferation are located laterally and not inferiorly (compared with a more limited retinectomy, e.g., from 5 to 7 o'clock position). Recurrence of PVR usually occurs at the vulnerable edges, and placement of a scleral buckle protects these areas. Regarding the anterior residual retina, we perform meticulous dissection and removal all the way to the ora serrata, minimizing the likelihood of inflammation and reproliferation. We also perform adequate diathermy to the edge of the intended retinectomy, thus minimizing hemorrhage during retinal excision and minimizing subsequent fibrous proliferation in areas of hemorrhage. In cases of significant anterior PVR, we prefer to perform lensectomy as the lens can serve as a scaffold for subsequent proliferation. One surgeon-based, self-reported questionnaire study done in Europe[39] reported the outcomes of patients who underwent PPV with or without scleral buckling for retinal detachment with PVR Grade B and C. For PVR Grade C detachments (637 patients), eyes treated with scleral buckle and vitrectomy had higher failure rates (8.9%) compared with those who were treated with vitrectomy alone (3.0%). However, the nature of the study does not permit us to draw conclusions regarding the role of scleral buckle as an adjunct to vitrectomy as the study was not randomized and more complicated cases were more likely to undergo scleral buckle placement. In a more recent study,[40] single-surgery attachment rate was 75.0% in the PPV and scleral buckle group (27 of $n = 36$ patients) versus 48.3% (14 of $n = 29$) in the PPV alone group with a follow-up of at least 3 months.

Controversial Points

- Scleral buckle can be an important adjunct to vitrectomy in eyes with PVR. Studies have shown a probable benefit of scleral buckle placement in addition to vitrectomy in eyes with PVR, but larger, controlled, randomized studies are needed.

Regarding the tamponade agent used for retinal detachment associated with PVR, the Silicone Oil Study Group showed that silicone oil was associated with better visual and anatomic success rates when compared to SF_6[41] but not C_3F_8.[42] However, more recently, there is a tendency by many surgeons to use silicone oil more frequently than gas in eyes with PVR. Surgeons have the option to instill either 1,000 or 5,000 cs silicone oil. Oil emulsification usually begins to occur at 13 months after oil instillation and occurs more frequently with 1,000 cs silicone oil.

Controversial Points

- The Silicone Oil Study Group reported no difference in visual and anatomic outcomes in eyes with retinal detachment and PVR repaired using C_3F_8 or silicone oil tamponade. However, many surgeons today prefer to use silicone oil in eyes with PVR-associated retinal detachment.

Various pharmacologic agents have been employed with limited success for the prevention or treatment of PVR and none of them has been widely adopted in clinical practice. These agents include intravitreal triamcinolone,[43] prednisone,[44] dexamethasone,[45] low-molecular-weight heparin,[46] 5-fluorouracil,[46] isotretinoin,[47,48] and daunorubicin.[49] The results from these studies are variable, and the heterogeneity of the studies in terms of the design, patient population, and follow-up makes it hard to draw conclusions regarding the relative efficacy of these agents. Currently, the best treatment for PVR is meticulous surgery.

> **Pearls**
>
> - Meticulous dissection of preretinal and subretinal membranes is critical for successful repair of retinal detachment with PVR. Retinectomy is needed in some cases.
> - Removal of the crystalline lens can improve surgical outcomes in patients with anterior PVR.

40.5.2 Giant Retinal Tears

GRTs are retinal breaks extending circumferentially more than 3 clock hours (equal to or greater than 90 degrees), and they occur in the presence of a PVD.[50] GRTs can be classified into three categories based on their location: (1) equatorial, (2) equatorial with posterior extension, and (3) oral.[51] It is important to differentiate GRTs from retinal dialysis, as the latter carries a different natural history and is managed in a different manner. The state of the vitreous can help in making this distinction. In eyes with GRT, there is a PVD, while in eyes with retinal dialysis the vitreous remains attached.[51,52]

GRTs are associated with trauma,[53] previous eye surgery,[54] myopia,[55] and hereditary vitreoretinopathies such as Wagner's,[56] Stickler's,[57] and Marfan's syndromes.[58] Retinal detachments associated with GRTs are challenging cases, and success rates were historically poor. Prior to the introduction of PPV, GRTs were managed with scleral bucking combined with intraocular tamponade with either air or silicone oil, and the success rate was 51 to 65%.[59,60] These cases were technically and physically challenging for the retinal surgeon as they required the use of specially designed operating tables with the surgeon operating in a supine "car-mechanic" fashion.

The introduction of vitrectomy revolutionized the treatment of GRTs and the introduction of heavy liquids was associated with increased retinal reattachment rates. PFCL has become invaluable in GRTs with an inverted anterior retinal flap. Kreiger and Lewis[61] proposed meticulous vitreous base shaving and showed that retinal reattachment can sometimes be achieved without the use of adjunctive scleral buckling. Primary retinal reattachment rates with vitrectomy alone range between 77 and 94%[55,61,62,63,64,65] and between 68 and 96% when vitrectomy is combined with scleral buckle.[53,55,66,67,68,69,70,71,72] Based on the current literature, it is difficult to determine the impact of adjunctive scleral buckling to vitrectomy in GRTs. Visual acuity improved postoperatively in at least half of the patients in most studies, and vision deteriorated in up to 40% when compared with the presenting visual acuity. Factors associated with higher redetachment rates were age below 30 years, female gender, prior vitrectomy, GRT extent greater than 180 degrees, and the presence of preoperative PVR.[69]

40.5.3 Retained Lens Fragments and Dislocated Intraocular Lenses

Retained lens fragment is one of the most common complications during cataract surgery, occurring in approximately 1% of phacoemulsification procedures.[73] Patients with retained lens fragments can develop increased IOP, inflammation, corneal edema, cystoid macular edema, and retinal detachment.[74] When this complication occurs, the cataract surgeon should remove all the lens material in the capsular bag and perform a thorough anterior vitrectomy. Maneuvers involving phacoemulsification posterior to the capsular bag or attempts to elevate the dropped material and remove it through an anterior approach are generally not recommended as they can result in serious complications such as GRT and/or retinal detachment.[54] It is advised that the anterior segment surgeon perform an anterior vitrectomy to remove the vitreous anterior to the pupillary plane and ensure that there is no vitreous in contact with the cataract wound, thus minimizing the risk of postoperative complications such as endophthalmitis, retinal breaks, and cystoid macular edema. Staining with triamcinolone is very helpful in identifying the presence of vitreous in the anterior chamber. If there is adequate capsular support, an IOL can be placed in the sulcus. The patient should then be referred for vitreoretinal consultation.

Small cortical fragments not causing inflammation or increased IOP can be observed.[75,76] Postoperative steroid and nonsteroidal anti-inflammatory drops may be administered to decrease the likelihood of cystoid macular edema. Indications for PPV include presence of larger lens fragments (e.g., =25% of the entire lens or a fragment =2 mm in diameter), significant intraocular inflammation, uncontrolled IOP, or coexisting pathology such as retinal detachment or corneal edema due to lens touch. After the core vitrectomy is performed, the presence of a PVD should be confirmed, and if not already present, a PVD is usually induced.[77] Subsequently, the vitreous base is usually shaved with the assistance of scleral depression to reduce vitreous traction and to facilitate removal of small lens particles. Cortical material, as well as small nuclear fragments, can usually be removed with the 23- or 25-gauge cutter.[78] When harder and larger lens material is present, the fragmatome can be used by enlarging one of the small-gauge sclerotomies to 20 gauge.

The timing of the vitrectomy has been a topic of debate. Studies have reported that there is no difference in the final visual outcome or complication rate if vitrectomy is performed the same day as the cataract surgery or at a later time.[79,80,81,82,83] If there is prompt availability of a vitreoretinal surgeon in the facility where the cataract surgery is performed, a same-day approach may be followed for logistical purposes, saving the patient another visit to the operating room. For cases in which the retained lens material is not removed the same day as the cataract surgery, the timing of PPV depends on the individual patient's clinical situation. Although a delay in PPV may be preferable in some cases in order to permit clearing of corneal edema, ocular congestion, and acute postoperative inflammation before proceeding with a second surgical procedure, PPV is usually performed within 2 weeks of the cataract surgery in order to expedite visual rehabilitation, avoid chronic glaucoma, and break the cycle of progressive lens-associated inflammation.[83] Outcomes with either approach (PPV and removal of retained lens fragments on the same day as the cataract surgery or at a later time) are generally good with approximately 60% of the patients achieving a visual acuity of 20/40 or better.[79,83]

There are various choices for placement of an IOL. If there is adequate iris support, an anterior chamber IOL or an iris sutured IOL can be placed. In cases of absent capsular support, an anterior chamber or scleral sutured IOL can be used. Further, one may employ the more recently introduced IOL technique where the haptics are externalized and inserted into scleral tunnels buried under partial thickness scleral flaps in a sutureless fashion.

Dislocated IOLs usually occur in cases of previous trauma or when complications occurred during cataract surgery. Thorough vitrectomy is performed around the IOL until it is freely mobile in the vitreous cavity. There are many ways to retrieve the IOL. Some surgeons use PFCL to elevate the IOL, while others use aspiration with a soft-tipped cannula and/or posterior segment forceps. After the IOL is moved into the anterior chamber, it can be either removed or fixated with one of the aforementioned techniques.

40.5.4 Macular Hole

Kelly and Wendel were the first to propose vitrectomy for the treatment of idiopathic macular holes in their seminal paper in 1991.[84] A subsequent study[80] reported that 69% of patients with stage 3 or 4 macular holes achieved hole closure after vitrectomy compared to 4% with observation alone. Since then, many studies have been published reporting favorable outcomes after vitrectomy for macular hole, with the hole closure rate varying from 85 to 100%.[81,82,83]

It is essential to evaluate macular hole patients preoperatively with spectral-domain optical coherence tomography (SD-OCT) in order to stage the macular hole. Surgery is recommended for macular hole stages 2, 3, and 4 according to the Gass classification. Most vitreoretinal surgeons today prefer a 23- or 25-gauge vitrectomy system for macular hole surgery. More recently, 27-gauge systems were introduced and are favored by some surgeons. A key step of the surgery is to separate the posterior hyaloid from the retina if a PVD is not already present, and then any ERM is removed. Many surgeons favor peeling the ILM as this ensures that any residual adherent cortical vitreous remnants and any associated fibrocellular membranes are removed.[85,86] The initial flap of ILM is created with various instruments such as a diamond-dusted silicone scraper, MVR blade, or ILM forceps. The membrane peeling is usually carried out with ILM forceps. The ILM is usually peeled to approximately 1 disc diameter around the hole, although some surgeons have proposed broader ILM peeling.[87] As the ILM is a thin transparent layer, a variety of dyes can be used to aid in its visualization. The most commonly used dyes are ICG, trypan blue, and brilliant blue. The dyes are usually in contact with the retinal surface for less than a minute and then washed out to minimize potential toxic effects. More specifically, there is some debate regarding the potential toxicity of ICG.[8] Following ILM peeling, the peripheral retina is examined carefully for any tears and then a fluid–air exchange is carried out, followed by an air-gas exchange. C_3F_8 and SF_6 gases are usually used to facilitate hole closure. Historically, face-down positioning has been recommended after the surgery, but it has recently been reported that face-down positioning may not be necessary, especially with smaller macular holes.[88] There is controversy regarding ILM peeling in macular hole surgery. The FILM[89] study reported that there were no differences in visual acuity at 3 and 6 months after macular hole surgery between patients in whom the ILM was peeled compared to patients in whom the ILM was not peeled. A recent Cochrane review concluded that ILM peeling increases the likelihood of hole closure with a single surgical procedure.[90] However, there are potential complications with ILM peeling, such as retinal thinning in the area of the ILM peel. Another point of debate is whether ILM peeling is necessary in eyes with small macular holes. Tadayoni et al showed that ILM peeling does not offer any additional benefit to vitrectomy in macular holes less than 400 µm in diameter.[91]

Pearls

- Removal of the ILM may assist with macular hole closure, especially for stage 3 and 4 macular holes.

Controversial Points

- ILM peeling has been shown to increase the rate of macular hole closure. However, there is no definite evidence that ILM peeling offers any additional visual benefit compared to vitrectomy alone with gas tamponade.

40.5.5 Submacular Surgery

Submacular surgery was performed in the 1990s for patients with wet age-related macular degeneration (AMD) as there was no other effective treatment for these patients. In 2004, the Submacular Surgery Trials research group reported the outcomes of submacular surgery in patients with wet AMD.[87] Of 454 patients enrolled, 228 study eyes were assigned to observation and 226 to surgery. There was no benefit from submacular surgery compared to observation over a 2-year period; the median change in visual acuity from baseline to the 2-year examination was a worsening of 2.1 lines (10.5 letters) in the observation arm and a worsening of 2.0 lines (10 letters) in the surgery arm. In addition, the impressive results achieved with anti-VEGF agents have rendered this procedure almost obsolete. However, submacular surgery may play a role in eyes with large submacular hemorrhage most commonly from trauma or wet AMD. Removing the blood with the vitrector has been shown to offer no benefit,[92] but pneumatic displacement of the blood with the use of subretinal tissue plasminogen activator with[93] or without air[94] has shown promising results, and many surgeons perform this procedure in patients with large submacular hemorrhage.

40.5.6 Diabetic Vitrectomy

Vitreous Hemorrhage

The Diabetic Retinopathy Vitrectomy Study showed the benefit of early vitrectomy in patients with vitreous hemorrhage in the setting of proliferative diabetic retinopathy.[95] Early vitrectomy was defined as surgery 1 to 4 months after the occurrence of vitreous hemorrhage and late vitrectomy was defined as surgery 12 to 18 months after the vitreous hemorrhage. Recovery of visual acuity to 10/100 or greater was significantly better for early surgery compared to late surgery (at 3 months, 50 vs. 17%, respectively). At 2 years, there was a benefit in the percentage of eyes recovering a visual acuity of 10/20 or better (25% in the early group vs. 15% in the late group). The benefits were better for patients with type 1 diabetes compared to patients with type 2 diabetes. Given the results of this trial, the prevailing practice in the retina community was to observe type 1 diabetics with vitreous hemorrhage for 1 to 3 months, and if the blood had not cleared, then proceed to vitrectomy. The observation period for type 2 diabetics was recommended to be 3 to 6 months. However, it should be noted that this trial was performed in an era with less advanced vitrectomy, illumination, and viewing systems than are available currently. Given the sophisticated minimally invasive systems utilized in modern vitrectomy, there is a trend toward much earlier intervention in eyes with diabetic vitreous hemorrhage. It is crucial in these cases to separate the adherent posterior hyaloid which serves as a scaffold for fibrovascular proliferation and to perform thorough 360-degree panretinal photocoagulation. The curved lighted endolaser probe is very useful in these cases, especially in phakic patients. Favorable prognostic factors include a preoperative vision > 5/200, no neovascular glaucoma or rubeosis, no or minimal cataract, and preexisting panretinal photocoagulation in at least one quadrant.[96] Rebound hemorrhage in the postoperative period is common but usually resolves spontaneously and rarely requires reoperation.[97]

Diabetic Macular Edema

It was proposed in the early 1990s by many authors to induce vitreomacular separation in patients with persistent diabetic macular edema not responsive to laser photocoagulation.[98,99,100] This was based on the observation that a PVD was less common in patients with diffuse diabetic macular edema compared to patients without edema.[98,99] Subsequently, many studies evaluated the role of vitrectomy in eyes with diabetic macular edema that was unresponsive to prior laser or anti-VEGF therapy or associated with a taut posterior hyaloid. While the results following vitrectomy for eyes with an attached hyaloid are generally favorable, there are limitations to the studies in that they are retrospective, uncontrolled, and lack homogeneous inclusion criteria. In addition, the ILM peeling that has been advocated by some authors is controversial. Until a randomized controlled study is performed, the role of vitrectomy for diabetic macular edema is unclear.

Diabetic Tractional Retinal Detachment

Visual improvements of =2 lines have been reported in 60 to 75% of eyes treated with PPV for diabetic tractional retinal detachment, with a mean postoperative visual acuity of =20/200 in 47 to 57% of patients, or =5/200 in 69 to 77% of patients.[101] Complete retinal reattachment may be achieved in 82% of patients with restoration of the macular anatomy in 80 to 100%.[102,103] Mean retinal reattachment rates for eyes with diabetic tractional retinal detachments are approximately 56%.[104] The results for combined rhegmatogenous and tractional retinal detachments are worse than for tractional retinal detachments, and encircling bands and silicone oil tamponade are important adjuncts which may increase the likelihood of anatomic success. The functional results are usually not as good as the anatomic results mainly because of long-standing macular ischemia. Other conditions that negatively influence surgical outcomes are neovascular glaucoma, lack of panretinal photocoagulation, anterior hyaloidal fibrovascular proliferation, and vitreous hemorrhage. Anti-VEGF agents should be used with caution in patients with extensive neovascular membranes as it has been shown that they may worsen the traction.[105]

References

[1] Landers MB, III, Stefánsson E, Wolbarsht ML. The optics of vitreous surgery. Am J Ophthalmol. 1981; 91(5):611–614

[2] Bovey EH, Gonvers M. A new device for noncontact wide-angle viewing of the fundus during vitrectomy. Arch Ophthalmol. 1995; 113(12):1572–1573

[3] Peyman GA. Improved vitrectomy illumination system. Am J Ophthalmol. 1976; 81(1):99–100

[4] van den Biesen PR, Berenschot T, Verdaasdonk RM, van Weelden H, van Norren D. Endoillumination during vitrectomy and phototoxicity thresholds. Br J Ophthalmol. 2000; 84(12):1372–1375

[5] Rossi T, Boccassini B, Iossa M, Rossi A, Mutolo A, Tamburrelli C. Wedge-shaped light pipe aperture for pars plana vitrectomy. Retina. 2009; 29 (8):1201–1206

[6] Rodrigues EB, Meyer CH, Kroll P. Chromovitrectomy: a new field in vitreoretinal surgery. Graefes Arch Clin Exp Ophthalmol. 2005; 243(4):291–293

[7] Kadonosono K, Itoh N, Uchio E, Nakamura S, Ohno S. Staining of internal limiting membrane in macular hole surgery. Arch Ophthalmol. 2000; 118 (8):1116–1118

[8] Gandorfer A, Haritoglou C, Kampik A. Toxicity of indocyanine green in vitreoretinal surgery. Dev Ophthalmol. 2008; 42:69–81

[9] Fujii GY, De Juan E, Jr, Humayun MS, et al. A new 25-gauge instrument system for transconjunctival sutureless vitrectomy surgery. Ophthalmology. 2002; 109(10):1807–1812, discussion 1813

[10] Eckardt C. Transconjunctival sutureless 23-gauge vitrectomy. Retina. 2005; 25(2):208–211

[11] Oshima Y, Wakabayashi T, Sato T, Ohji M, Tano Y. A 27-gauge instrument system for transconjunctival sutureless microincision vitrectomy surgery. Ophthalmology. 2010; 117(1):93–102.e2

[12] Machemer R, Buettner H, Norton EW, Parel JM. Vitrectomy: a pars plana approach. Trans Am Acad Ophthalmol Otolaryngol. 1971; 75(4):813–820

[13] Douvas NG. Pars plana vitrectomy. Microsurgical pars plana lensectomy. Trans Sect Ophthalmol Am Acad Ophthalmol Otolaryngol. 1976; 81(3, Pt 1):371–381

[14] O'Malley C, Heintz RM, Sr. Vitrectomy with an alternative instrument system. Ann Ophthalmol. 1975; 7(4):585–588, 591–594

[15] Machemer R. The surgical removal of epiretinal macular membranes (macular puckers) [author's transl; in German]. Klin Monatsbl Augenheilkd. 1978; 173(1):36–42

[16] Machemer R. Retinotomy. Am J Ophthalmol. 1981; 92:768–774

[17] Verma LK, Peyman GA, Wafapoor H, Greve MD, Millsap CM, Adile SL. An analysis of posterior segment complications after vitrectomy using the perfluorocarbon perfluoroperhydrophenanthrene (Vitreon). Vitreon Collaborative Study. Ophthalmic Surg. 1995; 26(1):29–33

[18] Chang S. Low viscosity liquid fluorochemicals in vitreous surgery. Am J Ophthalmol. 1987; 103(1):38–43

[19] Cherfan GM, Michels RG, de Bustros S, Enger C, Glaser BM. Nuclear sclerotic cataract after vitrectomy for idiopathic epiretinal membranes causing macular pucker. Am J Ophthalmol. 1991; 111(4):434–438

[20] Van Effenterre G, Ameline B, Campinchi F, Quesnot S, Le Mer Y, Haut J. Is vitrectomy cataractogenic? Study of changes of the crystalline lens after surgery of retinal detachment [in French]. J Fr Ophtalmol. 1992; 15(8-9):449–454

[21] Thompson JT, Glaser BM, Sjaarda RN, Murphy RP. Progression of nuclear sclerosis and long-term visual results of vitrectomy with transforming growth factor beta-2 for macular holes. Am J Ophthalmol. 1995; 119(1):48–54

[22] Melberg NS, Thomas MA. Nuclear sclerotic cataract after vitrectomy in patients younger than 50 years of age. Ophthalmology. 1995; 102 (10):1466–1471

[23] Holekamp NM, Shui Y-B, Beebe DC. Vitrectomy surgery increases oxygen exposure to the lens: a possible mechanism for nuclear cataract formation. Am J Ophthalmol. 2005; 139(2):302–310

[24] Ho PC, Tolentino FI. Bacterial endophthalmitis after closed vitrectomy. Arch Ophthalmol. 1984; 102(2):207–210

[25] Aaberg TM, Jr, Flynn HW, Jr, Schiffman J, Newton J. Nosocomial acute-onset postoperative endophthalmitis survey. A 10-year review of incidence and outcomes. Ophthalmology. 1998; 105(6):1004–1010

[26] Eifrig CWG, Scott IU, Flynn HW, Jr, Smiddy WE, Newton J. Endophthalmitis after pars plana vitrectomy: Incidence, causative organisms, and visual acuity outcomes. Am J Ophthalmol. 2004; 138(5):799–802

[27] Sakamoto T, Enaida H, Kubota T, et al. Incidence of acute endophthalmitis after triamcinolone-assisted pars plana vitrectomy. Am J Ophthalmol. 2004; 138(1):137–138

[28] Kunimoto DY, Kaiser RS, Wills Eye Retina Service. Incidence of endophthalmitis after 20- and 25-gauge vitrectomy. Ophthalmology. 2007; 114 (12):2133–2137

[29] Scott IU, Flynn HW, Jr, Dev S, et al. Endophthalmitis after 25-gauge and 20-gauge pars plana vitrectomy: incidence and outcomes. Retina. 2008; 28 (1):138–142

[30] Scott IU, Flynn HW, Jr, Acar N, et al. Incidence of endophthalmitis after 20-gauge vs 23-gauge vs 25-gauge pars plana vitrectomy. Graefes Arch Clin Exp Ophthalmol. 2011; 249(3):377–380

[31] Shimada H, Nakashizuka H, Hattori T, Mori R, Mizutani Y, Yuzawa M. Incidence of endophthalmitis after 20- and 25-gauge vitrectomy causes and prevention. Ophthalmology. 2008; 115(12):2215–2220

[32] Parolini B, Romanelli F, Prigione G, Pertile G. Incidence of endophthalmitis in a large series of 23-gauge and 20-gauge transconjunctival pars plana vitrectomy. Graefes Arch Clin Exp Ophthalmol. 2009; 247(7):895–898

[33] Wu L, Berrocal MH, Arévalo JF, et al. Endophthalmitis after pars plana vitrectomy: results of the Pan American Collaborative Retina Study Group. Retina. 2011; 31(4):673–678

[34] Pastor JC. Proliferative vitreoretinopathy: an overview. Surv Ophthalmol. 1998; 43(1):3–18

[35] The classification of retinal detachment with proliferative vitreoretinopathy. Ophthalmology. 1983; 90(2):121–125

[36] Lean JS, Stern WH, Irvine AR, Azen SP, The Silicone Study Group. Classification of proliferative vitreoretinopathy used in the silicone study. Ophthalmology. 1989; 96(6):765–771

[37] Machemer R, Aaberg TM, Freeman HM, Irvine AR, Lean JS, Michels RM. An updated classification of retinal detachment with proliferative vitreoretinopathy. Am J Ophthalmol. 1991; 112(2):159–165

[38] Khan MA, Brady CJ, Kaiser RS. Clinical management of proliferative vitreoretinopathy: an update. Retina. 2015; 35(2):165–175

[39] Adelman RA, Parnes AJ, Sipperley JO, Ducournau D, European Vitreo-Retinal Society (EVRS) Retinal Detachment Study Group. Strategy for the management of complex retinal detachments: the European vitreo-retinal society retinal detachment study report 2. Ophthalmology. 2013; 120(9):1809–1813

[40] Storey P, Alshareef R, Khuthaila M, et al. Wills PVR Study Group. Pars plana vitrectomy and scleral buckle versus pars plana vitrectomy alone for patients with rhegmatogenous retinal detachment at high risk for proliferative vitreoretinopathy. Retina. 2014; 34(10):1945–1951

[41] Vitrectomy with silicone oil or sulfur hexafluoride gas in eyes with severe proliferative vitreoretinopathy: results of a randomized clinical trial. Silicone Study Report 1. Arch Ophthalmol. 1992; 110(6):770–779

[42] Vitrectomy with silicone oil or perfluoropropane gas in eyes with severe proliferative vitreoretinopathy: results of a randomized clinical trial. Silicone Study Report 2. Arch Ophthalmol. 1992; 110(6):780–792

[43] Jonas JB, Hayler JK, Panda-Jonas S. Intravitreal injection of crystalline cortisone as adjunctive treatment of proliferative vitreoretinopathy. Br J Ophthalmol. 2000; 84(9):1064–1067

[44] Koerner F, Koerner-Stiefbold U, Garweg JG. Systemic corticosteroids reduce the risk of cellophane membranes after retinal detachment surgery: a prospective randomized placebo-controlled double-blind clinical trial. Graefes Arch Clin Exp Ophthalmol. 2012; 250(7):981–987

[45] Banerjee PJ, Bunce C, Charteris DG. Ozurdex (a slow-release dexamethasone implant) in proliferative vitreoretinopathy: study protocol for a randomised controlled trial. Trials. 2013; 14:358

[46] Charteris DG, Aylward GW, Wong D, Groenewald C, Asaria RH, Bunce C, PVR Study Group. A randomized controlled trial of combined 5-fluorouracil and low-molecular-weight heparin in management of established proliferative vitreoretinopathy. Ophthalmology. 2004; 111(12):2240–2245

[47] Chang Y-C, Hu D-N, Wu W-C. Effect of oral 13-cis-retinoic acid treatment on postoperative clinical outcome of eyes with proliferative vitreoretinopathy. Am J Ophthalmol. 2008; 146(3):440–446

[48] Fekrat S, de Juan E, Jr, Campochiaro PA. The effect of oral 13-cis-retinoic acid on retinal redetachment after surgical repair in eyes with proliferative vitreoretinopathy. Ophthalmology. 1995; 102(3):412–418

[49] Wiedemann P, Hilgers RD, Bauer P, Heimann K, Daunomycin Study Group. Adjunctive daunorubicin in the treatment of proliferative vitreoretinopathy: results of a multicenter clinical trial. Am J Ophthalmol. 1998; 126(4):550–559

[50] Freeman HM. Fellow eyes of giant retinal breaks. Trans Am Ophthalmol Soc. 1978; 76:343–382

[51] Scott JD. Giant tear of the retina. Trans Ophthalmol Soc U K. 1975; 95 (1):142–144

[52] Leaver PK, Lean JS. Management of giant retinal tears using vitrectomy and silicone oil/fluid exchange. A preliminary report. Trans Ophthalmol Soc U K. 1981; 101(1):189–191

[53] Ghosh YK, Banerjee S, Savant V, et al. Surgical treatment and outcome of patients with giant retinal tears. Eye (Lond). 2004; 18(10):996–1000

[54] Aaberg TM, Jr, Rubsamen PE, Flynn HW, Jr, Chang S, Mieler WF, Smiddy WE. Giant retinal tear as a complication of attempted removal of intravitreal lens fragments during cataract surgery. Am J Ophthalmol. 1997; 124(2):222–226

[55] Ang GS, Townend J, Lois N. Epidemiology of giant retinal tears in the United Kingdom: the British Giant Retinal Tear Epidemiology Eye Study (BGEES). Invest Ophthalmol Vis Sci. 2010; 51(9):4781–4787

[56] Richards AJ, Martin S, Yates JR, et al. COL2A1 exon 2 mutations: relevance to the Stickler and Wagner syndromes. Br J Ophthalmol. 2000; 84(4):364–371

[57] Stickler GB, Hughes W, Houchin P. Clinical features of hereditary progressive arthro-ophthalmopathy (Stickler syndrome): a survey. Genet Med. 2001; 3 (3):192–196

[58] Sharma T, Gopal L, Shanmugam MP, et al. Retinal detachment in Marfan syndrome: clinical characteristics and surgical outcome. Retina. 2002; 22 (4):423–428

[59] Norton EW, Aaberg T, Fung W, Curtin VT. Giant retinal tears. I. Clinical management with intravitreal air. Am J Ophthalmol. 1969; 68(6):1011–1021

[60] Freeman HM, Schepens CL, Couvillion GC. Current management of giant retinal breaks. II. Trans Am Acad Ophthalmol Otolaryngol. 1970; 74(1):59–74

[61] Kreiger AE, Lewis H. Management of giant retinal tears without scleral buckling. Use of radical dissection of the vitreous base and perfluoro-octane and intraocular tamponade. Ophthalmology. 1992; 99(4):491–497

[62] Ambresin A, Wolfensberger TJ, Bovey EH. Management of giant retinal tears with vitrectomy, internal tamponade, and peripheral 360 degrees retinal photocoagulation. Retina. 2003; 23(5):622–628

[63] Batman C, Cekiç O. Vitrectomy with silicone oil or long-acting gas in eyes with giant retinal tears: long-term follow-up of a randomized clinical trial. Retina. 1999; 19(3):188–192

[64] Chang S, Lincoff H, Zimmerman NJ, Fuchs W. Giant retinal tears. Surgical techniques and results using perfluorocarbon liquids. Arch Ophthalmol. 1989; 107(5):761–766

[65] Rofail M, Lee LR. Perfluoro-n-octane as a postoperative vitreoretinal tamponade in the management of giant retinal tears. Retina. 2005; 25(7):897–901

[66] Goezinne F, LA Heij EC, Berendschot TT, et al. Low redetachment rate due to encircling scleral buckle in giant retinal tears treated with vitrectomy and silicone oil. Retina. 2008; 28(3):485–492

[67] Ie D, Glaser BM, Sjaarda RN, Thompson JT, Steinberg LE, Gordon LW. The use of perfluoro-octane in the management of giant retinal tears without proliferative vitreoretinopathy. Retina. 1994; 14(4):323–328

[68] Mathis A, Pagot V, Gazagne C, Malecaze F. Giant retinal tears. Surgical techniques and results using perfluorodecalin and silicone oil tamponade. Retina. 1992; 12(3) Suppl:S7–S10

[69] Scott IU, Murray TG, Flynn HW, Jr, Feuer WJ, Schiffman JC, Perfluoron Study Group. Outcomes and complications associated with giant retinal tear management using perfluoro-n-octane. Ophthalmology. 2002; 109(10):1828–1833

[70] Sirimaharaj M, Balachandran C, Chan WC, et al. Vitrectomy with short term postoperative tamponade using perfluorocarbon liquid for giant retinal tears. Br J Ophthalmol. 2005; 89(9):1176–1179

[71] Unlü N, Kocaoglan H, Acar MA, Sargin M, Aslan BS, Duman S. The management of giant retinal tears with silicone oil. Eur J Ophthalmol. 2003; 13 (2):192–195

[72] Verstraeten T, Williams GA, Chang S, et al. Lens-sparing vitrectomy with perfluorocarbon liquid for the primary treatment of giant retinal tears. Ophthalmology. 1995; 102(1):17–20

[73] Pande M, Dabbs TR. Incidence of lens matter dislocation during phacoemulsification. J Cataract Refract Surg. 1996; 22(6):737–742

[74] Margherio RR, Margherio AR, Pendergast SD, et al. Vitrectomy for retained lens fragments after phacoemulsification. Ophthalmology. 1997; 104 (9):1426–1432

[75] Gilliland GD, Hutton WL, Fuller DG. Retained intravitreal lens fragments after cataract surgery. Ophthalmology. 1992; 99(8):1263–1267, discussion 1268–1269

[76] Blodi BA, Flynn HW, Jr, Blodi CF, Folk JC, Daily MJ. Retained nuclei after cataract surgery. Ophthalmology. 1992; 99(1):41–44

[77] Garg SJ. Use of a suction pick in small-gauge surgery facilitates induction of a posterior vitreous detachment. Retina. 2008; 28(10):1536

[78] Ho LY, Walsh MK, Hassan TS. 25-Gauge pars plana vitrectomy for retained lens fragments. Retina. 2010; 30(6):843–849

[79] Modi YS, Epstein A, Smiddy WE, Murray TG, Feuer W, Flynn HW, Jr. Retained lens fragments after cataract surgery: outcomes of same-day versus later pars plana vitrectomy. Am J Ophthalmol. 2013; 156(3):454–9.e1

[80] Freeman WR, Azen SP, Kim JW, el-Haig W, Mishell DR, III, Bailey I, The Vitrectomy for Treatment of Macular Hole Study Group. Vitrectomy for the treatment of full-thickness stage 3 or 4 macular holes. Results of a multicentered randomized clinical trial. Arch Ophthalmol. 1997; 115(1):11–21

[81] Wakely L, Rahman R, Stephenson J. A comparison of several methods of macular hole measurement using optical coherence tomography, and their value in predicting anatomical and visual outcomes. Br J Ophthalmol. 2012; 96 (7):1003–1007

[82] Passemard M, Yakoubi Y, Muselier A, et al. Long-term outcome of idiopathic macular hole surgery. Am J Ophthalmol. 2010; 149(1):120–126

[83] Krishnan R, Tossounis C, Fung Yang Y. 20-gauge and 23-gauge phacovitrectomy for idiopathic macular holes: comparison of complications and long-term outcomes. Eye (Lond). 2013; 27(1):72–77

[84] Kelly NE1, Wendel RT. Vitreous surgery for idiopathic macular holes. Results of a pilot study. Arch Ophthalmol. 1991 May; 109(5):654–9

[85] Wollensak G, Spoerl E, Grosse G, Wirbelauer C. Biomechanical significance of the human internal limiting lamina. Retina. 2006; 26(8):965–968

[86] Smiddy WE, Flynn HW, Jr. Pathogenesis of macular holes and therapeutic implications. Am J Ophthalmol. 2004; 137(3):525–537

[87] Hawkins BS, Bressler NM, Miskala PH, et al. Submacular Surgery Trials (SST) Research Group. Surgery for subfoveal choroidal neovascularization in age-related macular degeneration: ophthalmic findings: SST report no. 11. Ophthalmology. 2004; 111(11):1967–1980

[88] Nadal J, Delas B, Piñero A. Vitrectomy without face-down posturing for idiopathic macular holes. Retina. 2012; 32(5):918–921

[89] Lois N, Burr J, Norrie J, et al. Full-thickness Macular Hole and Internal Limiting Membrane Peeling Study (FILMS) Group. Internal limiting membrane peeling versus no peeling for idiopathic full-thickness macular hole: a pragmatic randomized controlled trial. Invest Ophthalmol Vis Sci. 2011; 52 (3):1586–1592

[90] Spiteri Cornish K, Lois N, Scott N, et al. Vitrectomy with internal limiting membrane (ILM) peeling versus vitrectomy with no peeling for idiopathic full-thickness macular hole (FTMH). Cochrane Database Syst Rev. 2013; 6: CD009306

[91] Tadayoni R, Gaudric A, Haouchine B, Massin P. Relationship between macular hole size and the potential benefit of internal limiting membrane peeling. Br J Ophthalmol. 2006; 90(10):1239–1241

[92] Bressler NM, Bressler SB, Childs AL, et al. Submacular Surgery Trials (SST) Research Group. Surgery for hemorrhagic choroidal neovascular lesions of age-related macular degeneration: ophthalmic findings: SST report no. 13. Ophthalmology. 2004; 111(11):1993–2006

[93] Martel JN, Mahmoud TH. Subretinal pneumatic displacement of subretinal hemorrhage. JAMA Ophthalmol. 2013; 131(12):1632–1635

[94] Chang W, Garg SJ, Maturi R, et al. Management of thick submacular hemorrhage with subretinal tissue plasminogen activator and pneumatic displacement for age-related macular degeneration. Am J Ophthalmol. 2014; 157 (6):1250–1257

[95] The Diabetic Retinopathy Vitrectomy Study Research Group. Early vitrectomy for severe vitreous hemorrhage in diabetic retinopathy. Two-year results of a randomized trial. Diabetic Retinopathy Vitrectomy Study report 2. Arch Ophthalmol. 1985; 103(11):1644–1652

[96] Thompson JT, de Bustros S, Michels RG, Rice TA, Glaser BM. Results of vitrectomy for proliferative diabetic retinopathy. Ophthalmology. 1986; 93 (12):1571–1574

[97] Novak MA, Rice TA, Michels RG, Auer C. Vitreous hemorrhage after vitrectomy for diabetic retinopathy. Ophthalmology. 1984; 91(12):1485–1489

[98] Nasrallah FP, Van de Velde F, Jalkh AE, Trempe CL, McMeel JW, Schepens CL. Importance of the vitreous in young diabetics with macular edema. Ophthalmology. 1989; 96(10):1511–1516, discussion 1516–1517

[99] Nasrallah FP, Jalkh AE, Van Coppenolle F, et al. The role of the vitreous in diabetic macular edema. Ophthalmology. 1988; 95(10):1335–1339

[100] Lewis H. The role of vitrectomy in the treatment of diabetic macular edema. Am J Ophthalmol. 2001; 131(1):123–125

[101] Ryan SJ, Schachat AP, Wilkinson CP, et al. 2012

[102] Helbig H. Diabetic tractional retinal detachment [in German]. Klin Monatsbl Augenheilkd. 2002; 219(4):186–190

[103] Helbig H, Kellner U, Bornfeld N, Foerster MH. Limits and possibilities of vitreous body surgery in diabetic retinopathy [in German]. Ophthalmologe. 1996; 93(6):647–654

[104] La Heij EC, Tecim S, Kessels AG, Liem AT, Japing WJ, Hendrikse F. Clinical variables and their relation to visual outcome after vitrectomy in eyes with diabetic retinal traction detachment. Graefes Arch Clin Exp Ophthalmol. 2004; 242(3):210–217

[105] Arevalo JF, Maia M, Flynn HW, Jr, et al. Tractional retinal detachment following intravitreal bevacizumab (Avastin) in patients with severe proliferative diabetic retinopathy. Br J Ophthalmol. 2008; 92(2):213–216

Index

Note: Page numbers set **bold** or *italic* indicate headings or figures, respectively.

1

13q deletion syndrome 404

A

ABC trial 218, 222
abetalipoproteinemia, *see* Bassen–Kornzweig syndrome
Accurus (Alcon) 600
acetazolamide (Diamox) 298
acetazolamide retinopathy 514, *515*
acquired retinal astrocytoma 428
acquired retinal macroaneurysm
- characterization 197
- clinical features *197*, 197, *198*
- differential diagnosis 198
- fluorescein angiography *197*, 198
- management, course 198
- pathogenesis, histopathology 198
- visual prognosis 198
acquired vasoproliferative tumor 425, 425, *426*
acute necrotizing herpetic retinitis 354, *354*
acute ophthalmic artery occlusion 106, *107*
acute posterior multifocal placoid pigment epitheliopathy (APMPPE) 370, 371–372, *374*
acute retinal pigment epitheliitis 371–372
adalimumab 384
adaptive optics 92, *94*
Addison-Schilder's disease 326, 336
adenocarcinoma 431
adenoma 431
adrenoleukodystrophy 326, 336
adult-onset foveomacular vitelliform dystrophy 280, *281*
aflibercept
- age-related macular degeneration 220
- branch retinal artery occlusion 124
- clinical studies 222
- cystoid macular edema 166
- diabetic macular edema 151, 165
- macular edema 131
- nonproliferative diabetic retinopathy 142
age-related macular degeneration
- anti-VEGF therapy 218, 220, 221–222
- cataract surgery and 212
- characterization 206
- choroidal neovascularization 227, 229
- classification 206
- diagnosis 206
- encapsulated cell technology 571, *572*
- exudative form 463
- genetic risk factors 211
- genetic testing 211
- laser photocoagulation 587
- neovascular
-- anti-VEGF therapy 218, 220, 221–222
-- central serous chorioretinopathy *216*, 216
-- characterization 213
-- choroidal neovascularization patterns 213, *214*
-- classification 213, *213*
-- clinical features *213*, 213
-- CNV treatment 216
-- diagnosis 213
-- disciform scar 214, *214*
-- exudative, differential diagnosis 216
-- laser photocoagulation 217
-- macular translocation 217
-- management 221
-- management, course 216
-- OCT monitoring 221
-- outer retinal tubulations 214
-- photodynamic therapy 217
-- pigment epithelial detachments 213, 214, *215*
-- polypoidal choroidal vasculopathy 216, *217*
-- submacular surgery 217
- non-neovascular
-- AREDS2 formulation 212
-- basal laminar (cuticular) drusen 209, *210*
-- clinical features 206
-- differential diagnosis 208
-- drusen 206, 207, *207*
-- fundus autofluorescence 208, *210*
-- geographic atrophy 208, *209–210*
-- lutein supplementation 212
-- management, course 210
-- ophthalmoscopy 210
-- pattern dystrophy 209, *210*
-- progression risk grading 213
-- reticular pseudodrusen 208
-- RPE abnormalities *208*, 208
-- vitamin, mineral supplementation 212
-- zeaxanthin supplementation 212
- nongenetic risk factors 211
- photodynamic therapy 222, 587, 589
- progression risk factors 211
- risk modification 212
- smoking and 211
- treatment 206
- treatments trials comparisons 220
- treatments under development 221
- UV light exposure and 212
AIDS retinopathy 116, *116*, 140
AIDS, ocular infections and 355, 357
AMD, *see* age-related macular degeneration
amikacin, endophthalmitis 525
amino acid disorders 326, 331
aminoglycosides
- endophthalmitis 524, 525
- toxicity 113
AMN 371–372
amphotericin B, Candida infection 363
anakinra 385
anatomy
- choroid *10*, 10, *11*
- cystoid degeneration 9–10
- enclosed oral bay 9, *10*
- fovea 8, *8*
- foveola 8, *8*
- fundus 11
- giant teeth 9
- Haller's layer 11
- macula *8*, 8
- macula lutea 8
- meridional folds, complex 9, *9*
- ora serrata 9, *9*
- ora serrata pearls 9
- retina 3
- retinal circulation *7*, 7
- retinal periphery *9*, 9
- retinal pigment epithelium, *see* retinal pigment epithelium
- retinal tufts 10
- Sattler's layer 11
- sensory retina *5*, 5
- vitreous *2*, 2
ANCHOR study 219, 221–222, 231
aneurysmatic telangiectasia 192
angioid streaks
- anti-VEGF therapy 236
- characterization 234, 316
- clinical features *234*, 234, *235*
- diagnosis 235
- Ehlers–Danlos syndrome 236
- laser photocoagulation 236
- management, course 236
- Paget's disease 236
- pathogenesis, histopathology 236
- pseudoxanthoma elasticum *235*, 235
- sickle hemoglobinopathies and 316
angiomatosis retinae 190
aniridia 425
anti-VEGF therapy, *see* specific medications
- adverse events 152, 177
- angioid streaks 236
- branch retinal artery occlusion 123
- central serous chorioretinopathy 247
- clinical studies 152, 222
- Coats' disease 191
- cystoid macular edema 166
- diabetic macular edema 151, 165
- diabetic retinopathy 136, 142
- idiopathic choroidal neovascularization 238
- intravitreal injection technique 153
- macular edema 130, 142, 151
- outcomes 153
- pathologic myopia 231
- presumed ocular histoplasmosis syndrome 234
- proliferative diabetic retinopathy *149*, 149
- retinitis pigmentosa 298
- retinopathy of prematurity 177, 179
- sickle cell hemoglobinopathies 321
antibiotics, prophylactic 494
anticoagulation, central retinal venous occlusion 129
antiphospholipid antibody syndrome 201, *201*
AREDS study 212
AREDS2 study 212
argon green laser photocoagulation 580
argon laser technique 146
arterial occlusive diseases
- acute ophthalmic artery occlusion 106
- branch retinal artery occlusion 113
- cardiovascular disease and 111
- central retinal artery occlusion 107
- central retinal artery, vein occlusion 112
- cilioretinal artery occlusion 114
- cotton-wool spots 114
- disease entities associated with 110
- mortality 111
- ocular ischemic syndrome 99
- overview 99
arteriolosclerosis 186
arteriovenous malformations, retinal 546, *546*, 547, *547*
Aspergillus infection 352, *363*, 363
asteroid hyalosis 69, *70*
astrocytic hamartoma
- characterization 426
- clinical features *427*, 427
- diagnosis 427
- differential diagnosis 407, 427
- genetics 427
- histopathology 428
- management, course 428
atherosclerosis 104, 111
atovaquone, toxoplasmic chorioretinitis 359
autosomal dominant central areolar chorioretinal dystrophy 290
autosomal dominant microcornea rod-cone dystrophy, cataract with staphyloma 279
autosomal dominant neovascular inflammatory vitreoretinopathy (ADNIV) 308
autosomal dominant vitreoretinochoroidopathy (ADVIRC) *279*, 279, 280, 308
autosomal recessive bestrophinopathy *279*, 279, 280, *280*
azathioprine 381–382, 382
azithromycin, toxoplasmic chorioretinitis 359
AZOOR 371–372

B

bacterial endogenous endophthalmitis 352–353, *353*, 362
Bardet–Biedl Syndrome 300
Barr, C. C. 259
Bartonella henselae infection (cat-scratch disease) 352, 361, *362*
basal encephalocele 552, *553*
basal laminar (cuticular) drusen 209, *210*
Bassen–Kornzweig syndrome 300, 326, 337
Batten's disease 300, 334
BB pellets 491
BEAT-ROP trial 177
Beaver Dam Eye Study 211
Beh?et's disease 201, 372, *375*, 375

benign reactive lymphoid hyperplasia 460
Bergmeister's papilla 544, *545–546*
Berkley Bioengineering Ocutome 800 600
Best's disease 89–90, *276*, 276, *277–278*, 280
Best's vitelliform macular dystrophy 19

bevacizumab
- adverse events 177
- age-related macular degeneration 218
- branch retinal artery occlusion 124
- central serous chorioretinopathy 247
- clinical studies 222
- Coats' disease 191
- diabetic macular edema 151, 165
- idiopathic choroidal neovascularization 238
- macular edema *131*, 131
- pathologic myopia 231
- presumed ocular histoplasmosis syndrome 234
- retinopathy of prematurity 177, 179
- sickle cell hemoglobinopathies 321
- treatments trials comparisons 220

Bietti's crystalline retinopathy 306, *307*
biodegradable implants 570
birdshot retinochoroidopathy 371–372, 377, *379*
black sunburst lesion *315*, 315
Blodi, B. A. 532–533
blunt trauma 479, *480*
Bonnet-Dechaume-Blanc syndrome 424
Borne, M. J. 532–533
Borrelia burgdorferi infection 362
branch retinal artery occlusion
- aflibercept 124
- anti-VEGF therapy 123
- bevacizumab 124
- characterization 113
- clinical features 113, *114*
- coagulopathy testing 123
- corticosteroids, intravitreal 124
- cystoid macular edema 166
- dexamethasone implant 125
- differential diagnosis 140
- intraocular neovascularization 122
- intravitreal pharmacotherapy 123
- isovolemic hemodilution 127
- laser photocoagulation *126*, 126
- management, course 113, *115*, 123
- OCT evaluation 113, *114*
- pharmacotherapy 123
- ranibizumab 123
- surgery 126
- systemic anticoagulation 126
- triamcinolone acetonide 124

branch retinal vein occlusion
- clinical features, diagnosis 121, *122*
- epidemiology 121
- laser photocoagulation 586
- pathogenesis 121
- pathophysiology 121
- risk factors 121

BRAVO study 122–123
British Xenon Arc Coagulation Study 585
BRVO, *see* branch retinal artery occlusion
butterfly-shaped pigment dystrophy *282*, 282

C

canakinumab 385
cancer-associated retinopathy 21
candidal endophthalmitis 352, 362, *363*
cannula-trocar systems *600*, 600, *601*
canthaxanthin retinopathy 512, *514*
carboplatin, for retinoblastoma 411, 416
carmustine (BCNU) toxicity 509–510
carotid endarterectomy 104–106
cat-scratch disease (Bartonella henselae infection) 352, 361, *362*
cataract surgery
- age-related macular degeneration and 212
- cystoid macular edema and 162
- diabetic macular edema and 162
- diabetic retinopathy and 157
- endophthalmitis, *see* endophthalmitis
- extraction, with macular holes surgery 258
- globe, needle penetration of 529
- intraocular lens dislocation 532, 537
- intraocular lens repositioning *534*, 534
- iris suture fixation 534
- retained lens fragments 529, *531*, 532–533
- retinal detachment following 527
- scleral suture fixation 534, *535–536*
- scleral sutureless fixation 536

CATT study 220–222
ceftazidime, endophthalmitis 496, 524, 525
cellophane maculopathy 267
central retinal artery occlusion
- ancillary studies 108
- characterization 107
- cilioretinal sparing *108*, 108
- clinical features 107
- demographics 107
- differential diagnosis *109*, 109
- electroretinography 109
- emboli *108*, 108, *109*
- fluorescein angiography 108
- history 107
- management, course 111
- ocular sequelae 108
- ophthalmoscopy *108*, 108
- systemic associations 109
- vision 107

central retinal artery, vein occlusion
- ancillary studies 112, *113*
- clinical features *112*, 112
- differential diagnosis 112, 113
- iris neovascularization 112
- management, course 113
- symptoms 112

Central Retinal Vein Bypass Study 130
central retinal venous occlusion
- aflibercept 131
- anti-VEGF therapy 130
- anticoagulation 129
- as OIS etiology 101
- bevacizumab *131*, 131, *132*
- clinical course 128
- clinical features, diagnosis 101, 104, *128*, 128, *129*
- coagulation disorders and 127
- cystoid macular edema 166
- dexamethasone implant 125, *132*, 133
- differential diagnosis 102, 106, 140
- disc collaterals 128, *129*
- intravitreal steroids 132
- iris neovascularization 129, *129*
- ischemic complications treatment 133
- laser photocoagulation 586
- laser-induced chorioretinal anastomosis (L-CRA) 130
- macroaneurysms 128, *129*
- management, course 129
- optic nerve sheath decompression 130
- pathophysiology 127
- radial optic neurotomy 129
- ranibizumab 130
- risk factors 127
- therapies 129
- triamcinolone acetonide 124, *132*, 132

central serous chorioretinopathy
- anti-VEGF therapy 247
- bullous 242
- characterization *216*, 216, 241, 459
- chronic 241
- clinical features 241, 457
- differential diagnosis 245, 459
- enhanced depth imaging OCT 243
- fluorescein angiography *241–242*
- fundus angiography 47, *47*, 242
- fundus autofluorescence *243*
- laser photocoagulation 246, 459
- management, course 246
- multifocal electroretinography, microperimetry 245
- observation 246
- optical coherence tomography 243, *244–245*
- pathophysiology 246
- photodynamic therapy 247, 459
- recurrences 246
- treatment modalities 246, 247
- typical *241*, 241

Central Vein Occlusion Study 129, 586
ceroid lipofuscinoses 326, 333
cestodes 365
Chan, C. L. 537
chlorambucil 383
chloroquine (Aralen) toxicity 506, *507*
chlorpromazine (Thorazine) toxicity 506
chlorthalidone retinopathy 514, *515*
chorioretinitis 354
chorioretinitis sclopetaria 481, *483*
choroid
- anatomy *10*, 10, *11*
- melanoma *80*, 80
- metastatic carcinoma *80*, 80
- ultrasound evaluation 77

choroidal detachments 77, 78, *79*
choroidal hemangioma
- characterization 432
- clinical features *432*, 432, *433*
- diagnosis 433
- genetics 433
- histopathology 434
- indocyanine green angiography 47, *50*
- management, course 434
- ultrasonography 68, 80, *81*

choroidal leiomyoma 436
choroidal metastasis *433–434*, 434, 435, *435*
choroidal neovascularization
- differential diagnosis 463
- idiopathic, *see* idiopathic choroidal neovascularization
- indocyanine green angiography 47, *48–49*
- laser photocoagulation 584, 587
- optic disc coloboma 549, *552*
- photodynamic therapy 286

choroidal neurilemoma 437
choroidal nevus
- characterization 402
- clinical features *392*, 392, *393*
- demographics 392
- diagnosis *394*, 394, *395*
- differential diagnosis *396*, 396
- growth detection factors 395
- halo nevus 393, *393*
- management, course 395
- visual acuity decrease, causes of 392

choroidal osteoma *81*, 81, 407, 435, *436*
choroidal rupture *481*, 481, *482*
choroidal thickening, ultrasonography 77, *78*
choroideremia *304*, 304, *305*
choroiditis areata 291
chromovitrectomy 599
cidofovir (Vistide) retinopathy 514
cilioretinal artery occlusion
- characterization 114, *115*
- clinical features 114, *115*
- treatment 114

cinchonism 508
cisplatin (Platinol) toxicity 509–510
clarithromycin, toxoplasmic chorioretinitis 359
clindamycin, toxoplasmic chorioretinitis 359
clinically significant macular edema (CSME) 150, *150*, 154, 584, 586
- *See also* diabetic macular edema

clofazimine toxicity 508
CME, *see* cystoid macular edema
CMV retinitis 352–353, *353*, 355, *355*, 355, *356*
CMV retinitis, pharmacotherapy 356
Coats' disease
- ancillary testing 190
- anti-VEGF therapy 191
- characterization 187
- clinical features 187, 187, *188–189*, 190
- corticosteroids 192
- diagnosis 187, *188*
- differential diagnosis 187, *189*, 190, 190, 192, 346, 407, 409, 463
- diseases associated with 187, 425
- fluorescein angiography *188*, 189
- laser photocoagulation complications 191
- management, course 191
- pathogenesis, histopathology 191

cobblestone degeneration 11
coccidioidomycosis 363

Collaborative Ocular Melanoma Study (COMS) 399–400
collagen vascular diseases 199
coloboma
- differential diagnosis 407
- of optic disc 549, *550–553*
color vision
- retinal physiology 24, *25*
- testing 90
Colyer, M. H. 532–533
combined hamartoma 407, 430
commotio retinae *480*, 480
cone dystrophy 303
confocal scanning laser ophthalmoscope 90–91, *91*
congenital cataract 407
congenital hypertrophy of the RPE (CHRPE) 428, *429*
congenital pit of optic disc *547*, 547, *548–550*
congenital retinal telangiectasis, *see* Coats' disease
congenital stationary night blindness
- defined 24, 308
- fundus albipunctatus 309, *309–310*
- with abnormal fundi *309*, 309, *310*
- with normal fundi 308, *309*
COPERNICUS Study 131
corneal lacerations 486, *486*, 487, *487*, 488, *488*
corticosteroids
- branch retinal artery occlusion 124
- complications of 373
- cystoid macular edema 163
- diabetic macular edema 153, 165
- endophthalmitis 525
- implants, sustained-release 387
- periocular injections 568
- retinitis pigmentosa 298
- toxoplasmic chorioretinitis 360
- uveitis 369–370, 372
cotton-wool spots
- diabetic retinopathy 138, *139*
- differential diagnosis 115, *116*
- disease entities associated with 116
- hypertensive retinopathy 184, 186
- interferon therapy 117
- management, course 117
- ophthalmoscopy 114, *116*
- systemic workup 117
CRAO, *see* central retinal artery occlusion
Crohn's disease 201
CRUISE Study 130–131
CRVO, *see* central retinal venous occlusion
CRYO-ROP study 176
cryotherapy
- retinoblastoma 417
- retinopathy of prematurity *174*, 176, 178
- trauma 494
cryptococcosis 363
crystalline retinopathy 511
cyclophosphamide 381, 383
cycloplegics, endophthalmitis 525
cyclosporine 381, 382
cystinosis 326, 331
cystoid degeneration 9–10
cystoid macular edema
- anti-VEGF therapy 166
- cataract surgery and 162
- classification, diagnosis *160*, 160, *161*
- comorbidities 378
- dexamethasone implant 570
- diabetic retinopathy and *164*, 164
- differential diagnosis 192, 296
- dominant 292
- drug toxicity and 168
- epinephrine toxicity 511
- fingolimod (Gilenya) toxicity 511
- fundus angiography 46, *47*
- latanoprost (Xalatan) 511
- nicotinic acid maculopathy 511, *512*
- overview 160
- paclitaxel, docetaxel toxicity 511, *513*
- pathophysiology *161*, 161, 162
- radiation retinopathy and 165, *166*
- retinal dystrophies and *167*, 167
- retinal venous occlusion 166
- uveitis and 163

D

Daniel, E. 381
dark adaptometry 90
deferoxamine (Desferal) toxicity 509
degenerative retinoschisis
- clinical features 450, *450*, 469, *470*, *472*
- definitions 469
- diagnosis 469
- differential diagnosis 450, *450*
- histology *469*, 469
- management 471, 473
- prognosis 470
- retinal detachments vs. 471, 473
- schisis detachment 469, *472*, 473
dexamethasone implant
- ADRs 387
- branch retinal artery occlusion 125
- diabetic macular edema 165–166
- dose 387
- endophthalmitis 525
- evidence *387*, 387
- indications 387
- macular edema *132*, 133
- mechanism of action 387
- uveitis 163
Diabetes Control and Complications Trial (DCCT) 142
diabetes mellitus type 1 156
diabetic macular edema
- anti-VEGF therapy 142, 151, 165
- cataract surgery and 162
- characterization 150
- clinical features *150*, 150, *151*
- corticosteroids 153, 165
- dexamethasone implant 570
- diffuse 150, *151*
- FAZ abnormalities 151, *151*
- focal 150, *151*
- focal, grid macular laser treatment, *see* focal, grid macular laser treatment
- intravitreal injection technique 153
- laser photocoagulation 584
- management, course 151
- mixed focal and diffuse 150, *151*
- pathophysiology 164
- sub-Tenon's injections 568–569
- vitrectomy 609
- vitrectomy surgery 165
diabetic papillopathy 139, *139*, 140
diabetic retinopathy
- anti-VEGF therapy 136, 142
- aspirin therapy 142
- cataract surgery and 157
- clinical features 103, *137*, 137, *138–139*
- clinical trials 136
- cotton wool spots 138, *139*
- cystoid macular edema and *164*, 164
- diagnosis, staging 140
- differential diagnosis 103, 106, 115, 140, 192
- epidemiology 136
- exudates 138, *139*
- focal, grid macular laser treatment 153, *154*
-- *See also* focal, grid macular laser treatment
- full-field ERG testing 86
- fundus angiography 46, *46*
- indirect ophthalmoscopy 37, *38*
- intraretinal microvascular abnormalities (IRMAs) 138, *138*, 143
- laser treatment technique recommendations 146
- macular edema in 137
- microaneurysm 137, *137*
- nonproliferative, *see* nonproliferative diabetic retinopathy
- overview 136, 157
- pregnancy and 142
- proliferative, *see* proliferative diabetic retinopathy
- retina preclinical molecular, pathophysiologic changes 137
- surgery 156
- vitrectomy indications 156
Diabetic Retinopathy Study (DRS) 136, 145, 148
Diabetic Retinopathy Vitrectomy Study 136, 608
diabetic vitrectomy 608
dideoxyinosine toxicity 509, *510*
diffuse unilateral subacute neuroretinitis *364*, 364
diode (infrared) laser photocoagulation 581
diphenhydramine, for retinoblastoma 411
dislocated intraocular lenses 607
dislocated lens, ultrasonography 74, *76*
disseminated intravascular coagulation 463
docetaxel toxicity 511, *513*
docosahexaenoic acid (DHA), retinitis pigmentosa 298
doxycycline, toxoplasmic chorioretinitis 359
Doyne's honeycomb macular dystrophy *286*, 286, *287–288*
DRCR.net 136, 149, 152–153, 568, 582
drug delivery, posterior segment
- biodegradable implants 570
- dexamethasone implant, *see* dexamethasone implant
- encapsulated cell technology (ECT) 571, *572*
- implantable drug pumps 571, *573*
- nonbiodegradable implants *569*, 569
- overview 568
- periocular injections 568
drug toxicity, cystoid macular edema and 168
dye yellow laser photocoagulation 581
dye-enhanced laser photocoagulation 588
- *See also* fluorescein angiography, indocyanine green angiography

E

Eales' disease
- characterization 195
- clinical features 195, *196*
- differential diagnosis 192, 195
- management, course 197
- pathogenesis, histopathology 195
Early Treatment Diabetic Retinopathy Study (ETDRS) 123, 136, 142, 145–146, 148, 154, 165, 230–231, 584
echinococcus 365
eclipse burn 515, *516*
Ehlers–Danlos syndrome 236
electrooculography 88, *89*
electroretinography
- central retinal artery occlusion 109
- full-field
-- accuracy in diagnosis 84
-- cone responses 85, *85*
-- disorders affecting 84, 86, 86
-- equipment 83
-- interpretation 84
-- oscillatory potentials 85, *85*
-- overview 83
-- practical considerations 83
-- purpose 84
-- retinal function testing 86
-- rod-isolated response 84, *85*
- multifocal
-- clinical applications 88
-- interpretation 87, *88*
-- overview 86
-- practical considerations 86
- negative ERG 86, *87*
- ocular ischemic syndrome 103, *105–106*
- principles 83
- retinitis pigmentosa 297
- trauma 479
elevated IOP 261
encapsulated cell technology (ECT) 571, *572*
endogenous endophthalmitis 407
endophotocoagulation 580, *604*, 604
endophthalmitis
- acute onset 522, *523*
- aminoglycosides 524, 525
- antibiotic regimens 496, 525
- antibiotic resistance 525
- causative organisms 562
- corticosteroids 525
- culture media 523
- delayed-onset *523*, *526*, 526
- diagnosis, confirmation of 522
- filtering blebs-associated 526
- glaucoma drainage implant-associated 526
- noninfectious 565, 566
- postoperative 606
-- categories of, miscellaneous 525–526
-- clinical features 522, *523*
-- diagnosis 522
-- epidemiology 522, 522

-- factors associated with 522
-- management, course 523, 525
- posttraumatic 495, 496
- risk following 562, 564
- ultrasonography 69, *70*
Endophthalmitis Vitrectomy Study (EVS) 523, 525
Endpoint Management software 590
enhanced depth imaging (EDI) *54*, 54
enhanced S-cone syndrome *303*, 303
enlarged vessels, in optic disc 545, *546*
enucleation
- for retinoblastoma 418
- traumatic 496
EOG, *see* electrooculography
Epidemiology of Diabetes Interventions and Complications (EDIC) study 142
epinephrine toxicity 511
epipapillary veil 544, *545*
epiretinal membrane
- characterization 267
- clinical features 267, *268*
- diagnosis 267, *268*
- epidemiology 267
- fluorescein angiography 268, *269*
- ICG staining 271
- management, course 271
- optical coherence tomography 267, *268*
- pathogenesis, pathology 269, *270*
- posterior vitreous detachment and 268–269
- preoperative evaluation 271
- primary vs. secondary 268, *269*
- progressive nuclear cataract 272
- recurrence 272
- surgical complications 272
- surgical procedure 271, *272*
- visual impairment mechanisms 270
ERG, *see* electroretinography
ergot alkaloids toxicity 511
ERM, *see* epiretinal membrane
ESBA1008 (Alcon) 221
etanercept 385
ethoxyzolamide retinopathy 514, *515*
etoposide, for retinoblastoma 411
ETROP study 176, 179
European Society of Cataract and Refractive Surgery 525
EXCITE study 219
expulsive choroidal detachment 460
external beam radiotherapy 418
exudative retinal detachment, *see* specific conditions
- characterization 457
- clinical features *457*, 457
- diagnostic testing 457
- differential diagnosis 451, 458
- hematologic, vascular 462
- idiopathic entities 459
- infectious 464
- inflammatory 460
- medications 464
- neoplastic 464
- pathogenesis 458
- post-surgical 460

F

FAF, *see* under fundus
FAME study 165
familial adenomatous polyposis 429, *429*
familial colonic cancer 429
familial exudative vitreoretinopathy
- characterization 344
- clinical features 345, *345–346*
- differential diagnosis 345, 346, 407
- diseases associated with 425
- management, course *347*, 347
- pathogenesis, genetics 346
Fastenberg, D. M. 532–533
fat embolism syndrome 503
FEVR, *see* familial exudative vitreoretinopathy
fibromuscular dysplasia 111
FILM study 608
fingolimod (Gilenya) toxicity 511
fingolimod, for macular edema 168
flash visual evoked potential studies 479
fluocinolone acetonide implants, inserts 387–388, 569, *569*, 570
fluorescein angiography
- acquired retinal macroaneurysm *197*, 198
- central retinal artery occlusion 108
- central serous chorioretinopathy *241–242*
- Coats' disease *188*, 189
- dye adverse reactions 41, 42
- dye transit times *42*, 43, *44*
- epiretinal membrane 268, *269*
- hyperfluorescence 45, *46*
- hypertensive retinopathy 185, *185–186*
- interpretation of 42
- macular degeneration 47, *48*
- macular holes 252, *252*
- principles 40, *42*, 42
- retinal angiomatous proliferation *49*
- retinopathy of prematurity 174, *175*
- sodium fluorescein
-- adverse reactions 41–42
-- properties 40, *41*
- vascular filling defects 45, *45*
Flynn, H. W., Jr. 537
focal, grid macular laser treatment
- choroidal neovascularization 155
- clinical studies 165
- complications, avoiding 155
- complications, side effects 155
- follow-up 155
- grid treatment 155
- principles 153, *154*
- technique 146, 154, *155*
ForeseeHome device 211
Foscarnet, CMV retinitis 356
fovea anatomy 8, *8*
foveola anatomy 8, *8*
foveomacalar retinitis 515, *516*
Fovista 221
Freeman, W. R. 259
fundus 11, 34, *35*
fundus albipunctatus 16, 21, 309, *309–310*
fundus angiography
- abnormal 43
- autofluorescence 43
- deeper choroidal fluorescence blockage 45
- dye adverse reactions 41, 42
- dye properties 40, 40, *41*
- dye, transit times *42*, 43, *44*
- fluorescein angiography 40, *42*, 42
- hyper-autofluoresce in abnormal findings 43
- hyperfluorescence 45, *46*
- hypofluorescence 44, *45*
- indocyanine green angiography 40, 43, *44*
- interpretation of 42, 42
- normal *42*, 42
- overview 40
- photosensitivity 41
- pseudofluorescence 43
- technique 41
- vascular filling defects 45, *45*
fundus autofluorescence
- central serous chorioretinopathy *243*
- described 91, *93*, *210*
- retinal pigment epithelium 208
fundus flavimaculatus, *see* Stargardt's disease
fundus pulverulentus 282, *283*

G

GALILEO Study 131
ganciclovir, CMV retinitis 356
Gangaputra, S. 381
ganglion cell layer analysis 54, *55*, *62*
Gardner's syndrome 429
gas ion lasers 577
Gaucher's disease
- characterization 327
- clinical features 327, *327*, 327
- diagnosis 328
- differential diagnosis 329
- genetic etiologies 326
- management, course 328
- pathogenesis, histopathology 328
GEFAL study 220
gentamicin, endophthalmitis 496
geographic choroidopathy 371–372, 377, *378*
gevokizumab 385
giant retinal tears 607
Gilliland, G. D. 532–533
glassblower's cataract 516
GM1 gangliosidosis
- characterization 326
- clinical features 326
- diagnosis 327
- differential diagnosis 327
- genetic etiologies 326
- management, course 327
- pathophysiology, histopathology 327
GM2 gangliosidoses
- characterization 324
- clinical features 325
- diagnosis 325
- management, course 326
- pathogenesis 325
Goldmann's fundus contact lens 38
Goldmann's three-mirror lens 36
Goldmann-Favre's disease 303, 343, *344*, 349
gyrate atrophy 305, *306*, 326, *332*, 332

H

hamartoma
- astrocytic, *see* astrocytic hamartoma
- combined 407, 430
- differential diagnosis 407
hand-held lens 38
Harada disease 77, *78*
helicoid choroidopathy 371–372, 377, *378*
hemangioma 407
hemiretinal vein occlusion 133
hemorrhage
- differential diagnosis 198
- suprachoroidal 527, *528*
- vitreous, *see* vitreous hemorrhage
heredopathia atactica polyneuritiformis, *see* Refsum's disease
Histoplasma capsulatum 231–232
histoplasmosis 425
HIV infection 355, *360*
Ho, L. Y. 532–533
Home Monitoring of Eye (HOME) study 211
Hruby lens 37
Hunter's syndrome, *see* under mucopolysaccharidosis, type II
Hurler's syndrome, *see* under mucopolysaccharidosis, type I
Hutton, W. L. 532–533
hydrochlorothiazide retinopathy 514, *515*
hydroxychloroquine (Plaquenil) toxicity 507, *508–509*
hypercoagulable syndrome 201, *201*
hypertension, malignant *463*, 463
hypertensive choroidopathy 184, *186*
hypertensive retinopathy
- clinical features 184, *185*
- cotton-wool spots 184, 186
- differential diagnosis 185
- fluorescein angiography 185, *185–186*
- grading 184
- in pregnancy 184
- management, course 186
- pathogenesis 186

I

idiopathic choroidal neovascularization
- anti-VEGF agents 238
- characterization 237
- clinical features 237
- diagnosis 237
- laser photocoagulation 238
- management, course *238*, 238
- pathogenesis, histopathology 238
- subfoveal, laser photocoagulation 238
idiopathic choroiditis 425
idiopathic macular telangiectasia (IMT) type 1
- characterization 187, 192
- clinical features 190, 192, *193–194*
- differential diagnosis 187, 192
- management, course 195
- pathogenesis, histopathology 193
idiopathic peripheral retinal vasculitis 425
implantable drug pumps 571, *573*
incontinentia pigmenti
- characterization 347
- clinical features 347, *348*
- diagnosis 348
- differential diagnosis 346, 349, 407
- management, course 349
- pathogenesis, genetics 349

indirect ophthalmoscopy
- fundus drawing 34, *35*
- Goldmann's fundus contact lens 38
- Goldmann's three-mirror lens 36
- hand-held lens 38
- Hruby lens 37
- macular examination 37, *38*
- Mainster posterior pole lens 38
- pearls 30, 34, 36
- principles, advantages *30*, 30, *31*
- scleral depression 34, 35–36, *36–37*
- scleral depression contraindications 35
- technique *30*, 30, *31–34*
- wide-field contact lenses 36
indocyanine green
- adverse reactions 41–42
- interpretation of 42
- properties 40, *41*
indocyanine green angiography
- abnormal 43
- choroidal hemangiomas 47, *50*
- choroidal neovascularization 47, *48–49*
- hypofluorescence 44, *45*
- principles 40, 43, *44*
- retinal angiomatous proliferation *49*
infantile Refsum's disease 334
infectious endophthalmitis 261
inflammatory chorioretinopathies 371–372
inflammatory pseudotumor 460
infliximab 384
interferon 385
interferon toxicity 510, *511*
intermediate uveitis *60*
intra-arterial chemotherapy (IAC) *415*, 415
intraocular foreign body
- BB pellets 491
- external magnet approach 490, *490*
- posterior vitreous detachment 491
- retinal detachment 491
- traumatic, management 489, *490–491*
- ultrasonography 74, 74, *77*
- vitrectomy 491, *491*
intraocular lens dislocation 532, 537
intraocular lens repositioning *534*, 534
intraocular steroids 386
intraocular tumor evaluation 78
intravitreal chemotherapy (IVC) 416, *417*
intravitreal injection
- antibiotics 564
- endophthalmitis risk following 562, 564
- endophthalmitis, causative organisms 562
- endophthalmitis, noninfectious 565, 566
- needle gauge 565
- overview 562
- personal protective equipment 564
- post-injection management, follow-Up guidelines 565
- procedure guidelines 563
- site of injection 565
- technique, anti-VEGF therapy 153
iridescent spots 314, *315*
iris suture fixation 534
IVAN study 220

J

Jansen's disease 308
Jansky–Bielschowsky disorder 333
juvenile xanthogranuloma 407

K

Ka?maz, R. O. 381
Kapusta, M. A. 532–533
Kearns–Sayre syndrome (mitochondrial myopathy) 301
Kelly, N. E. 259
Kim, J. E. 532–533, 537
krypton red laser photocoagulation 581

L

Lambrou, F. H., Jr. 532
lampalizumab 223
laser indirect ophthalmoscope 580
laser photocoagulation
- age-related macular degeneration 217, 587
- angioid streaks 236
- argon green 580
- branch retinal artery occlusion *126*, 126
- branch retinal vein occlusion 586
- central retinal vein occlusion 586
- central serous chorioretinopathy 246, 459
- choroidal neovascularization 587
- complications 583
- delivery systems 579
- diabetic macular edema 584
- diode (infrared) 581
- dye yellow 581
- dye-enhanced 588
- endophotocoagulation 580
- gas ion lasers 577
- history of 576
- idiopathic choroidal neovascularization 238
- image-guided, planned laser application 589, *590*
- indications 584
- krypton red 581
- laser indirect ophthalmoscope 580
- laser–tissue interactions 578
- liquid lasers 578
- macular treatment principles 583
- media 577
- microaneurysms, modified ETDRS guidelines 585
- micropulse laser 591
- mode locking 577
- MPS treatment protocol 587
- ocular complications 178
- output modes 577
- pathologic myopia 230–231
- peripheral circumferential scatter 320
- power 581
- presumed ocular histoplasmosis syndrome 234
- principles 576, *577*
- proliferative diabetic retinopathy 585
- pulse duration
-- clinical studies 589
-- improving selectivity of *589*, 589, *590*
-- modifications 590
-- morphology restoration 590, *591*
-- principles, applications of 581
-- selective retinal therapy with 591, *592*
- Q-switching 577
- response to 585
- retinal tear 588
- retinal tears 449
- retinoblastoma 417
- retinopathy of prematurity 176, *178*, 178
- scatter photocoagulation, *see* scatter (panretinal) laser photocoagulation
- selective retinal therapy 591, *592*
- semiconductor lasers 578
- settings 580
- sickle cell hemoglobinopathies *320*, 320
- slit-lamp biomicroscope 579
- solid-state lasers 577
- spot size 581
- techniques
-- post-treatment 583
-- pre-surgical workup 582
-- treatment 582
- tissue variables 578, *579*
- transpupillary thermotherapy 590
- types of 588
- wavelength 580, 581
laser-induced chorioretinal anastomosis (L-CRA) 130
laser-pointer exposure 516, *517*
latanoprost (Xalatan) 511
lattice retinal degeneration 445, *447*
Laurence–Moon–Bardet–Biedl syndrome 300
Leber's amaurosis 21
Leber's congenital amaurosis *302*, 302
leiomyoma, choroidal 436
lens rupture, implantation *494*, 494
lensectomy 493, *493*, *601*, 601
leukemia 246, 439
light response of the standing potential 19
light toxicity 514
lightning maculopathy 503
lipemia retinalis 109, *109*
lipidoses 324, 326
lipofuscin 92
lipopigment storage disorders
- characterization 333
- clinical features 333
- diagnosis 334
- pathogenesis, histopathology 334
liquid lasers 578
LUCAS study 220
lupus retinopathy, *see* systemic lupus erythematosus
lymphoma *438*, 438

M

macula
- anatomy *8*, 8
- choroidal ruptures 481, *481–482*
- coarse pigment mottling in 282, *283*
- cube scans *53*, 53, *58*, *63*
- examination, indirect ophthalmoscopy 37, *38*
- laser treatment principles 583
- sickle cell hemoglobinopathies 315, *316*
macula lutea 8
macular degeneration 47, *48*
- *See also* specific conditions
macular edema
- aflibercept 131
- anti-VEGF therapy 130, 142, 151
- bevacizumab *131*, 131, *132*
- characterization 122, *122–123*
- cystoid, *see* cystoid macular edema
- dexamethasone implant *132*, 133
- diabetic, *see* diabetic macular edema
- focal, grid macular laser treatment, *see* focal, grid macular laser treatment
- in diabetic retinopathy 137
- ocular ischemic syndrome 102, *103*
- optical coherence tomography *59*, 122
- radiation retinopathy-associated *518*, 518, *519*
- ranibizumab 130
- therapies 130
- triamcinolone acetonide *132*, 132
macular holes
- anatomic, visual results 259, *260*
- categories 253
- characterization 250
- chronic 253–254, *254*, 260
- classification 252, *252*
- clinical features *250*, 250
- clinical studies 259
- development stages 250, *251*
- diagnosis 250, *250*
- differential diagnosis *253*, 253
- fluorescein angiography 252, *252*
- full-thickness 61, *61*, 252
- ICG staining 257
- imaging 252, *252*
- intraocular gas selection 257
- management, course 253
- myopic 261
- nonsurgical treatment 258
- nuclear sclerotic cataracts 263
- operculum 252
- pathophysiology 250
- persistent, recurrent 253–254, 258, 259, 261, 263
- postoperative prone positioning 257
- preoperative considerations 253, 253
- pseudoholes 253, *253*
- retinal detachment 254
- retinal detachments, rhegmatogenous and 262
- retinal tears and 262
- RPE alterations and *262*, 262
- secondary 253, 255, *255*
- Stage 1 *251*, 251
- Stage 2 *251*, 251
- Stage 3 *251*, 252
- Stage 4 *252*, 252
- surgery
-- adjunctive agents 257
-- cataract extraction with 258
-- complications 261
-- indications 255
-- technique *256*, 256
- traumatic 253, 255, *255*, 261
- visual field loss and 262
- vitrectomy 608

Macular Photocoagulation Study 217, 234, 238, 587
macular sparing 6
macular translocation 217
Mainster posterior pole lens 38
malattia leventinese *286*, 286, *287–288*
malignant hypertension *463*, 463
MANTA study 220
MARINA study 218, 221–222, 231
medulloepithelioma 407
megalopapilla 556, *557*
melanocytoma, optic disc *437*, 437
melanoma
- characterization 402
- choroidal *396*, 397, 450, *451*
- choroidal, enlarged vessels 545, *546–547*
- classification 398, 398, 400
- clinical features *396*, 397
- demographics 397
- diagnostic testing 398
- differential diagnosis 198, 246, *396*, 396, 450, *451*, 461
- diffuse 400
- histopathology, cytogenetics 396, 400
- management 399
- metastasis risk 400
- ocular melanocytosis 400
- predisposing factors 397
- prognosis 399
- pseudomelanoma *401*, 401, 402
- symptoms 397
- ultrasonography 68, *80*, 80
Mello, M. O., Jr. 537
melphalan, for retinoblastoma 411, 416
meridional folds, complex 9, *9*
metabolic diseases, *see* specific diseases
- cherry-red spots 324, *324*, 324
- eccentric cherry-red spot 324, *325*
- genetic etiologies of 326
- pigmentary retinopathy 324, *324*, 324
- retinal expression 324
metastasis, choroidal *433–434*, 434, 435, *435*
metastatic carcinoma *80*, 80, 246
methotrexate 380, 381–382, 411
methoxyflurane (Penthrane) retinopathy 513
mfERG, *see* under electroretinography
microaneurysms, modified ETDRS guidelines 585
micropulse laser 591
Millenium Microsurgical System (Bausch & Lomb) 600
mitochondrial myopathy (Kearns–Sayre syndrome) 301
Mittendorf's dot 544, *545*
Mizuo–Nakamura phenomenon 309
Modi, Y. S. 532–533
morning glory disc anomaly 407, *552*, 552
Morquio type B disease 327
Moyamoya disease 111
mucolipidosis IV
- characterization 333
- clinical features 333
- diagnosis 333
- genetic etiologies 326
- pathogenesis, histopathology 333
mucopolysaccharidosis
- characterization 329
- type I
-- characterization 329
-- clinical features 329
-- diagnosis 330
-- genetic etiologies 326
-- management, course 330
-- pathogenesis, histopathology 330
- type II
-- clinical features 330
-- diagnosis 330
-- genetic etiologies 326
-- incidence 330
-- pathogenesis, histopathology 330
- type III
-- clinical features 331
-- diagnosis 331
-- genetic etiologies 326
-- incidence 331
-- pathogenesis, histopathology 331
multifocal choroiditis 232, 371–372, 378, *379–380*
multifocal ERG (mfERG) 26
multifocal pattern dystrophy simulating fundus flavimaculatus *282*, 282, *283*
multiple evanescent white dot syndrome (MEWDS) 370, 371–372, *373*
multiple sclerosis-related vasculitis 201, *202*
mycophenolate mofetil 380, 381
myelinated nerve fibers 407, 556, *557*

N

nanophthalmos 459
NAVILAS 592
necrotizing herpetic retinitis 352, 356, *357*
neonatal adrenoleukodystrophy 334
neurilemoma, choroidal 437
neurofibromatosis type 2 (NF2) 431, 431
neuronal ceroid lipofuscinosis (Batten's disease) 300, 334
nicotinic acid maculopathy 511, *512*
Niemann–Pick disease
- characterization 328
- clinical features *328*, 328, 329
- diagnosis 329
- genetic etiologies 326
- pathogenesis, histopathology 329
- retinal changes 329
nocardiosis 361, *362*
nonbiodegradable implants *569*, 569
nonproliferative diabetic retinopathy
- anti-VEGF therapy 142
- clinical features 137–138, *138–139*
- diagnosis, staging 140, 140, *141*
- management, course 140, 142
- progression risk 141
Norrie's disease 346, 407, 465
North Carolina Carolina-like dominant macular dystrophy 289
North Carolina macular dystrophy *288*, 288, *289*
NP-207 (piperidyl chlorophenothiazine hydrochloride) 505
NSAIDs 163
nuclear sclerotic cataracts 263

O

occult macular dystrophy *291*, 291
ocriplasmin 258
OCT, *see* optical coherence tomography
ocular histoplasmosis syndrome 378, *379*
ocular infections, *see* specific conditions
- bacterial 360
- cestodes 365
- characterization 352
- diagnosis 354
- fungal 362
- helminthic 364
- host factors *355*, 355
- management 354
- nematode (intestinal roundworm) 364
- protozoal 358
- route of infection 352, *353*
- trematodes 365
- viral 355
ocular inflammation (noninfectious)
- alkylating agents 383
- antimetabolites 380
-- *See also* specific agents
- antimetabolites, comparative results of 382
- biologics 384–385
- calcineurin inhibitors 382
- characterization 369
- corticosteroid implants, sustained-release 387
- specific receptor antagonists 385
- TNF-a inhibitors 384
- topical steroids 386
- treatment 378, 381
ocular ischemic syndrome
- ancillary tests 102, 102, *105*
- anterior segment 99, *100*
- arterial pulsations 104
- associated systemic diseases 104
- background 99
- clinical features 102, 104, 106
- cotton-wool spots 102
- demographics 99
- differential diagnosis 103, 106, 140
- electroretinography 103, *105–106*
- etiologies 99
- external signs 99, *100*
- flow, presentation 99, *100*
- imaging 103
- macular edema 102, *103*
- management, course 104
- mortality 104
- neovascularization 101, *102*
- noninvasive testing 103
- posterior segment *101*, 101
- retinal hemorrhages 101, *101*
- spontaneous retinal arterial pulsations 102
- symptoms 99
- vision 99
ocular trauma, *see* trauma
Oguchi's disease 21, 309, *310*
OIS, *see* ocular ischemic syndrome
onchocerciasis 365
ondansetron, for retinoblastoma 411
operating room microscope toxicity 516, *517*
ophthalmomyiasis interna 365
optic disc abnormalities
- aplasia *556*, 556
- Bergmeister's papilla 544, *545–546*
- coloboma 549, *550–553*
- congenital pit *547*, 547, *548–550*
- double-ring sign 555, *556*
- enlarged vessels 545, *546*
- hypoplasia 555, *556*
- megalopapilla 556, *557*
- melanocytoma *437*, 437
- morning glory disc anomaly 407, *552*, 552
- myelinated nerve fibers 556, *557*
- peripapillary staphyloma *553*, 553
- persistent hyaloid artery 544, *545*
- persistent hyperplastic primary vitreous 73, *76*, 557, *558*
- prepapillary vascular loops *543*, 543, *544–545*
- tilted disc syndrome *553*, 553, 554, *554–555*
- tortuosity, congenital *558*, 558
optic disc neovascularization
- proliferative diabetic retinopathy 143, *143–144*
- recurrent 147, *148*
- treatment 146, 147
optic nerve
- avulsion 484, *485*
- sheath decompression 130
- swelling *60*
optical coherence tomography
- artifacts 62, *63*
- blink artifact 62, *63*
- branch retinal artery occlusion 113, *114*
- central serous chorioretinopathy 243, *244–245*
- cross line scan 54
- cube scans *53*, 53, *58*, *63*
- decentration *63*
- en face 55
- enhanced depth imaging (EDI) *54*, 54
- epiretinal membrane 267, *268*
- errors 62
- ganglion cell layer analysis 54, *55*, *62*
- grid scan 53
- high-definition line scan 54
- history of 52
- layer specific 54
- layers on *56*, 56
- line scans *54*, 54, 56
- mirror artifact 62, *64*
- misalignment 62, *63*
- motion artifact 63, *64*
- normal retinal 56
- pathology *58*, 58
-- intermediate uveitis *60*
-- macular edema *59*
-- macular hole, full-thickness 61, *61*
-- optic nerve swelling *60*
-- outer photoreceptor loss *59*
-- pigment epithelial detachment *59*
-- reflectivity profiles 58
-- retinal surface thickening, distortion *58*
-- vitreomacular adhesion 61, *61*
-- vitreomacular traction 61, *61*
- patient related errors 62, *63–64*
- principles 52
- qualitative analysis *54*, 56, *57*
- quantitative analysis 57, *58*

- radial scan 53
- raster scan 53
- retinal nerve fiber layer (RNFL) analysis 54, *55*
- retinitis pigmentosa 297, *297*
- retinopathy of prematurity 174, *175*
- reverse shadowing 57, *57*
- scan quality 62
- scans, types of 53
- shadowing 57, 60
- software error *62*, 62
- spectral-domain 52–53
- swept-source 52–53, 56
- time-domain 52
- types, comparison of 52
- vignetting artifact *64*, 64
- vitreoretinal interface 61
- windowing 57, *57*, 60

ora serrata 9, *9*
ora serrata pearls 9
oral contraceptive toxicity 510
ornithine 306
osteoma 407
osteoma, choroidal 435, *436*
outer photoreceptor loss *59*
Ozurdex 387

P

paclitaxel toxicity 511, *513*
Paget's disease 236
panretinal photocoagulation (PRP) 133
- *See also* scatter (panretinal) laser photocoagulation

Panton, R. W. 537
panuveitis 371–372, 372, 378
panuveitis with suspected infection, management 354
pars plana vitrectomy, *see* vitrectomy
pars planitis *369*, 370, 425
Pasadhika, S. 381
PASCAL (Topcon Corp) 589
pathologic myopia
- anti-VEGF therapy 231
- choroidal neovascularization 227, *228–229*
- clinical features *227*, 227
- CNV recurrence risk factors 231
- diagnosis 229
- epidemiology 227
- Fuchs' spot 227, *228*
- lacquer cracks 227, *227–228*
- laser photocoagulation 230–231
- management, course *228–230*, 230
- pathogenesis, histopathology 229
- photodynamic therapy 229
- prognosis 227–228

patter scan laser technique 146
pattern dystrophy
- adult-onset foveomacular vitelliform dystrophy 280, *281*
- butterfly-shaped pigment dystrophy *282*, 282
- characterization 209, *210*, 280
- classification 283
- fundus flavimaculatus, *see* Stargardt's disease
- fundus pulverulentus 282, *283*
- histopathology 283
- multifocal simulating fundus flavimaculatus *282*, 282, *283*
- reticular dystrophy of RPE 282
- systemic diseases associated 283
- visual prognosis 283, *283*

pegaptanib 151, 218
penetrating injuries 485
penetrating, perforating injury 74, *76*
penicillin G, syphilitic chorioretinitis 361
perfluorocarbon liquid 604, *605*
perforating injuries *489*, 489
periocular injections 568
periocular steroids 386
peripapillary staphyloma *553*, 553
peripheral circumferential scatter laser photocoagulation 320
peripheral disciform degeneration 463
peripheral exudative hemorrhagic chorioretinopathy (PEHCR) 401
peripheral uveoretinitis 407
peroxisomal disorders 326, 334
persistent fetal vasculature
- differential diagnosis 407
- traction retinal detachment 466
- ultrasonography 73, *76*

persistent hyaloid artery 544, *545*
persistent hyperplastic primary vitreous 73, *76*, 557, *558*
pharmacotherapy
- CMV retinitis 356
- retinoblastoma protocols 411
- syphilitic chorioretinitis 361
- toxoplasmic chorioretinitis 359

phenergen, for retinoblastoma 411
phenothiazines toxicity 505
photodynamic therapy
- age-related macular degeneration 217, 222, 587, 589
- amelanotic melanoma 399
- astrocytic hamartoma 428
- central serous chorioretinopathy 247, 459
- choroidal hemangioma 434
- choroidal metastasis 435
- choroidal neovascularization 286
- choroidal osteoma 436
- clinical trials 217
- exudative AMD 206
- history of 576
- pathologic myopia 229
- principles, applications 588
- retinal detachments 463
- retinal hemangioblastoma 421, *422*, 423
- vasoproliferative tumor 425–426, *426*

PIER study 219, 222
pigment epithelial detachment *59*
pigmented ocular fundus lesions (POFLs) 429, *429*
pinealoblastoma, chemoreduction prevention of 414
pioglitazone, ADRs 168
plaque radiotherapy 417
pneumocystis choroiditis 360
POHS, *see* presumed ocular histoplasmosis syndrome
polyarteritis nodosa 201
polypoidal choroidal vasculopathy 216, *217*
Port Delivery System (Genentech) 572, *573*
Posterior MicroPump Drug Delivery System (PMP) 571, *573*
posterior scleritis 460, *461*
posterior vitreous detachments
- characterization 443
- clinical features 443
- degenerative retinoschisis and 471
- differential diagnosis *443*, 443
- intraocular foreign body 491
- management, course 444
- pathogenesis 444, *445*

prednisone
- endophthalmitis 525
- toxoplasmic chorioretinitis 360
- uveitis 372

pregnancy
- diabetic retinopathy and 142
- hypertensive retinopathy in 184
- toxoplasmic chorioretinitis, pharmacotherapy 359

prepapillary vascular loops *543*, 543, *544–545*
preproliferative retinopathy, *see* see nonproliferative diabetic retinopathy
presumed ocular histoplasmosis syndrome
- anti-VEGF therapy 234
- choroidal neovascularization 231, *233*, 234
- clinical features 231, *232–233*
- CNV recurrence risk 234
- diagnosis 232
- differential diagnosis 232, 364
- Histoplasma capsulatum 231–232
- laser photocoagulation 234
- management, course 233
- multifocal choroiditis 232
- pathogenesis, histopathology 232

primary hyperoxaluria type I 326, 336
probenecid, syphilitic chorioretinitis 361
proliferative diabetic retinopathy
- anti-VEGF therapy *149*, 149
- characterization 143
- clinical features 136–137
- diagnosis of *143*, 143, *144*
- diagnosis, staging 140
- follow-up 147, *148*
- high-risk characteristics 145
- intraretinal microvascular abnormalities (IRMAs) 143
- laser photocoagulation 585
- laser treatment technique recommendations 146
- management, course 144
- optic disc neovascularization 143, *143–144*
- optic disc neovascularization, recurrent 147, *148*
- optic disc neovascularization, treatment 146, 147
- pars plana vitrectomy *156*, 156
- pathophysiology 144
- scatter (panretinal) laser photocoagulation ADRs 148
- scatter (panretinal) laser photocoagulation technique 145, *147*
- traction retinal detachment 465, *465*

proliferative vitreoretinopathy
- characterization 452
- classification 454–455
- clinical features 453
- diagnosis *454*, 454
- management, course 454
- pathogenesis 454
- risk factors for 453
- vitrectomy 606

PrONTO study 219, 221–222
Protocol B study 153
Protocol E study 568
Protocol I study 151, 153
Protocol S study 149
Protocol T study 152
pseudomelanoma *401*, 401, 402
- *See also* choroidal nevus

pseudophakia 165
pseudoretinoblastomas 406
pseudotumor, inflammatory 460
pseudoxanthoma elasticum *235*, 235, 283
- *See also* angioid streaks

Pujari, S. S. 381
pulse duration laser photocoagulation
- clinical studies 589
- improving selectivity of *589*, 589, *590*
- modifications 590
- morphology restoration 590, *591*
- principles, applications of 581
- selective retinal therapy with 591, *592*

punctate inner choroiditis (PIC) 371, 371, 372, *374*
Purtscher's retinopathy *499*, 499
PVD, *see* posterior vitreous detachments
pyrimethamine, toxoplasmic chorioretinitis 359

Q

quinine toxicity 508, *509*

R

racemose angiomas, hemangiomas 546

radial optic neurotomy 129
RADIANCE study 231
radiation retinopathy 165, *166*, *518*, 518, *519*
ranibizumab
- age-related macular degeneration 218
- branch retinal artery occlusion 123
- clinical studies 222
- Coats' disease 191
- cystoid macular edema 166
- diabetic macular edema 151, 165
- macular edema 130
- nonproliferative diabetic retinopathy 142
- pathologic myopia 231
- proliferative diabetic retinopathy 149
- treatments trials comparisons 220

Refsum's disease
- characterization 301
- clinical features 335
- diagnosis 335
- genetic etiologies 326
- management, course 336
- pathogenesis, histopathology 335

renal failure 463
Replenish PMP 571, *573*
retained lens fragments 529, *531*, 532–533, 607
reticular dystrophy of RPE 282

reticular pseudodrusen 208
retina
- anatomy 3
- arteriovenous malformations 546, *546*, 547, *547*
- circulation *7*, 7
- degeneration, ERG evaluation of 84
- surface thickening, distortion *58*
- tufts, anatomy 10
- ultrasound evaluation 70, *72*
retinal capillary hemangioma 407
retinal cavernous hemangioma
- characterization 423
- clinical features *423*, 423
- diagnosis 423
- genetics 423
- histopathology 424
- management, course 424
retinal degenerations
- deafness and, syndromes associated with 300
- hereditary, *see* specific conditions
retinal detachments
- cataract surgery, following 527
- chemoreduction outcomes 413
- degenerative retinoschisis vs. 471, 473
- differential diagnosis 246
- diseases associated with 425
- intraocular foreign body 491
- localized, ultrasonography 71
- macular holes 254
- nonrhegmatogenous, differential diagnosis 407
- optic disc coloboma 549, *551–552*
- photodynamic therapy 463
- rhegmatogenous, *see* rhegmatogenous retinal detachments
- schisis detachment 469, *472*, 473
- total, ultrasonography 72, *75*
- traction, *see* traction retinal detachment
- trauma-associated 483, *484*, 493
- X-linked juvenile retinoschisis 343–344
retinal dystrophies, cystoid macular edema and *167*, 167
retinal folds, medication-induced 514, *515*
retinal hemangioblastoma
- characterization 421
- clinical features 421, *422*
- diagnosis 422
- genetics, pathogenesis 422
- histopathology 423
- management, course 422
retinal lasers, *see* laser photocoagulation, photodynamic therapy
retinal nerve fiber layer (RNFL) analysis 54, *55*
retinal periphery anatomy
- cystoid degeneration 9–10
- described *9*, 9
- enclosed oral bay 9, *10*
- giant teeth 9
- meridional folds, complex 9, *9*
- ora serrata 9, *9*
- ora serrata pearls 9
- retinal tufts 10
- sensory retinal detachments 10
retinal physiology
- adaptation 21
- arrestin 21
- color vision 24, *25*
- contrast recognition *22*, 22, *23*
- disease susceptibility 25
- electrical responses of 25, *26*
- Mach bands 23, *24*
- on- and off-pathways 24
- on-center cells, off-center cells 22, *22*
- oscillatory potentials 25
- phosphodiesterase 20–21
- photoreception *17*, 19, *20*
- receptive field 22
- receptor potential 20, 25
- recoverin 21
- retinal integration *22*, 22
- rhodopsin 5, 16, *17*, 20–21
- selected functions of 19
- transducin 20
- transduction 19, *20*
retinal pigment epithelium
- A2E 15, 17
- anatomy 3, *4*
- basement membrane 4, *4*
- blood–retinal barrier 15
- Bruch's membrane 4, *4*
- carbonic anhydrase inhibitors 18
- congenital hypertrophy, diseases associated with 425
- electrical activity of 19, *26*
- hypertrophy 5
- interphotoreceptor matrix 18, *18*, 18
- lipofuscin 5, 14
- melanin pigment 5
- melanin, melanosomes 14
- melanolipofuscin granules 5
- optical functions 14
- organelles, mitochondria 5
- outer blood–retinal barrier 4, 15
- outer segment phagocytosis *17*, 17
- PEDF, VEGF secretion 19
- photoreceptor regeneration 17
- physiology 14, *15*
- pigments 14
- proliferation 4
- protein adhesions 5
- retinal adhesion 18
- selected functions of 14
- serous detachments 16, *16*
- shed material 5
- structural junctions 5
- subretinal space control 15
- transport mechanisms 15
- tumors of 428
- visual pigment regeneration 16, *17*
- zonula occludens 4, *4*
retinal racemose hemangioma 424, 424, *425*
retinal tears
- characterization 444
- clinical features 444, 446, *446–448*
- cobblestone, paving stone degeneration and 446, *447*
- cryopexy 449
- diagnosis 446
- dialysis vs. 446, *448*, 483, *484*
- giant, vitrectomy 607
- laser photocoagulation 449, 588
- lattice retinal degeneration and 445, *447*
- macular holes and 262
- management, course 448
- pathogenesis 448
- retinal detachment risk factors 448
- trauma-associated 483, *484*, 493
- ultrasonography 70, *73*
retinal telangiectasis, congenital, *see* Coats' disease
retinal tumors 421
retinal venous occlusive disease
- branch retinal vein occlusion 121
- hemiretinal vein occlusion 133
- ischemic complications treatment 133
- macular edema, *see* macular edema
- overview 121
- sickle hemoglobinopathies and 316
retinitis pigmentosa
- case report 301
- characterization 296
- childhood-onset 302, *303*
- clinical features *296*, 296, *297*
- deafness and, systemic diseases associated 300
- defective components in 21, 296
- diagnostic testing 297
- differential diagnosis 296, 344, 463
- diseases associated with 187, 425
- electroretinography 297
- follow-up 298
- full-field ERG testing 86, *87*
- fundus angiography 43, *44*
- gene, stem cell therapy 298
- management, course 298
- multifocal ERG 88
- optical coherence tomography 297, *297*
- posterior subcapsular cataracts 298
- syndromic 299
- systemic diseases associated 299
- vitamin therapy 298
- X-linked recessive 297, *297*, 298
retinitis sclopetaria 481, *483*
retinoblastoma
- 13q deletion syndrome 404
- advanced groups D or E, chemoreduction outcomes 413
- chemoreduction 410, 411, *413–414*
- chemoreduction outcomes 411
- chemotherapy indications 412
- chemotherapy outcomes 412
- chemotherapy protocols 411
- classification of 406, 407
- clinical features 405
- cryotherapy 417
- diagnosis 406
- diagnostic testing 406, *410*
- differential diagnosis 190, 407, 409, 463
- enlarged vessels 545, *546–547*
- enucleation 418
- epidemiology 404
- external beam radiotherapy 418
- focal therapies 417
- genetic counseling 405, 405
- genetics of 404
- histopathology 418
- intra-arterial chemotherapy *415*, 415
- intravitreal chemotherapy 416, *417*
- laser photocoagulation 417
- life-threatening problems 405
- management 409
- metastasis risk 405
- metastasis, chemoreduction prevention of 414
- neuroblastic intracranial malignancy risk 405
- new cancer development risk 405
- pinealoblastoma, chemoreduction prevention of 414
- plaque radiotherapy 417
- pseudoretinoblastomas 406
- retinal detachment, chemoreduction outcomes 413
- sub-tenon's fascia chemotherapy 416
- thermotherapy 417
- trilateral 405
- ultrasonography *81*, 81
- visual acuity preservation by chemoreduction 414
retinopathy, *see* diabetic retinopathy
retinopathy of prematurity
- aggressive posterior ROP 172, *174*
- anti-VEGF therapy 177, 179
- characterization 171
- clinical features 171
- cryotherapy *174*, 176, 178
- diagnosis, classification *172*, 172, *173–174*, 175
- differential diagnosis 345–346, 407
- diseases associated with 425
- fluorescein angiography 174, *175*
- initial findings, oxygen role 171
- laser photocoagulation 176, *178*, 178
- laser photocoagulation, ocular complications 178
- optical coherence tomography 174, *175*
- pathogenesis 171
- plus disease 172, *174*
- preplus disease 172, *174*
- prevalence 171
- scleral buckle 179
- screening examination schedule 174
- sequelae, signs of previous history 175
- telemedical screening 176
- type 1 175–176
- type 2 175–176
- ultrasonography 72, *76*
- vitrectomy 179
retinoschisis, *see* degenerative retinoschisis
retinotomy, retinectomy 603
retrolental fibrosis 407
rhegmatogenous retinal detachments
- choroidal detachment 451, *451*
- clinical features 449
- diagnosis 449, *450*
- differential diagnosis 407, *450*, 450, 451, *451–452*
- epidemiology 449
- macular holes and 262
- management, course 452, *453*
- pathogenesis 451
- posterior vitreous 443
- risk factors for 449
- suprachoroidal hemorrhage 527, *528*
rheumatoid arthritis 201
rifabutin (Mycobutin) retinopathy 514
Riggs syndrome 308
rituximab 385
rosiglitazone, ADRs 168
RPE, *see* retinal pigment epithelium

S

SAILOR study 219
salmon patch hemorrhage 314, *315*
SANA trial 218
Sandhoff's disease
- characterization 324
- clinical features 325
- diagnosis 325
- genetic etiologies 326
- management, course 326
- pathogenesis 325
Sanfilippo's syndrome, *see* under mucopolysaccharidosis, type III
Sarrafizadeh, R. 537
scanning laser ophthalmoscopy 90
scatter (panretinal) laser photocoagulation
- adverse effects 148
- complications 583
- peripheral circumferential 320
- principles 582, *583*
- sickle cell hemoglobinopathies *320*, 320
- technique 145, *147*
Schaal, S. 259
Scheie's syndrome, *see* under mucopolysaccharidosis, type I
Schubert–Bornschein syndrome 308
sclera
- buckle, retinopathy of prematurity 179
- buckling, prophylactic 494
- depression 34, 35–36, *36–37*
- depression, contraindications 35
- folds, ultrasonography 77, *77*, 77
- rupture 484
- suture fixation 534, *535–536*
- sutureless fixation 536
SCORE Study 125, 132
SCORE-BRVO trial 125
Scott, I. U. 532–533
selective retinal therapy 591, *592*
semiconductor lasers 578
sensory retina anatomy
- axons synapse 6
- ellipsoid 6
- external limiting membrane 6
- ganglion cell layer 6
- inner nuclear layer 6
- junctions 6
- macular sparing 6
- MÃ¼ller's cells 6
- myoid 6
- overview 5, 5
- pedicle 6
- photoreceptor cells 5
- spherule 6
- synapses 6
sensory retinal detachments 10
serous retinal detachment, *see* exudative retinal detachment
serpiginous choroidopathy 371–372, 377, *378*
SFU 371
shaken baby syndrome 501, *501*, 501
sickle cell hemoglobinopathies
- anti-VEGF therapy 321
- black sunburst lesion *315*, 315
- choroidal occlusions 316
- clinical features 314
- differential diagnosis 319
- epidemiology 313
- histopathology 314
- hyphema and 314
- iridescent spots 314, *315*
- laser photocoagulation *320*, 320
- macula 315, *316*
- management, course 319
- nonproliferative 314
- optic disc 315
- pathogenesis, genetics 313
- proliferative
-- characterization 313–314
-- clinical classification 317
-- retinal manifestations *317*, 317
-- Stage I *317*, 317
-- Stage II 317, *318*
-- Stage III 317, *318*
-- Stage IV 318
-- Stage V 319
-- treatment guidelines 320
- retinal vessels 316
- salmon patch hemorrhage 314, *315*
- surgical management 321
- treatment guidelines 320
- treatment, indications for *318*, 319
- vitreoretinal interface 316
sickle cell hemoglobinopathy 236
Silicone Oil Study Group 606
SITE study 380–381
slit-lamp biomicroscope 579
small-cell carcinoma metastases 80
Smiddy, W. E. 259, 537
sodium fluorescein, *see* fluorescein angiography
- adverse reactions 41–42
- interpretation of 42
- properties 40, *41*
solar retinopathy 515, *516*
solid-state lasers 577
Sorsby's fundus dystrophy *290*, 290
sphingolipidoses 326
sphingomyelin lipidoses 326, 328
Spielmeyer–Vogt disease 334
spiramycin, toxoplasmic chorioretinitis 359
Squalamine Lactate Ophthalmic Solution 223
Stargardt's disease
- characterization *284*, 284, 303
- Group 1 284
- Group 2 *285*, 285
- Group 3 285
- Group 4 286
- pattern dystrophy simulating *282*, 282, *283*
- RPE alterations 15, 21
Stargardt's macular dystrophy 21
Steward, M. W. 532
Stickler's syndrome
- characterization 307, 349
- clinical features *348–349*, 349
- differential diagnosis 348, *348*, 349
- management, course 350
- pathogenesis, genetics 350
Sturge–Weber syndrome 433–434
sub-tenon's fascia chemotherapy 416
sub-Tenon's injections 568–569
subhyaloid hemorrhage 70, *71*
submacular surgery 217, 608
Submacular Surgery Trials (SST) Research Group 217
sulfa antibiotics retinopathy 514, *515*
sulfadiazine, toxoplasmic chorioretinitis 359
suprachoroidal hemorrhage 527, *528*
Susac's syndrome 113, *115*
SUSTAIN study 220, 222
Sveinsson's helicoid peripapillary chorioretinal dystrophy 291
sympathetic ophthalmia 375, *376*, 462, *496*, 496
syphilitic chorioretinitis 201, 352, 355, *360*, 360, 361
systemic arterial hypertension 116
systemic lupus erythematosus
- clinical features 199, *199–200*
- differential diagnosis 185, 199
- pathogenesis 201
- treatment *200*, 201
systemic vasculitic syndromes *201*, 201, *202*

T

tacrolimus 383
talc retinopathy 513, *515*
tamoxifen (Nolvadex) retinopathy 511, *514*
tamoxifen, for macular edema 168
Tay–Sachs disease
- characterization 324
- clinical features 325
- diagnosis 325
- differential diagnosis 327, 329
- genetic etiologies 109, 326
- management, course 326
- pathogenesis 325
tears, *see* retinal tears
Terson's syndrome *500*, 500
thermotherapy 417
thiazolidinediones, ADRs 168
thioridazine (Mellaril) toxicity *505*, 505, *506*
Thompson, J. T. 259
ticlopidine 126
tilted disc syndrome *553*, 553, 554, *554–555*
TNF-a inhibitors 384
tocilizumab 385
Tognetto, D. 259
topiramate retinopathy 514, *515*
topotecan, for retinoblastoma 411
tortuosity, congenital *558*, 558
toxicity, *see* specific drugs
- chloroquine derivatives 506
- crystalline retinopathy 511
- light 514
- medication 505
- operating room microscope 516, *517*
- overview 505
- retinal folds, medication-induced 514, *515*
- solar retinopathy 515, *516*
- vascular damage 510
toxocariasis *350*, 350, *364*, 364, 407, 466, *466*
toxoplasmic chorioretinitis *358*, 358, *360*
toxoplasmic chorioretinitis, pharmacotherapy 359
toxoplasmosis 352, 407, 425
traction retinal detachment, *see* specific conditions
- characterization 457
- clinical features *464*, 464
- conditions causing 465, 465
- congenital 466
- congenital pit of optic disc *547*, 547, *548–550*
- diabetic, vitrectomy 609
- differential diagnosis 451, *452*
- hereditary 465
- inflammatory 466
- neovascular 465
- pathogenesis 465
- trauma *466*, 466
- ultrasonography 71, *74*
transpupillary thermotherapy 590
trauma
- ancillary tests 477, *477*, 477, *478*
- antibiotics, prophylactic 494
- B-scan ultrasonography *478*, 478, *479*
- BB pellets 491
- blunt trauma 479, *480*
- choroidal rupture *481*, 481, *482*
- classification 475–476
- commotio retinae *480*, 480
- corneal lacerations 486, *486*, 487, *487*, 488, *488*
- cryotherapy 494
- electroretinogram 479
- endophthalmitis, *see* endophthalmitis
- enucleation 496
- epidemiology 475
- examination 476
- eye injury zones 476
- flash visual evoked potential studies 479
- foreign bodies, *see* intraocular foreign body
- lens rupture, implantation *494*, 494
- lensectomy 493, *493*
- MRI 479
- optic nerve avulsion 484, *485*
- patient history 476
- penetrating injuries 485
- perforating injuries *489*, 489
- plain roentgenograms *479*, 479
- preoperative management 479
- retinal tears, detachments 483, *484*, 493
- retinitis sclopetaria 481, *483*
- scleral buckling, prophylactic 494
- scleral rupture 484
- secondary procedures 491, *492–493*
- traction retinal detachment *466*, 466
- ultrasonography 73
- visual recovery predictors 475–476
- vitrectomy 491, *493*
- vitreous hemorrhage, *see* vitreous hemorrhage
Treatment of Age-Related Macular Degeneration With Photodynamic Therapy (TAP) trial 217
trematodes 365
triamcinolone
- branch retinal artery occlusion 124
- cystoid macular edema 166
- diabetic macular edema 165
- intravitreal 386
- macular edema *132*, 132
triamterene retinopathy 514, *515*
trimethoprim-sulfamethoxazole, toxoplasmic chorioretinitis 359
troxerutin 126
Tsipursky, W. S. 259

tuberculosis 352, 361
tuberous sclerosis complex (TSC) 427

U

UAIM 371–372
ultrasonography
- asteroid hyalosis 69, *70*
- choroid evaluation 77
- choroidal detachments 77, *79*
- choroidal detachments, hemorrhagic 78, *79*
- choroidal hemangiomas 80, *81*
- choroidal osteoma *81*, 81
- choroidal thickening 77, *78*
- dislocated lens 74, *76*
- endophthalmitis 69, *70*
- indications 66
- internal reflectivity, mass-like lesions 68
- intraocular foreign body 74, 74, *77*
- intraocular tumor evaluation 78
- kinetic properties evaluation 69
- mass-like lesion evaluation 68
- melanoma *80*, 80
- metastatic carcinoma *80*, 80
- pathology detail, obtaining 67
- penetrating, perforating injury 74, *76*
- persistent fetal vasculature 73, *76*
- principles 66, *66*
- retina evaluation 70, *72*
- retinal detachment (localized) 71
- retinal detachment (total) 72, *75*
- retinal detachment (traction) 71, *74*
- retinal tears 70, *73*
- retinoblastoma *81*, 81
- retinopathy of prematurity 72, *76*
- scleral folds 77, *77*, 77
- screening techniques 66, *67–68*
- special considerations 66
- subhyaloid hemorrhage 70, *71*
- traumatized eye evaluation 73
- vitreous evaluation 66, 69
- vitreous hemorrhage 69, *71*
- vitreous, normal *66*, *69*, 69

Usher's syndrome 299
uveal effusion syndrome 77, *78*, 459, 459
uveitis
- acute posterior 371–372, 372
- cidofovir (Vistide) retinopathy 514
- corticosteroids 369–370, 372
- cystoid macular edema and 163
- host factors 358, 362
- intermediate *369*, 369
- management 354, 369–370, 372
- noninfectious 369
- posterior, chronic treatment 375
- retinal complications 370
- rifabutin (Mycobutin) retinopathy 514
- self-limiting posterior 370, 371–372

uveoretinitis, peripheral 407

V

valganciclovir, CMV retinitis 356
Valsalva retinopathy 501, *501*
- characterization 201
- clinical features *202*, *203*
- differential diagnosis 202
- management, course 202

vancomycin, endophthalmitis 496, 524, 525
vasculitic syndromes, systemic *201*, 201, *202*
vasoproliferative tumor 407
verteporfin 217–218, 230–231
Verteporfin in Photodynamic Therapy (VIP) study 217
VIBRANT study 124
VIEW 1, 2 studies 220–222
Vilar, N. F. 532–533
vincristine, for retinoblastoma 411
VIP Study 230
VISION trial 218
Visulas 532 s VITE (Carl Zeiss Meditec) 589
vitelliform macular dystrophy, *see* Best's disease
vitiliginous chorioretinitis, *see* birdshot retinochoroidopathy
vitrectomy
- background 597
- complications 604
- diabetic 608
- diabetic macular edema 165, 609
- dislocated intraocular lenses 607
- giant retinal tears 607
- in diabetic eye *156*, 156
- indications 598
- intraocular foreign body 491, *491*
- macular hole 608
- outcomes 606
- PCIOLs, outcomes 536, 537
- preoperative considerations 597
- proliferative vitreoretinopathy 606
- retained lens fragment 607
- retained lens fragments 529, *531*, 532–533
- retinopathy of prematurity 179
- sickle cell hemoglobinopathies 321
- submacular surgery 608
- surgical techniques
-- cannula-trocar systems *600*, 600, *601*
-- chromovitrectomy 599
-- endophotocoagulation *604*, 604
-- epiretinal membrane dissection *602*, 602, *603*
-- general procedure 602
-- illumination 599, *600*
-- perfluorocarbon liquid 604, *605*
-- retinotomy, retinectomy 603
-- systems 600
-- visualization 597, *599*
- trauma 491, *493*

vitreomacular adhesion 61, *61*
vitreomacular traction syndrome
- characterization 272, *273*
- classification 273, *273*
- clinical features 274
- OCT pathology 61, *61*, *273*

vitreoretinal tuft 407
vitreous abnormalities, disorders associated with 307
vitreous anatomy
- anterior cortical gel 2
- area of Martegiani 2
- attachments 3
- base 3
- Berger's space 2
- Cloquet's canal 2
- collagen 2
- hyaluronic acid 3
- overview *2*, 2
- white-without-pressure, white-with-pressure 3

vitreous evaluation, ultrasonography 66, 69
vitreous hemorrhage
- diabetic vitrectomy 608
- differential diagnosis 407
- trauma 482
- ultrasonography 69, *71*

VMTS, *see* vitreomacular traction syndrome
Vogt-Koyanagi-Harada's syndrome 376, *377*, 459, *462*, 462
von Hippel–Lindau (VHL) syndrome
- diagnosis 421
- enlarged vessels 545, *546–547*
- genetics, pathogenesis 422
- management, course 422
- traction retinal detachment 465

voriconazole 363
Vote, B. J. 537

W

Wagner's disease 307, 349
Wegener's granulomatosis 201
welding arc retinopathy 516
Wendel, R. T. 259
whiplash maculopathy 503
Whipple's disease 201
white dot syndromes 371–372
wide-field contact lenses 36
Williamson, T. H. 259
Wyburn-Mason syndrome 424, 547

X

X-linked retinoschisis
- characterization 342
- clinical features *342*, 342, *343*
- diagnosis 343
- differential diagnosis 343, *344*, 346, 407
- management, course 344
- pathogenesis, genetics 344
- retinal detachment 343–344
- stellate maculopathy 342
- traction retinal detachment 465
- vitreous hemorrhage 343–344

XLJR, *see* X-linked retinoschisis

Y

YAG laser therapy 111

Z

Zellweger spectrum disorders 326, 334